Second Edition

NEUROLOGICAL SURGERY *Volume 3*

A Comprehensive Reference
Guide to the
Diagnosis and Management of
Neurosurgical Problems

Edited by

JULIAN R. YOUMANS, M.D., Ph.D.

Professor, Department of Neurological Surgery,
School of Medicine, University of California
Davis, California

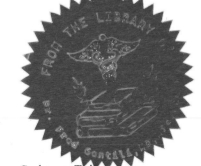

W. B. SAUNDERS COMPANY
Philadelphia • London • Toronto • Mexico City • Rio de Janeiro • Sydney • Tokyo

W. B. Saunders Company: West Washington Square
                            Philadelphia, PA 19105

                            1 St. Anne's Road
                            Eastbourne, East Sussex BN21 3UN, England

                            1 Goldthorne Avenue
                            Toronto, Ontario M8Z 5T9, Canada

                            Apartado 26370—Cedro 512
                            Mexico 4, D.F., Mexico

                            Rua Coronel Cabrita, 8
                            Sao Cristovao Caixa Postal 21176
                            Rio de Janeiro, Brazil

                            9 Waltham Street
                            Artarmon, N.S.W. 2064, Australia

                            Ichibancho, Central Bldg., 22-1 Ichibancho
                            Chiyoda-Ku, Tokyo 102, Japan

Library of Congress Cataloging in Publication Data

Youmans, Julian Ray, 1928–
  Neurological surgery.

  1. Nervous system—Surgery.   I. Title.
[DNLM: 1. Neurosurgery.   WL368 N4945]
RD593.Y68   1980   617'.48
ISBN 0-7216-9662-7 (v. 1)   80-21368

Volume 1   ISBN   0-7216-9662-7
Volume 2   ISBN   0-7216-9663-5
Volume 3   ISBN   0-7216-9664-3
Volume 4   ISBN   0-7216-9665-1
Volume 5   ISBN   0-7216-9666-X
Volume 6   ISBN   0-7216-9667-8
Neurological Surgery—Volume Three   Six Volume Set   ISBN   0-7216-9658-9

Last digit is the print number: 9   8   7   6   5   4   3   2

Contributors

MARSHALL B. ALLEN, JR., M.D., F.A.C.S.

Intracerebral and Intracerebellar Hemorrhage, Sympathectomy

Chairman of Department of Neurological Surgery, Medical College of Georgia. Chief of Neurological Surgery, Eugene Talmadge Memorial Hospital; Consultant, University Hospital and Veterans Administration Hospital, Augusta, Georgia; Dwight D. Eisenhower Army Medical Center, Fort Gordon, Georgia; and Central State Hospital, Milledgeville, Georgia.

NANCY JANE AUER, M.D.

Extracranial Arterial Occlusive Disease

Associate Resident in Neurological Surgery, Baptist Memorial Hospital, Memphis, Tennessee.

GILLES G. P. BERTRAND, M.D., F.R.C.S.(C.)

Anomalies of Craniovertebral Junction

Professor of Neurological Surgery, McGill University Faculty of Medicine. Neurological Surgeon-in-Chief, Montreal Neurological Institute and Hospital, Montreal, Quebec.

PETER McL. BLACK, M.D., Ph.D.

Hydrocephalus in Adults

Assistant Professor of Surgery, Harvard Medical School. Assistant in Neurosurgery, Massachusetts General Hospital, Boston, Massachusetts.

CHARLES E. BRACKETT, M.D., F.A.C.S.

Pulmonary Care and Complications, Arachnoid Cysts, Subarachnoid Hemorrhage, Post-Traumatic Arachnoid Cysts, Cordotomy

Professor of Neurological Surgery, Chairman of Department of Neurological Surgery, University of Kansas Medical Center, College of Health Sciences and Hospital. Chief of Neurological Surgery Service, University of Kansas Medical Center; Attending Staff, Kansas City Veterans Administration Hospital, Kansas City, Missouri.

DONALD DEANE BURROW, M.B., B.S., F.R.A.C.P.

Pathophysiology and Evaluation of Ischemic Vascular Disease

Lecturer in Medicine, School of Medicine, University of Adelaide. Senior Visiting Neurologist, Royal Adelaide Hospital and Repatriation General Hospital, Adelaide, South Australia.

ARTHUR L. DAY, M.D., F.A.C.S.

Intracavernous Carotid Aneurysms and Fistulae

Assistant Professor of Neurological Surgery, University of Florida College of Medicine. Attending Neurological Surgeon, Shands Teaching Hospital; Assistant Chief, Section of Neurological Surgery, Veterans Administration Medical Center, Gainesville, Florida.

CHARLES G. DRAKE, M.D., F.R.C.S.(C.), F.A.C.S.

Aneurysms of Posterior Circulation

Professor of Surgery, Chairman of Department of Surgery, Faculty of Medicine, The University of Western Ontario. Chief of Surgery, Victoria and St. Joseph's Hospitals, London, Ontario.

ALAN S. FLEISHER, M.D.

Carotid Artery Occlusion for Aneurysms

Associate Professor of Neurological Surgery, Emory University School of Medicine. Chief of Neurological Surgery, Grady Memorial Hospital, Atlanta, Georgia.

BARRY N. FRENCH, M.D., F.R.C.S.(C.), F.A.C.S.

Midline Fusion Defects

Associate Professor of Neurological Surgery, University of California, School of Medicine at Davis, Davis, California. Attending Staff, University of California Davis Medical Center at Sacramento and Sutter Community Hospitals of Sacramento, Sacramento, California; Consultant in Neurological Surgery, Veterans Administration Hospital, Martinez, California.

TAHER EL GAMMAL, M.B., Ch.B., F.F.R.

Intracerebral and Intracerebellar Hemorrhage

Professor of Radiology, Medical College of Georgia. Chief of Neuroradiology, Eugene Talmadge Memorial Hospital; Attending Staff, Veterans Administration Hospital, Augusta, Georgia.

MUTAZ B. HABAL, M.D., F.R.C.S.(C.), F.A.C.S.

Craniofacial Malformations

Adjunct Professor, University of Florida, Gainesville, Florida; Courtesy Professor, University of South Florida, Tampa, Florida. Director, Tampa Bay Center for Craniofacial Surgery; Attending Surgeon, Tampa General Hospital and University Community Hospital, Tampa, Florida; All Children's Hospital, St. Petersburg, Florida.

LEONARD I. MALIS, M.D., F.A.C.S.

Arteriovenous Malformations of Brain and Spinal Cord

Professor of Neurological Surgery, Chairman of Department of Neurological Surgery, City University of New York, Mount Sinai School of Medicine. Neurosurgeon-in-Chief, Department of Neurological Surgery, Mount Sinai Hospital, New York, New York.

JACK E. MANISCALCO, M.D., F.A.C.S.

Craniofacial Malformations

Clinical Assistant Professor of Surgery, University of South Florida College of Medicine. Attending Neurological Surgeon, St. Joseph's Hospital and Tampa General Hospital, Tampa, Florida.

ROBERT A. MORANTZ, M.D., F.A.C.S.

Special Problems with Subarachnoid Hemorrhage

Associate Professor of Neurological Surgery, University of Kansas School of Medicine. Attending Staff, University of Kansas Medical Center; Consulting Staff Neurological Surgeon, Kansas City Veterans Administration Hospital, Kansas City, Missouri.

MARK STEPHEN O'BRIEN, M.D., F.A.C.S., F.A.A.P.

Hydrocephalus in Children

Professor of Surgery, Emory University School of Medicine. Chief of Neurological Surgery, Henrietta Egleston Hospital for Children, Atlanta, Georgia.

ROBERT G. OJEMANN, M.D., F.A.C.S.

Hydrocephalus in Adults

Professor of Surgery, Harvard Medical School. Visiting Neurological Surgeon, Massachusetts General Hospital, Boston, Massachusetts.

S. J. PEERLESS, M.D., F.R.C.S.(C.)

Aneurysms of Posterior Circulation

Professor of Neurological Surgery, The University of Western Ontario. Chairman of Division of Neurological Surgery in the Department of Clinical Neurological Sciences, University Hospital and Victoria Hospital; Chief of Division of Neurological Surgery, University Hospital, London, Ontario.

DAVID GEORGE PIEPGRAS, M.D.

Operative Management of Intracranial Occlusive Disease, Meningeal Tumors of Brain

Assistant Professor of Neurological Surgery, Mayo Medical School. Consultant, Department of Neurological Surgery, Mayo Clinic; Attending Neurological Surgeon, St. Marys Hospital and Rochester Methodist Hospital, Rochester, Minnesota.

O. HOWARD REICHMAN, M.D., F.A.C.S.

Extracranial to Intracranial Arterial Anastomosis

Professor of Neurological Surgery. Chief of Division of Neurological Surgery, Loyola University of Chicago. Chief of Neurological Surgery, Foster G. McGaw Hospital of Loyola University, Maywood, Illinois; Consulting Physician, Hines Veterans Administration Hospital, Hines, Illinois.

SETTI S. RENGACHARY, M.D.

Arachnoid Cysts, Post-Traumatic Arachnoid Cysts

Associate Professor of Neurological Surgery, The University of Kansas Medical Center, College of Health Sciences. Chief, Neurological Surgery Service at Kansas City Veterans Administration Hospital, Kansas City, Kansas.

ALBERT L. RHOTON, JR., M.D., R.D., F.A.C.S.

Micro-Operative Technique, Intracavernous Carotid Aneurysms and Fistulae

Keene Family Professor of Neurological Surgery, University of Florida College of Medicine. Chairman of Department of Neurological Surgery, University of Florida Teaching Hospitals and Clinics; Consultant, Veterans Administration Hospital, Gainesville, Florida.

JAMES THOMAS ROBERTSON, M.D.

Ventriculography, Extracranial Arterial Occlusive Disease

Professor of Neurological Surgery, Chairman of Department of Neurological Surgery, University of Tennessee Center for the Health Sciences. Chief of Neurological Surgery Service, Baptist Memorial Hospital and City of Memphis Hospitals, Memphis, Tennessee.

JOHN SHILLITO, JR., M.D., F.A.C.S.

Craniosynostosis

Professor of Surgery, Harvard Medical School. Associate Chief of Neurosurgery, Children's Hospital Medical Center; Neurological Surgeon, Peter Bent Brigham Hospital, Boston, Massachusetts.

ROBERT R. SMITH, M.D., F.A.C.S.

Pathophysiology and Nonoperative Treatment of Subarachnoid Hemorrhage

Professor of Neurological Surgery, Chairman of Department of Neurological Surgery, University of Mississippi School of Medicine. Chief of Neurological Surgery Services, University Hospital and Veterans Administration Hospital; Consultant, Methodist Rehabilitation Center, Jackson, Mississippi.

ROGER D. SMITH, M.D.

Aneurysms of Anterior Circulation

Assistant Professor of Neurological Surgery, Department of Neurosurgery, Louisiana State University School of Medicine, New Orleans. Visiting Neurological Surgeon, Charity Hospital, Hotel Dieu Hospital, Southern Baptist Hospital, and West Jefferson Hospital, New Orleans, Louisiana.

THORALF M. SUNDT, JR., M.D., F.A.C.S.

Electroencephalography, Operative Management of Intracranial Occlusive Disease

Professor of Neurological Surgery, Mayo Medical School. Consultant, Department of Neurological Surgery, Mayo Clinic; Attending Neurological Surgeon, St. Marys Hospital and Rochester Methodist Hospital, Rochester, Minnesota.

GEORGE T. TINDALL, M.D.

Carotid Artery Occlusion for Aneurysms

Professor of Neurological Surgery, Emory University School of Medicine. Chief of Department of Neurological Surgery, Emory University Hospital, Atlanta, Georgia.

ALEXANDER B. TODOROV, M.D.

Genetic Aspects of Anomalies

Associate Professor of Neurology, College of Community Health Sciences, The University of Alabama. University, Alabama.

JAMES FRANCIS TOOLE, M.D., L.L.B., F.A.C.P.

Pathophysiology and Evaluation of Ischemic Vascular Disease

Professor of Neurology, Chairman of Department of Neurology, Bowman Gray School of Medicine, Wake Forest University. Chief of Neurology, North Carolina Baptist Hospital, Winston-Salem, North Carolina.

FARIVAR YAGHMAI, M.D., F.C.A.P.

Intracerebral and Intracerebellar Hemorrhage

Associate Professor of Pathology (Neuropathology), Medical College of Georgia. Attending Staff, Eugene Talmadge Memorial Hospital; Consulting Staff, University Hospital, Veterans Administration Hospital, Dwight David Eisenhower Army Medical Center, Augusta, Georgia, Milledgeville Central State Hospital, Milledgeville, Georgia.

M. GAZI YAŞARGIL, M.D.

Aneurysms of Anterior Circulation

Professor of Neurological Surgery, Chairman of Department of Neurological Surgery, University of Zurich, Chief of Neurological Surgery, Clinic Hospital, Zurich, Switzerland.

Contents

ix

VI

DEVELOPMENTAL AND ACQUIRED ANOMALIES

GENETIC ASPECTS
OF NEUROSURGICAL
PROBLEMS

A "birth defect" can be defined as a condition resulting from an insult to the embryo during pregnancy or from transmission of a hereditary trait. This broad definition includes conditions such as those resulting from the effects of teratogenic agents or secondary to chromosomal aberrations. The bulk of genetically transmissible disorders is due to single gene defects, and of 2336 listed in McKusick's *Mendelian Inheritance in Man*, a third are of importance in the field of neurological genetics.[71]

Neurological genetics embraces both delineation and clinical management of birth defects affecting the nervous system. It elucidates the clinical picture and provides knowledge of potential complications necessary for proper management. It also seeks to define the risk of recurrence of a defect and to provide the family or disabled person with genetic counseling. Neurological surgeons can complement medical management by operative correction of a birth defect, and this can lead to fruitful collaboration between neurosurgeons and neurogeneticists. In this chapter, birth defects are described with emphasis on problems that neurosurgeons may encounter. Only a brief description of basic genetic principles is given.

NEUROLOGICAL GENETICS

Basic Mendelian Traits

The usual assumption in mendelian genetics is that the trait to be studied is under the control of a single genetic "locus" and obeys the laws of mendelian inheritance. The assumption is sufficient for applying mendelian rules derived from study of large populations to particular clinical situations. Mendel described transmission of traits from one generation to another and defined them as "dominant" or "recessive" on the basis of their modes of inheritance. In Mendel's words,

Those characters which are transmitted entirely, or almost unchanged in the hybridization, and therefore in themselves constitute the characters of the hybrid, are termed dominant; and those which become latent in the process, recessive.[71]

Mendel also developed "rules" by which the geneticist can predict, or at least expect, the transmission of known characteristics from parents on through succeeding generations. Although it is not the purpose of this chapter to provide extensive detail concerning the transmission of heritable characteristics, a few basic points permit ready understanding of mendelian principles and their application to populations, families, and individuals.

In meiosis, paired parental genes are segregated so that each gene has a 50 per cent chance of being transmitted to the germ cell. Each offspring normally receives a single set of genes from one parent and a complementary set from the other parent. If one or both genes of the pair are dominant, the trait governed will be expressed to at least some degree in the offspring. If a recessive gene is paired with a dominant gene the recessive gene normally will be "masked" by

A. B. TODOROV

the dominant gene. Only when both of the paired genes are recessive will the recessive trait be expressed in the offspring. As applied to genetics, the terms "dominant" and "recessive" refer only to the interactions among genes at the same locus and their expression in the phenotype. The terms carry no implication of fitness or lethality. The transmission of a character can further be related to certain chromosomes, the class of autosomal chromosomes and the X-chromosome.

Autosomal Dominant Transmission

An autosomal dominant trait is suggested when a particular phenotype is expressed through several successive generations, affects both males and females, and is transmitted from either of the parents and notably from father to son. The segregation of the autosomal dominant trait is also independent of the sex of the offspring and follows the classic rule of 50 per cent, assuming only one of the particular parents carries the dominant trait. When both parents carry the same dominant trait, 25 per cent of their children will receive two dominant genes for the trait. If the dominant trait in such instances is deleterious, the phenotype will be incompatible with life in the homozygote (e.g., achondroplasia, von Recklinghausen disease, Huntington chorea).

Autosomal Recessive Transmission

In autosomal recessive segregation, phenotypically normal parents may produce a rare phenotype in a sibship. Consanguinity of parents and geographical or cultural isolation are factors that increase the incidence of recessive traits, especially the very rare ones. The usual situation arises from mating between phenotypically unaffected parents (carriers), which results in 25 per cent of descendants of both sexes being affected. Recessive disorders usually manifest themselves earlier in life than do dominant conditions, and in several instances the recessive conditions are genetically lethal. Genetic lethality has no relation to the longevity of the individual. It means that as a result of the inherited condition an affected individual does not have descendants. It must be stressed that carriers for a strictly autosomal recessive trait are phenotypically normal. Detection of such heterozygotes by special tests is the rationale for screening programs, such as that for Tay-Sachs disease.

X-Linked Transmission

At present no genetic pathological trait is known to be transmitted on the Y chromosome, and therefore the designation of "X-linked" is more appropriate terminology than "sex-linked." Because of having but one X chromosome, the male phenotype for any trait carried on this chromosome corresponds exactly to his genotype. The critical element by which X-linked heredity (recessive or dominant) is recognized is the absence of father-to-son transmission. In X-linked recessive heredity (e.g., hemophilia, Fabry disease) all sons of an affected male are phenotypically and genotypically normal. All daughters of such a father are phenotypically normal but carriers of the trait. On the average, a female carrier of the X-linked trait will transmit the disorder to half her sons. Also on average, one of two of her daughters will carry the trait, the others having a normal genotype. Situations that are difficult to interpret may occur if an affected male and a female carrier have children.

X-linked transmission differs from sex-limited heredity. In sex-limited inheritance, the condition occurs only in one sex, whereas in X-linked heredity, the transmission is through the X chromosome, and the trait may appear in both males and females.

Variability and Heterogeneity

A major concern in medical genetics is to delineate the relationship between a given phenotype and an already identified clinical entity. The same genetic defect may produce different phenotypes (variable expression, or variability), or identical phenotypes may be produced by different genes (genetic heterogeneity).

Variability exists because a gene operates in combination with the environment and the genetic background of the individual. It is most evident in conditions exhibiting marked pleiotropy or multiplicity of effects.

Heterogeneity exists when segregation occurs according to two different transmission models, as with Hurler (recessive) and Hunter (X-linked) diseases. The present inability to distinguish clinically between different phenotypes does not contradict the principle of heterogeneity. Charcot-Marie-Tooth disease is certainly a heterogeneous condition, as shown by the existence of dominant, recessive, and X-linked forms. In very general terms, if several transmission models are known, the clinical picture is mildest in the dominant form, most severe in the recessive model, and intermediate in its effects in the X-linked form. Another clinical clue that suggests heterogeneity is variation in the age of onset and mode of evolution of the disease. Werdnig-Hoffmann disease was thought to be homogeneous until it appeared that some patients became disabled in their teen-age years and had a protracted course of evolution.

Genetic Counseling

Valuable advice can be given to concerned parents regarding their chances of producing a child with a disability and the possibilities for its treatment. Numerous advances in surgical and medical techniques offer affected individuals and their families options that hold promise of a normal or nearly normal life despite conditions that once were beyond the skills of the practitioner.

Applications of genetic information that would be impossible, if not inhumane, when applied to populations are an entirely different matter when applied at the level of the individual family to prevent the burden of a severe phenotype. Genetic counseling provides the family with accurate risk figures and, for individuals, defines the chance of manifesting a given condition. Furthermore, greater awareness of the potentials on the part of individuals, families, and physicians will also improve the likelihood of earlier detection and management of disorders.

Geneticists use three types of information to arrive at decisions: empirical, modular, and particular. Empirical information is that accumulated through experience—mutation rates, gene frequencies, penetrance coefficients, and their relationships to age, sex, and age at onset of the disease. Empirical data derive from statistics collected from a given population at a given period of time. If used with caution, the empirical approach can provide a definite basis for modifying risk estimates for the occurrence of a condition.

Modular information is knowledge of the mode of inheritance of the condition derived from genetic analyses and from the nature of the condition. For example, it has been observed that dominant conditions tend to be disorders of structure, having relatively late onset, and are mild enough to permit transmission of the trait; and recessive conditions are more likely disorders of function with earlier onset, tending to be more disabling.

The third source of information is that "particular" to the person seeking advice, who is termed the "consultand." Information from this source derives from the family pedigree, including history of similarly disabled individuals in the particular family.

A basic step in counseling is to determine whether the genotypes of the parents are known. If the genotypes are known, and assuming complete penetrance of the gene, the classic percentages of mendelian transmission can be invoked. If the genotypes of the parents are unknown, then computation of the probability for transmission of a trait is more complex. The method for estimating probabilities is of little interest in itself. Some authors prefer a precise estimate of the probability; others are satisfied with a quotation of "high," "low," or "no" risk. Parents of an affected child take little note of the mathematics. What concerns them is the combination of the risk and the burden of the genetic condition. Under the term, "burden," Murphy introduced the notion of the "price" of the genetic condition.[77] The price of a birth defect is not merely the financial cost of treatment; it also includes the emotional investment over the span of the condition. The burden can be intense and of short duration, as in the birth of an anencephalic child. Or it can be long-standing and of small significance, as with color blindness. Curiously enough, the concept of the burden of birth defects has seemed too trivial for exploration except by a few geneticists, whereas it is by far the greatest concern of parents. A distinction should be made as well between the burden for parents and the burden for the disabled individual.

Referral to a neurogenetic unit should take into account the limitation in human nature on the amount of "bad news" that can be absorbed at one time. A three-stage approach is more likely to succeed. In the first stage, a referral to a neurogenetic unit will help delineate the problem and the possibilities of operative treatment. In the second, correction of the birth defect can be accomplished. In the third, a referral to a neurogenetic unit for medical follow-up and genetic counseling will be rewarding even though, knowing that operative management is under way, parents are likely to be unable or unwilling to accept counseling on the risk potential for successive children.

As with other aspects of medical and surgical care, attention should be given to legal implications, including appropriate referral, management, and informed consent. Von Hippel-Lindau disease is a good example of a condition in which failure to refer a family for follow-up and genetic counseling may have serious consequences. With this condition, proper evaluation and, eventually, neurosurgical treatment can be helpful for the patient and for 50 per cent of the cases in his family.

CONGENITAL MALFORMATIONS

Epidemiology of Congenital Malformations

Estimates of the incidence of birth defects vary widely, depending upon the definition of the term, the sources of the sample, and the age of the groups studied. Among stillborn infants, the incidence may reach 31.5 per cent; it may be 17.8 per cent in those who die during the first week of life.[80] Among surviving newborn children the incidence is estimated to be 5.4 to 7.4 per cent.[110] Major congenital anomalies show a frequency of 2 to 3.3 per cent, and minor variants and structural abnormalities[31] one of up to 9.6 per cent. The usual figure quoted to parents for the risk of birth of a congenitally malformed child is 2 per cent. Other factors such as the age of the parents and the family history should also be considered when giving a recurrence risk figure for congenital malformation.

Central nervous system anomalies are underreported. Malformations such as polydactyly do not escape attention, but minor central nervous system malformations do despite their much greater implications for the useful life of the child. From the data in the British Columbia register of handicapped children it is possible to compute the incidence of some birth defects.[81] Strabismus and club foot are the leading diagnoses; however, spina bifida, meningocele, and hydrocephalus are frequent also (Table 34–1). In a World Health Organization study of 24 centers in which there were 417,000 single births during the years 1961 to 1967, the incidence of central nervous system anomalies was 2.66 per 1000 births.[109] The most frequent malformations were anencephaly (0.92), hydrocephalus (0.61), and spina bifida with or without meningocele (0.55). Central nervous system malformations are cited infrequently as cause of death. Of 1196 death certificates listing congenital malformation as one of the causes of death, only 6.7 per cent mention a malformation of the central nervous system as the primary cause. There are also variations in the geographic distributions of central nervous system defects that are reported. The lowest rate was reported by Japan (0.5 average annual age-adjusted death rate per 100,000 population) and the highest by Ireland (6.8 per 100,000 population). The average of incidence rates reported by most countries participating in the World Health Organization study was within the range of 3.0 malformations per 100,000 population.[95] Over the past 20 years there has been a steady decrease in the number of deaths attributed to central nervous system birth conditions. In the United States the rate declined from 24.1

TABLE 34–1 INCIDENCE OF SOME BIRTH DEFECTS*

CONDITION	PER 1000 BIRTHS
Strabismus	2.30
Club foot	2.29
Cardiac malformation	1.70
Cleft palate and harelip	1.70
"Cerebral palsy"	1.40
Mongolism	1.00
Spina bifida and meningocele	0.94
Hydrocephalus	0.59

* After Newcombe, H. B.: Population genetics: Population records. *In* Burdette, W. J., ed.: Methodology in Human Genetics. San Francisco, Holden-Day, Inc., 1962, pp. 92–113. Data from the British Columbia Register of Handicapped Children.

TABLE 34–2 APPROXIMATE TIMING OF VARIOUS MALFORMATIONS DURING HUMAN MORPHOGENESIS

MOMENT OF INJURY	TYPE OF MALFORMATION	EXAMPLE
Blastogenesis	Defective separation of twins	Craniopagus twins
Embryogenesis		
24th day	Defects of neural tube closure	Anencephaly
26th day		Meningomyelocele
5th week	Anterior midline defects	Arhinencephaly
5th week	Failure in development of pontine flexure	Arnold-Chiari malformation
6th week	Defective development of rostral membraneous area	Dandy-Walker syndrome
6th week	First visceral arch syndromes	Craniofacial anomalies
7th week		Cleft palate
Fetogenesis		
11 to 13th week	Defects in neuronal migration and layering	Agyria
13th week		Pachygyria
16th week		Microgyria
20th week		Neuronal periventricular heterotopias
5th to 8th month	Defects in commissuration	Agenesis of corpus callosum

per 1000 deaths in 1950 to 17.8 per 1000 deaths in 1967, with major declines noted for spina bifida and hydrocephalus. Such declines parallel the decrease in national live birth rates during the same period, and more data are needed to ascertain whether there has been any impact of better neurosurgical management.

Various teratological and embryological studies have shown a relationship between the period of injury to the embryo and some types of malformations (Table 34–2). An injury during the early stages of blastogenesis may induce defective separation of twins and result in malformations such as craniopagus twins. Spinal dysraphias are engendered during the third to fourth week of embryogenesis. Defects in neuronal maturation and failures in commissuration may result from insults during the last trimester of pregnancy. Warkany's *Congenital Malformations*, Bergsma's *Birth Defects. Atlas and Compendium,* and Smith's *Recognizable Patterns of Human Malformation* are comprehensive reference textbooks that may be consulted for further discussion of these matters.[8,106,120]

Craniopagus Twins

Craniopagus twins are an object of curiosity to laymen and physicians alike. From various reports it appears that the site of the junction is the most important criterion for successful operative treatment. The site can be frontal, parietal, or occipital. Concomitantly there can be rotation of the heads in the coronal plane and various degrees of angulation between the longitudinal axes of twins' bodies. The coronal plane rotation can result in the heads' facing in the same or opposite directions. The angulation in longitudinal axis may result in alignment of the twins' bodies as in vertex parietal junction, or in formation of an acute angle in lower frontal or parietal junctions. The interface of the junction is most important, being relatively small in frontal junctions and larger in parietal junctions.

Problems encountered during operative procedures are related to four aspects of the malformation.

Plane of Cleavage

In only 1 case of 14 was there a thin sheet of bone between the heads.[117] In frontal craniopagus twins, a dural leaf delineating a plane of cleavage is likely to be present. In more posterior junctions, a dural shelf may be present on one side of the junction, a leptomeningeal coverage on the other. Only leptomeningeal separation can be expected in most cases, but it can be very dense, as described by Baldwin and Dekaban.[4]

Venous Connections

Common sagittal sinus is frequent in parietal and occipital junctions. Other venous connections are numerous. The dural shelf may contain the sagittal sinus, and the survival of one of the twins may depend on to which the sinus is allocated.

Cerebral Connections

These are not a problem in frontal junctions. In more posterior junctions there is often interdigitation and deformity of cerebral hemispheres. True cerebral connections were encountered by Baldwin and Dekaban and by O'Connell.[4,83,84] In the cases of O'Connell the frontal lobes formed a tower, the tip of each child's right frontal tower being in contact with her sister's tentorium.[84]

Skull and Skin Defects

Defects of skull and skin are the rule in all cases, and again they are most difficult to manage in parietal junctions.

Craniopagus twins are in poor condition during the first weeks of life and have a high perinatal mortality rate. Operative procedures are more successful when performed after three months of age. Neurosurgical results are excellent in frontal types of craniopagus, but in parietal junctions the outlook is that one or both children may die during the operation or at least be severely disabled mentally, although gratifying results are possible. Normal development after separation for parietal junction was reported by Voris and co-workers and by O'Connell.[84,117] The malformation is compatible with life, and a case is known of 23-year-old craniopagus twins who are well adjusted to their disability.[115]

Skull and Facial Structural Anomalies

Numerous "syndromes" that include craniofacial anomalies have been reported, often as isolated case reports, in the pediatric literature. As a reference source, the Goodman and Gorlin *Atlas of the Face in Genetic Disorders* is a comprehensive textbook of those conditions.[43]

The terms dysostosis and dysplasia are used interchangeably in the literature to denote anomalous skeletal features. There is some overlap between the two terms. Dysostosis implies a defect in the normal ossification of fetal cartilages. Dysplasia refers to abnormal skeletal development.

Craniosynostoses

A clinical discussion of craniosynostosis is given in Chapter 39. Onset is prenatal, and the condition may behave as a dominant trait, especially in bilateral coronal synostosis.[56] In a series of 519 cases, Shillito and Matson reported nine families in each of which two sibs were affected.[103] A recessive craniosynostosis is encountered among the Amish.[26] Other malformations are present in almost one fifth of cases and include spina bifida, meningocele, platybasia, arhinencephaly, internal hydrocephalus, aplasia of the corpus callosum, hypertelorism, cervical vertebral fusions, hare lip, and congenital heart defects.[30,38] Mental retardation may be encountered in cases with multiple synostosis. Craniosynostosis is part of birth defects such as acrocephalopolysyndactyly and acrocephalosyndactyly; cloverleaf skull, or Kleebattschädel syndrome; Crouzon craniofacial dysostosis; cranioectodermal dysplasia, involving short-limb dwarfism, dental abnormalities, thin hair, dolichocephaly, and craniosynostosis; craniosynostosis with fibular aplasia; craniosynostosis with radial defects, involving oxycephaly, absence of radii, ulnar hypoplasia, and oligodactyly; and mandibulofacial dysostosis.[44,63,66]

Acrocephalopolysyndactyly and Acrocephalosyndactyly

Patients with acrocephalopolysyndactyly and acrocephalosyndactyly are a heterogenous class in whom there is involvement of the skull (acrocephaly) and the extremities (syndactyly or polysyndactyly). The craniosynostosis is the primary reason for bringing these children to neurosurgical attention. There are two types of acrocephalopolysyndactyly (Noak syndrome and Carpenter syndrome) and five types of acrocephalosyndactyly (typical Apert syndrome; Apert-Crouzon syndrome; Saethre-Chotzen acrocephaly with skull asymmetry and mild syndactyly; Waardenburg type; and Pfeiffer syndrome). The best known are Carpenter and Apert syndromes.

Carpenter Syndrome

Carpenter syndrome is a recessive condition characterized by acrocephaly, peculiar facies, brachysyndactyly of the fingers with brachymesophalangy, preaxial polydactyly and syndactyly of the toes, hypogenitalism, obesity, and mental retardation.[113] Additional features are coxa valga, genu valgum, pes cavus, congenital heart defect, and abdominal hernias.

Apert Syndrome

Apert syndrome is relatively common, estimated to affect 1 in 160,000 births. There is evidence of autosomal dominant inheritance. The disorder is characterized by acrocephaly and syndactyly of the hands and feet. The syndactyly and interdigital osseous union give undifferentiated spoon-like hands with complete digital fusion. Progressive synostosis involves not only the skull but also the cervical vertebrae, feet, and hands. Polyhydramnios may be present at delivery of children with acrocephalosyndactyly. The condition is recognized at birth. Strabismus, dental malposition, high-arched palate, cardiac anomalies, tunnel chest, hydronephrosis, imperforate anus, and absence of corpus callosum may be observed. Deafness, hydrocephalus, and mental retardation are common complications.[48]

Delayed Ossification of the Cranial Vault

Several conditions may present with delayed ossification of the cranial vault. Radiography of the skull reveals membraneous calvaria with numerous wormian bones (Fig. 34–1).

Cleidocranial Dysplasia

Cleidocranial dysplasia is a dominant condition in which one third of the cases represent new mutations.[51] It may first be suspected because of the patient's ability to approximate the shoulders. The patients are of short stature (in the 150-cm range) and have coarse facial features, moderate maxillary hypoplasia, brachycephalic skull, and parietal bossing ("Arnold's head"). Palpation of the head discloses widely open fontanelles. Eruption of deciduous teeth is delayed, and they may still be present at middle age. Retention and impaction of permanent and supernumerary teeth is common.

The neck is short, and vertebral scoliosis is present. The clavicles are partially or completely absent. Mental retardation, seizures, hydrocephalus, deafness, and spinal cord involvement may occur. Radiographi-

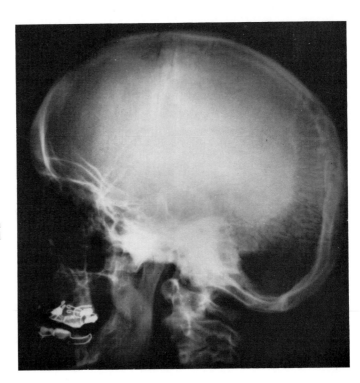

Figure 34–1 Multiple wormian bones in a patient with cleidocranial dysplasia.

cally there is a striking delay in ossification of the skull. The fontanelles are open, and multiple wormian bones can be seen. Basilar impression may occur. In the spine, multiple clefts may bisect the cervical laminae. The phalanges are usually short and have an Erlenmeyer flask appearance. The long bones and pelvis also show severe modeling disturbance.

Delayed skull ossification can also be encountered in pycnodysostosis, mandibuloacral dysplasia, and acro-osteolysis.[19,32,69]

Osteogenesis Imperfecta

Another hereditary condition in which there is delayed ossification of the cranial vault is osteogenesis imperfecta.[70] The condition can be described as camptomelic dwarfism. Clinical appearance is characteristic. Because of their propensity to fractures after trivial trauma, the patients present with severe skeletal deformities. Generalized osseous fragility is only one of the manifestations of the disease. The poorly ossified cranium has decreased vertical dimension, overhanging occiput, frontal bossing ("helmet head"), and platybasia. Radiologically the skull vault has a parchment-like appearance and is filled with wormian bones. The vertebrae have "codfish" or "hourglass" shape. Compression fractures involving the spinal cord are common. Herniation of the nucleus pulposus into the substance of the vertebral body may occur. Deafness usually begins by the teens and consists of conduction or perception hypoacusis. Two varieties of osteogenesis imperfecta are recognized. The congenital form is usually lethal owing to the numerous fractures and intracranial hemorrhages sustained by the fetus in utero and during delivery. The tardive form is usually a dominant trait, and its severity of expression is fairly variable, occasionally being limited to the presence of blue sclerae.

Other Syndromes with Craniofacial Involvement

Acrodysostosis

Acrodysostosis consists of progressive growth failure, nasal and maxillary hypoplasia, brachycephaly, and peripheral dysostosis. Frequently there are collapsed vertebral bodies and deformed end-plates in the thoracic and lumbar spine, with resultant kyphosis. Neurologically, one may encounter mental retardation, hydrocephalus, optic atrophy, seizures, choreoathetosis, and hearing loss.[94]

Costovertebral Dysplasia

Besides spine and rib anomalies, the characteristics of costovertebral dysplasia (spondylocostal or spondylothoracic dysplasia) are a short-trunk dwarfism with normal length extremities; short, webbed neck; increased anteroposterior diameter of the chest; and protuberant abdomen. Radiography of the spine reveals partial absence of or reduction in the number of vertebrae. Hemivertebrae, bifid vertebral bodies, and other segmentation defects can be present throughout the entire spinal column. The condition may be confused initially with Morquio disease or with spondyloepiphyseal dysplasia.[82]

Craniodiaphyseal Dysplasia

Craniodiaphyseal dysplasia (diaphyseal endostosis) features enlargement of the head secondary to cranial and facial hyperostosis. Optic atrophy, deafness, and other cranial nerve involvement are very common. As in the milder variant—Camurati-Engelmann disease—poor muscle development is striking. Correction of the lower extremity skeletal deformity may significantly improve the mobility of these patients.[22] Bone overgrowth is also present in osteopetrosis and in sclerosteosis.[6] In sclerosteosis a variable degree of syndactyly is present. Progressive enlargement of clavicles and mandible, deformity of the face, and overall gigantism point to the diagnosis. Optic, facial, and acoustic nerves are involved. Involvement of other cranial nerves and of the brachial plexus may occur. Neurosurgical management is directed toward relief of the bony overgrowth in the skull and intervertebral foramina.

Larsen Syndrome

Larsen syndrome consists of anomalies of the articulations, hands, face, and cervical and thoracic spine. Patients have dislocations of knee, hip, and elbow articulations. The hands have short metacarpals and long cylindrical fingers. The face features a prominent forehead, widely spaced eyes, and depressed nasal bridge. Patients with Larsen syndrome have midcervical kyphosis and cervicothoracic lordosis. Radiologically, abnormal segmentation of vertebral bodies is present. Hypoplasia of vertebral bodies, spina bifida, platybasia, and occipitalization of the atlas are usual findings. Impairment of the spinal canal may result in sudden death, tetraplegia, or paraplegia. A semirigid cervical collar worn until the child is old enough to sustain spinal fusion may be beneficial.[73] These patients have proportionate dwarfism, relative macro- and acrobrachycephaly, synostosis of the coronal suture with delayed closure of the anterior fontanelles, and mild mental retardation. The tubular bones are uniformly small, bone maturation is reduced, and the medullary cavities stenosed.

Skull and Scalp Defects

The management of defects of scalp and calvarium is discussed in Chapter 69 and by Lynch and Kahn.[67] A defect of the scalp and frequently of the calvarium can be seen in aplasia cutis congenita. The defect may vary from pinpoint to extensive size and is usually found in the midsagittal parietal region. The scalp presents variably shaped lesions ranging from parchment-like healed scars to raw granulation tissue with islands of normal skin. The skull and meninges may be absent. Associated defects such as polydactyly, cleft palate, and cardiac or kidney defects are common. Operative management consists of rotating scalp flaps. Aplasia cutis behaves as a dominant trait. It can be encountered in isolated patients or in children with chromosomal defects (trisomy 13–15). Differential diagnosis includes consideration of epidermolysis bulbosa. Ulcerated scalp lesions overlying a skull defect have been described in a family with limb malformations.[2]

Defects of Craniovertebral Junction, Spinal Column, and Related Structures

Craniovertebral Junction Anomalies

Pathological conditions of the craniovertebral junction may be congenital or ac-quired. The following discussion is limited to junctional anomalies in birth defects. Malformations such as basilar impression, platybasia, assimilation of the atlas, occipital vertebrae, odontoid process dysplasia, and related atlantoaxial dislocation may occur as isolated findings. As a rule, however, they are a part of a more generalized birth defect, as discussed further in Chapter 41.

Anomalies of Spinal Column and Related Structures

Klippel-Feil Syndrome

A relatively common anomaly, the Klippel-Feil malformation is found in 6.0 per cent of spinal roentgenograms.[12] Often referred to as "fusion," it is strictly speaking not an acquired process. It is basically a nonsegmentation of the mesodermal somites resulting in a mass of spine with no recognizable vertebrae. Klippel-Feil anomaly is highly variable. It can involve only two cervical vertebrae or, in extreme cases, may present as a nonsegmentation of the entire spine. Most often it is found in the cervical region. Thoracic and lumbar vertebrae are less often involved.

The Klippel-Feil syndrome can be divided into three categories. In the first there is a massive block of cervical and upper thoracic vertebrae. Anomalies in other organs are the rule. In the second there may be involvement of only one or two interspaces (C2–C3; C5–C6). Hemivertebrae, atlanto-occipital fusion, and other anomalies may be encountered. This is the most commonly seen type of Klippel-Feil anomaly. The third type is the presence of Klippel-Feil anomaly in both cervical and thoracolumbar regions.

Patients with cervical defects present with short neck, low posterior hairline, and occasionally with pterygium colli. The neck movements are reduced chiefly in lateral directions. More than 50 per cent of patients with a Klippel-Feil anomaly have scoliosis, and more than 30 per cent have a hearing deficit.[47] Renal abnormalities and congenital heart disease may be encountered.[75] The anomaly can remain asymptomatic or be lethal in extreme cases. Osteoarthritis and spinal root compression develop above and below the osseous block. Neurological symptoms are related to corresponding nerve root involvement and more exceptionally to spinal cord compression. A curious association is the presence of bimanual synkinesias (mirror movements) in children with the Klippel-Feil syndrome. The synkinesias tend to improve with age. The anomaly has been recognized as early as the seventh gestational week, and it is not surprising to find it in conjunction with many other birth defects.

Cervical Rib

Cervical ribs are common and occur in 0.5 per cent of the population.[91] They can be transmitted as a dominant trait. The anomaly is overincriminated as the culprit of entrapment neuropathy; in three quarters of the patients it remains asymptomatic.[25]

Developmental Segmental Anomalies of the Spine

Embryologically the vertebrae derive from the sclerotomes. During the fourth to seventh week of development the centers of chondrification appear around the notochord. Each vertebra has two ossification

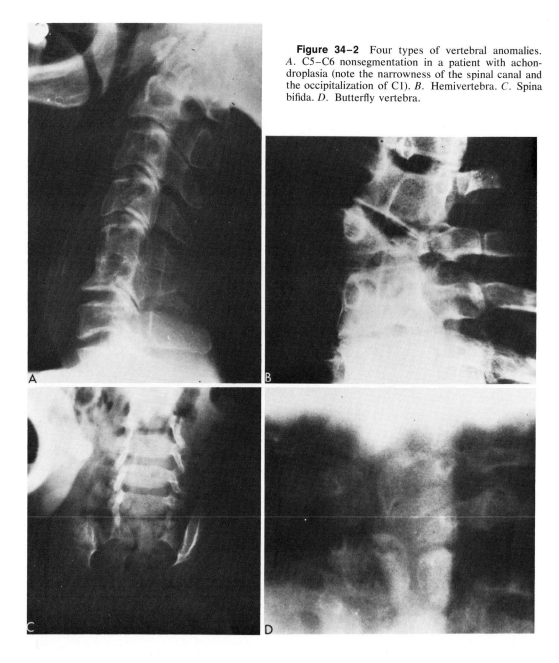

Figure 34–2 Four types of vertebral anomalies. *A*. C5–C6 nonsegmentation in a patient with achondroplasia (note the narrowness of the spinal canal and the occipitalization of C1). *B*. Hemivertebra. *C*. Spina bifida. *D*. Butterfly vertebra.

centers for the body and one for each side of the arch. Dysplasia in those centers may lead to absence of vertebrae, hemivertebrae, cleft and butterfly vertebrae, block vertebrae, or other segmentation anomalies (Fig. 34–2). It may involve only one vertebral segment or all levels of the spine.

The presence of anomalous vertebrae may result in severe kyphoscoliosis. Vertebral anomalies can be detected in half the cases of congenital scoliosis, especially in the cervical region. Other anomalies in congenital scoliosis include bifid posterior arch of the atlas, basilar impression, and the Arnold-Chiari malformation.[27]

Neural Tube Closure Defects

Defects of the neural tube are common malformations. Grouped under the term "dysraphia," these malformations represent a disturbance in the closure of the neural groove and defects in its skeletal investment. Embryologically the neural groove appears in presomite embryos of 18 postovulatory days.[88] The neural tube starts to form by 7 somites, and by 10 somites it is closed except at the ends. By the fourth week of embryogenesis it is fully closed, the cranial (rostral) neuropore closing two days before the caudal end. The caudal end has an embryological origin distinct from the rest of the neural formation. A dysraphia of the neural tube represents a close interaction between the ectoderm and mesoderm. The abnormally exposed neural plate leads to disorganized overgrowth of neural tissue, followed by epithelization from the periphery and degeneration of the nervous tissue. Finally, scar tissue replaces the original medullovasculosa. Early dysraphias are expressed by major cerebral dyscephalies such as iniencephaly, exencephaly, or anencephaly. Later insult to the neural groove leads to myelomeningocele or meningocele (encephalocele in the rostral portion). Minor defects in closure of the supporting structure may be manifest as spina bifida occulta or cranium bifidum. A dysraphic state can express itself at one part of the rachis. More commonly—in 83 per cent of all patients with neural-type dysraphia—additional anomalies are encountered.[13] The embryology of these problems is discussed in greater detail in Chapter 35.

Epidemiology and Etiology of Dysrhaphias

Numerous epidemiological data have been accumulated over the past decade in the hope of providing some clues to the etiology of dysraphias. The very diversity of the findings points to the lack of understanding of why dysraphia occurs. There is no simple explanation for the following facts or hypotheses:

Secular trend—a decrease in the incidence of dysraphias in various parts of the world has been noted in England and Wales, New York State, and Rhode Island.[33,52,125]

Seasonal variations—a greater number of dysraphias occur during the winter months in the northern hemisphere; the reverse is true in the southern hemisphere.[17]

Ethnic background—the incidence is 0.85 in Ireland; 0.08 in Japan.[33,79] In Boston higher than usual rates of anencephaly and spina bifida were reported among those of Irish descent than among the offspring of Jewish mothers.[78] A high incidence of anterior encephalocele is found in Nigerian Igbos.[87] The rate of anencephaly is six times as high in whites as in blacks, but the incidence of spina bifida cystica is the same in those two groups.[59]

Infections—an epidemic of rubeola in 1944 was reflected in a higher incidence of dysraphias in Rochester, Minnesota.[46] Toxoplasmosis, rickettsial infections, and influenza have also been suspected, but this association has not been substantiated.[58,96]

Toxins—potato blight was thought to be the culprit in Ireland, but this idea has now been discarded.[16,92]

Metabolic diseases (diabetes); hormonal imbalance; vitamin deficiencies; increased amounts of oligoelements in the drinking water.

Chromosomal aberrations—13–15 translocations are found in some cases.

Drugs—Aminopterin, analgesics, clomiphene have been suspected.

Moment of conception—conception in the postovulatory phase was suggested and denied.[57] Consecutive pregnancies within 12 to 18 months of one another may result in a higher incidence of defects caused by the presence of residual trophoblastic tissue. Abnormalities of the placenta or of the vascular supply to the placenta may be involved.

TABLE 34-3 OCCURRENCE OF DYSRAPHIAS IN SIBS OF PATIENTS WITH SPINA BIFIDA, ANENCEPHALY, AND HYDROCEPHALUS

	TYPE OF LESION		
	*SPINA BIFIDA**	*ANENCEPHALY**	*HYDROCEPHALUS†*
Number of index cases	423	361	187
Number of sibs	845	708	338
Per cent of sibs affected			
Spina bifida	3.7	1.8	1.2
Anencephaly	2.3	2.3	1.2
Hydrocephalus			1.4
Total percentage of affected sibs	6.0	4.1	3.8

* From Laurence, K. M.: The recurrence risk in spina bifida cystica and anencephaly. Develop. Med. Child Neurol., *11*:suppl. 20:23–30, 1969.

† From Lorber, J., and De, N. C.: Family history of congenital hydrocephalus. Develop. Med. Child Neurol., *6*:suppl. 22: 94–100, 1970.

Abortions and miscarriages are more likely a manifestation than a cause of anencephaly and spina bifida.[62] Only 79 per cent of infants with spina bifida are liveborn.[33]

Age of parents—there is a U-shaped curve of incidence of dysraphia, most cases occurring in the 15 to 19 or 40 to 44 maternal age groups.[17]

Birth order—this factor can be related to the previous age group observation. More often a dysraphic child is the product of the first or the fifth pregnancy. Twinning may predispose to dysraphia.[36]

Sex of the child—the incidence of spina bifida cystica is higher in females than in males.[17]

Genetic predisposition—there is a greater incidence of dysraphias in sibs or cousins of an affected child than in the general population.[61]

Genetic Considerations

Genetic counseling can be beneficial for families in which dysraphia has occurred. Counseling must be done at the earliest possible time, and the family needs several follow-up visits. The counseling must deal with two aspects of the problem, providing the family with recurrence risk figures and monitoring the next pregnancy. There are few families with strong evidence of a hereditary component. Most often, no single gene trait can be established, and counseling is based mainly on empirical data. The incidence of dysraphias in sibs and first cousins of affected persons is higher than in the general population. There is also a close association between the risk for recurrence of spina bifida and the risk for the occur-

rence of other dysraphias such as anencephaly (Table 34–3).

The total percentage of affected sibs is definitely higher than the percentage of the population with dysraphias, and the figure increases if more than one sib has been disabled by dysraphia. The empirical risks are summarized in Table 34–4.

Parents should be informed of the opportunities for monitoring a pregnancy with ultrasound and amniocentesis by 16 to 18 weeks of pregnancy. Amniocentesis makes it possible to measure the α-fetoproteins in the amniotic fluid. The α-fetoprotein level is raised in early pregnancy in association with anencephaly and open spina bifida. Open defects occurring after 24 weeks of pregnancy and closed defects, including skin-covered encephalocele and hydrocephalus, are associated with normal levels of α-fetoprotein. Twinning and especially triplets are associated with increased levels of α-fetoprotein. A disadvantage of relying exclusively on the α-fetoprotein determination is the possibility of false positive results; of 2495 such analyses, 4.8 per cent were false positives and one was a false negative.[74] Selective abortion of normal fetuses has occurred under the false diagnoses of dysraphias. The risks of amniocen-

TABLE 34-4 EMPIRICAL RECURRENCE RISK FOR DYSRAPHIAS

NUMBER OF AFFECTED SIBS	RECURRENCE RISK (PER CENT)
No previously affected child	0.08 to 0.85
One affected sib	4.0 to 6.0
Two affected sibs	11.0 to 13.0

tesis are slight, but it should not be undertaken without due regard to its hazards.[11] Determination of amniotic α-fetoprotein has an advantage over ultrasound imaging for neural tube defects. In 28 cases of fetal dysraphia, ultrasound gave correct diagnoses in 25 and missed the diagnosis in 3, while amniotic α-fetoprotein levels gave correct diagnoses in all 28. There were also four false positive tests out of 313 examinations.[14]

The risk of an affected descendant of a dysraphic parent seems greater than the expected incidence in the general population. A study of 106 persons with dysraphia having a total of 208 children revealed that 7 (3.3 per cent) of the children were disabled by spina bifida or anencephaly.[17]

Specific Dysraphic Syndromes

Cranium Bifidum Occultum

Cranium bifidum occultum has been described in a mother and her two children.[114]

Spina Bifida Occulta

Present in a significant percentage of the population, spina bifida occulta is more common in younger individuals and in males. Its incidence at L5 in children aged 7 to 8 years was estimated to be 16.1 per cent and decreased to 2.2 per cent in adults. At the S1 level the incidence was 51.6 per cent in the 7- to 8-year-olds and 26.4 per cent in the adults.[112] Lorber and Levick found spina bifida occulta in 14.3 per cent of mothers and 26.8 per cent of fathers of dysraphic patients as compared with 5 per cent in the control group.[65]

Spinal Extradural Cysts

Spinal extradural cysts, congenital lymphedema, and distichiasis (double rows of eyelashes) was encountered in three sibs.[7] The author has followed two sisters with extradural cysts at the same lower thoracic level.

Iniencephaly

An extreme dysraphia, iniencephaly is characterized by retroflexion of the head, abnormal segmentation of cervicothoracic vertebrae, and occipital exencephalocele and enlargement of the foramen magnum permitting parts of the brain and cerebellum to protrude into the spinal canal.[21]

Anencephaly

There is marked tendency for recurrence of anencephaly in the same sibship. The recurrence risk mentioned in Table 34–4 for spina bifida cystica is valid also for anencephaly. Younger mothers seem to be more prone to have an anencephalic child than older ones. The condition can be suspected from prenatal radiographs, which reveal absence of the skull vault and unusually dense and disorderly arrangement of the basilar and facial bones. Ultrasound testing and amniocentesis for α-fetoprotein determination are indicated in families with a previous history of anencephaly.

Occipital Encephalocele

Occipital encephalocele, progressive vitreoretinal degeneration, and high myopia is a triad transmitted as an autosomal recessive trait.[55]

Meningocele

Intrasacral meningocele may be manifest late in life.[107] Defects of the sacrum and coccyx with *anterior sacral meningocele* have been encountered in females.[23] Neurologically there was disturbance in sphincter control, and three of six patients had congenital anal canal stenosis. The same dysraphia with anal canal duplication cyst and covered anus was also observed in two brothers and a sister.[1]

Intrathoracic meningocele is commonly associated with neurofibromatosis and kyphoscoliosis but can also occur independently. The anomaly is a protrusion of the meninges through a defect in the vertebrae and the intervertebral foramina into the chest cavity.[123]

Lacunar Skull of the Newborn

Craniolacunae are defects in the inner wall of the cranial vault. They present radiologically as variable areas of decreased vault density with interlacing ridges of increased ossification outlining the lacunae. Lacunar skull of the newborn is usually associated with spinal dysraphia. Craniolacunia is present in utero and tends to disappear by 6 months of age.

Neurenteric Canal

In early embryological life, the neurenteric canal connects the primitive alimentary canal and the neural groove at its caudal end. Persistence of the canal may produce midline defects connecting the gastrointestinal tract with the spinal canal, and even with an opening in the back. Remnants of the neurenteric canal may give rise to teratomas. Diastematomyelia and diplomyelia may originate in faulty disappearance of the neurenteric canal. The occurrence of diastematomyelia among members of the same sibship has been described. A review of the question is provided by Maroun and associates.[68]

Deviation in Head Size

Head size is the result of interaction between brain size and the bony structures of the skull. Skull capacity is not a static figure. It parallels closely the brain growth during childhood. In senescence, the reverse occurs to some extent.

Microcephaly

Microcephaly may be an expression of lack of brain development but, alone, does not imply mental retardation. Especially when proportional to body size, microcephalic children may achieve the same academic performance as "normal"-headed students. Microcephaly can be defined as head circumference three standard deviations below the values of a control age group. There may be various causes for microcephaly, such as rubella, toxoplasmosis (chorioretinitis, periventricular calcifications, cataract, congenital heart disease, deafness), cytomegalic inclusion body disease, intrauterine irradiation of the embryo, pituitary dwarfism, chromosomal aberrations (cat-cry syndrome), or inborn errors of metabolism (phenylketonuria). Microcephaly is also a component of other birth defect syndromes.

Macrocephaly

Macrocephaly (large head) is of direct interest to pediatric neurosurgeons as a prime symptom of intracranial space-occupying lesions. It may result from skull thickening by bony overgrowth as in craniodiaphyseal and craniometaphyseal dysplasia, osteopetrosis, pycnodysostosis, and the like. Besides hydrocephalus, hemorrhages, tumors, and similar expanding lesions, there may be other causes for increased head size: leukodystrophies (e.g., Canavan spongy degeneration, Alexander disease, Krabbe globoid leukodystrophy); lipidoses and mucopolysaccharidoses (e.g., Tay-Sachs disease, Hurler and Hunter diseases); phakomatoses (e.g., von Recklinghausen neurofibromatosis, tuberous sclerosis); achondroplasia from a combination of hydrocephalus, subarachnoid hygroma, and true megalencephaly; idiopathic cerebral gigantism (Sotos disease); and idiopathic benign familial megalencephaly.

Sotos Disease

Clinically patients with Sotos disease present with symmetrically enlarged heads, prominent foreheads, coarse facial features, and congenital gigantism.[108] Advanced bone age is detected on skeletal x-ray survey. Neurologically, patients with Sotos disease are mentally retarded and delayed in acquisition of speech functions. Seizures, hypotonia, lack of fine motor control, and clumsiness are other symptoms. Sexual development and endocrine function is usually normal. Enlarged ventricles are seen on air studies. Postmortem examination in one case failed to reveal any significant central nervous system anomalies.[111] The condition is transmitted as a recessive trait, but in three families with 11 affected members there was dominant inheritance.[126]

Idiopathic Megalencephaly

In *idiopathic megalencephaly* ("large brain"), as in Sotos disease, there is an increased head volume.[28] Other disorders may occur concomitantly: adrenal cortical hyperplasia or adrenal insufficiency, pseudohermaphroditism, and myopathy. Patients may be intelligent or mentally retarded. Communicating hydrocephalus, optic atrophy, and progressive neurological deficit can be indicative of a more evolutionary condition than benign familial megalencephaly. Anatomically, there may be marked neuronal disarray with diffuse glial overgrowth. In some cases the impression is of a neoplastic tendency described as diffuse glioblastomatosis or diffuse gangliocytoma. Like microcephaly, megalencephaly seems to affect a heterogeneous group. A strong dominant character has been demonstrated in several families.[100]

An unusual and rare presentation is *unilateral megalencephaly*. Like bilateral megalencephaly, the condition has variously been interpreted as a neoplastic tendency or as a developmental disorder.[116]

Hydrocephalus and Related Malformations

Hydrocephalus

Congenital hydrocephalus is reported in about 0.1 per cent of all newborn children. Once it occurs the empirical risk of having a second child with hydrocephalus or another dysraphia increases to 4.2 per cent.[64] In a few families congenital hydrocephalus behaves as an X-linked character.[49] In X-linked cases associated findings include an irregular cranium, asymmetrical face, thumbs held across the palm of the hand, spasticity of the lower extremities, and abnormal plantar response.[53] Amniocentesis is of no value for prenatal diagnosis. Ultrasound imaging is the best method (Fig. 34–3).

In hydrocephalus the "burden" of the defect can be decreased by proper operative care. Genetic counseling is highly recommended for families with a history of congenital hydrocephalus. The empirical risk figures are similar to those for dysraphia. The X-linked form deserves special attention.

Hydrocephalus is a complication of a number of birth defect patterns: achondroplasia; the Klippel-Feil syndrome and anomalies of the occipitocervical junction such as platybasia; spinal dysraphias; phakomatoses such as tuberous sclerosis and von Recklinghausen disease; mucopolysaccharidoses such as Hurler disease; osteopetrosis, chondrodystrophies; the Dandy-Walker and Arnold-Chiari malformations; chromosomal anomalies (trisomy 13–15); prenatal infections (syphilis, toxoplasmosis, cytomegalic inclusions); absence of the corpus callosum; and cerebral mantle layering malformations such as micropolygyria.

Hydranencephaly

Hydranencephaly is an extreme degree of hydrocephalus.[37] The cerebral cortex is represented by a thin membrane, more plethoric in the basal regions. The corpus striatum is absent, the thalami are underdeveloped, the brain stem and cerebellum are grossly intact. The injury to the embryo is thought to occur between the second and third week after conception.

Syringomyelia, syringobulbia, and the Arnold-Chiari malformation are congenital malformations that are discussed in Chapter 41.

Dandy-Walker Malformation

The Dandy-Walker malformation is a dysgenesis of the cerebellar vermis with

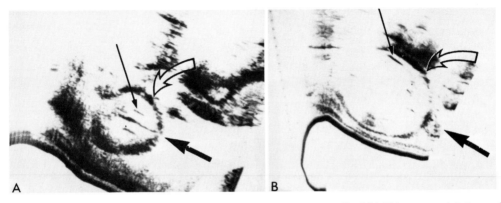

Figure 34–3   Ultrasound imaging. *A*. In a normal child. *B*. In hydrocephalic child. Thin arrow points to margins of thalami in normal fetus, to lateral margin of grossly enlarged lateral ventricle in the hydrocephalic child. In the hydrocephalic child, the biparietal distance is 9.9 cm as compared with 6.1 cm for the chest. (Courtesy of S. Arnon, M.D.)

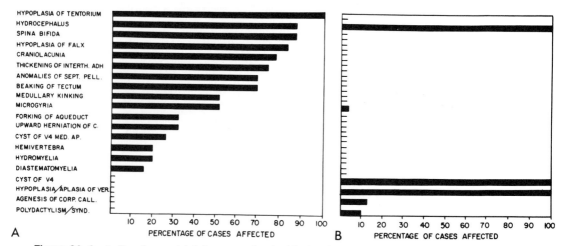

Figure 34–4 A. Developmental defects associated with Arnold-Chiari malformation. B. Defects associated with the Dandy-Walker malformation. (From Gardner, E., O'Rahilly, R., and Prolo, D.: The Dandy-Walker and Arnold-Chiari malformations. Arch. Neurol. (Chicago), 32:393–407, 1975. Copyright 1975, The American Medical Association. Reprinted by permission.)

cystic dilatation of the fourth ventricle and high-positioned tentorium cerebelli. The pattern of malformations seen in the Dandy-Walker syndrome is quite different from the Arnold-Chiari pattern, as illustrated by Figure 34–4. The most commonly associated features, besides posterior fossa findings, are hydrocephalus, agenesis of the corpus callosum, and mental retardation.[15,40] The Dandy-Walker syndrome has occurred in sibs; in one family the condition was associated with polycystic kidneys. In another family it was associated with lissencephaly, congenital cataracts, retinal dysgenesis, and choroid coloboma.[18] Of practical importance is the possibility of congenital heart disease, as a ventriculoperitoneal rather than a ventriculoatrial shunt should be considered in such cases to avoid the cardiopathy.

Failure of Commissuration and Defects in Neuronal Layering

Agenesis of Corpus Callosum

A major failure of commissuration is agenesis of the corpus callosum, found once in two to three thousand neuroradiological examinations. Embryologically the defect probably occurs within the second week after conception. Not surprisingly, other structures bordering the corpus callosum—anterior commissure, septum pellucidum, gyrus cinguli—may also be in-

volved. Porencephaly and microgyria are other findings. The main radiographic features of absence of the corpus callosum are dorsal extension and dilatation of the third ventricle and marked separation of the lateral ventricles, which have dilatated posterior horns, angular dorsal margins, and concave mesial borders.

Clinically, patients may present with mental deficiency, seizures, long tract symptoms, optic atrophy, and colobomas of optic nerve or iris. Precocious puberty, hydrocephalus, and microcephaly are additional features. Often the corpus callosum agenesis is an innocuous finding. Interhemispheric lipomas must be searched for. Families have been described in which agenesis of the corpus callosum was X-linked and recessive.[72] Agenesis of the corpus callosum is a feature of arhinencephaly and other syndromes.

SEIZURE DISORDERS

There are suggestions of a familial tendency in some seizure disorders. In a selected group of 74 patients with temporal lobe epilepsy who underwent temporal lobectomy, the family history was positive for epilepsy in 30 per cent. The operative outcome, however, was the same in patients with or without a familial history of epilepsy.[54]

Attention should be given to the teratogenic effects of anticonvulsant medications. The incidence of malformations in children born to mothers taking antiepileptic medication is 6.7 per cent as compared with 2.9 per cent in epileptic mothers not receiving such drugs. There is a question whether the antiepileptic drug is the teratogenic factor. It has been suggested that the greater incidence of malformations in children born to epileptic mothers is due to the basic condition of the mother (epilepsy), and not necessarily to the medication.[102] Until definitive information becomes available, caution is advisable in therapy during pregnancy of epileptic mothers.

Congenital malformations occur with any anticonvulsant drug. Most common are digital and skeletal anomalies, cleft lip, and cardiac defects. Neurological defects include microcephaly, cebocephaly, meningomyelocele, and anencephaly. Fatal neonatal hemorrhages seem to occur more frequently in infants of these mothers than in a control population.[9]

Hydantoins are likely to be responsible for the "fetal hydantoin syndrome." Such a clinical picture is found in 11 per cent of children prenatally exposed to hydantoins, and in addition, 31 per cent may exhibit some features of the syndrome.[45] The fetal hydantoin syndrome is characterized by prenatal delay in growth and craniofacial anomalies such as microcephaly, low-set ears, low nasal bridge, hypertelorism, and gingival hypertrophy. Fontanels are enlarged. Limb defects, especially hypoplasia of nails and distal phalanges, may become less prominent with advancing age. Other malformations also can be seen. A major concern is a potential for impairment of intellectual abilities.

The "fetal hydantoin syndrome" may have causes other than the anticonvulsant and resembles the effects of alcohol abuse during pregnancy. In the "fetal alcohol syndrome" also there are intrauterine growth retardation, microcephaly, facial dysplasia, and cardiac defects. Short palpebral fissure, micrognathia, low nasal bridge, convex upper lip, narrow vermilion border, and epicanthal folds are elements of the facial dysplasia. Neurologically these neonates may have symptoms of withdrawal such as irritability, tremor, opisthotonos, hyperacusia, and seizures.[90] Failure to thrive, delay in development, and fine motor dysfunction are other clinical elements.

During pregnancy, the dosages of hydantoins and phenobarbiturates required to maintain therapeutic levels are increased, and consequently the risk of teratogenicity may be greater.[60] Switching from hydantoins to phenobarbital may decrease the risk of malformed children. Neurosurgeons are mostly involved with short-term follow-ups for post-traumatic seizure disorders. In such cases, the problem of teratogenicity may be avoided by suggesting delay of pregnancy until antiepileptic medication can be discontinued. In any event an epileptic patient must continue to take her medication during pregnancy.

DEFECTS OF CRANIAL NERVES AND PERIPHERAL NERVOUS SYSTEM

Cranial Nerves

The *olfactory sense* can be completely absent as a dominant trait or as part of such syndromes as hypogonadotropic hypogonadism with anosmia.[105] Anosmia for more than 20 varieties of substances such as freesia flowers, musk, isovaleric or isobutyric acid, *n*-butylmercaptan, or cyanide can also be present as a hereditary trait.

Optic nerve involvement is seen in hereditary degenerations such as Behr or Leber optic atrophy. Optic atrophy may be encountered in hereditary spinocerebellar degenerations and other clinical syndromes.

Duane Syndrome

In the Duane syndrome (dominant) there is progressive retraction of the eyeball. The condition shows predilection for the left side but can be bilateral. The abduction of the eye is disturbed, and if several muscles are involved the eye is pulled backward. Transmission of the Duane syndrome and congenital thenar hypoplasia involving primarily the abductor pollicis brevis as a dominant trait has been reported in a family.[86]

Adie Syndrome

A totally harmless trait is the Adie syndrome of pupillotonia (usually unilateral) and absence of tendon reflexes.[3]

Marcus Gunn Phenomenon

The Marcus Gunn jaw-winking phenomenon is a congenital or dominant trait in 93 per cent of cases. In the remaining 7 per cent it appears after trauma or infections. It is characterized by slight ptosis of one eyelid and associated movements of the eyelid on opening or closing the jaw. Protrusion or lateral movements of the jaw result in elevation of the affected lid. Males are more commonly affected than females, and the left side more often than the right.

Peripheral Nervous System

Neuropathies with *predominantly sensory involvement* can be grouped as indifference to pain or insensibility to pain.

Congenital Indifference to Pain

In congenital indifference to pain the child perceives sensory stimuli but is unable to perceive them as "pain" at the level of higher cortical function. In hereditary sensory neuropathy, involvement of the peripheral sensory neuron (receptor) and the peripheral nerves are the substrata for abnormal perception of some or all sensations.[85]

The patient with congenital indifference to pain can perceive hot and cold, sharp and dull. However, no sensation is considered painful. The peripheral axon reflex is intact, and no histological abnormalities are found in the peripheral nerves. These patients have numerous cutaneous and oral mucosal burns, and repeated fractures and neurotrophic joints are common. They make no complaint, however, of headache, toothache, visceral, or labor pains. The condition is usually transmitted as a recessive trait, but has a dominant character in a few families.[24]

VASCULAR MALFORMATIONS

Intracranial Berry Aneurysms

Familial occurrence of berry aneurysms has been reported by several authors. They are more likely than other aneurysms to be present at a younger age. Also the incidence of anterior communicating an-

eurysms is less common, whereas right internal carotid aneurysms are more frequent.[95] A family history of berry aneurysms constitutes an indication for more aggressive approach to individuals with minor symptoms. Increased frequency of berry aneurysms is found in association with coarctation of the aorta, polycystic kidneys, fibromuscular dysplasia of the renal arteries, biliary fibroangiomatosis, and the Ehlers-Danlos syndrome. These aneurysms are discussed in greater detail in Chapters 46 and 53.

Angiomatosis

Various angiomatoses affecting the central nervous system are summarized in Table 34–5.

Von Hippel-Lindau Disease

Von Hippel-Lindau disease is an angiomatosis of the retina and hemangioblastoma in the cerebellum (66 per cent of cases subjected to autopsy), brain stem (14 per cent), and spinal cord (28 per cent). Cutaneous hemangiomas and visceral cysts are common (kidney, pancreas, liver, skeleton, spleen). Syringomyelia is found in 24 per cent of cases at autopsy and may represent an equivalent of the cystic hemangioblastoma found in the cerebellum. The first symptoms are mainly related to posterior fossa tumor (in 55 per cent of all cases) or to visual loss (18 per cent). Renal tumor and pheochromocytoma are first symptoms in 10 per cent. In another 12 per cent of patients the condition is diagnosed in asymptomatic individuals. The age at diagnosis is mostly by the early thirties, but some cases are known among children and the elderly. Patients coming to attention because of a malignant tumor (e.g., renal cell carcinoma) are usually older. The cause of death is usually the cerebellar hemangioblastoma (71 per cent). Renal cell carcinoma (14 per cent) and other malignant tumors such as pheochromocytoma, glioma conus medullaris, and ependymoma are the remaining causes of death.[50]

Hemangioblastoma of the cerebellum represents 2 per cent of all tumors and between 7 and 10 per cent of all posterior fossa tumors. The Lindau tumor is a typically unilateral large cyst with a small,

TABLE 34–5 CENTRAL NERVOUS SYSTEM INVOLVEMENT IN HEREDITARY ANGIOMATOSIS

CONDITION	HEREDITY	AGE AT DETECTION	VASCULAR MALFORMATION	REMARKS
Von Hippel-Lindau	Dominant	Adult	Hemangioblastoma (cerebellum, retina, spinal cord, other organs)	Syringomyelia, neoplasia (pheochromocytoma, renal cell carcinoma, glioma conus medullaris, ependymoma)
Sturge-Weber	Not proved	Birth	Facial nevus, meningeal angiomatosis (parieto-occipital)	Cortical blood vessel calcifications Epilepsy, mental retardation, variable neurological deficit
Hereditary hemorrhagic telangiectasia	Dominant	Adult	Telangiectasias (skin, mucosa, internal organs) Intracerebral telangiectasias and arteriovenous malformations	Bleeding diathesis, headaches, seizures, alternating hemiparesis, brain abscesses
Ataxia-telangiectasia	Recessive	2 years	Conjunctival telangiectasias	Cerebellar ataxia, IgA immunodeficiency, neoplasia, choreoathetosis
Klippel-Trenaunay-Weber	Not proved	Childhood	Extensive cutaneous hemangiomas, spinal cord angioma	Osseous and muscular hypertrophy, varices
Nevus flammeus	Dominant	Birth	Cutaneous nevi, metameric epidural angiomatosis	
Familial non-calcifying meningeal angiomatosis*	Sex-linked recessive	Childhood	Corticomeningeal angiomatosis, skin telangiectatic network (marbled skin)	Epilepsy, dementia, demyelination of centrum ovale
Cutaneous and spinal cord hem-angiomatosis†	?Recessive	Childhood	Cutaneous hemangioma, spinal cord hemangioblastoma	Acrocyanosis, articular hyperlaxity, vertebral body abnormalities, hypertelorism
Facial and brain stem angiomatosis‡	?Dominant	Childhood	Facial nevus, brain stem arteriovenous malformation	

* From Divry, P., and Van Bogaert, L.: Une maladie familiale caractérisée par une angiomatose diffuse cortico-méningée non-calcifiante et une démyélinisation progressive de la substance blanche. J. Neurol. Neurosurg. Psychiat., 9:41–54, 1946.

† From Gluszcz, A., Polis, Z., and Waleszkowski, J.: Familial syndrome of general dysplasia of the connective tissue and of the vascular system associated with angioblastoma of the spinal cord. Pol. Med. J., 2:924–936, 1963.

‡ From Wyburn-Mason, R.: Arteriovenous aneurysm of mid-brain and retina, facial naevi and mental changes. Brain, 66:163–203, 1943.

highly vascular mural nodule. One fifth of the patients have solid tumors. The lesions are usually unilateral. The recurrence risk is not precisely known but seems to be slight. The results of radiotherapy have been inconclusive. The spinal cord lesions are similar to those of syringomyelia, and the vascular tumor is more difficult to locate. The eye fundi lesions are striking, with pinkish vascular tumor and marked tortuosity of dilated arteriovenous pairs. Indirect ophthalmoscopy and fluorescein angiography can detect minute retinal lesions. The prognosis of retinal angiomatosis is excellent if treated early.[121] Long before there are any clinical signs of loss of sight, these lesions can be treated by photocoagulation with uniform success and few or no complications. Failure to recognize early lesions may result in loss of the eye by reactive retinal inflammation, detachment, or glaucoma. Blood dyscrasia may be present in von Hippel-Lindau disease.[97] The disease has an autosomal dominant pattern of inheritance, and the vascular lesions tend to occur in the same location in members of the same family. Neurological evaluation and intensive follow-up of all family members can be lifesaving. Prospective family evaluation has high return. For example, Christoferson and co-workers were able to locate nine cases among 90 persons in one family who were examined.[20] A major effort is made in follow-up of patients with von Hippel-Lindau disease to detect malignant disease such as renal cell carcinoma. The incidence of malignant tumors is also higher among unaffected members of von Hippel-Lindau families.

Sturge-Weber Syndrome

The clinical features of Sturge-Weber syndrome (encephalotrigeminal angioma-

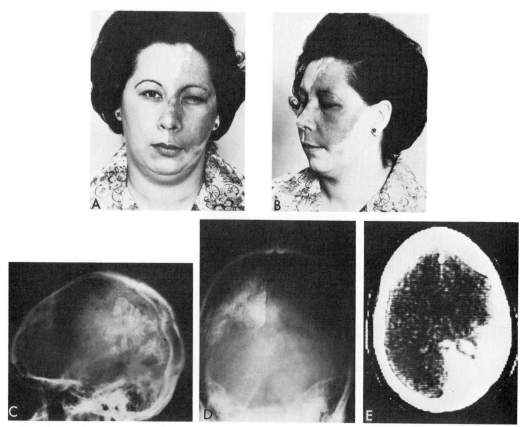

Figure 34–5 Sturge-Weber disease. *A* and *B*. Facial nevus. The patient lost the vision of her left eye owing to glaucoma. *C*, *D*, and *E*. Intracranial calcifications.

tosis) are facial nevus, seizures, and intracranial calcifications. The facial nevus usually is a unilateral port wine stain, primarily in the distribution of the ophthalmic division (Fig. 34–5). The nevoid lesions can extend to the scalp, neck, trunk, and extremities, following the distribution of sensory cutaneous nerves. Ipsilateral angiomatosis of the retina and glaucoma can be present. The seizures are mainly focal, secondarily generalized. The typical intracranial calcifications are in the ipsilateral parieto-occipital cortex underlying the angiomatous malformation of the meninges. In 16 per cent of cases the calcifications are bilateral.[10] Neurological deficits, such as spastic hemiparesis, are highly variable in severity and localization. On pathological examination the main lesion is found to be leptomeningeal venous angiomatosis, most often in the posterior parietal and occipital regions. The angiomatosis also affects other mesenchymal derivatives such as the lungs, gastrointestinal tract, or ovary. The leptomeningeal venous proliferation is concomitant to a reactive vascularity in the underlying cortical and subcortical regions, the latter having no tendency to angiomatosis. There is cortical atrophy with deposition of calcium predominantly in the second and third cortical layers. The subintimal calcium deposits are in the cerebral surface capillaries that are not part of the angiomatosis. On plain skull films one can see calcifications following cerebral convolutions, appearing as double curvilinear densities (tram lines); they are usually not apparent until after age 2. Long-standing acute lymphocytic leukemia in remission may present the same skull x-ray appearance. Computed tomography can permit early detection of intracranial calcifications before they become apparent on plain skull films. The leptomeningeal angiomatoses may be visualized with contrast enhancement.

Operation, even hemispherectomy, has been attempted, mainly for uncontrollable seizures.[34] Most patients with Sturge-Weber disease will live to the fourth or fifth decade, or even a normal life span. Seizure control is difficult and is the main object of therapy. Glaucoma can be controlled, and this may avoid loss of vision. Subarachnoid hemorrhage is not a frequent complication in this syndrome.

Intracranial Calcifications

Intracranial calcifications can be detected in the following birth defects: Sturge-Weber disease (curvilinear calcifications following the pattern of cerebral gyri); cytomegalic inclusion body disease (bilateral, stippled, or curvilinear, periventricular calcifications); toxoplasmosis (bilateral intracortical calcifications and linear streaks of calcifications in the basal ganglia); tuberous sclerosis (nodular calcifications in the ventricular walls); teratoma, craniopharyngioma, and other tumors; and retinoblastoma (intraorbital calcifications).

TUMORS

Tumors of the nervous system have occasionally been reported in families. Such reports have been published for most brain neoplasms, including glioma, astrocytoma, medulloblastoma, cerebral sarcoma, oligodendroglioma, meningioma, and neuroblastoma.*

Von Recklinghausen neurofibromatosis has a definite dominant character. Dominance has also been suggested for bilateral acoustic neuroma, bilateral retinoblastoma, and in some families, tuberous sclerosis. There are racial differences in the occurrence of brain tumors—gliomas are more common in blacks than in whites, and the reverse is true of pituitary adenomas.[35] Congenital defects such as dysraphias may be associated with a greater incidence of malignant disease. Also, a group of diseases called phakomatoses show a predisposition to develop multiple primary neoplasms, including tumors in the central nervous system (Table 34–6).

---

* See references: glioma, 98, astrocytoma, 76; medulloblastoma, 124; cerebral sarcoma, 39; oligodendroglioma, 89; meningioma, 101; neuroblastoma, 93.

TABLE 34–6 NERVOUS SYSTEM NEOPLASIAS IN PHAKOMATOSES

DISEASE	ASSOCIATED NEOPLASMS
Von Recklinghausen disease	Sarcoma, leukemia, glioma, squamous cell carcinoma
Tuberous sclerosis	Renal cell carcinoma, pheochromocytoma, glioma conus medullaris
Bilateral retinoblastoma	Gliomas
Ataxia-telangiectasia	Lymphoreticular neoplasms, leukemia, carcinoma of stomach, gliomas
Hereditary hemorrhagic telangiectasia	Hepatocellular carcinoma
Familial intestinal polyposis	Glioblastoma, medulloblastoma

Besides the conditions mentioned in Table 34–6, birth defects such as Down's syndrome, xeroderma pigmentosum, or progeria have also proclivity to malignant disease.

The aggregation of familial cases of brain tumors may result from exposure to a common noxious agent. It may also represent a yet-undefined genetic predisposition to develop malignant neoplasms. The main point is that neoplasia is not a random event, and particular genetic structure may be necessary for its development.

Von Recklinghausen Neurofibromatosis

The minimal diagnostic criterion is the presence of six café-au-lait spots larger than 1.5 cm. The rugged appearance of café-au-lait spots in Albright polyostotic fibrous dysplasia ("Coast of Maine" contour) is to be distinguished from the smoother appearance of these spots in neurofibromatosis ("Coast of California" contour). Von Recklinghausen disease involves multiple systems, and no organ is spared by the process.

Besides manifestations related to neurofibromas, patients with von Recklinghausen disease are to some degree mentally retarded. Anatomically the mental defect can be related to developmental anomalies of the brain architecture, and is suggestive of in utero onset of the disease. One can find neuronal heterotopias, pachymicrogyria, and disorganization of cortical layering with disarray of normal lamination. Constitutional defects such as a giant extremity, hemihypertrophy, macrocrania, sphenoid bone defect, spina bifida, and cerebral meningocele can also be found.

Tuberous Sclerosis

The incidence of tuberous sclerosis is higher than commonly believed. A minimal incidence figure for Los Angeles county is 24 new cases per 120,000 persons. The condition is characterized by a triad of skin lesions, epilepsy, and mental retardation.

The earliest diagnostic sign can be depigmented ash leaf–shaped areas on the skin, seen in 80 per cent of patients by age 2 (Fig. 34–6). Best seen under a Wood's lamp, the leukoderma appears earlier than the facial sebaceous adenoma or the sharkskin patch (shagreen skin). On the proximal nail fold

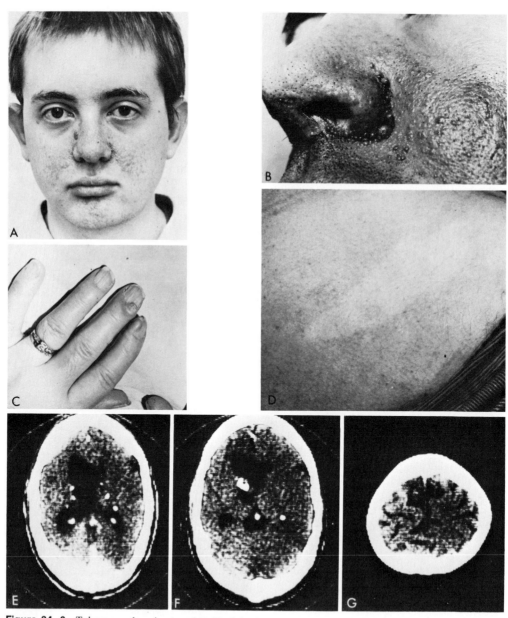

Figure 34–6 Tuberous sclerosis. *A* and *B*. Facial sebaceous adenoma. *C*. Subungual angiofibroma. *D*. Ash leaf–shaped depigmented spot. *E*. Ventricular dilatation and periventricular calcifications. *F*. Deeply situated tumor near the left foramen of Monro. *G*. Cortical atrophy.

subungual angiofibromas (Koenen tumors) occur. Pit-shaped tooth enamel defects are characteristic. The seizures, occasionally flexion spasms with hypsarrhythmia on the electroencephalogram in early childhood, may progress to common generalized convulsive epilepsy. Mental retardation occurs in most cases of tuberous sclerosis but is not necessarily profound. Most patients have an intelligence quotient within the range of 60 to 70. The brain lesions are mainly of two types—dense astrocytic fibrosis in cortical tubers and periventricular "candle guttering." The gliotic cortical plaques are not visualized by technetium brain scanning or computed tomography. The subependymal tumors, however, calcify and are easily detected on CT scan. They are present in 35 per cent of patients by age 4. The periventricular tumors are of astrocytic type. Electron microscopic studies show the presence of gliofilaments, beta-type glycogenic particles, and evidence of increased metabolic activity.

A major complication in tuberous sclerosis is malignant degeneration (glioma, sarcoma) in otherwise benign tumors. Massive hemorrhage in periventricular giant cell astrocytoma may occur.[118] The management of patients with tuberous sclerosis focuses on seizure control and operation for central nervous system, kidney, or other tumors. Renal transplants have been successfully done. In the long run, mental retardation and psychotic behavior put major strains on family and treating physicians.

CONNECTIVE TISSUE DISORDERS

Ehlers-Danlos Syndrome

Patients with the Ehlers-Danlos syndrome present with hyperextensibility, fragile skin, easy bruisability, and "cigarette-paper" scarring. The ligamentous laxity and hypermobility of joints are remarkable. These patients are able at will to luxate any of the major articulations, possibly causing injury to nearby nervous structures. Kyphoscoliosis and low back pain are common, and spondylolisthesis may require spinal fusion. The basic defect is in the organization of collagen fibers that leads to generalized organ friability. Patients with Ehlers-Danlos disease may rup-

ture—either spontaneously or after minor trauma—the great vessels, stomach, bowel, lungs, or eyeballs. Potentially lethal complications are related to pathological changes in blood vessels. Intracerebral and subarachnoid hemorrhages are common. Multiple intracranial aneurysms are found in a significant number of patients. Spontaneous development of carotid-cavernous fistulae have been reported.[5] The friability of arterial vessels requires special care in the performance of any invasive procedure. Death from a tear in the ascending aorta has been described after angiography for intracranial arteriovenous fistula.[99] Hemostasis is difficult. During operation the vessels do not contract and may continue to bleed. There are seven recognized entities of Ehlers-Danlos syndrome. The type I (gravis, dominant trait) and type IV (ecchymotic, arterial, or Sack's-type recessive trait) have the greatest potential for complications.

Diastrophic Dwarfism

The salient features of diastrophic dwarfism have been summarized by Walker and co-workers.[119] Diastrophic dwarfism is a short-micromelic dwarfism. There is progressive scoliosis, sometimes associated with kyphosis and responsible in a few patients for spinal cord compression. The kyphosis may decrease spontaneously by the time the child begins to walk, or its persistence and progression may result in ventral compression of the spinal cord by protrusion of a wedged vertebra. Removal of the posterior portion of the vertebra encroaching on the spinal cord and posterior laminectomy are procedures used with success.

Achondroplasia

Achondroplasia is a distinctive type of short-limb rhizomelic dwarfism. The clinical manifestations are fairly pathognomonic, and diagnosis is made early in life. Eighty per cent of cases result from new mutations, and the condition is transmitted as an autosomal dominant characteristic. The main neurological deficits encountered in achondroplasia are related to the smallness of the spinal cord and to the development of hydrocephalus. Besides those two major complications, achondroplasts may have any other nervous system disorder such as cerebral hemorrhage related to aneurysm or arteriovenous malformations.[41]

Constitutionally small spinal canal has been reported as an occasional finding in persons of normal stature. The persons most severely disabled by neurological deficit secondary to small spinal canal, however, are achondroplastic dwarfs. The anatomical basis for the spinal cord involvement in achondroplasia is the spade-shaped constriction of the canal related to premature closure of the ossification centers of the vertebral pedicles (neurosomatic growth plate). The constriction may be demonstrated by computed tomography. In lateral x-rays of the spine there is shortness of the pedicles, and in the anteroposterior view there is diminished interpediculate distance. Measurement of the interpediculate distance in symptom-free achondroplasts and in achondroplasts with neurological deficit severe enough to justify a decompressive laminectomy showed it to be significantly smaller in the lumbar area among the latter (Fig. 34–7).

Neurologically it is possible to identify three types of deficit: compression of the nerve roots, compression of the lower spinal cord, and compression at the cervical spinal canal level and the foramen magnum.

In the first type, radicular symptoms are (1) weakness of dorsiflexion and eversion or plantar flexion (or both) of the foot; in a few cases the quadriceps femoris is involved with weakness of extension and ''giving away'' of the knee; (2) hypoactivity or absence of osteotendinous reflexes of the lower extremities; and (3) complaints by the patient of painful paresthesias. After walking a few blocks these patients are obliged to stop and usually squat. The sensory changes range from patchy loss of cutaneous sensation to clearly delineated radicular hypoesthesia. Frequently there is definite proprioceptive loss. Although the radicular deficit most frequently involves the L5 and S1 roots bilaterally, followed by the L3 and L4 roots, it may also involve the entire cauda equina and produce sphincter disturbances. Involvement of the cervical roots may also occur.

The second type, lower spinal cord compression, is characterized by (1) muscular deficit ranging from mild paraparesis to severe spastic paraplegia; (2) presence of hyperactive osteotendinous reflexes, clonus, and a cutaneous plantar reflex in extension; (3) superficial sensory deficit usually below the lower costal margin (T9–T10 level), preserving often the lowest sacral dermatomes; and (4) marked deficit of posture and vibratory sensation.

The third type, compression at the level of the upper spinal canal and foramen mag-

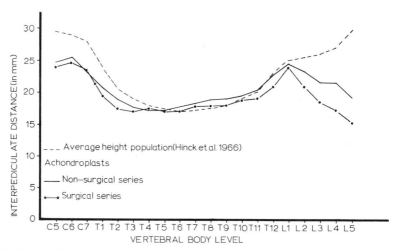

Figure 34–7 Interpediculate distance in average-height population (-----), and in 8 operative (•—•) and 30 randomly selected (—) patients with achondroplasia. The Mann-Whitney U test strongly suggests a statistically significant difference ($p < 0.05$) in the interpediculate distance between the operative and nonoperative series of achondroplasts. All operative patients underwent laminectomy for small spinal canal symptoms.

num, is difficult to recognize in the early stages. Vague complaints such as occipital headache may be the only initial symptom. Later, one can find tetraparesis, usually spastic (sometimes flaccid), manifested by osteotendinous hyperreflexia, spasticity, clonus, and an upgoing plantar response. There is no definite pattern of sensory changes. An injury may precede the appearance of symptoms.

The compression at the upper cervical canal level and the foramen magnum is severe. Extreme hypoplasia of the foramen magnum and segmental malacia of the upper cervical cord is seen in the homozygous form of achondroplasia. Histologically there are diffuse gliosis and moderate vascular proliferation. Large swollen and vacuolated axons are present. The gray matter is poorly demarcated, and only a few shrunken neurons are seen in the anterior horn. The lesions can be related to a direct compression of the spinal cord and even more to a compromised vascular supply.

Decompressive laminectomy gives definite improvement in most cases of radicular involvement. In those cases with spinal cord involvement, a decompressive laminectomy is beneficial to over half the patients. It has to be extensive to avoid a recurrence of the neurological symptoms. An extreme case may need a laminectomy from C4 to the sacrum. Lateral foraminotomy may be combined with laminectomy in the treatment of the radicular type of compression.

Shortly after laminectomy, a few achondroplasts develop symptoms of cord compression at a level higher than the previous one. At reintervention the neurostructures may protrude through the previously decompressed area. The upper border of the window continues to constrict the underlying cord and may be responsible for the

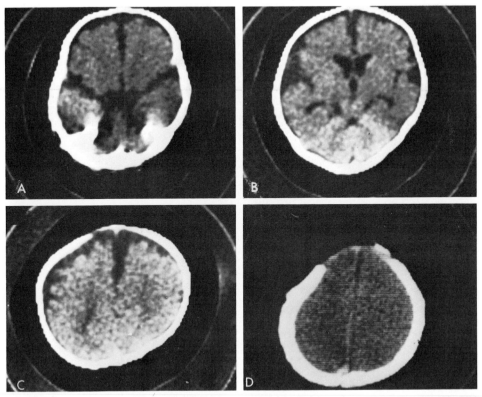

Figure 34–8 *A, B,* and *C.* Mild ventricular dilatation and subdural hygromas in a 6-month-old child with achondroplasia. The accumulated subdural effusions were initially drained by subdural taps, and eventually the left side was treated with membrane stripping. After an uneventful course for four months, the child was admitted in deep coma with a three-day history of decrease in level of consciousness. Subdural taps for subdural effusions were done with little success. *D.* Increased intracranial pressure did not respond to treatment and the child died.

neurological deficit. A fibrous string may be found near the first complete neural arch, and this may add to the compression.

Pantopaque myelography performed by lumbar puncture is, in general, useless. The dye accumulates against the posterior border of the scalloped vertebral bodies and does not permit correct visualization of the stenosis. Introduction of the dye through a ventricular puncture seems to be far less dangerous than suboccipital puncture and may give more precise information about the upper level of compression.

There is no spinal instability consequent to extensive laminectomies in achondroplasts if the facets are spared at operation. A brace is recommended after extensive laminectomies.

The *macrocephaly* in achondroplasia is present from birth and is readily apparent because of the hypoplasia of the facial structures.[104] The head circumference reaches the ninety-seventh percentile, with the greatest increase during the first year of life. The macrocephaly is related to some megalencephaly, but mainly, if not exclusively, to internal and external hydrocephalus (Fig. 34–8). A likely explanation for the development of hydrocephalus is a disturbance in the normal cerebrospinal fluid flow due to the particular skull structure. In achondroplasia there is abnormal ossification of the preformed cartilage bones at the base of the skull. The foramen magnum is small, flattened on both sides, with the plane of the foramen at an abnormal angle to the clivus. A shunting procedure is not a sine qua non for achondroplastic children, and careful evaluation is essential. The decision to perform a shunting procedure has to take into account not only the velocity of the increase in head size and the computed tomographic findings but also the motor and mental development of the child. Most achondroplastic children are delayed in achieving milestones as compared with others. The bulk of children in need of shunting procedures are below the fiftieth percentile in reaching their milestones in comparison with other achondroplasts. An important complication in these children is development of subdural hygroma. Repeated subdural taps may alleviate the acute stage, but a shunting procedure is in-dicated if there is no improvement within a few days.

REFERENCES

1. Aaronson, I.: Anterior sacral meningocele, anal canal duplication cyst and covered anus occurring in one family. J. Pediat. Surg., 5:559–563, 1970.
2. Adams, F. H., and Oliver, C. P.: Hereditary deformities in man due to arrested development. J. Hered., 36:3–7, 1945.
3. Adie, W. J.: Tonic pupils and absent tendon reflexes: A benign disorder sui generis: its complete and incomplete forms. Brain, 55:98–113, 1932.
4. Baldwin, M., and Dekaban, A.: The surgical separation of Siamese twins conjoined by the heads (cephalopagus frontalis) followed by normal development. J. Neurol. Neurosurg. Psychiat., 21:195–202, 1958.
5. Bannerman, R. M., Ingall, G. B., and Graf, C. J.: The familial occurrence of intracranial aneurysms. Neurology (Minneap.), 20:283–292, 1970.
6. Beighton, P., Durr, L., and Hamersma, H.: The clinical features of sclerosteosis. A review of the manifestations in 25 affected individuals. Ann. Intern. Med., 84:393–397, 1976.
7. Bergland, R. M.: Congenital intraspinal extradural cyst. Report of three cases in one family. J. Neurosurg., 28:495–499, 1968.
8. Bergsma, D.: Birth Defects. Atlas and Compendium. Baltimore, The National Foundation—March of Dimes; Williams & Wilkins Co., 1973.
9. Bleyer, W. A., and Skinner, A. L.: Fatal neonatal hemorrhage after maternal anticonvulsant therapy. J.A.M.A., 235:626–627, 1976.
10. Boltshauser, E., Wilson, J., and Hoare, R. D.: Sturge-Weber syndrome with bilateral intracranial calcification. J. Neurol. Neurosurg. Psychiat., 39:429–435, 1976.
11. Brinsmead, M. W.: Complications of amniocentesis. Med. J. Aust., 1:379–385, 1976.
12. Brown, M. W., Templeton, A. W., and Hodges, F. J.: The incidence of acquired and congenital fusions in the cervical spine. Amer. J. Roentgen., 92:1255–1259, 1964.
13. Brown, S. F.: Congenital malformations associated with myelomeningocele. J. Iowa Med. Soc., 65:101–104, 1975.
14. Campbell, S.: Early prenatal diagnosis of neural tube defects by ultrasound. Clin. Obstet. Gynec., 20:351–359, 1977.
15. Carmel, P. W., Antunes, J. L., Hilal, S. K., and Gold, A. P.: Dandy-Walker syndrome: Clinico-pathological features and reevaluation of modes of treatment. Surg. Neurol., 8:132–138, 1977.
16. Carter, C. O.: Diet and congenital defects. Brit. Med. J., 1:290–291, 1973.
17. Carter, C. O.: Clues to aetiology of neural tube malformations. Dev. Med. Child. Neurol., 16: suppl. 32:3–15, 1974.

18. Chemke, J., Czernobilsky, B., Mundel, G., and Barishak, Y. R.: A familial syndrome of central nervous system and ocular malformations. Clin. Genet., 7:1–7, 1975.

19. Cheyney, W. D.: Acro-osteolysis. Amer. J. Roentgen., 94:595–607, 1965.

20. Christoferson, L. A., Gustafson, M. B., and Petersen, A. E.: Von Hippel-Lindau's disease. J.A.M.A., 178:280–282, 1961.

21. Cimino, C. V., and Painter, J. W.: Iniencephaly. Radiology, 79:942–944, 1962.

22. Clawson, D. K., and Loop, J. W.: Progressive diaphyseal dysplasia (Engelmann's disease). J. Bone Joint Surg., 46-A:143–150, 1964.

23. Cohn, D., and Bay-Nielsen, E.: Hereditary defect of the sacrum and coccyx with anterior sacral meningocele. Acta Paediat. Scand., 58:268–274, 1969.

24. Commings, D. E., and Amromin, G. D.: Autosomal dominant insensitivity to pain with hyperplastic myelinopathy and autosomal dominant indifference to pain. Neurology (Minneap.), 24:838–848, 1974.

25. Coury, C., and Delaporte, J.: Les anomalies congénitales des côtes; formes anatomo-radiologiques et incidences pratiques (à propos de 288 cas). Sem. Hôp. Paris, 30:2656–2681. 1963.

26. Cross, A. E., and Opitz, J. M.: Craniosynostosis in the Amish. J. Pediat., 75:1037–1045, 1969.

27. Decking, D., and Heine, J.: Röntgenologische Veränderungen der Halswirbelsäule bei Missbildungen. Z. Orthop., 114:294–304, 1976.

28. DeMyer, W.: Megalencephaly in children. Neurology (Minneap.), 22:634–643, 1972.

29. Divry, P., and Van Bogaert, L.: Une maladie familiale caractérisée par une angiomatose diffuse cortico-méningée non-calcifiante et une démyélinisation progressive de la substance blanche. J. Neurol. Neurosurg. Psychiat., 9:41–54, 1946.

30. Duggan, C. A., Keener, E. B., and Gay, B. B.: Secondary craniosynostosis. Amer. J. Roentgen., 109:277–293, 1970.

31. Ekelund, H., Kullander, S., and Kallen, B.: Major and minor malformations in newborns and infants up to one year of age. Acta Paediat. Scand., 59:297–302, 1970.

32. Elmore, S. M.: Pycnodysostosis: A review. J. Bone Joint Surg., 49-A:153–162, 1967.

33. Elwood, J. H.: Major central nervous system malformations notified in Northern Ireland, 1969 to 1973. Develop. Med. Child Neurol., 18:512–520, 1976.

34. Falconer, M. A., and Rushworth, R. G.: Treatment of encephalotrigeminal angiomatosis (Sturge-Weber disease) by hemispherectomy. Arch. Dis. Child., 35:433–447, 1960.

35. Fan, K. J., Kovi, J., and Earle, K. M.: The ethnic distribution of primary central nervous system tumors: Armed Forces Institute of Pathology, 1958 to 1970. J. Neuropath. Exp. Neurol., 36:41–49, 1977.

36. Field, B., and Kerr, C.: Twinning and neural tube defects. Lancet, 2:964–965, 1974.

37. Fowler, M., Dow, R., White, T. A., and Greer, C. H.: Congenital hydrocephalus—hydrencephaly in five siblings with autopsy studies: A new disease. Develop. Med. Child. Neurol., 14:173–188, 1972.

38. Freeman, J. M., and Borkowf, S.: Craniostenosis: A review of the literature and report of thirty-four cases. Pediatrics, 30:57–70, 1962.

39. Gainer, J. V., Chou, S. M., and Chadduck, W. M.: Familial cerebral sarcomas. Arch. Neurol. (Chicago), 32:665–668, 1975.

40. Gardner, E., O'Rahilly, R., and Prolo, D.: The Dandy-Walker and Arnold-Chiari malformations. Arch. Neurol. (Chicago), 32:393–407, 1975.

41. Gendell, H. M., Barmada, M. A., Maroon, J. C., and Wisotzkey, H.: Intracranial hemorrhage in achondroplasia. Surg. Neurol., 8:283—285, 1977.

42. Gluszcz, A., Polis, Z., and Waleszkowski, J.: Familial syndrome of general dysplasia of the connective tissue and of the vascular system associated with angioblastoma of the spinal cord. Pol. Med. J., 2:924–936, 1963.

43. Goodman, R., and Gorlin, R. J.: Atlas of the Face in Genetic Disorders. St. Louis, C. V. Mosby Co., 1977.

44. Greitzer, L. J., Jones, K. L., Schnall, B. S., and Smith, D. W.: Craniosynostosis—radial aplasia syndrome. J. Pediat., 84:723–724, 1974.

45. Hanson, J. W., Myrianthopoulos, N. C., Harvey, M. A., and Smith, D. W.: Risks to the offspring of women treated with hydantoin anticonvulsants with emphasis on the fetal hydantoin syndrome. J. Pediat., 89:662–668, 1976.

46. Haynes, S. G., Gibson, J. B., and Kurland, L. T.: Epidemiology of neural-tube defects and Down's syndrome in Rochester, Minn., 1935–1971. Neurology (Minneap.), 24:691–700, 1974.

47. Hensinger, R. N., Lang, J. E., and MacEwen, G. D.: Klippel-Feil syndrome. A constellation of associated anomalies. J. Bone Joint Surg., 56-A:1246–1253, 1974.

48. Hogan, G. R., and Bauman, M. L.: Hydrocephalus in Apert's syndrome. J. Pediat., 79:782–787, 1971.

49. Holmes, L. B., Nash, A., ZuRhein, G. M., Levin, M., and Opitz, J. M.: X-linked aqueductal stenosis: Clinical and neuropathological findings in two families. Pediatrics, 51:697–704, 1973.

50. Horton, W. A., Wong, V., and Eldridge, R.: Von Hippel-Lindau disease. Clinical and pathological manifestations in nine families with 50 affected members. Arch. Intern. Med. (Chicago), 136:769–777, 1976.

51. Jackson, W. P. U.: Osteo-dental dysplasia (cleidocranial dysostosis). The "Arnold Head." Acta Med. Scand., 139:292–307, 1951.

52. Janerich, D. T.: Epidemic waves in the prevalence of anencephaly and spina bifida in New York state. Teratology, 8:253–256, 1973.

53. Jansen, J.: Sex-linked hydrocephalus. Develop. Med. Child. Neurol., 17:633–640, 1975.

54. Jensen, I.: Genetic factors in temporal lobe epilepsy. Acta neurol. Scand., 52:381–394, 1975.

55. Knobloch, W. H., and Layer, J. M.: Retinal detachment and encephalocele. J. Pediat. Ophthal., 8:181–184, 1971.

56. Kosnik, E. J., Gilbert, G., and Sayers, M. P.: Familial inheritance of coronal craniosynostosis. Develop. Med. Child Neurol., 17:630–633, 1975.

57. Kuhr, M. D.: Neural tube defects and mid-cycle abstinence: A test of the "over-ripeness" hypothesis in man. Develop. Med. Child Neurol., 19:589–592, 1977.

58. Kurent, J. E., and Sever, J. L.: Perinatal infections and epidemiology of anencephaly and spina bifida. Teratology, 8:359–361, 1973.

59. Kurtzke, J. F., Goldberg, I. D., and Kurland, L. T.: Congenital malformations of the nervous system. In Kurland, L. T., Kurtzke, J. F., and Goldberg, I. D., eds.: Epidemiology of Neurologic and Sense Organ Disorders. Cambridge, Mass., Harvard University Press, 1973, pp. 169–210.

60. Lander, C. M., Edwards, V. E., Eadie, M. J., and Tyrer, J. H.: Plasma anticonvulsant concentrations during pregnancy. Neurology (Minneap.), 27:128–131, 1977.

61. Laurence, K. M.: The recurrence risk in spina bifida cystica and anencephaly. Develop. Med. Child. Neurol., 11:suppl. 20:23–30, 1969.

62. Laurence, K. M., and Roberts, C. J.: Spina bifida and anencephaly: Are miscarriages a possible cause? Brit. Med. J., 2:361–362, 1977.

63. Levin, L. S., Perrin, J. C., Ose, L., Dorst, J. P., Miller, J. D., and McKusick, V. A.: A heritable syndrome of craniosynostosis, short thin hair, dental abnormalities and short limbs: Cranioectodermal dysplasia. J. Pediat., 90:55–61, 1977.

64. Lorber, J., and De, N. C.: Family history of congenital hydrocephalus. Develop. Med. Child Neurol., 6:suppl. 22:94–100, 1970.

65. Lorber, J., and Levick, K.: Spina bifida cystica: Incidence of spina bifida occulta in parents and in controls. Arch. Dis. Child., 42:171–173, 1967.

66. Lowry, R. B.: Congenital absence of the fibula and craniosynostosis in sibs. J. Med. Genet., 9:227–229, 1972.

67. Lynch, P. J., and Kahn, E. A.: Congenital defects of the scalp. A surgical approach to aplasia cutis congenita. J. Neurosurg., 33:198–202, 1970.

68. Maroun, F. B., Jacob, J. C., and Heneghan, W. D.: Diastematomyelia. St. Louis, Warren H. Green, Inc., 1976.

69. McKusick, V. A.: New syndrome manifested by mandibular hypoplasia, acroosteolysis, stiff joints, and cutaneous atrophy (mandibuloacral dysplasia) in two unrelated boys. In The Clinical Delineation of Birth Defects. Vol. VII, No. 7, Part XI, Orofacial Structures. Baltimore, The National Foundation, Williams & Wilkins, 1971, pp. 291–296.

70. McKusick, V. A.: Heritable disorders of connective tissue. 4th Ed. St. Louis, C. V. Mosby Co., 1972.

71. McKusick, V. A.: Mendelian Inheritance in Man. 4th Ed. Baltimore and London, Johns Hopkins University Press, 1975.

72. Menkes, J. H., Philippart, M., and Clark, D. B.:

Hereditary partial agenesis of corpus callosum. Arch. Neurol. (Chicago), 11:198–208, 1964.

73. Micheli, L. J., Hall, J. E., and Watts, H. G.: Spinal instability in Larsen's syndrome. J. Bone Joint Surg., 58-A:562–565, 1976.

74. Milunsky, A., and Alpert, E.: Prenatal diagnosis of neural tube defects. I. Problems and pitfalls: Analysis of 2495 cases using the alpha-fetoprotein assay. Obstet. Gynec., 48:1–5, 1976.

75. Morrison, S. G., Perry, L. W., and Scott, L. P.: Congenital brevicollis (Klippel-Feil syndrome) and cardiovascular anomalies. Amer. J. Dis. Child., 115:614–620, 1968.

76. Motz, I. P., Bots, G., and Endtz, L. J.: Astrocytoma in three sisters. Neurology (Minneap.), 27:1038–1041, 1977.

77. Murphy, E. A.: Genetic counseling. In Medicine in the University and Community of the Future. Proceedings of the Scientific Sessions Marking the Centennial of the Faculty of Medicine, Dalhousie University. Halifax, Nova Scotia, Dalhousie University Press, 1969, pp. 143–148.

78. Naggan, L., and MacMahon, B.: Ethnic differences in the prevalence of anencephaly and spina bifida in Boston, Mass. New Eng. J. Med., 277:1119–1123, 1967.

79. Neel, J. V.: A study of major congenital defects in Japanese infants. Amer. J. Hum. Genet., 10:398–445, 1958.

80. Nelson, M. M., and Forfar, J. O.: Congenital abnormalities at birth: Their association in the same patient. Develop. Med. Child Neurol., 11:3–16, 1969.

81. Newcombe, H. B.: Population genetics: Population records. In Burdette, W. J., ed.: San Francisco, Holden-Day, Inc., 1962, pp. 92–113.

82. Norum, R. A.: Costovertebral anomalies with apparent recessive inheritance. In The Clinical Delineation of Birth Defects. Vol. V, No. 4, Part IV, Skeletal Dysplasias. Baltimore, The National Foundation, Williams & Wilkins, 1969, pp. 326–329.

83. O'Connell, J. E. A.: Surgical separation of two pairs of craniopagus twins. Brit. Med. J., 1:1333–1336, 1964.

84. O'Connell, J. E. A.: An operation to separate craniopagus twins. Brit. J. Surg., 55:841–850, 1968.

85. Ohta, M., Ellefson, R. D., Lambert, E. H., and Dyck, P. J.: Hereditary sensory neuropathy, type II. Arch. Neurol. (Chicago), 29:23–37, 1973.

86. Okihiro, M. M., Tasaki, T., Nakano, K. K., and Bennett, B. K.: Duane syndrome and congenital upper limb anomalies. A familial occurrence. Arch. Neurol. (Chicago), 34:174–179, 1977.

87. Onuigob, W. I.: Encephaloceles in Nigerian Igbos. J. Neurol. Neurosurg. Psychiat., 40:726, 1977.

88. O'Rahilly, R., and Gardner, E. D.: The timing and sequence of events in the development of the human nervous system during the embryonic period proper. Z. Anat. Entwicklungsgesch., 134:1–12, 1971.

89. Parkinson, D., and Hall, C. W.: Oligodendrogliomas; simultaneous appearance in frontal lobes of siblings. J. Neurosurg., 19:424–426, 1962.

90. Pierog, S., Chandavasau, O., and Wexler, I.: Withdrawal symptoms in infants with the fetal alcohol syndrome. J. Pediat., *90*:630–633, 1977.

91. Pionnier, R., and Depraz, A.: Les anomalies costales d'origine con génitale (étude statistique d'après 10,000 radiographies). Radiol. Clin. (Basel), *25*:170–186, 1956.

92. Renwick, J. H.: Hypothesis: Anencephaly and spina bifida are usually preventable by avoidance of a specific but unidentified substance present in certain potato tubers. Brit. J. Prev. Soc. Med., *26*:67–88, 1972.

93. Roberts, F. F., and Lee, K. R.: Familial neuroblastoma presenting as multiple tumors. Radiology, *116*:133–136, 1975.

94. Robinow, M., Pfeiffer, R. A., Gorlin, R. J., McKusick, V. A., Renuart, A. W., Johnson, G. F., and Summitt, R. L.: Acrodysostosis. A syndrome of peripheral dysostosis, nasal hypoplasia, and mental retardation. Amer. J. Dis. Child., *121*:195–203, 1971.

95. Sakai, N., Sakata, K., Yamada, H., Yamamoto, M., Aiba, T., and Takeda, F.: Familial occurrence of intracranial aneurysms. Surg. Neurol., *2*:25–29, 1974.

96. Saxen, L., Klemetti, A., and Haro, A. S.: A matched-pair register for studies of selected congenital defects. Amer. J. Epidem., *100*:297–306, 1974.

97. Scherrer, J. R., Hausser, E., and Berney, J.: Thrombocytopénie associée à un hémangioblastome cérébelleux. Schweiz. Med. Wschr., *95*:1456–1459, 1965.

98. Schoenberg, B. S., Glista, G. G., and Reagan, T. J.: The familial occurrence of glioma. Surg. Neurol., *3*:139–145, 1975.

99. Schoolman, A., and Kepes, J. J.: Bilateral spontaneous carotid-cavernous fistulae in Ehlers-Danlos syndrome; case report. J. Neurosurg., *26*:82–86, 1967.

100. Schreier, H., Rapin, I., and Davis, J.: Familial megalencephaly or hydrocephalus. Neurology (Minneap.), *24*:232–236, 1974.

101. Sedzimir, C. B., Frazer, A. K., and Roberts, J. R.: Cranial and spinal meningiomas in a pair of identical twin boys. J. Neurol. Neurosurg. Psychiat., *36*:368–376, 1973.

102. Shapiro, S., Slone, D., Hartz, S. C., Rosenberg, L., Siskind, V., Monson, R. R., Mitchell, A. A., and Heinonen, O. P.: Anticonvulsants and parental epilepsy in the development of birth defects. Lancet, *1*:272–275, 1976.

103. Shillito, J., and Matson, D. D.: Craniosynostosis: A review of 519 surgical patients. Pediatrics, *41*:829–853, 1968.

104. Siebens, A. A., Hungerford, D. S., and Kirby, N. A.: Curves of the achondroplastic spine: A new hypothesis. Johns Hopkins Med. J., *142*:205–210, 1978.

105. Singh, N., Grewal, M. S., and Austin, J. H.: Familial anosmia. Arch. Neurol. (Chicago), *22*:40–44, 1970.

106. Smith, D. W.: Recognizable Patterns of Human Malformation. Genetic, Embryologic and Clinical Aspects. Philadelphia, W. B. Saunders Co., 1970.

107. Sostrin, R. D., Thompson, J. R., Rouhe, S. A., and Hasso, A. N.: Occult spinal dysraphism in the geriatric patient. Radiology, *125*:165–169, 1977.

108. Sotos, J. F., Cutler, E. A., and Dodge, P.: Cerebral gigantism. Amer. J. Dis. Child., *131*:625–627, 1977.

109. Stevenson, A. C., Johnston, H. A., Stewart, M. I. P., and Golding, D. R.: Congenital malformations. A report of a series of consecutive births in 24 centers. Bull. W.H.O., *34*:suppl.:1–127, 1966.

110. Stewart, A. L., Keay, A. J., and Smith, P. G.: Congenital malformations: A detailed study of 2500 liveborn infants. Ann. Hum. Genet., *32*:353–360, 1969.

111. Sugarman, G. I., Heuser, E. T., and Reed, W. B.: A case of cerebral gigantism and hepatocarcinoma. Amer. J. Dis. Child., *131*:631–633, 1977.

112. Sutow, W. W., and Pryde, A. W.: Incidence of spina bifida occulta in relation to age. Amer. J. Dis. Child., 91:211–217, 1956.

113. Temtamy, S. A.: Carpenter's syndrome: Acrocephalosyndactyly. An autosomal recessive syndrome. J. Pediat., *69*:111–120, 1966.

114. Terrafranca, R. J., and Zellis, A.: Congenital hereditary cranium bifidum occultum frontalis. Radiology, *61*:60–66, 1953.

115. Todorov, A., Cohen, K. L., Landau, E., and Spilotro, V.: Craniopagus twins. J. Neurol. Neurosurg. Psychiat., *37*:1291–1298, 1974.

116. Townsend, J. J., Nielsen, S. L., and Malamud, N.: Unilateral megalencephaly: Hamartoma or neoplasm? Neurology (Minneap.), *25*:448–453, 1975.

117. Voris, H. C., Slaughter, W. B., Christian, J. R., and Cayia, E. R.: Successful separation of craniopagus twins. J. Neurosurg., *14*:548–560, 1957.

118. Waga, S., Yamamoto, Y., Kojima, T., and Sakakura, M.: Massive hemorrhage in tuberous sclerosis. Surg. Neurol., *8*:99–101, 1977.

119. Walker, B. A., Scott, C. I., Hall, J. G., Murdoch, J. L., and McKusick, V. A.: Diastrophic dwarfism. Medicine (Balt.), *51*:41–59, 1972.

120. Warkany, J.: Congenital Malformations. Chicago, Year Book Medical Publishers, 1975.

121. Welch, R.: Von Hippel-Lindau disease: The recognition and treatment of early angiomatosis retinae and the use of cryosurgery as an adjunct to therapy. Trans. Amer. Ophthal. Soc., *68*:367–424, 1970.

122. Wyburn-Mason, R.: Arteriovenous aneurysm of mid-brain and retina, facial naevi and mental changes. Brain, *66*:163–203, 1943.

123. Ya Deau, R. E., Clagett, O. T., and Divertie, M. B.: Intrathoracic meningocele. J. Thorac. Cardiovasc. Surg., *49*:202–209, 1965.

124. Yamashita, J., Handa, H., and Toyama, M.: Medulloblastoma in two brothers. Surg. Neurol., *4*:225–227, 1975.

125. Yen, S., and MacMahon, B.: Genetics of anencephaly and spina bifida. Lancet, *2*:623–626, 1968.

126. Zonana, J., Sotos, J. F., Romsche, C. A., Fisher, D. A., Elders, M. J., and Rimoin, D. L.: Dominant inheritance of cerebral gigantism. J. Pediat., *91*:251–256, 1977.

35

MIDLINE FUSION DEFECTS AND DEFECTS OF FORMATION

Two per cent of liveborn infants have major congenital anomalies, and an unknown percentage of embryos are spontaneously aborted with anomalies too serious to permit development and birth.[328,527,537] Unfortunately, 60 per cent of congenital defects of all types in both stillborn and liveborn infants involve the central nervous system.[510] Further, 64 per cent of all malformations of the central nervous system involve abnormal closure and development of the neural tube and neighboring tissues along the posterior midline of the body. Varieties of these malformations important to the neurosurgeon may be grouped under the general terms "cranial dysraphism" and "spinal dysraphism" (Table 35–1). Dysraphism (Greek: raphe, seam) means defective fusion of parts that normally unite.[710] The meaning of the term has been extended through use to encompass all forms of anomalous development of the tissues associated with the various malformations, whether or not actual malfusion has occurred.[430,431] The occurrence of these malformations in a newborn may be particularly destructive to the family, an unrewarding challenge to the medical profession, and a drain on the financial resources of the family and society. In contrast to a pyloric stenosis or a cleft lip, which can be corrected by an operation, dysraphism has ill effects that are apt to be permanent. Further, quite often these defects of the central nervous system deprive the victim of those qualities held in high esteem by our society—independence, physical prowess, and intelligence.

The goal of this chapter is threefold; first to provide a background of normal embryology of the nervous system, its coverings, and the surrounding tissues in conjunction with a review of the theories of abnormal embryology that may lead to a malformation; second, to review the pathological and clinical continuum from mild to severe forms of a malformation, which indicates that the tendency to categorize patients into one pigeonhole, all good or all bad, is incorrect; and third, to detail clinically useful information that may assist with development of a plan of management for the patient with the malformation.

Despite the tenor of pessimism regarding malformations of the central nervous system that pervades the literature and the medical community, many malformations are as challenging, and their treatment as rewarding, as any problem a neurological surgeon encounters. Correction of a defect before irreparable damage has occurred in a developing child with decades of life ahead is admirable compensation for one's efforts.

EMBRYOLOGY OF THE NERVOUS SYSTEM

Traditionally, the development of the central nervous system is divided into the embryonic period from conception to 8½

B. N. FRENCH

TABLE 35–1 CLASSIFICATION OF CRANIAL AND SPINAL DYSRAPHISM

Spina bifida aperta
  Myeloschisis
  Myelomeningocele
  Hemimyelomeningocele
  Syringomyelomeningocele
  Spinal meningocele
Arnold-Chiari malformation
Dandy-Walker malformation
Cranium bifidum
  Cranial meningocele
  Encephalomeningocele
Occult cranial dysraphism
  Cranial dermal sinus
Occult spinal dysraphism
  Spinal dermal sinus
  Tethered cord syndrome
  Lumbosacral lipoma
  Diastematomyelia
  Neurenteric cyst
  Combined anterior and posterior spina bifida
  Anterior sacral meningocele
  Occult intrasacral meningocele
Nondysraphic malformations
  Perineurial (Tarlov) cyst
  Spinal extradural cyst
  Nondysraphic spinal meningocele
  Caudal regression syndrome
  Sacrococcygeal teratoma

weeks of development, the fetal period from 8½ to 40 weeks of development, and the postnatal period. Embryologists divide the embryonic period into 23 stages, or horizons, according to the time of onset of certain major developmental features. The age of the fetus during the fetal period is often described by the crown-rump length.[420,536] In this chapter, however, significant developments in either period are described by gestational age in days, weeks, or months rather than by using the unfamiliar terminology of the embryologist.

Formation of the Embryonic Disc

Repeated cellular division after fertilization creates a hollow sphere of cells called the blastocyst. This early developmental period characterized by proliferation of cells blends into a period of differentiation and specialization of the flattened, oval embryonic disc with three clearly differentiated germ layers of entoderm, ectoderm, and mesoderm by 14 days. Initially a longitudinal groove, the primitive streak, forms on the caudal end of the embryonic disc and is the first indication of the longitudinal axis of the embryo. Hensen's node is a heaped-up collection of cells surrounding an opening called the primitive pit and is located at the cephalic end of the primitive streak. At this stage, the embryonic disc is composed of an outer layer of ectoderm and an inner layer of entoderm. Cells migrate inwardly and in a cephalic direction from each side of the primitive streak and insinuate themselves between the ectoderm and the entoderm to form the paraxial intraembryonic mesoderm.

By 17 days, surface cells, which originate from Hensen's node, migrate cephalically between the sheets of paraxial mesoderm on either side and the ectoderm above and the entoderm below to form a midline longitudinal cord of cells, the notochordal process. The solid notochord changes to a hollow cylinder of cells and, by day 18, temporarily become incorporated into the underlying entoderm, which forms the future gastrointestinal and respiratory tracts (intercalation of the notochord). Also at this stage, the neurenteric canal located at the primitive pit of Hensen's node temporarily penetrates through the embryonic disc and joins the amniotic cavity dorsal to the disc, with the yolk sac ventral to the disc. The neurenteric canal disappears after only one or two days, the notochord separates from the entoderm (excalation of the notochord), and the entoderm is reconstituted as a continuous layer of cells. As the embryo elongates, Hensen's node and the primitive streak regress caudally toward the future coccygeal region, presumably because of reduction in the cell mass secondary to the massive migration.

Formation of the Neural Tube

By 18 days of development, the embryo is a flattened oval disc with a longitudinal axis of 1.5 mm established by the primitive streak caudally and the notochord cephalically. The three germ layers of ectoderm, mesoderm, and entoderm are clearly differentiated. The subsequent development of the neural tube can be divided into three phases: neurulation occurring from 18 days to 28 days; canalization of the tail bud occurring from 28 days to 40 days; and regression, or dedifferentiation, in the caudal region occurring from 41 days throughout embryonic and fetal life (Fig. 35–1).[419]

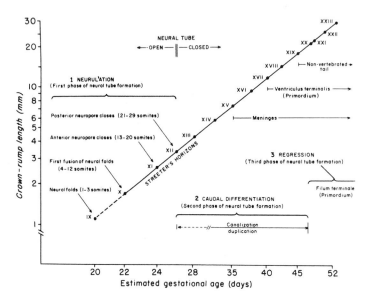

Figure 35–1 The three phases of neural tube development during the embryonic period are neurulation, caudal differentiation or canalization, and regression. The timing of the events is recorded in terms of the gestational age, crown-rump length, and somite development. The Roman numerals refer to Streeter's horizons in development. (From Lemire, R. J.: Variations in development of the caudal neural tube in human embryos (horizons XIV–XXI). Teratology, 2:361–370, 1969. Reprinted by permission.)

Neurulation

The midline ectoderm cephalic to Hensen's node thickens to form the neural plate and is destined to form the central nervous system. By 18 days a central longitudinal depression, the neural groove, appears in the neural plate, and the plate margins heap up to form the neural folds. The middorsal region of the embryo is relatively precocious in development, and this process precedes similar activity of the neural plate and surrounding tissues in the cephalic and caudal regions. The cephalic neural folds are always larger and anticipate the location of the future brain.

While the notochord and neural plate are developing, the paraxial mesoderm thickens on either side of the notochord, and cells in the mesodermal rod condense to form paired segments of mesoderm called somites, which flank the notochord in the middorsal area at approximately 16 days.[536] Two or three pairs of somites are added caudal to the first formed each day until approximately 30 somite pairs have formed by 28 days. A cavity called the myocoele forms within each somite to create a hollow sphere of mesoderm. The dorsomedial portion of the sphere is called the myotome and forms the skeletal muscle at that segmental level. The ventromedial portion is called the sclerotome and will condense around the notochord and future neural tube to form the vertebral body and posterior elements. The ventrolateral por-

tion is called the dermatome and forms the connective tissue and muscles of the body wall.

By 22 days, the neural groove has deepened, and the prominent neural folds meet in the dorsal midline at the level of the future lower rhombencephalon at the level of somites 1 through 7.[537] Fusion of the folds begins the transformation of the flat neural plate into a hollow neural tube; the entire process is called neurulation. The superficial ectoderm attached at the lateral edge of the neural plate is pulled toward the midline by the fusing neural folds and also fuses dorsal to the neural tube. Shortly thereafter the surface ectoderm, destined to form the epidermis, separates from the neural tube, and mesoderm interposes itself between the two layers. This entire process of fusion of tissues that begins in the middorsal region of the embryo then proceeds simultaneously in both cephalad and caudal directions. Thus, all stages of the neurulation process may be examined in a single embryo between 22 and 28 days, depending on the level studied.

A temporary delay in closure of the neural tube occurs at the cephalic end (rostral neuropore) and at the caudal end (caudal neuropore), the final closure taking place at approximately 24 days and 26 to 28 days respectively.[536,554] Thus, by 28 days the neural tube is completely formed, five subdivisions of the future brain are recognizable, and 30 pairs of somites are arranged along the neural tube and notochord, prepared to form vertebral units, intervertebral discs, and paraspinous muscles. The caudal neuropore is probably located at the level of the twenty-fifth somite, which corresponds to the junction of the first and second lumbar vertebral segments. In other words, the process of neurulation forms the spinal cord only to the level of L1–L2, and caudally, a process of canalization is believed to occur.

Canalization of the Tail Bud

The entire neural tube is covered by surface ectoderm when the caudal neuropore closes. Just caudal to the neuropore, Hensen's node and the primitive streak form an undifferentiated caudal cell mass. Unlike neurulation, the process of canalization of this cell mass occurs under intact surface ectoderm. The process has been well described in the chick and rat embryo, but its full import in human embryogenesis is unknown.[419] Central vacuolization of the cell mass creates a tube of neural ectoderm, which then merges with the neural tube formed by neurulation at the level of L1 or L2.[38,420] The process of canalization appears to be less precise than neurulation, and numerous morphological variations of structures derived from the caudal cell mass can be found in otherwise normal human embryos.[420] Normal children and children with nonneural congenital anomalies show a 45 per cent and 57 per cent incidence respectively of central canal forking or duplication in the region of the conus medullaris, ventriculus terminalis, and filum terminale.[425]

Regression

The vertebral column and developing spinal cord match segment for segment, and the spinal nerve roots exit via the intervertebral foramina directly opposite their point of origin until nine weeks of development. Thereafter, the neural tube "ascends" within the vertebral column (Fig. 35–2). Two processes are involved in the ascension of the spinal cord and the associated development of the cauda equina and the filum terminale.[401] The first process is a regression, or dedifferentiation, of already formed structures, which causes a portion of the distal neural tube formed by canalization to undergo cellular necrosis between 40 and 48 days to form the future filum terminale.[420,721] The central canal immediately cephalic to the area of necrosis dilates to form the ventriculus terminalis, which lies at the entry zone of the fifth sacral nerve root and marks the caudal limit of the conus medullaris and the beginning of the filum terminale. A rudimentary ependymal cavity, called the coccygeal medullary vestige, is located at the distal end of the future filum attached to the posterior aspect of the fifth coccygeal vertebral segment. The second process is the mechanical effect of disproportionate growth of the vertebral column and the neural tube. Since the cephalic portion of the neural tube is fixed in position, a relative cephalad migration of the caudal cord occurs.[36] The lumbosacral spinal nerves have attached to the cord by this time and thus lengthen to form the cauda equina. The filum terminale lengthens because of growth of its fibrous components

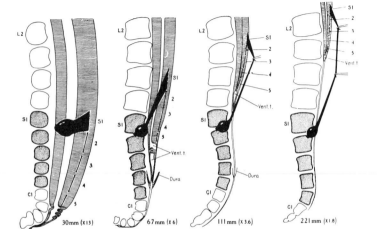

Figure 35–2 The relationship of the caudal end of the developing spinal cord to the vertebral column during the fetal period from the eighth through the twenty-fifth week. The increase in length of the S1 nerve root and the filum terminale reflects the "ascension" of the conus medullaris by a combination of regression and disproportionate elongation of the vertebral column. (From Streeter, G. L.: Factors involved in the formation of the filum terminale. Amer. J. Anat., 25:1–12, 1919. Reprinted by permission.)

30 mm (x13)   67 mm (x 6)   111 mm (x 3.6)   221 mm (x 1.8)

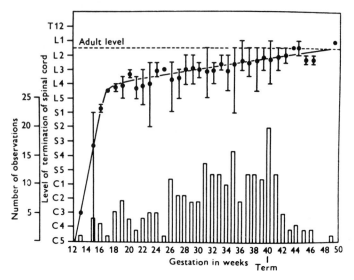

Figure 35–3 The level of the conus medullaris in the human shows a relatively rapid "ascent" from 12 weeks to 17 weeks of age and a slower "ascent" throughout the remainder of fetal life to term. The conus reaches the adult level of L1–L2 two months after birth on the average and sooner in some fetuses. (From Barson, A. J.: The vertebral level of termination of the spinal cord during normal and abnormal development. J. Anat., *106*:489–497, 1970. Reprinted by permission.)

in addition to the stretching mechanism. The tip of the conus medullaris lies at the level of the first to third coccygeal segments up to nine weeks of development.[721] Between 9 and 17 weeks, the conus rapidly "ascends" to the fourth lumbar vertebral body. Thereafter, ascent slows, and the conus reaches the third lumbar vertebral body by term and the adult level of the L1–L2 intervertebral disc space (variation from T12 to L3) by two months' postnatal development (Fig. 35–3).[38,595]

Comparative growth rates of the different levels of the vertebral column and spinal cord change during gestation and postnatal life. The lumbar spine grows faster than the cervical or thoracic spine during the last trimester and in childhood. During the same time periods, the lumbar spinal cord grows faster than the cervical or thoracic cord, but not as rapidly as the lumbar spine, which accounts for the continued ascension of the conus in the later stages of gestation and in infancy. Since the adult cord level may be achieved by two months after birth, both the spinal cord and the vertebral column must grow at equivalent rates throughout childhood.[38]

Formation of the Meninges

The pia, arachnoid, and dura begin to form after closure of the posterior neuro-

pore. The pia is recognizable by 37 days and is well defined on the dorsal neural tube by 52 days. The dura initially forms ventral to the neural tube at 40 days and surrounds the entire neural tube by 52 days. The intervening arachnoid does not begin to separate from the dura until the second half of gestation and may still not be completely separated until after birth. The caudal dural sac extends to approximately the fourth sacral vertebral body in the fetus, but lies at the second sacral level in the adult. Thus, far less change occurs in the relationship of the dura and the vertebral column than in that of the spinal cord and the vertebral column.[721]

Development of the Neural Crest

Neural crest cells originate from the neural ectoderm at the apices of the neural folds and form bilateral cell columns on the dorsolateral aspect of the neural tube. Ultimately the columns segment, and the neural crest cells give rise to the dorsal root ganglia of the cranial and spinal nerves, the sympathetic ganglia of the autonomic nervous system and the chromaffin system including the adrenal medulla and carotid bodies, and the pigment layers of the retina and the integumentary system. The cells also contribute to the pia, the arachnoid, and the sheath of Schwann of the peripheral nerves. Anomalous neural crest influences may be responsible for the frequent cutaneous hemangiomatous and pigmentation malformations that occur in both spina bifida aperta and occult spinal dysraphism.[689]

Formation of the Vertebrae and Ribs

The vertebral unit is composed of the vertebral body, posterior elements, and intervertebral disc, which form from the ventromedial sclerotome in three stages: the period of membrane formation from 22 to 26 days, the period of cartilage formation from 40 to 64 days, and the period of bone formation.[653] The notochord is the important influence in formation of the vertebral body, and the neural tube appears to direct formation of the posterior elements.[41]

Period of Membrane Formation

The sclerotome cells on each side of the notochord and neural tube migrate medially from the somite, but the segmental arrangement is altered. The dense midline cell cluster that finally surrounds the notochord to form the centrum of the vertebral body is composed of cells from adjacent sclerotome pairs. Cells from the caudal half of the cranial sclerotome condense with cells from the cephalic half of the adjacent caudal sclerotome. Thus, each vertebral body is composed of portions of four somites. The intervening sclerotome cells form the anulus fibrosus of the intervertebral disc, and the notochord persists as the nucleus pulposis. The notochord within the primitive vertebral body disappears. Paired cell masses extend dorsolaterally from each centrum to outline the future neural arch, which forms the posterior elements and the medial rib structures.

Period of Cartilage Formation

Conversion to cartilage first begins around the chondrification center in the centrum and later in separate centers in each neural arch and in each rib process. The centra and arches are chondrified by 47 days, but the arches are incomplete dorsal to the neural tube. The process of arch clo-sure is progressive, and by nine weeks the arches are complete in the thoracic and upper lumbar regions but remain open in the cervical and the lower lumbar area.[653] If these neural arches fail to fuse later, a spina bifida is formed. The chondrification process eventually forms a confluent cartilaginous vertebral unit and rib process with no lines of demarcation between the prior chondrification centers.

Period of Bone Formation

Endochondral ossification centers develop in the centrum and in each of the neural arch processes and the costal processes. The neural arch processes extend dorsally and medially to form the laminae, and with fusion and further dorsal prolongation, the spinous process is formed. The ventral extension of each neural arch process fuses with the vertebral body; the lateral extension forms the transverse process with which the rib articulates. The shafts of the ribs are formed by extension of their primary ossification centers. Thus, any process that interferes with the development and growth of the primordial vertebral unit may produce malformations such as aplasia of one or more ribs, fused ribs, hermivertebrae, fused vertebrae, or anterior or posterior spina bifida.

Formation of the Brain

Elevation of the head fold distinguishes the future brain from the slender neural tube of the spinal cord, and by 25 days the forebrain (prosencephalon), the midbrain (mesencephalon), and the hindbrain (rhombencephalon) are recognizable. By 35 days, the prosencephalon has subdivided into the telencephalon (future cerebral hemispheres) and diencephalon while the rhombencephalon has formed the metencephalon (future pons) and myelencephalon (future medulla oblongata).

The embryo gradually assumes the shape of the letter C by a process of flexion. By 20 days the cephalic (mesencephalic) flexure, and by 28 days the cervical flexure, have formed curves that are convex dorsally, and by 30 days the pontine flexure has formed a curve that is convex ventrally.

The future choroid plexus can be identified by 40 days. Near the end of the embryonic period at eight and one half weeks, the cerebral hemispheres are thin-walled and smooth on the surface. The major fissures and gyral patterns do not develop until two and one half to five and one half months of gestation. Thus, many of the embryological abnormalities of the cerebral hemispheres, in contrast to malformations of the spinal cord, are products of the fetal period of development.

Formation of the Skull

A concentration of cells around the cephalic end of the notochord lying ventral to the rhombencephalon is the first evidence of the skull base, appearing between five and six weeks of development. Cephalic extension of the process forms a "floor" for the developing brain, first in cartilage and later in bone by endochondral bone formation. Four bones constitute the base of the skull. The occipital bone around the foramen magnum has four endochondral ossification centers, which create the occipital arch and the supraoccipital part of the occipital bone below the inion and the superior nuchal line. The interparietal part of the occipital bone, which lies above the superior nuchal line, is formed by the intramembranous process of bone formation, as are all the bones of the cranial vault and the facial bones. The frontal bone appears early in the ninth week and the parietal bones in the tenth week. The supraoccipital and interparietal portions of the occipital bone unite in approximately the third month. The other three bones of the skull base are the sphenoid bone; the ethmoid bone including the crista galli, cribriform plate, ethmoidal labyrinth, and cartilaginous nasal septum; and the petrous portion of the temporal bone. The endochondral skull base has its own intrinsic growth potential and, in contrast to the passive intramembranous bone of the cranial vault, is subject to abnormal osseous development independent of the influence of the overlying neural structures.[179,294] The bones around the foramen magnum are particularly prone to abnormal development, as in occipitoatlantal fusion, platybasia, basilar impression, and hypo-plasia of the skull base such as occurs in achondroplasia.[398]

GENETIC AND ENVIRONMENTAL INTERACTION IN NEURAL TUBE MALFORMATIONS

A multifactorial genetic background is more likely to be responsible for neural tube malformations than are abnormalities of a single gene or aberrations in chromosome number or morphology.[748] A combination of several genes and several environmental factors may interact to trigger the underlying hereditary predisposition that manifests itself as a form of cranial or spinal dysraphism. The risks of occurrence or recurrence of neural tube malformations are clear only for the severe malformations such as anencephaly, exencephaly, encephalocele, and spina bifida aperta. Although a family may have one child with spina bifida aperta and a second with a form of occult spinal dysraphism, the association is unusual. Families with several members suffering from one or a variety of forms of occult spinal dysraphism are also rare.

The risk of having an infant with a neural tube malformation depends on the incidence in the general population, the number of previous cases in the family, the degree of kinship to a previously afflicted child, and many other factors. The epidemiology of neural tube malformations shows a distinct geographic variation, the highest incidence of eight per thousand births being found in the north and west of the British Isles with lower rates of two to three per thousand births in the southern and eastern parts of the country.[74] The incidence is much lower, at one to two per thousand births, in the United States and Canada. It is lower in Negroes than in Caucasians, and females predominate two to one over males. The general risk of having an afflicted infant in a previously unaffected family in North America is 1 in 400, but the risk of recurrence rises to 1 in 20 births (5 per cent) after one afflicted infant and increases to 10 to 15 per cent after two. Other interesting factors such as a variation in incidence over the years; seasonal variation; the influence of socioeconomic class, of maternal age, and of birth order; and the potential influence of teratogens are discussed in Chapter 34 and have been reviewed by Brocklehurst and by Thompson and Rudd.[80,748]

The causes of neural tube malformations must operate through certain mechanisms of teratogenesis such as arrest of development, anomalous structural or functional development, or abnormalities of degeneration of formed structures.[420] As well, the time when a teratogenic agent acts during development is important, as the maximum disruptive effect occurs during the time of differentiation and formation of the organ systems. Thus, an agent acting during the second to fourth weeks may cause defects in more than one system because the critical period of one organ system often coincides with that of another. The clinical importance of this fact is that more than one congenital anomaly may be present in a defective newborn.[245]

SPINA BIFIDA APERTA

Definition

"Spina bifida aperta" is preferable to "spina bifida cystica" or "myelodysplasia" as a general term for the "open" forms of spinal dysraphism (see Table 35–1).[80,289,469] "Aperta" derives from the Latin "aperio, apertus," meaning "open." These lesions are most often open to the environment or threatening to be open, which means that decisions with long-term ramifications for the patient and the family and society must be made on short notice and cannot be deferred until some convenient time. Thus, the term amplifies one feature that contributes greatly to the controversies over management. The term "spina bifida cystica" describes the protruding cystic form but not the frequently occurring open, leaking, flat neural plaque. "Myelodysplasia" implies a malformation of structure of the spinal cord, which may be found in the open, the covered, and the occult forms.

Infants with spina bifida aperta present a continuum of clinical and pathological features. The form of the neural malformation depends upon the time during embryological development that the teratogenic insult acts. For example, a malformation initiated

prior to or just at 28 days of gestation is likely to induce gross defects in the process of neurulation and involve a high level of the cord and spine; later than 28 days, neurulation has already occurred, the cord is formed, and the malformation will most likely involve the lower levels of the cord and spine.[537] The earlier the insult occurs, the more likely the neural malformations are to be widespread and of greater complexity and severity.[38] Clinically the infant has a localized defect of the skin, vertebral column, and spinal cord in the thoracolumbar, lumbar, or sacral region, and a neurological deficit the severity of which depends upon the anatomical level of the neural malformation and its pathological nature. A neural malformation may undergo secondary degeneration from intrauterine exposure to amniotic fluid and from many postnatal factors such as exposure, mechanical distortion, syringohydromyelia, and ischemia from compression. All these factors may increase the severity of the neurological deficit beyond that due to the primary malformation. Although the clinician can frequently differentiate a myeloschisis from a myelomeningocele, the term "myelomeningocele" is the most practical for day-to-day use and is used throughout this chapter where applicable. The hemimyelomeningocele and syringomyelomeningocele are relatively distinct on clinical grounds and should be considered specific entities.

If the embryological insult occurs still later in gestation, then the spinal cord and proximal nervous system have completed many critical phases in development. The lower spinal malformation may involve only the meninges and take the form of a spinal meningocele, which is considered separately since the prognosis is vastly different from the previously mentioned forms.

Myeloschisis

This earliest embryological form of spina bifida aperta manifests a gross defect in neurulation involving either a failure of the neural folds to fuse or a reopening of a just-fused neural tube. Depending on the applicable mechanism, myeloschisis forms before or just after 28 days of gestation. Myeloschisis is commonly found in the

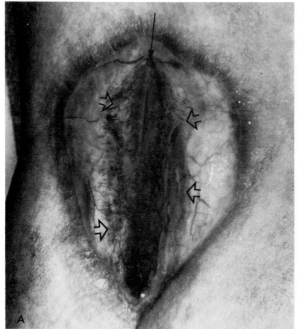

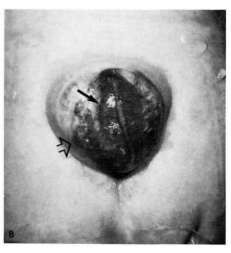

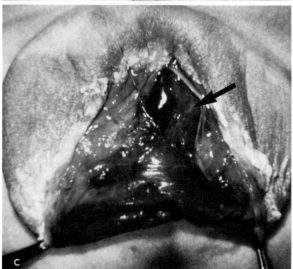

Figure 35–4 *A*. Myeloschisis of the thoracolumbar area showing the open neural plaque (area medullovasculosa) with the central neural groove merging into the central canal at the upper end of the plaque (*arrow*). The dura is splayed over the ridges of the pedicles (*open arrows*) to fuse with the edge of the skin defect (zona cutanea). Cerebrospinal fluid leaked from the central canal, and air was present in the ventricles. *B*. More typical cystic form with the neural plaque ballooned posteriorally by ventral cerebrospinal fluid accumulation. The zona epitheliosa fuses with the edge of the neural plaque (*arrow*) and the zona cutanea (*open arrow*). This plaque appeared to have undergone neurulation, but with marked posterior degeneration (see Fig. 35–6*B*). *C*. Myelomeningocele of lumbosacral area with a ruptured sac, cerebrospinal fluid leakage, and exposure of an abnormally low, but well-formed, spinal cord (*arrow*). The anal sphincter is patulous.

thoracolumbar region at the junctional area of the cord between the part formed by neurulation and that formed by canalization. The accompanying posterior spina bifida involves the entire lumbar and sacral spine.[38,39,420] The open, flat plaque of neural tissue displays a central neural groove merging with an opening representing the central canal of the neurulated cord at the cephalic end of the plaque (Fig. 35–4*A*). Cerebral spinal fluid may leak from the opening of the central canal, which may be patent along the entire cord to the ventri-

cles.[23,183] Experimental myeloschisis suggests that the open neural plate forms anterior horn cells and nerve roots medially and posterior horn cells laterally despite the failure of the plate to close.[782] Exposure of the neural tissue to amniotic fluid, however, and stretching of the plaque in the cystic form lead to secondary degeneration and progressive destruction of the plaque. As a result, the neurological deficit is usually complete below the level of the lesion. A myeloschisis is virtually always incompletely epithelialized and leaking cerebral spinal fluid, presenting the imminent danger of meningitis and ventriculitis after birth.

Myelomeningocele

Neurulation has occurred in this form and the malformation must develop after 28 days of gestation. The neural malformation ranges from severe to slight involvement of cord structure (Fig. 35–4B and C). As a result, the neurological deficit may vary below the level of the lesion. Myelomeningocele tends to spare the thoracolumbar junction and usually occurs in the lumbar, lumbosacral, or sacral area. The extent of the posterior spina bifida may be localized to as few as two or three levels compared with the extensive spina bifida in myeloschisis.[39] Occasionally the neural malformation is completely covered by membranes, but more commonly the neural tissue is exposed or the sac has ruptured. Occasionally fluid that appears to leak from the dome of a cystic sac may be an exudate from the ulcerated surface rather than a true cerebrospinal fluid leak.[691]

Hemimyelomeningocele

This rare form occurs in fewer than 10 per cent of unselected patients with spina bifida aperta.[187,199,200] Initial inspection suggests a myelomeningocele located slightly off the midline. The neurological deficit is more pronounced in one leg than the other, in contrast to the usual symmetrical deficit, because diastematomyelia is always pres-ent. The relatively intact hemicord, corresponding to the good leg, lies protected within its own dural sheath and is usually covered by a deformed lamina extending from the pedicle to a midline bony or fibrocartilaginous septum. The involved hemicord, corresponding to the bad leg, is usually set off to one side and appears as a typical myelomeningocele. Often the split cord reunites below the open lesion. Plain roentgenograms may display characteristic features of diastematomyelia such as hemivertebrae formation or a narrowed intervertebral disc or a midline ossified septum.[187]

Syringomyelomeningocele

This rare malformation of the spinal cord is usually found in the cervical or thoracic area (Fig 35–5). The lesion suggests a spinal meningocele because the skin and membrane coverage is usually complete and the neurological deficit is slight, if present at all.[537] The malformation is a herniation of the dilated central canal and dysplastic neural tissue between the dorsal columns of a normally fused spinal cord through a localized posterior spina bifida.[755] Cystic lesions on the cervical or thoracic area, called meningoceles clinically, may be properly classified as syringomyelomeningoceles on the basis of pathological examination of the tissue in the walls of the sac.

The infant with spina bifida aperta has more than a localized malformation of skin, skeleton, and spinal cord. Most infants have abnormalities of the brain and skull; these are discussed separately in the sec-

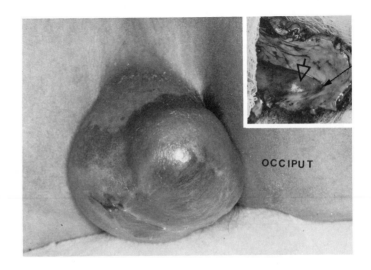

Figure 35–5 Syringomyelomeningocele of the cervical region in a 3-day-old, neurologically normal infant. The inset shows the interior of the opened sac with a mass of dysplastic neural tissue (*open arrow*) and the tiny opening leading into the region of the central canal (*solid arrow*). The infant remains normal without hydrocephalus three years after operation.

OCCIPUT

tion on the Arnold-Chiari malformation. In addition, congenital anomalies in other organ systems may coexist with the obvious central nervous system lesion and require individual management.

Abnormal Embryology

Numerous investigators have formulated theories of abnormal embryogenesis to explain spina bifida aperta. The theories fall into four general groups: the theory of developmental arrest attributed to von Recklinghausen, the overgrowth hypothesis associated with Patten and Barry and co-workers, the hydrodynamic theory associated with Gardner, and the theory of neuroschisis proposed by Padget.* The developmental arrest and overgrowth theories postulate an effect on the neural plate so early in development that neurulation never occurs at the affected level. The hydrodynamic and neuroschisis theories hypothesize rupture of an already formed neural tube at the affected site. Whether a dysraphic lesion is due to a failure to form a neural tube or due to rupture of a previously closed neural tube has practical importance. Nonclosure indicates that dysraphic abnormalities develop by 28 days of gestation at the latest, whereas rupture of the formed neural tube suggests that events as late as the second or third month of development might initiate the abnormality. The theories do not address the process of canalization of the caudal tail bud, which is responsible for formation of the neural tube distal to L1.[537] The pathology of spina bifida aperta is so diverse that no single theory is likely to explain all forms of spinal dysraphism. Too often, one theory cannot explain a particular feature of the dysraphism or a unique theory is invoked to explain but a single facet of the abnormality.

Developmental Arrest

In 1886, von Recklinghausen suggested that myeloschisis begins as a simple failure of the embryonic neural plate to close due to an arrest of normal development with subsequent secondary changes in surrounding tissues.[770,782] Myeloschisis and presumably myelomeningocele and spinal meningocele are explained by arrest of development later in gestation. Many of the distant malformations of the central nervous system cannot be explained adequately on the basis of arrest of development, however, and other mechanisms must be invoked to account for the pathological diversity of spina bifida aperta.

The Overgrowth Hypothesis

Lebedeff, in 1881, and Cleland, in 1883, suggested that the neural tube failed to close during early development owing to overgrowth of the neural tissue everting the neural folds and preventing fusion.[80,118] Lebedeff's observations concerned excessive neural tissue development in the open neural plate of chick embryos. More recently, Patten reported similar overgrowth in human dysraphic embryos.[551–553] The youngest embryo of five weeks' development had an excessive amount of neural plate tissue at the site of a lumbosacral myeloschisis.[553] Although Patten considered that the marked overgrowth of neural tissue could be a secondary reaction to failed fusion, he preferred to interpret the overgrowth as a primary phenomenon interfering with the normal closure of the neural tube and causing a secondary spina bifida. Older dysraphic embryos lacked overgrowth, which suggested that the exposed neural tissue suffered secondary degeneration.

In 1957, Barry, Patten, and Stewart determined that neural overgrowth was not limited to the area of myeloschisis.[36] They calculated that the cord segments immediately cephalic to the myeloschisis had an increased volume suggestive of overgrowth despite the normal external form and structure. Overgrowth was also considered the primary cause of the Arnold-Chiari malformation that so frequently accompanies spina bifida aperta, but the finding is disputed by Brocklehurst.[77]

Overgrowth of neural tissue can be produced experimentally in the chick embryo by mechanically opening the closed neural tube.[234] Chemical teratogens such as trypan blue and excessive vitamin A administered to pregnant rats can result in offspring with myeloschisis showing overgrowth followed by degeneration of the neural tissue.[80]

---

* See references 36, 247, 538–541, 552, 553, 770.

Whether overgrowth of neural tissue is the primary cause or a secondary phenomenon in spina bifida aperta has yet to be determined.

The Hydrodynamic Theory

Several theories involving hydrodynamic principles as the causative agent in spinal dysraphism have been discussed over the years. Morgagni noted the association of hydrocephalus and spina bifida aperta in 1761.[80] The suggestion that he considered the relationship causal was probably an overstatement, as the circulation of the cerebrospinal fluid was unknown at that time.[80,247] In 1863, Virchow suggested that excessive fluid within the central canal, or hydromyelia, could lead to a cystic dilatation of the lower spinal cord with protrusion through the posterior bone and soft-tissue elements. If the central canal were obstructed more proximally, then the dilatation and protrusion at more cephalic levels could explain cervical syringomyelomeningocele or encephalocele.[80] The hydrodynamic mechanism has been developed to its fullest in the writings of Gardner and is summarized in his monograph, *The Dysraphic States*, published in 1973.[247] All dysraphic states are explained by a series of ingenious mechanical steps consequent to the inadequate escape of cerebrospinal fluid from the neural tube in early development or from the subarachnoid space during later development.

Weed's study of the pig embryo in 1917 showed that the neural tube is filled with a proteinaceous fluid immediately after closure of the posterior neuropore long before the choroid plexus appears during the sixth week.[785,786] With the appearance of the choroid plexus in the fourth ventricle and secretion of cerebrospinal fluid, the lumen of the neural tube begins to distend, producing a physiological hydrocephalus and hydromyelia, according to Gardner. Normally the fluid finds its way into the primitive subarachnoid space through the semipermeable roof plate of the rhombencephalon, which differentiates into the area membranacea superior and the area membranacea inferior.[785,786] The area membranacea superior lies between the developing cerebellum above and the paired choroid plexuses below, is lined with cells similar to

ependyma, and is the first route of escape for fluid from the distended neural tube. The area membranacea inferior extends caudally from the choroid plexus to the obex; has a thinner, nonependymal structure; and is the site of the future foramen of Magendie. The area membranacea superior thickens as the rostral cerebellum develops, and the area membranacea inferior becomes the second permeable area and eventually ruptures to form the midline foramen as the lateral ventricular choroid plexus develops and begins its secretory function.

The developmental chronology of the communication between the neural tube through the rhombencephalic roof plate and the primitive subarachnoid space is controversial and critical to the hydrodynamic theory. Weed suggested that the area membranacea superior became permeable to a tracer dye as early as six weeks in the pig embryo.[247,785-787] Early reports suggested that the true midline foramen becomes patent at 12 to 16 weeks, but Brocklehurst and Padget have observed an open foramen as early as eight or nine weeks of development in the human.[78,540,735,761] The lateral foramina of Luschka open at four to six months of development or even later, if at all, in man.[78,540,735]

Gardner presumes that too rapid accumulation of fluid within the neural tube or too little escape will lead to overdistention and bulging of the neural tube at some site followed by rupture to produce anencephaly or myeloschisis and many other malformations. The theory has been criticized on several points. Experimental animal models suggest that the severe forms of anencephaly and myeloschisis result from failure of the neural tube to close rather than from opening of the closed tube. As well, myeloschisis has been found in human embryos before the choroid plexus has formed.[422,537] Assuming that cerebrospinal fluid production is required to produce the necessary overdistention for rupture of the neural tube, the theory is deficient. Gardner believes, however, that the excessive proteinaceous fluid present before choroid plexus formation and cerebrospinal fluid production is sufficient to rupture the tube.[247] Extensive open lesions of the entire neural tube are probably not due to overdistention, since the inital point of rupture should decompress the neural tube and limit the extent of the lesion. The theory depends, in part, on the validity of Weed's view that the rhombencephalon is burst by the secretory pressure of the cerebrospinal fluid. Brocklehurst suggests that the development of the roof plate of the rhombencephalon including the midline foramen may be an active process of sequential development rather than a mechanistic blowout.[78]

The objections should not be interpreted as an indication that hydrodynamic factors are not important in spina bifida aperta. Substantial evidence suggests that hydrodynamic disturbances contribute to many of the malformations associated with spina bifida aperta such as syringohydromyelia, Arnold-Chiari malformation, aqueduct stenosis, and other abnormalities. Even authorities who consider the hydrodynamic theory as ''simplistic'' and ''mechanistic'' agree.[245]

Neuroschisis Theory

On the basis of observations in monkey and human embryos, Padget developed a theory that postulates reopening of the closed neural tube.[538-541] A cleft develops in the dorsal midline of the neural tube for no explained reason. The opening permits the proteinaceous fluid within the neural tube to escape into the surrounding mesoderm, and the cutaneous ectoderm covering the previously closed neural tube is elevated. Padget likened the elevation of the cutaneous ectoderm to a dermatological blister and named the lesion a neuroschistic bleb. The bleb fluid could rupture capillaries and produce leakage of red cells and adhesions upon healing. The bleb wall may rupture and expose the open area of the neural tube to the amniotic fluid, and some redundancy of the neural tissue could superficially resemble the overgrowth suggested by Patten. Degeneration of the exposed neural tissue may follow. The edges of the ruptured cutaneous ectodermal bleb may become applied to the everted edge of the open neural tube and establish secondary cutaneous-neural ectodermal continuity. Thus, the spina bifida aperta is transformed into a typical ''never closed'' neural tube, which concurs with the prevailing theory of nonclosure.

Neuroschisis may occur anywhere along the neural tube, be it dorsal, lateral, or ventral, at any time during development; may be a partial or total division of the neural tube wall; and may even heal completely. Thus, the sequelae of bleb formation may vary greatly and thus explain all forms of cranial and spinal dysraphism and many of the features of the Arnold-Chiari malformation. Objections to the theory are few, as it is a relatively recent proposal. No etiology for the cleft in the neural tissue has been suggested, however, and the possibility that neuroschistic blebs are artifacts is mentioned.[537]

Pathology

The Neural Malformation

The distribution of myelomeningocele is listed in Table 35–2. The high incidence in the thoracolumbar region is most likely related to the early embryological disturbance of caudal neuropore closure at the L1 or L2 level resulting in myeloschisis. Rarely are two or more open malformations present in one infant.[486]

The spinal cord at, above, and below the level of the neural plaque shows considerable pathological variation, and numerous associated intraspinal abnormalities may coexist, as revealed in postmortem studies by Emery and Lendon and by Cameron.[98,199,200,379] While such detailed information may appear to be academic, the knowledge provides a better understanding of the clinical manifestations and anatomical variations found at operation.

TABLE 35–2 DISTRIBUTION OF MYELOMENINGOCELE AND SPINAL MENINGOCELE*

LEVEL	MYELO-MENINGOCELE (PER CENT)	SPINAL MENINGOCELE (PER CENT)
Cervical	3	10
Thoracic	5	15
Thoracolumbar	26	4
Lumbar	26	37
Lumbosacral	30	19
Sacral	10	15

* Data from Barson, A. J.: Brit. J. Radiol., *38*:294–300, 1965; Lorber, J.: Develop. Med. Child Neurol., *13*:279–303, 1971; Shulman, K., and Ames, M. D.: N.Y. State J. Med., *68*:2656–2659, 1963; Stark, G. D.: Spina Bifida. Problems and Management. Oxford, Blackwell, 1977.

At Level of the Neural Plaque

Thirty-five per cent of the plaques showed a form of myeloschisis with an open neural plate lacking a central canal (Fig. 35–6A). Twenty-five per cent had a formed spinal cord containing a central canal with varying degrees of degeneration of the dorsal cord (Fig. 35–6B). Thirty-one per cent had a form of diastematomyelia, with nine per cent showing a typical hemi-myelomeningocele (Fig. 35–6C). Eight per

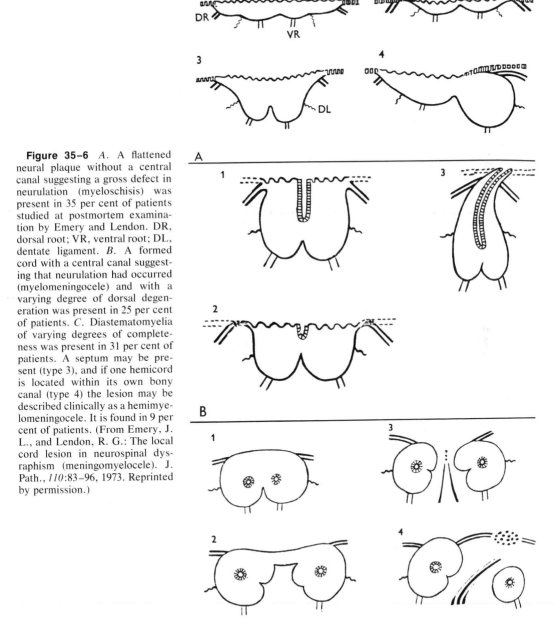

Figure 35–6 *A*. A flattened neural plaque without a central canal suggesting a gross defect in neurulation (myeloschisis) was present in 35 per cent of patients studied at postmortem examination by Emery and Lendon. DR, dorsal root; VR, ventral root; DL, dentate ligament. *B*. A formed cord with a central canal suggesting that neurulation had occurred (myelomeningocele) and with a varying degree of dorsal degeneration was present in 25 per cent of patients. *C*. Diastematomyelia of varying degrees of completeness was present in 31 per cent of patients. A septum may be present (type 3), and if one hemicord is located within its own bony canal (type 4) the lesion may be described clinically as a hemimyelomeningocele. It is found in 9 per cent of patients. (From Emery, J. L., and Lendon, R. G.: The local cord lesion in neurospinal dysraphism (meningomyelocele). J. Path., *110*:83–96, 1973. Reprinted by permission.)

cent of the plaques were unclassified owing to extensive necrosis, and only one per cent had virtually normal structure.[200]

Above the Plaque

Syringohydromyelia was present in 43 per cent of the cords studied by Emery and Lendon (Fig. 35–7).[199,200] Distention of the central canal, or hydromyelia, was twice as common as distention of the central canal plus a separate longitudinal cavitation in the cord substance, or syringohydromyelia. All the latter cases had a demonstrated communication between the central canal and the separate syrinx. Diastematomyelia within a single dural tube extended craniad from the plaque in 31 per cent. A surprising 6 per cent of patients had compression of the cord by a ventral arachnoid cyst.

Spina bifida aperta develops prior to the stage of ascent of the cord at 9 to 25 weeks of development, and the cord is tethered low in the spinal canal. As a result, the spinal cord segments maintain their segmental relationship to the vertebral body level below T10 in contrast to the normal state, in which the cord segments between T10 and the tip of the conus are confined between vertebral body levels T10 to L2. Thus, the spinal cord segments are longer than normal near the plaque because of the tethering effect. The elongation of cord segments is, however, dissipated within five to seven levels above the plaque.[36,518]

Below the Plaque

Diastematomyelia extended caudal to the plaque in 25 per cent, whereas 42 per cent showed only two or more central canals within a single cord. Eighteen per cent of specimens were unclassified because no organized neural tissue could be identified, and fifteen per cent of the distal cords appeared to be normal.

Associated Intraspinal Abnormalities

Emery and Lendon also described various forms of intraspinal lipomatous malformations occurring in 74 per cent of patients with spina bifida aperta studied at postmortem examination.[198] Fibrolipomas of the filum terminale below the ventriculus terminus occurred in 50 per cent; dural fibrolipomas separate from the cord near the plaque or a diastematomyelia occurred in 26 per cent; and 8 per cent had an admixture of fat, neural tissue, and dense connective tissue called a leptomyelolipoma involving the conus area.

Rarely, other abnormalities may occur in association with spina bifida aperta at other sites in the spinal canal such as epidermoid or dermoid tumors.[159,386] Inclusion of epithelial remnants in the original closure of the open lesion may be responsible for the occasional case of dermoid tumor developing at the operative site.[89,445]

Neuronal Content

The neuron population of the spinal cord is usually related to the degree of cord malformation and secondary damage, but even a normal appearing thoracic cord segment may have decreased cell content.[423,424] In general, cell content is proportional to the

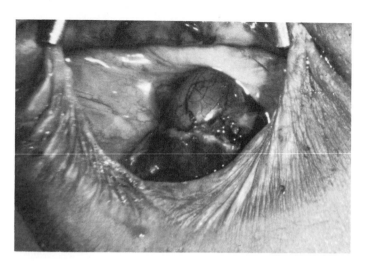

Figure 35–7 A lumbosacral myelomeningocele shows gross hydromyelia of the cord proximal to the neural plaque, which has been separated from the zona epitheliosa. After placement of a shunt for the marked hydrocephalus, the level of motor function improved from L2 to L5, which was compatible with the true anatomical level of the neural plaque.

cord weight.[43] The dorsal root ganglia derive from the neural crest and are normally formed with only slight decrease of the cell population of those near the plaque.[204,205] As a result, the sensory nerves are usually intact because of the normal dorsal root ganglion cells, as indicated by a preserved axon reflex test to intradermal histamine (0.1 per cent) injection.[573]

The Skin and the Meninges

Closure of the neural tube sets the stage for development of normal epithelial cover and a circumferential envelope of dura and arachnoid. In spina bifida aperta, however, the degree of skin and meningeal covering of the neural malformation depends, in part, on the time at which the lesion forms during development. Generally, the skin margins remain at the periphery of the neural plaque, usually separated by a zone of modified leptomeninges and parchmentlike epithelium (zona epitheliosa) (see Fig. 35–4B). The open neural plaque prevents the dura or arachnoid from enclosing the neural tissue. The dura does develop ventral to the plaque and extends laterally over the everted pedicles and laminae of the posterior spina bifida onto the fascia of the paraspinous muscles to attach to the edge of the skin defect (zona cutanea). The dura is lightly adherent to the fascia and densely adherent to the skin edge. The arachnoid also develops ventral to the neural plaque and attaches to the area of the skin margin and to the neural tissue, thus contributing to the zona epitheliosa. In essence, the arachnoid may form a cystlike chamber ventral to the neural tissue and in continuity with the subarachnoid space, with the neural tissue forming part of the dorsal wall of the cyst. If the subarachnoid space fills with cerebrospinal fluid and does not rupture, then the neural plaque balloons posteriorly; hence the term "spina bifida cystica" (cf. Fig. 35–4B). Rupture or aspiration of the arachnoid "balloon" collapses the sac and produces a flat myeloschisis-like appearance. The skin coverage and redundancy of the sac is usually greater if a myelomeningocele has developed later in gestation (cf. Fig. 35–4C). Regardless of the size of the sac, the relationships of the dura, arachnoid, and skin margin are fairly similar. The dural sac re-forms its normal tubular structure at the upper end of the open

neural plaque and occasionally below, depending on the site and extent of the neural plaque. The skin margins are usually hemangiomatous, which produces the reddish discoloration in the dysplastic skin edge.

Incompletely covered forms constitute approximately 80 per cent of all cases according to experience with large clinical series and according to the results of amniocentesis for alpha-fetoprotein determination.[74,691] In perhaps 20 per cent of cases, parchment skin derived from the meninges and the epithelial margin, or occasionally modified skin, covers the area of the neural plaque, reducing the risk of infection after birth and rendering amniocentesis for antenatal detection of spina bifida aperta falsely negative. Of course, any lesion that was completely covered in utero may rupture during or after birth—with the subsequent risk of meningitis and ventriculitis.

The Vertebral Unit

The hallmark of spina bifida aperta is the defective development of the posterior elements of the vertebral unit, but the skeletal defect is often more complicated than a simple posterior spina bifida. The abnormal neural tube development not only prevents formation of the laminae and spinous processes but may also result in a lateral or even anterolateral displacement of the pedicles and laminar rudiments in severe myeloschisis. A widened spinal canal at the level of the defect results, and the everted pedicle-laminar rudiments can be palpated as a "sawtooth ridge" lateral to the neural plaque. The ridge is covered by the paraspinous muscle fascia, the splayed dura, and occasionally the skin, depending upon the size of the skin deficiency. The extent of the posterior spina bifida usually exceeds that of the skin deficiency.[39] The T12–L1 bony level is critical. If a posterior spina bifida involves these levels, the entire lumbar and sacral spine is also bifid, regardless of localization of the skin defect to the thoracolumbar or lumbar area (Fig. 35–8; çf. Fig. 35–10). On the other hand, if T12 and L1 have normal posterior elements, the posterior spina bifida may be quite localized to either the lumbar or sacral spine or to the thoracic spine.

The thoracolumbar or high lumbar spina bifida aperta with paralysis below L3 and with posterior spina bifida involving T12 or

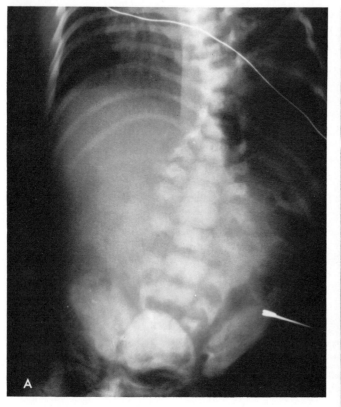
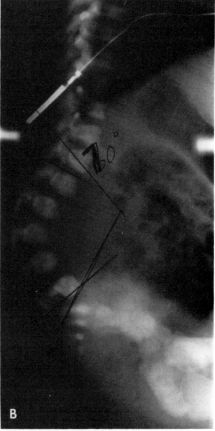

Figure 35–8 *A*. Congenital lumbar kyphosis with a thoraco-lumbar myelomeningocele. There is posterior spina bifida from T10 through the sacrum with widening of the interpedicular diameter. The pedicles are everted to the extent that the intervertebral foramina are seen on the anteroposterior film. *B*. Lateral view shows the lumbar kyphosis extending from T12 to L5 with wedge-shaped lumbar vertebral bodies near the apex of the curve.

L1 may be associated with a congenital lumbar kyphosis (Figs. 35–8 and 35–9).* The five lumbar vertebrae are usually wedge-shaped but may be incomplete on one side (hemivertebrae).[39],[783] Typically the pedicles and laminar rudiments are widely separated and everted with anterior rotation of the transverse processes, as shown in Figure 35–9. The erector spinae muscles lose their extensor function as they are displayed lateral and anterior to the spine. Psoas major and the displaced posterior muscles then act as flexors to mold the primitive cartilaginous lumbar spine into a rigid kyphotic curve with the apex at approximately L2 or L3. The crura of the diaphragm insert onto the apical vertebrae of the kyphus.

The lumbar aorta is reduced in caliber below the mesenteric vessels and spans the

kyphus from the lower thoracic spine to the lumbosacral spine like a bowstring.[783] The aorta is relatively safe in operations on the anterior surface of the kyphotic spine because of this fortuitous anatomical arrangement.

Other abnormalities of the thoracic or lumbar vertebral bodies may occur and lead to other varieties of progressive spinal curvature in later life.[618] Failure of formation of the vertebral body may be complete (aplasia) or incomplete (wedge vertebrae, hemivertebrae); failure of segmentation of contiguous vertebral bodies may be complete (solid bony bar involving two or more levels) or incomplete (unilateral unsegmented bar involving two or more levels). The malformations may occur singly or in combination and may be associated with absence or fusion of ribs if the thoracic spine is involved.

Diastematomyelia with an ossified or fi-

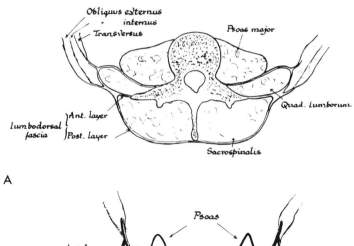

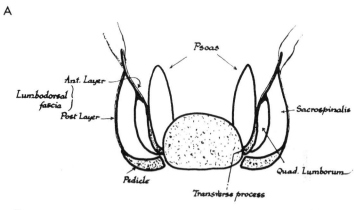

Figure 35–9 *A.* Transverse section of the normal lumbar spine and paraspinous muscles. *B.* In congenital lumbar kyphosis, the transverse processes, pedicles, and paraspinous muscles are displaced anterolaterally, and the displaced paraspinous muscles function as flexors of the spine. (From Drennan, J. C.: The role of muscles in the development of human lumbar kyphosis. Develop. Med. Child. Neurol., *12*:suppl. 22:33–38, 1970. Reprinted by permission.)

brocartilaginous septum may be suggested by typical vertebral body deformities such as a narrowed or fused intervertebral disc space, a shortened anteroposterior diameter of the vertebral bodies, and a central bony density in the spinal canal at that level (Fig. 35–10).[336,462]

Muscles of the Lower Extremities

The morphology of the lower extremity muscles is highly variable owing to a number of factors: the integrity of the lower motor neuron, whether the lower motor neuron damage occurred in utero prior to the formation of normal muscle or after muscle had already developed, the duration of lower motor neuron denervation, secondary changes of disuse atrophy or local pressure necrosis in paralyzed limbs, and intraneural hemorrhage at the time of breech delivery. Breech delivery occurs in 3 to 4 per cent of all normal deliveries, but the rate increases to 18 to 24 per cent for children with spina bifida aperta. Damage to soft tissues, including the sciatic nerve, may occur and add neurological deficit to the already existing damage to the infant.[585]

The Arnold-Chiari Malformation

Virtually all infants with spina bifida aperta have a hindbrain anomaly popularly known as the Arnold-Chiari malformation. This malformation is a complex of deformities contributing to hydrocephalus, syringohydromyelia, respiratory difficulties, and mental retardation, to mention a few important features. The problem merits separate discussion, which follows the section on spina bifida aperta, but one element of the deformity, craniolacunia, should be mentioned at this time.[436,677] Craniolacunia is most likely a temporary developmental disturbance of ossification that begins in utero and that is erased by a continuation of the slowed ossification of the membrane bone of the skull. Patchy areas of thinned bone are separated by intervening ridges of more developed bone in an arborizing pattern. The majority of the lacunae consist of thinned bone, but areas in which bone is absent (craniofenestria) may occur. Both the pericranial and endocranial layers of the periosteum remain intact, so true herniation of the brain and the dura do not occur, but the underlying cerebral tissue may

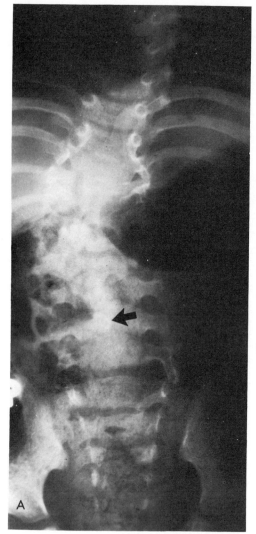

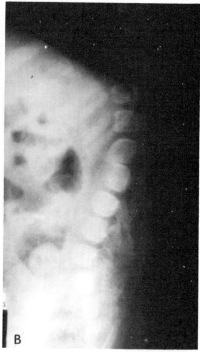

Figure 35–10 *A.* Posterior spina bifida from T10 through the sacrum with widening of the interpedicular diameter and eversion of the pedicles. A midline bony density overlying the L4 vertebral body corresponds to an ossified septum (*arrow*). *B.* Lateral view of a different child with a hemimyelomeningocele. The roentgenogram at birth shows the intervertebral disc space at L1–L2 narrowed and the anteroposterior diameter shortened. A septum was not seen at birth, but appeared faintly ossified at 1 year of age on the anteroposterior views.

bulge into the lacuna and produce a small elevation on the cortical surface.[559] Craniolacunia is associated with myelomeningocele and encephalocele, and has also been reported in uncomplicated aqueductal stenosis, arthrogryposis multiplex congenita, and phenylketonuria, and in a few apparently normal newborns.[377,581,712]

Associated Congenital Anomalies

Genitourinary malformations appear to be more frequent in infants with spina bifida aperta than in normal infants. Hypospadias, cryptorchidism, extrophy of the bladder, imperforate rectum, double ureters, and horseshoe kidney have been reported.[341,469,691,707] Congenital heart disease, cleft palate, and other anomalies do occur, but no more frequently than in random births. Approximately 7 per cent of infants have a facial conformation at birth suggesting Down's syndrome, but chromosome studies are normal and the children develop normal facial appearance with increasing age.[645,684,707]

Clinical Evaluation and Initial Management

The assessment of a newborn infant with myelomeningocele consists of a detailed general and neurological examination to determine whether the spinal lesion is open or closed, is within the time limits, is sufficiently clean, and is anatomically suitable for early closure. The neurological function of the extremities and sphincters, the nature of the limb deformities, the presence of early spinal deformities, the severity of hydrocephalus, and the presence of other congenital anomalies are detailed. The clinical examination is supplemented by roentgenograms of the skull, chest, entire spine, pelvis, hips, and lower extremities. Correlation of the clinical, radiological, and laboratory investigation permits an estimate of the prognosis for the infant, which may be of considerable importance in formulating a plan of management.

Treatment is begun in the nursery even before the infant is examined by following a routine level of care for the new infant with myelomeningocele. The infant is not fed and is nursed in the prone or lateral position in an incubator warmed sufficiently to produce normal body temperature. The open lesion is kept moist by a Telfa patch overlain by wet gauze frequently moistened with Ringer's lactate solution. Gauze is not placed directly on the lesion, as it tends to adhere to the neural tissues even when wet. If the lesion is cystic and protruding, then a ring of sterile gauze is constructed to surround the lesion and prevent mechanical irritation of the exposed neural tissue. Drying or mechanical damage can aggravate the existing neurological deficit, and mechanical stimulation of the exposed neural tissue can produce movements in the lower limbs that confuse the neurological examination.

The Spinal Lesion

The physician wears a mask, cap, and sterile gloves while dressing or examining the open lesion. The exposed area is swabbed to obtain specimens for culture and sensitivity tests, and if the lesion is leaking, cerebrospinal fluid is sent for Gram stain, culture and sensitivity tests, cell and differential counts, and protein and sugar determinations. An intact sac should be left unviolated until operation, at which time cerebrospinal fluid can be aspirated and sent for the studies. Cerebrospinal fluid from the sac has a higher protein content and leukocyte count than normal fluid, but no correlation exists between these two parameters and subsequent infection.

The process of bacterial colonization of the newborn infant begins at birth, and the first bacteria to become established may be those from the mother's vagina or perineum.[796] The umbilicus is colonized with *Staphylococcus aureus* within a few hours of birth, and later the entire skin surface is covered by anaerobic bacteria and *Staphyloccus aureus* and *S. epidermidis*. The gastrointestinal tract is sterile for four to eight hours, but then a variety of organisms is found such as micrococci, staphylococci, streptococci (*S. faecalis* and *S.viridans*), and yeast such as *Candida albicans*. The colonization of the gastrointestinal tract may be independent of the initial feeding, but the bacterial content of the infant's food is important for the subsequent pattern of colonization. Thus, the infant should not be fed until the plan of management has been decided.[469]

The spinal level of the lesion is estimated, and the appearance of the skin, membranes, and exposed neural tissue is documented and photographed. The size of the skin defect is measured, and the paraspinous area is palpated for protruding pedicles, as both factors are important in skin closure. A skin defect greater than half the width of the back will most likely require special techniques for closure. The surgeon should not count on the parchment skin of the zona epitheliosa for any part of the skin closure, but can use the hemangiomatous skin at the edge of the zona cutanea. A lesion slightly to one side of the midline suggests a hemimyelomeningocele that may be confirmed by the neurological examination.

The Neurological Examination

The infant must be metabolically stable prior to examination because a low body temperature, impaired respiration, or sedation by drugs administered to the mother during labor may falsely increase the neurological deficit.[703,707]

Motor Function

Patterns of motor function in the lower limbs fall into three general groups.* The first group consists of a lower motor neuron deficit with flaccid paralysis, areflexia, and

---

* See references 662, 664, 665, 703, 705, 707.

hypotonia distal to the last functioning cord segment. In the second group, the reflex arc in some isolated cord segments distal to the upper segmental level of the lesion is preserved, and the limbs display reflex activity, hypertonia, and occasionally hyperreflexia. Usually the voluntary motor deficit below the upper segmental level of the lesion is complete in either group. The majority of infants evidence patterns of the third group, a combination of a lower and an upper motor neuron deficit, which may produce a confusing clinical picture of normal voluntary movement, involuntary reflex movement, and flaccid paralysis.[665,703,707] The neurological level is usually symmetrical in the lower limbs within one or two segments; widely disparate function suggests hemimyelomeningocele. Sharrard's study of the lower limb innervation in man shows that usually more than one segmental level supplies each muscle.[662,664] It follows that each muscle group that controls a particular movement in a joint will be subserved by several segmental levels (Table 35-3). Generally, movement can be assessed only in the muscle groups, but if possible, individual muscle function is recorded. The segmental level of the spinal lesion is charted simply as voluntary movement present (+), movement present but probably involuntary and reflex in nature (+/R), or no movement at all (0).

The infant should be observed at rest, and spontaneous movements should be noted. Next, movements of the lower limbs in the Moro response and asymmetrical tonic neck reflex are elicited; normal responses indicate intact corticospinal tracts.[703] Then the effects of a painful stimulus applied to the upper limbs, lower limbs, and perineum are observed, and movements must be judged as voluntary or reflex by their character. Generally a brisk, stereotyped, reproducible movement obtained by pinprick applied to the lower extremities and unaccompanied by crying can be considered reflex. Although the reflex arc has been actuated, the painful stimulus has not been transmitted through the cord lesion to consciousness, and the movements cease when the stimulus ceases. Lower extremity movements that follow a painful stimulus applied to the trunk or upper limbs and are associated with crying are more likely to be voluntary, especially if the movements are repeated beyond the application of the stimulus.[238,664] Faradic stimulation has been used to predict future function in muscle groups, but early enthusiasm waned as the technique has failed to be an accurate predictor of voluntary function.[186,708,715,811-813] Similarly, electrical stimulation of the neural plaque may produce movements, but the only implication is that an intact anterior horn cell and motor root are present, not that they are under voluntary control.[708]

TABLE 35-3   INNERVATION OF LOWER EXTREMITY MUSCLE GROUPS IN APPROXIMATE DESCENDING SEGMENTAL ORDER*

Hip flexion	L1-L3
Hip adduction	L2-L4
Knee extension	L2-L4
Ankle inversion	L4
Ankle dorsiflexion	L4-L5
Ankle eversion	L5-S1
Toe extension	L5-S1
Hip abduction	L5-S1
Hip extension	L5-S2
Knee flexion	L5-S2
Ankle plantar flexion	S1-S2
Toe flexion and intrinsic muscles of foot	S2-S3
Perineal muscles	S2-S3

* Data from Sharrad, W. J. W.: The segmental innervation of the lower limb muscles in man. Ann. Roy. Coll. Surg. Eng., 35:106-122, 1964, and Neuromotor evaluation of the newborn. In American Academy of Orthopaedic Surgeons: Symposium on Myelomeningocele. St. Louis, C. V. Mosby Co., 1972, pp. 26-40.

Sensory Function

The segmental level of the sensory deficit usually correlates with the motor level within one or two segments. The sensory level is more often higher than the motor level, possibly owing to the greater exposure and degeneration of the dorsal aspect of the cord than of the ventral aspect. Sensory function can only be tested by observing the infant's response to a painful stimulus. Thus, the infant must be quiet or sleeping so that the relationship between the pinprick and the grimacing, crying, or Moro response is clear. Testing begins in the lowest sensory dermatomes in the perianal region and is continued proximally until the interface between absence and presence of sensation is located.

Sensory loss aggravates the motor handicap, since there is no proprioceptive feedback. Skin breakdown over pressure points at the ankles or toes or gluteal regions occurs more frequently with anesthetic skin, and sensory loss in the perianal skin may lead to maceration of the skin secondary to urinary incontinence.[573] Painless pathological fractures of the anesthetic lower extremities may occur and go undetected until a warm mass of callus simulating osteomyelitis appears at the fracture site.

Sphincter Function

Normal bladder function requires a balance between storage and emptying controlled by sacral spinal cord segments two, three, and four. Over 90 per cent of infants with myelomeningocele will have bladder dysfunction.[702,704] Only those infants with a hemimyelomeningocele who have a good leg intact to the S2 level or below, or those who have an incomplete upper motor neuron deficit, can hope to be spared. Normal renal function and competent ureteral valves without reflux are present in 90 per cent of newborns, but many difficulties follow as the type of neurogenic bladder becomes manifest.[361,704] The appearance of the natal cleft and the anal sphincter reveals the motor function of the pelvic floor. A flat or protruding natal cleft and patulous anal sphincter without anal reflex indicates a lesion of the lower motor neuron to the pelvic floor. A deep cleft, tight anal sphincter with anal reflex, and the absence of voluntary motor activity and sensation distal to the S1 level indicate a lesion of the upper motor neuron to the pelvic floor. Examination of bladder function in the newborn is limited to observation of detrusor function as suggested by spontaneous voiding, the ability to manually express urine with suprapubic pressure, suggesting a flaccid bladder with a lower motor neuron lesion, and assessment of perianal sensation and tone in the anal sphincter and pelvic floor. Approximately one third of children have flaccid, insensitive external sphincters and absence of detrusor contraction indicating a lower motor neuron deficit.[702] Urine may be expressed easily, but the tendency toward trabeculation of the bladder, retention of residual urine, and ureteral reflux appears to be less than in the next two groups. In one group, incomplete voluntary function may produce variable activity in the detrusor muscle, and the striated external sphincter may actively contract in either a reflex or voluntary manner. The bladder tends to be distended, and it is difficult to express urine. The last group has isolated functioning sacral cord segments with active reflex detrusor and external striated sphincter function. Both groups may have uncoordinated detrusor-sphincter action (sphincter-detrusor dyssynergia) and tend to develop bladder trabeculation, residual urine, and ureteral reflux. The Credé maneuver (suprapubic pressure to expel urine) can safely be performed only if the pelvic floor and external sphincter are flaccid. If the external sphincter is hyperactive, the maneuver may cause high intravesical pressure and ureteral reflux.[592] An intravenous pyelogram is not an essential preoperative evaluation unless an anomaly that might influence treatment such as agenesis of the kidneys or massive hydronephrosis is suspected.

An accurate prognosis of bladder function cannot be determined early after birth. The operative procedure may convert a future upper motor neuron bladder to a flaccid receptacle. As well, the newborn's bladder may appear flaccid until upper motor neuron reflexes develop weeks to months after birth.

The bowel is controlled through the same sacral segmental area, S3–S4, and its function parallels the neurogenic dysfunction of the bladder. Although only 10 to 20 per cent of patients may achieve reliable urinary control, 50 per cent can achieve satisfactory bowel control.[647] Fecal continence is maintained by the anterior angulation of the rectum in the puborectalis sling. A lower motor neuron deficit produces a loss of tone in the sling, an abnormal anorectal angulation, and a tendency to rectal prolapse, constipation, and incontinence. An upper motor neuron lesion of the pelvic floor leads to constipation but may allow relatively normal defecation and satisfactory continence.

Relationship of Neurological Level to Limb and Spine Deformities

The spine and limb deformities that are observed in the newborn or that develop in later life have several contributing factors, but the most important factor is muscle imbalance secondary to the neurological deficit.[104,660,663,666-670] Three varieties of imbalance between the agonist and the antagonist muscle groups may occur: a normal muscle acting against a flaccid antagonist, a normal muscle acting against a spastic antagonist, or a spastic muscle acting against a flaccid antagonist. An imbalance may culminate in a fixed deformity of a joint because the strong contraction of agonist muscles is not countered by the contraction of weak or flaccid antagonist muscles.

Occasionally a fixed and rigid deformity of the ankle or knee is present at birth with no obvious evidence of muscle imbalance. Such deformities are most likely due to in utero muscle imbalances shaping the joint structure as early as 16 weeks of gestation.[703] The lack of obvious muscle imbalance at birth suggests that a progressive decrease in neurological function can occur in utero because of degeneration of the exposed neural tissue. More often, the joint deformity present at birth correlates with detectable muscle imbalance, is elastic, and can be manually corrected, but assumes the deformed position at rest. This elastic type of joint deformity develops late in utero and is the same type that develops during the later years of infancy and childhood. Occasionally a true primary congenital deformity of a joint or a deformity secondary to in utero fetal positioning may be superimposed upon the deformities related to the neurological level. Table 35–4 summarizes the more common patterns of limb and spine deformities related to various segmental levels. The clinical picture may not fit the suggested pattern because of gradations in power in a particular functioning muscle group, the balancing effect of a spastic paralyzed muscle group as opposed to a flaccid group, a change in the neurological deficit such as the development of spasticity in a previously flaccid muscle group, the effects of intrauterine pressure on paralyzed limbs, and the effects of orthopedic treatment that alters the forces at play. Thus, extremity and spine deformities may evolve during infancy and childhood rather than remaining static.

Scoliosis of the spine is either congenital or developmental.[618] Congenital curves are due to structural abnormalities of the vertebral units such as failure of formation or failure of segmentation at and above the level of the myelomeningocele. The incidence of congenital scoliosis in myelomeningocele is approximately 30 per cent, and virtually all can be expected to progress. The second group of patients with developmental scoliosis usually have a straight spine at birth, and the vertebral unit abnormalities are limited to a posterior spina bifida at the level of the open lesion. Approximately 50 per cent of such children with straight spines at birth will develop scoliosis between 5 and 10 years of age. A thoracic or thoracolumbar scoliosis is usually associated with kyphosis, whereas the lower lumbosacral spinal curvature is usually a lordoscoliosis. Scoliosis is more likely to develop in the presence of an asymmetrical paralysis of the lower limbs, as with a hemimyelomeningocele, but the direction of the curvature is not determined by the side of the worst leg.[187]

Lumbar lordosis is usually absent at birth and develops as a compensatory mechanism to maintain an upright posture of the trunk in the presence of fixed flexion contractures at the hip with L1 or L2 motor levels (see Table 35–4). After 10 years of age, the deformity may increase rapidly if the child spends a great deal of time sitting.[666] Scoliosis frequently accompanies the lordosis.

Congenital lumbar kyphosis is a fixed, rigid spinal deformity present at birth in infants with thoracolumbar or thoracolumbosacral myelomeningocele with innervation to the L3 or L4 level (cf. Table 35–4 and Figs. 35–8 and 35–9). The kyphosis is attributed to the wide separation and eversion of the pedicles and rudimentary laminae of the involved vertebrae and the anterior rotation of the transverse processes, which displace the erector spinae muscles laterally and anterior to the spine.[182] The displacement changes the spinal extensor function of these muscles to one of spinal flexion, and when combined with functioning psoas muscles, the deformity tends to progress with time. The absence of posterior bony elements and their supporting ligaments permits the kyphosis to develop to the extreme. With levels of paralysis above L3, there is insufficient power in unbalanced lumbar and hip flexion to produce the severe kyphosis. Innervation below L4 limits hip flexion be-

TABLE 35–4 NEUROMUSCULOSKELETAL EXAMINATION IN MYELOMENINGOCELE

LOWERMOST FUNCTIONING SEGMENTAL LEVEL OF SPINAL CORD	FUNCTIONING MUSCLE GROUPS IN LOWER EXTREMITIES	NATURE OF LIMB DEFORMITY	PROGNOSIS FOR AMBULATION	PROGNOSIS FOR EXTREMITIES AND SPINE
T12	None	Minimal	Wheelchair	Developmental scoliosis
L1	Hip flexors, external rotators	Flexion, external rotation of hip	Wheelchair	Developmental scoliosis; lumbar lordosis; flexion–lateral rotation deformity of hip
L2	Hip flexors, adductors, external rotators	Flexion, adduction of hip	Wheelchair; household ambulation	Developmental scoliosis; lumbar lordosis; flexion-adduction deformity of hip with early or late dislocation
L3	Hip flexors, adductors, external rotators; knee extensors	Genu recurvatum	Wheelchair; walking with long leg braces and crutches	Congenital lumbar kyphosis; flexion-adduction deformity of hip with early or late dislocation
L4	Hip flexors, adductors, external rotators; knee extensors; ankle dorsiflexors, invertors	Flexion, adduction, external rotation of hip; genu recurvatum dorsiflexion, inversion of ankle, calcaneus deformity of foot	Walking with short leg braces and crutches	Congenital lumbar kyphosis; flexion-adduction contracture of hip with early or late dislocation; extension contracture of knee; calcaneovarus deformity of foot
L5	Hip flexors, adductors, external rotators, abductors but not extensors; knee flexors, extensors; ankle dorsiflexors, invertors, evertors	Flexion of hip; semi-flexion of knee; dorsiflexion of ankle, gross calcaneus deformity of foot	Walking with short leg braces	Flexion contracture of hip with low incidence of dislocation; calcaneovalgus deformity of foot
S1	Normal except for paralysis of toe flexors and intrinsic muscles of foot	Clawing of toes, flattening of sole of foot	Walking unaided	Vertical talus
S2	Virtually normal	Progressive clawing of toes	Walking unaided	Pes cavus and claw toes

cause of activity of the balancing hip extensors and prevents congenital lumbar kyphosis. The kyphotic protuberance leads to skin ulceration and infection, difficulty in fitting braces and abdominal appliances, and compression of the abdominal contents against the diaphragm leading to inadequate respiratory exchange as well as to development of a compensatory thoracic lordosis.*

Hydrocephalus and Craniolacunia

Approximately 90 per cent of children with myelomeningocele have active or arrested hydrocephalus at birth or within a few weeks after birth owing to obstruction of cerebrospinal fluid circulation associated with the Arnold-Chiari malformation (Fig. 35–11).† A normal head circumference at birth does not rule out hydrocephalus, since at least 34 per cent of such infants have ventriculomegaly.[442,656] Often, split sutures and a full fontanelle indicate raised intracranial pressure even with a normal head circumference. If the head circumference is over the ninetieth percentile, in virtually every case there is active hydrocephalus and usually of severe degree.[338,444]

Roentgenograms of the skull show craniolacunia (lacunar skull deformity, Lückenschädel skull deformity) in at least 77 per cent of children with myelomeningocele.‡ The characteristic radiological appearance is a general thinning of the vault of the skull with patchy areas of rarefaction sharply circumscribed by ridges of dense bone in a branching pattern. The defects tend to cluster high in the parietal and frontal bones near suture lines. The defects can

---

* See references 37, 39, 171, 172, 182, 330, 618, 663, 670.

† See references 307, 308, 416, 442, 691, 707.

‡ See references 97, 338, 440, 558, 559, 712.

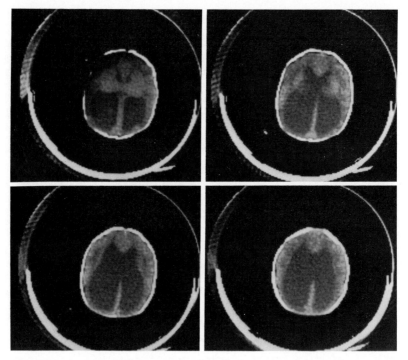

Figure 35–11   Cranial computed tomography three days after birth in an infant with a lumbosacral myelome-ningocele shows marked hydrocephalus. The head circumference was just over the fiftieth percentile, and the sutures were not spread.

be seen on antenatal roentgenograms and are already receding by the time of birth.[298,457,484,665] The more severe grades of deformity are seen in younger infants, but all defects are fading by 3 to 6 months of age, disappearing from the parietal bone last, and have completely resolved by 1 year of age.[436,558,559]

Craniolacunia is unrelated to the presence of hydrocephalus or elevated intracranial pressure, and may disappear while the hydrocephalus worsens. Skull markings secondary to increased intracranial pressure are more linear with less distinct edges and the intervening bone neither is dense nor has an arborizing pattern. As well, the digital markings are more widespread and involve the lower half of the cranial vault.

The Historical Perspective of Treatment

The newborn with myelomeningocele must withstand numerous life-threatening challenges throughout life. The immediate danger after birth is from meningitis and ventriculitis until the open area heals spontaneously or is closed by operation. Thereafter, progressive hydrocephalus threatens neurological function and life. During and after the first year, paralysis of the bladder with urinary stasis threatens frequent and occasionally overwhelming episodes of infection. Over the years, repeated episodes of upper tract infection and ureteral reflux lead to fatal chronic renal failure. Severe spinal deformities may contribute to impairment of respiratory function and frequent episodes of pneumonia.

Until the turn of the century, untreated myelomeningocele had a mortality rate of 80 to 90 per cent in the first year of life and a further 10 per cent over the next three to four years.[236,658,659] Operative treatment was introduced in the late 1800's to counter the dreadful natural history.[79,80,476,596] Throughout this early period to the 1960's, certain patients were selected for operation and, therefore, selected to live.* The lack of effective treatment for hydrocephalus

* See references 47, 124, 136, 278, 342, 346, 645, 659, 688.

was recognized as a limiting factor in survival, and some authors believed early hydrocephalus was a contraindication to operation on the spinal lesion, but opinion was not uniform.* Even the surgically adventurous authors, however, agreed with the majority that extensive paralysis of the legs and sphincters was a contraindication for operation.[659] Only 37 per cent of patients were considered suitable for operation.[278,342,346,645,688] The timing of operation was controversial only in terms of how long the surgeon should wait. Operation in the first few days after birth was considered inadvisable by the majority, except for a leaking lesion in a patient with no hydrocephalus and good neurological function.[342,346] Generally, operation was deferred until the lesion had epithelialized and the hydrocephalus had been arrested, and in essence, followed a test of viability.† The operative mortality rate was approximately 50 per cent before the turn of the century, but was reduced to approximately 10 per cent over the next 50 years.[342,346,504,645] Infection and hydrocephalus were the leading causes of death of both treated and untreated patients.

The first 50 years of operative treatment of myelomeningocele involved limited referral to the surgeon, selection of infants without hydrocephalus or severe neurological deficit for operation, and delayed operation on patients who had passed a test of viability. This plan of management permitted 20 to 30 per cent of patients to lead a relatively normal life unencumbered by retardation or physical defects; another 30 per cent were mildly disabled, and the remainder were moderately to severely disabled.[341,342,346,645] The inclusion of an unknown number of patients with meningocele in these series improves the results considerably.

The development of effective shunting procedures in the 1950's and, to a lesser extent, antibiotic therapy radically altered the possible therapeutic effort that could be expended upon the infant with myelomeningocele, and a new enthusiasm for treatment developed.‡ Hydrocephalus was no longer

a limiting factor in survival, although a new cause of morbidity and death was introduced. Virtually all infants are now transported to a center for consideration of treatment, and today the surgeon is requested to evaluate a greater proportion of severely involved infants.

The controversies over treatment revolved around two issues: early closure within 48 hours after birth, and selective care of infants with a better prognosis versus unselective total care of every infant irrespective of the severity of the lesion.

Early Closure of the Spinal Lesion

Early closure of the spinal lesion within 24 to 48 hours after birth received its greatest boost from Sharrard, Zachary, Lorber, and Bruce, from Sheffield, England, in 1963. A controlled trial between early and late closure was terminated before a statistically significant result had been obtained because improved leg function and a decreased mortality rate were believed to follow early closure.[671] Other authors have denied that neurological improvement occurs after operation.§ The conclusion that neurological function could be improved was gradually modified by the Sheffield group in subsequent publications over the years to a conclusion that deterioration in neurological function due to infection, direct trauma, desiccation, chemical injury from antiseptic solutions, and stretching from cystic distention of the subarachnoid space is prevented by early closure.[96,308,665,812,813] Survival is improved by early closure according to the majority of authors, and initial treatment of the hydrocephalus followed by delayed closure of the back is currently favored by only a minority.¶

Selective Versus Unselective Total Care

The stimulus to unselective total care also derived from the Sheffield group and was taken up by other units in the United Kingdom, North America, and Sweden.** The benefits of early closure, shunting for

---

* See references 47, 124, 136, 278, 342, 346, 659.
† See references 47, 236, 342, 346, 504, 659, 771.
‡ See references 177, 413, 446, 528, 529, 579, 580, 693, 706.

§ See references 81, 186, 228, 469, 697, 798.
¶ See references 21, 228, 283, 439, 468, 469, 474, 603, 681, 691, 697.
** See references 16, 23, 188, 228, 230, 238, 473, 474, 588, 603, 681.

hydrocephalus, and extensive orthopedic reconstruction were extended to all patients without regard to the severity of the neuromusculoskeletal deficit or the hydrocephalus. The raw survival rate was increased over the natural history, but the number of severely disabled children was also increased.[414,444,445] Lorber withdrew his support for unselective care in two papers in 1971 and 1972, and attempted to develop retrospective criteria by analysis of those cases in which there were undesirable results from total care.[444,445] The criteria were then applied prospectively to select infants for no treatment.[446-448] The following criteria were offered: (1) severe paraplegia at or above the third lumbar segmental level with only hip flexion, adduction, and knee extension present; (2) thoracolumbar or thoracolumbosacral lesions related to vertebral (not skin) levels; (3) kyphosis or scoliosis; (4) grossly enlarged head with a maximal head circumference 2 cm or more above the ninetieth percentile in relation to birth weight; (5) associated gross congenital anomalies such as cyanotic heart disease, ectopia of the bladder, or Down's syndrome; (6) intracerebral birth injuries; and (7) neonatal ventriculitis occurring prior to back closure. An infant fulfilling one or more of these criteria would receive no treatment, and the child, the family, and society would be spared a great burden upon the infant's death.

Selection of infants with a better prognosis for operation was not new and had always been practiced. Many physicians had continued the time-honored process of selection throughout the period of enthusiasm for unselective total care.* Others evaluated their personal results and suggested selection criteria of their own.† However, the emphasis had shifted from selection of infants to live, as practiced in the past, to selection of infants to die based on the denial of potentially effective and lifesaving treatment. Inability to treat does not involve ethical, moral, or religious considerations; withholding potentially effective treatment does, and therein lie the seeds of controversy.[279]

Objections to the selection of infants to die are directed toward the reliability of selection criteria, the fate of the infant selected for nontreatment, and ethical considerations.[162]

Selection for nontreatment based on severe paraplegia or on the bony level of the lesion or the presence of kyphosis or scoliosis has been criticized because none of these factors is necessarily a cause of death, and the sequelae can be corrected or controlled by intensive treatment.[16,188,228] Severe hydrocephalus at birth, whether manifested by a head circumference more than 2 cm above the ninetieth percentile, or by a frontal cortical mantle less than 1 cm in thickness, or by a parietal cortical mantle less than 2.5 cm in thickness, is not necessarily related to the intellectual outcome of the child if the hydrocephalus is treated early and effectively.‡ An attempt by Stein and co-workers to relate craniolacunia to the ultimate intellect of the child and give the deformity the status of a prognostic feature has been relatively unsuccessful, since over 20 per cent of infants with craniolacunia develop normal intelligence.[712] Thus, craniolacunia cannot be supported as an index of future retardation.[337,440,712] The assertion that the severely involved children tend to die of other complications in later childhood despite total care may not be supported by the survival rates in the 1970's.[238,709,713]

Some physicians can accept the idea that a few patients are going to die regardless of the effort expended to save them and that many patients who live because of that effort will be retarded and physically incapacitated. They cannot, however, accept rigid criteria that select patients to be allowed to die despite their having the potential for normal mental function. Examination of the group selected retrospectively for nontreatment by Lorber's criteria reveals severe physical deficit but normal intellect in 19 per cent.[444]

The fate of the child who is not operated on is a concern of every author.[239] Early reports suggest that 11 to 30 per cent of infants given supportive treatment will survive for 1 to 16 years.[219,414,607,684] Analysis shows that the care was decidedly supportive, with shunting procedures performed in

---

* See references 315, 468, 469, 684, 703, 707, 709.
† See references 16, 230, 231, 337, 414, 607, 693, 712, 713.

‡ See references 308, 338, 444, 445, 583, 684.

a number of the survivors, and that some infants did not meet specific criteria for delegation to the supportive treatment group. The figures can, therefore, be interpreted as the results of partial treatment rather than no treatment. Selection of patients for no treatment by relatively rigid criteria definitely limits survival.[445,709] The treatment must, however, be limited to no intensive care, feeding on demand, no tube feeding, no antibiotics for infection, and analgesics as required.[446,447] Adherence to a strict no treatment plan should result in a survival rate of no more than 3 to 4 per cent at 2 years of age.* Nevertheless, some infants may survive even ventriculitis without antibiotic treatment.[684] Less strict authors suggest that shunting for hydrocephalus and back closure, if still required, can be performed sometime after the first month of age in the child who survives. In this case essentially the treatment plan of the pre-1960's is followed.[693,707]

The ethical, religious, and social implications of a selection process may be discussed ad infinitum. In 1975, a group in Great Britain studied the ethics of selective treatment and came to the following conclusion:

The doctor has no ethical obligation to treat cases in which the likely benefits are very dubious. Thus, in the present state of medical knowledge, the policy of selection for the treatment of spina bifida is, in our opinion, justified . . . but we recognize that these criteria change and should be subject to constant

---

* See references 315, 447, 603, 607, 693, 707, 709.

scrutiny in the light of medical advance and the conflict of ethical principles. . . .[405]

Active steps to shorten the infant's life span were condemned by the group. Whether a selection process is or is not used in a center depends on so many circumstances that, at least in the United States, no uniform policy is likely in the foreseeable future.

Current Treatment of Myelomeningocele

The plan of management for an infant with myelomeningocele depends on the infant's viability as determined in the initial evaluation and the time the infant is received. No single plan of management is correct. Any unit treating such patients must consider three options (Fig. 35–12).

Early Closure of the Spinal Lesion

Early closure of the spinal lesion is preferred if the operation can be commenced before 36 hours after birth. The chance of ventriculitis is reduced and the possibility of maintaining the initial level of neurological function is enhanced.[84] Early operation in the full-term, otherwise healthy infant is preferred when the surgeon and the anesthesiologist are experienced.

Control of Hydrocephalus and Delayed Closure of the Spinal Lesion

The back lesion is certain to be colonized in patients received later than 36 hours after

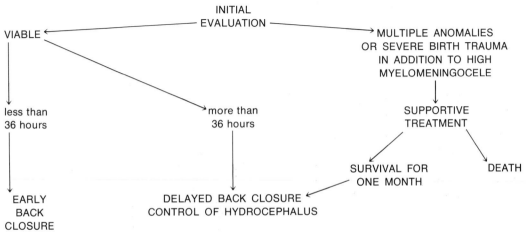

Figure 35–12 Management of the infant with myelomeningocele.

birth, and repair at that time is associated with increased rates of mortality and morbidity.* Operation should be deferred until a later date. Superficial infection can be cleared by frequent Ringer's lactate dressing changes, the application of topical antibiotics selected according to the results of cultures, and systemic antibiotics for infections that do not respond to local care. Ventricular cerebrospinal fluid should be cultured at any time the child shows the slightest suggestion of sepsis. Cerebrospinal fluid leakage from the sac due to hydrocephalus confirmed by cranial computed tomography is controlled by external ventricular drainage or placement of an indwelling shunt. Progressive hydrocephalus in the absence of leakage is also treated by external drainage or placement of a shunt. The method selected depends on the degree of infection of the open lesion and the results of culture of ventricular cerebrospinal fluid and its chemistry. An indwelling shunt should never be placed until the cerebrospinal fluid is proved free of infection by a three-day culture. When the back lesion is clean and free of infection, delayed closure can be performed if still required.[228]

Supportive Treatment

A very few infants are so severely afflicted with a high paralysis, spine and limb deformities, hydrocephalus, and other congenital or traumatic abnormalities that no realistic benefit can follow aggressive operative treatment. In such a patient, the treatment is supportive to the extent that the back lesion is dressed as for delayed closure, and oral feedings are commenced, but no antibiotics are given for infection. The family should not be held in suspended animation waiting for the infant to die, and if the infant survives an arbitrary period of one month, then it is integrated into the delayed-closure treatment plan.

The neurosurgeon usually carries the burden of developing the initial relationship with the family. It is not appropriate for the decision for life or death to be dumped into the lap of the family. The emotionally devastated parents cannot make a satisfactory decision following the physician's long recitation of problems and possible prognoses.

Thus, a viable infant received earlier than 36 hours after birth is regarded as meriting early closure. A viable infant arriving later than 36 hours after birth is regarded as requiring early control of hydrocephalus if it occurs and delayed closure of the back; an infant so critically afflicted that survival of early operative treatment is in question is regarded as requiring supportive treatment with the expectation that the child may die within the first month. Survival to one month, however, would indicate integration into a full treatment plan.

Technique for Operative Care of the Back Lesion

The thermostat of the operating room is set at 80° Fahrenheit, and a heating lamp is directed on the infant during initial prepara-

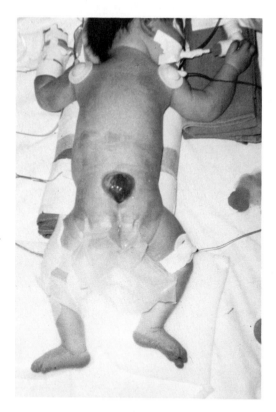

Figure 35–13 The infant is prone on bolsters with a heating blanket beneath the white sheet. Endotracheal intubation, an umbilical vein cannula, and a peripheral intravenous line are in place. Plastic draping excludes the anus from the open lesion and covers the rectal temperature probe. A heat lamp warms the infant during the operation. The legs are visualized through a sterile transparent bowel bag placed over the legs at the time of draping.

---

* See references 81, 307, 469, 661, 671, 707.

tions. An umbilical cannula is placed by the neonatologists, or a saphenous vein cutdown is performed if the anesthesiologist cannot place a reliable intravenous catheter (Fig. 35–13). General intubation anesthesia is preferred, since a better closure is obtained if both the patient and the surgeon are comfortable during the procedure.* The infant is placed in the prone position on small bolsters overlying a heating blanket, and his temperature is monitored by a rectal probe. A sterile plastic drape is attached to the medial thighs and over the anus to exclude the anal region from the operative site. A larger transparent plastic drape can be placed over the legs so movements are readily visible during stimulation of nerve roots during closure. The buttocks and posterior thighs, the flanks to the level of the bolsters, the back to the level of the scapulae, and the skin surrounding the open area are prepared with an iodine-based solution. No preparation solution is placed on the neural tissue, and a nurse is delegated to gently irrigate the neural plaque to prevent desiccation under the heating element during the preparation period. The back and thighs are widely draped so the surgeon can see the contour of the back and the color of the skin during closure. If the lesion is cystic and unruptured, a fine needle is passed into the sac laterally, and fluid is aspirated for Gram stain and the usual cerebrospinal fluid studies.

---

* See references 32, 81, 177, 286, 308, 467, 641, 681.

Magnification may be useful for dealing with a complex lesion with nerve roots adherent to the walls of the sac or when dissecting the upper or lower ends of the neural plaque. The bipolar coagulator is mandatory.

The surgeon must consider the neural tissue, closure of the dura, management of a complicating spinal deformity, and closure of the skin.

The Neural Tissue

Most experienced surgeons have observed a few instances of an apparent improvement in neurological function after closure of the defect. The improvement is not due to the operation but rather to return of function in segments that seemed paralyzed on the first examination. Thus, all neural tissue should be preserved (Fig. 35–14). Dissection begins at the lateral aspect of the lesion at the junction between the zona epitheliosa and the hemangiomatous skin edge (Fig. 35–15A). The tissue is opened and the interior of the sac is inspected. Laterally, the floor of the sac is formed by the glistening white dura, and medially, nerve roots can be seen passing from the neural tissue on the dome of the sac down into the spinal canal. The junctional interface is dissected cranially and caudally to the upper and lower ends of the neural plaque on one side and then on the other. At the upper end of the neural plaque, a virtually normal spinal cord can

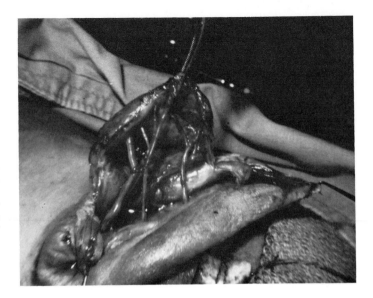

Figure 35–14 An "overgrown" lumbosacral neural plaque has been untethered from the skin edge at its caudal tip. Large nerve roots are seen diving down into the spinal canal to their exit foramina. No neural tissue was sacrificed, although the plaque was too large to be accommodated in the spinal canal. The preoperative motor level changed from L2 to L4 postoperatively, which was compatible with the anatomical level of the lesion and the ankle deformities present at birth.

be seen entering the re-formed dural tube lying under the upper intact lamina. Filamentous adhesions often bind the cord to the dural tube, and these bands should be divided. Just caudal to the normal cord and dural tube, the plaque is usually densely adherent to the zona epitheliosa and often to the hemangiomatous skin edge. Careful dissection is essential at this level, and magnification is helpful. Dissection of the upper and lower ends of the neural plaque is important, since the upper end is functioning neural tissue and, at both ends, adhesions may occur between the neural tissue and the surrounding tissues. Such adhe-

sions may produce tethering of the spinal cord with late neurological deterioration.[21] The surgeon should look for a bony or fibrocartilaginous spur near the level of the first intact lamina if the patient has a unilateral paralysis as in a hemimyelomeningocele or if the spinal roentgenogram shows a narrowed intervertebral disc space or a midline septum.[187] Occasionally laminectomy of one or two proximal levels will facilitate the procedures necessary at the upper end of the plaque. The lower end of the cord and cauda equina should be carefully dissected free; a nerve stimulator may be helpful at this stage to distinguish con-

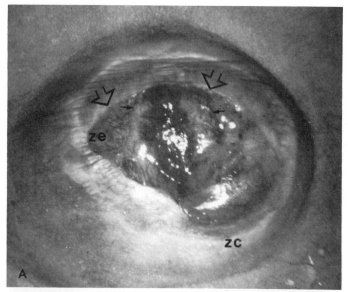

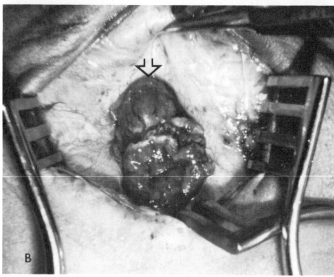

Figure 35–15 *A.* Lumbar myelomeningocele with the edges of the neural plaque (*small arrows*) attached to the zona epitheliosa (ze), which is attached to the hemangiomatous zona cutanea (zc). Wrinkled parchment skin extending in from the zona cutanea contributes to the zona epitheliosa and partially covers the neural plaque (*open arrows*). The parchment skin cannot be used for skin closure. *B.* The neural plaque has been separated from the zona cutanea. The inner lining of the sac held in the forceps is the splayed dura running up to the edge of the zona cutanea. The spinal cord enters the reformed dural tube within the spinal canal at the upper end of the sac (*open arrow*).

Illustration continued on opposite page

ducting motor nerve elements from fibrous tissue strands.[81,467] An identifiable filum terminale should be divided.

The edge of the neural plaque should be debrided of the membranous tissue of the zona epitheliosa and thin parchment skin originating from the zona cutanea to preclude the formation of an inclusion dermoid cyst at a later date.[89,445] The tissue is sent for culture and sensitivity tests.

All neural tissues should be replaced within the open spinal canal. Often, the bulk of the neural tissue is more than the shallow spinal canal can accommodate, but no tissue should be sacrificed at this time (cf. Fig. 35–14).

Closure of the Dura

One of the keys to a successful operation is a watertight reconstruction of the dural sac. The normal dural tube is encountered

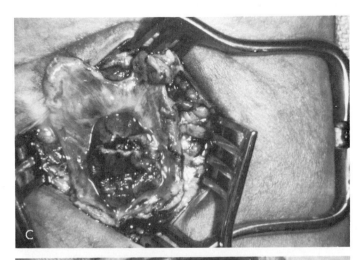

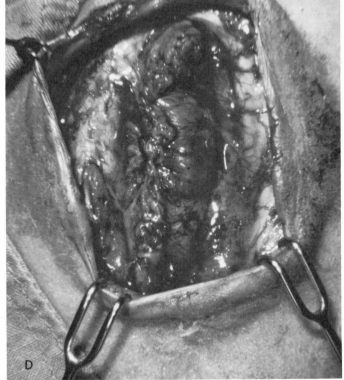

Figure 35–15 (*continued*) *C.* The dura has been mobilized, leaving a rim attached to the zona cutanea for placement of deep skin sutures. *D.* The closed dura is shown in a different patient. The exposed paraspinous fascia is seen overlying the ridges of the widened pedicles. Fascial flaps may be closed over the spinal canal for reinforcement.

at the upper end where the neural plaque has been separated from the dural cuff. Below this level, the dura is splayed over the everted pedicles of the posterior spina bifida and is lightly adherent to the paraspinous fascia and tightly adherent to the edge of the hemangiomatous skin. The dural tube may or may not be reconstituted at the lower end, depending on the level and extent of the neural lesion. Initially, the dura at the upper end of the sac is defined, and then the open dura is dissected laterally on each side and easily separated from the paraspinous fascia until sufficient tissue is available on both sides to permit direct closure over the neural tissue without producing strangulation (Fig. 35–15B and C). A small rim of dura is left attached to the hemangiomatous skin edge to form a tough, avascular layer for placement of deeper sutures approximating the skin edge.[812,813] The dura is closed with a running 5-0 vascular nylon that will not fray the dural edge (Fig. 35–15D). A paraspinous fascial patch is used as a dural graft if insufficient dural coverage is available. The anesthesiologist produces a Valsalva maneuver to test the integrity of the dural closure.

A second, imbricated layer of paraspinous fascia is closed over the spinal canal when possible, but the fascia is usually insufficient in the lumbosacral area. Widely everted pedicles may prevent mobilization of sufficient fascia to bridge the gap. The everted pedicles can be fractured and bent medially on either side after the fascial flaps are fashioned, and usually this maneuver will permit closure of the fascia attached to the pedicles.[236,512,513] Occasionally, the displaced paraspinous muscles lateral to the fractured pedicles can now be sutured over the midline to offer a third layer, but the author does not attempt this in patients with leg function for fear of compressing the neural tissue.[307,469]

Management of a Complicating Spinal Deformity

Everted pedicles can form a prominent bony ridge on either side of the open spinal canal and can impair skin healing postoperatively or be a site of pressure ulceration in later life. Prominent pedicles can be fractured and rotated medially, or they may be removed.

A severe congenital lumbar kyphosis can create difficulties with skin closure, impair postoperative skin healing, and lead to pressure ulceration in later life in addition to problems with fitting of braces. Primary vertebrectomy and wiring of the spine to correct the kyphosis can be performed at the initial operation. The procedure is formidable in the neonate and may be followed by nonunion and recurrence of a progressive deformity. Nevertheless, it can provide healthier skin over the kyphus, which facilitates a definitive corrective procedure in later life if the curvature does progress.[171,172,663,670]

Closure of the Skin

The two most important factors contributing to poor wound healing are tension on the skin edges and the use of poor quality skin. All the skin surrounding the open area may be used, including the peripheral rim of hemangiomatous skin, but the parchment skin does not heal and should be removed. If the debrided skin defect is less than half the width of the back, then direct closure may be obtained by extensive circumferential undermining with the line of closure in the horizontal, oblique, or vertical direction. The direction of closure is not important to ultimate healing.[310] Gentle undermining is performed on the level of the fascial plane, following the curvature of the back around the flanks and the buttocks. If the plane of dissection enters the subcutaneous tissue the blood supply to the overlying skin flap will be amputated. Blunt finger dissection is preferable where possible, as blood vessels are stretched rather than cut. Division of the tight fibrous band tethering the subcutaneous tissue and skin along the line of the iliac crest bilaterally provides greater mobility of the skin. The skin is closed in two layers with a layer of interrupted 3-0 absorbable suture in the subcutaneous tissue. If these sutures are placed in the tough dural cuff left attached to the zona cutanea, then the hemangiomatous skin edge and subcutaneous tissue can be approximated without the sutures tearing out of the delicate tissues. The skin is closed with interrupted vertical mattress sutures of 5-0 nylon or 5-0 stainless steel. If the skin edges blanch along the line of closure, then the blood supply is inadequate

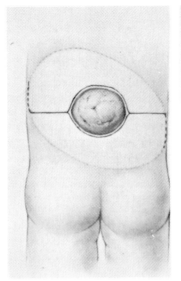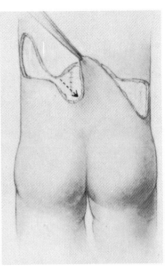

Figure 35–16 The S-shaped rotation flap will often suffice for skin defects that cannot be closed directly after extensive undermining but is inadequate for very large defects. (From Matson, D. D.: Surgical repair of myelomeningocele. J. Neurosurg., 27:180–186, 1967. Reprinted by permission.)

and revision of the closure is necessary. The skin may have to be approximated two or three times in different directions before a satisfactory tension-free closure is accomplished. Intravenous fluorescein can demonstrate the blood supply to the skin and indicate nonviable areas that should be debrided, but the technique has not been found necessary by the author.[767]

A satisfactory closure may not be made possible by undermining if the width of the skin defect exceeds half the width of the back. Special techniques are required, and a surgeon should become adept at one particular technique for closing large defects rather than trying a different one each time. Occasionally, relaxing incisions in the flank will allow direct closure of undermined skin.[308,812,813] Use of S-shaped rotation flaps

is a popular technique, but it may be inadequate for large defects (Fig. 35–16).[275,467,555,691] For larger lesions, bipedicle flaps with a rostral and a caudal base may be raised (Fig. 35–17). The width of each flap must be at least half the width of the defect to obtain adequate closure, and the length of the flap should be no greater than twice the width. The bipedicle flaps may be closed immediately over the neural repair for early closure, or the flaps may be raised and their transfer delayed two or three weeks for delayed closure of the spinal lesion.[166,286,815] The flank defects may be sutured to the deep tissues and the area allowed to granulate, or skin grafts may be placed to accelerate healing.

Whether the closure is direct or by flaps, tension on the skin margins may be relieved

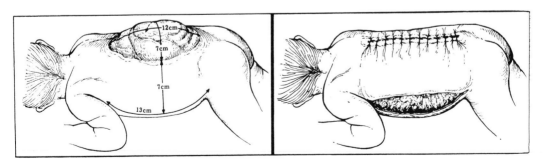

Figure 35–17 Large skin defects can be closed immediately or by the delay method with bipedicle flaps. The length of the flap is no greater than twice the width. The flank defects may be left to granulate or be skin grafted. (From Zook, E. G., Dzenitis, A. J., and Bennett, J. E.: Repair of large myelomeningoceles. Arch. Surg. (Chicago), 98:41–43, 1969. Copyright 1969, American Medical Association. Reprinted by permission.)

by placing stainless steel retention sutures remote from the skin edge. The wire is passed subcutaneously beneath the skin flaps and fixed over ordinary sterile white plastic buttons on the skin surface to prevent the wire from pulling through.[310] Meticulous hemostasis is necessary in any form of closure to prevent a subcutaneous hematoma from placing additional tension on the incision. Such care will obviate the need for a subcutaneous drain.

The Postoperative Period

Routine Care

A light noncompressive dressing is placed over the operative site, and a fresh sterile plastic drape turned over the dressing excludes the anus and keeps the dressing dry. The patient is nursed in a 20-degree head-down prone position in the incubator to reduce the hydrostatic pressure exerted by the cerebrospinal fluid on the repair site. If the repaired defect was large, the infant is suspended by an abdominal sling hung from the cover of the incubator to stretch the abdominal skin toward the back and relieve tension on the suture line.[812,813] Urine must be expressed every two or three hours from an atonic bladder to prevent stasis, particularly when the head-down position or the sling is used. Neonatal ureteral peristalsis may be weak, and hydroureter and hydronephrosis can develop on a postural basis and be aggravated further by the bladder paralysis. Intermittent catheterization may be necessary if the pelvic floor and external sphincter are spastic. A baseline intravenous pyelogram is performed within one week of closure of the back.

Delayed Wound Healing

The dressing is changed daily and the wound inspected for areas of skin necrosis, subcutaneous hematoma or effusion, wound infection, or cerebrospinal fluid leak. Delayed wound healing has been reported in up to 40 per cent of patients, particularly if no selection is practiced and many large lesions are closed.[681] An effusion or hematoma that stretches the skin incision should be aspirated. If wound breakdown occurs owing to ischemia of the skin edges without superimposed infection or cerebrospinal fluid leak, then Telfa–

Ringer's lactate dressings and time may produce healing by granulation, or skin grafting of the granulating surface can hasten healing of large areas of skin slough. Wound breakdown with cerebrospinal fluid leak is usually associated with progressive hydrocephalus and is best treated by external ventricular drainage rather than by an attempt to resuture the incision or to find and close the site of the dural leak. Infection at the site of the repair is usually due to *Staphylococcus aureus* or coliform organisms, and appropriate antibiotics are selected on the basis of culture and sensitivity tests.

Meningitis and Ventriculitis

Prophylactic antibiotics are not used routinely in the postoperative period. Should the cultures of the neural plaque or zona epitheliosa or the cerebrospinal fluid obtained at operation become positive, however, then appropriate antibiotics are started. Despite closure, the risk of meningitis and ventriculitis is 10 to 25 per cent.[449] The ventricle is routinely tapped 24 to 48 hours after operation, and the cerebrospinal fluid is cultured regardless of the infant's clinical course, as neonates may have well-established infection for several days before clinical manifestations are evident. The ventricular tap is repeated if there is jaundice or increased intracranial pressure with irritability, vomiting, poor feeding, seizures, pyrexia, or hypothermia.[812,813] If the back becomes infected, then the ventricular tap is repeated. The importance of early detection of cerebrospinal fluid infection is twofold. The primary cause of death in both the child with myelomeningocele who has been operated on and the one who has not is infection. In addition, therapy with intraventricular antibiotics and external ventricular drainage to control hydrocephalus may result in a decrease in morbidity and death from ventriculitis.

Hydrocephalus

Cranial computed tomography is performed in the first week after operation as a baseline study of ventricular size, whether or not hydrocephalus is symptomatic or the head circumference is increasing. If the hydrocephalus is progressive, then a ventriculoperitoneal shunt may be placed, but only if the back is healing well and after a ventricular cerebrospinal fluid culture shows no growth over a 72-hour period. Omitting the cerebrospinal fluid culture may lock the patient and the surgeon into the vicious circle of shunt infection.

Closure of the back lesion may exacerbate the hydrocephalus for three reasons.[342,346,442] Leakage of cerebrospinal fluid may be decompressing an otherwise active hydrocephalus, and closure of the safety valve results in rapid head expansion. A bulging cystic lesion may forestall progressive ventriculomegaly by a damping effect on elevated intracranial pressure. Acute loss of cerebrospinal fluid from the lesion during operation may cause further impaction of the Arnold-Chiari malformation in the foramen magnum and increase the degree of obstruction to cerebrospinal fluid circulation. The concept of the sac as a source of cerebrospinal fluid absorption has been long laid to rest.[560]

Occasionally the Arnold-Chiari malformation will become symptomatic during the first month after birth and cause respiratory stridor or apneic episodes or lower cranial nerve paresis. The presentation and management of these complications are discussed separately in the section on the Arnold-Chiari malformation.

Results and Prognosis

The overall results of treatment and the prognosis for an infant with myelomeningocele vary greatly. The decade of the study, the level and severity of the defect, the timing of closure, the enthusiasm for treatment of hydrocephalus and infective complications, the duration of follow-up, the philosophy of the unit, and the rehabilitation facilities available for aftercare are a few of the factors influencing outcome.

Overall Survival

The overall survival rate in the early years of life has been improving in the units practicing unselective total care, as indicated in Table 35–5. Currently, most units can obtain a minimum rate of 80 per cent over the first two years in infants free of other major congenital defects. In the past,

TABLE 35–5 OVERALL SURVIVAL IN MYELOMENINGOCELE WITH UNSELECTIVE TOTAL CARE

AUTHOR	STUDY PERIOD	FOLLOW-UP (YEARS)	SURVIVAL (PER CENT)
Lorber*	1959–1963	7–11	41
Lorber*	1967–1968	2–4	63
Hemmer†	1961–1966	1–5	67
Hunt et al.‡	1963–1971	1–7	71
Ames and Schut§	1963–1968	3–8	80
French	1975–1979	1–4	93

* Results of treatment of myelomeningocele. An analysis of 524 unselected cases, with special reference to possible selection for treatment. Develop. Med. Child Neurol., 13: 279–303, 1971.
† Meningoceles and myeloceles. Progr. Neurol. Surg., 4:192–226, 1971.
‡ Predictive factors in open myelomeningocele with special reference to sensory level. Brit. Med. J., 4:197–201, 1973.
§ Results of treatment of 171 consecutive myelomeningoceles—1963 to 1968. Pediatrics, 50:466–470, 1972.

units practicing selection have reported survival of 70 to 78 per cent of the selected patients with similar follow-up periods, and currently the rate should be even greater.[691,693,709]

Hydrocephalus reduces overall survival because of the complications of shunting.[228,444] Foltz reported survival to 15 years of age in 89 per cent of children without hydrocephalus or with inactive hydrocephalus in contrast to 50 per cent for a comparable group with active hydrocephalus.[228]

The higher the level of the lesion, the lower the survival rate, but considerable improvement has occurred over the years for all levels, as shown in Table 35–6.[16,228,307,444] The cause of death is often a combination of factors. Approximately 70 per cent of all deaths occur in the first two years of life, with meningitis and ventriculitis accounting for 24 to 45 per cent, uncontrolled hydrocephalus and shunt complications for 19 to 30 per cent, pneumonia for

TABLE 35–6 MYELOMENINGOCELE LEVEL AND SURVIVAL

LEVEL	EARLY SERIES (PER CENT)	LATER SERIES (PER CENT)
Thoracolumbar	25	52–65
Lumbar	45	75
Lumbosacral	42	89
Sacral	70	over 90

22 per cent, renal complications for 11 per cent, and miscellaneous factors for the remainder.[190,449,693] Shunt complications cause the majority of deaths after one year of life, with renal diseases accounting for approximately 10 per cent of deaths.[190,445,693].

Hydrocephalus

The incidence of hydrocephalus is 80 to 90 per cent in myelomeningocele, but an important variation in incidence occurs with the level of the lesion. Hydrocephalus occurs in over 90 per cent of patients with a thoracolumbar lesion, in almost 90 per cent of those with a lesion in the lumbar area, in 75 per cent of those with a lesion in the lumbosacral area, and in 50 per cent or less of those with a lesion in the sacral area.[16,228,238,442,693] The higher lesions are associated with not only an increased incidence of hydrocephalus but also a greater incidence of active hydrocephalus.[228] Both the absence of hydrocephalus and the presence of inactive or arrested hydrocephalus give a better prognosis in terms of morbidity and mortality rates. Approximately 30 per cent of patients either develop arrested hydrocephalus and do not require a shunt despite clinical evidence of ventriculomegaly or will become independent of a shunt in the future.[228,231,707]

Intellectual Development

The level of intellectual development is one of the more controversial issues in the treatment of myelomeningocele and is also the most difficult to evaluate (Table 35–7). The measured intelligence quotient (IQ) is frequently overestimated in infants and young children, may be an unreliable indicator of ultimate self-sufficiency, and does not always correlate with school performance. The intellectual potential is reduced when combined either with a high lesion or with active hydrocephalus.[228] Ventriculitis, shunt infection, or episodes of shunt obstruction can reduce intellectual potential independently of other factors.[444]

The normal IQ is usually considered to be 80 or higher, with 74 as the lower limit of educability.[228] Thirty to forty per cent of all children treated unselectively will be retarded to some degree compared with approximately twenty per cent in a selectively treated group.[707]

Hydrocephalus decreases the intellectual potential.* Although the mean IQ of an unselectively treated hydrocephalic group may be in the normal range, 41 to 54 per cent of the children may have an IQ below 80.[445,602] Even selectively treated patients with hydrocephalus will have an incidence of retardation of 34 per cent.[709] The currently published morbidity and mortality statistics may be improved by early diagnosis and effective shunting of progressive hydrocephalus and aggressive management of shunt infection and obstruction.[228,583] The child without hydrocephalus or whose hydrocephalus is arrested has a better prognosis for normal IQ, the incidence of retardation being 23 to 26 per cent with unselective treatment compared with only 3 per cent in those selectively treated.†

The fact that children from an unselected group with no hydrocephalus or with arrested hydrocephalus had a higher incidence of retardation than those from a selected group indicates that other factors must be important in poor intellectual attainment. Indeed, the likelihood of retardation increases with the higher lesions.‡ Of survivors with thoracolumbar lesions, 30 per cent are retarded compared with a maximum of 25 per cent with lumbar or lower lesions. The difference is more striking if the excessive mortality rate among patients with higher lesions, many of whom would have been retarded had they survived, is considered.

Children with myelomeningocele may

TABLE 35–7 INTELLECTUAL DEVELOPMENT IN MYELOMENINGOCELE

PARAMETER	EDUCABLE (IQ > 74) (PER CENT)
Level	
Thoracolumbar	70
Lumbar and below	75
Overall	
Unselective care	60–70
Selective care	80
Hydrocephalus	
Unselective care	46–59
Selective care	66
No hydrocephalus	
Unselective care	74–77
Selective care	97

---

* See references 177, 228, 308, 445, 583, 602, 683, 693.
† See references 177, 308, 445, 602, 693, 707.
‡ See references 228, 338, 415, 441, 684, 703.

have serious learning difficulties and poor school achievement over and above the incidence of frank retardation.[707] Seventy to eighty per cent may require specialized schooling to reach acceptable education levels. The Wechsler test may show a good verbal quotient but a poor performance quotient, which indicates brain damage. Good word recall, not necessarily equated with meaningful use, gives rise to the so-called "cocktail party chatter syndrome." Poor performance scores on subtests of visuospatial perception and body image are common. When significant social and physical disabilities and long absences from school for operations and illnesses are added, the requirement for specialized schooling is not surprising.

Ambulation

The outlook for ambulation is based on the segmental level of motor function, as listed in Table 35–4. Motor function at L3 would seem to be the highest possible level compatible with a form of ambulation other than a wheelchair, but many such patients rely on a wheelchair for many of their daily activities. The ambulatory capacity at any motor level decreases with age as body weight increases more than muscle power.[72] Often the motor level does not relate directly to the prognosis for ambulation because so many other factors affect the ability to ambulate—such as intelligence, coordination, spinal curvature, orthopedic deformities, trophic ulceration, lower limb fractures, aggressiveness of the rehabilitation program, and motivation of the patient and family, to mention a few.[321] In an unselected group of patients, as many as 60 per cent may require a wheelchair for all or part of their day compared with 25 per cent of patients from a selected group.[445,709] The orthopedic care of the spine and lower limb deformities is beyond the scope of this chapter.*

Sphincter Function

Eighty to ninety per cent of patients will be incontinent of urine with the lifelong risks of urinary stasis and infection, trabeculation and diverticulae of the bladder, ureteral reflux, and chronic renal failure,

depending on the nature of the neurogenic bladder.† Reliance on early urinary diversion with implantation of the ureters into an isolated segment of the ileum or colon or to the skin or via a cutaneous vesicostomy has given way to use of intermittent catheterization.[174,175,361,564,592] A perineal urethrostomy may be necessary in the male to prevent urethral stricture from catheter use.[592] Implantable electrical stimulation devices to gain control of voiding and artificial sphincters to permit urinary continence are still in the developmental stages.[492,493,648] External collecting devices may provide social urinary control in males but, unfortunately, are not suitable for females.[388]

Control of defecation can be achieved in 50 per cent of children with the assistance of the postprandial gastrocolic reflex combined with a rectal suppository or enema.[140,647] Poor control of defecation can lead to perianal excoriation or rectal prolapse.[96,140,308]

Sexual Function

Sacral segments S2 to S4 are involved with erection and ejaculation in the male. A lower motor neuron lesion of these segments prevents erection and ejaculation. An upper motor neuron lesion with reflex activity in S2 to S4 may permit reflex erections, but effective ejaculation is unlikely. In both males and females, complete lesions of upper or lower motor neuron type will produce genital anesthesia. Despite the abnormal function in these segments, satisfactory sex play is possible, since gratification is a combination of both psychological and physical factors.[128,682,703]

Psychosocial Adaptation

Potential problems within the family are numerous and revolve around financial stress; dependence of the afflicted child on the parents with consequent social isolation, physical and emotional drain of frequent hospital visits, illnesses, operative procedures, guilt feelings, and inability to plan for the future; poor self-image on the part of the child; and marital discord, to mention a few.[392,577,601] The social worker can do a great deal to empathize with and counsel the parents and children and draw

---

* See references 215–217, 532, 663, 666–670.

† See references 188, 209, 231, 308, 445, 691, 693.

attention to problems that the family may not mention to the physicians.

Other Problems

Ten to thirty per cent of patients have epilepsy of either an idiopathic nature or secondary to meningitis and ventriculitis, hydrocephalus, shunt insertion, or shunt complications.[231,445,707]   Ophthalmological complications such as abducens paresis, secondary optic atrophy related to increased intracranial pressure, primary optic atrophy, skew deviation, and horizontal or vertical or downbeat nystagmus secondary to meningitis and ventriculitis or to the Arnold-Chiari malformation occur in 30 per cent of patients.[272,295,616]

Delayed Neurological Complications

Neurological function in a child with myelomeningocele requires sequential monitoring over the years, since the postoperative neurological examination is subject to change. The Arnold-Chiari malformation may cause bulbar compression with apneic episodes or laryngeal nerve paresis, symptomatic syringohydromyelia, or acute medullary compression following a lower spine operation in later life.[164,288,289,784] A change from a lower motor neuron to an upper motor neuron deficit, an increasing spasticity, or a rise in segmental neurological deficit may herald a symptomatic lesion in the spinal canal such as tethering of the spinal cord at the level of the previous repair like that shown in Figure 35–18, an inclusion dermoid cyst from epithelial tissue incorporated in the original repair, a diastematomyelia with septum, or a lipomatous mass or arachnoid cyst or intramedullary dermoid tumor unrelated to the prior lesion.*

Antenatal Detection of Myelomeningocele

An open neural tube malformation can be diagnosed in the antenatal period with posi-

---

* See references: tethering of cord, 349, 594; inclusion dermoid cyst, 89, 445; diastematomyelia with septum, 446; lipomatous mass, arachnoid cyst, intramedullary dermoid tumor, 159, 198, 203, 387.

tive accuracy more than 90 per cent of the time by the combination of ultrasonography and amniocentesis to detect elevated alpha-fetoprotein levels at 16 weeks' gestation.[266,575] The fundamental work by Brock and Sutcliffe in 1972 showed that the alpha-fetoprotein level in the amniotic fluid was elevated in fetuses with anencephaly and open myelomeningocele but not in those with skin-covered lesions, which represent 5 to 20 per cent of all neural tube malformations.[11,74,75,514] Elevated alpha-fetoprotein level is not specific for neural tube malformations and may be found in other conditions.[252]

Parents at risk for recurrence of myelomeningocele in subsequent pregnancies are prime candidates for pregnancy monitoring, and therapeutic abortion may be offered when test results are positive. However, over 90 per cent of infants with neural tube malformations are born to families without previously affected children that would not, therefore, be candidates for pregnancy monitoring by amniocentesis. The maternal serum alpha-fetoprotein level, however, is also elevated, and in Great Britain all pregnancies are monitored by serum alpha-fetoprotein assessment, and amniocentesis is performed in women with elevated serum levels. Similar programs may not be cost effective in countries with lower incidence rates, but trial programs are under way in the United States.†

The neurological surgeon is just as responsible as any other physician for informing the parents of a child with a neural tube malformation that future pregnancies may be screened to detect a severe defect before birth. This information should be provided to the parents before the infant is discharged from the hospital to reassure them that they will not have to be at the mercy of mere chance with each succeeding pregnancy.

SPINAL MENINGOCELE

Definition

A spinal meningocele is a herniation of a sac of dura and arachnoid filled with cere-

---

† See references 73, 74, 76, 498, 773, 774.

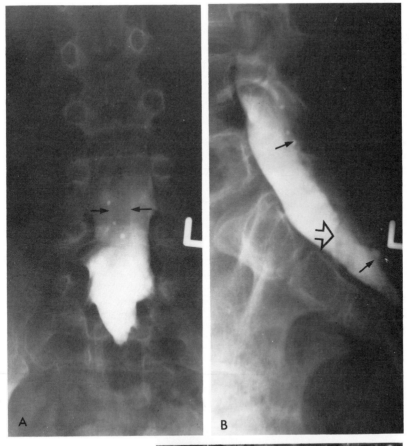

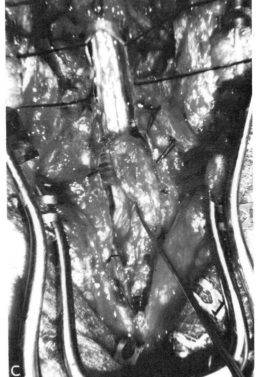

Figure 35–18 A 9-year-old child with a lumbosacral myelomeningocele closed at birth developed progressive spasticity and weakness in both lower limbs. *A.* The posteroanterior view of the metrizamide (Amipaque) myelogram shows the low spinal cord (*arrows*) with exiting nerve roots. *B.* The lateral view shows the spinal cord shadow (*arrows*) tethered posteriorly in the spinal canal and ventrally passing nerve roots (*open arrow*). *C.* Operative view of the spinal cord tethered in the sacrum plus a dorsal lipoma of the conus. Untethering dramatically reversed the spasticity.

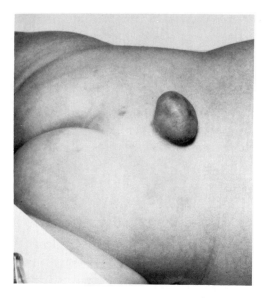

Figure 35–19 A skin-covered cystic mass over the upper sacrum in a 1-month-old infant with no neurological deficit and no hydrocephalus was confirmed to be a meningocele at operation.

bral units suffers delayed development and permits herniation of the meninges through the deficient area. Gardner's hydrodynamic theory suggests that delayed patency of the subarachnoid space produces an increase in the subarachnoid cerebrospinal fluid pressure and an external hydrocephalus.[247] The meninges bulge, produce a posterior spina bifida, and herniate further to produce a meningocele. Padget's theory of neuroschisis proposes that a local neuroschistic bleb damages the epithelial capillaries and healing produces neuroectodermal-epithelial adhesions.[538–540] Interposition of the mesoderm necessary to form laminae is retarded, a posterior spina bifida results, and the meninges herniate to form the sac. The neural cleft that originally produced the bleb heals, and the spinal cord forms normally. Patten's theory of overgrowth of the neural tissue has not been advanced as an explanation of the origin of spinal meningocele.[552,553]

brospinal fluid outside the confines of the spinal canal through a localized posterior spina bifida (Fig. 35–19). The external covering of the sac varies from a shiny translucent membrane derived from modified skin and meninges to a covering of normal skin. Cerebrospinal fluid leakage is uncommon, and the risk of meningitis is low. Hemangiomatous skin and long black hairs frequently surround the base of the sac. The spinal cord and nerve roots are located within the spinal canal rather than herniating into the sac, and the neurological examination is normal. If a neurological deficit is detected or neural elements are seen within the sac on transillumination or at operation, the lesion should be classified as a myelomeningocele.[469]

Abnormal Embryology

The abnormal processes that result in spinal meningocele either do not involve the neuroectoderm or occur after 28 days of development, since the spinal cord develops normally.[537] Forms bridging myelomeningocele and pure spinal meningocele do occur, however. The theory of arrested development would suggest that the mesoderm that forms the laminae of the verte-

Pathology

The incidence of spinal meningocele, as compared with myelomeningocele, varies over the years, partly because of changing referral practices with time and partly perhaps because of inaccurate use of the term. Prior to 1960, meningoceles formed about 25 per cent of all cases of spina bifida aperta treated by neurological surgeons.[645] After 1960, the incidence was around 12 per cent.[48,177,412,691] In the 1970's, the incidence of meningocele is 5 per cent or less, as virtually every living infant with spina bifida aperta is referred for assessment, irrespective of the severity of the defect.[486] Females predominate by approximately 1.2 to 1, as for myelomeningocele.

The distribution of posterior spinal meningocele is listed in Table 35–2. The differing pathogenesis of meningocele and myelomeningocele is suggested by the high frequency of thoracolumbar myelomeningocele (26 per cent) compared with the paucity of meningoceles at that level (4 per cent). On the other hand, the incidence of the two types is comparable in the lumbar and sacral spine (myelomeningocele 66 per cent, spinal meningocele 71 per cent).

Pathological studies of spinal meningocele are rare, reflecting the good prognosis for survival. Overt dysplasia of the spinal cord is rare, as suggested by the absence of neurological deficit. Other dysraphic lesions such as diastematomyelia with septum, or a tethered cord syndrome due to adhesions or a thick filum terminale may accompany the meningocele.[177] The incidence of hydrocephalus is only 5 to 20 per cent, which can be attributed to a similar low frequency of the Arnold-Chiari malformation in spinal meningocele.[495,707]

Clinical Evaluation and Investigation

The protruding sac is usually covered with a translucent membrane of modified meninges and skin. The lesion is soft, but the fluid usually cannot be compressed easily from the sac into the spinal canal owing to the small communication with the subarachnoid space. Transillumination produces a brilliant glow. The neurological examination is normal. The head circumference is usually normal, and the anterior fontanelle is relaxed because active hydrocephalus is rare in the immediate neonatal period.

A totally skin-covered meningocele must be differentiated from a lumbosacral lipoma or lipomyelomeningocele or hamartoma.[749] A midline location favors meningocele, whereas a lipoma is frequently off the midline.[184] A sacral meningocele must be differentiated from a sacrococcygeal teratoma. The lipoma and teratoma are firmer to palpation, and transillumination produces little or no glow in the tissue-filled masses.[421]

Plain roentgenograms of the spine should show a localized posterior spina bifida and normal vertebral bodies. The spinal canal should be widened only at the level of the laminal defect, if at all. Widening of the spinal canal over a longer length or abnormalities of the vertebral bodies may indicate that the meningocele is combined with more complex intraspinal abnormalities such as diastematomyelia or lipoma, or that the provisional diagnosis of meningocele is incorrect. Plain roentgenograms of the skull will not show craniolacunia, and the sutures are not spread, since

hydrocephalus is unusual. Other procedures such as myelography or spinal computed tomography are indicated if the diagnosis of simple meningocele is in question.

Treatment

The meningocele sac should be removed to prevent ulceration and infection and for cosmesis. Operation should be deferred in infants with low birth weight or coexisting illnesses until the infant has matured over several months. In healthy infants, however, modern pediatric anesthesia permits operation in the first week of life prior to discharge from hospital. The parents can then take home a normal child, and anxiety over a future separation and operation is obviated. Only the rare leaking or poorly covered meningocele need be removed within a few hours after birth.

The operation usually is uncomplicated because adequate skin is present for a tension-free closure and hydrocephalus is absent, which reduces the risk of postoperative cerebrospinal fluid leakage. The general preparations are the same as for myelomeningocele. A transverse or vertical incision is begun near but not on any portion of the sac. The paraspinous muscle fascia is located, and then the incision is directed toward the neck of the sac that herniates through the midline defect. The incision deviates on each side of the sac to provide enough skin for closure, and the neck is defined circumferentially at the level of the paraspinous fascia. The sac is usually pedunculated with a small neck rather than sessile with a broad neck. It is opened laterally to inspect the contents. An incision in the dorsal midline or at the neck of the sac endangers neural elements at two sites of potential adherence. The sac may be multiloculated. After insuring that neural elements are absent or after dissecting adherent neural elements free under magnified vision, the surgeon enlarges the neck of the sac to inspect the interior of the spinal canal. Nerve roots or the filum terminale may be adherent to the inside of the neck and should be freed to prevent later tethering. The dura is closed with a running 5-0 vascular nylon suture, a second layer of paraspinous fascia is then turned over the defect, and a two-layer skin closure is performed. No special postoperative care is required unless the meningocele is unusually complicated.

Results and Prognosis

The neurological examination should be normal postoperatively, barring the finding of an unsuspected myelomeningocele with adherent neural elements that have been damaged during dissection. Such a complication should be rare if magnified vision and nerve stimulation are used. The head circumference is followed closely to detect hydrocephalus, which will occur in 10 to 20 per cent of patients. The risk of hydrocephalus is less with lower-level meningoceles.[486] The spine develops normally without scoliosis or kyphosis, assuming the vertebral bodies are normal. The incidence of late deterioration of neurological function is lower than in myelomeningocele, particularly if care is taken to relieve tethering at the original operation. Genetic counseling should be arranged for the parents.

THE ARNOLD-CHIARI MALFORMATION

Historical Background and Definition

The term "Arnold-Chiari malformation" has been reinforced by 70 years of use, although it does ignore the contribution of Cleland in 1883 and exaggerates the contribution of Arnold in 1894.[25,118] Cleland described an elongation of the vermis of the cerebellum lying in a prolongation of the fourth ventricle in a child with hydrocephalus and myeloschisis in 1883.[118] He commented on beaking of the collicular plate, a membrane in the region of the median aperture of the elongated fourth ventricle, and dilation of the central canal of the spinal cord. In 1891 and 1896, Chiari described four types of abnormality found in hydrocephalus associated with spina bifida.[101,114,115,763] In type I, the cerebellar tonsils of the inferior lobe of each cerebellar hemisphere extend into the upper cervical spinal canal with no involvement of the brain stem. In type II, a hypoplastic inferior vermis plus tonsils of the cerebellum, a pocket-shaped elongation of the fourth ventricle and choroid plexus, and the medulla oblongata are displaced into the upper cervical canal. A dorsal protuberance is present at the cervicomedullary junction, the cervical spinal cord is shortened, with the roots close together, and syringohydromyelia may be found in the distal spinal cord. Cleland's 1883 description corresponds to the Chiari type II deformity. The current definitions of types I and II are listed in Table 35–8. In type III, the entire cerebellum is displaced into the cervical canal, with the fourth ventricle emptying into a cervical hydroencephalocele. The criteria for type III have been modified in recent times to include extension of the fourth ventricle into an occipital encephalocele.[167,374] Type IV involves hypoplasia of the cerebellum and is not now considered a form of dysraphism. In 1894, Arnold had described multiple anomalies in a newborn infant with spina bifida, but devoted most of the description to details of the visceral and lung abnormalities. The description and illustration of the cerebellar and hind-

TABLE 35–8   PATHOLOGY OF TYPE I AND TYPE II ARNOLD-CHIARI MALFORMATION*

FEATURE	TYPE I	TYPE II
Age group	Adult	Infant
Caudal displacement of cerebellar tonsils	Yes	Yes
Caudal displacement of inferior vermis and fourth ventricle	No	Yes
Caudal displacement of medulla oblongata	No	Yes
Dorsal kink of cervicomedullary junction	No	Yes
Course of upper cervical nerve roots	Normal	Usually cephalad
Spina bifida aperta	Usually absent	"Always" present
Hydrocephalus	May be present; frequently nonprogressive	"Always" present; frequently progressive
Syringohydromyelia	May develop late	May develop early

* After Carmel, P. W., and Markesbery, W. R.: Early descriptions of the Arnold-Chiari malformation: The contribution of John Cleland. J. Neurosurg., 37:543–547, 1972.

brain deformities were incomplete, but only the cerebellum appears to have been involved and not the medulla, in keeping with Chiari's type I anomaly.[101] In 1907, while studying in Arnold's laboratory in Heidelburg, Schwalbe and Gredig reviewed the cerebellar and hindbrain anomalies associated with spina bifida. They elected to add Arnold's name to the type II anomaly and referred to the cerebellar deformity as Arnold's malformation and the hindbrain deformity as Chiari's malformation. Thus, the term "Arnold-Chiari malformation" was born.[643] While the term has been used to describe all severities of deformity, many authors restrict the full eponym to the type II anomaly and use the term "Chiari type I" for the simpler anomaly of the cerebellar tonsils. Other authors prefer to ignore Arnold totally and refer exclusively to Chiari type I and type II anomalies.

The adult form of the Arnold-Chiari malformation, with or without bony anomalies (basilar impression and invagination, occipitalization of the atlas, Klippel-Feil deformity, scoliosis), is discussed in Chapter 41.[247]

Normal Embryology of the Cerebellum

The ventrally convex pontine flexure of the rhombencephalon is established at the future level of the trigeminal nerve by five weeks of development. The apex and rostral limb of the flexure is the metencephalon, from which the cerebellum and pons develop. The caudal limb of the flexure is the myelencephalon, from which the medulla oblongata develops. The buckling of the neural tube at the flexure spreads apart the lateral walls of the rhombencephalon at its lateral margins, and the roof plate is thinned as a result. The thin rhombic roof merges laterally with thick lateral plates called the rhombic lips. As the pontine flexure buckles further, lateral bulges of the primitive fourth ventricle are squeezed between the rhombic lips to form the future lateral recesses of the fourth ventricle or foramina of Luschka. The roof plate is invaginated by tufts of capillaries on either side to form the paired choroid plexuses of the fourth ventricle by the sixth week. The choroid plexuses divide the roof plate into the areae membranaceae superior and in-

ferior, as already mentioned. Rostral to the lateral recesses and to the area membranacea superior, the walls of the rhombencephalon form dorsal plates called the corpus cerebelli on each side. They enlarge and fuse in the midline to form the future midline cerebellar vermis at approximately eight weeks. The area membranacea superior forms the posterior medullary velum, and the area membranacea inferior forms the future midline foramen of Magendie. In these early stages of development, the cerebellum lies within the fourth ventricle and the choroid plexus is essentially dorsal to the cerebellum. Brocklehurst noted that a meshwork of mesenchymal cells and blood vessels surrounds the dorsal aspect of the rhombencephalon where the roof plate is thin or deficient.[78] The inferior portion of the cerebellar vermis undergoes a process of involution so that the choroid plexus lying within the fourth ventricle is incorporated under the cerebellum, with the foramen of Magendie becoming hidden between the cerebellar tonsils. The primitive cerebellum develops rapidly with formation of the lobules and fissures between one and one half and four months of gestation.

Normal Embryology of the Venous Sinuses

The development of the venous drainage of the brain is a complex process that is of importance to neurosurgeons primarily in the region of the torcular, lateral sinuses, and foramen magnum.[720] Abnormally large venous sinuses are present in the dura at the level of the foramen magnum in the Arnold-Chiari malformation and present a danger at the time of posterior fossa decompression. The position of the posterior venous sinuses is of diagnostic importance in the Dandy-Walker malformation. Venous sinuses may congregate near the neck of an occipital encephalocele and present a danger at the time of operation.

The eventual anatomical location of the posterior dural sinuses appears to be dependent to a great extent on the development of the brain.[720,735] As the cerebral hemispheres enlarge and fold backward in early development, the sagittal and lateral sinuses are displaced posteriorly from their position on the surface of the telencephalon. By the third month of development, the torcular lies just above the superior margin of the squama occipitalis, and the transverse sinuses lie on the parietal bones. With further development of the cerebral hemispheres, the torcular and lateral sinuses migrate further posteriorly to reach their normal position on the occipital bone at the level of the inion and the superior nuchal line. Only after 1 year of age is the inner table of the occipital bone sufficiently molded by the lateral sinuses to form a visible groove on a plain roentgenogram of the skull.

Abnormal Embryology

Five major theories have been proposed to explain the Arnold-Chiari malformation and the frequently associated malformations listed in Table 35–9: the traction theory, the hydrodynamic theory, the overgrowth hypothesis, neuroschisis, and arrested development.

The Traction Theory

This theory is of historical interest and presents a simplistic mechanical explanation for a very complex abnormality. The theory presumes that adherence of the

TABLE 35–9 ANATOMICAL ANOMALIES ASSOCIATED WITH THE ARNOLD-CHIARI MALFORMATION TYPE II

STRUCTURE	ANOMALY
Cerebellum	Caudal displacement of tonsils, vermis and fourth ventricle; cerebellum smaller than normal
Brain stem	Caudal displacement of pons, medulla, and basilar artery; stretching of lower cranial nerves; cervicomedullary kink
Cervical cord	Compression of upper segments; hydromyelia or syringohydromyelia
Lower spinal cord	Hydromyelia or syringohydromyelia
Skull and cervical spine	Craniolacunia; enlarged foramen magnum, small posterior fossa, scalloped petrous bone; enlarged upper cervical canal
Meninges	Hypoplasia of falx cerebri; low-set tentorium cerebelli with large incisura; large venous sinuses in dura of foramen magnum; thickened, adherent, obliterative, compressive leptomeninges at level of foramen magnum
Midbrain	Tectal "beak"; aqueduct stenosis or forking
Cerebral hemispheres and third ventricle	Polymicrogyria; cortical heterotopia; large massa intermedia; Meynert's commissure; hydrocephalus

lower end of the spinal cord at the site of the myelomeningocele prevents upward migration beginning at the ninth week. Traction occurs as the vertebral column elongates, and the cerebellum and hindbrain are "pulled down" into the cervical spinal canal.[430,431,560]

The traction theory is deficient for several reasons. The traction force caused by fixation at the myelomeningocele is dissipated within five segments above the fixation.[36,203,537] The cervicomedullary kink and the short cervical spinal cord segments to the C7 level suggest, rather, that the cervicomedullary area has been "pushed down" from above.[36,97,201–203,270] The dorsal aspect of the pons, medulla, and upper cervical cord is displaced more than the ventral, which would not be the case with traction from below.[201] The cord is characteristically tethered low in the spinal canal in occult spinal dysraphism, but the Arnold-Chiari malformation is not found.[270] Similarly, the malformation may be absent in some cases of lumbosacral or sacral myelomeningocele when the traction forces might be considered to be maximal.[97] Traction is unable to account either for the associated malformations of the Arnold-Chiari malformation or for the occurrence of the type II deformity with a normal spine or for the development of the deformity in embryos before the spinal cord begins to ascend.[185,245,270,556,743] Experimental tethering of the spinal cord in animals fails to produce any changes remotely suggestive of the hindbrain deformity.[270] Thus, the traction theory should never be invoked as an explanation for the Arnold-Chiari malformation.

The Hydrodynamic Theory

This theory suggests that a pressure gradient from above is the primary cause of the displacement of the cerebellum and hindbrain into the cervical spinal canal. Gardner suggests that the interplay between the pulsatile choroid plexuses in the fourth ventricle and the larger plexuses in the lateral ventricles contributes to the normal posterior migration of the tentorium cerebelli and its contained venous sinuses (Bering effect).[247] Overaction of the anterior choroid plexuses will push the tentorium too far inferiorly, diminish the size of the posterior fossa, extrude the cerebellum and hindbrain, kink the cervicomedullary junction, and further aggravate the embryonic hydrocephalus. Progression of the hydrocephalus then creates the associated malformations listed in Table 35–9. Other authors have advanced alternate versions of a hydrodynamic theory.[97,202,761] While many authors discount hydrodynamic explanations as the primary cause of the Arnold-Chiari malformation, it is undeniable that a pressure gradient from hydrocephalus may have important secondary influences such as increasing the degree of caudal displacement, forming some of the associated malformations, and precipitating clinical manifestations.*

The Overgrowth Hypothesis

Patten, Kapsenberg and Van Lookeren Campagne, and Barry and co-workers extended their studies of overgrowth at the site of embryonic myeloschisis to other areas of the nervous system.[36,373,551–553] Overgrowth of the cerebral hemispheres is believed to displace the tentorium inferiorly to create a small posterior fossa. The only recourse for the overgrown cerebellum and medulla oblongata is caudal displacement.

Subsequent authors criticized the method of assessing the volume of the structures in the region of the Arnold-Chiari malformation and have been unable to duplicate the findings of increased volume or have suggested that the small posterior fossa gave the appearance of increased volume of the neural tissue.[77,203] The cerebellum in infants with the Arnold-Chiari malformation weighs uniformly less at all ages than the cerebellum of normal infants, which supports the critics of the overgrowth hypothesis.[763]

Neuroschisis

Padget indicated that one sequela of a neural cleft allowing escape of fluid from the neural tube was a decrease in the size of the primitive brain, producing an embryonic microcephaly.[540] Premature approximation and fusion of the cerebellar primordia occur in the midline in a posterior fossa already small. Subsequent development of the cerebellum in the abnor-

mally small posterior fossa leads to herniation into the upper cervical spinal canal. Hydrocephalus follows folding and fusion at the mesencephalon, producing aqueduct stenosis and forking, or follows failure of formation of the fourth ventricle apertures for similar reasons. Support for the theory of embryonic microcephaly with secondary hydrocephalus is provided by the frequent observation of a normal head circumference in infants with myelomeningocele in association with marked hydrocephalus.[558,559] The head circumference reverts to an abnormally small size following a shunting procedure.

Developmental Arrest

Daniel and Strich, Emery and Levick, and Peach suggested that a primary dysgenesis of the brain stem might impair the formation of the pontine flexure.[153,201,558,559] The resulting elongated brain stem would herniate into the upper cervical spinal canal. This theory explains only one component of the entire Arnold-Chiari complex.

Pathology

Over 90 per cent of infants with myelomeningocele have an Arnold-Chiari malformation, usually type II, and conversely, virtually all type II anomalies occur in infants with myelomeningocele (see Tables 35–8 and 35–9).[518] Only rarely does the type II anomaly present in adulthood unassociated with myelomeningocele, and rarely does an infant with myelomeningocele have a type I anomaly or no anomaly at all.[97,115,544,733] The tendency to adhere to rigid descriptions of a type I and a type II form may be a mistake, since pathological and clinical studies indicate a gradation in the severity of the anomaly.† In addition, the hydrodynamic effects of hydrocephalus may modify many of the features of the Arnold-Chiari malformation, including the degree of caudal displacement of the brain stem and cerebellum, the molding of the collicular plate, the shape and size of the aqueduct, the degree of syringohydromyelia, and the clinical manifestations. De-

---

* See references 4, 118, 194, 202, 245, 460, 465, 764.

† See references 101, 153, 202, 249, 558, 559.

scriptions of the apparently static anomaly should be read with the dynamic contribution of hydrocephalus in mind.

Hydrocephalus

Ventriculomegaly occurs in at least 90 per cent of patients with myelomeningocele. Russell and Donald reintroduced the importance of the Arnold-Chiari malformation in the pathogenesis of the hydrocephalus into the English language literature in 1935.[621] The cerebrospinal fluid obstruction is traditionally believed to occur at the foramen magnum or at the level of an aqueduct stenosis, but in actual fact, the site of obstruction may be quite variable and there may be more than one.[108,480] Obstructive

hydrocephalus will follow a block at the aqueduct or at the fourth ventricular outlets.[432,454,621,679] The cerebral aqueduct is shorter than normal, laterally compressed, and posteriorly kinked owing to compression of the midbrain by the dilated ventricles above.[195] The fourth ventricular foramina may be congenitally occluded with remnants of the rhombencephalic roof or obliterated by fibrovascular connective tissue typically found around the brain stem at the level of the foramen magnum. Communicating hydrocephalus may follow obliteration of the subarachnoid pathways around the displaced brain stem by fibrovascular connective tissue. The fourth ventricle then discharges cerebrospinal fluid directly into the spinal subarachnoid space,

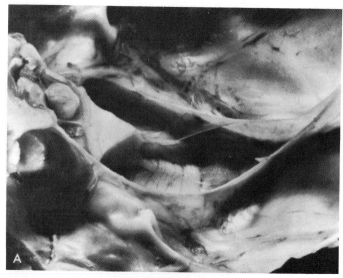

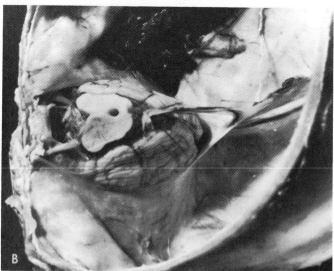

Figure 35–20 The hydrodynamic effects of hydrocephalus at the level of the tentorial incisura. *A.* Without a shunt, the dilated ventricles have herniated over the tentorium, depressing the superior cerebellum and compressing the brain stem into a wedge, obliterating the aqueduct. *B.* A second child who received a shunt prior to death shows upward herniation of the cerebellum through the incisura. The aqueduct is widely patent. (From Emery, J. L.: Pathology of the brain associated with myelomeningocele, including the Cleland-Arnold-Chiari deformity. *In* The American Academy of Orthopaedic Surgeons: Symposium on Myelomeningocele. St. Louis, C. V. Mosby Co. 1972. Reprinted by permission.)

from which it has no escape.[345] The small posterior fossa is filled to capacity by the cerebellum, even to the point of upward herniation of the superior surface of the cerebellum.[97,541] Thus, the basal cisterns may be obliterated as well. Rarely, a congenital cyst lying within the third ventricle may cause hydrocephalus.[111]

The hydrodynamic effect of the hydrocephalus is suggested by the appearance of the superior aspect of the cerebellum at the enlarged incisura. In active hydrocephalus, the ballooned ventricles herniate over the edge of the tentorium, indent the cerebellum, and compress the hindbrain (Fig. 35–20A). After successful shunting, the superior part of the cerebellum tends to herniate upward through the incisura (Fig. 35–20B).[764] Generally, the more severe the hydrocephalus, the smaller the posterior fossa, the greater the aqueduct stenosis, and the more pronounced the caudal displacement of the hindbrain and cerebellum.[465] All these changes appear to be less marked after successful ventricular shunting.[764]

The Hindbrain, Cerebellum, and Spinal Cord

Emery classified patients with the Arnold-Chiari malformation into five groups on the basis of a pathological study of 100 specimens (Fig. 35–21).[202] In group A (4 per cent of cases), the fourth ventricle had not descended below the foramen magnum but the upper part of the cervical cord was slightly displaced caudally. In group B (26 per cent of cases), the fourth ventricle had descended below the foramen magnum with linear compression of the upper cervical cord segments but no dorsal dislocation of the medulla. Groups C, D, and E (70 per cent of cases) showed progressive caudal displacement of the cerebellar vermis, pons, and medulla below the foramen magnum, an increasingly prominent dislocation of the medulla dorsal to the upper cervical cord segments, and a more apparent upward course of the cervical nerve roots. Generally, the more extensive the myelomeningocele, e.g., a thoracolumbar or thoracolumbosacral lesion, the more severe the deformity.[201] The relationship between the degree of deformity and hydrocephalus was not studied. The cranial nerves exiting from the brain stem may be elongated and

stretched as a result of the caudal displacement of the pons and medulla.

The medullary kink occurs just caudal to the level of the cuneate and gracile nuclei (Fig. 35–22).[558,559] The dentate ligaments attach to and fix the upper segments of the cervical spinal cord and thereby influence the development of the medullary kink. The displaced pons and medulla initially compress the upper cervical segments in a linear fashion, and dorsal displacement over the fixed upper cervical segments follows to form a flattened S-shaped deformity. The C3 and C4 cord segments are severely compressed dorsoventrally in groups C, D, and E, with less compression further caudally until the cord assumes a normal shape in the lower cervical region.[455] In more severe deformities, the first and second cervical segments are displaced dorsally with the medulla so that the posterior nerve roots of

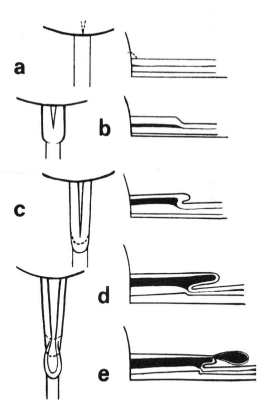

Figure 35–21 Variations occur in the degree of caudal displacement of the fourth ventricle and the cervicomedullary kink in patients with myelomeningocele and the Arnold-Chiari malformation. (From Emery, J. L., and MacKenzie, N.: Medullo-cervical dislocation deformity (Chiari II deformity) related to neurospinal dysraphism (meningomyelocele). Brain, 96:155–162, 1973. Reprinted by permission.)

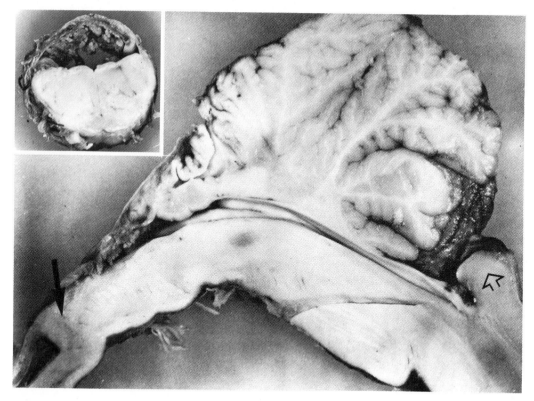

Figure 35–22   Midsagittal section of an Arnold-Chiari malformation showing the tectal beak (*open arrow*), the elongated pons and medulla, and the cervicomedullary kink (*solid arrow*). The inset shows the malformed vermis and fourth ventricle extending caudally with the extraventricular choroid plexus forming the roof of the fourth ventricle. (From McAdams, A. J.: The Arnold-Chiari malformation: Pathology and developmental considerations. *In* McLaurin, R. L., ed.: Myelomeningocele. New York, Grune & Stratton Inc., 1977, pp. 197–207. Reprinted by permission.)

C2 often arise from the ventral aspect of the kink. The neuronal count in the upper cervical cord may be reduced.[423]

The central canal may be narrowed at the C3 and C4 level owing to the compression at the dorsal kink, but is totally obliterated in only 2 per cent of cords. As a result of the compression, hydromyelia usually spares the upper segments, but is progressively more severe in the distal segments. Forty-eight per cent of cords show hydromyelia, and almost half of those have a smooth-lined syrinx in the dorsal spinal cord tissue separate from the central canal. All cavities were found to communicate with the central canal at some point, however, suggesting that Gardner's term "syringohydromyelia" is preferable.[247]

The abnormal leptomeninges at the foramen magnum are important to the pathogenesis of the hydrocephalus and to the foramen magnum compression syndrome in the Arnold-Chiari malformation. Failure of involution of the vermis could lead to persistence of the intraventricular position of the caudal vermis with matted fibrous and vascular tissue surrounding the tongue of cerebellar vermis and lateral brain stem (see Fig. 35–22).[78,153,722,761] The arachnoid and pia are characteristically thickened, opaque, and vascular. The displaced inferior vermis is atrophic and sparsely cellular, and clefts in the tissue may connect with the displaced fourth ventricle. The fourth ventricle lies dorsal to the C3 and C4 segments and may form a cystlike extension if the foramen of Magendie fails to become perforated or is occluded by adhesions.[557] The choroid plexus usually extends distal to the tongue of cerebellar vermis, and both may be intimately adherent to the floor of the fourth ventricle and preclude safe separation of the tissues at operation.[477]

The adhesions of the pia and arachnoid layer may obliterate the subarachnoid space around the brain stem as well as one or more of the three apertures of the fourth ventricle, which are abnormally crowded along with the displaced cerebellum and brain stem into the upper cervical spinal canal.[541,558,559]

The dura in the region of the occipitoatlantal membrane and between C1 and C2 is often adherent to the underlying thickened arachnoid. This dural indentation may continue to compress the neural structures at the foramen magnum and below even after removal of the overlying bone. The dura must be opened to decompress the malformation satisfactorily, but large anomalous venous channels coursing through the dura render the opening hazardous.[323,345,469]

The cerebellum, in the Arnold-Chiari malformation, weighs less than normal throughout postnatal life, and the greater the size of the displaced tongue of cerebellar vermis, the greater the disparity.[763,764] The less-than-normal weight may be due to necrosis of the caudal cerebellar lobules, general growth arrest, ischemic damage, or a combination of these. The cell content of the internal granular layer is reduced in the central lobules, particularly in the nodule, pyramid, and uvula.[196]

Although the length of the basilar artery is normal, the origin may be displaced so far below the level of the foramen magnum that the vertebral arteries must make a downward loop after they enter the dura between the occiput and the arch of C1. Thus, an angiographic diagnostic feature for the Arnold-Chiari malformation could be the visualization of the origin of the basilar artery below the level of the foramen magnum. The cranial loop of the posterior inferior cerebellar artery is displaced below the level of the foramen magnum.[110,201,409]

The Mesencephalic Spur

In 1883 Cleland mentioned the deformity of the superior and inferior colliculi that occurs in approximately 75 per cent of patients with the Arnold-Chiari malformation.[118,558,559] First the inferior and, with more severe deformity, the superior colliculi undergo a progressive fusion and flattening into a ''beak,'' which progresses to fusion of all four colliculi into a conical mass with the apex lying between the cerebellar hemispheres. Mechanical deformation between the hydrocephalic ventricles above and the cerebellum below may contribute to the molding.[4]

Massa Intermedia, Meynert's Commissure, Microgyria, Cortical Heterotopia

The massa intermedia lies within the third ventricle and connects the medial aspects of the thalami. In the Arnold-Chiari malformation, the diameter of the massa increases from a normal of approximately 8 mm to 12 mm, and at times the volume of the third ventricle may be considerably decreased.[271]

A transverse tract called Meynert's commissure connects the globus pallidus on each side with additional fibers going to the subthalamic nucleus. The tract is enlarged in the Arnold-Chiari malformation and may be seen in the anterior wall of the third ventricle between the anterior commissure above and the suprachiasmatic recess below.[271]

Microgyria is present in over 50 per cent of patients and consists of an increase in the number of cerebral gyri but a decrease in the width, particularly in the lateral occipital lobe.[345,558] The cortex in these areas has only four layers compared with the normal six.

Heterotopic gray matter, consisting of neurons separated from the surface cortex by a band of white matter and from the ventricular lumen by a layer of ependyma, may bulge into the walls of the ventricles.[97,558] Similarly, islands of heterotopic cerebellar cortex may lie in the white matter of the displaced inferior vermis.[97]

The Dura

The falx cerebri is abnormal in virtually every patient in that the anterior two thirds often penetrates only a short distance into the longitudinal fissure between the cerebral hemispheres, while the posterior portion may be fenestrated. Where the falx is deficient, the gyri of the medial surfaces of the hemispheres may interdigitate and fuse with one another and partially obliterate the longitudinal fissure.[97,558]

The tentorium cerebelli is displaced abnormally low on the occipital bone and may be less than 2 cm above the margin of the foramen magnum. As a result, the posterior fossa is markedly reduced in size.[153,558] The lateral sinuses and torcular are also close to the foramen magnum, rendering occipital craniectomy hazardous. Characteristically the tentorial incisura is large because the leaves of the tentorium are hypoplastic. The combination of a small posterior fossa and a large incisura permits the cerebellum to herniate rostrally.[97,541]

Anomalies of the Skull and Cervical Spine

Craniolacunia of the vault, which has been discussed, and several abnormalities of the base of the skull permit diagnosis of the Arnold-Chiari malformation on the basis of plain roentgenograms. The foramen magnum is enlarged in all dimensions and is rounder than normal in 71 per cent of patients.[399] A small notch or incisura is occasionally seen in the posterior rim of the foramen, and the lateral margins may be everted in an "inferior cone."[387] Sixty-five per cent of patients have scalloping of the posteromedial aspects of the petrous bones increasing with age owing to forcible wedging of the cerebellum between the tentorium and the petrous bone.[301,399] The occipital bone is normally convex externally, but in 41 per cent of patients with the Arnold-Chiari malformation and an especially small posterior fossa, the inion is low set and the occipital bone is flat.[399] The clivus may be concave and thinned near the basion as a result of pressure from the cerebellum and brain stem being jammed into the foramen magnum.[810] The sagittal diameter of the cervical spinal canal, in contrast to the interpedicular diameter, is significantly increased at the level of C2 and C3 to accommodate the displaced hindbrain and cerebellum.[516,517,519] Platybasia and basilar impression, occipitalization of C1, and abnormal fusion of the bodies of C2 and C3 (Klippel-Feil anomaly) may occur but are not considered to be so intimately related to the Arnold-Chiari malformation as the previously mentioned skeletal changes.

Management of the Arnold-Chiari Malformation

An Arnold-Chiari malformation becomes symptomatic most frequently by producing hydrocephalus and less commonly is a source of respiratory insufficiency, a foramen magnum compression syndrome, or syringohydromyelia.

Hydrocephalus

The predominant approach to control of hydrocephalus prior to the advent of reliable shunting procedures was occipital craniectomy and upper cervical laminectomy with dural opening to decompress the presumed site of obstruction to cerebrospinal fluid circulation.[345,469,711] The results were poor, as would be expected from the variable pathogenesis of the hydrocephalus. Direct operation has no place in the treatment of hydrocephalus associated with the Arnold-Chiari malformation except in rare circumstances. Current methods for the control of hydrocephalus in children are discussed in Chapter 36.

Abductor Vocal Cord Paresis and Episodic Apnea

Bilateral abductor vocal cord paresis and episodic apnea are two forms of respiratory insufficiency related to the interplay of the Arnold-Chiari malformation and hydrocephalus in neonates with myelomeningocele.*

Bilateral abductor vocal cord paresis is more common and is usually related to increased intracranial pressure due to untreated hydrocephalus or shunt obstruction. The vocal cords become paretic in an adducted position, and although the cry may be normal, upper airway obstruction is indicated by inspiratory stridor and hoarseness.[326] Severe stridor and life-threatening obstruction may occur suddenly. Direct laryngoscopy without anesthesia reveals the cords resting in the paramedian or median position with loss of abductor function. The inadequate airway can be corrected only by intubation. The most likely mechanism is stretching of the vagus nerves secondary to uncontrolled hydrocephalus and increased caudal displacement of the brain stem. The sometimes transient and reversible episodes of stridor are supportive evidence. Another mechanism, ischemia of the medulla related to the same factors, receives slight support from the postmortem observation of the caudal displacement of the vertebral-basilar circu-

---

* See references 6, 60, 62, 225, 226, 323, 326, 387, 395, 397, 632, 657.

lation and a report of medullary hemorrhage in two patients with the syndrome.[201,507] Primary dysgenesis of the nucleus ambiguus producing subclinical respiratory insufficiency accentuated by elevated intracranial pressure is not confirmed either by the clinical course or by the demonstration of normal respiratory function in the asymptomatic period.[395,397]

Episodic apnea is less frequent than cord paralysis but is a greater threat to life and more difficult to treat. The period of apnea may cease spontaneously or with application of a noxious stimulus, or may require intubation and assisted ventilation. Such infants require an apnea monitor in the hospital and at home if unexpected deaths are to be avoided.[326] Medullary compression at the foramen magnum aggravated by increased intracranial pressure secondary to uncontrolled hydrocephalus is believed to produce the episodic cessation of respiration.

In either situation, respiratory sufficiency must be guaranteed by intubation, and immediate steps must be taken to control the increased intracranial pressure by ventricular drainage or by placement or revision of a shunt. The sooner the intracranial pressure is restored to normal, the better the prognosis for rapid resolution of the problem.[60,387] Failure of an early return of function in the case of abductor vocal cord paralysis will necessitate a tracheostomy for as long as one or two years before cord function is sufficient to permit removal of the tracheostomy.

In a few patients, cord paralysis or apneic spells will develop in the absence of elevated intracranial pressure or will fail to respond or will recur despite control of elevated intracranial pressure. Such patients may have local compression at the foramen magnum and warrant occipital craniectomy, cervical laminectomy, and dural decompression.[322,323,387] Other lower cranial nerve palsies may develop, such as impairment of the gag reflex resulting in dysphagia and aspiration or facial paralysis or atrophy of the tongue.[323,326,685,766]

Foramen Magnum Compression Syndrome and Syringohydromyelia

Patients over the age of 1 year may present with variations of a foramen magnum compression syndrome, syringohydromyelia, or both.[288,289,323,632] The investigation is directed to detection of uncompensated hydrocephalus and the presence of syringohydromyelia. Positive-contrast or radioisotope ventriculography may confirm a communication between the enlarged ventricles and the dilated central canal, assuming the hydrocephalus is not due to aqueduct stenosis.[288,289,599] Syringohydromyelia and the Arnold-Chiari malformation may be demonstrated by air or positive-contrast myelography, which reveal an expanded or collapsing cord and the displaced hindbrain and cerebellum (Fig. 35–23).

If the ventricles are enlarged in the presence of communicating syringohydromyelia or a foramen magnum syndrome, a functioning shunt may produce improvement. Even if the hydrocephalus is due to an aqueduct stenosis, a shunt may help a fora-

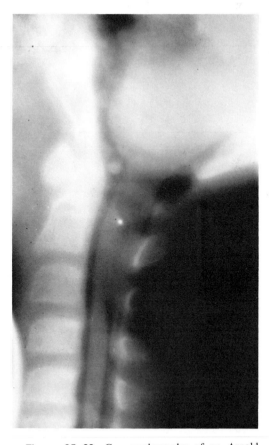

Figure 35–23 Gas myelography of an Arnold-Chiari malformation shows displacement of the caudal tail of the cerebellar vermis and fourth ventricle to the level of C4. (Courtesy of David C. Hemmy, M.D., Medical College of Wisconsin.)

men magnum syndrome by reducing the caudal displacement of the Arnold-Chiari malformation, but it will not be likely to improve a noncommunicating syringohydromyelia. Thus posterior fossa craniectomy, upper cervical laminectomy, and dural opening may be indicated in three circumstances: symptomatic foramen magnum syndrome or syringohydromyelia with normal ventricles; noncommunicating syringohydromyelia; and progressive deterioration after establishment of a functioning shunt in communicating syringohydromyelia or foramen magnum syndrome. The thickened arachnoid over the cerebellar tissue and cervical cord must be opened to show normal cord to insure that the laminectomy extends far enough distally to decompress the malformation completely, since the symptomatic compression may be restricted to the upper part of the cervical cord on occasion.[323]

Few reports of the results of treatment of these rarely identified problems are available.[288,323,632] Hoffman and his associates obtained improvement in 12 of 15 patients treated by decompression; there were two postoperative deaths from meningitis.[323] In the series reported by Hall and co-workers, two of five patients treated by a shunt improved, whereas two patients were unchanged and one died during the investigative stage.[288]

The delayed development of a spastic paraparesis, flaccid paraparesis, or flaccid monoparesis in a lower limb should also suggest the possibility of a tethered cord at the site of the myelomeningocele as well as a foramen magnum syndrome or syringohydromyelia.[288]

THE DANDY-WALKER MALFORMATION

Definition

The Dandy-Walker malformation is a developmental abnormality of the rostral portion of the embryonic roof of the fourth ventricle associated with a varying degree of hypoplasia of the cerebellar vermis and the medial aspects of the cerebellar hemispheres. The fourth ventricle forms a large cyst, and the exit foramina may or may not be atretic. The cystic expansion enlarges the posterior fossa and is associated with elevation of the tentorium cerebelli and lateral sinuses onto the parietal bones. Hydrocephalus and other neuroanatomical and systemic abnormalities occur frequently. A degree of overlap occurs with the posterior fossa extra-axial arachnoid cyst associated with a normal-sized but compressed fourth ventricle and hydrocephalus.

Abnormal Embryology

Four main theories have been proposed to explain the disturbed formation of the rhombic roof and corpus cerebelli: congenital atresia of the foramina of Magendie and Luschka, dysraphism of the corpus cerebelli, neuroschisis, and the hydrodynamic theory.

Congenital Atresia of the Foramina of Magendie and Luschka

In 1914, Dandy and Blackfan reported a case of hydrocephalus presumed due to inflammatory obstruction of the foramina of Magendie and Luschka. A greatly dilated fourth ventricle separated the lateral lobes of the cerebellum.[151] In 1917, they reported a similar case with congenital closure of the foramina and postulated that an intrauterine inflammatory process had caused a condition similar to the case reported in 1914.[152] In 1921, Dandy reviewed congenital occlusion of the foramina of Magendie and Luschka as a specific cause of hydrocephalus and concluded that ". . . this type of hydrocephalus results from the failure of these foramina to develop, rather than a secondary closure after development."[149]

In 1942, Taggart and Walker also stated that congenital atresia of the foramina of Magendie and Luschka was the primary factor producing the dilated fourth ventricle with secondary maldevelopment of the cerebellar vermis and hydrocephalus.[735] They proposed several theories that might explain the presence or absence of hydrocephalus. The abnormally small choroid plexuses might produce less fourth ventricular fluid; the cyst wall might act as a semipermeable membrane permitting passage of ventricular fluid into the subarachnoid space; the cyst wall contains vessels and might absorb some of the cerebrospinal fluid. Thus, hydrocephalus might not be present at all or might become compensated unless some later factor upset the delicate balance of cerebrospinal fluid circulation.

In 1955, however, Gibson found the foramina of Luschka open in some cases and postulated that a partial communicating hydrocephalus might be present.[257] This fact would explain the failure of attempts to reestablish normal cerebrospinal fluid circulation by creating a communication between the fourth ventricle and subarachnoid spaces by excising a portion of the cyst membrane. He also found remnants of the vermis in the cyst wall and postulated that the vermis was compressed and distorted rather than absent. Thus, midline fusion of the corpus cerebelli might have occurred normally at eight weeks of development with later secondary compression by the expanded fourth ventricle.

Dysraphism of the Corpus Cerebelli

In 1954, Benda applied the eponym "Dandy-Walker syndrome," thus ignoring the contribution of Blackfan and Taggart.[50,51] He believed atresia of the foramina was not the essential feature, although it might well be present, and considered the malformation to be a failure of fusion of the corpus cerebelli comparable to myeloschisis. He did not address the problem of the lack of cranium bifidum in the vast majority of cases.

Neuroschisis

A neuroschistic cleft and bleb formation involving the roof of the fourth ventricle in the region of the corpus cerebelli without rupture of the cutaneous ectoderm might produce adhesions with the inner dural layer and inhibit complete development of the vermis.[540,541] Thus, failure of perforation of the caudal membranous roof at the site of the foramen of Magendie is not the cause, but is only a part, of the Dandy-Walker malformation.

The Hydrodynamic Theory

Two somewhat similar theories postulate that an abnormal distention of the fourth ventricle leads to maldevelopment of the cerebellar vermis. In 1959, Brodal and Hauglie-Hanssen reported a strain of hydrocephalic mice with changes similar to the Dandy-Walker malformation.[82] Prior to the expected time of perforation of the foramina, some undetermined process increased the intraventricular pressure and caused the area membranacea superior to bulge, which impaired development of the vermis and displaced the primitive choroid plexus caudally.

Gardner, on the other hand, considers that delayed permeability of the area membranacea superior leads to an increase in the physiological embryonic encephalohydromyelia and causes the area membranacea superior to bulge and form an incipient Dandy-Walker malformation.[247,248] The bulging coincides with the development of the posterior choroid plexus, but occurs before the appearance of the anterior choroid plexus. The interplay between the distending forces created by the posterior and anterior primitive choroid plexuses determines the size of the posterior fossa and the final position of the tentorium and venous sinuses. If the earlier developing posterior choroid plexus produces excessive distending forces, then a dilated fourth ventricle, a large posterior fossa, and a high location of the tentorium result. The opposite situation results in the Arnold-Chiari malformation.

Gardner also described a variant of the Dandy-Walker malformation that he calls the Dandy-Walker cyst. He suggests that the ependymal layer of the rhombic roof is more permeable to ventricular fluid than the outer layer of the glia and pia, with the result that ventricular fluid pumped through the ependymal layer may accumulate to form a true cyst or so-called "arachnoid cyst" between the two layers. This loculated cyst between the layers of the rhombic roof distends the fourth ventricle and may bulge between the spread cerebellar hemispheres into the enlarged aqueduct. Gardner believes that noncommunication between the lateral ventricles and an "enlarged fourth ventricle" containing high-protein fluid in a suspected Dandy-Walker malformation is, in reality, a Dandy-Walker cyst.[584,735]

Several authors have attempted to relate the Arnold-Chiari and Dandy-Walker malformations by a similar mechanism of formation or by similar morphological features.* Gardner, O'Rahilly, and Prolo

---

* See references 51, 165, 247, 248, 250, 540, 541, 695.

concluded that the malformations are different and separate disorders, since the only major pathological feature in common is hydrocephalus, which is a frequent result of any teratogenic insult to the central nervous system.[245] Not even hydrocephalus can be used as a unifying concept, as both the Arnold-Chiari and Dandy-Walker malformations may occur without hydrocephalus.[147,558]

Pathology

The Posterior Fossa Cyst

The Roof

The thin, translucent membrane attaches to the calamus scriptorius inferiorly, to the medial edge of the cerebellar hemispheres laterally, and to the remnants of the vermis superiorly.[735] The cyst wall is separate from the dura of the posterior fossa. The outer layer of the wall is arachnoid overlying occasional small blood vessels, and the inner lining is ependyma. A layer of tissue derived from the cerebellum lies between. In the thinnest areas of the wall, only a few myelinated nerve fibers or glial remnants are present, but as the membrane blends with the cerebellum superiorly and laterally, the middle layer may consist of recognizable compressed and distorted lobules of the inferior vermis.[257] The cyst may bulge through the foramen magnum into the subarachnoid space of the upper cervical spinal canal or may protrude through the incisura posterior to the quadrigeminal plate.[469]

The Foramina of Luschka and Magendie

Although Dandy and Taggart and Walker believed all three foramina must be imperforate, other authors have found the lateral foramina patent at postmortem examination or have demonstrated a communication between the posterior fossa cyst and the subarachnoid space to lumbar air injection or to radioactive tracer or at pathological examination.* Forty-three per cent of the cases reported in the literature had some degree of patency of the cyst wall.

---

* See references 82, 102, 147, 149, 151, 152, 245, 290, 297, 339, 624, 719, 735.

Thus, atresia of the foramina of Magendie and Luschka, once considered the hallmark of the Dandy-Walker malformation, is absent so frequently that no direct correlation exists between atresia, the cyst, and the hydrocephalus.

The Choroid Plexus of the Fourth Ventricle

The choroid plexus is usually hypoplastic and may be displaced caudally near the brain stem or in the dilated lateral recesses or even higher on the ependymal surface of the widely separated cerebellar hemispheres.[147,466,735,777]

The Cerebellum

The degree of involvement of the inferior vermis varies greatly, and although a cursory examination may suggest that the inferior portion or all of the vermis is replaced by the cyst wall, microscopy may show many of the divisions to be present though hypoplastic.[50,82,149,257,624] The remaining superior vermis is often displaced superiorly by the cyst and may herniate through the incisura into the quadrigeminal cistern and cause secondary compression of the aqueduct.[82,584] The cerebellar hemispheres are usually displaced laterally and dorsally and show the effects of hypoplasia and secondary atrophy due to chronic pressure from the cyst. The dentate, emboliform, globose, and fastigial nuclei are variably involved, depending on the size of the cyst and the degree of vermal hypoplasia.[50,82,257,735] More often, the dentate nucleus is preserved and the medial nuclei are deformed or absent.

The Brain Stem

The pons and medulla may be flattened in the anteroposterior diameter.[82] Histologically, the medial accessory olivary nucleus is more often depleted of cells than any other nucleus, and the tracts traversing the brain stem are spared except with severe associated cerebral malformation.[50,82,297,735] The cuneate and gracile nuclei, which lie just caudal to the attachment of the cyst wall, may be displaced downward, and the obex is usually closed.[257] The ninth and tenth nerves may be stretched by distention of unperforated lateral recesses.[584]

Hydrocephalus

Enlargement of the lateral and third ventricles is present, but for rare exceptions.[102,245,297] The mechanism may involve one or a combination of aqueduct stenosis, fourth ventricular outlet occlusion, and incompetence of subarachnoid pathways.

The aqueduct was patent in 87 per cent of the reported cases determined by postmortem examination, intraoperative visualization, or investigative procedures. The aqueduct may be incorporated into the cyst when the superior vermis is severely hypoplastic.[802] The aqueduct may be anatomically occluded on the basis of stenosis or forking, or functionally occluded by compression from the herniated superior vermis or from extension of the cyst into the incisura.[102,147,245,584] In the latter case the aqueduct may appear occluded on air ventriculography but patent to positive-contrast or radioisotope ventriculography or at postmortem examination.[133,290,584] Functional occlusion may have been responsible for several sudden deaths following ventriculography.[82,339,584] Lack of communication between the lateral ventricles and the cystic fourth ventricle may be suggested by a normal protein level in ventricular cerebrospinal fluid and an elevated level in the cyst fluid.[410,584] Such a finding should, however, raise the possibility of an isolated, noncommunicating, extra-axial posterior fossa arachnoid cyst rather than a Dandy-Walker malformation.

Since 43 per cent of patients had a communication of some sort between the posterior fossa cyst and the subarachnoid space, an element of communicating hydrocephalus due to incompetence of the subarachnoid pathways or absorptive capacity may also exist as in other forms of congenital hydrocephalus.[149,257,339,469,495] Thus, competent pathways and an adequate absorptive capacity must be demonstrated prior to planning a direct attack on the cyst for the purpose of creating communication between it and the subarachnoid pathways.[149,339,495]

Hart and co-workers observed that there is ". . . no correlation between the degree of hydrocephalus and the size of the posterior fossa cyst, the extent of vermal attenuation, or the patency or non-patency of the foramina."[297] The interaction of several factors may account for the observation.

Delayed opening of the foramina in development may have contributed to a marked degree of cyst formation and severe hydrocephalus, and the fact that the foramina became patent later cannot be correlated with clinical or pathological findings after birth. The wall of an imperforate cyst may have been permeable to cerebrospinal fluid, or an apparently patent foramen may have been occluded by surrounding structures in life. The hypoplastic choroid plexuses may produce less ventricular fluid than normal, or vessels in the wall of the cyst may absorb a small amount of fluid.[735] In addition, the etiology of the hydrocephalus as determined at postmortem examination may not reflect the situation in life.

The Dura and Venous Sinuses

Formation of a large cyst early in embryological development results in a large posterior fossa and retarded descent of the tentorium cerebelli and venous sinuses. The finding is not pathognomonic of Dandy-Walker malformation, as any congenital space-occupying lesion in the posterior fossa will have similar features. The dural structures are otherwise normal, in contrast to the Arnold-Chiari malformation.

Associated Anomalies

Other anomalies in the central nervous system or elsewhere occurred in 39 per cent of patients in a predominantly clinical series and in 68 per cent of patients in a detailed pathological series.[102,297]

Central Nervous System

Agenesis of the corpus callosum occurs in approximately 30 per cent of patients, but the intellectual development may still be normal.* Nonspecific abnormalities of the gyri in the cerebral hemispheres, microcephaly, heterotopic glial tissue in the subarachnoid space around the brain stem, porencephaly, heterotopic cerebellar cortex in the cerebellum, agenesis of the anterior commissure and cingulate gyrus, and occipital encephalocele have been reported.† The Dandy-Walker malformation

---

* See references 133, 147, 245, 297, 301, 369, 584, 760, 793.
† See references 102, 147, 222, 297, 369, 482, 584, 640.

has been reported with syringohydromyelia on rare occasions, but examination of the spinal cord has been neglected over the years.[51,297,772]

Systemic Anomalies

Renal cysts and ureteral stenosis with hydronephrosis, congenital cardiac defects, cleft palate, Klippel-Feil syndrome, Cornelia de Lange syndrome, polydactyly-syndactyly, and occasionally, a syndrome of polydactyly with macrostomia, macroglossia, and micro-ophthalmia have been reported.[102,147,297,339,719] Craniolacunia, atlanto-occipital fusion, platybasia, and myelomeningocele are not generally associated with the Dandy-Walker malformation.

Clinical Evaluation

The Dandy-Walker malformation accounts for less than 4 per cent of all cases of hydrocephalus in several large series, and as of 1978, reports of only 159 cases can be found in the English language literature.[*] The age distribution is as follows: birth to 1 year (62 per cent), 1 to 5 years (17 per cent), 6 to 10 years (5 per cent), 11 to 20 years (11 per cent), and over 21 years (5 per cent). Females show a slight preponderance.[83]

The clinical manifestations of the Dandy-Walker malformation depend upon the effects produced by the cyst, the accompanying hydrocephalus, and any associated abnormalities. Increased intracranial pressure is the predominant presenting symptom under 2 years of age and is accompanied by vomiting, full fontanelle, split sutures, and paresis of the abducens nerve. After 2 years of age, headache and papilledema may occur, and other deficits become apparent as the child reaches or fails to reach certain milestones in development. Of patients 2 years of age or older, 60 per cent manifested ataxia, predominantly of gait, and 40 per cent had mental retardation.[†] Cranial nerve palsies, brain stem signs, and cerebellar deficits other than ataxia are infrequently reported except for abducens palsy as a nonlocalizing sequela of hydrocephalus, nystagmus, and occasionally upper extremity incoordination.[‡] Overt signs of brain stem compression may occur during investigative procedures or after ineffective treatment or as complications of treatment.[§] Motor signs such as hemiparesis or spastic paraparesis are usually associated with other congenital defects of the brain related to the hydrocephalus.[102,777] Seizures may occur as in any other nervous system malformation.[82,151,257,339,624] A common feature that spans all age groups is macrocephaly that is usually associated with hydrocephalus but can be due to the enlarged posterior fossa alone.[102]

The physical examination is helpful in making the diagnosis. The occipital region is prominent, and the head is frequently dolicocephalic, but in the majority of patients there is only nonspecific macrocephaly.[50,102,369,409,466] In an infant with active hydrocephalus, the lambdoid sutures may be split more than in other forms of hydrocephalus, even to the extent that the occipital bone feels as if it were floating.[584]

Transillumination of the occipital region of the skull in infants under 1 year of age may allow a presumptive differentiation between the Dandy-Walker malformation and an extra-axial arachnoid cyst of the posterior fossa.[290,339,369,469,802] The Dandy-Walker malformation has a triangular appearance with the sides corresponding to the lateral attachments of the elevated tentorium, the apex marking the elevated torcular, and the base delineating the inferior border of the posterior fossa. Absence of the vertical midline shadow of the sagittal sinus over the superior occipital bone indicates that the transilluminated space is entirely within an enlarged posterior fossa. An arachnoid cyst shows an oval transillumination pattern with rounded or lobulated lateral borders rather than straight borders.[290]

If a shunt for hydrocephalus is placed in a patient with an unrecognized Dandy-Walker malformation and the cyst and ventricles do not communicate, then signs of a posterior fossa mass such as nystagmus,

---

* See references 82, 102, 121, 126, 133, 147, 151, 160, 222, 245, 257, 290, 297, 334, 339, 368, 369, 396, 410, 458, 469, 584, 624, 633, 680, 719, 735, 756, 758, 777, 802.

† See references 82, 121, 126, 133, 147, 245, 257, 624, 735, 777, 802.

‡ See references 22, 126, 147, 151, 245, 369, 410, 584, 624, 719, 735, 802.

§ See references 82, 121, 339, 396, 458, 584.

lower cranial nerve palsies, slurred speech, truncal ataxia, and dysmetria of the upper limbs may develop. In infants, the anterior fontanelle may be soft and the coronal sutures approximated following insertion of the shunt, but the lambdoid sutures may remain split and the occipital bone "floating," suggesting a persistent high-pressure mass in the posterior fossa.[584]

Investigation

Many of the investigative procedures will help to differentiate a Dandy-Walker malformation from a posterior fossa extra-axial cyst, which usually requires different treatment (Table 35–10). Plain skull roentgenograms may show a disproportionate amount of splitting of the lambdoid sutures and prominence of the posterior fontanelle, an increased distance between the occiput and the ears, and thinning of the occipital and posterior parietal bones up to the level of the attachment of the elevated tentorium.[50,233,301,466] The groove of the transverse sinuses is usually not visible before the age of 1 year and is seen in only 50 per cent of children 1 to 2 years old. After 2 years of age, the groove is usually detectable on the occipital bone, almost parallel to the hard palate. In the Dandy-Walker

malformation, the groove may be elevated to the level of the lambdoid suture or onto the posterior parietal bone, and extends vertically downward from the elevated inion.[301,466,735] A posterior fossa cyst may be present despite a normally situated torcular and lateral sinuses, which suggests that the cyst was less significant during early development.[126,257]

Several radiological lines have been described to determine whether the posterior fossa is abnormally large. The Bucy line is drawn from the orbital floor to the external auditory meatus. The lateral sinus groove usually lies above this line in the Dandy-Walker malformation. Juhl and Wesenberg described the lambdoinnominate line drawn on a lateral skull roentgenogram from the lambda (midpoint of the posterior fontanelle) to the innominate synchondrosis, a radiolucent line in the occipital bone 1 to 2 cm posterior to the foramen magnum.[369] The skull posterior and inferior to the line is the squamous portion of the occipital bone and shows a marked increase in size in the infantile form of the Dandy-Walker malformation. If the posterior fossa is quite large, the inferior portion of the occipital bone is flattened and displaced inferiorly. Wolpert and co-workers described a ratio of the circumferential distance of the skull from the nasion to the inion (NI) and from the inion

TABLE 35–10   DIFFERENTIAL DIAGNOSIS OF DANDY-WALKER MALFORMATION AND POSTERIOR FOSSA EXTRA-AXIAL ARACHNOID CYST

FEATURE	DANDY-WALKER MALFORMATION	POSTERIOR FOSSA EXTRA-AXIAL ARACHNOID CYST
Relation to fourth ventricle	Cyst is the fourth ventricle	Posterior to normal or compressed fourth ventricle
Malformation of inferior vermis	Yes	Rarely
Patency of foramina of Magendie and Luschka	Occasional	Usually patent
Associated agenesis of corpus callosum	30 per cent	Normal
Cranial computed tomography	Vallecula absent	Normal vallecula
Lumbar pneumoencephalography	Occasionally fills cyst	Usually fills cyst, may fill displaced fourth ventricle
Ventriculography (air or positive-contrast)	Usually fills cyst except for functional aqueduct occlusion	Usually fills displaced fourth ventricle except for functional aqueduct occlusion, may fill cyst
Ventriculography (radioisotope)	Fills cyst but not subarachnoid space	Fills subarachnoid space and usually cyst
Cisternography (radionuclide)	Rarely fills	Usually fills
Cerebral angiography (posterior circulation)	Posterior inferior cerebellar artery absent or hypoplastic, displaced downward	Posterior inferior cerebellar artery normal, displaced anterosuperiorly
	Vermian branch of posterior inferior cerebellar artery absent	Vermian branch of posterior inferior cerebellar artery displaced anterosuperiorly
	Inferior vermian veins absent or widely separated	Inferior vermian veins displaced anterosuperiorly

to the posterior lip of the foramen magnum (IM).[802] The normal value of the ratio, NI/IM, is 6. If the torcular is elevated, the inion is also elevated and the ratio is decreased.

Radioisotope Studies

A nuclear brain scan can demonstrate the elevated position of the lateral sinuses and the torcular.[133,339] Conway and associates defined the torcular angle seen on the posterior view of the radioisotope scan.[133] The routine posterior view may not show the elevated transverse sinuses, and the elevated torcular is seen as a single "blob" of increased uptake that has been termed the "cyclops" sign in a Dandy-Walker malformation. If this picture is seen, the head should be repositioned to place the torcular in the center of the posterior field so that lateral sinuses can be visualized and the torcular angle can be measured. Normal sagittal and lateral sinuses form an inverted T configuration on the posterior view, whereas an inverted Y configuration is seen in the Dandy-Walker malformation. The mean torcular angle in normal subjects is 162 degrees (range 135 to 182 degrees). In Dandy-Walker malformation, the mean torcular angle is 110 degrees (range 88 to 117 degrees). Elevation of the transverse sinuses may be seen on the lateral view, but the finding is less reliable.

Radioisotope ventriculography or lumbar cisternography may show communication of the ventricles with the cyst or communication of the cyst with the subarachnoid spaces even though a prior procedure with air or positive contrast suggested obstruction of the pathways.[133] If both the cyst and the subarachnoid spaces contain isotope after its injection from above or from below, a posterior fossa extra-axial arachnoid cyst may more likely be the diagnosis than a Dandy-Walker malformation. However, the fact that 43 per cent of Dandy-Walker malformations may communicate with the subarachnoid space suggests that this conclusion may be an overgeneralization.[102,290,719] Radioisotope cisternography should be performed prior to a direct fourth ventriculostomy. If there is no filling of the basal cisterns or the absorption of isotope into the sagittal sinus is deficient, then a direct operation is very likely to fail to control the hydrocephalus.

Computed Tomography

Cranial computed tomography greatly simplifies the diagnosis of hydrocephalus and a posterior fossa cyst (Fig. 35–24). Absence of the vallecula suggests a Dandy-Walker malformation, whereas a normal vallecula and a compressed fourth ventricle suggests an arachnoid cyst. The compressed hypoplastic cerebellar hemispheres

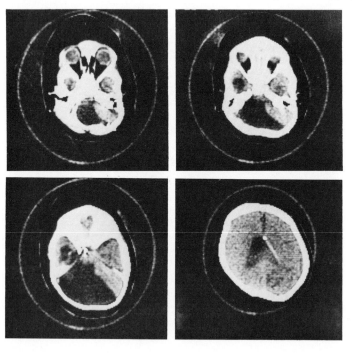

Figure 35–24 Cranial computed tomography of a Dandy-Walker malformation treated by a ventriculoperitoneal shunt, Marked asymmetrical hypoplasia of both cerebellar hemispheres and the absence of the vallecula are demonstrated on the posterior fossa cuts.

lie against the petrous bones.[102] Computed tomography does not, however, adequately display communication of the cyst with the ventricles or with the subarachnoid space. The combination of cranial computed tomography with meglumine iothalamate (Conray) ventriculography or lumbar instillation of metrizamide (Amipaque) may provide additional information, but the traditional studies still have considerable merit.

Air Studies

Ventriculography when Dandy-Walker malformation is suspected should always be performed frontally, as the elevated tentorium may be a hazard with a parietal approach. The ventriculogram usually shows enlarged lateral and third ventricles and a large cyst in the posterior fossa if the aqueduct is patent (Fig. 35–25). Characteristically,· the air is visualized immediately under the elevated tentorium in a triangular pattern similar to that described for transillumination.[82,83,802] The occipital horns are elevated in keeping with the elevated tentorium.[369,466,719] A misdiagnosis of aqueduct stenosis may be made if there is an anatomical or functional occlusion of the aqueduct unless the elevation of the occipital horns is appreciated.* The contrast agent in the cyst lies directly adjacent to the occipital bone and occasionally extends through the foramen magnum into the upper cervical canal

---

* See references 102, 121, 126, 147, 466, 584, 735.

or through the incisura posterior to the quadrigeminal plate.[369,466] Associated abnormalities such as agenesis of the corpus callosum may be present.

Lumbar pneumoencephalography is not a preferred procedure because many of the patients have increased intracranial pressure, the Dandy-Walker malformation frequently does not communicate with the subarachnoid space, and the cisterna magna is usually small or obliterated. Lumbar air studies may, however, confirm the presence of an extra-axial arachnoid cyst by filling both the cyst and a compressed and displaced fourth ventricle.

Angiography

Cerebral angiography of the anterior circulation in cysts of the posterior fossa may show the nonspecific signs of hydrocephalus and elevation of the posterior branches of the middle cerebral and posterior cerebral arteries associated with the elevated tentorium.[369,410,584,802] In the anteroposterior view, the posterior cerebral arteries may be abnormally separated and the medial occipital branches may fail to approach the midline posteriorly because of the upward herniation of the superior vermis or the superior extension of the cyst.[584] In the venous phase, the torcular and lateral sinuses are elevated, the lateral sinuses make a steep descent to the sigmoid sinuses, and the torcular and transverse sinuses form an inverted Y rather than an inverted T.[369] The

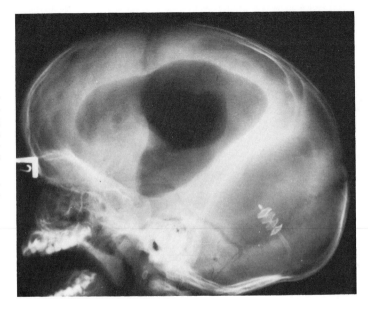

Figure 35–25 Air ventriculography in a Dandy-Walker malformation treated by a cystoperitoneal shunt. Elevation of the tentorium onto the parietal bones is associated with elevation of the occipital horns of the lateral ventricles. (Courtesy of Cully A. Cobb III, M.D., University of California, Davis.)

superficial cerebral draining veins normally angle anteriorly as they enter into the superior sagittal sinus, but the restricted posterior migration of the hemispheres causes the veins to drain in a retrograde or right-angle relationship to the sinus.[802] The thalamus is displaced in a superior and anterior direction as indicated by the internal cerebral, the thalamostriate, and the basilar veins of Rosenthal. As a result, the vein of Galen is elongated and the straight sinus is elevated along with the tentorium.[133,254,584,802] Anterior circulation angiography does not differentiate the Dandy-Walker malformation from an extra-axial arachnoid cyst.

Posterior circulation angiography shows a considerable variation in arterial development, depending upon the severity of the Dandy-Walker malformation, but may differentiate it from an arachnoid cyst (see Table 35–10).[802] The basilar artery may be displaced anteriorly and superiorly, producing a secondary redundancy of the posterior communicating artery; the superior cerebellar arteries may be displaced antero-superiorly and appear redundant if the herniated superior vermis is hypoplastic; and a large avascular area is demonstrated in the posterior fossa.[369,410,584] These findings are not specific for the Dandy-Walker malformation, but may occur with any posterior fossa mass.[410] Usually, the anterior inferior cerebellar artery is normal in origin and distribution. The posterior inferior cerebellar artery (PICA) is more important in the differentiation of the two types of cyst.

In the normal lateral view, the choroidal arc indicates the roof of the fourth ventricle and the midline vermian branch designates the posterior vermis.[410] In a Dandy-Walker malformation, the posterior inferior cerebellar artery may be displaced downward and the choroidal arc backward, indicating an enlarged fourth ventricle, and the vermian branch may be absent, indicating absence of the posterior vermis. In a severe Dandy-Walker malformation, the posterior inferior cerebellar artery may be totally absent or shortened.[254,802] Although some authors have reported forward and upward displacement of a normal artery, La Torre and co-workers consider this finding to be typical of an arachnoid cyst displacing normal cerebellar hemispheres and fourth ventricle anteriorly and superiorly.[410,802] The capillary blush may show small cerebellar hemispheres displaced anterosuperiorly, but this is not pathognomonic of a Dandy-Walker malformation.

The venous phase will display the inferior vermian vein in 85 per cent of normal pediatric angiograms.[410] These veins may be absent or widely separated and draining directly into the vein of Galen in a Dandy-Walker malformation, but are displaced anterosuperiorly by an arachnoid cyst.[102,410]

Treatment

Direct Fourth Ventriculostomy

Dandy introduced direct posterior fossa exploration and excision of the cyst membrane to create communication between the cyst and the subarachnoid space.[149] He recognized that normal patency of the subarachnoid spaces and normal absorption of cerebrospinal fluid were critical to the success of the procedure. Although the procedure was occasionally curative, the great frequency with which unresolved hydrocephalus necessitated postoperative ventricular shunting became apparent.* Fifty-five fourth ventriculostomies reported in the literature have been associated with a mortality rate of 11 per cent and a failure to control hydrocephalus in 64 per cent for a total failure rate of 75 per cent.† Perhaps the only indication for fourth ventriculostomy is mild hydrocephalus in the older child or adult, which suggests that the cerebrospinal fluid dynamics have been in reasonable balance over the years. If isotope cisternography demonstrates patency of the pathways and adequate absorption of cerebrospinal fluid, then a standard suboccipital craniectomy with removal of the posterior arch of C1 to expose the entire cyst may be indicated.[222,758] The dura is opened widely and the cyst wall is generously removed. Hemostasis must be meticulous. Postoperative lumbar punctures or ventricular drainage reduces the chance of cerebrospinal fluid leakage through the incision. A shunting procedure should fol-

---

* See references: curative, 121, 634, 777; shunt required, 102, 222, 466, 469, 584.
† See references 102, 126, 147, 222, 245, 339, 369, 458, 469, 624, 735, 777.

low without delay in the event that the hydrocephalus is not controlled.

Direct operation is advisable for a defined posterior fossa extra-axial arachnoid cyst or when the nature of the lesion is in doubt. Prior to sophisticated neuroradiological techniques, posterior fossa exploration was often required to determine the exact nature of the disorder, but such a situation should be unusual at the present time.

Shunting Procedures

Ventricular shunting was originally the second step following a failed fourth ventriculostomy but has become the preferred primary treatment.* The question of the patency of the aqueduct must be answered by ventriculography prior to placement of a shunt. If the lateral, the third, and the dilated fourth ventricles communicate, then a single ventriculoperitoneal shunt is placed. If the cyst does not communicate because of an anatomical or functional block of the aqueduct, then a lateral ventricular shunt alone may be inadequate and hazardous. Potentially fatal brain stem compression or symptoms suggestive of shunt malfunction may be caused by the entrapped posterior fossa cyst.[339,584] Not all authors have experienced this complication, nor do they agree that ventricular shunting alone will lead to disaster, even in the presence of aqueductal occlusion.[102,222] However, if ventriculography shows an occluded aqueduct, a double shunt from the lateral ventricles and the cyst connected to a single peritoneal catheter is the safer alternative. Raimondi and his associates suggested that

---

* See references 102, 222, 245, 339, 369, 410, 469, 584, 758.

a double shunt be inserted at the first operation in all patients with the Dandy-Walker malformation to avoid complications from an entrapped posterior fossa cyst.[584] Other authors have inserted double shunts, but usually in two stages.[102,758] The child with two shunts may be at additional risk if one shunt fails, since a high-pressure and a low-pressure compartment are created, one on either side of the incisura, which may aggravate upward or downward herniation of neural structures.

If the ventricles are of normal size or only slightly enlarged and if the aqueduct is patent, then a single cystoperitoneal shunt is placed.[102] Experience with cystoperitoneal shunting is limited, but it may be the simplest procedure to perform for any Dandy-Walker malformation with a patent aqueduct.[102,222,584]

Results and Prognosis

The overall results from various modalities of treatment in three series consisting of 51 patients are listed in Table 35–11.[102,222,584] The series were collected since 1947, and half of the cases have been diagnosed and treated since 1962. Adults and older children have a better prognosis, as the malformation has been more stable for longer and has fewer associated malformations than is the case with the infantile form. Control of hydrocephalus is one of the most important factors determining the intellectual development of survivors.[222] Supratentorial anatomical abnormalities such as agenesis of the corpus callosum or cortical dysgenesis may, however, be associated with retardation despite excellent control of the hydrocephalus.[102,222] Disabilities in the survivors consist of mental retar-

---

TABLE 35–11 RESULTS AND PROGNOSIS IN DANDY-WALKER MALFORMATION

MODE OF TREATMENT	NUMBER OF PATIENTS	MORTALITY RATE (PER CENT)	SURVIVAL (PER CENT)	NORMAL INTELLECT (PER CENT)	INTELLECTUAL/ PHYSICAL IMPAIRMENT (PER CENT)	NOT RECORDED (PER CENT)
Various*	51	39	61	58	42	—
Primary shunt†	47	26	74	46	29	25
Secondary shunt‡	22	55	45	60	30	10

* See references 102, 222, 584.
† See references 83, 102, 222, 339, 369, 410, 584.
‡ See references 102, 222, 339, 369.

dation, nystagmus, ocular palsies, ataxia, and spasticity. Blindness due to optic atrophy as a result of delayed diagnosis or failure to control intracranial pressure is, it is to be hoped, a complication of the past.

An analysis of 69 patients collected from the literature who were treated by a shunting procedure suggests a lower mortality rate for primary as opposed to secondary shunt operations (see Table 35–11). No significant difference exists in the outcome of treatment, considering the small number of patients and the incomplete follow-up.

ENCEPHALOCELE

Definition

An encephalocele is a protrusion of cranial contents beyond the normal confines of the skull, and the term embodies cranial meningocele (meninges and cerebrospinal fluid), encephalomeningocele (brain tissue and meninges), and hydroencephalomeningocele (a portion of the ventricle, brain tissue, and meninges). All forms protrude through a cranial defect called cranium bifidum, which is the counterpart of the spina bifida of spinal dysraphism. ''Encephalocele'' is a useful general term to refer to common features of the various forms of the anomaly, but considerable differences exist in the pathology, treatment, and prog-

---

TABLE 35–12 CLASSIFICATION OF ENCEPHALOCELE ACCORDING TO SITE OF INTRACRANIAL DEFECT*

Occipital
Cranial vault
  Posterior fontanelle
  Interparietal
  Anterior fontanelle
  Interfrontal
  Temporal
Frontoethmoidal
  Nasofrontal
  Nasoethmoidal
  Naso-orbital
Cranial base
  Transethmoidal (intranasal)[†]
  Sphenoethmoidal } (sphenopharyngeal or
  Transsphenoidal } nasopharyngeal)[†]
  Frontosphenoidal or } orbital encephalocele[†]
    spheno-orbital }

---

* After Suwanwela, C., and Suwanwela, N.: A morphological classification of sincipital encephalomeningoceles. J. Neurosurg., 36:201–211, 1972.
† Common terms based on the external location of the encephalocele sac.

nosis of encephaloceles at each anatomical location (Table 35–12). Each, therefore, is discussed separately.

Cranial dysraphism is less common than its spinal counterpart in the experience of most neurological surgeons and accounts for only 8 to 19 per cent of all cases of cranial and spinal dysraphism combined.* The population incidence has been estimated at 1 per 3000 to 1 per 10,000 live births.[109,374,443,487] The occipital and frontobasal regions are the two most frequent locations. In the Western Hemisphere, 80 to 90 per cent of all encephaloceles occur in the occipital area in contrast to an equivalent predominance of the frontobasal location in Thailand, Africa, and other regions in the Eastern Hemisphere.[469,487,534,726,727] Seventy per cent of cases of occipital encephalocele occur in the female, but no sex preference is noted for the frontobasal location.[281,443,487]

Abnormal Embryology

As is the case with spina bifida aperta, no one theory adequately explains all the anatomical variations known collectively as ''encephalocele.'' The complex relationship of exencephalus and anencephalus and encephalocele, the considerable pathological diversity of encephalocele, and the important feature of secondary herniation of normally developed cerebral tissues indicate that direct comparisons with spina bifida aperta are not adequate.

Developmental Arrest

The anterior neuropore at the cephalic end of the neural tube should close at the level of the foramen cecum of the frontal bone by approximately 24 days of development.[420] Failure of this neuropore to close usually results in a lethal malformation and spontaneous abortion, in contrast to failure of the posterior neuropore to close, which causes myeloschisis.[142] The malformation may be termed anencephalus, exencephalus, acrania, cranioschisis, or craniorachischisis if the spine is involved, as it is in approximately 50 per cent of cases.[242] The essential nature of the defect is that the un-

---

* See references 35, 189, 223, 469, 487, 645.

fused cephalic neural folds are exposed to the amniotic fluid because the dura, cranium, and skin fail to cover the neural tissue. The brain forms a mass of protruding neural tissue that degenerates during gestation until only a hemorrhagic mass of glial scar, ependyma, choroid plexus, neuronal elements, and meninges remains at birth (anencephalus).[262] The "hemorrhagic" tissue has been termed the area cerebrovasculosa and is similar in structure to the area medullovasculosa in myeloschisis.[242] Failure of the neural tube to close may explain anencephalus, but it does not explain most of the clinical cases of encephalocele in which there is no evidence of dysraphism of the brain.[197]

The Hydrodynamic Theory

Gardner attributes encephalocele to an overdistention of the primitive neural tube due to delayed permeability of the roof of the fourth ventricle, but does not detail the pathogenesis as he does for other forms of cranial and spinal dysraphism.[247]

Neuroschisis

Neuroschisis of the closed neural tube with the formation of a bleb and, upon healing, adhesions between the overlying cutaneous ectoderm and the neuroectoderm can explain all the varieties of encephalocele seen in man.[538–541] An adhesion could produce the neural malformation and prevent the mesoderm from forming normal cranium, thus creating the defect through which the meninges and brain tissue herniate. St. Hillaire first proposed this mechanism with the publication of his adhesive theory in 1827.[503]

The Influence of Secondary Herniation

The cranial defect is created before the developing cerebral hemispheres crowd posteriorly and carry the tentorium and dural sinuses to their normal position. Encephalocele at all sites may contain well-developed brain tissue that had not yet formed when the neural-cranial defect developed. These findings can be explained only by displacement and herniation of cerebral tissues through the cranial defect late in fetal development. The herniated tissue may suffer pathological changes secondary to compression and ischemia.[197]

Occipital Encephalocele

The occipital location predominates in the Western Hemisphere and is more common in females in a ratio of 2.3 to 1. The pathological changes of occipital encephalocele show a gradation from little or no alteration but for a sac, as in cranial meningocele, to a moderate involvement of brain structures, as in an encephalomeningocele, to the severe deformities of brain structures incompatible with a good result or even with survival, as in the occipitocervical form.

Pathology

The Skull Defect

The midline, circular occipital cranial defect is usually located just below, rather than at or above, the external occipital protuberance.[541,737] The severe occipitocervical form manifests a midline cleft from the occipital protuberance to the foramen magnum with associated spina bifida of the upper cervical spine (Fig. 35–26*B*).[197,374,535] Craniolacunia is present only in the severe forms and the rare cases of simultaneous cranial and lower spinal dysraphism.*

The Dura and Venous Sinuses

The hypoplastic tentorium cerebelli runs from the petrous part of the temporal bone to the margins of the occipital defect, and thus, the location of the occipital defect may influence the size of the posterior fossa.[109,541] The falx cerebri may be hypoplastic and deviated from the midline if the posterior cerebral hemispheres herniate asymmetrically into the encephalocele.[374] The neck of the sac is in close relationship to the sagittal sinus, torcular, and occipital sinus, any of which may split to surround the bony defect.[281,737] The lateral sinuses are rarely, if ever, found within the sac, but are in a normal location or run obliquely across the occipital cortex above the bony defect.[109,197] Occasionally, the lateral sinuses may not exist as such, and the superior sagittal sinus drains into large intradural veins that empty into the cavernous sinuses.[541] The straight sinus may run toward or into the sac in the occipitocervical form or may even be absent. If it is ab-

---

* See references 35, 109, 281, 374, 443, 487.

sent, a dense network of venules surrounds the brain stem and upper cervical cord.[197,374]

The Encephalocele Sac

The encephalocele is usually completely covered by normal or modified skin that has only rudimentary or no secondary structures and hemangiomatous discoloration and hypertrichosis around the base (Fig. 35–26A). The cranial meningocele contains no neural elements, and the intracranial structures are usually normal. An apparent cranial meningocele may be lined by nodules of dysplastic neural tissue containing neuronal and glial elements, and is better considered a mild form of encephalomeningocele.[197,443,487] The nodules may appear as slightly thickened areas in the wall on palpation or on transillumination or at operation. An encephalomeningocele may contain a variable amount of brain tissue. The vermis of the cerebellum is the most frequently involved brain structure and may be variably hypoplastic or even aplastic

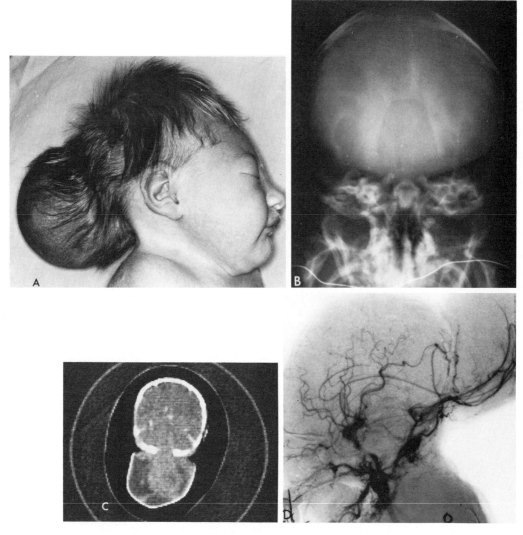

Figure 35–26 *A.* Large sessile occipitocervical encephalomeningocele associated with primary microcephaly and a sloping forehead. *B.* Towne's view showing the cleft occipital bone and spina bifida occulta of C1. Lückenschädel is also present. *C.* Cranial computed tomography shows tissue of brain density in the sac communicating intracranially through the cleft occipital bone. No hydrocephalus was present. No visual evoked responses could be recorded from the occipital area or from the sac. *D.* Superimposed anterior and posterior cerebral angiograms show branches of all three major arteries passing into the sac and a wide separation between the clivus and the basilar artery.

with relative sparing of the cerebellar hemispheres. Rarely the entire cerebellum is aplastic.[197,374,695]

In more severe cases, the brain stem is partially cleft in the midline and is displaced toward or even herniated into the sac along with herniation or aplasia of the midbrain tectum.[541,695] The separated cerebellar hemispheres may be displaced anteriorly between the clivus and the brain stem and basilar artery, causing stretching of the cranial nerves.[109,374,541,695] The medial temporal lobes may herniate through the enlarged incisura to fill the superior space between the clivus and the displaced brain stem.

A large encephalomeningocele often contains portions of one or both occipital lobes and occasionally of the lateral ventricles to form a hydroencephalocele.[30,374] If one hemisphere herniates more than the other, then the less involved cerebral hemisphere may encroach across the midline of the cranial cavity onto the side of the herniated hemisphere and be associated with a displacement of the falx cerebri.[374] The orbital portion of the frontal lobe may herniate over the sphenoid wing and form a pseudotemporal lobe.[541] The cranial cavity is microcephalic if large portions of the cerebral hemispheres herniate, and the anterior and middle fossae of the skull base are hypoplastic.[374] Rarely, a cystic portion of an encephalomeningocele may extend intracranially above or below the tentorium cerebelli.[469,737] The cortex of the herniated occipital lobe may be histologically normal or show microgyria with four-layered cortex, indicating damage between the sixth and seventh months of development.[109,197] In addition, herniated brain tissue may show secondary changes compatible with recent or remote infarction due to compressive and ischemic effects at the neck of the sac.[197,374] The fact that normal brain tissue can herniate into the sac is important clinically because a surgeon cannot assume that all the contents within an encephalomeningocele are nonfunctional. These observations also confirm that the formation of an encephalomeningocele may span virtually all of gestation rather than the restricted early time period as in spinal dysraphism.

Hydrocephalus

Intrauterine or perinatal hydrocephalus is far less common in encephalocele than in spinal dysraphism. The underlying cause may be aqueduct stenosis or forking, but more commonly the obstruction is at the level of the fourth ventricular outflow or basal subarachnoid spaces and is due to dense networks of venules and nodules of fibrous tissue surrounding the brain stem, upper spinal cord, and opening of the sac.[35,197,374]

Associated Anomalies

CENTRAL NERVOUS SYSTEM. Many of the complex neuroanatomical malformations found in the severe forms of encephalomeningocele help explain the variety of neurological deficits in survivors. The optic nerves, chiasm, and tracts may be elongated, atrophic, or absent; in addition there may be damage to the herniated occipital visual cortices.[206,374,541] The corpora quadrigemina may be absent.[695] The involvement of the fiber tracts in the brain stem depends upon agenesis, hypoplasia, dyplasia, or secondary degeneration of the cerebral, cerebellar, and brain stem structures. The nuclei with cerebellar connections are most frequently involved, e.g., the inferior olive, the spinocerebellar tract, the red nucleus, the dentatorubral tract, and the dentatothalamic tract.[109,374] The corpus callosum is usually normal even in severe cases, but the anterior commissure, septum pellucidum, or fornix may be deficient.[109,301,374,541,695] The Arnold-Chiari malformation (type II and type III) has been reported rarely, presumably owing to the high frequency of vermis hypoplasia.[35,97,558,559] The combination of the Dandy-Walker malformation and encephalomeningocele has been reported on several occasions.[109,584,640,725]

SYSTEMIC ANOMALIES. The association of arhinencephaly, occipital encephalocele, and polydactyly has been reported with and without a 13–15 trisomy syndrome.[496] Micrognathia, cleft palate, subglottic stenosis, and cardiac malformations such as ventricular septal defect or patent ductus arteriosus have also been noted.[143,281,443]

Clinical Evaluation

An occipital encephalocele usually presents as a pedunculated or sessile midline swelling over the occipital bone totally covered with normal or dysplastic skin. The size of the mass gives no indication of its contents. The sessile lesions, however, more often involve a cleft of the occipital bone and first cervical arch and contain brain tissue than do pedunculated lesions (cf. Fig. 35–26). Transillumination may show a fluid-filled sac typical of a cranial meningocele or dark areas indicative of brain tissue in an encephalomeningocele.[469] Although the size of an encephalocele does not correlate with a poor prognosis, the head circumference (omitting the encephalocele) may be of prognostic importance in the absence of hydrocephalus. A microcephalic cranium combined with a large sessile encephalocele suggests that a good proportion of the cerebral tissue is in the sac and virtually no hope exists for normal mental and physical development.[281,443,487]

Hydrocephalus occurs less commonly with encephalocele than with spinal dysraphism and is rarely present at birth.[109,374,541,695] Hydrocephalus may artificially increase the head circumference into the normal range, and the prognosis is poor if the head circumference decreases into the microcephalic range after shunting.[443] Hydrocephalus at birth or later is a distinctly unfavorable prognostic indicator in both cranial meningocele and encephalomeningocele.[281,443,469,487]

The majority of infants with cranial meningocele or mild encephalomeningocele manifest no obvious neurological abnormalities at birth as do patients with the severe occipitocervical encephalomeningocele that contains portions of the cerebellum, brain stem, and cerebrum.[469,541] These children may show poor crying and sucking, regurgitation or aspiration of feedings, increased tone in the limbs, and poor temperature regulation.[143,374,541] An abnormal neurological examination at birth is a poor prognostic indicator for mental and physical development.

Investigation

As well as the neurological status of the infant, the anatomy of the encephalocele and its contents and the presence of hydrocephalus or other central nervous system malformations are important parameters affecting prognosis and treatment.[737]

Plain roentgenograms of the skull usually show a localized midline circular defect with a sclerotic everted margin between the external occipital protuberance and the foramen magnum except for the cleft occi-

put in the severe occipitocervical encephalomeningocele (see Fig. 35–26B).[109] The frontal bone may slope posteriorly on the lateral view if a large amount of brain tissue has herniated into the encephalomeningocele, and the finding correlates with hypoplasia of the anterior and middle cranial fossae.[374]

Cranial computed tomography readily reveals the contents of the sac, hydrocephalus, and associated brain malformations (see Fig. 35–26C). Ventriculography is restricted to clarification of the communication between the cerebrospinal fluid pathways and the sac or to better delineation of associated cerebral malformations.

Cerebral angiography supplements computed tomography by showing the vascular supply of the contents of the sac, thus revealing the anatomical region of the extracranial brain (see Fig. 35–26D). Anterior and posterior circulation angiography may show the pericallosal artery, branches of the middle cerebral artery, and all the branches of the vertebral-basilar circulation passing into the sac in severe occipitocervical forms. Resection of such complicated lesions may result in death or unacceptable morbidity.[259] The venous phase of the angiogram may detail the anatomy of the venous sinuses, or retrograde jugular venography may be required.

Little attention has been focused on the preoperative investigation of potential or actual function of the herniated brain tissue. Herniated brain stem structures certainly function, as evidenced by changing vital signs with manipulation of the tissue and by the sudden death of patients during or shortly after operative injury.[197,281,695] Surgeons have considered the contents to be functional, and preserve and replace brain tissue within the cranial cavity when possible.[281,469,487] Electroencephalographic recordings from the sac suggest that electrically active tissue may be present.[206] Visual evoked responses recorded from the sac may indicate the location and function of the visual cortex of the occipital lobe.[206] The absence of visual evoked responses may indicate defective visual cortex or dysplasia of the optic pathways.[109,374]

Treatment

Fortunately, an occipital encephalocele is usually skin covered, and immediate operation is rarely required. A delay of several days insures that the infant's condition is stable and the anatomy of the malformation can be evaluated. Virtually all encephaloceles can be excised, but not all need to or can be treated by operation. A microcephalic infant with neurological deficit and a sac containing cerebrum, cerebellum, and brain stem structures as shown by computed tomography and angiography may be better left without operation.*

The purposes of the operation are to remove the sac, to preserve neural function, and to obtain a watertight dural closure. The anatomy of the encephalocele is usually simpler when the cranial defect is small and circular and the sac is pedunculated and fluid-filled. On the other hand, a sessile, tissue-filled sac associated with a cleft of the occiput and C1 posterior arch may have complicated venous anatomy at the neck of the sac and contain potentially functional brain stem and cerebral structures.

General intubation anesthesia in the prone position with controlled ventilation and close temperature monitoring is preferred.[143] A reliable intravenous catheter is mandatory, since sudden blood loss from the venous sinuses may occur. A horizontal incision encompassing the neck of the sac is appropriate for the majority of encephaloceles associated with a circular defect in the occipital bone. A vertical incision permits exposure above and below the posterior fossa and may be preferable for the complicated occipitocervical sac. Particular care must be taken at the neck of the sac, since the sagittal sinus, torcular, transverse sinuses, and occipital sinus are in the vicinity. Initially, the neck of the sac is defined at the bony defect, and then the wall is opened away from the neck; sufficient dura for an imbricated closure is preserved. The contents of the sac are inspected, and it is decided whether to resect or preserve the tissue. The bony opening may have to be enlarged to allow clear definition of all the structures at the neck and to permit the contents to be replaced intracranially. If the brain tissue appears normal and cannot be placed within the cranium, the cranial defect should be enlarged and the dura and skin closed over the tissue in preference to sacrifice of normal tissue.

---

* See references 206, 259, 281, 409, 443, 469, 487, 737.

An intracranial extension of the encephalocele above or below the tentorium may have been revealed by the preoperative studies, and the posterior fossa or supratentorial area may require exploration.[469,737] Once the contents of the sac have been excised or replaced, the dura is closed in an imbricated fashion and tested by a Valsalva maneuver. Occasionally, a periosteal flap can be swung over the defect for additional support. The skin is then closed in two layers. The sac and excised contents are sent for pathological examination.

A shunt should be placed prior to excision of the sac in the rare instance of early hydrocephalus to forestall intraoperative and postoperative complications such as sudden ventricular collapse or cerebrospinal fluid leakage. Acute hydrocephalus or cerebrospinal fluid leakage following excision of the sac necessitates continuous external ventricular drainage. A shunt is placed after the incision is healed and the cerebrospinal fluid is proved free of infection.

Results and Prognosis

Firm conclusions regarding the results and prognosis of occipital encephalocele are lacking, since the lesion is relatively uncommon. Few large series have been collected during the period in which reliable shunting procedures have been available, and the lesion presents a spectrum in severity.[35,281,443,487] A few basic observations can be made, however, by grouping series collected between 1948 and 1967. These series consist of 74 patients with cranial meningocele and 122 patients with encephalomeningocele followed for a minimum of 1½ years to a maximum of 20 years.

Mortality Rates

The long-term mortality rate of cranial meningocele is only 14 per cent. Postoperative infection accounts for most early deaths and shunt complications for most late deaths. The long-term mortality rate for encephalomeningocele is at least 52 per cent. Early deaths after operation are usually due to injury to vital brain stem centers in occipitocervical malformations or to postoperative infection.[443] Late deaths are due to shunt complications, untreated hydrocephalus, or systemic factors such as infection in severely incapacitated survivors.

If all cases of severe encephalomeningocele unsuitable for operation were included, then the overall mortality rate would be higher. For example, without operation, severe encephalomeningocele has a mortality rate of 90 per cent in the first few months of life with death primarily due to systemic factors such as infection rather than uncontrolled hydrocephalus.[487]

Morbidity

An infant with a pure cranial meningocele or a sac containing dysplastic neural nodules in the wall has a relatively good prognosis for normal mental and physical development.[281,487] Fifty-three per cent will be physically and mentally normal, twenty-eight per cent mentally normal but physically impaired, and nineteen per cent retarded, with the majority having physical handicaps as well. Hydrocephalus plays an important role in the latter group.

The survivors in the encephalomeningocele group tend to have the simpler malformations, and 36 per cent of the survivors will have normal mental development, but one third to one half of these patients will have physical disabilities. Sixty-four per cent of the survivors will be mentally and physically disabled. Both the survivors and the fatalities should be considered to characterize the prognosis for encephalomeningocele properly because those infants with the worst prognosis tend to die over the years, making the results of the surviving group tend to look better than they are. When all cases of encephalomeningocele are considered, only 17 per cent of patients have normal mental development and 83 per cent will be mentally retarded and physically impaired, or dead. Infants with primary microcephaly before or after shunting, and a large encephalomeningocele, virtually never develop normally whether they are treated operatively or nonoperatively.[281,443,487,737] Hydrocephalus reduces the slim likelihood of a good prognosis even further.

The physical disabilities vary in severity and include epilepsy, degrees of visual impairment extending to blindness, strabismus, deafness, motor disability such as monoparesis or hemiparesis or quadriparesis, impaired coordination, and dysarthria.[143,281,434,443,487]

Hydrocephalus

Early hydrocephalus in encephalocele that has not been operated on is unusual, but acute postoperative hydrocephalus is well known.[291,443,487] Hydrocephalus occurs in no less than 36 per cent of patients with cranial meningocele and 31 per cent of patients with encephalomeningocele. The lower incidence in encephalomeningocele may be artifactual, as some patients died of other causes prior to developing hydrocephalus or did not have investigation for hydrocephalus when the prognosis was obviously poor.

Encephalocele at Other Sites

Encephalocele of the cranial vault, frontoethmoidal region (sincipital), and cranial base contributes 10 to 20 per cent of all cases of encephalocele in the Western Hemisphere, with an incidence ranging from 1 in 50,000 to 1 in 100,000 births.[176,469,487] Encephaloceles at these sites are generally nonhereditary and nonfamilial with no apparent sex preference, but the incidence does vary with the anatomical location and the racial and geographic origin of the patient.[176,727,762] The incidence is higher in Russia, in African natives, in eastern Asia, and specifically in Thailand, where it is estimated at 1 in 5000 live births.[161,534,726,727]

Encephalocele of the Cranial Vault

Encephalocele at Posterior Fontanelle

An encephalocele at the posterior fontanelle is likely to be considered a high occipital or posterior interparietal encephalocele. No author has clearly described an encephalocele through the junctional area of the occipital and parietal bones.

Interparietal Encephalocele

In the Western Hemisphere, the interparietal site is the most common location of cranial vault encephalocele and accounts for approximately 11 per cent of all encephaloceles.* The encephalocele is usually lo-

---

* See references 35, 223, 434, 469, 482, 487.

cated in the midline or immediate paramedian posterior parietal region 1 or 2 cm anterior to the posterior fontanelle. The lesion may be sessile or pedunculated, large or small, and is covered with normal or modified skin. Occasionally, the encephalocele is farther forward, in which case the prognosis is less favorable because of a greater incidence of associated brain malformation such as agenesis of the corpus callosum. Three types of lesion may occur.[482] The heterotopic glial rest has no connection with the intracranial contents and is comparable to the nasal glioma.[157] Presumably, the coverings of the nervous system were restored after displacement of the neural tissue. These patients may develop normally if no other intracranial abnormality occurs. The cranial meningocele contains only cerebrospinal fluid or neural elements in the wall of the sac, and the prognosis is good, with approximately 70 per cent of patients developing normally.[434,482,487] Interparietal encephalomeningocele has a poor prognosis, with only 15 per cent of patients developing normally and the remainder having mental or physical disabilities or dying because of associated cerebral malformations.[482,487]

Plain roentgenograms of the skull show a midline or paramedian circular cranial defect. Cranial computed tomography in the coronal plane helps to distinguish a cranial meningocele from an encephalomeningocele. Cerebral angiography may show the pericallosal arteries deviated toward or into the sac, and the location of the sagittal sinus should be determined on the venous phase. Operative repair hazards injury to the sagittal sinus if it is not displaced from the midline.[482] Ventriculography may show a communication between the ventricles and the sac.

Interparietal encephalocele must be distinguished from congenital parietal foramina on plain roentgenograms. The latter are characterized by two circumscribed posterior parietal areas of lucency symmetrically situated on either side of the sagittal suture approximately 3 cm anterior to the lambdoid suture and 1 cm lateral to the sagittal suture. These familial anomalous foramina may transmit the parietal branches of the occipital artery and vein, but the blood vessels have no effect on the size of the foramina. The larger foramina may have a transverse suture connecting the two defects. Large parietal foramina may be palpated as soft defects that suggest abnormally situated fontanelles, and no cerebral tissue protrudes as with an encephalocele, although the brain may bulge during crying.[436] The defects may decrease in size with early growth, but they remain stable after 3 years of age. They are of no clinical significance unless unusually large. Cranioplasty is indicated if the foramina are more than 3 cm in diameter after 3 years of age, since spontaneous obliteration by normal bone growth does not occur.[469]

Interparietal encephalocele must also be distinguished from congenital defects of the scalp, skull, and dura in the parietal area.[235,469] The simplest defect of the scalp appears as a superficial ulceration in the posterior parietal area near the vertex and is termed aplasia cutis congenita. Excision and early closure may be preferable for smaller lesions, but if left alone, the open area will epithelialize and leave an atrophic area devoid of hair.[235,436] Occasionally the skin covering the area is thin and parchmentlike with surrounding hemangiomatous discoloration and local overgrowth of hair. Rarely, the scalp and skull are deficient, and intact dura is exposed. Direct closure of small defects is preferable. Such areas may epithelialize completely if kept clean, however, and the defect can be covered by full-thickness scalp flaps at a later date. Rarely, scalp, bone, and dura are absent, and the brain is exposed. If the area of exposure is large, fatal infection or hemorrhage from drying and cracking of the exposed brain can occur. The open area must be kept moist at all times. A small defect may be covered by full-thickness scalp flaps, but large defects must be conservatively managed until epithelialization is complete.[469] Cranioplasty and full-thickness scalp coverage can be provided when the infant is older.

Encephalocele at Anterior Fontanelle

An anterior fontanelle encephalocele occurs through the junctional area of the two parietal and two frontal bones.[342,637] Only one case of encephalomeningocele with displacement of the pericallosal arteries and ventricles toward the skull defect and probable absence of the corpus callosum has been reported in detail.[637] Congenital dermoid cysts without intracranial extension may form at the anterior fontanelle, particularly in Nigerians, and must be differentiated from an encephalocele.[5,531]

Interfrontal Encephalocele

An interfrontal encephalocele in the middle of the forehead occurs through a bony defect in the frontal bones in the region of the metopic suture.[161,728] The frontal bone inferior to the bony defect that borders the nasal bones is intact, whereas the bony defect may merge into the anterior fontanelle superiorly. Cerebral and systemic abnormalities may be associated.

Temporal Encephalocele

A temporal encephalocele protrudes just behind the lateral orbital margin through the pterion or anterolateral fontanelle, which is the junctional area of the frontal, parietal, and temporal bones and the greater wing of the sphenoid.[515] Fewer than 1 per cent of all cases of encephalocele are located at the pterion, and they show a 3 to 1 preference for females.[26] The encephalocele is usually sessile and tends to enlarge, producing progressive deformity of the ipsilateral eye and ear as it spreads over the zygoma onto the face. Neurological deficit is present in 25 per cent of patients, but the prognosis for normal development is generally good.

Plain roentgenograms reveal the bony defect at the pterion and may also show deformity of the ipsilateral bony orbit and sphenoid wing. On pneumoencephalography, air may not fill the encephalocele or the ipsilateral subarachnoid space and ventricle, whereas the contralateral ventricle is filled.[515] Arteriography has not been reported, but would show herniation of temporal and parietal cortical branches of the middle cerebral artery into the defect if the lesion is an encephalomeningocele. The operative repair is similar to that of occipital encephalocele. In the few patients reported, cranial meningocele is as frequent as encephalomeningocele into which the temporal or parietal lobe herniates. Hydrocephalus has not been reported as a complication before or after operation.

Frontoethmoidal and Basal Encephalocele

Encephaloceles in the frontoethmoidal (sincipital) and basal regions share a few common features: a variable terminology, an internal cranial defect that may not correspond with the external bony defect, and generally, the fact that an intracranial operative approach is preferable to an extracranial route. The terminology suggested by Suwanwela is valuable, since it is based on the anatomy of the cranial defect rather than on the descriptive location of the external sac (see Table 35–12).[113,726–731]

Frontoethmoidal Encephalocele

Pathological Anatomy

The three types of frontoethmoidal encephalocele, the nasofrontal, nasoethmoidal, and naso-orbital forms, have in common an internal cranial defect between the frontal and ethmoid bones; hence, the characterization, frontoethmoidal (Fig. 35–27). Approximately 50 per cent of patients have a single midline opening corresponding to the foramen cecum, with the crista galli located at the posterior rim of the defect. Approximately 25 per cent of patients have an opening on either side of the midline anterior to the cribriform plate, with the crista galli again located at the posterior aspect of the bridge of bone between the two defects. The remaining 25 per cent of patients have a single lateralized opening anterior to the cribriform plate. All forms may be associated with an element of hypertelorism. The external defect viewed from the facial aspect is different for each of the three types.

NASOFRONTAL TYPE. The nasofrontal encephalocele has an external defect located at the nasion between the frontal bone above and the depressed nasal and ethmoid bones below (Fig. 35–27B). The nasal bones, the nasal cartilage, and the frontal processes of the maxillary bone have a normal relationship, but the medial wall of the orbit may be displaced laterally, and the root of the nose widened. The anterior cranial fossa is unusually deep in its midportion owing to inferior displacement of the ethmoid bones in relation to the orbital roof on either side. The internal and external cranial defects are close together, and the passageway between the openings is correspondingly short.[113,727,728] The single external sac is usually pedunculated and is located at the glabella or at the root of the nose.

NASOETHMOIDAL TYPE. The external bony opening is located between the nasal bone above and the depressed nasal cartilage below (Fig. 35–27C). The passageway through the neck of the sac is long, since the internal and external defects are separated.[113,728] The bony canal is formed by the nasal bones and the frontal process of the maxillary bone superiorly, the nasal cartilage and nasal septum attached internally to the ethmoid bone inferiorly, and the medial wall of the orbit laterally. The orbital wall may be membranous instead of bony. The external sac is located lower than the nasofrontal sac and may extend into the inner

canthus of both eyes, producing a bilobed mass. The nasoethmoidal form is more often sessile than pedunculated.

NASO-ORBITAL TYPE. The external bony opening is located at the anterior and inferior portion of the medial wall of one or both orbits in the naso-orbital form (Fig. 35–27D). The frontal and nasal bones and the nasal cartilage are in a normal relationship. The passageway for the neck of the sac is long. The frontal process of the maxillary bone forms the anterior wall of the canal, whereas the lacrimal bone and lam-

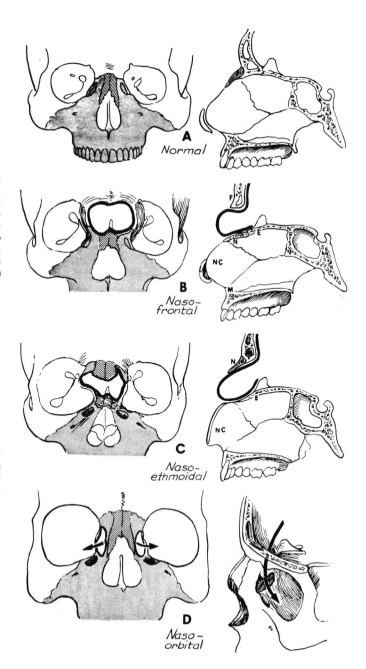

Figure 35–27 A. Normal anterior and median views of the cranial and facial bones to show the relationship of the frontal, nasal, and ethmoid bones. B. The nasofrontal encephalocele has a close relationship between the internal and external openings between the frontal bone (F) above and the displaced nasal (N) and ethmoid (E) bones below; NC, nasal cartilage; M, maxillary bone. C. The nasoethmoidal variety has a long separation between the internal and external openings between the frontal and nasal bones above and the depressed ethmoid bone below. D. The naso-orbital variety has the same internal opening as B and C, but two external openings in the medial orbital wall may occur. The frontal and nasal bones are in a normal position. Both C and D may present as bilateral masses. (From Charoonsmith, T., and Suwanwela, C.: Frontoethmodial encephalomeningocele with special reference to plastic reconstruction. Clin. Plast. Surg., 1:27–47, 1974. Reprinted by permission.)

A
Normal

B
Naso-
frontal

C
Naso-
ethmoidal

D
Naso-
orbital

ina papyracea of the ethmoid bone form the posterior margin of the defect. The external mass may be single or bilateral, and appears as a fullness in the anterior and inferior aspect of the orbit, displacing the eye superiorly and laterally.[208,727]

THE ENCEPHALOCELE SAC AND ASSOCIATED CEREBRAL MALFORMATIONS. Encephalomeningocele is the most common form of encephalocele in the frontoethmoidal group, while the nasofrontal form is more likely to be a cranial meningocele.[737] As a generalization, the brain tissue contained in a frontoethmoidal encephalocele is not critical to function, and approximately 75 per cent of patients will have normal mental and physical development.[434,487] The frontal lobes are more frequently involved in the routine frontoethmoidal encephalocele with herniation of the olfactory apparatus and stretching of the olfactory tracts. The inferior frontal lobe and third ventricle may be displaced anteriorly with the anterior communicating artery at the level of the crista galli, and as a result, the optic nerves may recurve in a posterior direction to enter the optic canals. The internal carotid arteries are similarly deformed. In severe forms, the sac may contain both frontal lobes and the intervening falx cerebri, and there may also be associated cerebral malformations.[113,727,728] Holoprosencephaly, elongation of the quadrigeminal plate, angulation of the aqueduct producing hydrocephalus, elongation of the brain stem and hypothalamus, herniation of the temporal lobe over the sphenoid wing into the anterior cranial fossa, agenesis of the corpus callosum, microgyria, and agyria may occur.[728] The prognosis is just as grave as for occipital encephalomeningocele in these complicated lesions.

Hydrocephalus occurs in approximately 10 to 20 per cent of patients with frontoethmoidal encephalocele and at an even higher rate in patients with severe malformations.*

Clinical Evaluation

A frontoethmoidal encephalocele is clinically obvious as a single or bilateral mass in the region of the glabella, nose, or orbits.

---

* See references 434, 469, 487, 728, 729, 731, 737.

Skin coverage is usually complete except for the severe malformation. In particular, the naso-orbital form bulges from behind the intact skin of the lower eyelid in the medial orbit. Investigation and treatment are required because the encephaloceles tend to enlarge with time and produce greater cosmetic deformity of the developing facial bones.

Investigation

Plain roentgenograms of the skull (including a basal view), paranasal sinuses, and orbits, and tomography are required.[299] The bony defect is smooth and well circumscribed without sclerosis of the margins. The nasofrontal form may show a V-shaped defect in the frontal bone, lateral displacement and bowing of the superomedial orbital wall, a gap between the frontal and ethmoid bones, and depression of the cribriform plate and attached nasal bones, which are located below the single, midline soft-tissue mass. The nasoethmoidal form shows a circular defect between the orbits, an increased interorbital distance, and elevation of the nasal bone and frontal bones above the frequently bilobed soft-tissue mass. The naso-orbital variety may show a bilateral soft-tissue mass lateral to the nasal bone, overlying a defect in the frontal process of the maxilla and medial orbital wall. The cribriform plate and ethmoid, frontal, and nasal bones are in a relatively normal relationship. Cranial computed tomography will confirm the presence of tissue in the sac and show hydrocephalus and associated brain malformations.

Frontoethmoidal encephalocele must be differentiated from other mass lesions associated with hypertelorism such as nasal glioma, dermoid cyst, hemangioma, or sinus pericranii. No treatment or a simpler operation may suffice if the lesion is not an encephalocele.[56,426,452] Invasive tests may be necessary to confirm the diagnosis in questionable cases by proving that the tissue in the mass has a cerebral blood supply or that there is communication between the subarachnoid space and the mass. Cerebral angiography has been rarely reported but may show the inferior frontal artery passing through the defect into the extracranial sac. Ventriculography or pneumoencephalography may clarify the neck of the sac but actually fills a portion of the sac in only 13 per cent of patients because of adhesions around the neck of the cranial opening.[730] Isotope cisternography more reliably shows a communication between the mass and subarachnoid space, and should precede the other invasive studies.[730]

Encephalocele of the Cranial Base (Transethmoidal, Spheno-Ethmoidal and Transsphenoidal Encephalocele)

Pathological Anatomy

In the Western Hemisphere, encephaloceles of the cranial base constitute only 5 per cent of all encephaloceles.[35,434,469,487] The terminology appears complicated because authors have referred to the lesions both by the site of the bony defect and by the location of the sac. Table 35–12 records Suwanwela's classification according to the site of the bony defect, which is self-explanatory. It also includes the popular terminology found in the literature.[728] An encephalocele through a defect in the ethmoid bone (transethmoidal) tends to locate within the nasal cavity and is usually termed an intranasal encephalocele but has also been called a nasopharyngeal and a sphenopharyngeal encephalocele.* An encephalocele through a more posterior bony defect between the ethmoid and the sphenoid bones (sphenoethmoidal) or through the sphenoid bone (transsphenoidal) tends to locate in the epipharynx and is variably termed a sphenopharyngeal or nasopharyngeal encephalocele.†

Cleft palate and eye abnormalities such as enlargement of the optic disc, microphthalmia, coloboma, and optic atrophy may occur with the transsphenoidal encephalocele.‡ Cerebral malformations such as agenesis of the corpus callosum are also more frequent with posterior defects, presumably because more important areas of the brain are involved.[500,762] A single case of pituitary insufficiency has been reported with a transsphenoidal encephalocele.[794]

Clinical Evaluation

A basal encephalocele gives little or no external evidence of its presence except for broadening of the bridge of the nose or, occasionally, frank hypertelorism and a broad bitemporal skull diameter.[176,746] The presenting symptoms of an encephalocele in the nasal cavity or the epipharynx may be obstructed or noisy respiration, frequent respiratory "infection" associated with nasal discharge, and rarely cerebrospinal fluid leakage with or without meningitis.§ Occasionally, excision of a presumed nasal polyp is followed by a postoperative cerebrospinal fluid leak, and on pathological examination the excised-polyp is found to contain brain tissue.

Examination of the nasopharynx reveals a mass covered by nasal mucous membrane lying medial to the middle turbinate bone next to the nasal septum, particularly if the encephalocele is the transethmoidal type.[639] Ordinary nasal polyps lie lateral to the middle turbinate bone except for very posterior polyps and are more obviously pedunculated than the typical encephalocele. A probe can be passed freely both medial and lateral to a nasal polyp but fails to pass medial to an encephalocele because of the intimate relationship of the nasal septum and the encephalocele sac. The mass may fluctuate synchronously with the patient's pulse or respiration, or enlarge with straining or deliberate obstruction of the jugular veins (Furstenberg sign). Nasal polyps are rare in infants and young children, and thus, a mass in the nose in this age group should raise the suspicion of encephalocele.[155,176,639,746]

Investigation

Plain roentgenograms of the skull including a basal view and tomography of the anterior fossa may show widening of the affected side of the nose, a defect in the ethmoidal, sphenoethmoidal, and sphenoidal area and a mass in the nasal cavity or pharynx.[27,268,794] The edges of the bony defect are beveled downward, the sinus air cells may be opacified, and the turbinate bones may be deformed or absent. Cranial computed tomography in the coronal plane will be useful to evaluate the contents of the mass, hydrocephalus, associated malformations, and perhaps the bony defect.

---

* See references 17, 155, 176, 220, 344, 505, 639.
† See references 27, 411, 500, 571, 762, 794.
‡ See references 27, 176, 268, 344, 411, 571, 762.

§ See references 176, 220, 344, 500, 746, 762, 779, 794, 814.

Invasive procedures are necessary to confirm the presence of brain tissue within the sac or a communication between the subarachnoid space and the sac to differentiate a basal encephalocele from lesions requiring simpler or different treatment such as a nasal glioma, mucocele of the paranasal sinuses, or neurogenic tumor of the nasal cavity (neuroepithelioma).* Cerebral angiography shows the proximal anterior cerebral artery displaced inferiorly toward the neck of a transsphenoidal encephalocele, whereas the anterior inferior frontal artery extends extracranially into a transethmoidal encephalocele below the plane of the ophthalmic artery and the lamina cribrosa.[411] Pneumoencephalography or ventriculography only occasionally shows air filling the encephalocele or delineates the neck of the transethmoidal sac, but the anterior-inferior portion of the frontal horn of the lateral ventricle may taper inferiorly.[639] The third ventricle, however, may herniate into the posteriorly situated sphenoethmoidal and transsphenoidal encephalocele.[27,268,411,571,794] Radioisotope cisternography can demonstrate a communication between the subarachnoid space and the sac more reliably than air and may even confirm cerebrospinal fluid leakage.[569] Metrizamide (Amipaque) cisternography with computed tomography may also confirm a communication.

Frontosphenoidal and Spheno-Orbital Encephalocele

Pathological Anatomy

A frontosphenoidal encephalocele extends through a defect between the frontal and sphenoid bones, whereas a spheno-orbital encephalocele extends through a normal foramen (superior orbital fissure, optic foramen) or a defect in the sphenoid wing. Either form is usually termed an orbital encephalocele and is very rare.† Differentiation of the naso-orbital encephalocele (frontoethmoidal group) from the spheno-orbital or frontosphenoidal encephalocele (basal group) is important because the intracranial operative approach is slightly different. The literature fails to stress the essential differences between the two types other than

that the former is located anteriorly and the latter posteriorly in the orbit. The general terms "orbital meningocele" and "orbital encephalocele" are applied loosely to both.‡ Occasionally cerebral malformations such as agenesis of the corpus callosum will be present.[212]

Clinical Evaluation

The anterior naso-orbital encephalocele is externally visible as a swelling in the anteroinferior aspect of one or both orbits, causing superior and lateral displacement of the globe. A spheno-orbital or a frontosphenoidal encephalocele causes exophthalmos as well as a lateral displacement of one globe, depending on the actual site of the mass. The posterior encephalocele is more likely to cause a pulsating exophthalmos that may be reducible because the route from the subarachnoid space is more direct and the neck is often broad.[54,150,546] Enlargement of the orbit and prominence of the temporal region may develop. The involved eye is usually normal, but microphthalmos, coloboma, hydrophthalmos, anophthalmos, microcornea, and enophthalmos have been reported.[123,131,212,546,718] Except for the eye signs, the neurological examination is usually normal.[212]

A posterior orbital encephalocele must be differentiated from a congenital cystic eye, which does not require an intracranial operation, and from tumors of the eye such as a teratoma, which may occasionally be associated with a bony defect.[155,212] Unilateral congenital agenesis of the sphenoid bone and the orbital plate of the frontal bone also may produce pulsating exophthalmos. Over 50 per cent of the patients will have von Recklinghausen's disease.[469,617]

Investigation

The investigation of an "orbital encephalocele" should accurately localize the defect in the orbital wall so that the operative approach can be planned. Plain roentgenograms of the skull (including basal views and optic foramina) and tomography of the anterior fossa and sphenoid wing are required. Cranial computed tomography of

---

* See references 107, 155, 157, 176, 376, 479, 488.
† See references 54, 123, 150, 212, 546, 718.

‡ See references 123, 131, 208, 273, 546, 718.

the orbit may aid the differential diagnosis of the orbital lesions and show the sphenoid wing defect. Invasive procedures are necessary to prove that the lesion is an encephalocele and to direct the operative approach. Cerebral angiography may show the abnormally low and anteriorly displaced internal carotid siphon and ophthalmic artery origin and a sphenoid wing defect. Similarly the air study may show prolongation of the temporal horn of the ventricle or subarachnoid space into the orbit, confirming the presence of an encephalocele.[54] Encephaloceles associated with small defects or enlarged normal foramina show lesser degrees of abnormality on angiography and air study.[212]

Treatment of Frontoethmoidal and Basal Encephalocele

The majority of these encephaloceles are skin covered, and operation is elective.[727] Early operation may, however, minimize the facial deformity, enhance the likelihood of normal binocular vision, and prevent further damage to brain tissue herniated through a broad-necked defect.[208,727] Untreated encephaloceles tend to enlarge with time and increase the facial and orbital deformities during the growing phase. Occasionally, a basal encephalocele requires urgent neurosurgical management after extracranial excision of a "nasal polyp" has resulted in a cerebrospinal fluid fistula.[17,155,176,263] Operation on the posterior basal encephalocele such as the transsphenoidal and sphenoethmoidal lesion may be contraindicated, since the herniated brain tissue may consist of the anterior cerebral arteries, the optic nerves and chiasm, and the anterior portion of the third ventricle. Intracranial repair may have to be abandoned because of the complexity of the lesion or may result in death.*

The operation must achieve three goals: a watertight closure of the dural defect to eliminate the possibility of postoperative cerebrospinal fluid fistula, meningitis, and death that characterized early operative results; repair of the cranial defect, if necessary, with autogenous bone, tantalum mesh, tantalum plate, or acrylic; and creation of the best possible milieu for normal skeletal and soft-tissue growth of the face, which is particularly important in frontoethmoidal encephalocele. Although the prognosis for mental and physical development may be good, the patient may be incapacitated by cosmetic deformity.[487] Hydrocephalus is not unusual in association with a frontal or basal encephalocele and may necessitate a shunt prior to an intracranial repair of the defect.[569] Tapping the mass percutaneously, particularly in the orbital and intranasal locations, as a diagnostic or therapeutic maneuver risks cerebrospinal fluid leakage and meningitis.[155]

Dural Closure

The intracranial approach is preferred for repair of frontoethmoidal and basal encephalocele.† Extracranial repair is feasible only for the purely frontal encephalocele and the nasofrontal type of the frontoethmoidal group.[113,155,728,737] The bony canal for the neck of the sac is short because the intracranial and the extracranial defects are contiguous, whereas the two defects may be considerably separated in all other forms. Successful closure of the dural and cranial defects is unlikely if the neck of the sac is long.[728] Extracranial repair of the nasoethmoidal, naso-orbital, and basal forms is frequently followed by cerebrospinal fluid fistula, and a secondary corrective intracranial operation is required under less than ideal circumstances. On occasion, a satisfactory closure without leakage is obtained by the extracranial route, but may be followed by a recurrence of the encephalocele because the dural repair was inadequate.[155,487,727]

A coronal incision and a bifrontal bone flap are necessary to expose midline cranial defects in the anterior fossa. A unilateral frontotemporal craniotomy is adequate for a lateralized bony defect, particularly the spheno-orbital or frontosphenoidal "orbital" encephalocele. Preoperative localization of the defect is important because these rare posterior orbital forms may require exposure through both the middle and anterior fossae. Intradural exploration to identify the tongue of brain tissue extending into the encephalocele avoids multiple tears of the dura that may occur in separating the

---

* See references 27, 268, 411, 500, 571, 762, 794.

† See references 17, 155, 243, 509, 520, 791.

dura from the abnormal bony structure of the anterior fossa surrounding the cranial defect.[469] The herniated brain may be pulled into the intracranial cavity if the neck of the sac is broad and the tissue is considered functional. In most cases, the bony defect is small and the sac contains nonfunctional tissue. Returning this tissue to the intracranial cavity is difficult, if not impossible, and attempts to do so may be undesirable because if the sac ruptures there is greater risk of postoperative cerebrospinal fluid leak. Amputation of the stalk of brain tissue flush with the neck of the sac is safer in this situation. If the extracranial mass is large and a source of respiratory obstruction, the contents can be removed in pieces through the neck of the sac; care must be taken not to rupture the extracranial portion. A watertight closure of the dural defect with a flap of falx cerebri, temporalis muscle fascia, or fascia lata is performed. The external portion of the encephalocele should be left untouched after the intracranial repair is completed.* The external sac often shrivels to the point at which no second operation is required, or if an extracranial removal is later necessary, the dural closure will be healed with no risk of cerebrospinal fluid fistula.

A special exception is the older child with a severe craniofacial deformity and midline encephalocele. Both the encephalocele and the craniofacial malformation may be corrected in one sitting by the craniofacial team.

Cranial Defect

The size and location of the cranial defect influences the management. Small defects fill in with fibrous tissue and are cosmetically acceptable. Large cranial defects may predispose to recurrence of the encephalocele or be cosmetically repulsive. Cranial bone may be harvested from the temporal region of the skull to repair the cranial defect. The donor site is subtemporal and regenerates quickly in the infant and young child. If for some reason it is not feasible to use this site, then the outer cranial table or autogenous rib may be used. Large defects in an infant may require a sheet of tantalum

mesh to bridge the defect and support the dural repair.

Facial Deformity

Facial deformities—hypertelorism, orbital deformity, or a cleft nose, lip, or palate—may be the most important lingering difficulty for the child with a frontoethmoidal or basal encephalocele.[487] Radical craniofacial reconstructive procedures may offer new hope for the child with normal intelligence and physical ability who is incapacitated by facial deformity.[113,132]

Results and Prognosis

Successful repair of frontoethmoidal and basal encephalocele by the intracranial route is the rule with rare instances of cerebrospinal fluid fistula and a minimal incidence of recurrence over the years, most frequently in the nasoethmoidal form.[452,737] The prognosis for intellectual and physical development is better than for occipital or interparietal encephalocele. The association of a poor prognosis with the encephalomeningocele form does not hold except for large herniations of brain tissue and for the transsphenoidal and sphenoethmoidal varieties. Early and late hydrocephalus occur less frequently than with encephalocele at any other cranial site, which further enhances the likelihood of normal development.[727,729,731]

CONGENITAL CRANIAL DERMAL SINUS

Definition

A congenital cranial dermal sinus is an epithelium-lined tract that forms a potential communication between the scalp and the deeper tissues within the cranial cavity. The tract may form anywhere from the nasion to the foramen magnum, but is more frequently near the external protuberance of the occipital bone. It may terminate in the subcutaneous tissues or on the skull, or may penetrate the skull through a cranial defect to end in the epidural or intradural space or on brain tissue. A portion of the tract may expand to form an inclusion tumor. The lesion may present as local infection and drainage from the skin orifice,

---

* See references 35, 176, 344, 434, 469, 727, 779, 791.

meningitis, or a mass lesion causing cerebellar and brain stem compression or hydrocephalus, or as a combination of these. The cranial dermal sinus is only a small part of the spectrum of intracranial inclusion tumors (epidermoid, dermoid, teratoid, teratomatous) that more often develop without a communication with the external surface of the body.

Abnormal Embryology

All authors concur that the failure of the neural ectoderm to separate from the overlying cutaneous ectoderm by the time neurulation is completed at 28 days may initiate a series of abnormalities.* If the epithelial-neural ectoderm adhesion remains intact throughout development, then the adhesion may impair mesoderm formation and result in a defect in the bone and meninges. As the neural structures migrate posteriorly during development, relative to the initial site of the adhesion, the string of epithelial cells may elongate and maintain communication between the external surface and the intracranial structures. If the epithelial string forms a real or potential tube, then organisms from the skin surface may colonize any portion of the tube down

---

* See references 145, 227, 435, 464, 736, 754, 757, 776.

to the deepest attachments. As well, any portion of the epithelial tube may expand to form an inclusion tumor. More commonly, the external portion of the epithelial string regresses and disappears, so the skin surface rarely communicates with the deeper neural structures. Mesoderm may form normally, and no cranial defect develops. Many variations of sinus formation and location of an inclusion tumor can occur, depending on the portion of the epithelial string that regresses and the portion that expands to form a tumor (Fig. 35–28). A similar series of events explains the many variations of sinus and inclusion tumor seen along the spinal column. Only the neuroschisis theory of Padget accounts for the initial adhesion of the epithelial and neural ectoderm layers that could lead to a combination of a dermal sinus and an inclusion tumor of the cranium or spine.[540,541]

The cranial dermal sinus with an associated inclusion tumor occurs along the dorsal midline, whereas the more frequent location of such tumors without an associated dermal sinus is off the midline near the orbit and in the cerebellopontine angle. Presumably a brief adhesion of the epithelium and neural ectoderm could pull loose a few epithelial cells that might develop into central nervous system inclusion tumors elsewhere than along the midline of the developing neural tube. On the other hand, inclusion tumors in these lateral locations could be due to infolding of epithelial cells

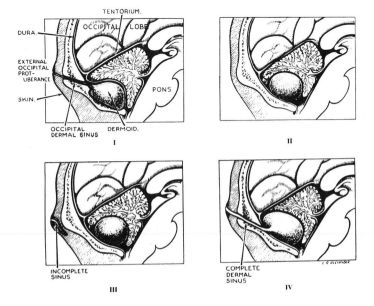

Figure 35–28 Several combinations of an occipital cranial dermal sinus and an intracranial inclusion tumor are possible, according to the portion of the epithelial-neural ectodermal adhesion that regresses and the portion of the epithelial string that forms a tumor. (From Logue, V., and Till, K.: Posterior fossa dermoid cysts with special reference to intracranial infection. J. Neurol. Neurosurg., Psychiat., *15*:1–12, 1952. Reprinted by permission.)

at the sites of the secondary optic and otic vesicles.

Whether an epidermoid, dermoid, or very rarely, teratoid or teratomatous tumor develops is very likely related to slight differences in the time of inclusion of the epithelial cells, the potential for development of the included cells, and the developmental influence of the surrounding normal tissues on the misplaced epithelial cells.

Pathology

Seventy-three patients with congenital cranial dermal sinus have been reported in the literature since Ogle, in 1855, first described an occipital dermal sinus associated with meningitis and a posterior fossa dermoid tumor in a 2½-year-old boy.*

Eighty-four per cent of the sinuses were located near the external protuberance of the occipital bone, eleven per cent at the nasion, and five per cent in the posterior parietal area. The epithelial tract in the occipital area always extends caudally from the skin opening toward the fourth ventricle owing to the posterior displacement of the neural structures during the development of the cerebral hemispheres. If the occipital dermal sinus extends intracranially the tract virtually always crosses below the tentorium cerebelli, whether or not the opening of the sinus appears to be at or even above the external occipital protuberance.[438,508] Tumors associated with an occipital dermal sinus may be extradural or subdural, between the cerebellar hemispheres or within the fourth ventricle.[438] A dermal sinus tract at the nasion may be associated with an extradural tumor within the ethmoid sinuses.[46,736] If the tract extends intracranially through the cribriform plate the tumor may develop near the anterior third ventricle or anterior horn of the lateral ventricle. A parietal dermal sinus is quite rare. One extradural tumor and a single case of a midparietal sinus extending to the subarachnoid space beneath the tentorium cerebelli have been reported.[146,582]

Eighty-nine per cent of dermal sinuses at all sites were associated with an inclusion tumor. The tumor was extradural in 18 per cent and subdural or deeper in 82 per cent. All reported tumors were dermoids except for three that were classified as epidermoid tumors.[523,582,736]

The frequency of intracranial infection or inflammation is important to the clinical presentation and management. Forty-three per cent of all cases had one or more forms of infection—infection in the cutaneous opening or meningitis or infection of the associated tumor. Meningitis may be bacterial or aseptic and secondary to leakage of tumor contents into the cerebrospinal fluid. The fatty acids rather than the cholesterol in the tumor are probably responsible for the aseptic meningeal reaction.[438,629] Thirty-two per cent of all the tumors were infected, as determined by gross appearance, histological study, or results of culture.[13,438,692] Of all cultures, 30 per cent grew *Staphylococcus aureus,* 10 per cent *Escherichia coli,* and 5 per cent *Streptococcus.* From only 5 per cent of the patients was more than one organism cultured from the cerebrospinal fluid.[757] Fifty-five per cent of the cultures showed no growth.

Associated neural or systemic anomalies are unusual, although the Klippel-Feil deformity, hemivertebrae and fused laminae, hypoplasia of the vermis of the cerebellum, and one case of occipital encephalocele have been reported.[146,438,608,757] Cranial dermal sinus is rarely associated with other forms of craniospinal dysraphism in the same patient or in other family members.[13,692]

Clinical Evaluation

Cranial dermal sinus presented between birth and 5 years of age in 84 per cent of patients, between 6 and 10 years in 4 per cent, between 11 and 20 years in 6 per cent, and later than 21 years of age in 6 per cent. The sex incidence is approximately equal.

The dermal sinus may be seen in 79 per cent of patients as a visible opening or dimple, occasionally with local thickening of the scalp due to a small dermoid tumor. A small area of scalp devoid of hair or discolored by hemangiomatous malformation may surround the mouth of the sinus from which project a few hair shafts (Fig. 35–29). Occasionally a cord can be palpated, extending from the dimple to the underlying skull.[438,508]

---

* See references 13, 46, 135, 146, 264, 402, 427, 438, 464, 469, 470, 490, 508, 523, 582, 608, 692, 736, 745, 757, 805.

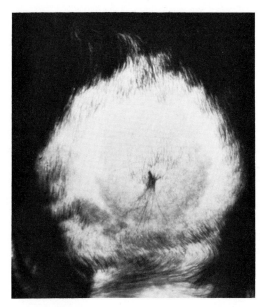

Figure 35-29 A shaven occiput shows long hairs projecting from an occipital dermal sinus surrounded by hemangiomatous discoloration of the skin. (Courtesy of H. Hoffman, M.D., F.R.C.S. (C), The Hospital for Sick Children, Toronto.)

The patients may present in one of four ways: relatively asymptomatic, with meningitis, with a mass lesion, or with a combination of meningitis and a mass lesion.

Relative Absence of Symptoms

Thirty per cent of all patients were "relatively asymptomatic" at the time of presentation. The sinus declared itself by local drainage of uninfected sebaceous debris or by localized purulent drainage or a frank scalp abscess.* Many patients presenting with meningitis or a mass lesion or a combination of the two had local warning symptoms for years before the fulminant presentation. Despite the relatively asymptomatic state, all these patients had an associated tumor at operation or at postmortem examination, and one tumor grew *Bacillus proteus*.[438] Occasional patients have an epithelial tract that extends intracranially and terminates in a tumor but has no obvious external opening.[469,470,582,736]

Meningitis

Nineteen per cent of the patients presented with symptoms of meningeal irritation. Only three patients had more than one episode of meningitis.[13,490,608]

Mass Lesion

Thirty-six per cent of the patients presented with signs of a mass lesion manifested by increased intracranial pressure due to hydrocephalus with or without cerebellar deficit. A few patients had a combination of an abscess and a tumor.[438,508,692]

Combination of Meningitis and Mass Lesion

Fifteen per cent of the patients presented with both meningitis and symptoms of a mass lesion.†

Thus, infection in an extracranial or intracranial site or both was a feature in 43 per cent of all patients, and a mass lesion occurred in 51 per cent of all patients with cranial dermal sinus. Under the age of 5 years, meningitis was the presenting feature in 42 per cent and a mass lesion in 21 per cent. In contrast, no patient over the age of 10 years presented with meningitis, but 67 per cent presented with a mass lesion.

A search should be made for a dermal sinus over the occipital region and the spine in any patient with meningitis. If more than one episode of *Staphylococcus aureus* meningitis occurs, the occiput should be shaved in the region of the external occipital protuberance.[469,470,490]

Investigation

Cerebrospinal fluid should be sent for cytological examination as well as for culture if a congenital dermal sinus is found along the craniospinal axis during the physical examination of a patient with meningitis. Epithelial debris may indicate an unsuspected tumor combined with the dermal sinus or may provide the reason for an aseptic chemical meningitis if the culture produces no causative organism.

Plain roentgenograms of the skull may be interpreted as normal in 17 per cent of patients, particularly in the young. In older children, special coned views of the occiput or tomography may show a defect corre-

---

* See references 46, 438, 464, 469, 470, 508, 582, 692, 757.

† See references 13, 438, 508, 608, 692, 757.

sponding to the dermal sinus tract or show secondary signs of increased intracranial pressure.[438,469,470,490,508] The bony changes depend upon the size and course of the epithelial tract as well as the anatomical location of the tumor relative to the calvarium. A circular defect in the occipital bone from 1 mm to 1 cm in diameter near the external occipital protuberance usually transmits the dermal sinus. A small tract may, however, pass obliquely through the thick bone of the inion and not create a visible bony defect. If the sinus is thickened by tumor near the point of entry through the dura, the bony defect is correspondingly larger. A visible defect usually forms a short channel 1 to 1.5 cm in length by 3 to 6 mm in diameter, expanding into a larger oval groove that accommodates the expanded tail of the sinus as it fuses with the tumor. An extradural tumor may erode the inner table of the occiput and produce scalloped edges over an area as large as 5 cm in diameter.

Other conditions producing a midline defect in the occipital bone must be differentiated from a dermal sinus. The defect with a dermal sinus lies in the midline and passes obliquely through the bone and is only faintly visible. The bony defects of both an emissary vein and an occipital encephalocele run horizontally and create a punched-out defect through the full thickness of the occipital bone.[438] A dermal sinus at the nasion is frequently associated with widening of the interorbital distance or frank hypertelorism and deformity and opacification of the ethmoid sinuses.

Cranial computed tomography is the most useful procedure to display an inclusion tumor, associated abscess or hydrocephalus, and even the cranial defect. A normal scan should, however, never lead to the conclusion that a dermal sinus does not extend intracranially. Angiography, ventriculography, and occasionally, pneumoencephalography are performed only if there is doubt about the diagnosis or location of the lesion.

Treatment

An asymptomatic cranial dermal sinus should be excised prophylactically

throughout its full extradural and intradural extent. Excision of the external sinus to the level of the bone is inadequate, may not prevent later meningitis, and does not reduce the risk of developing a deeper tumor.* Delaying the operation until symptoms develop may permit a neurologically damaging or fatal episode of meningitis to occur. Adhesions after the infection decrease the chance for total removal of the tumor capsule from the adjacent brain and increase the risk of complications as well. Symptomatic forms require initial management of the presenting problem of meningitis or hydrocephalus before definitive removal of the sinus and associated tumor.

Every operation for an occipital dermal sinus is designed for total excision and may require an occipital craniectomy and exploration of the fourth ventricle. Otherwise a small intradural tumor may be missed. The incision for excising the external sinus opening should be a vertical elipse that allows extension for the posterior fossa exploration. The epithelial tract always extends inferiorly toward the occipital bone. A localized craniectomy around the tract keeps the tract intact so the location of dural penetration can be found. The tract always passes below the torcular, and no problems with venous sinus bleeding have been reported. Rarely, the tract penetrates the dura at a distance from the bony defect, even extending as low as the foramen magnum.[757] When the site of penetration through the dura is found, a larger occipital craniectomy is performed and any intradural extension is removed completely.

An apparently incomplete dermal sinus still may be associated with an intradural tumor even in the presence of a normal occipital bone (cf. Fig. 35–28). Thus a craniectomy, dural opening, and inspection of the cerebellar midline should be performed whether or not the preoperative investigation was normal if the patient has a prior history of meningitis or cerebellar deficit or hydrocephalus.[438] A prior episode of meningitis may cause tenacious adhesions between the tumor capsule and surrounding brain tissue. A conservative debridement of all keratinous contents within the tumor capsule is preferable to attempts to remove

---

* See references 135, 438, 464, 469, 470, 757.

a capsule adherent to the floor of the fourth ventricle or vermis of the cerebellum.

After excision of the lesion, portions of the cutaneous opening, the deeper tract, and the terminal tumor should be sent separately for culture. In the event of postoperative meningitis, the results of the culture already growing will give the best indicator of preferred antibiotic therapy. An organism may be grown from an apparently asymptomatic lesion, in which case a course of appropriate antibiotics will be determined by the clinical status of the patient.[438] If the patient has recently had a culture-proved meningitis, antibiotic prophylaxis may be indicated, especially if the tumor spills during the operation or if a remnant of the capsule must be left attached to the brain.

Results and Prognosis

The neurological deficits produced by damaging meningitis or a late discovered tumor can be totally prevented by prophylactic excision of a cranial dermal sinus. Incomplete excision is unacceptable because meningitis and tumor formation can still occur.* The outlook for a child who has had a symptomatic cranial dermal sinus completely excised is excellent provided irreversible sequelae of infection or tumor compression have not occurred, because associated central nervous system and systemic anomalies are rare.[135,464,508,736] Rarely, excision of a dermal sinus and tumor may be followed by bacterial or chemical meningitis or a cerebellar abscess.[438,490,692]

SIMPLE SPINA BIFIDA OCCULTA

The term "simple spina bifida occulta" describes the common occurrence of a failure of complete formation of the laminae and spinous process of a vertebral unit in the absence of orthopedic, urological, or neurological deficit. Simple spina bifida occulta is usually an incidental finding on plain roentgenograms, in contrast to occult

spinal dysraphism, which entails embryological maldevelopment of neural ectoderm, notochord, mesoderm, cutaneous ectoderm, and occasionally entoderm that may predispose to orthopedic, urological or neurological deficits. Many of the forms of occult spinal dysraphism have an associated posterior spina bifida of variable extent and occasionally vertebral body anomalies. The term "spina bifida occulta" is frequently applied to the more complex and frequently symptomatic bony and neural malformations, but fails to characterize either their primary cause or their variability and complexity.

The neural arches and spinous process that form the posterior elements of the vertebral unit are formed first in cartilage and are later ossified by the activity of the paired neural arch endochondral ossification centers. The time of completion of ossification varies with the level of the spine. The lumbar spinous processes are ossified by the third year and the sacrum by the seventh year, according to anatomical studies, and fusion is detected radiographically by 7 years of age.[261,320,792] If the cartilaginous stage is abnormal, a persistent defect in the neural arch is created. Such defects are secondary to the abnormal embryological development of the neural ectoderm and notochord, according to prevailing theories of embryogenesis.[371] On the other hand, the cartilaginous precursor may form, but if one or both ossification centers are abnormal or delayed, failed or incomplete or delayed ossification may occur.

The incidence of simple spina bifida occulta varies with the level of the spine; the age, sex, ethnic, and racial origin of the patient; and whether the defect is detected by anatomical dissection or by radiography. The defect occurs at transitional levels of the spine in descending order of frequency as follows: lumbosacral, occipitocervical, thoracolumbar, and cervicothoracic.[429] In children less than 8 years of age, the radiographically identified incidence is as high as 49 per cent at S1, 13.5 per cent at L5, and 9.1 per cent at both S1 and L5, with a male predominance of 3 to 1.[375,723,724,778] The greater incidence of simple spina bifida occulta in males is in contrast to the greater incidence of occult spinal dysraphism in females. In adults, S1 is defective in 4.4 per cent and L5 in 1.7 per cent, and rarely are

---

* See references 135, 438, 464, 469, 470, 757.

L5 and S1 both defective.* The lower incidence in adults implies that most childhood defects are instances of developmental delay in ossification rather than a complete failure of the cartilaginous stage of formation. After the age of 7 years, however, simple spina bifida occulta in the lumbosacral region indicates a definite failure of ossification or cartilage formation. The incidence at other junctional sites of the spine is 1 per cent or less except for minor racial variations.†

The importance of a posterior element defect can only be determined in context with the clinical evaluation of the patient. The finding is of no importance if the individual is normal but may be quite important if combined with an orthopedic, urological, or neurological deficit. Widening of the spinal canal indicated by an increased interpedicular diameter further supports the possibility of intraspinal abnormality. On the other hand, normal posterior elements do not reduce the significance of a lumbar congenital dermal sinus, which still may penetrate intraspinally and be a source of meningitis or tumor.[19]

OCCULT SPINAL DYSRAPHISM

Occult spinal dysraphism is an entity composed of a variety of malformations of embryological development varying from the very simple to the very complex (see Table 35-1). Not all the abnormalities are "dysraphic" in the same sense as spina bifida aperta. The intrathoracic meningocele occurs predominantly with von Recklinghausen's neurofibromatosis and is not a midline fusion defect. Similarly, the caudal regression syndrome and sacrococcygeal teratoma do not blend with the rest of the malformations but are included because they may create problems in differential diagnosis for the neurosurgeon. Many authors discuss all the abnormalities of occult spinal dysraphism as if they were variations on a theme, and in a general sense, that concept is valid.‡ Indeed, this introductory

overview of occult spinal dysraphism reviews the features common to many of the malformations to avoid repetition. No one would dispute, however, that an infant born with a neurological deficit due to a large lumbosacral lipomyelomeningocele is different from an older child with recent onset of pes cavus due to a tethered cord syndrome or a normal child with meningitis due to a lumbar spinal dermal sinus. Although each is representative of a form of occult spinal dysraphism, little is gained by lumping such cases together. In the present state of development of pediatric neuroradiology, a refined diagnosis of the complexity of the intraspinal abnormality can be made preoperatively in many patients.

Pathogenesis of the Clinical Presentation

The development of the lower spinal cord from the time of fertilization to its ascent to the level of the intervertebral disc between L1 and L2 spans all of gestation and, at least, the first two postnatal months. (cf. Figs. 35-1, 35-2, and 35-3).[38] The clinical presentation of occult spinal dysraphism is usually a product of one or a combination of factors such as traction, compression, true myelodysplasia, and rarely, inflammation.

Traction

The processes of regression and "ascent" of the conus are abnormal in occult spinal dysraphism, resulting in a spinal cord fixed more caudally within the spinal canal than usual. For example, a thick, short filum terminale representing abnormal regression may prevent ascent; the conus medullaris or filum terminale may be fused into a sacral intraspinal lipoma that is continuous with an overlying subcutaneous lipoma; a bony or cartilaginous septum may penetrate the area of a diastematomyelia and prevent ascent. The cord is certainly stretched, as shown by taut, straight vessels on the lower cord rather than relaxed, tortuous vessels.[170,316,366,594] The lumbar and sacral nerve roots may run a horizontal or even upward course to their foramina of exit, and no cauda equina may form if the cord is tethered into the sacrum. Neurological dysfunction may result from the combination of stretching and repetitive trauma to the fixed cord that may occur during the process of normal flexion and extension of the spine in day-to-day activity.[67,593] Many children with occult spinal dysraphism first show symptoms when beginning to walk or during early adolescence, and the deterioration may be attributable to increased stretching of the cord during phases of rapid growth and to the child's increased activity.[366,469] The rare instance of sudden aggravation of symptoms following exercise or injury lends support to this mechanical concept.[141,700,808] More recently, Yamada has confirmed that the tethered cord is ischemic, and release of the tethering improves oxidative metabolism within the caudal cord.[806]

Compression

Compression of the neural structures may be the entire or a contributing cause of the clinical presentation of occult spinal dysraphism. Any lesion may compress or deform the neural structures directly—an intraspinal lipoma, a dermoid tumor, a neurenteric cyst, a bony septum in a diastematomyelia, or the first intact lamina proximal to a lipomyelomeningocele.[184,358]

Myelodysplasia

The neural elements may be malformed in some forms of occult spinal dysraphism such as the lipomyelomeningocele. The child is born with an existing deficit that may or may not increase with time because of traction or compression. If the initial deficit is due to myelodysplasia, then no improvement can be brought about by an operation, although progression from the secondary effects of traction or compression may be halted or even reversed.

Inflammation

Meningitis due to a congenital dermal sinus may create or aggravate a neurological deficit as a result of acute inflammation, abscess formation, tumor enlargement, or postinflammatory fibrosis.

Historical Background

The basic concepts of occult spinal dysraphism were well formulated over 50 years ago. Johnson described a child with a sacral lipoma with tethered cord who improved after operation in 1857.[362] Virchow coined the term "spina bifida occulta" in 1875 to describe the bony defect hidden by intact skin, and in 1886, von Recklinghausen suggested that hypertrichosis was an indicator of an underlying spina bifida occulta.[70] Spiller in 1916 and Brickner in 1918 stressed the association of a cutaneous malformation overlying a bony defect in patients with abnormal motor, sensory, and sphincter function and deformities of the foot and ankle.[70,700] Spiller suggested that the flexed position might increase symptoms by stretching the lower sacral roots, and Brickner believed that improvement might occur after operation if "traction and pressure" could be relieved. Brickner suggested roentgenograms of the lower spine in any patient with the described symptoms, whether or not a cutaneous malformation was present, as well as "prophylactic operation for lumbosacral lipoma to prevent future symptoms." Thus, by 1930, these and a few other papers had described many of the clinical features, the pathogenesis, and the essentials of treatment that have been refined over the following 50 years.[168,491,610,642,804]

Clinical Evaluation

In many instances the presentation of all the types is remarkably similar, and one or a combination of five features may be seen in a single patient (Fig. 35–30 and Table 35–13). Features of the clinical presentation special to a particular malformation are discussed separately in each subsection. Generally, most forms of occult spinal dysraphism show a female predominance of three to one.[19,343,358,469,752]

The developmental history of the child is an important background upon which the various clinical presentations are superimposed. The infant may have an obvious abnormality at birth that may remain stable or appear to progress. Progression can be difficult to confirm because the pre-existing deficit may hamper development, and only an appearance of progression is created. In reality, the impaired functions were always impaired but could not be assessed until the child became older. On the other hand, the infant may have been considered normal at

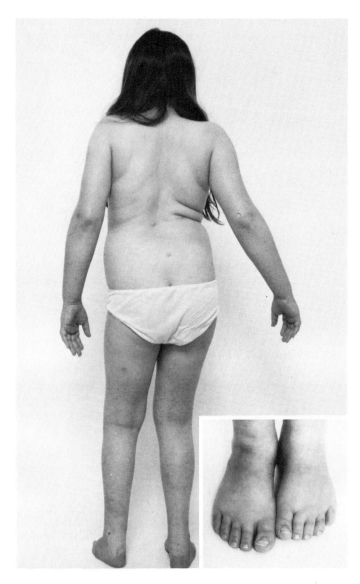

Figure 35-30 A 9-year-old girl with a lumbosacral lipoma and progressive neuromusculoskeletal syndrome. Bilateral lower limb weakness, more marked in the left, with atrophy of the calf muscles, a smaller left foot (*inset*), and thoracolumbar lordoscoliosis are present. Sphincter function was normal.

TABLE 35-13   CLINICAL PRESENTATION OF OCCULT SPINAL DYSRAPHISM*

FEATURE	PER CENT
Cutaneous malformation	83
Neuromusculoskeletal syndrome	67
Sphincter disturbance	30
Spinal curvature	12
Back pain	4

* Data from Anderson, F. M.: Pediatrics, *55*:826–835, 1975; Ingraham, F. D., and Lowrey, J. J.: New Eng. J. Med., *228*:745–750, 1943; James, C. C. M., and Lassman, L. P.: Spinal Dysraphism. London, Butterworth, 1972; Matson, D. D.: Neurosurgery of infancy and Childhood. 2nd Ed. Springfield, Ill., Charles C Thomas, 1969; Till, K.: Pediatric Neurosurgery for Paediatricians and Neurosurgeons. Oxford, Blackwell, 1975.

birth, but walking and sphincter control are delayed. Are these delays manifestations of a subtle deficit present from birth or a new deficit of recent origin? Planning the management of a child with either of these development histories is difficult. In contrast, proved regression in a previously attained function simplifies decisions regarding management.[469]

Cutaneous Malformation

An abnormality of the overlying skin is present in 83 per cent of all patients with occult spinal dysraphism, although some forms such as the tethered cord syndrome show a lesser incidence, on the order of 50 per cent.[19,343,358,469,752] The abnormalities consist of a subcutaneous lipoma; hypertrichosis, telangiectasia, or hemangioma; pigmentation; atrophic skin; or an accessory appendage (Fig. 35–31).[333,742] No particular cutaneous malformation reliably indicates the underlying abnormality, and a subcutaneous lipoma may overlie a diastematomyelia with septum, or an area of hypertrichosis may overlie an intraspinal lipoma. The absence of a cutaneous marker should never rule out consideration of occult spinal dysraphism in a patient with an appropriate clinical presentation.

Neuromusculoskeletal Syndrome

The presenting deficit is frequently a combination of neurological and orthopedic abnormalities, and the term "neuromusculoskeletal syndrome" is preferred to the term "orthopedic syndrome" introduced by James and Lassman.[358] Some variation of foot or ankle deformity, short leg, weakness, distal reflex loss, muscle atrophy, sensory loss, or trophic change, and occasionally, proximal reflex acceleration, an extensor plantar response, and spasticity occur in 67 per cent of patients, usually in one lower extremity. The combination of lower and upper motor neuron signs is frequent. Local involvement of the roots or anterior horn cells of the tethered conus medullaris accounts for the distal lower motor neuron deficit, and the stretched proximal spinal cord accounts for the upper motor neuron signs. Sensory loss in the young child may be declared by a poorly healing ulceration of a toe or maceration of the skin in the diaper area as well as by a difference in temperature between the two limbs. The involved leg may be shorter, the foot smaller, and the muscles wasted; and progressive changes in the posture of the foot and ankle are common. The shoe on the involved foot may be worn at the toe more than the shoe on the normal foot. Occasionally the involved foot requires a smaller shoe size. The earliest change in foot posture is adduction of the forefoot, which is seen best when the child is walking and may be inapparent at rest.[353,354,358] Later a frank pes cavovarus develops, and with time a cavovalgus deformity may supervene. An evolving deformity or a relapse during treatment of the foot and ankle deformity should suggest the possibility of a neurological lesion. However, occult spinal dysraphism accounts for only a few of all patients with pes cavovarus.[69,313]

Sphincter Disturbance

Bladder function is abnormal in at least 30 per cent of patients, but the abnormality rarely presents alone and is usually combined with some element of the neuromusculoskeletal syndrome. True neurogenic incontinence is usually continuous rather than interspersed with intervals of normal control and is frequently associated with evidence of perianal sensory loss or anal sphincter relaxation if a lower motor neuron deficit is present. An atonic bladder may be palpably distended, and urine may be expressed immediately after voiding.[469] On the other hand, upper motor neuron bladder dysfunction may not be associated with appropriate sensory loss or anal sphincter laxity. Thus, normal perianal sensation and anal sphincter tone cannot exclude neurogenic bladder dysfunction.[795]

Spinal Curvature

Scoliosis or other acquired progressive spinal curvatures may accompany the neuromusculoskeletal syndrome or present alone in 12 per cent of patients. The occult dysraphic lesion may be at the site of the curvature, as in a case of diastematomyelia with septum, or may be remote from the curvature, as in the tethered cord syndrome.[324] Occult spinal dysraphism should be considered in the evaluation of any new patient with scoliosis even in the absence of a cutaneous manifestation or the neuromusculoskeletal syndrome.

Back or Leg Pain

Only 4 per cent of patients have pain as part of their syndrome, and it is rarely the only symptom. Inability to touch the toes because of pain and spasm in the back region may be an early sign of deterioration.

Photographs of the feet and ankles, the entire lower extremities, and the back are useful for following the child with occult spinal dysraphism.

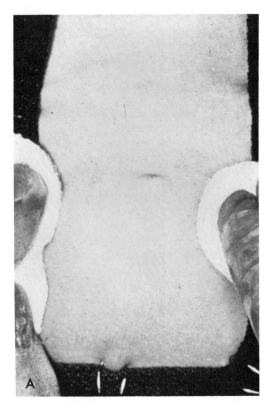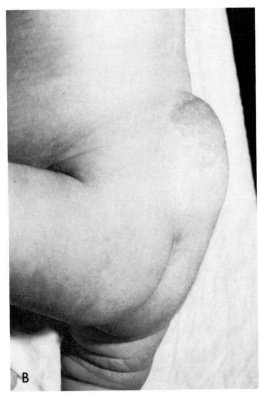

Figure 35–31 A variety of cutaneous malformations occur in occult spinal dysraphism and are frequently combined in a single patient. *A*. A lumbar congenital dermal sinus. *B*. A lumbosacral lipoma with overlying hemangiomatous discoloration.   *Illustration continued on the opposite page*

Investigation

Only general features of the investigative procedures are presented here, and specific points for each malformation are discussed in the pertinent subsection.

Plain roentgenograms are abnormal in 95 per cent of patients, but bony defects are particularly difficult to appreciate in infants. Posterior spina bifida and widening of the spinal canal are apt to be least impressive in congenital dermal sinus and the tethered cord syndrome.[19,103] Lumbosacral lipoma and diastematomyelia with septum may be accompanied by vertebral body abnormalities such as failure of segmentation, hemivertebrae, narrowed intervertebral disc space, or an ossified septum in addition to posterior spina bifida and canal widening. The normal interpedicular diameter in millimeters from birth to 5 years of age is as follows: L1, 15 to 18; L2, 16 to 18; L3, 16 to 18; L4, 17 to 19; and L5, 18 to 21; from 5 to 10 years of age: L1, 19 to 23; L2, 20 to 23, L3, 20 to 24; L4, 21 to 25; and L5, 22 to

26.[241,303] A fusiform widening of the spinal canal and a normal convex inner cortical margin to the pedicles suggest a congenital widening. A localized expansion with decalcification, flattening, or frank erosion of the medial margin of the pedicles suggests an intraspinal space-occupying lesion with rare exceptions.[139] Vertebral body abnormalities with normal posterior elements occur in neurenteric cyst and anterior sacral meningocele, whereas portions of the entire vertebral unit of the sacrum are absent in the caudal regression syndrome.

Tomography may clarify the bony abnormalities but is rarely indicated because the radiation dose is excessive and definitive myelography is indicated for the symptomatic patient.

Myelography must clarify several important points in occult spinal dysraphism: (1) the level of the conus medullaris, (2) the direction of the nerve roots, (3) the diameter of the filum terminale (normal 2 mm or less), (4) the size of the caudal sac, (5) the presence of a space-occupying le-

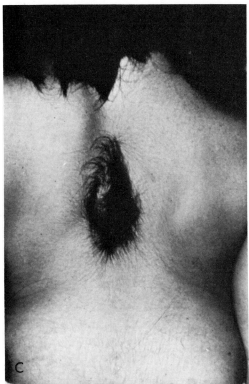

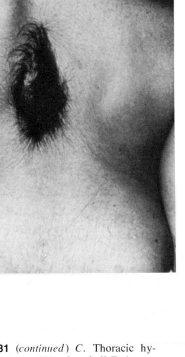

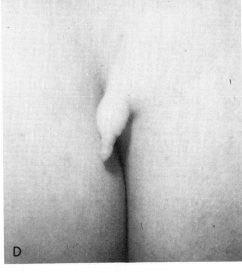

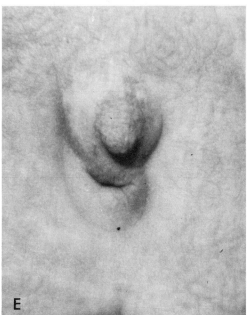

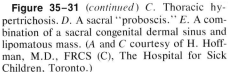

Figure 35–31 (*continued*) *C*. Thoracic hypertrichosis. *D*. A sacral "proboscis." *E*. A combination of a sacral congenital dermal sinus and lipomatous mass. (*A* and *C* courtesy of H. Hoffman, M.D., FRCS (C), The Hospital for Sick Children, Toronto.)

sion, (6) the presence of a midline septum or division of the dural tube into two compartments, (7) the presence of bands or adhesions between the dura and the neural elements or a posterior meningocele, and (8) the demonstration of multiple abnormalities. Special techniques and determination are necessary to confirm or exclude every point.* General anesthesia is usually necessary in a child under 10 years of age, particularly if air is the contrast agent, since the discomfort and duration of the procedure are greater than with positive-contrast myelography with iophendylate (Panto-

paque). The recent introduction of the water-soluble positive-contrast agent metrizamide (Amipaque), which can be combined with spinal computed tomography, may obviate the need for general anesthesia. Only a lumbar puncture is required, and the contrast medium diffuses throughout the cerebrospinal fluid without requiring aspiration at the end of the procedure. A lumbar puncture off the midline with a short-beveled nee-

---

* See references 169, 224, 280, 300, 301, 366, 451, 614, 615, 635, 716, 808.

dle risks damage to the low-lying neural elements but is preferred by Harwood-Nash and Fitz.[224,300,301] A cisternal or lateral cervical puncture avoids the spinal abnormality and is safe in occult spinal dysraphism because the Arnold-Chiari malformation does not occur.*

Prone and supine positions are necessary with positive-contrast myelography and may increase the information yield of air myelography, since in most forms of occult spinal dysraphism there is a low cord tethered toward the posterior dural sac. For many years, prone myelograms with Pantopaque were interpreted as normal because the contrast agent layers out in the capacious caudal sac anterior to the posterior lesion.[18,141,366,808] Although the anterior spinal artery shadow on the prone view may help to localize the conus, it will not do so accurately if the cord is pulled out of the anteriorly pooled contrast medium. In the supine view, the contrast layers directly over the posteriorly displaced conus, filum, and nerve roots. The conus should be considered abnormally low if it is at or below the level of the third lumbar vertebra in a child less than 5 years of age, at or below the intervertebral disc between the second and third lumbar vertebrae in one between 6 and 12 years of age, and at or below the midpoint of the second lumbar vertebra in a person over 12 years of age. The filum terminale is normally 2 mm or less in width. The spinal puncture needle should not be removed for the supine views in children, since the water-soluble contrast agent can escape from the dural puncture site into the extradural space. A sponge doughnut will protect the projecting needle. Use of a very small-diameter needle may permit its removal for the supine views. The combination of metrizamide myelography with spinal computed tomography not only aids localization of the neural elements and intraspinal abnormality but also allows a reasonably accurate diagnosis of the nature of the intraspinal lesion on the basis of density measurements. Lateral views of the spine in the prone and supine positions during air myelography may also show posterior tethering.[134,635,716] Normally the conus moves anteriorly in the canal in the prone position. Failure to do so suggests the presence of bands or adhesions, but the sign is not infallible.

Spinal computed tomography without metrizamide is not as informative but may display bony detail, a fibrous septum. lipomatous material, an anterior sacral meningocele, a lateral meningocele, or a neurenteric cyst.[293,360,734,789,803]

Treatment

Operation is clearly indicated for the patient with progressive deterioration, but is controversial in the patient with an apparently fixed deficit or no deficit at all except for a spinal dermal sinus. The pros and cons of operation are discussed in each subsection on the basis of the experience with the particular lesion.

The goal of the operation is relief of tethering and compression. Important requisites for a successful operation are: (1) general intubation anesthesia without chemical paralysis; (2) isolation of the perineum from the incision with a plastic drape; (3) visualization of the legs through a sterile plastic drape; (4) monitoring of the bladder by a cystometrographic apparatus made from a central venous pressure set-up; (5) magnified vision, bipolar coagulation, and nerve stimulation, which are essential; (6) a practice of always working from normal to abnormal areas; (7) maintenance of sinuses, bands, and lipomas intact as the exposure deepens toward the spinal canal; (8) avoidance of the assumption that a lesion ends extradurally; (9) expectation and correction of anomalies not revealed by preoperative investigation; (10) avoidance of heroic resection of a lipoma or dermoid tumor adherent to the conus or cauda equina; and (11) watertight closure of the dura with or without an autogenous graft.[469,751]

Results and Prognosis

Most authors stress that the purpose of the operation is to prevent further progression of existing deficits rather than to produce improvement.[469,751] Nevertheless, experienced neurosurgeons dealing with large numbers of patients indicate that pain is ameliorated in virtually all patients and that bladder function is improved in 52 per cent, sensory appreciation in

---

* See references 19, 92, 280, 300, 469, 716, 808.

44 per cent, and motor power in 34 per cent.[19,356,358,469,752] Many such improvements are minor, however, and do not alter the abilities of the child significantly. Deficits present at the time of birth that may be due to myelodysplasia, or long-standing deficits such as urinary incontinence, usually do not improve. Foot and ankle deformities remain stable at best, and at least 28 per cent of patients require further orthopedic procedures for the pre-existing or progressive deformity. Approximately 6 per cent of patients are made permanently worse by operation or suffer delayed deterioration that may or may not be remediable by additional operations.

CONGENITAL SPINAL DERMAL SINUS

Definition

A congenital spinal dermal sinus is an epithelium-lined tract that forms a potential communication between the skin surface in the midline along the spine and the deeper tissues. These tracts are found from the coccyx to the cervical area and may terminate in the subcutaneous tissues, on the posterior elements of the spine, in the epidural or intradural space, or in the neural elements. Posterior spina bifida may be present. An inclusion tumor may develop anywhere along the length of the tract with a preference for the intraspinal location. Presenting features may be meningitis, intraspinal abscess, or compression of the spinal cord or cauda equina. A congenital dermal sinus of the sacrococcygeal area rarely, if ever, extends intraspinally.

A pilonidal sinus is an acquired epithelium-lined tract resulting from penetration of the skin surface by the ends of broken hairs. There is a preference for the intergluteal area in hirsute adult males. Acute or chronic infection may occur. Bony defects and intraspinal extension do not occur. A pilonidal sinus is not the same lesion as the congenital sacrococcygeal dermal sinus.

Normal Embryology of the Sacrococcygeal Region

A simple sac called the coccygeal medullary vestige is the distal tip of the canalized neural tube and lies opposite the third or fourth coccygeal vertebral segment. The neural tube above this level forms the filum terminale. The extradural filum terminale is bifid in the adult, with one limb attached to the ventral sacral spinal canal and the other limb recurving to the skin surface from the region of the sacrococcygeal joint. In early development, the terminal neural tube and last coccygeal vertebral segment are intimately related and perhaps fused to the overlying epithelium. As the spine begins to elongate faster than the surrounding tissues, the overlying skin is "displaced" cranially, since it is unable to keep pace with the downward growth of the tip of the spine, and a fibrous ligament joins the periosteum over the coccygeal segments to the displaced skin. Whether the ligament is derived from a dedifferentiated portion of the neural tube or from a prolongation of connective tissue surrounding the last coccygeal vertebral segment has not been clarified.[401,459,533] The traction effect of the ligament produces a depression or dimple in the skin in the sacrococcygeal area that may be pulled in deeper to form a sinus as the buttocks develop.

Abnormal Embryology

The term "congenital spinal dermal sinus" was coined by Walker and Bucy in 1934 to describe defective separation of the epithelial ectoderm from the neural ectoderm resulting in an epithelial tract penetrating a variable distance into the deeper tissue.[778] The mesoderm may migrate normally if the tract is small, and an insignificant defect or even no bony defect will result. If a tract in the lumbar or sacral area terminates on or in the neural tube, the tract may "ascend" with the conus medullaris during 9 to 25 weeks of development. Thus, a marked discrepancy between the level of the skin opening and the terminal portion of the tract can occur. The relationship of the intraspinal level of an inclusion tumor to the skin opening may be influenced in the same manner. If the conus is tethered by the tract or by an associated form of occult spinal dysraphism, the discrepancy in levels is minimized.[*] Padget's theory of neuroschisis could apply

---

* See references 100, 221, 358, 629, 644, 775, 808.

to spinal dermal sinus, but other theories that do not involve adhesion of the two ectodermal layers have been proposed.[53,68,538,539]

Pathology

A congenital spinal dermal sinus above the sacrococcygeal level is quite rare and the incidence is unknown. In contrast, the sacrococcygeal dimple or sinus, the so-called postanal dimple, is present in 2 to 4 per cent of newborns.[304,574] The sex incidence for the benign sacrococcygeal dimple is equal, whereas males predominate over females 1.4 to 1 in the reported cases of the higher sinuses. A familial occurrence of spinal dermal sinus and other forms of cranial or spinal dysraphism is rarely reported.[13,692]

Among 92 patients reported in the literature, 87 per cent had a spinal dermal sinus above the sacrococcygeal junction.* The sinus was located in the cervical area in 1 per cent, in the thoracic area in 10 per cent, in the lumbar area in 41 per cent, in the lumbosacral area in 12 per cent, in the sacrum in 23 per cent, and at the sacrococcygeal junction in 13 per cent. The paucity of reported cases of sacrococcygeal sinus, in contrast to their everyday occurrence, indicates the benign nature of the lesion at the sacrococcygeal location. Only three cases near that level have been associated with meningitis, and some doubt exists whether the sinuses were actually of the low sacral rather than the sacrococcygeal type.[605,674,701] Rarely, two dermal sinuses are present.†

The outer portion of the tract is usually lined by stratified squamous epithelium with dermal appendages accounting for the small hairs frequently seen projecting from the orifice of the sinus. The lining of the deeper tract is simpler, and dermal appendages disappear in deeper portions of the tract.[435] Of the reported sinuses, 7 per cent terminated in the extraspinal tissues; 21 per cent in the extradural space or attached to the dura; 7 per cent in the subdural space; 31 per cent in the subarachnoid space; and

27 per cent attached to either the filum terminale, nerve roots, or spinal cord; for 7 per cent the terminal point was not stipulated.

Fifty per cent of the patients with dermal sinus had an inclusion tumor. These tumors were classified as epidermoid in 13 per cent, dermoid in 83 per cent, and teratoma in 4 per cent. Epidermoids are composed strictly of the epidermal layer and are filled with keratinous debris; dermoids contain dermal appendages such as hair follicles and sebaceous and sweat glands in addition to the epidermal cells; teratomas are composed of derivatives of all three embryonic germ layers.[57] Forty-two per cent of all tumors were asymptomatic as far as neural compression was concerned and were found incidentally at operations performed when the diagnoses had not been made preoperatively. Inclusion tumors in the lumbar region are located in the subarachnoid space among the roots of the cauda equina but frequently attach to the conus medullaris. Above the level of L1 and L2, the tumor is often intimately related to, if not frankly within, the thoracic spinal cord. Fewer than 20 per cent of all intraspinal inclusion tumors are associated with a dermal sinus, and usually the posterior elements of the spine are normal in the absence of an accompanying dermal sinus.[28,180,319,453]

Infection is one of the most serious risks of congenital dermal sinus, and 61 per cent of all patients had one or a combination of infections: meningitis (54 per cent of all patients), intraspinal abscess (23 per cent of all patients), infected tumor (30 per cent of all tumors). In patients with meningitis, the responsible organism was *Escherichia coli* in 18 per cent, *Staphylococcus aureus* in 16 per cent, anaerobic gram-negative organisms in 15 per cent, *Proteus* in 10 per cent, *Hemophilus influenzae* in 6 per cent, pneumococcus in 4 per cent, streptococcus in 3 per cent, and meningococcus in 1 per cent; there was no growth in 27 per cent. Nineteen per cent of patients had more than one organism cultured. Thus, gram-negative organisms (49 per cent) predominate over gram-positive organisms (24 per cent) as a cause of meningitis in spinal dermal sinus in contrast to the reverse situation in cranial dermal sinus. Multiple organisms as well are more frequently found in spinal dermal sinus. The abscesses were extradural in 14 per cent, subdural in 43 per cent, within a

---

* See references 15, 19, 55, 57, 63, 64, 100, 117, 119, 129, 229, 241, 251, 260, 291, 292, 304, 318, 358, 385, 393, 435, 441, 471, 502, 508, 530, 561, 565, 566, 574, 586, 589, 605, 623, 629, 636, 644, 650, 659, 674, 701, 744, 753, 757, 775, 778, 780, 781.

† See references 304, 358, 586, 644, 781, 808.

tumor in 5 per cent, within the spinal cord in 24 per cent, and not specified in 14 per cent. Twenty-nine per cent of all abscesses occurred without a prior history of meningitis. Intraneural abscesses tend to dissect a great distance up and down the cord rather than remaining localized. On occasion, an abscess may develop in the conus from infection spreading up a patent filum terminale from a sacral or lumbosacral dermal sinus.[260,508,674,780] Intraspinal infection increases the operative risk because tenacious adhesions develop between the neural elements and the tract or the abscess wall or the tumor.[469]

Dimples or sinuses may occur with any form of occult spinal dysraphism and are not pathognomonic of an epithelial tract extending intraspinally. Cutaneous dimples or sinuses frequently accompany a lumbosacral lipoma that extends intraspinally, and sinuses have been reported with diastematomyelia with and without a septum, with an arachnoid cyst, with a lumbar meningocele, and with the tethered cord syndrome.*

All the dermal sinuses reported have occurred along the dorsal midline except for a single case of recurrent meningitis due to a ventral tract extending from the perineum through the vertebral body of L5 to expand into an intraspinal teratoma.[221]

---

* See references, 15, 57, 137, 291, 319, 358, 471, 472 475, 586, 674, 716.

Clinical Evaluation

Sacrococcygeal Region

A dimple or sinus in the sacrococcygeal area does not communicate with the dura or subarachnoid space or neural structures except for rare reported cases (Fig. 35–32).†
If traction is put on skin above the sinus and the tract relaxes, then the sinus is directed cranially. If the sinus tightens, then it extends caudally. A caudally directed sinus in the sacrococcygeal region conforms to the description of the ligament between the tip of the coccyx and the overlying skin and will not pass intraspinally.[533] More frequently, the sacrococcygeal sinus points cranially but attaches to the tip of the coccyx or the sacrococcygeal junction. Intradural extension would be rare indeed, since the dural sac ends at the level of the second sacral segment.[805] Conceivably, local infection in the depths of a sacrococcygeal dermal sinus could lead to a sacral abscess and subsequent meningitis, but such an occurrence is a rarity, considering the overall incidence of sacrococcygeal sinus.[304]

Above the Sacrococcygeal Region

The higher sinuses are of greater clinical importance, and 79 per cent of patients reported in the literature have presented

---

† See references 304, 574, 605, 674, 701, 744.

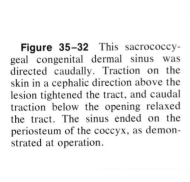

Figure 35–32 This sacrococcygeal congenital dermal sinus was directed caudally. Traction on the skin in a cephalic direction above the lesion tightened the tract, and caudal traction below the opening relaxed the tract. The sinus ended on the periosteum of the coccyx, as demonstrated at operation.

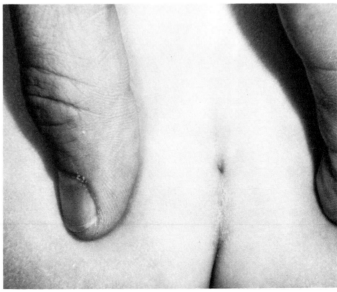

between birth and 5 years of age, 8 per cent between 6 and 10 years, 9 per cent between 11 and 20 years, and only 4 per cent over 20 years of age.

The external appearance of the dermal sinus varies according to the accompanying epidermal and mesodermal abnormalities (see Fig. 35–31A and E). The sinus may be an almost invisible pimple with or without a few hairs projecting from the orifice, or the opening may be obvious. Some other cutaneous abnormality such as hemangiomatous discoloration, hypertrichosis, or pigmentation may distract the eye, and the sinus opening must be diligently searched for within the cutaneous marker. Examination with the plus 10 lens of an ophthalmoscope may be helpful.[55] A palpable cord may extend deep from the orifice or other cutaneous malformation.[508]

The patients present in one of four ways: relatively asymptomatic, with meningitis, with a mass lesion, or with a combination of meningitis and a mass lesion.

Relative Absence of Symptoms

Twenty-four per cent of the patients were either totally or relatively asymptomatic with symptoms restricted to local drainage of sebaceous material or to localized purulent drainage. Mild local symptoms may precede symptoms of meningitis or a mass lesion for weeks to years. Of the patients who ultimately developed meningitis, however, 38 per cent did not have preceding local inflammation or drainage.

Meningitis

Thirty-six per cent of the patients reported in the literature presented with meningitis. An infant who has repeated episodes of meningitis or from whom an organism out of keeping with his age or multiple organisms have been cultured must be searched carefully for a dermal sinus. A dermal sinus or intraspinal abscess or infected tumor should be suspected if purulent meningitis does not respond to appropriate antibiotics or relapses after an adequate course of antibiotics.[566]

Mass Lesion

Twenty-one per cent of patients presented with a neurological deficit signifying an intraspinal mass lesion. In these patients and in those with a mass lesion and meningitis, the neurological deficit was of the lower motor neuron type in 49 per cent, of the upper motor neuron type in 27 per cent, and there were combined signs in 16 per cent; 8 per cent were not described. These percentages reflect the preponderance of dermal sinuses in the lumbar and sacral regions. The neural compression was due to tumor alone in 35 per cent, to intraspinal abscess alone in 30 per cent, to tumor and meningitis in 21 per cent, and to intraspinal abscess in addition to or within a tumor in 14 per cent.* Patients with a simple inclusion tumor usually present in older childhood and frequently have a history of several years of episodic exacerbation and remission of neurological deficit. On the other hand, an intraspinal abscess or infected tumor is more likely to present acutely and progress rapidly.

Combination of Meningitis and Mass Lesion

Nineteen per cent of patients presented with a combination of meningitis and an intraspinal mass lesion.

Thus, clinically evident infection was a feature in 55 per cent of all patients, and a mass lesion in 40 per cent of all patients. Under the age of 5 years, meningitis or abscess was the reason for presentation in 86 per cent, and a tumor in 14 per cent of patients. Over the age of 6 years, meningitis or abscess was the reason for presentation in 53 per cent, and a tumor in 47 per cent.

Investigation

The lumbar puncture performed in a case of meningitis with spinal dermal sinus may be confusing. The puncture may be "dry" if a tumor fills the spinal canal, or keratinous debris may be obtained on aspiration.[319,530,589] Purulent material from the lumbar area and clearer fluid from the cisternal area suggest an intraspinal abscess. Cytological examination of cerebrospinal fluid for epithelial debris should be requested for any patient with a dermal sinus to detect an unsuspected tumor.

Probing the sinus to assess its depth and

---

* See references 229, 260, 385, 508, 530, 644, 674, 753, 778, 780, 781.

direction, or the injection of positive-contrast material into the orifice for roentgenography, or the injection of a dye at operation to outline the extent of the sinus will give inaccurate information and is potentially dangerous. Epithelial debris may fill the deeper portions of the sinus and prevent passage of the injected material or probe to the full depth of the sinus. Forceful injection or probing may force contaminated debris intraspinally to cause infection. A sinus that is not anatomically patent may still cause meningitis. Furthermore, a sinus must always be explored to its full extent under direct vision, regardless of the results of any investigative procedure.

Plain roentgenograms of the spine are of little help in deciding whether a dermal sinus should be explored, but they may guide the extent of the procedure or indicate associated abnormalities. No fewer than 34 per cent of patients reported in the literature had normal roentgenograms of the spine. At operation, a small percentage of those patients were found to have minor posterior element defects. Normal spine roentgenograms do not rule out intraspinal extension of the dermal sinus nor do they rule out an associated inclusion tumor. Numerous accounts of a dermal sinus passing through the interspinous ligament or the ligamentum flavum or a sacral hiatus have been published.[*] In addition, a posterior element defect in the region of the dermal sinus does not necessarily mean that the sinus extends into the intraspinal space through that defect.[508,778] Widening of the interpedicular diameter, erosion of the medial aspects of the pedicles, scalloping of the posterior vertebral bodies, or anomalies of the vertebral bodies suggest either an intraspinal inclusion tumor or an associated form of occult spinal dysraphism such as lipoma, diastematomyelia, or meningocele.[†] Since the intraspinal portion of a dermal sinus that is attached to the neural structures may ascend within the spinal canal, the roentgenographic abnormalities may be several segments higher than the level of the sinus.

Myelography has been performed in only 20 per cent of the patients with dermal sinus who have been reported in the literature, which reflects the time period and the operative principle that intradural exploration is indicated by the course of the sinus. Even a normal myelogram does not exclude either an intradural extension of the sinus or a small inclusion tumor.[471,744,751,805] Metrizamide myelography and spinal computed tomography should, however, be performed for several reasons. If the dermal sinus is tenuous and does not appear to extend through the dura at operation, the surgeon is certainly encouraged to limit the scope of his exploration to avoid needless removal of multiple lumbar laminae and the risk of late spinal curvatures. In this situation, the surgeon and the patient will benefit if the myelogram has shown the site of penetration of the dermal sinus into the spinal canal as a filling defect on the supine views, or rarely, as contrast filling the extraspinal sinus, or has shown an asymptomatic tumor higher in the spine.[19,441,465] Myelography may clarify whether a neurological deficit is due to an inclusion tumor with a smooth, lamellated, or flaky surface or to an unsuspected form of occult spinal dysraphism at the level of the sinus or higher. Either situation may require a modified operative plan.[‡] Myelography is not advisable in the presence of an infected dermal sinus or during or soon after an episode of meningitis.[19]

Treatment

All authors agree that prophylactic removal of a dermal sinus located above the sacrococcygeal region is indicated as soon as it is discovered. On the other hand, the management of the more common sacrococcygeal sinus is controversial. Since they so rarely extend intraspinally, operation is not indicated in the majority of cases.[358,586] Some authors have suggested that a sacrococcygeal sinus should be excised if the bottom cannot be seen despite pressure on the surrounding skin.[304,574,674] Considering that 2 to 4 per cent of newborns have a sacrococcygeal deep dimple or sinus, prophylactic removal to prevent possible local infection is unreasonable in view of the number of patients involved. The depth of a

---

* See references 15, 129, 251, 304, 393, 435, 508, 565, 586, 623, 629, 644, 744, 775, 778.

† See references 57, 241, 291, 303, 438, 469, 471, 744.

‡ See references 31, 119, 291, 358, 435, 808.

sinus visualized externally should not be a criterion for excision, since both meningitis and tumor may be associated with a sinus whether or not its depths are visualized. If there is any question that the sinus is actually over the lower sacrum or has a lipomatous element or is associated with sacral bony defects, then the sinus should be excised (see Fig. 35–31E).

If local infection of the dermal sinus or meningitis is present when the patient is first seen, the sinus opening and cerebrospinal fluid should be sterilized by appropriate antibiotic therapy prior to operation. If the cerebrospinal fluid cannot be sterilized or an immediate relapse occurs after appropriate antibiotic therapy, it is likely that a repository of sepsis such as an abscess or infected tumor exists in the intraspinal space. In this difficult situation, operation must be performed under cover of appropriate antibiotics in spite of the infection.[441,566,636]

The goal of operation is total removal of the lesion, and only a surgeon prepared to perform laminectomy and intradural neurological operations should explore a congenital dermal sinus. A culture from a locally discharging dermal sinus is sent three days prior to operation to serve as a guide to the local bacterial colonization. The operation is performed under general anesthesia in the prone position with preparation made for a cephalad extension of the incision. The mouth of the sinus is excised in an ellipse, and the underlying fibrous tract kept intact down through the fascia to the posterior bony elements or to the fibrous tissue bridging the spina bifida. The dura is exposed, and the attachment of the tract to the dura is excised in an ellipse. The dura is opened more widely to visualize the subdural and subarachnoid spaces immediately under the fibrous tract. If the tract extends beneath the dura or if a tumor is identified, the incision and laminectomy are carried as far cephalad as required to expose the entire lesion. Aggressive attempts at total excision may cause neural damage if adhesions between the tumor capsule and neural tissue are dense.[180,435,469,586,753]

A portion of the sinus and the tumor, if present, and cerebrospinal fluid are sent for culture, especially when there is a history of prior infection.[441,469] Prophylactic antibiotics are controversial but are advised if the operation follows a recent episode of meningitis, the antibiotic being selected on the basis of the previous organism. Prophylactic antibiotics are not used for a prophylactic operation unless the sinus is locally discharging.

Results and Prognosis

A prophylactic operation should result in minimal morbidity, no deaths, and an excellent prognosis for normal development. Occasionally, meningitis may occur postoperatively after excision of an infected or even an asymptomatic lesion.[15,441,781] Incomplete superficial cosmetic removal of a dermal sinus is condemned. Numerous examples of inadequate operations followed by later episodes of meningitis or neural compression by an unrecognized tumor have been reported.*

PILONIDAL SINUS

Hodges coined the term "pilonidal sinus" in 1880 to describe a congenital dimple in the sacrococcygeal region that secondarily fills with hair and produces local infection. The term has, however, also been used to describe an acquired sinus secondary to the penetration of ends of broken hair into the skin followed by a granulomatous inflammatory reaction in the deeper tissues. This mechanism is postulated to explain the intergluteal pilonidal sinus in hirsute adult males and similar sinuses seen at other areas of the body such as the axilla, the web space of the hand in barbers, and the perineum.[9,335,549,550,696] Some authors believe, however, that most pilonidal sinuses in adults represent secondary infection of a congenital sacrococcygeal dermal sinus present from infancy rather than an acquired lesion.[304,335,549,550] The term "congenital sacrococcygeal dermal sinus" should be applied to all dimples or sinuses in this area seen in infancy and childhood. The term pilonidal sinus should be restricted to the acquired sinuses in adults, since the term conveys no understanding of the embryological origin of the lesion in the pediatric age group.

---

* See references, 15, 229, 241, 304, 358, 385, 471, 508, 565, 586, 659, 805.

THE TETHERED CORD SYNDROME

Definition

The tethered cord syndrome consists of an abnormally low conus medullaris tethered by one or more forms of intradural abnormality such as a short, thickened filum terminale, fibrous bands or adhesions, or a totally intradural lipoma. The clinical distinctions merit separating this heterogeneous group from the other forms of occult spinal dysraphism listed in Table 35–1. Cutaneous manifestations occur in only 54 per cent of patients; the bony defects are simpler, and the frequency of remote scoliosis as a presenting symptom is as great as for diastematomyelia with septum. The tethered cord syndrome has been known by many names such as the tethered conus, tight filum terminale, filum terminale syndrome, meningocele manqué, and the preferred form, the tethered cord syndrome.*

Abnormal Embryology

The embryological origin of the various forms of the tethered cord syndrome are unknown. Tethering of a sacral cord to the caudal dural sac by a lipoma presumably involves an inclusion of adipose cells during early development similar to the formation of the more complex lumbosacral lipoma. An abnormality of cannalization and regression must contribute to the isolated, short, thick, tethering filum terminale. The source of bands and adhesions fixing the cord or roots to the dura is not clear. James and Lassman suggest the possibility that a meningocele sac that failed to develop fully or atrophied soon after formation, resulting in adhesions of nerve roots or the filum terminale near the neck of the sac (atretic meningocele, meningocele manqué), is responsible.[358,359]

Pathology

The intradural disorder in the tethered cord syndrome is generally simpler than in other forms of occult spinal dysraphism such as lumbosacral lipoma or diastematomyelia with septum, and more frequently

occurs with no cutaneous anomaly. The common intradural abnormality of a short filum terminale, bands or adhesions, and intradural lipoma may overlap in any single patient. For example, the filum terminale may be short and thickened, located in the midline, and be the only source of the cord tethering, or may blend into adhesions to the dural sac off the midline.[18,141,324,358,366] The short filum may be enlarged by a lipoma or fuse with a small lipoma in the caudal dural sac. Fibrous bands may tether the conus or portions of the cauda equina to the dura, or the neural structures may be adherent directly to the dura. In the case of a short filum or bands or adhesions, the conus is usually at L5 or above. On occasion the conus is fused into the sacral dural sac by a lipoma so that no cauda equina ever develops.[324]

A cutaneous anomaly is present in approximately half the patients but generally has no connection with the intradural abnormality. A subcutaneous lipoma that penetrates all the tissue planes to fuse with the neural structures is usually considered a form of lumbosacral lipoma. The true importance of the tethered cord syndrome lies in the frequent absence of a cutaneous anomaly, the simpler bony defects, and the remote scoliosis as a presenting feature.

Clinical Evaluation

The tethered cord syndrome has been clarified only recently, and its true incidence in the overall picture of occult spinal dysraphism is unknown. The frequency may be higher than the early reports of the 1950's and 1960's might suggest because of improved prone and supine myelographic technique, metrizamide myelography with spinal computed tomography, and an increased awareness of the syndrome.† The sex ratio appears to be approximately two to one for females, as for other forms of occult spinal dysraphism.[18,141,244,366,451]

Of the 48 patients reported in the literature, 31 per cent presented between birth and 5 years of age, 21 per cent between 6 and 10 years, 42 per cent between 11 and 20 years, and 6 percent over 21 years of age.‡

---

* See references, 224, 244, 324, 358, 366, 451, 751, 808.

† See references 18, 141, 224, 244, 302, 324, 366, 451, 751.

‡ See references 18, 141, 244, 276, 324, 366, 451, 776.

Cutaneous manifestations are absent in 46 per cent of patients and cannot be relied upon as a clue.[322] The patients with cutaneous manifestations showed hypertrichosis in 22 per cent, subcutaneous lipoma without intraspinal extension in 15 per cent, and hemangiomatous discoloration, congenital dermal sinus, or multiple manifestations in 17 per cent. Gait difficulty with weakness of one or occasionally both legs occurred in 93 per cent of patients, with visible muscle atrophy, a short limb, or ankle deformity in 63 per cent. Sensory deficit was present in 70 per cent and bladder dysfunction in 40 per cent of patients. Only 4 per cent of the patients presented with bladder dysfunction in the absence of motor, sensory, or skeletal abnormalities. Pain in the back or leg or in the arches of the feet occurred in 37 per cent. Hoffman and associates noted that inability to touch the toes was an early sign, as well as the development or the progression of signs during growth spurts. A relatively high rate of occurrence of scoliosis or kyphosis was noted in 29 per cent, predominantly because of including Hoffman's patients.[324]

Investigation

Plain roentgenograms showed posterior spina bifida of the low lumbar and sacral spine in 98 per cent, but the interpedicular distance is frequently normal and vertebral body anomalies are unusual. The presence or absence of bony malformations in the region of the spinal curvature higher in the spine has not been clarified adequately in the literature. Prone and supine myelography and more recently metrizamide myelography with spinal computed tomography show the low conus, which is a necessary feature of the syndrome, and a variety of abnormalities that may be difficult to characterize. A filum more than 2 mm in width is pathological and suggests a short, thick filum terminale. On occasion, the distal spinal cord is so attenuated and tapered owing to traction that it appears as a thick filum or a filum with adherent roots. The cord shadow may extend into the sacral dural sac in a sacralized cord with or without a filling defect of a lipoma, and this picture may be simulated by an intrafilar lipoma widening the filum terminale. In the former case, nerve roots originate from the shadow, which indicates that the structure is the spinal cord. The myelogram may appear normal, even with excellent myelographic technique, and the clinical presentation would decide the advisability of operation.[324]

Treatment

The complexity of the operation varies with the complexity of the lesion. A short filum terminale without other associated abnormality can be exposed through a limited lumbosacral laminectomy through the area of the spina bifida to display the thickened filum tenting the dorsal dural sac. The filum is stimulated to insure proper identification and then is divided between two clips. When the filum is the significant tethering mechanism, the divided ends may separate up to 2.5 cm.[324] Operation in the presence of bands, adhesions, or a sacralized cord with lipoma may be more difficult. Meticulous separation of the neural tissue adherent to the dural sac or adhesive bands between dura and neural tissue may relax the cord and nerve roots. The filum terminale should be sectioned as well. A sacralized cord and lipoma can be untethered by exposing the caudal sacral dural sac and separating the lipoma from the dura, as opposed to separating the lipoma from the conus. On occasion, the myelogram may suggest a sacralized cord, but a lipoma of the filum terminale is found. If the nerve roots are easily separated, the filum and its lipoma can be excised.

Results and Prognosis

In contrast to the earlier literature on the tethered cord syndrome, recent reports note earlier diagnosis when deficits are less severe and improvement is more likely. The 48 patients reported in the literature had improved motor function in 84 per cent, improved bladder function in 87 per cent, and cessation of pain in virtually every patient. The less complicated abnormality and lower incidence of primary myelodysplasia may also contribute to the good results.

The spinal curvature is an important feature of the tethered cord syndrome. Thirty per cent of the patients reported by Hoffman and co-workers had scoliosis either as a primary presenting complaint or as a secondary feature and were being considered for an operation for scoliosis.[324] Of these patients, 33 per cent had arrest or improvement of their scoliosis after operation and required no spinal fusion. The remaining two thirds of the patients had spinal fusion either under the same anesthetic or at a later date because the scoliosis progressed.

LUMBOSACRAL LIPOMA

Definition

A subcutaneous lipoma, which commonly overlies the lumbar or sacral spine, may extend through a posterior spina bifida to an extradural or intradural location to attach to a low-lying conus medullaris, the cauda equina, or the filum terminale. A neuromusculoskeletal syndrome may be due to primary myelodysplasia of the involved neural structures or to secondary traction or compression. A subcutaneous lipoma does not always extend intraspinally itself and may be associated with another form of occult spinal dysraphism such as a congenital dermal sinus or a diastematomyelia with septum or a thickened filum terminale.[358,383,407,586,747]

Abnormal Embryology

A confluent subcutaneous and intraspinal lipoma probably develops in a manner analogous to a congenital dermal sinus and an intraspinal dermoid tumor. Inclusion of adipose cells from the overlying mesodermal tissues into the neural tube or the caudal cord developing by canalization can explain the typical lipoma that transgresses several tissue planes.[19,40] Tethering through the tissue planes occurs during early embryological development and restricts the ascent of the conus, resulting in a low-lying, stretched spinal cord.[644,808] The presence of an abnormal amount of fat within the spinal canal at levels of intact laminae may lead to compression of the neural elements.

Pathology

Intraspinal lipoma unassociated with spinal dysraphism accounts for 1 per cent of primary intraspinal tumors, shows no sex preference, becomes symptomatic in a mature age group, and occurs commonly in the thoracic region.[99,191,586,611,747]

Lumbosacral lipoma, on the other hand, accounts for 32 per cent of all cases in large series of occult spinal dysraphism and usually presents in infancy or childhood. A two to one preference for the female sex is shown in 135 cases reported in the literature.* Transitional forms between lumbosacral lipoma associated with occult spinal dysraphism and intradural lipomas unassociated with spinal dysraphism have been reported in the cervical, thoracic, and lumbar regions.[91,99,363,714]

The subcutaneous mass is composed of normal adipose tissue without a capsule and lies over the defect in the lumbodorsal fascia above the spina bifida like the cap on a mushroom. On occasion, the subcutaneous mass is small, with a narrow intraspinal communication. The stalk of the lipoma passing intraspinally merges with the dura and usually either the filum terminale, the cauda equina, the conus medullaris, or even the more proximal spinal cord (Fig. 35–33).[184,358,437,644,768] If the cord is tethered in the sacrum, the caudal nerve roots may run directly lateral to their intervertebral foramina of exit, and the cauda equina and filum terminale do not exist. The intraspinal extension may vary from a small area of fusion of the stalk to the neural elements to a large mass filling the entire lumbar and sacral spinal canal with the neural elements embedded within or compressed by the lipoma (Fig. 35–34).[407] The neural elements remain within the spinal canal, however.

The lipomyelomeningocele is more complex. The subcutaneous fat has a broad area of fusion with the neural elements through deficient dura, and like the neural plaque in a myelomeningocele, the spinal cord herniates out of the spinal canal into the lipoma (Fig. 35–35). This lesion is more likely to be associated with primary myelodysplasia and a congenital neuromusculoskeletal syndrome. The first intact lamina above the lipoma may be a fibrous or cartilaginous band that can compress the herniating spinal cord and contribute to a progressive neurological

---

* See references 19, 44, 184, 267, 342, 346, 358, 383, 407, 437, 469, 511, 586, 612, 698, 732, 747, 752, 768, 809.

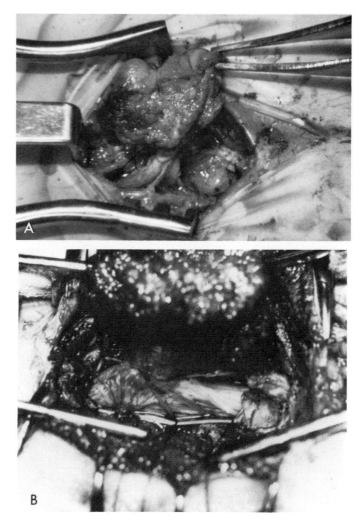

Figure 35–33 *A*. A small subcutaneous sacral lipoma fuses intradurally with a filum terminale thickened by lipoma. *B*. A subcutaneous lipoma fuses with a low conus over a small area at the level of the dura. (*B* from Villarejo, F. J., Blazquez, M. G., and Gutierrez-Diaz, J. A.: Intraspinal lipomas in children. Child's Brain, *2*:361–370, 1976. Reprinted by permission.)

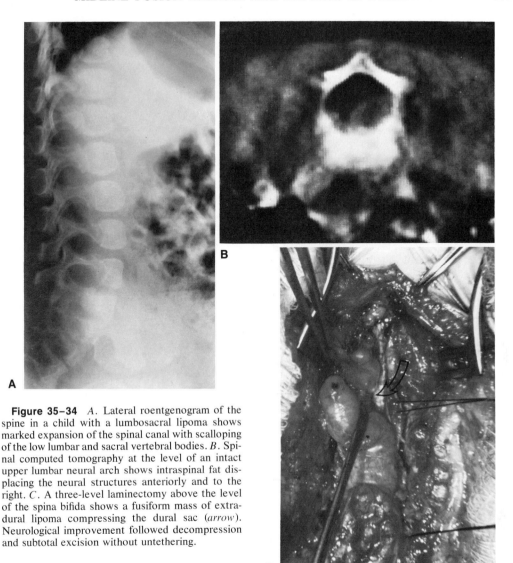

Figure 35–34 *A.* Lateral roentgenogram of the spine in a child with a lumbosacral lipoma shows marked expansion of the spinal canal with scalloping of the low lumbar and sacral vertebral bodies. *B.* Spinal computed tomography at the level of an intact upper lumbar neural arch shows intraspinal fat displacing the neural structures anteriorly and to the right. *C.* A three-level laminectomy above the level of the spina bifida shows a fusiform mass of extradural lipoma compressing the dural sac (*arrow*). Neurological improvement followed decompression and subtotal excision without untethering.

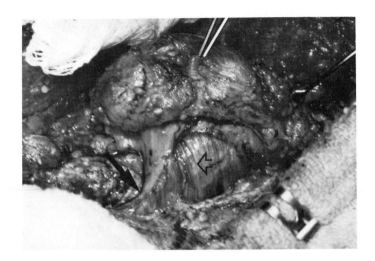

Figure 35–35 This lumbosacral lipomyelomeningocele herniated from the spinal canal around the first intact neural arch above the spina bifida (*level indicated by solid arrow*). The extraspinal cord is capped by the subcutaneous lipoma, and the nerve rootlets are draped over the lipomatous tissue anterior to the cord (*open arrow*). Proximal muscle power improved postoperatively.

deficit after birth.[184] As a result of the variation in complexity of the lipoma, the associated bony abnormalities of the posterior elements and the vertebral bodies vary greatly.

Histologically, the intraspinal lipoma is normal adipose tissue laced by connective tissue bands, and rarely other tissue elements are present such as islands of cartilage, anomalous bone, striated muscle, or endometrial tissue.[44,274,383,407,809] The site of attachment of the lipoma to the neural tissue consists of an intermingling of fat pannicles and dense collagenous connective tissue that may penetrate deeply into the neural tissue. The clinical implication is that total removal of a lipoma from the neural elements may be hazardous.[198]

Clinical Evaluation

The subcutaneous lipoma is located in the lumbosacral area in over 90 per cent of patients and is usually apparent at birth. The mass rarely enlarges with time unless there is some other tissue element within the lipoma, such as a meningocele or teratoma, or a general increase in body fat occurs.[44,809] Full-thickness normal skin covers the mass in 50 per cent of cases, and the remainder show variations of hemangiomatous discoloration, dimpling or sinus formation, hypertrichosis, or rarely, a projecting appendage over the subcutaneous lump (see Figs. 35–30 and 35–31 B, D, and E). The lesion is usually midline, soft, compressible but not cystic, and dense to transillumination. A lipomatous mass lateral to the midline that can be transilluminated suggests a component of meningocele or myelomeningocele within the lipoma.[184,407] The underlying spina bifida may be palpable. Since a degree of sacral agenesis is present in 24 per cent of patients, the sacrum should be palpated posteriorly and anteriorly by rectal examination.[184,612]

The majority of patients with lumbosacral lipoma are asymptomatic at birth.[184,732] The few children who evidence a form of the neuromusculoskeletal syndrome at birth are likely to have primary myelodysplasia with a lipomyelomeningocele or a complicated intraspinal lipoma. The lipoma may produce a neurological deficit or worsen an existing deficit after birth by traction or by compression from the lipoma or the first proximal lamina in a lipomyelomeningocele. All authors are unanimous in their belief that the majority of asymptomatic lipomas will produce symptoms at some time in the future.* The number of patients who remain asymptomatic and never come to the physician's attention, however, is unknown.

The age at which symptoms develop and the rapidity of progression are unpredictable. Symptoms usually develop in early childhood but have been reported as early as at 3 weeks of age. Rarely the onset is in the late teens, early twenties, or even later.[184,407,747] The deficits usually progress over a period of years, but an abrupt deterioration to an incapacitating degree can occur and occasionally is related to trauma.[44,383,407,732,808] Approximately 70 per cent of the children manifest a form of the neuromusculoskeletal syndrome. Predominantly sacral sensory deficit is present in 62 per cent and bladder malfunction in 44 per cent. Three quarters of all patients with bladder malfunction also show some other evidence of motor, sensory, or reflex change. Only 9 per cent of all children with lumbosacral lipoma present with bladder dysfunction in isolation from any other symptoms or signs. The incidence of sensory deficit and bladder dysfunction may actually be higher, since these modalities are difficult to assess in infants and young children.† Anal sphincter dysfunction and the occurrence of spinal curvatures are rarely mentioned.[44,184,383] The presenting problem is more often bladder dysfunction or leg pain when symptoms begin after childhood.[407,747]

Clinical examination alone does not reveal the exact form or the complexity of the intraspinal abnormality. The physician cannot predict whether a child with a lumbosacral swelling will or will not develop neurological deficit, the exact nature of the neurological deficit, or whether the deficit will occur rapidly or slowly; and he certainly cannot predict the response to treatment once the deficit has developed. The unpredictability of these lesions has led the majority of authors to suggest prophylactic

---

* See references 44, 184, 267, 359, 407, 732, 768, 808.

† See references 44, 184, 383, 407, 732, 768.

investigation and operation for asymptomatic lumbosacral lipoma.*

Investigation

Plain roentgenograms show posterior spina bifida of varying extent in 86 per cent of patients.† Patients whose radiographs appear normal may have defects at operation or may have a superficial lesion with no intraspinal extension. Other abnormalities such as widening of the interpedicular diameter and scalloping of the posterior vertebral bodies suggest an intraspinal mass (see Fig. 35–34A).[267,644] Abnormal fusion and segmentation of vertebral elements, abnormality of the ribs, or scoliosis is unusual in lumbosacral lipoma unless a complicated form is present.[267,383] Asymmetry or partial agenesis of the sacrum has been found in 24 per cent of cases in which the sacrum has been specifically studied.[184,383,407,612]

Myelography by the lumbar route is rarely, if ever, associated with complications, but puncture may fail if the sac is entirely filled with fat. Cisternal or lateral cervical puncture is then indicated. The myelogram may appear normal in neurologically normal children without intraspinal extension. Extradural lipoma, may give the dural sac a tapered appearance due to lateral and posterior compression; intradural lipoma may cause irregularity of the walls of the dural sac or filling defects ranging from a small encroachment to obliteration of the terminal sac.[267] As in other forms of occult spinal dysraphism with a low conus, the cord shadow may be followed into the sacrum and the nerve roots may exit horizontally (Fig. 35–36A).[267,808]

Spinal computed tomography is particularly useful because an abnormal amount of intraspinal fat is readily localized and confirmed by density measurement (cf. Figs. 35–34B and 35–36B).[360]

---

* See references 44, 184, 267, 383, 407, 768.
† See references 184, 267, 383, 407, 612, 768.

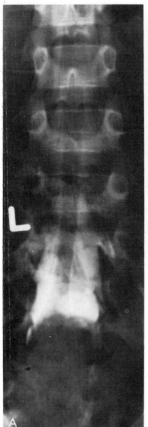

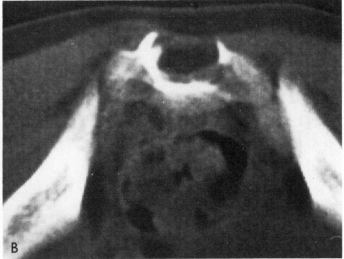

Figure 35–36 *A.* Metrizamide (Amipaque) myelogram shows a shadow extending into the sacrum and blending with a filling defect in the caudal dural sac. Nerve roots originate from the shadow, indicating that the structure is a sacralized spinal cord. *B.* Spinal computed tomography at the level of the sacral spina bifida and sacral filling defect confirms an intraspinal mass of fat density, which at operation was found to be continuous with a subcutaneous lipoma.

Treatment

The goal of operation is relief of traction and compression. Cosmetic removal of the superficial lipoma without exploration of the intradural space is inadequate, since future neurological deterioration is not prevented and future operation is made more difficult.[64,383,407,732,808] Whether the incision is vertical or transverse depends on the size and lateral extension of the subcutaneous lipoma, but laminectomy of at least one level proximal to the lipoma must be completed to determine the normal relationships of the dura, cord, and roots.[184,407] Preoperative studies may indicate the need for a more extensive laminectomy on occasion (see Fig. 35–34B).

The subcutaneous lipoma is normal adipose tissue but is often a slightly paler yellow than and can be demarcated from the normal subcutaneous tissue. The margins of the lipoma are defined to the level of the lumbodorsal fascia, and then medial dissection localizes the defect in the fascia through which the lipoma communicates with the intraspinal structures. At this point, the first normal lamina is removed to expose the normal dural sac and to clarify the proper plane of separation of the muscles and the fascia from the stalk of the lipoma and the caudal dural sac. The dura is opened proximally to expose normal neural contents and the intradural extension of the lipoma. If, over a small area, the stalk of the lipoma fuses with the neural contents, a simple division of the stalk at a safe distance from the neural structures is all that is required. Frequently the intraspinal lipoma fills the caudal dural sac and obscures the distal spinal cord and the cauda equina. The lipoma should be freed at its attachment to the caudal dural sac, which will not endanger the important sacral roots to the sphincters. The mass is then lifted craniad to see whether the roots of the cauda equina can be separated from the under surface of the lipoma and to see more clearly the area of adherence of the distal cord to the lipoma. The intermingling of fat, collagenous connective tissue, and the neural tissue of the cord produces a tougher, fibrous area that is apparent to the surgeon; dissection should terminate at this tissue or before it is reached.

Whether a lipoma can be removed completely and without difficulty depends on the complexity of the lesion.[184,407] In a lipomyelomeningocele, the spinal cord herniates into the lipoma, and complete removal without producing additional neurological deficit is impractical (see Fig. 35–35). Untethering may be impossible in the complex lesions. Removal of a compressive lamina at the upper end of the herniation or of masses of extradural or intradural fat separate from the cord may, however, provide adequate decompression for some patients.[184] All authors are unanimous that incomplete removal of the lipoma is preferable to a zealous dissection because decompression or untethering or both may provide a stable clinical course or even neurological improvement without the risk of producing iatrogenic deficit.[644]

Results and Prognosis

The literature supports the opinion that asymptomatic patients will develop symptoms and symptomatic patients will become worse as time passes, and recommends prophylactic operation for all patients with lumbosacral lipoma. An operation for a lumbosacral lipoma should never be taken lightly, however, since temporary worsening of neurological function occurs frequently after operation.[64,184,407,644] In the symptomatic patients reported in the literature motor function improved in 44 per cent, sensory function in 27 per cent, reflex function in 25 per cent, bladder function in 43 per cent, and pain in almost all patients. Some of the improvements may not be clinically significant to the patient. On the basis of these results, the physician must accept a rather poor likelihood of improvement in the deficit if an asymptomatic child is followed until symptoms develop. Many of the children in these series had long-standing neurological deficits, however, and the duration and severity of the deficits may account for the poor rate of improvement. The progression of the neurological deficit is halted and a stable state achieved in many patients, but the future is not necessarily free of difficulty.[732] Bladder dysfunction may be stable and still be followed by repeated urinary tract infections and the necessity for numerous urological procedures.[698] A deformity of the ankle may progress in spite of improvement in muscle function, and orthopedic corrective procedures may be required.[383] The true results of prophylactic or therapeutic operation will remain unknown until a large number of patients who have been operated on are followed into adulthood.

DIASTEMATOMYELIA

Definition

Diastematomyelia is a primary embryological malformation involving division of a variable length of the spinal cord into two hemicords of more or less equal caliber. The anomaly occurs in both occult spinal dysraphism and spina bifida aperta. The division may be partial or complete, and rarely may occur at two separate sites. Often a septum of bone, cartilage, or fibrous tissue is present between the hemicords, in which case each hemicord is surrounded by its own dural sheath, and abnormalities of the posterior elements or the vertebral bodies are usually present. On the other hand, the diastematomyelia may not be associated with a septum, in which case a single dural tube usually surrounds both hemicords and spinal column abnormalities may be minor. Fibrous bands may tether the hemicords to the dura whether a septum is present or not. Diastematomyelia is an intrinsic anomaly that requires no treatment in itself and is compatible with normal neurological function.[357,358] Spinal cord function is frequently compromised by traction or compression, however, as in other forms of occult spinal dysraphism. Diastematomyelia with or without septum may be associated with other manifestations of occult spinal dysraphism at the same or other levels of the spine.

The term "diastematomyelia" has been incorrectly applied to the septum and has been extended to include cases in which a septum passes through the nerve roots of the cauda equina rather than the spinal cord.[485,501] The term "diplomyelia" means a true doubling of the spinal cord and implies two fully formed spinal cords each with a full complement of nerve roots.[59,314,567] A true duplication has never been reported, and the pathological specimens examined to date merely represent different degrees of diastematomyelia. The terms "diplomyelia," "duplication," "reduplication," and "doubling" are pathologically superfluous and largely incorrect.

Abnormal Embryology

Diastematomyelia has intrigued authors for nearly a century, and several embryological theories have been proposed. Generally the theories involve a primary disturbance of the neural ectoderm or an extrinsic disturbance that results in secondary splitting of the neural ectoderm.

Primary Disturbance of the Neural Ectoderm

Twinning

In 1940, Herren and Edwards suggested that the neural folds might turn inward and fuse with the neural plate before fusing with one another and thus produce two neural tubes. The mesodermal tissues surrounding the neural tubes may form a separate bony canal for each tube, and in essence, the midline bony spicule would represent the fused medial pedicles of each bony canal.[314]

The Overgrowth Hypothesis

In 1949, Kapsenberg and Van Lookeren Campagne suggested that the overgrowth of the neural ectoderm observed by Patten in spina bifida aperta might also explain diastematomyelia.[373,553] The overgrown neural plate and folds are incapable of reaching one another to fuse into a single neural tube. Each fold bends inward independently, and two separate neural tubes form. Induction of the mesoderm by the two neural tubes then directs formation of the vertebral laminae, which curve inward medially and fuse in the midline to form a septum. Barson and Cole described a case of partial triplomyelia in a patient with von Recklinghausen's neurofibromatosis in 1967. Incomplete division must have occurred twice to give rise to three central canals, three posterior and four anterior horns. The amount of tissue in the area was greatly in excess of normal and more than seen in the usual form of diastematomyelia.[42]

The Hydrodynamic Theory

Gardner postulates that hydromyelic overdistention of the embryonic neural tube results in a rupture of the roof and floor plates of the neural tube without damage to the overlying cutaneous ectoderm or ventral entoderm. The upper and lower edges of the split neural tube unite on either side to form two small neural tubes. The line of fusion on the medial aspect of each tube explains the histological appearance of the "ventral" median fissure that develops on the medial aspect of each hemicord.[247]

Extrinsic Disturbance with Secondary Splitting of the Neural Ectoderm

Primary Mesodermal Abnormality

In 1940, Lichtenstein suggested that a primary mesodermal abnormality created the midline septum, which then splits the flat neural plate, with subsequent formation of two neural tubes.[430]

Accessory Neurenteric Canal

In 1952, Bremer suggested that the neural plate might become divided by an accessory neurenteric canal forming craniad to Hensen's node through which the neurenteric canal proper transiently joins the dorsal and ventral surfaces of the embryo at day 18.[68] Both the neural plate and the notochord are divided, leading to a double condensation of mesoderm that attempts to form two vertebral bodies. The mesodermal vertebral body precursors merge, but the medial portion of each condensation may fuse into a median septum projecting into the anterior spinal canal. If the dorsal portion of the accessory neurenteric canal fails to disappear, a congenital dermal sinus may lead to the dorsal tip of the septum.[137,148,158,462,475]

Split Notochord Syndrome

In 1960, Bentley and Smith suggested that a primary split of the notochord leads to a dorsal herniation of the entoderm through the split.[53] The neural plate responds with a similar split, creating a diastematomyelia. Subsequent growth and development obliterates the entodermal tract, but the gap between the hemicords fills with mesodermal tissue of the vertebral body to create the septum. Both the accessory neurenteric canal theory and the split notochord syndrome also apply to the formation of a neurenteric cyst.

Pathology

The features of diastematomyelia in 314 patients have been reported in the English literature.[*]

The Spinal Cord

Diastematomyelia occurs with or without a septum, but the general histological features of the spinal cord are common to both types. The cord is normal above the level of the diastematomyelia and usually reunites below the level of the split and again becomes normal. Because no true duplication of the cord occurs, each division represents an equal or unequal portion of one spinal cord.[314,562] The central canal bifurcates to extend into each hemicord and reunites below the split. The anterior spinal artery also bifurcates at the split so that each hemicord retains an anterior spinal artery. The artery may influence the formation of a central sulcus in each division, which enhances the resemblance to a "doubling" of the spinal cord.[†] Each hemicord appears to rotate inwardly 90 degrees so that the central sulci of both hemicords face one another. The paired anterior and posterior nerve roots, however, continue to exit from the lateral side of each hemicord. The more laterally located posterior horn in each hemicord is usually single, but the new central sulcus related to the anterior spinal artery tends to divide the more medially located anterior horn so that it resembles two anterior horns. Each hemicord has a separate pial and, usually, arachnoid covering. The two divisions of the cord are usually obvious even without an intervening septum, and only rarely are they so closely approximated as to resemble a normal cord.[355] Al-

---

* See references 22, 24, 59, 86, 87, 112, 122, 130, 137, 138, 148, 154, 156, 158, 207, 214, 240, 246, 253, 265, 276, 282, 284, 291, 314, 317, 327, 352, 357, 358, 360, 372, 380, 433, 450, 461–463, 469, 472, 475, 478, 501, 522, 562, 563, 567, 604, 606, 626, 628, 635, 651, 652, 675, 678, 734, 745, 759, 776, 789, 800.
† See references 86, 87, 122, 430, 553, 788.

though the spinal cord typically reunites below the split, occasionally the split continues through the conus and may even include a double filum terminale.[317,752] One division of the cord may be significantly smaller, and the roots hypoplastic. The smaller hemicord may correlate with the symptomatic lower extremity.[282,776] Interference with development of the neural tube may result in abnormal migrations of the neural crest cells that form the dorsal nerve roots and sensory ganglia. As a result, functioning and nonfunctioning roots may attach at a variety of sites on the hemicords, and degeneration of nonfunctioning nerve roots may create fibrous bands.[355]

The spinal cord was divided at a single level in 96 per cent of the patients reported in the literature, and there were rare separate divisions at two or even three distinct levels.[358] The cord always divides into two divisions. The single case of histologically documented "triplomyelia" in a patient with von Recklinghausen's neurofibromatosis did not involve actual division of the cord.[42] Partial diastematomyelia is an incomplete dorsal division of the spinal cord that leaves the anterior bridge intact. The dorsal split may contain a bony spur extending from the dorsal lamina, a fold of the posterior dura, a lipoma, or the termination of a congenital dermal sinus.[282,358,635,776]

Diastematomyelia Without Septum

A split cord without an intervening septum is a common feature of the spinal cord above a myelomeningocele.[199,200] In occult spinal dysraphism, however, diastematomyelia without a septum was found in only 10 per cent of the reported patients.[291,358,776] The dural tube is always single, and the contained hemicords may have fibrous bands, commissural bands, or aberrant nerve roots passing between them. The bands or adhesions may attach to the dura or even pass through the dura to attach to the overlying lamina or fibrous tissue bridging the spina bifida.[355,450] A few patients with diastematomyelia without septum have a normal spine, but the majority have at least a spina bifida.[86,87,358]

Diastematomyelia With Septum

A septum of some form was found between the hemicords of 90 per cent of the patients described in the literature. A single septum was present in 96 per cent, and two separate septa in 4 per cent, although frequently the septa were within the same diastematomyelia.*

The Septum

The septum is located in the cervical spine in 1 per cent,[214,265,358,745] in the thoracic spine in 28 per cent (3 per cent at T1 to T6 and 25 per cent at T7 to T12), in the lumbar spine in 70 per cent (16 per cent at L1, 22 per cent at L2, 16 per cent at L3, 13 per cent at L4, and 3 per cent at L5), and in the sacrum in 1 per cent.[148,317,380] The levels are only approximations, as the septum may span more than one vertebral level or may overlie the intervertebral disc space. The higher a septum is situated in the spine, the longer it tends to be in terms of the number of vertebral segments it spans.[317]

Since diastematomyelia with septum forms in early development when the spinal cord and the spine are of equal length, a penetrating septum may tether the cord and prevent cranial migration. Thus, a lumbar septum usually penetrates the distal spinal cord and is associated with a low conus.[92,317,752] Rarely the cord escapes penetration by a low lumbar septum that is found among the roots of the cauda equina. The higher the level of the septum in the spine, the less the restriction on cranial migration and the higher the conus may be located provided no secondary abnormality results in a low-lying conus.[317] The cleft in the spinal cord is virtually always longer than the penetrating septum and its dural sheath.[380]

Since the septum originates from mesoderm, the structure may vary from fibrous tissue or cartilage or fibrocartilage in 25 per cent to bone in 75 per cent of the patients (Fig. 35–37). The septum was attached to both the anterior and posterior vertebral elements in 68 per cent, to the posterior elements alone in 11 per cent, and to the anterior elements alone in 21 per cent. The posterior attachment of the septum may be to a deformed lamina or to the fibrous tissue bridging a spina bifida.[462] The anterior attachment varies from a broad to a narrow base, and occasionally a fibrocartilaginous

---

* See references 59, 148, 282, 317, 358, 450, 522, 651, 675.

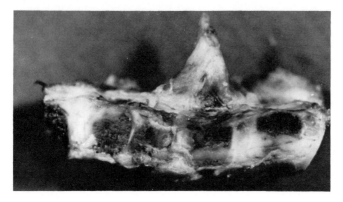

Figure 35–37 Lateral view of a specimen of the spine from a patient with diastematomyelia with septum. The bony septum is attached to the ventral spinal canal and is associated with narrowing of a nearby intervertebral disc. (From Maroun, F. B., Jacob, J. C., and Heneghan, W. D.: Diastematomyelia. St. Louis, Warren H. Green, Inc., 1976. Reprinted by permission.)

union of a bony spur permits easy disarticulation of the septum from the anterior spinal canal.[355]

The Dura

Each hemicord is surrounded by its own dural tube near the level of the septum. The two dural tubes reunite into a single tube above and below the septum, and thus the length of the diastematomyelia is usually greater than that of either the septum or the medial dural wall that encloses the septum and separates the hemicords.[355]

The Spine

Abnormalities of the posterior elements are the most common skeletal defects, and a multiple-level spina bifida, fusion of adjacent hemilaminae, or anomalous spinous processes are frequent.[373,469] The vertebral bodies are more frequently involved in diastematomyelia with septum than with any other form of occult spinal dysraphism with the exception of neurenteric cyst. The intervertebral disc space is characteristically narrowed, with or without partial or complete fusion of the bodies near the level of the septum, as shown in Figure 35–37. The transverse diameter of the vertebral bodies is usually widened and the anteroposterior diameter narrowed. Abnormalities of fusion such as hemivertebrae, butterfly vertebrae, and rarely, sagittal cleft vertebrae may occur. This combination of posterior and anterior skeletal abnormalities causes widening of the interpedicular diameter that is the most reliable indicator of the level of the septum as opposed to the level of the spina bifida. Congenital scoliosis is frequently associated with the vertebral body abnormalities.[317,800]

Pathogenesis of the Clinical Features

Symptoms and signs produced by diastematomyelia with or without septum are primarily due to traction by the septum, by the dura enclosing the septum, by adhesions between the divisions of the cord and the dura and extradural tissues, or by an abnormality at another site. The relationship of the septum to the caudal end of the cleft where the hemicords reunite and to the medial dural cuff enclosing the septum is important in the pathogenesis of the deficit. The septum and its surrounding dura are located at the distal end of the cleft in the majority of symptomatic patients, and the penetrating structures can exert both traction and a compressive force on the cord. When two septa are present in one cleft, then only the distal septum may be symptomatic.[148,522] A septum located above the caudal end of the cleft is unlikely to cause symptoms through a traction mechanism, and other mechanisms must be invoked. Adhesions between the hemicords and septum or between the hemicords and the dura could be responsible for traction symptoms, or a large eccentric septum may cause local compression of one or both hemicords, or there may be an associated abnormality located elsewhere in the spinal canal.

Associated Abnormalities

Diastematomyelia with or without a septum is not associated with the Arnold-Chiari malformation unless the patient has myelomeningocele or spinal meningocele. The septum may be at the same level as the myelomeningocele or meningocele or at a different level.* Other abnormalities that may occur intraspinally or extraspinally at the level of the diastematomyelia are epidermoid tumor, a congenital dermal sinus leading to the septum, a neurenteric cyst, an arachnoid cyst, a lipoma, or hydromyelia.† Occasionally a second form of occult spinal dysraphism is present at a different level, particularly tethering of the cord by a thick filum terminale, a sacral intraspinal meningocele, or a teratoma of the sacrum.‡ Diastematomyelia also occurs with anterior spina bifida and combined spina bifida.[53,630]

Clinical Evaluation

Diastematomyelia in occult spinal dysraphism occurs in females more often than in males in a ratio of three and one half to one of the reported cases. Other forms of cranial or spinal dysraphism may occur in the family, but their true incidence is unknown.[246,291,372,463,562] The ages at which patients presented were: between birth and 5 years, 57 per cent; between 6 and 10 years, 25 per cent; between 11 and 20 years, 12 per cent; and over 21 years, only 6 per cent.

Cutaneous manifestations were present in 77 per cent of the patients, with hypertrichosis in 50 per cent, congenital dermal sinus in 11 per cent, a subcutaneous lipoma in 10 per cent, and hemangiomatous discoloration or pigmentation in 6 per cent. Twenty-three per cent of patients had no cutaneous malformation.

Twenty per cent of the patients were asymptomatic and were evaluated because of a cutaneous manifestation or an incidental radiological finding. Even patients with a low lumbar septum transfixing a tethered cord can remain free of symptoms

throughout life or develop symptoms only in adulthood.[358] For example, among 14 patients ranging in age from 21 to 64 years, the septum was at L1 or below in 69 per cent.§ Of these older patients, 14 per cent were asymptomatic, 36 per cent presented primarily with back or leg pain suggestive of lumbar disc disease, and only 50 per cent had a long-standing neuromusculoskeletal syndrome. In the entire group, 80 per cent of the patients manifested some form of the neuromusculoskeletal syndrome (in one lower extremity in 52 per cent, in both lower extremities in 12 per cent, deformity of the ankle or foot in 26 per cent, sensory deficit in 15 per cent, bladder dysfunction in 14 per cent, pain in the back or legs in 8 per cent), and there was a remarkable 34 per cent incidence of scoliosis. The relatively low frequency of bladder dysfunction may reflect the young age of presentation before bladder control could be reliably assessed or the fact that the sphincter centers in the caudal cord are infrequently affected compared with other forms of occult spinal dysraphism. Twenty-six per cent of the patients had upper motor neuron signs such as spasticity, hyperreflexia, or an extensor plantar response.

The scoliosis that develops in diastematomyelia with septum is different from that occurring with the tethered cord syndrome. The vertebral body structure is often congenitally abnormal in the region of the curve in diastematomyelia, in contrast to mild posterior element defects remote from the curve in the tethered cord syndrome. The incidence of scoliosis is not influenced by the level of the septum, according to a review of the literature, although some authors suggest that thoracic septa are more likely to be so associated.[317] The incidence of vertebral body abnormalities in the patients with scoliosis is at least 43 per cent compared with 21 per cent for the entire group of patients. Although 40 per cent of the patients with scoliosis had no cutaneous manifestations, 85 per cent had some other element of the neuromusculoskeletal syndrome as a clue to the diagnosis. The incidence of diastematomyelia in a large series of patients with congenital scoliosis is at

---

* See references 52, 59, 122, 469, 501, 563, 606, 788, 789, 800.

† See references: epidermoid tumor, 22, 24, 57, 92, 138, 291, 380, 472, 475, 606; dermal sinus leading to septum, 137, 148, 158, 462, 475; neurenteric cyst, 92, 309; arachnoid cyst, 148, 563; lipoma, 22, 462; hydromyelia, 314, 408.

‡ See references: thick filum terminale, 158, 282, 317, 563, 635, 752; sacral meningocele, 282; teratoma of sacrum, 380.

---

§ See references 148, 207, 240, 314, 357, 380, 522, 628, 651, 734.

least 5 per cent and perhaps would be higher if all the patients had myelography.[380,800] Any patient with a widened interpedicular diameter in the area of the curve should have a myelogram prior to an operation for scoliosis.

Investigation

Plain roentgenograms of the spine are more striking in diastematomyelia than in most other forms of occult spinal dysraphism. Spina bifida was present in 93 per cent of patients and absent in only 7 per cent.* Spina bifida may occur at more than one level of the spine as a so-called "skip" lesion.[317] Rather than a complete spina bifida, there may be fusion of the posterior laminae at several levels on one side.[501,526,606] Abnormalities in the vertebral bodies occur in not less than 21 percent of all patients, with a decrease in the width of the intervertebral disc space or fusion of the bodies in 40 per cent and hemivertebrae, sagittal cleft vertebrae, or butterfly vertebrae in at least 21 per cent. A higher incidence, 43 per cent, of vertebral body abnormalities occurs in patients with scoliosis.[317,380,789,800] The interpedicular diameter was increased in 96 per cent of these patients and was normal in only 4 per cent, particularly in diastematomyelia without septum.† The pedicles are usually normal but can be hypoplastic in the widened area of the canal. Erosion of the pedicles, however, or scalloping of the posterior vertebral bodies should suggest other intraspinal abnormalities in addition to diastematomyelia.

Plain roentgenograms revealed the septum in 66 per cent. An ossified septum is best seen on the anteroposterior view and is usually, but not invariably, located in the area of the canal with the widest interpedicular diameter.[309,317,563,651,800] When present in the area of the spina bifida, it is often found attached to the side of the fused laminae.[317,358] The septum may undergo increased ossification with age, and sequential roentgenograms over several years may show "development" of the bony septum (see Fig. 35–10B).[352] Patients without a septum visible on plain films were found at op-

eration to have no septum in 12 per cent, a fibrous septum in 38 per cent, and bone in 21 per cent; no details were given for 29 per cent.

Tomography has been suggested to show a septum that is small or poorly ossified or a spine that is severely deformed. What may appear to be an abnormal spinous process is often proved to be a bony septum.[154,789] Lateral tomography may show the septum inclined in a cranial-to-caudal or caudal-to-cranial direction. Central ossification of the septum with no attachment anteriorly or posteriorly suggests that the septum has a separate center of ossification that has not ossified the fibrous anterior and posterior portions.[317] Generally, however, tomography exposes the child to unnecessary radiation, since the child with symptomatic occult spinal dysraphism warrants a myelogram regardless of the results of tomography.

Spinal computed tomography may show an ossified or fibrous septum and help to display deformities of the vertebral body and laminae.[734,789] The patient is even better evaluated with metrizamide myelography to outline the entire spinal canal combined with spinal computed tomography to focus on specific abnormalities. Positive contrast or air highlights the septum as a central fill-

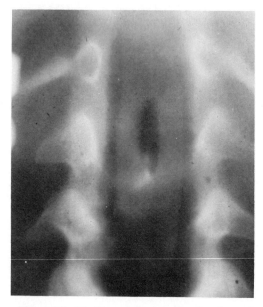

Figure 35–38 Gas myelogram showing the perimedullary space around each hemicord, the intermedullary cleft craniad to the small septum, and the tapered conus extending below L2. (Courtesy of David C. Hemmy, M.D., Medical College of Wisconsin.)

---

* See references 317, 380, 462, 501, 651, 734, 800.
† See references 92, 207, 317, 358, 462, 501.

ing defect in the contrast-filled spinal canal and shows the intermedullary cleft craniad to the level of the septum (Fig. 35–38). Lateral to the septum are the shadows of the two hemicords surrounded by the perimedullary space lateral to each division, showing nerve roots or perhaps adhesions between the hemicords and the dura.[317] If the intermedullary cleft is caudal to the septum, then other pathological conditions should be diligently searched for to explain the symptoms.

Positive contrast myelography in the prone position may falsely suggest a central septum in congenital kyphosis because the contrast column splits around the ventral protuberance of the vertebral body into the spinal canal. In the supine position the central area of lucency will disappear, and spinal computed tomography will not show a septum.[800] Diastematomyelia without septum has no central filling defect and may show no intermedullary cleft if the hemicords are attached by adhesions. Similarly, adhesions between the divisions of the cord and the dura and extradural tissues may not be visualized.[358] Thus, the true incidence of symptomatic diastematomyelia without septum cannot be determined with certainty because of the false negative myelogram.

Treatment

Guthkelch and his associates believe that asymptomatic children and those with an apparently stable neuromusculoskeletal syndrome should have a prophylactic operation within the first two years of life.[282,284] This conclusion followed his personal experience with 6 of 7 patients initially normal and 7 of 10 patients with an apparently stable neuromusculoskeletal syndrome who deteriorated under observation and required operation. He considered a young child to have a per-year risk of developing cord symptoms of 13 per cent, decreasing with age until adolescence, with an overall probability of developing cord symptoms of 83 per cent. Prophylactic operation is suggested by many, but not all, authors.* A more conservative approach is to consider the relationship of the septum to the caudal

---

* See references 59, 253, 358, 469, 522, 672.

intermedullary cleft. An asymptomatic patient may be followed closely if the septum is located in the midpoint of the intermedullary cleft. If the septum is at the caudal end of the intermedullary cleft, then a prophylactic operation is advised. Myelography and operation should be advised for a symptomatic patient, even if his condition is apparently stable, particularly if a sphincter abnormality is present. Bladder dysfunction is a potentially life-threatening complication, and the earlier the operation, the more likely the bladder dysfunction is to improve.

Patients with congenital scoliosis must have a myelogram to rule out diastematomyelia. If present, the septum must be removed prior to halo-pelvic traction or an attempt at operative correction of the curvature. Failure to do so may result in a neurological catastrophe.[587,800]

General anesthesia in the prone position with particular attention to freedom of the abdomen to reduce epidural venous congestion is necessary, since the extradural and intradural vascularity may be prominent.[148,462,469] A preoperative roentgenogram should be used to localize the level of the septum if no localizing mark has been placed on the back at the time of the myelogram because, owing to the deformed spine, intraoperative localization may be difficult.[562] At least one and possibly two segments should be exposed above and below the level of the septum to expose the entire dual enclosure around the septum, since it must be removed as well. The laminal arch is largely intact at the level of the septum with the spina bifida adjacent to it.[358] Great care must be taken not to twist the instrument if rongeurs are used for the laminectomy, since the septum is frequently attached posteriorly and the spur may be angulated into the cord.[309] A high-speed drill is the preferable alternative. Many authors suggest an initial extradural resection of the septum so that the intact medial dura on either side may act as a protective layer between the operator and the hemicords.[355,485] Adhesions or compression of one hemicord by the septum are not visualized in this blind procedure, however, and the dura should be opened separately over each hemicord and adhesions divided before the septum is manipulated. Even with the dura open, the dural envelope can act as a protective layer while the bony septum is burred down flush with the ventral surface of the spinal canal. Small arterial vessels within the septum cause nuisance bleeding, which can be controlled by bone wax or by the action of the high-speed burr. The central dural envelope is also resected to prevent it from acting as a tethering structure and to forestall the formation of adhesions or re-formation of the bony septum.[501] The anterior dural defect may be left open, but the posterior dura is closed to reconstruct a single dural tube over the relaxed hemicords. The filum terminale should be sectioned if the operation is in the lumbar region near the conus.[364,563]

Results and Prognosis

The early results after operation were mentioned for approximately one third of the patients described in the literature. Postoperative clinical assessment showed 53 per cent to be in stable condition, whereas 45 per cent had some degree of improvement. Only 2 per cent were permanently worse after operation.[207,472] Scoliosis may, however, continue to progress after operation.[282,327,606] Improvement in motor function or gait occurred in 44 per cent, in sensation in 66 per cent, and in bladder function in 47 per cent; and pain was relieved in virtually every patient.

Failure to improve or late deterioration after operation may be due to incomplete removal of the septum, failure to remove the central dural sleeve, failure to remedy another symptomatic abnormality at the operative level or at a different level, or rarely, a regrowth of the septum.[309,472,501]

NEURENTERIC CYST

Definition

A neurenteric cyst is located in an intramedullary or intradural extramedullary location in the ventral cervicodorsal spinal canal and may be a cause of spinal cord compression. Embryologically, the cyst derives from entodermal tissue displaced dorsally into the spinal canal ventral to the neural plaque through the interposed mesodermal layer that forms the vertebral bodies. Thus, abnormalities of the anterior vertebral unit are frequent, but the pos-

terior elements are usually intact. A transvertebral communication (anterior spina bifida) between the intraspinal neurenteric cyst and a posterior mediastinal cyst may persist in some cases. "Neurenteric cyst" is the preferred term, but the lesion has also been called an enterogenous cyst, a neuroenteric cyst, a foregut cyst, and a gastrocytoma.*

Abnormal Embryology

The entodermal tissue of the foregut region that gives origin to the esophagus and the respiratory system may be the source of cysts located in the anterior, middle, or posterior mediastinum. A brief review of the developmental cysts of the mediastinum puts the neurenteric cyst in perspective for the neurological surgeon unacquainted with these lesions. At four to five weeks of gestation, the ventral laryngotracheal groove appears in the floor of the pharynx, and over one week the tubular outgrowth of the future trachea extends anterior to the foregut. By six weeks, the caudal end of the trachea enlarges and bifurcates to form the lung buds. Simultaneously the esophagus elongates during the sixth and seventh weeks of development. The area where the tracheal bud originates may be the source of the intramural cyst of the esophagus, and the cyst becomes engulfed in the elongating esophagus. These cysts lie in the posterior mediastinum and contain a ciliated epithelial lining and occasionally cartilage in the wall but never develop an enteric epithelial lining. The more common bronchiogenic cyst most likely arises from the respiratory epithelium of the developing lung bud and is situated within the lung or in association with the main bronchi, especially on the left side. These latter cysts occupy the middle mediastinum, are lined by ciliated columnar epithelium, and have a wall containing smooth muscle and occasionally cartilage. Pericardial cysts develop in the anterior cardiophrenic angle in association with the diaphragm and are lined by a single layer of mesothelial cells and have a wall of smooth muscle and connective tissue.

---

* See references 178, 296, 325, 348, 391, 403, 428, 469, 525, 649, 686.

None of the cysts mentioned so far is associated with vertebral body abnormalities or with the intraspinal neurenteric cyst.[65,211,625] The enteric cyst that originates from the foregut and is located in the posterior mediastinum, however, is associated with cervicothoracic vertebral body abnormalities in at least 40 per cent of patients and, occasionally, with an intraspinal neurenteric cyst.* Twelve percent of all mediastinal masses in any location in infants and children are enteric cysts, and in the posterior mediastinum the enteric cyst is second in frequency to the neurogenic tumors (neuroblastoma, ganglioneuroblastoma, ganglioneuroma, neurofibroma) as a cause of a mass lesion.[65] The cysts tend to lie to the right of the spine and are very likely related to the developmental processes of gastric and gut rotation.[483] The enteric cysts have been referred to as esophageal, gastric, gastrogenic, alimentary, gastroenteric, enterogenous, and archenteric cysts as well as esophageal duplication and mediastinal enterocystoma.[211,600,765] The epithelium varies from a ciliated columnar lining suggestive of respiratory epithelium to a typical gastric or small intestinal lining. The type of epithelium is not specific for the origin of the cyst because the primitive esophagus is lined by ciliated columnar epithelium that is gradually converted to stratified epithelium by the time of birth.[211] The wall of the cyst has a well-developed muscularis mucosae, two or three smooth muscle layers, and occasionally, a Meissner's and an Auerbach's plexus.

Enteric cysts may occur in the abdominal cavity, since the foregut structures descend from the cervicodorsal region during embryological development. Thus, some abdominal enteric cysts may have little relationship to the level of the vertebral abnormalities, and vertebral abnormalities may be missed if the cervicothoracic spine is not included in the investigation.[211,277]

The posterior enteric cyst, the intraspinal neurenteric cyst, and the rare case of combined anterior and posterior spina bifida are all related in their abnormal embryology. The main theories postulate: (1) a primary split in the notochord, (2) abnormal excalation of the notochord from the entoderm, (3) a primary adhesion of entoderm and ectoderm anterior to the notochordal head process, and (4) arrest or delay of caudal migration of the neurenteric canal or the formation of an accessory neurenteric canal.† The four theories are variations on a theme and involve similar concepts. Prior to the formation of the somites, an abnormal communication or fusion occurs between the entoderm and the neural ectoderm so that a diverticulum of entoderm is pulled into the region of the developing notochord, developing mesodermal sclerotomes, and both neural and epithelial ectoderm. As a result, the notochord splits around the diverticulum and the mesodermal vertebral body sclerotomes are condensed in two halves with the potential of creating a central cleft in the vertebral bodies.[53,93,630] The ultimate form of the prevertebral, vertebral, and postvertebral abnormalities depends on the developmental behavior of the entoderm–neural ectoderm adhesion.[694] Conceivably, the communication could disappear completely and all structures derived from the three involved germ layers could develop normally. On the other hand, any portion of the communication might persist to form a number of potential diverticulae, sinuses, fistulae, or cysts in a variety of locations along the course of the communication, with normal development occurring in areas where the communication had disappeared. If the tract through the notochord and sclerotome condensations resolves, a partial fusion of the two halves of the spine could result in a single vertebral column but with various degrees of hemivertebrae and midline cleft formation. With slightly greater healing, the split in the vertebral bodies could be totally bridged with cartilage so that no connection would exist between the prevertebral and intraspinal structures.[598] Formation of a well-defined nucleus pulposus in both the right and left hemivertebrae of a split vertebral column has been suggested as proof of an original split in the notochord.[630]

The entoderm–neural ectoderm adhesion not only contributes to local disorganization of the vertebral precursors but may give rise to a neurenteric band or connec-

* See references: vertebral body abnormalities, 8, 45, 65, 211, 265, 521, 609, 765, 799; intraspinal neurenteric cyst, 178, 325, 348, 403, 525, 570, 686.

† See references 45, 49, 53, 68, 211, 247, 483, 630, 765.

tion with the alimentary tract. If the band does not elongate with growth, the development of the diaphragm may be impeded. Traction diverticulae may develop at the alimentary attachment and produce either an intrathoracic cyst extending from the abdomen into the thorax or a cyst restricted to the abdomen.

An intraspinal neurenteric cyst may result if the intraspinal portion of the entoderm–neural ectoderm communication persists. If the remainder of the communication through the vertebral bodies disappears, then the intraspinal neurenteric cyst may not be associated with a mediastinal cyst or a vertebral body abnormality.* Persistence of the entire communication in combination with a disturbance of the epithelial ectoderm in the dorsal midline of the embryo causes a combined anterior and posterior form of spina bifida.†

The so-called "teratomatous cysts" of the spinal canal lie posterior or posterolateral to the spinal cord or cauda equina and are not associated with vertebral body abnormalities, although posterior element defects occasionally occur. The terminology is not clear, and the abnormal embryology is believed to differ from that of the anteriorly located neurenteric cyst.‡

Pathology

Neurenteric cysts are rare, and only 20 cases have been reported in the literature with sufficient information for analysis.§ Unfortunately, Matson's 10 patients were not described in detail.[469]

Intraspinal neurenteric cysts are located ventral to the spinal cord in the cervical area (40 per cent), in the thoracic area (50 per cent), or at the cervicothoracic junction (10 per cent) within the boundaries of C3 above and T7 below. The cyst lies in an intramedullary or intradural extramedullary location in most patients. Seventeen patients had a cystic lesion containing fluid described variously as black, coffee-ground, brown, chocolate, yellow, and mucoid, and occasionally clear and colorless.

One patient had a solid intramedullary strawberry tumor.[391]

Histologically, the cyst consisted of a simple or pseudostratified columnar epithelium with no muscle layer in nine cases, and in seven of those patients there was no communication with the mediastinal cyst.¶ Nine cysts had muscle in the wall and an epithelial lining considered to be of esophageal, gastric, or intestinal origin, and in six of these patients there was communication with a mediastinal cyst.** Two patients had a fibrous cord and no cyst.[325,525]

Fifty-three per cent of the patients had a coexisting posterior mediastinal enteric cyst, one patient had an ileal enteric duplication, and two had cysts in the neck.[178,348,497] In all but one of these patients with a prevertebral cyst there was a direct communication through an anterior defect in the vertebral bodies.†† The single patient lacking a direct communication did have vertebral body anomalies.[403] In the 47 per cent of the patients without a mediastinal cyst there was a normal spine in three patients, minor evidence of an intraspinal space-occupying lesion in two patients, a Klippel-Feil deformity in one, and vertebral body defects in a single patient; for two patients no details were given.‡‡ Overall, 69 per cent of patients with a neurenteric cyst had vertebral body anomalies. Nonspecific widening of the interpedicular diameter and scalloping of the posterior vertebral body or erosion of the pedicles due to the cyst rarely occurred, and only two patients had posterior element defects.[348,686]

Associated malformations consisted of a myelomeningocele unrelated to the level of the neurenteric cyst in two patients and a dorsal congenital dermal sinus near the level of the neurenteric cyst in one patient.[88,497,598]

Clinical Evaluation

Sixty per cent of the patients presented between birth and 5 years of age, none

---

* See references 88, 106, 296, 391, 428, 649.
† See references 49, 213, 497, 578, 591, 630.
‡ See references 3, 90, 331, 400, 542, 597, 613, 807.
§ See references 88, 105, 106, 178, 296, 325, 348, 391, 403, 428, 497, 525, 568, 570, 598, 649, 686.

¶ See references 105, 106, 296, 348, 403, 428, 568, 649, 686.
** See references 88, 178, 325, 391, 497, 525, 570, 598.
†† See references 178, 325, 348, 497, 525, 570, 598.
‡‡ See references: normal spine, 106, 296, 568; minor evidence of intraspinal lesion, 105, 649; Klippel-Feil deformity, 428; vertebral body defects, 391; no details, 88, 598.

between 6 and 10 years, twenty per cent between 11 and 20 years, and twenty per cent over 20 years of age. The sex ratio was 3.8 males for every female. No familial cases have been reported.

Twelve patients presented with a variety of spinal cord compression syndromes such as the central cord syndrome, quadriparesis, paraparesis, or hemiparesis, but virtually all neurological deficits were of an upper motor neuron type, since all the cysts occurred above T7. Two patients presented with meningitis—due to *Streptococcus faecalis* in one and to *Escherichia coli* in the other.[348,497] Two patients presented with a myelomeningocele remote from the site of the neurenteric cyst.[88,598] Two patients had no symptoms of spinal cord compression and were brought to attention because of respiratory symptoms due to the associated mediastinal mass.[325,525] One patient had both respiratory distress and paraplegia.[570] One infant was stillborn.[598]

Patients under 10 years of age had a coexisting prevertebral cyst in 80 per cent of cases in contrast to a 25 per cent incidence in patients over 10 years of age. The incidence of vertebral body defects and a communication between the prevertebral and the intraspinal lesions also is greater in younger patients. Thus, the more complicated lesions present earlier in life.

Investigation

The investigation of a patient presenting with spinal cord compression is straightforward, and the initial studies should raise the possibility of a neurenteric cyst. Plain roentgenograms and tomograms of the chest and cervical and thoracic spine may reveal a posterior mediastinal mass and vertebral body abnormalities, a widened interpedicular diameter, and occasionally, evidence of an intraspinal expanding lesion. Although tomograms may suggest an anterior spina bifida, the defect may be closed with cartilage so that no communication exists between the prevertebral and the intraspinal spaces.[598]

More frequently, the neurological surgeon is called into consultation by the thoracic surgeon to answer the question of whether a neurologically normal patient with a mediastinal mass should have a myelogram to rule out an intraspinal communication or extension of the lesion. An enteric cyst in the posterior mediastinum rarely communicates with the spinal canal, as evidenced by the rarity of intraspinal neurenteric cysts compared with the large number of posterior mediastinal enteric cysts. Nevertheless, a posterior mediastinal mass, particularly on the right side, associated with cervicothoracic vertebral body malformations should raise the suspicion of an enteric cyst coexisting with an intraspinal neurenteric cyst. If plain roentgenograms including tomograms are abnormal, performing a myelogram is the safest course; if the myelogram is normal, a communication between the mediastinal mass and the spinal canal is very unlikely. Neurogenic tumors of the posterior mediastinum are more common than enteric cysts, and 10 per cent are so-called "dumbbell" forms that extend through an intervertebral foramen into the spinal canal. If foraminal enlargement or pedicle erosion is present, a myelogram is indicated.[10] The suggestion of a neurological deficit, however subtle, is an indication for myelography regardless of normal plain roentgenograms.

Spinal and body computed tomography may be helpful to demonstrate the relationship of the mediastinal mass to the vertebral bodies and the vertebral body defects.

Myelography demonstrated an intramedullary lesion in one patient with neurenteric cyst, an intradural extramedullary lesion in seven, and a complete block in three, and was falsely normal in one patient.

Treatment

No standard operative approach can be outlined for the neurenteric cyst because the spinal level, the associated vertebral body anomalies, and the presence or absence of a mediastinal prevertebral cyst all influence the care. Of the patients reported in the literature eight had a laminectomy, two had a thoracotomy, one had a laminectomy followed by a thoracotomy, two had a thoracotomy followed by a laminectomy, and one had a laminectomy followed by an anterior transcervical approach for a recurrent cyst; two patients had procedures unrelated to the neurenteric cyst, and three had no operation.

The intraspinal lesion can be corrected first at a separate operation or at the same sitting as the prevertebral lesion if a transthoracic anterior operation appears feasible. Since the lesions are cystic, a laminectomy with a more lateral approach than usual or a costotransversectomy in the thoracic region should be adequate, as cyst drainage and conservative resection of the cyst wall adherent to the spinal cord appears to eradicate the cyst successfully. An anterior dural defect leading through the spinal defect may be plugged with a muscle-fascial patch from a posterior approach or be ligated or sutured directly if the transthoracic approach is used.

Results and Prognosis

The outcome will depend on the severity of the neurological deficit and the associated malformations. Review of the literature reveals that 10 patients had improved motor function, 1 had no further episodes of meningitis, 1 was neurologically worse, 6 died after operation or from other malformations, and the results in 2 are unknown. Only one patient had a recurrence of the cyst, but the duration of the follow-up was limited in all cases.[178]

COMBINED ANTERIOR AND POSTERIOR SPINA BIFIDA

The combination of defects in the anterior and posterior spine may occur at the same level (true combined spina bifida) or remote from one another.

True Combined Spina Bifida

In the cervicothoracic spine, the defects frequently involve gross central nervous system defects such as anencephalus or total craniorachischisis posteriorly and marked derangement of the thoracic and abdominal organs anteriorly with communication through an anterior spina bifida. Such infants are stillborn and of only pathological interest.[49] In the low thoracic, lumbar, and sacral spines, the alimentary and central nervous system malformations may be less severe, and the infants may be born alive.* The spine is divided into two halves over several segments by a cleft with prolapse of intestinal duplications through the

cleft to the back.[630] The neural malformation may vary from a spina bifida aperta with myeloschisis to a diastematomyelia that brackets the herniated intestinal duplication. The intestinal duplication may open on the back and drain meconium if connected to the normal bowel, or may appear as a skin-covered swelling over the low thoracic, lumbar, or sacral region like a meningocele.

Defects at Remote Levels

Rarely, anterior spina bifida of the cervicothoracic region with neurenteric cyst is associated with spina bifida aperta at a lower level of the spine.[88,598] Such cases are not true combined spina bifida but rather separate and distinct defects.

Roentgenograms of the entire spine should be taken prior to any operative procedure for what appears to be a typical or atypical spina bifida aperta or occult spinal dysraphism. An obvious split spine or a subtle anterior vertebral body cleft should raise the suspicion of a combined "spina bifida," and further central nervous system and alimentary system investigations are needed to rule out these rare malformations.

ANTERIOR SACRAL MENINGOCELE

Definition

Anterior sacral meningocele is a form of anterior spina bifida usually presenting in the adult and not associated with posterior spina bifida, cutaneous manifestations, or neurological abnormalities. The sacral spinal meninges herniate into the pelvis through a defect in the anterior wall of the sacrum, producing local symptoms from pressure on the bladder and rectum and the pelvic organs in the female. The sacral malformation may be considered a variety of the caudal regression syndrome, but the bowel and bladder rarely have neurogenic dysfunction.[690]

Abnormal Embryology

Defective fusion of the sclerotomes that form the sacral vertebral bodies occurs at

---

* See references 53, 93, 213, 378, 578, 591.

several levels on one side to produce a hemisacrum of variable extent. The posterior elements of the sacrum and lumbar spine are formed normally in virtually all patients.[29,71,351] The meninges bulge through the defective hemisacrum to form the presacral intrapelvic meningocele. The spinal cord and cauda equina are anatomically and functionally normal, indicating that the process of canalization of the caudal tail bud occurred normally. The pelvic organs, however, are frequently malformed.[20,125,311] The müllerian ducts have yet to fuse to form the uterus and vagina when the caudal neural tube development is already complete, and the earlier-formed anterior sacral meningocele may affect development of the pelvic organs.

Pathology

Approximately 100 patients with anterior sacral meningocele have been reported in the literature since the first case was described in 1837.[20] Ninety per cent of these cases were in females, which suggests that women are more likely to have the diagnosis made because the meningocele impairs normal vaginal birth and because the pelvis is more accessible for examination than in the male. An alternate explanation is a hereditary predisposition of females to develop anterior sacral meningocele.*

The Sacrum

The size of the hemisacral defect is variable, but usually the entire coccyx and half of one or more segments of the sacrum are absent. The intact hemisacrum curves around the dome of the meningocele sac in a hooked fashion and creates the classic radiological picture of the scimitar sacrum. Approximately one fifth of patients have a midline sacral defect with the lateral wings of the sacrum draping either side of the defect.[20,34,218,418]

The Meningocele and the Neural Structures

The meningocele is filled with cerebrospinal fluid and is located in the presacral retroperitoneal space anterior to the defect in the sacrum. The wall consists of arachnoid, dura, and compressed fibrous tissue lined by a single layer of squamous or columnar epithelium with occasional mucous cells.[14] The sac usually communicates with the sacral subarachnoid space through a narrow neck that penetrates through the larger sacral defect. The remainder of the bony defect is bridged with relatively avascular fibrous tissue.[20,311,687] An anterior sacral meningocele rarely protrudes through an enlarged sacral foramen or through the sciatic foramen to present as a mass in the gluteal region.[12,14,127] Rarely, the sacral spinal canal may be enlarged by a coexisting intrasacral meningocele, or the meningocele can coexist with a solid dermoid or teratoma.[14,85,287,329]

The spinal cord, cauda equina, and filum terminale are usually normal, but adhesions tethering the cord to the sacral dura and a prominent filum terminale have been reported.[20,347,790]

The Pelvic Organs

Abnormalities of the uterus, vagina, rectum, anus, and urinary tract such as bicornuate uterus with vaginal septum, horseshoe kidney, and partial duplication of the ureters are frequent.† Rarely the meningocele communicates with a rectal diverticulum, producing pelvic abscess and meningitis if the combination is not recognized.[71,381,717]

Clinical Evaluation

An anterior sacral meningocele commonly presents in the second and third decades in both sexes as chronic constipation or obstipation, or as an obstetrical complication in women.[125,127,687] The more complex forms and occasionally overlapping conditions of occult spinal dysraphism or caudal regression syndrome present at a younger age, with structural and functional abnormalities of the urinary and lower alimentary systems.[1,20,654,790] The presenting symptoms are of three general types: (1) local pressure on the rectum (fecal soiling, constipation), bladder (incontinence, enuresis, urinary retention, recurrent bladder and upper tract infections), and uterus and vagina (dysmen-

---

* See references 1, 20, 125, 389, 631, 687.

† See references 20, 29, 125, 181, 287, 311, 329.

orrhea, dyspareunia, dystocia); (2) occasionally, headache that occurs with straining during defecation, presumably owing to the rapid displacement of cerebrospinal fluid from the sac into the subarachnoid space through a large communication between the meningocele and the subarachnoid space; and (3) neurological symptoms such as pain in the back or perianal area and occasionally radiating down one leg, which are produced by irritation of the sacral nerves and lumbosacral plexuses. True neurogenic dysfunction of the sphincters or lower extremities is unusual and likely to be associated with a transitional form of anterior sacral meningocele, occult spinal dysraphism, or caudal regression syndrome.[14,20,125,790]

No cutaneous manifestations are present over the sacrum, but the examination may show an anatomical malformation of the rectum or anus, particularly in children.[20] A portion of the sacrum and usually the entire coccyx are absent on rectal examination, but the meningocele may be large enough to prevent internal examination of the sacrum. The mass in the presacral space displaces the rectum, uterus, and vagina anterosuperiorly, and on abdominal examination this "mass" may be palpated arising out of the pelvis. Rectal or vaginal examination will confirm the presence of a smooth, mobile or fixed, noninflammatory mass that may transmit a pulsation with coughing or sneezing. The differential diagnosis of presacral masses is extensive and includes the presacral dermoid cyst, chondroma, chordoma, sacrococcygeal teratoma, and various tumors of the pelvic organs, to mention a few.[790]

Investigation

Plain roentgenograms of the pelvis and sacrum may reveal the classic sickle-shaped scimitar sacrum, which differs from any other form of occult spinal dysraphism. Occasionally the defect is in the midline or is quite minor if the anterior sacral meningocele is small.[218] Special views of the sacral foramina may be required for the rare transforaminal form. The posterior sacral elements are virtually always normal except for a rare coincidental simple spina bifida occulta. The diagnosis is virtually certain at this stage when combined with a compatible clinical presentation.

Ultrasound imaging may display a fluid-filled mass in the pelvic cavity, and computed tomography can detail the sacral abnormality, the communication between the subarachnoid space and the meningocele, the density of the contents of the mass, and the relationship to the surrounding pelvic organs.[29,803]

Myelography demonstrates a normal sacral sac and localizes the site and size of the communication with the meningocele. The meningocele usually fills immediately with contrast medium, unlike the occult intrasacral meningocele, which frequently fills after a delay and which, rarely, may coexist with an anterior sacral meningocele.[14,287,329,404] Metrizamide myelography plus computed tomography will define the full extent of the sac far more easily than Pantopaque myelography, which requires sequential positioning of the patient in six planes to define the limits of the meningocele. The myelographic findings may modify the operative approach if sacral or lumbar intraspinal abnormalities are visualized or the meningocele sac contains a solid tumor mass.[20]

The intravenous pyelogram and cystogram may reveal anterior displacement of the bladder and lateral displacement of the ureters by a large mass, as well as congenital anomalies of the urinary system such as duplication of the collecting system or a horseshoe kidney.[20,29,687] A barium enema will show anterior displacement, compression, and poor filling of the rectum. Hysterosalpingography may display congenital abnormalities of the cervix and uterus.[125] Arteriography of the pelvic vessels shows displacement by an avascular mass but is not required, since the diagnosis is certain by other methods.[29]

Treatment

Owing to increased understanding of the pathological changes and the availability of antibiotics to treat infection, operative cure of an anterior sacral meningocele can be achieved with a minimal mortality rate. Until 20 years ago, treatment was hazardous because the frequent misdiagnosis of the mass as a perirectal or pelvic abscess and transvaginal or transrectal needle aspiration led to meningitis and death.[676] On the other hand, primary laparotomy to remove a suspected neoplasm of the pelvic organs was also frequently followed by a cerebrospinal fluid fistula, meningitis, and death.[95,127,365,687] The general consensus was that the prognosis of anterior sacral meningocele was relatively benign, and operation should be deferred unless the symptoms were serious. Even a cesarean section and sterilization after pregnancy were considered preferable to removal of the meningocele.[127]

Two basic posterior approaches permit successful obliteration of the communication between the sacral dural sac and the meningocele.* A laminectomy of the hemisacrum and dural opening expose the neural contents, and any associated neural tethering can be corrected.[20] The communication with the meningocele is found through the anterior wall of the dural sac and is obliterated with a fascial graft. An alternative posterior approach is to incise the fibrous tissue bridging the anterior sacral defect to expose the posterior wall of the meningocele. The sac can then be opened, drained, and inspected for a solid component. The communication with the sacral dural sac is found over the posterior dome of the meningocele and is ligated. In either approach, the meningocele sac does not have to be removed, since it will gradually absorb the residual fluid, and the pelvic organs will return to their normal position after successful obliteration of the communication. Computed tomography may show persistent cerebrospinal fluid in the cyst for as long as three months after closure of the communication.[29]

An anterior transabdominal approach may be required if an undiagnosed solid-tissue mass lies within the sac or if the dura is extremely friable or the communication too large to be closed securely by the posterior approach. The rare occurrence of an intrasacral meningocele and anterior sacral meningocele may complicate the operation, as sacral nerve roots may be related to the neck of the intrasacral lesion and hamper closure of the anterior dural defect.[14]

Results and Prognosis

Rarely, an untreated anterior sacral meningocele can be fatal when it spontaneously ruptures into the rectum or produces obstetrical complications.[14] The main complications are postoperative spinal fluid fistula and meningitis, which rarely occur following a posterior transsacral approach. A symptomatic meningocele producing constipation, urinary retention or frequency, and back and perineal and leg pain can be cured in almost every patient by obliteration of the communication between the sacral dural sac and the meningocele. Patients with associated alimentary and renal malformations or neurological deficits due to overlapping forms of occult spinal dysraphism or the caudal regression syndrome will have lesser symptomatic improvement.

OCCULT INTRASACRAL MENINGOCELE

Definition

An occult intrasacral meningocele is an abnormally prolonged, space-occupying, single diverticulum of the meninges extending into the distal sacrum beyond the normal level of termination of the dural sac at S2. The anomaly is not an obvious form of occult spinal dysraphism, since the posterior elements of the spine are intact except for local erosion in 60 per cent of patients. The neural elements are free of direct involvement in 63 per cent. The occurrence of posterior spina bifida in 40 per cent, however, and the combination of occult intrasacral meningocele with typical cases of occult spinal dysraphism such as the tethered cord syndrome indicate that the entity should be classified with occult spinal dysraphism.† Other cystic lesions within the sacrum have been confused with or not differentiated from occult intrasacral meningocele, for example, the perineurial or Tarlov's cyst and ectasia of the caudal dural sac seen in the von Recklinghausen, Marfan, and Ehlers-Danlos syndromes and in some of the chondro-osseous dysplasias.[332,367,499,524] Occasionally the term has been misapplied to a typical form of occult spinal dysraphism such as the tethered cord syndrome, in which the dural sac is abnormally prolonged into the sacrum but is not, in itself, a space-occupying lesion.[370,572]

---

* See references 7, 20, 34, 85, 127, 311, 347, 687, 769.

† See references 2, 144, 367, 572, 590, 699.

Abnormal Embryology

The caudal dural sac extends the full length of the spinal cord and column in early embryonic life and later constricts around the filum terminale to "ascend" to the normal adult level of S2. Presumably persistent patency of the dural sac distal to the S2 vertebral body is due to an abnormality of reduction of the dural sac, but no specific cause has been proposed. The posterior skeletal elements form normally in 60 per cent of patients, since the neural tube is rarely involved in the area of abnormality.

Pathology

The distal sacral subarachnoid space communicates with the diverticulum through a narrow communication into a single chambered or, rarely, internally multiloculated meningocele.[404] The wall of the meningocele sac is dura or nonspecific fibrous tissue with or without a lining of flattened epithelium. The sacral and coccygeal nerve roots are anterior to and separate from the cyst wall in 79 per cent of cases, so the meningocele sac may be ligated or excised without division of the roots. In 21 per cent, however, the roots are densely adherent to the anterior wall of the sac, which precludes excision.[285,367,572] The filum terminale may be within the sac or contained in its wall and may be associated with a low conus.[367,572,699] The meningocele acts as a space-occupying lesion and expands the sacral spinal canal by pressure erosion. The overlying laminae are thinned, and the posterior aspects of the sacral vertebral bodies are scalloped. The sacral foramina may be enlarged by local protrusions of the meningocele sac.

Clinical Evaluation

The true occult intrasacral meningocele is rare.* The age at diagnosis varied from 14 to 75 years with 75 per cent of the symptomatic patients presenting between 20 and 40 years of age. The sex incidence is equal. The late age of presentation is most likely due to the slow expansion of the meningocele over several years, and typically, the

---

* See references 2, 144, 285, 367, 572, 590, 699.

symptoms and signs have been present for years prior to the diagnosis. Intermittent or progressively severe pain in the back, buttocks, or sciatic nerve distribution suggestive of lumbar disc disease was the initial symptom in 69 per cent of patients and was a feature in 80 per cent of all cases. The pain may be increased by the upright position, coughing, or straining, and relieved by lying down, which has been attributed to emptying and filling of the meningocele. Mild unilateral or bilateral lower extremity weakness was noted in 56 per cent, and diminished sensation primarily in the perineal area occurred in 50 per cent of patients. The distal motor and sensory areas are typically involved, and the upper motor neuron signs or proximal weakness is probably due to an associated form of occult spinal dysraphism.[572] Only one patient manifested a chronic neuromusculoskeletal syndrome.[404] Dysfunction of both bladder and bowel occurred in 44 per cent of patients and was the earliest symptom in 19 per cent. Cutaneous manifestations over the sacrum are rarely present.[332,699]

Investigation

Plain roentgenograms and tomograms of the sacrum show enlargement of the sacral spinal canal with thinning of the overlying laminae and scalloping of the sacral vertebral bodies in 80 per cent of patients, with posterior spina bifida in 40 per cent. The plain film abnormalities may be confused with the dilatation of the sacral canal seen with tumors such as a neurofibroma or ependymoma or with the syndromes previously mentioned.

Spinal computed tomography may demonstrate the cerebrospinal fluid–filled sac and the dilated sacral canal.

Myelography may show a virtually normal sac to the level of S1 or S2 with a narrow isthmus extending into the distal sacral canal and expanding into the meningocele. At the initial study, the meningocele filled in 74 per cent of patients, but the communication may be so small that the sac will not fill at the initial study. One should not assume that a solid space-occupying lesion is present or that the dural sac terminates at a normal level, but rather, the patient should be kept erect for 24 to 48 hours and repeat films should be taken to demonstrate delayed filling of the sac, which occurred in 26 per cent of the patients. Delayed filling is typical of Pantopaque myelography, and metrizamide may fill the narrow-necked meningocele more reliably, since it is water-soluble. If metrizamide does not fill the sac immediately, delayed films are not possible and spinal computed tomography becomes more important.[256] Occasionally an upward extension of the cyst posterior or lateral to the normal dural sac will cause tapering or a local defect of the distal dural sac on the myelogram.[144,285,404]

Treatment

Sacral laminectomy displays the termination of the normal dural sac and the distal meningocele. The dural sac and meningocele are opened to insure that no nerve roots are intimately associated with the site of communication and to localize the filum terminale. If feasible, the entire sac is separated from the anteriorly displaced sacro-coccygeal nerve roots and is ligated or excised, as was possible in 67 per cent of the reported patients. If the sac contains nerve roots or the nerve roots are adherent anteriorly, then the narrow communication can be enlarged by a graft to eliminate the ball-valve mechanism or can be plugged with tissue to close the communication. If the occult intrasacral meningocele is combined with the tethered cord syndrome or another form of occult spinal dysraphism, the operation must be modified accordingly by sectioning the filum or untethering a sacral lipoma.

Results and Prognosis

The reported results have been good, with relief of or improvement in pain in 12 of 14 patients, improved sensation in 7 of 8 patients, and improved sphincter function in all 7 affected patients. Recurrent pain in two patients was attributed to lumbar disc disease in one and to adhesions at the operative site in the other.

THE PERINEURIAL (TARLOV) CYST

The perineurial cyst described by Tarlov in 1938 develops as an outpouching of the perineurial space on the extradural portion of the posterior sacral or coccygeal nerve roots at the junction of the root and ganglion.[738-741] The posterior root fibers or ganglion or both are involved in the cyst wall, and the anterior root is compressed. The cysts are usually multiple and in an eccentric location within the sacral canal, thus differentiating this lesion from the occult intrasacral meningocele. Occasionally a similar cyst develops in the midline on the extradural portion of the filum terminale, which is more in keeping with the occult intrasacral form. Low back pain and sciatica have been attributed to the cyst, particularly if the communication with the subarachnoid space is poor and pressure erosion is present on plain roentgenograms. Contrast material does not readily enter symptomatic cysts at myelography with Pantopaque, and delayed filling is typical.

SPINAL EXTRADURAL CYST

The spinal extradural cyst that occurs in the thoracic and upper lumbar area is a diverticulum of the dural sac or a cystic protrusion of arachnoid through a dural defect, which may cause spinal cord compression. The cyst is usually composed of dura with or without a lining of flattened epithelium or arachnoidlike cells and is connected to the dural sleeve of a nerve root or to the midline dorsal dural sac by a pedicle. Kyphosis or scoliosis of the thoracic spine is frequently present in addition to spinal cord compression. Localized erosion compatible with a chronic space-occupying lesion may be seen on plain roentgenograms. Myelography usually reveals a partial or complete extradural compressive lesion, but occasionally the contrast agent fills the cyst, which lies posteriorly in the spinal canal.* The intradural arachnoid diverticulum or cyst may present with a similar clinical picture and have a common pathological basis with the spinal extradural cyst.[232,384]

NONDYSRAPHIC SPINAL MENINGOCELE

Protrusion of the meninges from the confines of the spinal canal can occur in the absence of spinal dysraphism, perhaps on the

---

* See references 120, 350, 543, 545, 586, 801.

basis of a heritable disorder of connective tissue affecting the ability of the dura and the osseous structures to resist the pulsatile force of the cerebrospinal fluid. As already mentioned, the syndromes of von Recklinghausen, Marfan, and Ehlers-Danlos, and some of the chondro-osseous dysplasias may show widening of the interpedicular diameter of the spinal canal with thinning of the laminae and pedicles, scalloping of the posterior vertebral bodies, and dural ectasia on myelography.[306,332,499,524] Enlargement of the intervertebral foramina may also occur and facilitates protrusion of the dural sac into the paraspinous area, creating a nondysraphic meningocele in the thoracic or, rarely, the pelvic cavity.[332,499] The paraspinous muscles most likely inhibit the formation of meningoceles in the lumbar region. Posterior element defects do not occur.

The intrathoracic (lateral) meningocele occurs predominantly in von Recklinghausen's neurofibromatosis in middle life.* In 60 per cent of patients, the lesion is an asymptomatic posterior mediastinal mass detected on a routine roentgenogram of the chest. Local changes of rib erosion, scalloping of several posterior vertebral bodies, widening of the transverse diameter of the spinal canal, enlargement of usually multiple intervertebral foramina, and kyphoscoliosis may be present on tomographic studies of the thoracic spine. The meningocele is frequently at the apex of the scoliosis on the convex side. Multiple meningoceles may occur or consecutive intervertebral foramina may have coalesced with a single broad-based meningocele. The meningocele tends to enlarge with the passage of time. In 23 per cent of patients, the meningocele is associated with pain, suggesting intercostal neuralgia, and very rarely with respiratory insufficiency. Neurological deficit does not occur because of the meningocele, but may develop because of the kyphoscoliosis that occurs in 67 per cent of patients.[494]

The main consideration in the differential diagnosis is a posterior mediastinal tumor such as a neurofibroma, but actually such neoplasms extending outside the spinal canal are uncommon in patients with neurofibromatosis, rarely cause changes in more

than one vertebral body, rarely are evident on the chest roentgenograms, and are less frequently associated with spinal curvature. The absence of vertebral body fusion abnormalities tends to exclude the diagnosis of a mediastinal enteric cyst. The diagnosis is made by spinal computed tomography, which shows a cystic lesion filled with fluid with the radiodensity of water, and myelography confirms the communication with the subarachnoid space.

Treatment is required only for unremitting pain or respiratory embarrassment, since the risk of spontaneous rupture is slight.[494,622] The operative approach varies, depending upon the size of the neck and the number of meningoceles, but thoracotomy with extrapleural dissection or costotransversectomy usually suffices.

CAUDAL REGRESSION SYNDROME

Definition

The caudal regression syndrome is a failure of formation of part or all of the coccygeal, sacral, and occasionally lumbar vertebral units and the corresponding segments of the caudal spinal cord. Since the coccygeal and sacral vertebral units are more often involved, the frequent presentation is a congenital neurogenic dysfunction of both bladder and bowel, sparing the lower extremities.[394] Overlap with true spinal dysraphism does occur, particularly in lumbosacral lipoma, anterior sacral meningocele, and spina bifida aperta.[690] The syndrome is also termed the caudal dysplasia syndrome or sacral agenesis.[576,612]

Abnormal Embryology

The cause of the "caudal regression" is unknown, although maternal diabetes has a striking association. Approximately 16 per cent of patients with the syndrome have a diabetic mother, and approximately 1 per cent of infants born to diabetic mothers will have a form of the syndrome.[210,547,548] Presumably, absence of both the neural ectoderm and the notochord is required to produce the syndrome, since the two structures have a mutual inductive influence.[371] If the notochord is absent and the

---

* See references 58, 94, 382, 417, 489, 494, 673.

neural tube is intact, posterior arches form but vertebral bodies do not. If the neural tube is absent (or abnormal) and the notochord intact, the vertebral bodies form but posterior arches do not. Absence of both is most likely associated with failure of the spine to form at those levels. The lack of the trophic influence of lower motor neurons may explain the grossly defective musculature in the area subserved by the cord segments that are absent with the lumbar forms. Neural crest development may proceed, however, and the sensory system may be relatively less affected.[627] The urogenital primordia (wolffian ducts) develop at the same time as the caudal neural tube, and disturbance of these processes contributes to the frequent urinary and bowel malformations.[340]

Pathology

Failure of one or all of the coccygeal and sacral vertebral units to form is considered rare and was noted in only 0.43 per cent of unselected roentgenograms in children, but approximately 200 cases have been reported in the literature.[576,655] Sacral agenesis may be classified as: agenesis (total —the entire sacrum is absent; subtotal— one to four whole sacral segments are absent) or hemisacrum (total—all sacral segments are present on one side, but the corresponding segments on the other side are absent; subtotal—all sacral segments are present on one side, but one to four corresponding segments on the other side are absent).[690] The scimitar sacrum of anterior sacral meningocele is considered a subclass of sacral agenesis but should be distinguished from true sacral agenesis because sphincter function is not impaired on a neurogenic basis.

In the rare lumbosacrococcygeal agenesis, the spinal cord and dural sac both terminate at the last intact vertebral segment. The spinal cord displays progressive dysplasia until it ends in a glial knot, and the dural sac may terminate in a meningocele-like dilation.[576,627] Usually no nerve roots are present below the last vertebral segment, but occasionally sensory fibers are well formed and rectal ganglion cells are present, indicating that the sensory system is less involved than the motor system.[33,340,627,690] The muscles supplied by the

affected segments are developmentally immature, with large amounts of fat and a few small muscle fibers. Rarely, caudal regression is combined with obvious features of spinal dysraphism in the cord above the deficient level such as hydromyelia and diastematomyelia, or may be combined with a form of occult spinal dysraphism such as lumbosacral lipoma.[184,407,612,795]

Fat and fibrous connective tissue replace the absent skeletal structures to fill the space between the skin and peritoneum in the abdominal area. Fibrous tissue binds the closely approximated ilia together when the sacrum is absent.[576,795]

Approximately 10 per cent of patients with true sacral agenesis have an imperforate anus at birth.[394,795] The low variety of anal malformation with a normal pelvic floor and some form of abnormal anal opening occurs more commonly. Incomplete formation of the levator ani occurs with three or four missing sacral segments.[795] The high variety of imperforate anus with the bowel ending above the pelvic floor is seen less frequently.[193] Agenesis of one kidney, duplication of the ureters, horseshoe kidney, and hypoplasia of the aorta below the affected level occurs in severely afflicted infants.*

Clinical Evaluation

The child with sacral caudal regression of at least two segments presents at 3 to 5 years of age with failure to develop sphincter control.[407,795] Continued urinary incontinence or frequent urinary tract infections and chronic constipation without a sense of rectal distention are the more common complaints. In occult spinal dysraphism isolated bladder dysfunction is unusual in the absence of signs of the neuromusculoskeletal syndrome. Just the opposite is true of distal sacral caudal regression. Bladder function is always abnormal, but neurological deficit or orthopedic deformities in the lower extremities are absent or mild. Similarly, bowel control is usually not a problem in occult spinal dysraphism even if the bladder is affected, but bowel dysfunction is a frequent complaint in caudal regression.[795] The type of neurogenic blad-

---

* See references 312, 340, 394, 619, 627, 690.

der appears to have no relationship to the type of bony deformity, and both flaccid and spastic bladders have been reported.[394,627,690,795] Neurological deficits may be present in the ankles with attendant delay in learning to walk and an abnormal gait thereafter if the upper sacral and lower lumbar spinal cord segments are involved. Delayed onset of gait difficulty or progressive deterioration does not occur and, if present, suggests an associated anomaly.

From the skeletal point of view, the gait is usually normal if the S1 vertebral segment or, at least, a sacralized L5 vertebral segment is present, since a complete bony pelvic ring is formed.[237] If no such support is available the iliac bones meet in the midline and assume a more vertical position that predisposes to dislocation of the hips and adds to the effect produced by muscle imbalance.[690]

External evidence of the anomaly is limited to flattening of the buttocks, a shallow natal cleft, and occasionally paragluteal dimpling, particularly if the entire sacrum is absent. Cutaneous manifestations of occult spinal dysraphism are rarely present.[33,163,255,340] Palpation of the sacral area may confirm the absence of vertebral segments, and the anal sphincter may be anatomically malformed and is usually lax. Perianal sensation is normal in one third to one half of patients with caudal regression limited to one or two sacral segments and thus cannot be used as a reliable indicator of the functional state of the bladder.[690,795]

Patients with severe total sacral or lumbosacrococcygeal caudal regression may manifest severe neurological and orthopedic deformities, thoracopelvic disproportion, Buddha position, kyphosis of the lower lumbar spine, paralysis and atrophy of the legs with bilateral equinovarus deformities, flexion contractures of the knees and hips, and dislocation of the hips.[620] No upper motor neuron features are present in these patients, as may occur with occult spinal dysraphism.

Investigation

Plain roentgenograms of the sacrum, pelvis, and lumbar spine frequently do not show the coccyx in infants, and coccygeal agenesis should be diagnosed with due care. The degree of sacral agenesis does not necessarily correlate with a neurological deficit in the extremities owing to errors in determining the exact number of missing segments because of fusion of adjacent segments or the cartilaginous structure of lower segments.[237,394] Hemivertebrae, fusions, or forked ribs may be seen above the level of the caudal regression.[627] Posterior spina bifida, widening of the interpedicular diameter of the spinal canal, or erosion of the pedicles should suggest the possibility of an associated form of occult spinal dysraphism.[612]

Myelography should be performed in any patient who has caudal regression overlapping with occult spinal dysraphism, as might be suggested by an atypical clinical history or neurological examination or plain roentgenograms. The myelogram may be normal if only the distal two sacral segments are absent, or the distal sacral sac may be truncated at an abnormally high level corresponding to the absent vertebral units.[61,312]

Investigation of the anatomy and function of the urinary tract by the pediatric urologist is the key to proper care. The diagnosis of neurological vesical dysfunction is often quite delayed, and renal deterioration from infection or ureteral reflux may have already occurred. Awareness of the caudal regression syndrome as a cause of isolated bladder dysfunction and confirmation by plain roentgenography can result in early referral rather than delay while waiting for the child to "outgrow" the incontinence.

Treatment

Treatment is directed toward gaining urinary continence, if possible, and protecting the upper renal tracts. In cases overlapping with occult spinal dysraphism, an appropriate operation such as untethering of the cord from a lumbosacral lipoma may be required.

SACROCOCCYGEAL TERATOMA

The sacrococcygeal region is a frequent location for the midline teratomas that occur in one of every 30,000 to 40,000 births as well as for many other forms of presacral and postsacral neoplasms.* The neurological surgeon must be aware of the numerous possible neoplastic and nonneoplastic lesions in the area and not assume that a sacral mass is simply a form of myelomeningocele, meningocele, or occult spinal dysraphism.[421] Otherwise, he may recommend an inappropriate operation and become involved in the unfamiliar presacral anatomy of the rectum.

The sacrococcygeal teratoma is believed to develop from the totipotential cells in the area of Hensen's node, which migrates caudally to lie within the coccyx. The neoplasm is composed of derivatives of all three germ layers, and a wide variety of tissue types may be found.[390] The tumor tends to develop caudal to the level of the sacrum and extend anteriorly into the pelvis between the sacrum and rectum.[421] Type I tumors are mostly external and distort or discolor the buttock. The tumors are highly vascular, and surface erosions may bleed. Although pelvic extension is minimal, a presacral mass may be felt on rectal examination in many cases. The differential diagnosis must rule out sacral meningocele or myelomeningocele, sacral lipoma, hemangioma, lymphangioma, duplication of the rectum, bone tumor, and epidermoid cyst, to list a few.[421,638] Type II tumors have more internal extension involving the pelvic structures, but the external mass still

* See references 116, 173, 192, 305, 390, 456, 638, 646.

predominates. A type III tumor has a small external mass with the intrapelvic extension predominating, and a type IV lesion is completely intrapelvic. Type IV masses must be distinguished from the anterior sacral meningocele and all other forms of neoplastic and nonneoplastic presacral masses.[790]

The sacrococcygeal teratoma may be cystic, solid, or mixed. Seventy to ninety per cent are benign and tend to be cystic and have radiographically visible calcification; malignant forms tend to be solid and to lack calcification. Exceptions to the general rule are frequent, however.[390,456,638] Females predominate four to one over males. Infant males and patients of either sex with tumors developing beyond the neonatal age range are more likely to have malignant forms.[638]

Overlying skin abnormalities such as a dimple or sinus, hair, discoloration, or dilated veins may be present.[421,646] The important feature is the combination of the coccygeal location caudal to the sacrum of a presacral mass and anterior displacement of the rectum identified by rectal examination (Fig. 35–39). Occasionally, an infant with a large sacrococcygeal teratoma in the perineal area will hold the legs immobile in a flexed position on the lower abdomen, which falsely suggests a neurological deficit.[390] The majority of patients are without neurological deficit, but tumor can extend intraspinally and cause lower motor neuron signs.

Plain roentgenograms usually show a

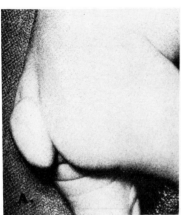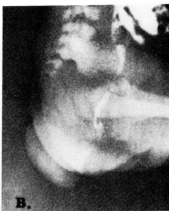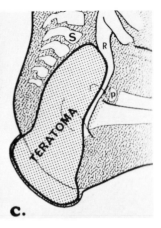

Figure 35–39   *A.* A clinically visible sacrococcygeal teratoma is located caudal to the sacrum. *B.* The barium enema shows anterior displacement of the rectum by a presacral mass. *C.* A drawing shows the predominance of the intrapelvic teratoma (type III). (From MacPherson, R. I., and Young, G.: Sacrococcygeal tumor. J. Canad. Ass. Radiol., *21*:132–142, 1970. Reprinted by permission.)

normal lumbar and sacral spine without erosion and without posterior or anterior defects, although exceptions do occur.[192,638] The mass extends posteriorly and inferiorly from the coccygeal region in type I, but displaces the rectal gas shadow anteriorly in types II, III, and IV. Involvement of the pelvic organs may be visualized on the intravenous pyelogram, cystogram, and barium enema. Ultrasound imaging or spinal computed tomography should be quite helpful in disclosing the sacral relationship of the mass and whether the lesion is cystic, solid, or calcified. Myelography is restricted to patients with neurological deficit. Aortography can demonstrate extreme neovascularity in the malignant forms, with blood supply chiefly from the internal iliac and middle sacral arteries.[481]

The key to successful treatment is early correct diagnosis, early radical operation in which removal of the coccyx is mandatory, radiotherapy and chemotherapy for malignant forms, and early detection and eradication of recurrent tumor.[390,456,638]

REFERENCES

1. Aaronson, I.: Anterior sacral meningocele, anal canal duplication cyst and covered anus occurring in one family. J. Pediat. Surg., 5:559–563, 1970.
2. Abbott, K. H., Retter, R. H., and Leimbach, W. H.: The role of perineurial sacral cysts in the sciatic and sacrococcygeal syndromes: A review of the literature and report of 9 cases. J. Neurosurg., 14:5–21, 1957.
3. Adams, R. D., and Wegner, W.: Congenital cyst of the spinal meninges as cause of intermittent compression of the spinal cord. Arch. Neurol. Psychiat., 58:57–69, 1947.
4. Adeloye, A.: Mesencephalic spur (beaking deformity of the tectum) in Arnold-Chiari malformation. J. Neurosurg., 45:315–320, 1976.
5. Adeloye, A., and Odeku, E. L.: Congenital subgaleal cysts over the anterior fontanelle in Nigerians. Arch. Dis. Child., 46:95–98, 1971.
6. Adeloye, A., Singh, S. P., and Odeku, E. L.: Stridor, myelomeningocele, and hydrocephalus in a child. Arch. Neurol. (Chicago), 23:271–273, 1970.
7. Adson, A. W.: Spina bifida cystica of the pelvis: Diagnosis and surgical treatment. Minn. Med., 21:468–475, 1938.
8. Ahmed, S., Jolleys, A., and Dark, J. F.: Thoracic enteric cysts and diverticulae. Brit. J. Surg., 59:963–968, 1972.
9. Aird, I.: Pilonidal sinus of axilla. Brit. Med. J., 1:902–903, 1952.
10. Akwari, O. E., Payne, W. S., Onofrio, B. M., Dines, D. E., and Muhm, J. R.: Dumbbell neurogenic tumors of the mediastinum: Diag-

11. nosis and management. Mayo Clin. Proc., 53:353–358, 1978.
12. Allan, L. D., Ferguson-Smith, M. A., Donald, I., Sweet, E. M., and Gibson, A. A.: Amniotic-fluid alpha-fetoprotein in the antenatal diagnosis of spina bifida. Lancet, 2:522–525, 1973.
13. Alexander, C. M., and Stevenson, L. D.: Sacral spina bifida, intrapelvic meningocele and sacrococcygeal teratoma. Amer. J. Clin. Path., 16:466–471, 1946.
14. Altman, R. S.: Dermoid tumor of the posterior fossa associated with congenital dermal sinus. J. Pediat., 62:565–570, 1963.
15. Amacher, A. L., Drake, C. G., and McLachlin, A. D.: Anterior sacral meningocele. Surg. Gynec. Obstet., 126:986–994, 1968.
16. Amador, L. V., Hankinson, J., and Bigler, J. A.: Congenital spinal dermal sinuses. J. Pediat., 47:300–310, 1955.
17. Ames, M. D., and Schut, L.: Results of treatment of 171 consecutive myelomeningoceles—1963 to 1968. Pediatrics, 50:466–470, 1972.
18. Anderson, F. M.: Intranasal (sphenopharyngeal) encephalocele; a report of a case with intracranial repair and a review of the subject. Arch. Otolaryng. (Chicago), 46:644–654, 1947.
19. Anderson, F. M.: Occult spinal dysraphism: Diagnosis and management. J. Pediat., 73:163–177, 1968.
20. Anderson, F. M.: Occult spinal dysraphism: A series of 73 cases. Pediatrics, 55:826–835, 1975.
21. Anderson, F. M., and Burke, B. L.: Anterior sacral meningocele: A presentation of three cases. J.A.M.A., 237:39–42, 1977.
22. Andersson, H., and Carlsson, C. A.: The surgical management of myelomeningocele with a preliminary report of 31 cases. Acta Paediat. Scand., 55:626–635, 1966.
23. Andersson, H., and Sullivan, L.: Diastematomyelia: Report of two cases submitted to laminectomy. Acta Orthop. Scand., 36:257–264, 1965.
24. Andersson, H., Carlsson, C. A., and Rosengren, K.: A radiological study of the central canal in myelomeningocele. Dev. Med. Child. Neurol. suppl., 13:96–102, 1967.
25. Arcomano, J. P., Sengstacken, R. L., and Wunderlich, H. O.: Diastematomyelia. Amer. J. Dis. Child., 104:393–396, 1962.
26. Arnold, J.: Myelocyste, Transposition von Gewebskeimen und Sympodie. Beitr. Path. Anat., 16:1–28, 1894.
27. Arseni, C., and Horvath, L.: Meningoencephalocele of the pterion. Acta Neurochir. (Wien), 25:231–240, 1971.
28. Avanzini, G., and Crivelli, G.: A case of sphenopharyngeal encephalocele. Acta. Neurochir. (Wien), 22:205–212, 1970.
29. Bailey, I. C.: Dermoid tumors of the spinal cord. J. Neurosurg., 33:676–681, 1970.
30. Balériaux-Waha, D., Osteaux, M., Terwinghe, G., deMeeus, A., and Jeanmart, L.: The management of anterior sacral meningocele with computed tomography. Neuroradiology, 14:45–46, 1977.
31. Ballantyne, J. W.: Manual of antenatal pathology and hygiene. In The Embryo. Edinburgh, W. Green & Sons, 1904.
32. Banna, M., and Talalla, A.: Intraspinal dermoids in adults. Brit. J. Radiol., 48:28–30, 1975.

32. Bannister, C. M.: A method of repair of myelomeningoceles. Brit. J. Surg., *59*:445–448, 1972.

33. Banta, J. V., and Nichols, O.: Sacral agenesis. J. Bone Joint Surg., *51A*:693–703, 1969.

34. Barlow, P., and Gracey, L.: Anterior sacral meningocele causing urinary retention. Brit. J. Surg., *50*:732–734, 1963.

35. Barrow, N., and Simpson, D. A.: Cranium bifidum: Investigation, prognosis and management. Aust. Paediat. J., *2*:20–26, 1966.

36. Barry, A., Patten, B. M., and Stewart, B. H.: Possible factors in the development of the Arnold-Chiari malformation. J. Neurosurg., *14*:285–301, 1957.

37. Barson, A. J.: Radiological studies of spina bifida cystica: The phenomenon of congenital lumbar kyphosis. Brit. J. Radiol., *38*:294–300, 1965.

38. Barson, A. J.: The vertebral level of termination of the spinal cord during normal and abnormal development. J. Anat., *106*:489–497, 1970.

39. Barson, A. J.: Spina bifida: The significance of the level and extent of the defect to the morphogenesis. Develop. Med. Child Neurol., *12*:129–144, 1970.

40. Barson, A. J.: Symptomless intradural spinal lipomas in infancy. J. Path., *104*:141–144, 1971.

41. Barson, A. J.: Differentiation, growth and disorders of development of the vertebrospinal axis. *In* Davis, J. A., and Dobbing, J., ed.: Scientific Foundations of Paediatrics, London, William Heinemann Medical Books Ltd., 1974.

42. Barson, A. J., and Cole, F. M.: Neurofibromatosis with congenital malformation of the spinal cord. J. Neurol. Neurosurg. Psychiat., *30*:71–74, 1967.

43. Barson, A. J., and Sands, J.: Physical and biochemical characteristics of the human dysraphic spinal cord. Develop. Med. Child Neurol. suppl., *35*:11–19, 1975.

44. Bassett, R. C.: The neurologic deficit associated with lipomas of the cauda equina. Ann. Surg., *131*:109–116, 1950.

45. Beardmore, H. E., and Wigelsworth, F. W.: Vertebral anomalies and alimentary duplications. Clinical and embryological aspects. Pediat. Clin. N. Amer., *5*:457–474, 1958.

46. Beau, A., Neimann, N., and Gosserez, M.: Kystes dermoides et fistules congénitales médians du dos du nez. Arch. Franc. Pédiat., *11*:1100–1108, 1954.

47. Beckman, E. H., and Adson, A. W.: Spina bifida: Its operative treatment. St. Paul. Med. J., *19*:357–363, 1917.

48. Beks, J. W. F., van Rootselaar, F. J., and Harms-Prosee, A. M.: Therapeutic results in 133 cases of spina bifida. Psychiat. Neurol. Neurochir., *69*:411–416, 1966.

49. Bell, H. H.: Anterior spina bifida and its relation to a persistence of the neurentric canal. J. Nerv. Ment. Dis., *57*:445–462, 1923.

50. Benda, C. E.: The Dandy-Walker syndrome or the so-called atresia of the foramen of Magendie. J. Neuropath. Exp. Neurol., *13*:14–29, 1954.

51. Benda, C. E.: Dysraphic states. J. Neuropath. Exp. Neurol., *18*:56–74, 1959.

52. Benstead, J. G.: A case of diastematomyelia. J. Path. Bact., *66*:553–557, 1953.

53. Bentley, J. F. R., and Smith, J. R.: Developmental posterior enteric remnants and spinal malformations: The split notochord syndrome. Arch. Dis. Child., *35*:76–86, 1960.

54. Bernasconi, V., Giovanelli, M., and Perria, C.: Meningoencephalocele of posterior part of orbit. Neurochirurgia (Stuttgart), *11*:19–20, 1968.

55. Bigler, J. A., and Gibson, S.: Conference at the Children's Memorial Hospital of Chicago. Case I: Congenital dermal sinus. J. Pediat., *35*:102–107, 1949.

56. Birnbaum, L. J., and Owsley, J. Q., Jr.: Frontonasal tumors of neurogenic origin. Plast. Reconstr. Surg., *41*:462–470, 1968.

57. Black, S. P. W., and German, W. J.: Four congenital tumors found at operation within the vertebral canal with observations on their incidence. J. Neurosurg., *7*:49–61, 1950.

58. Blewett, J. H., Jr., and Szypulski, J. T.: Double unilateral intrathoracic meningocele. Report of a case. J. Thorac. Cardiovasc. Surg., *67*:481–483, 1974.

59. Bligh, A. S.: Diastematomyelia. Clin. Radiol., *12*:158–163, 1961.

60. Bluestone, C. D., Delerme, A. N., and Samuelson, G. H.: Airway obstruction due to vocal cord paralysis in infants with hydrocephalus and meningomyelocele. Ann. Otol., *81*:778–783, 1972.

61. Blumel, J., Evans, E. B., and Eggers, G. W. N.: Partial and complete agenesis or malformation of the sacrum with associated anomalies. Etiologic and clinical study with special reference to heredity: A preliminary report. J. Bone Joint Surg., *41-A*:497–518, 1959.

62. Bokinsky, G. E., Hudson, L. D., and Weil, J. V.: Impaired peripheral chemosensitivity and acute respiratory failure in Arnold-Chiari malformation and syringomyelia. New Eng. J. Med., *288*:947–948, 1973.

63. Boldrey, E. G., and Elvidge, A. R.: Dermoid cysts of the vertebral canal. Ann. Surg., *110*:273–284, 1939.

64. Bouton, J. M., Martin, C. H., and Rickham, P. P.: Hamartoma and spina bifida. J. Pediat. Surg., *1*:559–565, 1966.

65. Bower, R. J., and Kiesewetter, W. B.: Mediastinal masses in infants and children. Arch. Surg. (Chicago), *112*:1003–1009, 1977.

66. Brailsford, J. F.: The Radiology of the Bones and Joints. 5th Ed. Baltimore, Williams & Wilkins Co., 1953.

67. Breig, A.: Overstretching of and circumscribed pathological tension in the spinal cord—a basic cause of symptoms in cord disorders. J. Biomech., *3*:7–9, 1970.

68. Bremer, J. L.: Dorsal intestinal fistula; accessory neurenteric canal; diastematomyelia. Arch. Path. (Chicago), *54*:132–138, 1952.

69. Brewerton, D. A., Sandifer, P. H., and Sweetnam, D. R.: ''Idiopathic'' pes cavus. An investigation into its aetiology. Brit. Med. J., *2*:659–661, 1963.

70. Brickner, W. M.: Spina bifida occulta. Amer. J. Med. Sci., *155*:473–502, 1918.

71. Brihaye, J., Gerard, A., Kiekens, R., and Retif, J.: Recto-meningeal fistulae in dysraphic states. Surg. Neurol., *10*:93–95, 1978.

72. British Medical Journal, Editorial: Perspectives in spina bifida. Brit. Med. J., *2*:909–910, 1978.

73. Brock, D. J. H.: α-Fetoprotein and the prenatal diagnosis of central nervous system disorders. A review. Child's Brain, 2:1–23, 1976.

74. Brock, D. J. H.: Alpha-fetoprotein and the pre-natal diagnosis of neural tube defects. J. Roy. Coll. Surg. Edinb., 23:184–192, 1978.

75. Brock, D. J. H., and Sutcliffe, R. G.: Alpha-feto-protein and the antenatal diagnosis of anen-cephaly and spina bifida. Lancet, 2:197–199, 1972.

76. Brock, D. J. H., Bolton, A. E., and Scrimgeour, J. B.: Prenatal diagnosis of spina bifida and an-encephaly through maternal plasma-alpha-fe-toprotein measurement. Lancet, 1:767–769, 1974.

77. Brocklehurst, G.: A quantitative study of a spina bifida foetus. J. Path., 99:205–211, 1969.

78. Brocklehurst, G.: The development of the human cerebrospinal fluid pathway with particular ref-erence to the roof of the fourth ventricle. J. Anat., 105:467–475, 1969.

79. Brocklehurst, G.: The pathogenesis of spina bi-fida: A study of the relationship between ob-servation, hypothesis, and surgical incentive. Develop. Med. Child Neurol., 13:147–163, 1971.

80. Brocklehurst, G.: Spina Bifida for the Clinician. London, William Heinemann Medical Books, Ltd., 1976.

81. Brocklehurst, G., Gleave, J. R. W., and Lewin, W.: Early closure of myelomeningocele with special reference to leg movement. Brit. Med. J., 1:666–669, 1967.

82. Brodal, A., and Hauglie-Hanssen, E.: Congenital hydrocephalus with defective development of the cerebellar vermis (Dandy-Walker syn-drome). Clinical and anatomical findings in two cases with particular reference to so-called atresia of the foramina of Magendie and Luschka. J. Neurol. Neurosurg. Psychiat., 22:99–108, 1959.

83. Brown, J. R.: The Dandy-Walker syndrome. In Handbook of Clinical Neurology, Vinken, P. J., Bruyn, G. W., eds.: Chapter 24 in Congeni-tal Malformations of the Brain and Skull, Volume 30, Part I, Amsterdam, Elsevier-North Holland Publishing Co., 1977.

84. Bruce, A., and Lorber, J.: Is antibiotic prophy-laxis necessary in spina bifida? Develop. Med. Child Neurol., 6:18–22, 1964.

85. Brown, M. H., and Powell, L. D.: Anterior sa-cral meningocele. J. Neurosurg., 2:535–538, 1945.

86. Bruce, A., McDonald, S., and Pirie, J. H. H.: A case of localized doubling of the spinal cord. Rev. Neurol. Psychiat. Edin., 3:709–718, 1905.

87. Bruce, A., McDonald, S., Pirie, J. H. H.: A second case of partial doubling of the spinal cord. Rev. Neurol. Psychiat. Edin. 4:6–19, 1906.

88. Brun, A., and Saldeen, T.: Intraspinal enter-ogenous cyst. Acta Path. Microbiol. Scand., 73:191–194, 1968.

89. Bryant, H., and Dayan, A. D.: Spinal inclusion dermoid cyst in a patient with a treated myelo-cystocele. J. Neurol. Neurosurg. Psychiat., 30:182–184, 1967.

90. Bucy, P. C., and Buchanan, D. N.: Teratoma of the spinal cord. Surg. Gynec. Obstet., 60:1137–1144, 1935.

91. Bucy, P. C., and Gustafson, W. A.: Intradural li-poma of the spinal cord. Neurochirurgie, 3:341–349, 1938.

92. Burrows, F. G. O.: Some aspects of occult spinal dysraphism: A study of 90 cases. Brit. J. Ra-diol., 41:496–507, 1968.

93. Burrows, F. G. O., and Sutcliffe, J.: The split no-tochord syndrome. Brit. J. Radiol., 41:844–847, 1968.

94. Byron, F. X., Alling, E. E., and Samson, P. C.: Intrathoracic meningocele. J. Thorac. Cardio-vasc. Surg., 18:294–303, 1949.

95. Calihan, R. J.: Anterior sacral meningocele. Ra-diology, 58:104–108, 1952.

96. Calvert, D. G.: Direct spinal anaesthesia for re-pair of myelomeningocele. Brit. Med. J., 2:86–87, 1966.

97. Cameron, A. H.: The Arnold-Chiari and other neuro-anatomical malformations associated with spina bifida. J. Path. Bact., 73:195–211, 1957.

98. Cameron, A. H.: Malformations of the neuro-spi-nal axis, urogenital tract and foregut in spina bifida attributable to disturbances of the blasto-pore. J. Path. Bact., 73:213–221, 1957.

99. Caram, P. C., Scarcella, G., and Carton, C. A.: Intradural lipomas of the spinal cord with par-ticular emphasis on the "intramedullary" li-pomas. J. Neurosurg., 14:28–42, 1957.

100. Cardell, B. S., and Laurance, B.: Congenital der-mal sinus associated with meningitis. Report of a fatal case. Brit. Med. J., 2:1558–1561, 1951.

101. Carmel, P. W., and Markesbery, W. R.: Early descriptions of the Arnold-Chiari malforma-tion: The contribution of John Cleland. J. Neurosurg., 37:543–547, 1972.

102. Carmel, P. W., Antunes, J. L., Hilal, S. K., and Gold, A. P.: Dandy-Walker syndrome: Clin-ico-pathological features and reevaluation of modes of treatment. Surg. Neurol., 8:132–138, 1977.

103. Carr, T. L.: The orthopaedic aspects of one hun-dred cases of spina bifida. Postgrad. Med. J., 32:201–210, 1956.

104. Carroll, N. C., and Sharrard, W. J. W.: Long-term follow-up of posterior iliopsoas transplan-tation for paralytic dislocation of the hip. J. Bone Joint Surg., 54-A:551–560, 1972.

105. Case records of the Massachusetts General Hos-pital (Case 46122). New Eng. J. Med., 262:623–627, 1960.

106. Case records of the Massachusetts General Hos-pital (Case 26-1975). New Eng. J. Med., 29:33–38, 1975.

107. Cassidy, W. A., and Wahl, J. W.: Congenital dis-placement of central nervous system tissue in the nasal fossae: Report of two cases. Arch. Otolaryng. (Chicago), 59:93–99, 1954.

108. Castellino, R. A., Zatz, L. M., and DeNardo, G. L.: Radioisotope ventriculography in the Ar-nold-Chiari malformation. Radiology, 93:817–821, 1969.

109. Caviness, V. S., Jr., and Evrard, P.: Occipital encephalocele: A pathologic and anatomic analysis. Acta. Neuropath. (Berlin), 32:245–255, 1975.

110. Cerulla, L., and Raimondi, A. J.: The neurora-diological evaluation of the Arnold-Chiari mal-formation. In McLaurin, R. L., ed.: Myelome-ningocele. New York, Grune & Stratton, 1977, pp. 227–239.

111. Chadduck, W. M., and Netsky, M. G.: Arnold-Chiari malformation with cyst of third ventricle: A case report. J. Neurosurg., 23:357–361, 1965.
112. Chambers, W. R.: Diastematomyelia: Report of a case diagnosed preoperatively. J. Pediat., 45:668–671, 1954.
113. Charoonsmith, T., and Suwanwela, C.: Frontoethmoidal encephalomeningocele with special reference to plastic reconstruction. Clin. Plast. Surg., 1:27–47, 1974.
114. Chiari, H.: Ueber Veränderungen des Kleinhirns infolge von Hydrocephalie des Grosshirns. Deutsch. Med. Wochenschr., 17:1172–1175, 1891.
115. Chiari, H.: Ueber Veranderungen des Kleinhirns, des Pons und der Medulla Oblongata infolge von congenitaler Hydrocephalie des Grosshirns. Denschr. Akad. Wiss. Wien, 63:71–116, 1896.
116. Christensen, E. R.: Presacral and sacral tumours in children. Danish Med. Bull., 5:25–32, 1958.
117. Clark, S. N.: Report of a case of spina bifida occulta in cervical region. J. Nerv. Ment. Dis., 48:201–205, 1918.
118. Cleland, J.: Contribution to the study of spina bifida, encephalocele, and anencephalus. J. Anat. Physiol., 17:257–292, 1883.
119. Cliffton, E. E., and Rydell, J. R.: Congenital dermal (pilonidal) sinus with dural connection. J. Neurosurg., 4:276–282, 1947.
120. Cloward, R. B., and Bucy, P. C.: Spinal extradural cyst and kyphosis dorsalis juvenilis. Amer. J. Roentgen., 38:681–706, 1937.
121. Cohen, I.: Agnesis of the cerebellum (verified by operation). J. Mount Sinai Hosp. N.Y., 8:441–446, 1942.
122. Cohen, J., and Sledge, C. B.: Diastematomyelia: An embryological interpretation with report of a case. Amer. J. Dis. Child., 100:257–263, 1960.
123. Cohen, M.: Orbital meningoencephalocele associated with microphthalmia. J.A.M.A., 89:746–749, 1927.
124. Cohn, G. A., and Hamby, W. B.: The surgery of cranium bifidum and spina bifida: A follow-up report of 64 cases. J. Neurosurg., 10:297–300, 1953.
125. Cohn, J., and Bay-Nielsen, E.: Hereditary defect of the sacrum and coccyx with anterior sacral meningocele. Acta Paediat. Scand., 58:268–274, 1969.
126. Coleman, C. C., and Troland, C. E.: Congenital atresia of the foramina of Luschka and Magendie with report of two cases of surgical cure. J. Neurosurg., 5:84–88, 1948.
127. Coller, F. A., and Jackson, R. G.: Anterior sacral meningocele. Surg. Gynec. Obstet., 76:703–707, 1943.
128. Comarr, A. E.: Neurological disturbances of sexual function among patients with myelodysplasia. In McLaurin, R. L., ed.: Myelomeningocele. New York, Grune & Stratton, Inc., 1977, pp. 797–808.
129. Connolly, N. K.: Congenital dermal sinuses in children. Lancet, 2:251, 1955.
130. Constantinou, E.: A case of diastematomyelia. J.A.M.A., 185:983–984, 1963.
131. Consul, B. N., and Kulshrestha, O. P.: Orbital meningocele. Brit. J. Ophthal., 49:374–376, 1965.
132. Converse, J. M., and Fleury, A. F.: A note on frontal encephalocele. Case report with a 20 year follow-up. Plast Reconstr. Surg., 49:343–345, 1972.
133. Conway, J. J., Yarzagaray, L., and Welch, D.: Radionuclide evaluation of the Dandy-Walker malformation and congenital arachnoid cyst of the posterior fossa. Amer. J. Roentgen., 12:306–314, 1971.
134. Cook, P. L.: Gas myelography in the investigation of occult spinal dysraphism. Brit. J. Radiol., 49:502–515, 1976.
135. Corkill, G., McCulloch, G. A. J., and Tonge, R. E.: Cranial dermal sinus: Value of plain skull x-ray examination and early diagnosis. Med. J. Aust., 1:885–887, 1974.
136. Coughlin, W. T.: Spina bifida: A clinical study with a report of 12 personal cases. Ann. Surg., 94:982–1006, 1931.
137. Cowie, T. N.: Diastematomyelia with vertebral column defects: Observation on its radiological diagnosis. Brit. J. Radiol., 24:156–160, 1951.
138. Cowie, T. N.: Diastematomyelia: Tomography in diagnosis. Brit. J. Radiol., 25:263–266, 1952.
139. Cowie, T. N.: Congenital spinal deformities of surgical importance. Acta Radiol. (Stockholm), 46:38–47, 1956.
140. Cox, J. A.: Care of the bowel. In McLaurin, R. L., ed.: Myelomeningocele. New York, Grune & Stratton, Inc., 1977, pp. 699–703.
141. Craig, W. McK., and Mulder, D. W.: Late neurologic symptoms of spina bifida occulta: Report of a case. Proc. Staff Meet. Mayo Clin., 31:98–100, 1956.
142. Creasy, M. R., and Alberman, E. D.: Congenital malformations of the central nervous system in spontaneous abortion. J. Med. Genet., 13:9–16, 1976.
143. Creighton, R. E., Relton, J. E. S., and Meridy, H. W.: Anaesthesia for occipital encephalocoele. Can. Anaesth. Soc. J., 21:403–406, 1974.
144. Crellin, R. Q., and Jones, E. R.: Sacral extradural cysts. A rare cause of low backache and sciatica. J. Bone Joint Surg., 55-B:20–31, 1973.
145. Critchley, M., and Ferguson, F. R.: The cerebrospinal epidermoids (cholesteatomata). Brain, 51:334–384, 1928.
146. Crue, B. L., Jr., Dudley, H. R., and Delaney, L. J.: Congenital dermal sinus and cyst. U.S. Armed Forces Med. J., 8:1765–1779, 1957.
147. D'Agostino, A. N., Kernohan, J. W., and Brown, J. R.: The Dandy-Walker syndrome. J. Neuropath. Exp. Neurol. (Chicago), 22:450–470, 1963.
148. Dale, A. J.: Diastematomyelia. Arch. Neurol. (Chicago), 20:309–317, 1969.
149. Dandy, W. E.: The diagnosis and treatment of hydrocephalus due to occlusions of the foramina of Magendie and Luschka. Surg. Gynec. Obstet. 32:112–124, 1921.
150. Dandy, W. E.: An operative treatment for certain cases of meningocele (or encephalocele) into the orbit. Arch. Ophthal. (Chicago), 2:123–132, 1929.
151. Dandy, W. E., and Blackfan, K. D.: Internal hydrocephalus: An experimental clinical and pathological study. Amer. J. Dis. Child., 8:406–482, 1914.
152. Dandy, W. E., and Blackfan, K. D.: Internal hy-

drocephalus. Amer. J. Dis. Child., *14*:424–443, 1917.

153. Daniel, P. M., and Strich, S. J.: Some observations on the congenital deformity of the central nervous system known as the Arnold-Chiari malformation. J. Neuropath. Exp. Neurol., *17*:255–266, 1958.

154. Davies, D. K. L., Jennett, W. B., and Hoskins, E. O. L.: A case of diastematomyelia. Brit. J. Radiol., *30*:326–327, 1957.

155. Davis, C. H., Jr., and Alexander, E., Jr.: Congenital nasofrontal encephalomeningoceles and teratomas. Review of seven cases. J. Neurosurg., *16*:365–377, 1959.

156. Davis, E. D.: Diastematomyelia with early Arnold-Chiari syndrome and congenital dysplastic hip. Clin. Orthop., *52*:179–185, 1967.

157. Davis, E. W.: Gliomatous tumors in the nasal region. J. Neuropath. Exp. Neurol., *1*:312–319, 1942.

158. Dawson, C. W., and Driesbach, J. H.: Diastematomyelia and acquired clubfoot deformity. J.A.M.A., *175*:569–572, 1961.

159. de Baecque, C., Snyder, D. H., and Suzuki, K.: Congenital intramedullary spinal dermoid cyst associated with an Arnold-Chiari malformation. Acta Neuropath. (Berlin), *38*:239–242, 1977.

160. Dekaban A., and Guin, G. H.: Clinical pathological conference. The Dandy-Walker syndrome. Clin. Proc. Child. Hosp. D.C., *20*:19–26, 1964.

161. De Klerk, D. J. J., and De Villiers, J. C.: Frontal encephaloceles. S. Afr. Med. J., *47*:1350–1355, 1973.

162. De Lange, S. A.: Selection for treatment of patients with spina bifida aperta. Develop. Med. Child. Neurol., *16*:suppl. 32:27–30, 1974.

163. Del Duca, V., Davis, E. V., and Barroway, J. N.: Congenital absence of the sacrum and coccyx. J. Bone Joint Surg., *33-A*:248–253, 1951.

164. DeLong, W. B., and Schneider, R. C.: Surgical management of congenital spinal lesions associated with abnormalities of the cranio-spinal junction. J. Neurol. Neurosurg. Psychiat., *29*:319–322, 1966.

165. De Reuck, J., and Thienpoint, L.: Fetal Chiari's type III malformation. Child's Brain, *2*:85–91, 1976.

166. De Reuck, J., and vander Eecken, H.: Transitional forms of Arnold-Chiari and Dandy-Walker malformations. J. Neurol. *210*:135–141, 1975.

167. Desprez, J. D., Kiehn, C. L., and Eckstein, W.: Closure of large meningomyelocele defects by composite skin-muscle flaps. Plast. Reconstr. Surg., *47*:234–238, 1971.

168. De Vries, E.: Spina bifida occulta and myelodysplasia with unilateral clubfoot beginning in adult life. Amer. J. Med. Sci., *175*:365–371, 1928.

169. Di Chiro, G., and Timins, E. L.: Supine myelography and the septum posticum. Radiology, *111*:319–327, 1974.

170. Di Chiro, G., Harrington, T., and Fried, L. C.: Microangiography of human fetal spinal cord. Amer. J. Roentgen., *118*:193–199, 1973.

171. Dickson, R. A., and Leatherman, K. D.: The kyphotic spine in myelomeningocele. *In* McLaurin, R. L., ed.: Myelomeningocele. New York, Grune & Stratton, Inc., 1977, pp. 609–620.

172. Dickson, R. A., and Leatherman, K. D.: Vertebral body resection for spinal deformity in myelomeningocele. *In* McLaurin, R. L., ed.: Myelomeningocele. New York, Grune & Stratton, Inc., 1977, pp. 621–633.

173. Dillard, B. M., Mayer, J. H., McAlister, W. H., McGavrin, M., and Strominger, D. B.: Sacrococcygeal teratoma in children. J. Pediat. Surg., *5*:53–59, 1970.

174. Diokno, A. C.: Intermittent self-catheterization. *In* McLaurin, R. L., ed.: Myelomeningocele. New York, Grune & Stratton, Inc., 1977, pp. 705–713.

175. Diokno, A. C.: Indications for cutaneous vesicostomy, technique and long term results. *In* McLaurin, R. L., ed.: Myelomeningocele. New York, Grune & Stratton, Inc., 1977, pp. 781–784.

176. Dodge, H. W., Jr., Love, J. G., and Kernohan, J. W.: Intranasal encephalomeningoceles associated with cranium bifidum. Arch. Surg. (Chicago), *79*:87–96, 1959.

177. Doran, P. A., and Guthkelch, A. N.: Studies in spina bifida cystica. I. General survey and reassessment of the problem. J. Neurol. Neurosurg. Psychiat., *24*:331–345, 1961.

178. Dorsey, J. F., and Tabrisky, J.: Intraspinal and mediastinal foregut cyst compressing the spinal cord. Report of a case. J. Neurosurg., *24*:562–567, 1966.

179. Dorst, J. P.: Functional craniology: An aid in interpreting roentgenograms of the skull. Radiol. Clin. N. Amer., *2*:347–365, 1965.

180. Dowling, J. L.: Dermoids, dimples and spinal meningitis. Med. J. Aust., *2*:751–754, 1956.

181. Drennan, A. M.: Anterior sacral meningocele. J. Path. Bact., *32*:843–844, 1929.

182. Drennan, J. C.: The role of muscles in the development of human lumbar kyphosis. Develop. Med. Child Neurol., *12*:suppl. 22:33–38, 1970.

183. Drummond, M. B., and Donaldson, A. A.: Air, Myodil and Conray studies in the hydrocephalus of myelomeningocele. Develop. Med. Child Neurol., *16*:suppl. 32:131–143, 1974.

184. Dubowitz, V., Lorber, J., and Zachary, R. B.: Lipoma of the cauda equina. Arch. Dis. Child., *40*:207–213, 1965.

185. Duckett, S.: Foetal Arnold-Chiari malformation. Acta Neuropath. (Berlin), *7*:175–179, 1966.

186. Duckworth, T., and Brown, B. H.: Changes in muscle activity following early closure in myelomeningocele. Develop. Med. Child Neurol., *12*:suppl. 22:39–45, 1970.

187. Duckworth, T., Sharrard, W. J., Lister, J., and Seymour, N.: Hemimyelocele. Develop. Med. Child Neurol. suppl., *16*:69–75, 1968.

188. Eckstein, H. B.: Myelomeningocele. Postgrad. Med. J., *48*:496–500, 1972.

189. Eckstein, H. B., and MacNab, G. H.: Myelomeningocele and hydrocephalus. Lancet, *1*:842–845, 1966.

190. Eckstein, H. B., Cooper, D. G. W., Howard, E. R., and Pike, J.: Cause of death in children with meningomyelocele or hydrocephalus. Arch. Dis. Child., *42*:163–165, 1967.

191. Ehni, G., and Love, J. G.: Intraspinal lipomas: report of cases; review of literature and clinical and pathological study. Arch. Neurol. Psychiat., *53*:1–28, 1945.

192. Eklöf, O.: Roentgenologic findings in sacrococ-

cygeal teratoma. Acta Radiol. [Diagn.] (Stockholm), *3*:41–48, 1965.

193. Elliott, G. B., Tredwell, S. J., and Eliott, K. A.: The notochord as an abnormal organizer in production of congenital intestinal defect. Amer. J. Roentgen., *110*:628–634, 1970.

194. Emery, J. L.: Kinking of the medulla in children with acute cerebral oedema and hydrocephalus and its relationship to the dentate ligaments. J. Neurol. Neurosurg. Psychiat., *30*:267–275, 1967.

195. Emery, J. L.: Deformity of the aqueduct of Sylvius in children with hydrocephalus and myelomeningocele. Develop. Med. Child Neurol., *16*:suppl. 32:40–48, 1974.

196. Emery, J. L., and Gadson, D. R.: A quantitative study of the cell population of the cerebellum in children with myelomeningocele. Develop. Med. Child Neurol., *17*:suppl. 35:20–25, 1975.

197. Emery, J. L., and Kalhan, S. C.: The pathology of exencephalus. Develop. Med. Child Neurol., *12*:suppl. 22:51–64, 1970.

198. Emery, J. L., and Lendon, R. G.: Lipomas of the cauda equina and other fatty tumors related to neurospinal dysraphism. Develop. Med. Child Neurol. suppl., *20*:62–70, 1969.

199. Emery, J. L., and Lendon, R. G.: Clinical implications of cord lesions in neurospinal dysraphism. Develop. Med. Child Neurol., *14*:suppl. 27:45–51, 1972.

200. Emery, J. L., and Lendon, R. G.: The local cord lesion in neurospinal dysraphism (meningomyelocele). J. Path., *110*:83–96, 1973.

201. Emery, J. L., and Levick, R. K.: The movement of the brain stem and vessels around the brain stem in children with hydrocephalus and the Arnold-Chiari deformity. Develop. Med. Child Neurol. suppl., *11*:49–60, 1966.

202. Emery, J. L., and MacKenzie, N.: Medullo-cervical dislocation deformity (Chiari II deformity) related to neurospinal dysraphism (meningomyelocele). Brain, *96*:155–162, 1973.

203. Emery, J. L., and Naik, D.: Spinal cord segment lengths in children with meningomyelocele and the "Cleland-Arnold-Chiari" deformity. Brit. J. Radiol., *41*:287–290, 1968.

204. Emery, J. L., and Singhal, R.: Changes associated with growth in the cells of the dorsal root ganglion in children. Develop. Med. Child Neurol., *15*:460–466, 1973.

205. Emery, J. L., Nunn, H., and Singhal, R.: The cell population of dorsal root ganglia in children with neurospinal dysraphism. Develop. Med. Child Neurol., *15*:467–473, 1973.

206. Engel, R., and Buchan, G. C.: Occipital encephaloceles with and without visual evoked potentials. Arch. Neurol. (Chicago), *30*:314–318, 1974.

207. English, W. J., and Maltby, G. L.: Diastematomyelia in adults. J. Neurosurg., *27*:260–264, 1967.

208. Esilä, R., Törmä, T., and Vannas, S.: Unilateral orbital anterior hydroencephalocele and bilateral atresia of the lacrimal passages. Acta Ophthal. (Kobenhavn), *45*:390–398, 1967.

209. Evans, A. T.: Infection of the urinary tract in patients with myelomeningocele. *In* McLaurin, R. L., ed.: Myelomeningocele. New York, Grune & Stratton, Inc., 1977, pp. 773–780.

210. Evrard, P., and Caviness, V. S.: Extensive developmental defect of the cerebellum associated with posterior fossa ventriculocele. J. Neuropath. Exp. Neurol., *33*:385–399, 1974.

211. Fallon, M., Gordon, A. R. G., and Lendrum, A. C.: Mediastinal cysts of fore-gut origin associated with vertebral abnormalities. Brit. J. Surg., *41*:520–533, 1954.

212. Fargueta, J. S., Menezo, J. L., and Bordes, M.: Posterior orbital encephalocele with anophthalmos and other brain malformations: Case report. J. Neurosurg., *38*:215–217, 1973.

213. Faris, J. C., and Crowe, J. E.: The split notochord syndrome. J. Pediat. Surg., *10*:467–472, 1975.

214. Fauré, C., Lepintre, J., Michel, J. R., and Nasselin, S.: Les fistules dermiques congénitales: à propos de 6 observations. J. Radiol. Electr., *39*:481–486, 1958.

215. Feiwell, E.: Paralytic calcaneus in myelomeningocele. *In* McLaurin, R. L., ed.: Myelomeningocele. New York, Grune & Stratton, Inc., 1977, pp. 447–460.

216. Feiwell, E.: Conservative treatment of hip dislocation in the myelomeningocele. *In* McLaurin, R. L., ed.: Myelomeningocele. New York, Grune & Stratton, 1977, pp. 513–522.

217. Feiwell, E.: The unstable hip: Infra-acetabular osteotomy. *In* McLaurin, R. L., ed.: Myelomeningocele. New York, Grune & Stratton, Inc., 1977, pp. 539–552.

218. Felson, B., and Spitz, H. B.: Pelvic mass in a 12-year-old girl. J.A.M.A., *237*:1255–1256, 1977.

219. Fernandez-Serrats, A. A., Guthkelch, A. N., and Parker, S. A.: Ethical and social aspects of treatment of spina bifida. (letter) Lancet, *2*:827, 1968.

220. Finerman, W. B., and Pick, E. I.: Intranasal encephalomeningocele. Ann. Otol., *62*:114–120, 1953.

221. Fisher, D. A.: Embryonal rest tumor of the central nervous system. Report of an unusual case with a communicating congenital dermal sinus and recurrent meningitis. J. Dis. Child., *99*:90–97, 1960.

222. Fisher, E. G.: Dandy-Walker syndrome: An evaluation of surgical treatment. J. Neurosurg., *39*:615–621, 1973.

223. Fisher, R. G., Uihlein, A., and Keith, H. M.: Spina bifida and cranium bifidum: Study of 530 cases. Mayo Clin. Proc., *27*:33–38, 1952.

224. Fitz, C. R., and Harwood-Nash, D. C.: The tethered conus. Amer. J. Roentgen., *125*:515–523, 1975.

225. Fitzsimmons, J. S.: Laryngeal stridor and respiratory obstruction associated with meningomyelocele. Arch. Dis. Child., *40*:687–688, 1965.

226. Fitzsimmons, J. S.: Laryngeal stridor and respiratory obstruction associated with myelomeningocele. Develop. Med. Child. Neurol., *15*:533–536, 1973.

227. Fleming, J. F. R., and Botterell, E. H.: Cranial dermoid and epidermoid tumors. Surg. Gynec. Obstet., *109*:403–411, 1959.

228. Foltz, E. L.: Myelomeningocele: Selection for treatment. *In* O'Brien, M. S., ed.: Pediatric Neurological Surgery. New York, Raven Press, 1978, pp. 105–124.

229. Forgrave, E. G., and Abbott, K. H.: Spinal (lumbosacral) epidermoid tumor, pilonidal sinus, and persistent meningitis. Bull. Los Angeles Neurol. Soc., *15–16*:244–247, 1951.

230. Forrest, D. M.: Early closure in spina bifida: Results and problems. Proc. Roy. Soc. Med., 60:763–767, 1967.

231. Forrest, D. M.: Spina bifida: Some problems in management. Proc. Roy. Soc. Med., 70:233–239, 1977.

232. Fortuna, A., La Torre, E., and Ciapetta, P.: Arachnoid diverticula: A unitary approach to spinal cysts communicating with the subarachnoid space. Acta Neurochir. (Nien), 39:259–268, 1977.

233. Fowler, F. D., and Alexander, E., Jr.: Atresia of the foramina of Luschka and Magendie: A cause of obstructive internal hydrocephalus. J. Dis. Child., 92:131–137, 1956.

234. Fowler, I.: Responses of the chick neural tube in mechanically produced spina bifida. J. Exp. Zool., 123:115–151, 1953.

235. Frank, L., and Ruby, A.: Familial congenital defect of the scalp. Arch. Derm. (Chicago), 75:266–267, 1957.

236. Frazier, C. H.: Surgery of the spine and spinal cord. New York, D. Appleton & Co., 1918.

237. Freedman, B.: Congenital absence of the sacrum and coccyx; report of a case and review of the literature. Brit. J. Surg., 37:299–303, 1950.

238. Freeman, J. M.: Practical Management of Meningomyelocele. Baltimore, University Park Press, 1974.

239. Freeman, J. M.: The shortsighted treatment of myelomeningocele: A long-term case report. Pediatrics, 53:311–313, 1974.

240. Freeman, L. W.: Late symptoms from diastematomyelia. J. Neurosurg., 18:538–541, 1961.

241. French, L. A., and Peyton, W. T.: Mixed tumors of the spinal canal. Arch. Neurol. Psychiat., 47:737–751, 1942.

242. Friede, R. L.: Developmental Neuropathology. New York, Springer-Verlag, 1975.

243. Funkhouser, W. L.: Encephalo-meningocele through the foramen cecum. Southern Med. J., 15:385–387, 1922.

244. Garceau, G. J.: The filum terminale syndrome (the cord traction syndrome). J. Bone Joint Surg. 35-A:711–716, 1953.

245. Gardner, E., O'Rahilly, R., and Prolo, D.: The Dandy-Walker and Arnold-Chiari malformations. Arch. Neurol. (Chicago), 32:393–407, 1975.

246. Gardner, W. J.: Diastematomyelia and the Klippel-Feil syndrome: Relationship to hydrocephalus, syringomyelia, meningocele, meningomyelocele and iniencephalus. Cleveland Clin. Quart., 31:19–44, 1964.

247. Gardner, W. J.: The Dysraphic States From Syringomyelia to Anencephaly. Amsterdam, Excerpta Medica, 1973.

248. Gardner, W. J.: Hydrodynamic factors in Dandy-Walker and Arnold-Chiari malformations. Child's Brain, 3:200–212, 1977.

249. Gardner, W. J.: and Goodall, R.: The surgical treatment of Arnold-Chiari malformation in adults: An explanation of its mechanism and importance of encephalography in diagnosis. J. Neurosurg., 7:199–206, 1950.

250. Gardner, W. J., Smith, J. L., and Padget, D. H.: The relationship of Arnold-Chiari and Dandy-Walker malformations. J. Neurosurg., 36:481–486, 1972.

251. Garg, B. K., and Mital, V. K.: Pyogenic meningitis secondary to a congenital sacral sinus. Indian J. Pediat., 36:389–395, 1969.

252. Garoff, L., and Seppälä, M.: Alpha fetoprotein and human placental lactogen levels in maternal serum in multiple pregnancies. J. Obstet. Gynaec. Brit. Comm., 80:695–700, 1973.

253. Gates, E. M., and Morton, J. A.: Diastematomyelia. J. Int. Coll. Surg., 22:100–102, 1954.

254. Geilfuss, C. J., and Puckett, S. E.: Radiographic diagnosis of the Dandy-Walker syndrome with the emphasis on angiography. Radiology, 92:255–258, 1969.

255. Gellis, S., and Feingold, M.: Caudal dysplasia syndrome (caudal regression syndrome). Amer. J. Dis. Child., 116:407–408, 1968.

256. Gelmers, H. J., and Go, K. G.: Intrasacral meningocele. Acta Neurochir. (Wien), 39:115–119, 1977.

257. Gibson, J. B.: Congenital hydrocephalus due to atresia of the foramen of Magendie. J. Neuropath. Exp. Neurol., 14:244–262, 1955.

258. Giles, R. G.: Vertebral anomalies. Radiology, 17:1262–1266, 1931.

259. Gilmor, R. L., Kalsbeck, J. E., Goodman, J. M., and Franken, E. A.: Angiographic assessment of occipital encephaloceles. Radiology, 103:127–130, 1972.

260. Gindi, S. E., and Fairburn, B.: Intramedullary spinal abscess as a complication of a congenital dermal sinus. J. Neurosurg., 30:494–497, 1969.

261. Girdany, B. R., and Golden, R.: Centers of ossification of the skeleton. Amer. J. Roentgen., 68:922–924, 1952.

262. Giroud, A.: Causes and morphogenesis of anencephaly. In CIBA Foundation Symposium on Congenital Malformations Wostenholme, G. E. W., and O'Connor, M., eds.: Boston, Little Brown & Co., 1960, pp. 199–218.

263. Gisselsson, L.: Intranasal forms of encephalomeningocele. Acta Otolaryng. (Stockholm), 35:519–531, 1947.

264. Giuffrè, R., and Curatolo, P.: Cranial dermal sinuses in childhood and adolescence. Neurochirurgia (Stuttgart), 21:72–75, 1978.

265. Gleeson, J. A., and Stovin, P. G. I.: Mediastinal enterogenous cysts associated with vertebral anomalies. Clin. Radiol., 12:41–48, 1961.

266. Globus, M. S., Loughman, W. D., Epstein, C. J., Halbasch, G., Stephens, J. D., and Hall, B. D.: Prenatal genetic diagnosis in 3000 amniocenteses. New Eng. J. Med., 300:157–163, 1979.

267. Gold, L. H. A., Kieffer, S. A., and Peterson, H. O.: Lipomatous invasion of the spinal cord associated with spinal dysraphism: Myelographic evaluation. Amer. J. Roentgen., 107:479–485, 1969.

268. Goldhammer, Y., and Smith, J. L.: Optic nerve anomalies in basal encephalocele. Arch. Ophthal. (Chicago), 93:115–118, 1975.

269. Golding, F. C.: Discussion of the significance of congenital abnormalities of the lumbosacral region. Proc. Roy. Soc. Med., 43:636–638, 1950.

270. Goldstein, F., and Kepes, J. J.: The role of traction in the development of the Arnold-Chiari malformation. An experimental study. J. Neuropath. Exp. Neurol., 25:654–666, 1966.

271. Gooding, C. A., Carter, A., and Hoare, R. D.:

New ventriculographic aspects of the Arnold-Chiari malformation. Radiology, *89*:626–632, 1967.

272. Goodner, E. K.: Myelomeningocele. Part II. Ophthalmologic problems. Western J. Med., *121*:291–292, 1974.

273. Gördüren, S.: Orbital encephalocele associated with acrocephaly. Brit. J. Ophthal., *36*:151–154, 1952.

274. Gowers, W. R.: Myo-lipoma of spinal cord. Trans. Path. Soc. London, *27*:19–22, 1876.

275. Greeley, P. W., Oldberg, G., and Curtin, J. W.: Plastic surgical repair of lumbar myelomeningocele. Ann. Surg., *142*:552–559, 1955.

276. Groff, R. A., and Yaskin, J. C.: Late occurrence of sphincter and other neurological disturbances associated with congenital malformations of the vertebral column. Trans. Amer. Neurol. Ass., 218–222, 1947.

277. Gross, R. E., Neuhauser, E. B. D., and Longino, L. A.: Thoracic diverticula which originate from the intestine. Ann. Surg., *131*:363–375, 1950.

278. Gross, S. W., and Sachs, E.: Spina bifida and cranium bifidum: A study of one hundred and three cases. Arch. Surg. (Chicago), *28*:874–888, 1934.

279. Grossman, J.: Spina bifida. Family Health, *10*:36–46, 1978.

280. Gryspeerdt, G. L.: Myelographic assessment of occult forms of spinal dysraphism. Acta Radiol. [Diagn.] (Stockholm), *1*:702–717, 1963.

281. Guthkelch, A. N.: Occipital cranium bifidum. Arch. Dis. Child., *45*:104–109, 1970.

282. Guthkelch, A. N.: Diastematomyelia with median septum. Brain, *97*:729–742, 1974.

283. Guthkelch, A. N.: The indications and contraindications for early operation in myelomeningocele. *In* Morley, T. P., ed.: Current Controversies in Neurosurgery. Philadelphia, W. B. Saunders Co., 1976.

284. Guthkelch, A. N., Jones, R. A. C., and Zierski, J.: Diastematomyelia. Develop. Med. Child Neurol., *13*:suppl. 25:137–138, 1971.

285. Haase, J.: Papilledema associated with a sacral intraspinal cyst. Surg. Neurol., *6*:360–362, 1976.

286. Habal, M. B., and Vries, J. K.: Tension free closure of large meningomyelocele defects. Surg. Neurol., *8*:177–180, 1977.

287. Haddad, F. S.: Anterior sacral meningocele. Report of two cases and review of the literature. Canad. J. Surg., *1*:230–242, 1958.

288. Hall, P. V., Campbell, R. L., and Kalsbeck, J. E.: Meningomyelocele and progressive hydromyelia. Progressive paresis in myelodysplasia. J. Neurosurg., *43*:457–463, 1975.

289. Hall, P. V., Kalsbeck, J. E., Wellman, H. N., Batnitzky, S., et al.: Clinical radioisotope investigations in hydrosyringomyelia and myelodysplasia. J. Neurosurg., *45*:188–194, 1976.

290. Haller, J. S., Wolpert, S. M., Rabe, E. F., et al.: Cystic lesions of the posterior fossa in infants; a comparison of the clinical, radiological and pathological findings in Dandy-Walker syndrome and extra-axial cysts. Neurology (Minneap.), *21*:494–506, 1971.

291. Hamby, W. B.: Pilonidal cyst, spina bifida oc-

culta and bifid spinal cord. Arch. Path. (Chicago), *21*:831–838, 1936.

292. Hamby, W. B.: Tumors of the spinal canal in childhood. Report of a case of meningitis due to an intramedullary epidermoid communicating with a dermal sinus. Analysis of the literature of a subsequent decade (1933–1942). J. Neuropath. Exp. Neurol., *3*:397–412, 1974.

294. Hammerschlag, S. B., Wolpert, S. M., and Carter, B. L.: Computed tomography of the spinal canal. Radiology, *121*:361–367, 1976.

295. Harcourt, R. B.: Ophthalmic complications of meningomyelocele and hydrocephalus in children. Brit. J. Ophthal., *52*:670–676, 1968.

296. Harriman, D. G. F.: An intraspinal enterogenous cyst. J. Path. Bact., *75*:413–419, 1958.

297. Hart, M. N., Malamud, N., and Ellis, W. G.: The Dandy-Walker syndrome. Neurology (Minneap.), *22*:771–780, 1972.

298. Hartley, J. B., and Burnett, C. W. F. A study of craniolacunia. J. Obstet. Gynec. Brit. Emp., *50*:1–12, 1943.

299. Harverson, G., Bailey, I. C., and Kiryabwire, J. W. M.: The radiological diagnosis of anterior encephalocoeles. Clin. Radiol., *25*:317–322, 1974.

300. Harwood-Nash, D. C.: Myelography in children. Seminars Roentgen., *7*:297–312, 1972.

301. Harwood-Nash, D. C., and Fitz, C. R.: Neuroradiology in Infants and Children. St. Louis, C. V. Mosby Co., 1976.

302. Hauge, T.: Myelography in a case of the occult form of spinal dysraphism. Acta. Radiol. [Diagn.] (Stockholm), *1*:718–720, 1963.

303. Haworth, J. B., and Keillor, G. W.: Use of transparencies in evaluating the width of the spinal canal in infants, children and adults. Radiology, *97*:109–114, 1962.

304. Haworth, J. C., and Zachary, R. B.: Congenital dermal sinus in children. Their relation to pilonidal sinuses. Lancet, *269*:10–14, 1955.

305. Head, H. D., Gerstein, J. D., and Muir, R. W.: Presacral teratoma in the adult. Amer. Surg., *41*:240–248, 1975.

306. Heard, G., and Payne, E. E.: Scalloping of the vertebral bodies in von Recklinghausen's disease of the nervous system (neurofibromatosis). J. Neurol. Neurosurg. Psychiat., *25*:345–351, 1962.

307. Heimburger, R. F.: Early repair of myelomeningocele (spina bifida cystica). J. Neurosurg., *37*:594–600, 1972.

308. Hemmer, R.: Meningoceles and myeloceles. Progr. Neurol. Surg., *4*:192–226, 1971.

309. Hendrick, E. B.: On diastematomyelia. Progr. Neurol. Surg., *4*:277–288, 1971.

310. Hendrick, E. G., Hoffman, H. J., and Humphreys, R. P.: A technique for repair of large spina bifida defects. *In* McLaurin, R. L., ed.: Myelomeningocele. New York, Grune & Stratton, Inc., 1977, pp. 191–196.

311. Henley, R. B., and Lawrence, L. B.: Pelvic meningocele. A case report. J. Neurosurg., *23*:206–207, 1965.

312. Herlinger, H.: Radiological investigation of a case of sacro-coccygeal agenesis. Brit. J. Radiol., *37*:376–379, 1964.

313. Heron, J. R.: Neurological syndromes associated

with pes cavus. Proc. Roy. Soc. Med., *62*:270–271, 1969.

314. Herren, R. Y., and Edwards, J. E.: Diplomyelia (duplication of the spinal cord). Arch. Path. (Chicago), *30*:1203–1214, 1940.

315. Hide, D. W., Williams, H. P., and Ellis, H. L.: The outlook for the child with myelomeningocele for whom early surgery was considered inadvisable. Develop. Med. Child Neurol., *14*:304–307, 1972.

316. Hilal, S. K., and Keim, H. A.: Selective spinal angiography in adolescent scoliosis. Radiology, *102*:349–359, 1972.

317. Hilal, S. K., Marton, D., and Pollack, E.: Diastematomyelia in children. Radiology, *112*:609–621, 1974.

318. Hipsley, P. L.: Dermoid cyst of the spinal canal. Aust. N.Z. J. Surg., *2*:421, 1932–1933.

319. Hirt, H. R., Zdrojewski, B., and Weber, G.: The manifestations and complications of intraspinal congenital dermal sinuses and dermoid cysts. Neuropaediatrie, *3*:231–247, 1972.

320. Hodges, P. C.: An epiphyseal chart. Amer. J. Roentgen., *30*:809–810, 1933.

321. Hoffer, M. M., Feiwell, E., Perry, R., Perry, J., and Bonnett, C.: Functional ambulation in patients with myelomeningocele. J. Bone Joint Surg. *55*–A:137–148, 1973.

322. Hoffman, H. J.: Personal communication, 1978.

323. Hoffman, H. J., Hendrick, E. B., and Humphreys, R. P.: Manifestations and management of Arnold-Chiari malformation in patients with myelomeningocele. Child's Brain, *1*:255–259, 1975.

324. Hoffman, H. J., Hendrick, E. B., and Humphreys, R. P.: The tethered spinal cord: Its protean manifestations, diagnosis and surgical correction. Child's Brain, *2*:145–155, 1976.

325. Holcomb, G. W., Jr., and Matson, D. D.: Thoracic neurenteric cyst. Surgery, *35*:115–121, 1954.

326. Holinger, P. C., Holinger, L. D., Reichert, T. J., and Holinger, P. H.: Respiratory obstruction and apnea in infants with bilateral abductor vocal cord paralysis, meningomyelocele, hydrocephalus and Arnold-Chiari malformation. J. Pediat., *92*:368–373, 1978.

327. Holman, C. B., Svien, H. J., Bickel, W. H., and Keith, H. M.: Diastematomyelia. Pediatrics, *15*:191–194, 1955.

328. Holmes, L. B.: Congenital malformations. New Eng. J. Med., *295*:204–207, 1976.

329. Holness, R. O., Hoffman, H. J., Mancer, K., and Armstrong, D.: Intracranial teratocarcinoma in a child with anterior sacral and intrasacral meningocele. Neurosurgery, *2*:143–147, 1978.

330. Hoppenfeld, S.: Congenital kyphosis in myelomeningocele. J. Bone Joint Surg. *49-B*:276–280, 1967.

331. Hosoi, K.: Intradural teratoid tumors of the spinal cord. Report of a case. Arch. Path. (Chicago), *11*:875–883, 1931.

332. Howieson, J., Norrell, H. A., and Wilson, C. B.: Expansion of the subarachnoid space in the lumbosacral region. Radiology, *90*:488–492, 1968.

333. Hsiao, Y. T., and Li, P.L.: Lumbosacral mammiform tumour (apparently supernumerary breast) associated with spina bifida occulta.

Report of a case. Chinese Med. J. suppl., *1*:131–134, 1936.

334. Hubbert, C. H., Faris, A. A., and Martinez, A. J.: Dandy-Walker syndrome: Spectrum of congenital anomalies. Southern Med. J., *67*:274–277, 1974.

335. Hueston, J. T.: The aetiology of pilonidal sinuses. Brit. J. Surg., *41*:307–311, 1953.

336. Humphry, M.: Six specimens of spina bifida with bony projections from the bodies of the vertebrae into the vertebral canal. J. Anat. Physiol., *20*:585–592, 1886.

337. Hunt, G., Lewin, W., Gleave, J., and Gairdner, D.: Predictive factors in open myelomeningocele with special reference to sensory level. Brit. Med. J., *4*:197–201, 1973.

338. Hunt, G. M., and Holmes, A. E.: Some factors relating to intelligence in treated children with spina bifida cystica. Develop. Med. Child Neurol., *17*:suppl. 35:65–70, 1975.

339. Huong, T. T., Goldbatt, E., and Simpson, D. A.: Dandy-Walker syndrome associated with congenital heart defects: Report of three cases. Develop. Med. Child Neurol., *17*:suppl. 35:35–41, 1975.

340. Ignelzi, R. J., and Lehman, R. A. W.: Lumbosacral agenesis: Management and embryological implications. J. Neurol. Neurosurg. Psychiat., *37*:1273–1276, 1974.

341. Ingraham, F. D.: Spina Bifida and Cranium Bifidum. Cambridge, Mass., Harvard University Press, 1943.

342. Ingraham, F. D., and Hamlin, H.: Spina bifida and cranium bifidum. II: Surgical treatment. New Eng. J. Med., *228*:631–641, 1943.

343. Ingraham, F. D., and Lowrey, J. J.: Spina bifida and cranium bifidum. III: Occult spinal disorders. New Eng. J. Med., *228*:745–750, 1943.

344. Ingraham, F. D., and Matson, D. D.: Spina bifida and cranium bifidum. An unusual nasopharyngeal encephalocele. New Eng. J. Med., *228*:815–820, 1943.

345. Ingraham, F. D., and Scott, H. W., Jr.: Spina bifida and cranium bifidum. V: The Arnold-Chiari malformation: A study of 20 cases. New Eng. J. Med., *229*:108–114, 1943.

346. Ingraham, F. D., and Swan, H.: Spina bifida and cranium bifidum. I: A survey of five hundred forty-six cases. New Eng. J. Med., *228*:559–563, 1943.

347. Ivamoto, H. S., and Wallman, L. J.: Anterior sacral meningocele. Arch. Neurol. (Chicago), *31*:345–346, 1974.

348. Jackson, F. E.: Neurenteric cysts. Report of a case of neurenteric cyst with associated chronic meningitis and hydrocephalus. J. Neurosurg., *18*:678–682, 1961.

349. Jackson, I. J., Thompson, I. M., Hooks, C. A., and Hoffman, G. T.: Urinary incontinence in myelomeningoceles due to a tethered spinal cord and its surgical treatment. Surg. Gynec. Obstet., *103*:618–624, 1956.

350. Jacobs, L. G., Smith, J. K., and Van Horn, P. S.: Myelographic demonstration of cysts of spinal membranes. Radiology, *62*:215–221, 1954.

351. Jaffee, R.: Anterior sacral meningocele. Report of a case. Obstet. Gynec., *28*:684–688, 1966.

352. James, C. C. M., and Lassman, L. P.: Diastematomyelia. Arch. Dis. Child., *33*:536–539, 1958.

353. James, C. C. M., and Lassman, L. P.: Spinal dysraphism: An orthopaedic syndrome in children accompanying occult forms. Arch. Dis. Child., 35:315–327, 1960.

354. James, C. C. M., and Lassman, L. P.: Spinal dysraphism: Spinal cord lesions associated with spina bifida occulta. Physiotherapy, 48:154–157, 1962.

355. James, C. C. M., and Lassman, L. P.: Diastematomyelia. A critical survey of 24 cases submitted to laminectomy. Arch. Dis. Child., 39:125–130, 1964.

356. James, C. C. M., and Lassman, L. P.: Results of treatment of progressive lesions in spina bifida occulta five to ten years after laminectomy. Lancet, 2:1277–1279, 1967.

357. James, C. C. M., and Lassman, L. P.: Diastematomyelia and the tight filum terminale. J. Neurol. Sci., 10:193–196, 1970.

358. James, C. C. M., and Lassman, L. P.: Spinal Dysraphism. Spina Bifida Occulta. London, Butterworth & Co. Ltd., 1972.

359. James, H. E., and Schut, L.: The spontaneous remission of a large sacrococcygeal lipomeningocele sac with presentation of a tethered cord syndrome. Neuropaediatrie, 5:340–343, 1974.

360. James, H. E., Oliff, M., and Mulcahy, J.: Spinal dysraphism: A comprehensive diagnostic approach. Neurosurgery, 2:15–21, 1978.

361. Jeffs, R. B.: Practical urological evaluation of neurogenic bladder in myelomeningocele. In McLaurin, R. L., ed.: Myelomeningocele. New York, Grune & Stratton Inc., 1977, pp. 667–676.

362. Johnson: Sacrum of a child containing a fatty tumor connected with the anterior of the spinal canal. Lancet, 2:35–36, 1857.

363. Johnson, D. F.: Intramedullary lipoma of the spinal cord. Bull. Los Angeles Neurol. Sci., 15:37–42, 1950.

364. Jones, J. B.: Diastematomyelia. Clin. Orthop., 21:164–168, 1961.

365. Jones, J. D. L., and Evans, T. G.: Anterior sacral meningocele. J. Obstet. Gynaec. Brit. Emp., 66:477–479, 1959.

366. Jones, P. H., and Love, J. G.: Tight filum terminale. Arch. Surg. (Chicago), 73:556–566, 1956.

367. Joseph, R. A., and McKenzie, T.: Occult intrasacral meningocele. J. Neurol. Neurosurg. Psychiat., 33:493–496, 1970.

368. Joubert, M., Eisenring, J. J., Robb, J. P., and Andermann, F.: Familial agenesis of the cerebellar vermis: A syndrome of episodic hyperpnea, abnormal eye movements, ataxia, and retardation. Neurology (Minneap.), 19:813–825, 1969.

369. Juhl, J. H., and Wesenberg, R. L.: Radiological findings in congenital and acquired occlusions of the foramina of Magendie and Luschka. Radiology, 86:801–813, 1966.

370. Kak, V. K., Chugh, K. S., and Sodhi, J. S.: Occult intrasacral meningocele. Neurochirurgia (Stuttgart), 15:148–152, 1972.

371. Källén, B.: Early embryogenesis of the central nervous system with special reference to closure defects. Develop. Med. Child Neurol. suppl., 16:44–53, 1968.

372. Kapsalakis, Z.: Diastematomyelia in two sisters. J. Neurosurg., 21:66–67, 1964.

373. Kapsenberg, J. G., and Van Lookeren Campagne, J. A.: A case of spina bifida combined with diastematomyely, the anomaly of Chiari and hydrocephaly. Acta Anat. (Basel), 7:366–388, 1949.

374. Karch, S. B., and Urich, H.: Occipital encephalocele: A morphological study. J. Neurol. Sci., 15:89–112, 1972.

375. Karlin, I. W.: Incidence of spina bifida occulta in children with and without enuresis. Amer. J. Dis. Child., 49:125–134, 1935.

376. Karma, P., Räsänen, O., and Kärjä, J.: Nasal gliomas. A review and report of two cases. Laryngoscope, 87:1169–1179, 1977.

377. Karshner, R. G., and Reeves, D. L.: Lacunar skull (Lückenschädel) of the newborn. Report of seven cases. Amer. J. Roentgen., 57:321–328, 1947.

378. Keen, W. W., and Coplin, W. M. L.: Sacrococcygeal tumor (teratoma) with an opening entirely through the sacrum and a sinus passing through this opening and communicating with the rectum, the sinus resembling a bronchus. Surg. Gynec. Obstet., 3:661–671, 1906.

379. Keiller, V. H.: A contribution to the anatomy of spina bifida. Brain, 45:31–103, 1922.

380. Keim, H. A., and Greene, A. F.: Diastematomyelia and scoliosis. J. Bone Joint Surg., 55-A:1425–1435, 1973.

381. Kennedy, R. L. J.: An unusual rectal polyp: Anterior sacral meningocele. Surg. Gynec. Obstet., 43:803–804, 1926.

382. Kessel, A. W. L.: Intrathoracic meningocele, spinal deformity and multiple neurofibromatosis. J. Bone Joint Surg. 33-B:87–93, 1951.

383. Kieck, C. F., and De Villiers, J. C.: Subcutaneous lumbosacral lipomas. S. Afr. Med. J., 49:1563–1566, 1975.

384. Kim, J. H., Shucart, W. A., and Haimovici, H.: Symptomatic arachnoid diverticula. Arch. Neurol. (Chicago), 31:35–37, 1974.

385. King, A. B., and Richter, C. P.: Spinal subdural abscess due to a congenital dermal sinus and accompanying changes in the autonomic nervous system. Bull. Johns Hopk. Hosp., 85:431–439, 1949.

386. Kirsch, W. M., and Hodges, F. J., III: An intramedullary epidermal inclusion cyst of the thoracic cord associated with a previously repaired meningocele. Case Report. J. Neurosurg., 24:1018–1020, 1966.

387. Kirsch, W. M., Duncan, B. R., Black, F. O., and Stears, J. C.: Laryngeal palsy in association with myelomeningocele, hydrocephalus, and the Arnold-Chiari malformation. J. Neurosurg., 28:207–214, 1968.

388. Klauber, G. T.: External devices for incontinence in children. In McLaurin, R. L., ed.: Myelomeningocele. New York, Grune & Stratton, Inc., 1977, pp. 725–732.

389. Klenerman, L., and Merrick, M. V.: Anterior sacral meningocele occurring in a family. J. Bone Joint Surg., 55-B:331–334, 1973.

390. Kling, S.: Sacrococcygeal teratoma. Canad. J. Surg., 12:22–26, 1969.

391. Knight, G., Griffiths, T., and Williams, I.: Gastrocytoma of the spinal cord. Brit. J. Surg., 42:635–638, 1954–1955.

392. Kolin, I. S., Scherzer, A. L., New, B., and Gar-

field, M.: Studies of the school-age child with meningomyelocele: Social and emotional adaptation. J. Pediat., *78*:1013–1019, 1971.

393. Kooistra, H. P.: Pilonidal sinuses occurring over the higher spinal segments with report of a case involving the spinal cord. Surgery, *11*:63–74, 1942.

394. Koontz, W. W., Jr., and Prout, G. R., Jr.: Agenesis of the sacrum and the neurogenic bladder. J.A.M.A., *203*:481–486, 1968.

395. Krieger, A. J.: Measurement of respiration in Arnold-Chiari malformation. Child's Brain, *2*:31–37, 1976.

396. Krieger, A. J., Detwiler, J., and Trooskin, S.: Respiration in an infant with the Dandy-Walker syndrome. Neurology (Minneap.), *24*:1064–1067, 1974.

397. Krieger, A. J., Detwiler, J. S., and Trooskin, S. Z.: Respiratory function in infants with Arnold-Chiari malformation. Laryngoscope, *86*:718–723, 1976.

398. Kruyff, E.: Occipital dysplasia in infancy. The early recognition of craniovertebral abnormalities. Radiology, *85*:501–507, 1965.

399. Kruyff, E., and Jeffs, R.: Skull abnormalities associated with the Arnold-Chiari malformation. Acta Radiol. [Diag.] (Stockholm), *5*:9–24, 1966.

400. Kubie, L. S., and Fulton, J. F.: A clinical and pathological study of two teratomatous cysts of the spinal cord containing mucus and ciliated cells. Surg. Gynec. Obstet., *47*:297–311, 1928.

401. Kunitomo, K.: The development and reduction of the tail and of the caudal end of the spinal cord. Contrib. Embryol., *8*:161–198, 1918.

402. Kwan, S. T.: Intracranial dermoid cyst. Arch. Neurol. Psychiat., *24*:1292–1293, 1930.

403. Laha, R. K., and Huestis, W. S.: Intraspinal enterogenous cyst: Delayed appearance following mediastinal cyst resection. Surg. Neurol., *3*:67–70, 1975.

404. Lamas, E., Lobato, R. D., and Armor, T.: Occult intrasacral meningocele. Surg. Neurol., *8*:181–184, 1977.

405. Lancet: Ethics of selective treatment of spina bifida. Lancet, *1*:85–88, 1975.

406. Lanier, R. R.: The presacral vertebrae of American white and Negro males. Amer. J. Phys. Anthrop., *25*:341–420, 1939.

407. Lassman, L. P., and James, C. C. M.: Lumbosacral lipomas: Critical survey of 26 cases submitted to laminectomy. J. Neurol. Neurosurg. Psychiat., *30*:174–181, 1967.

408. Lassman, L. P., James, C. C. M., and Foster, J. B.: Hydromyelia. J. Neurol. Sci., *7*:149–155, 1968.

409. La Torre, E., and Occhipinti, E.: Angiographic findings in some malformations of the brain. Report of seven cases. Europ. Neurol., *4*:210–225, 1970.

410. La Torre, E., Fortuna, A., and Occhipinti, E.: Angiographic differentiation between Dandy-Walker cyst and arachnoid cyst of the posterior fossa in newborn infants and children. J. Neurosurg., *38*:298–308, 1973.

411. Lau, B. P., and Newton, T. H.: Sphenopharyngeal encephalomeningocele. Radiol. Clin. Biol., *34*:386–393, 1965.

412. Laurence, K. M.: The natural history of spina bi-

fida cystica: Detailed analysis of 407 cases. Arch. Dis. Child., *39*:41–57, 1964.

413. Laurence, K. M.: The survival of untreated spina bifida cystica. Develop. Child Neurol. suppl., *11*:10–19, 1966.

414. Laurence, K. M.: Effect of early surgery for spina bifida cystica on survival and quality of life. Lancet, *1*:301–304, 1974.

415. Laurence, K. M., and Tew, B. J.: Natural history of spina bifida cystica and cranium bifidum cysticum: Major central nervous system malformations in South Wales, Part IV. Arch. Dis. Child., *46*:127–138, 1971.

416. Laws, E. R., Jr.: Neurosurgical management of meningomyelocele. *In* Freeman, J. M., ed.: Practical Management of Meningomyelocele. Baltimore, University Park Press, 1974.

417. Leech, R. W., Olafson, R. A., Gilbertson, R. L., and Shook, D. R.: Intrathoracic meningocele and vertebral anomalies in a case of neurofibromatosis. Surg. Neurol., *9*:55–57, 1978.

418. Leigh, T. F., and Rogers, J. V., Jr.: Anterior sacral meningocele. Amer. J. Roentgen., *71*:808–812, 1954.

419. Lemire, R. J.: Variations in development of the caudal neural tube in human embryos (Horizons XIV–XXI). Teratology, *2*:361–370, 1969.

420. Lemire, R. J.: Embryology of the central nervous system. *In* Davis, J. A., and Dobbing, J., ed.: Scientific Foundations of Paediatrics. London, William Heinemann Medical Books, Ltd., 1974.

421. Lemire, R. J., Graham, C. B., and Beckwith, J. B.: Skin-covered sacrococcygeal masses in infants and children. J. Pediat., *79*:948–954, 1971.

422. Lemire, R. J., Shepard, T. H., and Alvord, E. C., Jr.: Caudal myeloschisis (lumbo-sacral spina bifida cystica) in a five millimeter (Horizon XIV) human embryo. Anat. Rec., *152*:9–16, 1965.

423. Lendon, R. G.: Neuron population in the spinal cord of children with spina bifida and hydrocephalus. Develop. Med. Child Neurol. suppl., *15*:50–54, 1968.

424. Lendon, R. G.: Neuron population in the lumbosacral cord of myelomeningocele children. Develop. Med. Child Neurol. suppl., *20*:82–85, 1969.

425. Lendon, R. G., and Emery, J. L.: Forking of the central canal in the equinal cord of children. J. Anat., *106*:499–505, 1970.

426. Leone, C. R., Jr., and Marlowe, J. F.: Orbital presentation of an ethmoidal encephalocele. Report of a case of a 62 year old woman. Arch. Ophthal. (Chicago), *83*:445–447, 1970.

427. Lepintre, J., and Labrune, M.: Fistules dermiques congénitales communiquant avec le système nerveux central. 21 cas opérés chez l'enfant. Neurochirurgie, *16*:335–348, 1970.

428. Levin, P., and Antin, S. P.: Intraspinal neurenteric cyst in the cervical area. Neurology (Minneap.), *14*:727–730, 1964.

429. Levy, J. I., and Freed, C.: The incidence of cervico-thoracic spina bifida occulta in South African negroes. J. Anat., *114*:449–456, 1973.

430. Lichtenstein, B. W.: Spinal dysraphism, spina bifida and myelodysplasia. Arch. Neurol. Psychiat., *44*:792–810, 1940.

431. Lichtenstein, B. W.: Distant neuroanatomic

complications of spina bifida (spinal dysraphism); hydrocephalus, Arnold-Chiari deformity, stenosis of aqueduct of Sylvius, etc.; pathogenesis and pathology. Arch. Neurol. Psychiat., 47:195–214, 1942.

432. Lichtenstein, B. W.: Atresia and stenosis of the aqueduct of Sylvius. J. Neuropath. Exp. Neurol., 18:3–21, 1959.

433. Liliequist, B.: Diastematomyelia: Report of a case examined by gas myelography. Acta Radiol. [Diag.] (Stockholm), 3:497–502, 1965.

434. Lipschitz, R., Beck, J. M., and Froman, C.: An assessment of the treatment of encephalomeningoceles. S. Afr. Med. J., 43:609–610, 1969.

435. List, C. F.: Intraspinal epidermoids, dermoids and dermal sinuses. Surg. Gynec. Obstet., 73:525–538, 1941.

436. Lodge, T.: Developmental defects in the cranial vault. Brit. J. Radiol., 48:421–434, 1975.

437. Loeser, J. D., and Lewin, R. J.: Lumbosacral lipoma in the adult. Case report. J. Neurosurg., 29:405–409, 1968.

438. Logue, V., and Till, K.: Posterior fossa dermoid cysts with special reference to intracranial infection. J. Neurol. Neurosurg. Psychiat., 15:1–12, 1952.

439. Long, D. M.: Silver nitrate therapy as an adjunct in the treatment of myelomeningocele. J. Neurosurg., 36:769–772, 1972.

440. Lonton, A. P., Barrington, N. A., and Lorber, J.: Lacunar skull deformity related to intelligence in children with myelomeningocele and hydrocephalus. Develop. Med. Child Neurol., 17:suppl. 35:58–64, 1975.

441. Lorber, J.: Recurrent E. coli meningitis and persistent cauda equina syndrome due to congenital dermal sinus. Proc. Roy. Soc. Med., 48:332–333, 1955.

442. Lorber, J.: Systemic ventriculographic studies in infants born with meningomyelocele and encephalocele, the incidence and development of hydrocephalus. Arch. Dis. Child., 36:381–389, 1961.

443. Lorber, J.: The prognosis of occipital encephalocele. Develop. Med. Child Neurol. suppl., 13:75–86, 1967.

444. Lorber, J.: Results of treatment of myelomeningocele. An analysis of 524 unselected cases, with special reference to possible selection for treatment. Develop. Med. Child Neurol., 13:279–303, 1971.

445. Lorber, J.: Spina bifida cystica. Results of treatment of 270 consecutive cases with criteria for selection for the future. Arch. Dis. Child., 47:854–873, 1972.

446. Lorber, J.: Early results of selective treatment of spina bifida cystica. Brit. Med. J., 4:201–204, 1973.

447. Lorber, J.: Selective treatment of myelomeningocele: To treat or not to treat? Pediatrics, 53:307–308, 1974.

448. Lorber, J.: Some paediatric aspects of myelomeningocele. Acta Orthop. Scand., 46:350–355, 1975.

449. Lorber, J., Kalhan, S. C., and Mahgrefte, B.: Treatment of ventriculitis with gentamicin and cloxacillin in infants born with spina bifida. Arch. Dis. Child., 45:178–185, 1970.

450. Lourie, H., and Bierny, J. P.: Diastematomyelia with two spurs and intradural neural crest ele-

ments. Case report. J. Neurosurg., 32:248–251, 1970.

451. Love, J. G., Daly, D. D., and Harris, L. E.: Tight filum terminale. Report of condition in three siblings. J.A.M.A., 176:31–33, 1961.

452. Low, N. L., Scheinberg, L., and Andersen, D. H.: Brain tissue in the nose and throat. Pediatrics, 18:254–259, 1956.

453. MacCarty, C. S., Leavens, M. E., Love, J. G., and Kernohan, J. W.: Dermoid and epidermoid tumors in the central nervous system of adults. Surg. Gynec. Obstet., 108:191–198, 1959.

454. MacFarlane, A., and Maloney, A. F. J.: The appearance of the aqueduct and its relationship to hydrocephalus in the Arnold-Chiari malformation. Brain, 80:479–491, 1957.

455. MacKenzie, N. G., and Emery, J. L.: Deformities of the cervical cord in children with neurospinal dysraphism. Develop. Med. Child Neurol., 13:suppl. 25:58–67, 1971.

456. MacPherson, R. I., and Young, G.: Sacrococcygeal tumor. J. Canad. Ass. Radiol., 21:132–142, 1970.

457. Maier, R. H.: Prenatal diagnosis of lacunar skull (Lückenschädel). Radiology, 23:615–619, 1934.

458. Maloney, A. F. J.: Two cases of congenital atresia of the foramina of Magendie and Luschka. J. Neurol. Neurosurg. Psychiat., 17:134–138, 1954.

459. Mallory, F. B.: Sacro-coccygeal dimples, sinuses and cysts. Amer. J. Med. Sci., 103:263–277, 1892.

460. Margolis, G., and Kilham, L.: Experimental virus-induced hydrocephalus; relation to pathogenesis of the Arnold-Chiari malformation. J. Neurosurg., 31:1–9, 1969.

461. Maroun, F. B., Jacob, J. C., and Heneghan, W. D.: La diastématomyélie. Ses manifestations cliniques et son traitment chirurgical. Neurochirurgie, 18:285–316, 1972.

462. Maroun, F. B., Jacob, J. C., and Heneghan, W. D.: Diastematomyelia. St. Louis, Warren H. Green, Inc., 1976.

463. Marr, G. E., and Uihlein, A.: Diplomyelia and compression of the spinal cord and not of the cauda equina, by a congenital anomaly of the third lumbar vertebra. Surg. Clin. N. Amer., 24:963–968, 1944.

464. Martin, J., and Davis, L.: Intracranial dermoid and epidermoid tumors. Arch. Neurol. Psychiat., 49:56–70, 1943.

465. Masters, C. L.: Pathogenesis of the Arnold-Chiari malformation: The significance of hydrocephalus and aqueduct stenosis. J. Neuropath. Exp. Neurol., 37:56–74, 1978.

466. Matson, D. D.: Prenatal obstruction of the fourth ventricle. Amer. J. Roentgen., 76:499–506, 1956.

467. Matson, D. D.: Surgical repair of myelomeningocele. J. Neurosurg., 27:180–186, 1967.

468. Matson, D. D.: Surgical treatment of myelomeningocele. Pediatrics, 42:225–227, 1968.

469. Matson, D. D.: Neurosurgery of Infancy and Childhood. 2nd Ed. Springfield, Ill., Charles C Thomas, 1969.

470. Matson, D. D., and Ingraham, F. C.: Intracranial complications of congenital dermal sinuses. Pediatrics, 8:463–474, 1951.

471. Matson, D. D., and Jerva, M. J.: Recurrent men-

ingitis associated with congenital lumbosacral dermal sinus tract. J. Neurosurg., 25:288–297, 1966.

472. Matson, D. D., Woods, R. P., Campbell, J. B., and Ingraham, F. D.: Diastematomyelia (congenital clefts of the spinal cord): Diagnosis and surgical treatment. Pediatrics, 6:98–112, 1950.

473. Mawdsley, T., and Rickham, P. P.: Further follow-up study for early operation for open myelomeningocele. Develop. Med. Child Neurol. suppl., 20:8–12, 1969.

474. Mawdsley, T., Rickham, P. P., and Roberts, J. R.: Long-term results of early operation in open myelomeningoceles and encephaloceles. Brit. Med. J., 1:663–666, 1967.

475. Maxwell, H. P., and Bucy, P. C.: Diastematomyelia: Report of a clinical case. J. Neuropath. Exp. Neurol., 5:165–167, 1946.

476. Mayo-Robson, A. W.: A series of cases of spina bifida treated by plastic operation. Trans. Clin. Soc. London, 18:210–220, 1885.

477. McAdams, A. J.: The Arnold-Chiari malformation: Pathology and developmental considerations. In McLaurin, R. L., ed.: Myelomeningocele. New York, Grune & Stratton, Inc., 1977, pp. 197–207.

478. McCann, P.: Diastematomyelia. Irish J. Med. Sci., 6:155–160, 1966.

479. McCormack, L. J., and Harris, H. E.: Neurogenic tumors of the nasal fossa. J.A.M.A., 157:318–321, 1955.

480. McCoy, W. T., Simpson, D. A., and Carter, R. F.: Cerebral malformations complicating spina bifida. Radiological studies. Clin. Radiol., 18:176–182, 1967.

481. McDonald, P.: Malignant sacrococcygeal teratoma. A report of 4 cases. Amer. J. Roentgen., 118:444–449, 1973.

482. McLaurin, R. L.: Parietal cephaloceles. Neurology (Minneap.), 14:764–772, 1964.

483. McLetchie, N. G. B., Purves, J. K., and Saunders, R. L. deC. H.: The genesis of gastric and certain intestinal diverticula and enterogenous cysts. Surg. Gynec. Obstet., 99:135–141, 1954.

484. McRae, D. L.: Observation on craniolacunia. Acta Radiol. [Diag.] (Stockholm) 5:55–64, 1966.

485. Meacham, W. F.: Surgical treatment of diastematomyelia. J. Neurosurg., 27:78–85, 1967.

486. Meacham, W. F., and Dickens, R. D., Jr.: Midline fusion defects and defects of formation. In Youmans, J. R., ed.: Neurological Surgery. Philadelphia, W. B. Saunders Co., 1973, pp. 588–607.

487. Mealey, J., Jr., Dzenitis, A. J., and Hockey, A. A.: The prognosis of encephaloceles. J. Neurosurg., 32:209–218, 1970.

488. Mendeloff, J.: The olfactory neuroepithelial tumors: A review of the literature and report of six additional cases. Cancer, 10:944–956, 1957.

489. Mendelsohn, H. J., and Kay, E. B.: Intrathoracic meningocele. J. Thorac. Surg., 18:124–128, 1949.

490. Méndez-Cashion, D., and Cordero, R.: Recurrent meningitis associated with congenital dermal sinus. Ann. Intern. Med., 54:503–509, 1961.

491. Meredith, J. M.: Unusual congenital anomalies

of the lumbosacral spine (spina bifida) with a report of three cases. J. Nerv. Ment. Dis., 99:115–133, 1944.

492. Merrill, D. C.: Electrical stimulation of the bladder. In McLaurin, R. L., ed.: Myelomeningocele. New York, Grune & Stratton, Inc., 1977, pp. 715–723.

493. Merrill, D. C.: The treatment of urinary incontinence by electrical pelvic floor stimulation. In McLaurin, R. L., ed.: Myelomeningocele. New York, Grune & Stratton, Inc., 1977, pp. 733–743.

494. Miles, J., Pennybacker, J., and Sheldon, P.: Intrathoracic meningocele. Its development and association with neurofibromatosis. J. Neurol. Neurosurg. Psychiat., 32:99–110, 1969.

495. Milhorat, T. H.: Hydrocephalus and the Cerebrospinal Fluid. Baltimore, Williams & Wilkins Co., 1972.

496. Miller, J. Q., and Selden, R. F.: Arhinencephaly, encephalocele, and 13–15 trisomy syndrome with normal chromosomes. Neurology (Minneap.), 17:1087–1091, 1967.

497. Millis, R. R., and Holmes, A. E.: Enterogenous cyst of the spinal cord with associated intestinal reduplication, vertebral anomalies, and a dorsal dermal sinus. Case report. J. Neurosurg., 38:73–77, 1973.

498. Milunsky, A.: Maternal serum AFP screening. New Eng. J. Med., 298:738–739, 1978.

499. Mitchell, G. E., Lourie, H., and Berne, A. S.: The various causes of scalloped vertebrae with notes on their pathogenesis. Radiology, 89:67–74, 1967.

500. Modesti, L. M., Glasauer, F. E., and Terplan, K. L.: Sphenoethmoidal encephalocele. A case report with review of the literature. Child's Brain, 3:140–153, 1977.

501. Moes, C. A. F., and Hendrick, E. B.: Diastematomyelia. J. Pediat., 63:238–248, 1963.

502. Moise, T. S.: Staphylococcus meningitis secondary to a congenital sacral sinus. Surg. Gynec. Obstet., 42:394–397, 1926.

503. Mood, G. F.: Congenital anterior herniations of brain. Ann. Otol., 47:391–401, 1938.

504. Moore, J. E.: Spina bifida with a report of 385 cases treated by excision. Surg. Gynec. Obstet., 1:137–140, 1905.

505. Moore, P. M.: Intranasal encephalomeningocele. Report of a case. Laryngoscope, 62:659–677, 1952.

506. Morel, M. P.: A case of spina bifida occulta of the 12th dorsal and 1st lumbar vertebrae. Brit. J. Radiol., 15:154, 1942.

507. Morley, A. R.: Laryngeal stridor, Arnold-Chiari malformation and medullary haemorrhages. Develop. Med. Child Neurol., 11:471–474, 1969.

508. Mount, L. A.: Congenital dermal sinuses as a cause of meningitis, intraspinal abscess and intracranial abscess. J.A.M.A., 139:1263–1268, 1949.

509. Mulliken, J. B.: A large frontoethmoidal encephalomeningocele. Case report. Plast. Reconstr. Surg., 51:592–595, 1973.

510. Murphy, D. P.: The etiology of congenital malformations in light of biologic statistics. Amer. J. Obstet. Gynec., 34:890–897, 1937.

511. Murray, P. J., O'Gorman, A. M., and Blundell,

J. E.: Lumbosacral lipomata producing en-uresis. Trans. Amer. Neurol. Ass., *98*:287–290, 1973.

512. Mustardé, J. C.: Meningomyelocele: The problem of skin cover. Brit. J. Surg., *53*:36–41, 1966.

513. Mustardé, J. C.: Reconstruction of the spinal canal in severe spina bifida. Plast. Reconstr. Surg., *42*:109–114, 1968.

514. Nadler, H. L.: Present status of the prevention of neural tube defects. Pediatrics, *55*:751–753, 1975.

515. Nagulich, I., Borne, G., and Georgevich, Z.: Temporal meningocele. J. Neurosurg., *27*:433–440, 1967.

516. Naik, D. R.: Cervical spinal canal in normal infants. Clin. Radiol., *21*:323–326, 1970.

517. Naik, D. R.: A sign of spina bifida cystica on lateral radiographs of the spine. Clin. Radiol., *23*:193–195, 1972.

518. Naik, D. R., and Emery, J. L.: The position of the spinal cord segments related to the vertebral bodies in children with meningomyelocele and hydrocephalus. Develop. Med. Child Neurol. suppl., *16*:62–68, 1968.

519. Naik, D. R., and Emery, J. L.: Diagnosis of Cleland-Arnold-Chiari deformity on plain radiographs of the spine. Develop. Med. Child Neurol. suppl., *20*:78–81, 1969.

520. Nakamura, T., Grant, J. A., and Hubbard, R. E.: Nasoethmoidal meningoencephalocele. Arch. Otolaryng. (Chicago), *100*:62–64, 1974.

521. Nathan, M. T.: Cysts and duplications of neurenteric origin. Pediatrics, *23*:476–484, 1959.

522. Naylor, P. F. D.: Diastematomyelia with hairy haemangioma and connective tissue naevus. Proc. Roy. Soc. Med., *57*:319, 1964.

523. Neblett, C. R., Caram, P. C., and Morris, R.: Lateral congenital dermal sinus tract associated with an intradiploic dermoid tumor: Case report. J. Neurosurg., *33*:103–105, 1970.

524. Nelson, J. D.: The Marfan syndrome, with special reference to congenital enlargement of the spinal canal. Brit. J. Radiol., *31*:561–564, 1958.

525. Neuhauser, E. B. D., Harris, G. B. C., and Berrett, A.: Roentgenographic features of neurenteric cysts. Amer. J. Roentgen., *79*:235–240, 1958.

526. Neuhauser, E. B. D., Wittenborg, M. H., and Dehlinger, K.: Diastematomyelia: Transfixion of the cord or cauda equina with congenital anomalies of the spine. Radiology, *54*:659–664, 1950.

527. Nishimura, H. Takano, K. T., Tanimura, T., Yasuda, M., and Uchida, T.: High incidence of several malformations in the early human embryos as compared with infants. Biol. Neonat., *10*:93–107, 1966.

528. Nulsen, F. E., and Becker, D. P.: Control of hydrocephalus by valve-regulated shunt. J. Neurosurg., *26*:362–374, 1967.

529. Nulsen, F. E., and Spitz, E. B.: Treatment of hydrocephalus by direct shunt from ventricle to jugular vein. Surg. Forum, *2*:399, 1952.

530. O'Connell, J. E. A.: Congenital dermal sinus. Proc. Roy. Soc. Med., *35*:685, 1942.

531. Odeku, E. L.: Congenital malformations of the cerebrospinal axis seen in the Western Nigeria. The African child with "encephalocele." Int. Surg., *48*:52–62, 1967.

532. Odom, J. A., Jr., and Brown, C. W.: Surgical treatment of scoliosis in myelodysplasia. *In* McLaurin, R. L., ed.: Myelomeningocele. New York, Grune & Stratton, Inc., 1977, pp. 581–589.

533. Oehlecker, F.: Sakralabszesse bei kongenitalen Hauterverlagerungen. Deutsch. Z., *197*:262–279, 1926.

534. Onuigbo, W. I. B.: Encephaloceles in Nigerian Igbos. J. Neurol. Neurosurg. Psychiat., *40*:726, 1977.

535. O'Rahilly, R.: Anomalous occcipital apertures. Arch. Path. (Chicago), *53*:509–519, 1952.

536. O'Rahilly, R., and Gardener, E.: The timing and sequence of events in the development of the human nervous system during the embryonic period proper. Z. Anat. Entwicklungsgesh., *134*:1–12, 1971.

537. Osaka, K., Tanimura, T., Hirayama, A., and Matsumoto, S.: Myelomeningocele before birth. J. Neurosurg., *49*:711–724, 1978.

538. Padget, D. H.: Spina bifida and embryonic neuroschisis—a causal relationship; definition of postnatal confirmations involving a bifid spine. Johns Hopkins Med. J., *128*:233–252, 1968.

539. Padget, D. H.: Neuroschisis and human embryonic maldevelopment: New evidence on anencephaly, spina bifida and diverse mammalian defects. J. Neuropath, Exp. Neurol., *29*:192–216, 1970.

540. Padget, D. H.: Development of so-called dysraphism; with embryologic evidence of clinical Arnold-Chiari and Dandy-Walker malformations. Johns Hopkins Med. J., *130*:127–165, 1972.

541. Padget, D. H., and Lindenberg, R.: Inverse cerebellum morphogenetically related to Dandy-Walker and Arnold-Chiari syndromes: Bizarre malformed brain with occipital encephalocele. Johns Hopkins Med. J., *131*:228–246, 1972.

542. Page, R. E.: Intraspinal enterogenous cyst associated with spondylolisthesis and spina bifida occulta. J. Bone Joint Surg. *56-B*:541–544, 1974.

543. Papo, I., Longhi, G., and Caruselli, G.: Giant spinal extradural cyst. Surg. Neurol., *8*:350–352, 1977.

544. Parker, H. L., and McConnell, A. A.: Internal hydrocephalus resulting from a peculiar deformity of the hind-brain. Trans. Amer. Neurol. Ass., *1*:14–16, 1937.

545. Parkinson, D., Chaudhuri, A., and Schwartz, I.: Congenital intraspinal extradural cysts (intraspinal meningocele). Canad. J. Neurol. Sci., *3*:205–210, 1976.

546. Parsons, J. H., and Coats, G.: A case of orbital encephalocele with unique malformations of the brain and eye. Brain, *29*:209–226, 1906.

547. Passarge, E.: Congenital malformations and maternal diabetes. Lancet, *1*:324–325, 1965.

548. Passarge, E., and Lenz, W.: Syndrome of caudal regression in infants of diabetic mothers. Pediatrics, *37*:672–675, 1966.

549. Patey, D. H., and Scarff, R. W.: Pathology of postanal pilonidal sinus. Its bearing on treatment. Lancet, *2*:484–486, 1946.

550. Patey, D. H., and Scarff, R. W.: Pilonidal sinus

in a barber's hand with observations on post-natal pilonidal sinus. Lancet, 2:13–14, 1948.

551. Patten, B. M.: Embryological stages in the development of spina bifida and myeloschisis. Anat. Rec., 94:487, 1946.

552. Patten, B. M.: Overgrowth of the neural tube in young human embryos. Anat. Rec., 113:381–393, 1952.

553. Patten, B. M.: Embryological stages in the establishing of myeloschisis with spina bifida. Amer. J. Anat., 93:365–395, 1953.

554. Patten, B. M.: Patten's Human Embryology. Elements of clinical development. New York, McGraw-Hill, Inc., 1976.

555. Patterson, T. J. S., and Till, K.: The use of rotation flaps following excision of lumbar myelomeningoceles. An aid to the closure of large defects. Brit. J. Surg., 46:606–608, 1959.

556. Peach, B.: Arnold-Chiari malformation with normal spine. Arch. Neurol. (Chicago), 10:497–501, 1964.

557. Peach, B.: Cystic prolongation of the fourth ventricle; and anomaly associated with the Arnold-Chiari malformation. Arch. Neurol. (Chicago), 11:609–612, 1964.

558. Peach, B.: The Arnold-Chiari malformation: Morphogenesis. Arch. Neurol. (Chicago), 12:527–535, 1965.

559. Peach, B.: Arnold-Chiari malformation: Anatomic features of 20 cases. Arch. Neurol. (Chicago), 12:613–621, 1965.

560. Penfield, W., and Coburn, D. F.: Arnold-Chiari malformation and its operative treatment. Arch. Neurol. Psychiat., 40:328–336, 1938.

561. Perloff, M. M.: Congenital dermal sinus complication by meningitis. Report of a case. J. Pediat., 44:73–76, 1954.

562. Perret, G.: Diagnosis and treatment of diastematomyelia. Surg. Gynec. Obstet., 105:69–83, 1957.

563. Perret, G.: Symptoms and diagnosis of diastematomyelia. Neurology (Minneap.), 10:51–60, 1960.

564. Persky, L.: Indications for sigmoid conduit diversion: Technique and long term results. In McLaurin, R. L., ed.: Myelomeningocele. New York, Grune & Stratton, Inc., 1977, pp. 785–789.

565. Pettersson, G., and Werkmäster, K.: Intraspinal dermoid cysts in children. Acta Paediat. (Stockholm), 52:187–189, 1962.

566. Peyser, E., Cohen, W., and Joseph, A. Y.: Congenital dermal sinus complicated by B. proteus and nonhemolytic Streptococcus meningitis. Neurology (Minneap.), 7:296–298, 1957.

567. Pickles, W.: Duplication of the spinal cord (diplomyelia): An account of a clinical example with a consideration of other reports. J. Neurosurg., 6:324–331, 1949.

568. Pilz, P., Fischbach, R., and Brenneis, M.: Enterogene cyste des Halsmarkes mit Mucomyelie. Acta Neuropath. (Berlin), 40:277–278, 1977.

569. Pinto, R. S., George, A. E., Koslow, M., and Barasch, G.: Neuroradiology of basal anterior fossa (transethmoidal) encephaloceles. Radiology, 117:79–85, 1975.

570. Piramoon, A. M., and Abbassioun, K.: Mediastinal enterogenic cyst with spinal cord compression. J. Pediat. Surg., 9:543–545, 1974.

571. Pollock, J. A., Newton, T. H., and Hoyt, W. F.: Transsphenoidal and transethmoidal encephaloceles: A review of clinical and roentgenographic features in 8 cases. Radiology, 90:442–453, 1968.

572. Pool, J. L.: Spinal cord and local signs secondary to occult sacral meningoceles in adults. Bull. N.Y. Acad. Med., 28:655–663, 1952.

573. Porter, R. W.: Vasomotor control in the lower limbs of children with meningomyelocele. Develop. Med. Child Neurol. suppl., 15:62–69, 1968.

574. Powell, K. R., Cherry, J. D., Hougen, T. J., et al.: A prospective search for congenital dermal abnormalities of the craniospinal axis. J. Pediat., 87:744–750, 1975.

575. Powledge, T. M., and Fletcher, J.: Guidelines for the ethical, social and legal issues in prenatal diagnosis. New Eng. J. Med., 300:168–172, 1979.

576. Price, D. L., Dooling, E. C., and Richardson, E. P., Jr.: Caudal dysplasia (caudal regression syndrome). Arch. Neurol., 23:212–220, 1970.

577. Prince, B.: Myelomeningocele. Part IV. Psychosocial problems and social work interventions. West. J. Med., 121:297–298, 1974.

578. Prop, N., Frensdorf, E. L., and van de Stadt, F. R.: A postvertebral entodermal cyst associated with axial deformities: A case showing the "entodermal-ectodermal adhesion syndrome." Pediatrics, 39:555–562, 1967.

579. Pudenz, R. H.: The ventriculoatrial shunt. J. Neurosurg., 25:602–608, 1966.

580. Pudenz, R. H., Russell, F. E., Hurd, A. H., and Sheldon, C. H.: Ventriculoauriculostomy. A technique for shunting cerebrospinal fluid from the right auricle. Preliminary report. J. Neurosurg., 14:171–179, 1957.

581. Pullon, D. H. H.: Craniolacunia and phenylpyruvic oligophrenia. Brit. J. Radiol., 31:634–636, 1958.

582. Quade, R. H., and Craig, W. McK.: Unusual dermoid and epidermoid cranial cysts. Proc. Staff Meet. Mayo Clin., 14:459–462, 1939.

583. Raimondi, A. J., and Soare, P.: Intellectual development in shunted hydrocephalic children. Amer. J. Dis. Child., 127:664–671, 1974.

584. Raimondi, A. J., Samuelson, G., Yarzagaray, L., and Norton, T.: Atresia of the foramina of Luschka and Magendie. The Dandy-Walker cyst. J. Neurosurg., 31:202–216, 1969.

585. Rális, Z. A.: Traumatizing effect of breech delivery on infants with spina bifida. J. Pediat., 87:613–616, 1975.

586. Rand, R. W., and Rand, C. W.: Intraspinal Tumors of Childhood. Springfield, Ill., Charles C Thomas, 1960.

587. Ransford, A. O., and Manning, C. W. S. F.: Complications of halo-pelvic distraction for scoliosis. J. Bone Joint Surg. 57-B:131–137, 1975.

588. Ransohoff, J., and Mathews, E. S.: Neurosurgical management of patients with spina bifida and myelomeningocele. Med. Clin. N. Amer., 53:493–496, 1969.

589. Rao, S. B., and Dinakar, I.: Intraspinal dermoids. Neurol. India, 18:185–188, 1970.

590. Reddy, D. R., Sathyanarayana, K., and Krishnamurthi, D.: Occult intrasacral meningocele:

Report of a case. Aust. N.Z. J. Surg., *44*:273–275, 1974.

591. Reddy, D. R., Subrahmanian, M. J., Prabhakar, V., and Rao, B. D.: Neurenteric cyst. A case report. Neurol. India, *20*:221–223, 1972.

592. Rege, P. R.: Myelomeningocele-treatment modalities in perspective. *In* McLaurin, R. L., ed.: Myelomeningocele. New York, Grune & Stratton, Inc., 1977, pp. 677–697.

593. Reid, J. D.: Effects of flexion-extension movements of the head and spine upon the spinal cord and nerve roots. J. Neurol. Neurosurg. Psychiat., *23*:214–221, 1960.

594. Reigel, D. H., Scarff, T. B., and Woodford, J.: Surgery for tethered spinal cord in myelomeningocele patients. American Association of Neurological Surgeons, 1976.

595. Reimann, A. F., and Anson, B. J.: Vertebral level of termination of the spinal cord with report of a case of sacral cord. Anat. Rec., *88*:127–138, 1944.

596. Report of a Committee of the Society nominated November 10, 1882, to investigate spina bifida and its treatment by the injection of Dr. Morton's iodo-glycerine solution. Clin. Soc. Trans., *18*:339–418, 1885.

597. Rewcastle, N. B., and Francoeur, J.: Teratomatous cysts of the spinal canal with "sex chromatin" studies. Arch. Neurol. (Chicago), *11*:91–100, 1964.

598. Rhaney, K., and Barclay, G. P. T.: Enterogenous cysts and congenital diverticula of the alimentary canal with abnormalities of the vertebral column and spinal cord. J. Path. Bact., *77*:457–471, 1959.

599. Rhoton, A. L., Jr.: Microsurgery of Arnold-Chiari malformation in adults with and without hydromyelia. J. Neurosurg., *45*:473–483, 1976.

600. Richards, G. J., Jr., and Reeves, R. J.: Mediastinal tumors and cysts in children. Amer. J. Dis. Child., *95*:284–290, 1958.

601. Richards, I. D. G., and McIntosh, H. T.: Spina bifida survivors and their parents: A study of problems and services. Develop. Med. Child Neurol., *15*:292–304, 1973.

602. Richings, J. C., and Eckstein, H. B.: Locomotor and educational achievements of children with myelomeningocele. Ann. Phys. Med., *10*:291–298, 1970.

603. Rickham, P. P., and Mawdsley, T.: The effect of early operation on the survival of spina bifida cystica. Develop. Med. Child Neurol. suppl., *11*:20–26, 1966.

604. Rigault, P., Pouliquen, J. C., Guyonvarch, G., and Durand, Y.: Quatre cas de diastématomyélie. Rev. Chir. Orthop., *58*:33–50, 1972.

605. Ripley, W., and Thompson, D. C.: Pilonidal sinus as a route of infection in a case of Staphylococcus meningitis. Amer. J. Dis. Child., *36*:785–788, 1928.

606. Ritchie, G. W., and Flanagan, M. M.: Diastematomyelia. Canad. Med. Ass. J., *100*:428–433, 1969.

607. Robards, M. F., Thomas, G. G., and Rosenbloom, L.: Survival of infants with unoperated myeloceles. Brit. Med. J., *4*:12–13, 1975.

608. Roberts, A. P.: A case of intracranial dermoid cyst associated with Klippel-Feil deformity and recurrent meningitis. Arch. Dis. Child., *33*:222–225, 1958.

609. Roberts, K. D., and Weeks, M. M.: Two cases of spinal abnormality associated with duplication of the gut and melaena. Brit. J. Surg., *44*:377–383, 1956–1957.

610. Robertson, A. A.: Spina bifida occulta with spinal cord lesion. Med. Clin. N. Amer., *7*:1855–1866, 1924.

611. Rogers, H. M., Long, D. M., Chou, S. N., and French, L. A.: Lipomas of the spinal cord and cauda equina. J. Neurosurg., *34*:349–354, 1971.

612. Roller, G. J., and Pribram, H. F. W.: Lumbosacral intradural lipoma and sacral agenesis. Radiology, *84*:507–512, 1965.

613. Rosenbaum, T. J., Soule, E. H., and Onofrio, B. M.: Teratomatous cyst of the spinal canal. Case report. J. Neurosurg., *49*:292–297, 1978.

614. Roth, M.: Caudal end of the spinal cord. I. Normal pneumographic features, Acta. Radiol. [Diag.] (Stockholm), *3*:177–188, 1965.

615. Roth, M.: The caudal end of the spinal cord II. Abnormal pneumographic features: Lumbar intumescence artery syndrome and spinal dysraphism. Acta. Radiol. [Diag.] (Stockholm), *3*:297–304, 1965.

616. Rothstein, T. B., Romano, P. E., and Shoch, D.: Meningomyelocele. Amer. J. Ophthal., *77*:690–693, 1974.

617. Rovit, R. L., and Sosman, M. C.: Hemicranial aplasia with pulsating exophthalmos. An unusual manifestation of von Recklinghausen's disease. J. Neurosurg., *17*:104–121, 1960.

618. Rozen, M. J.: Pathophysiology and spinal deformity in myelomeningocele. *In* McLaurin, R. L., ed.: Myelomeningocele. New York, Grune & Stratton, Inc., 1977, pp. 565–579.

619. Rusnak, S. L., and Driscoll, S. G.: Congenital spinal anomalies in infants of diabetic mothers. Pediatrics, *35*:989–995, 1965.

620. Russel, H. E., and Aitken, G. I.: Congenital absence of sacrum and lumbar vertebrae with prosthetic management. J. Bone Joint Surg., *45-A*:501–508, 1963.

621. Russell, D. S., and Donald, C.: The mechanisms of internal hydrocephalus in spina bifida. Brain, *38*:203–215, 1935.

622. Ryttman, A.: Lateral intrathoracic meningocele with spontaneous rupture into the pleural cavity diagnosed with RIHSA myelography. Neuroradiology, *5*:165–168, 1973.

623. Sachs, E., Jr., and Horrax, G.: A cervical and a lumbar pilonidal sinus communicating with intraspinal dermoids. J. Neurosurg., *6*:97–112, 1949.

624. Sahs, A. L.: Congenital anomaly of the cerebellar vermis. Arch. Path. (Chicago), *32*:52–63, 1941.

625. Salyer, D. C., Salyer, W. R., and Eggleston, J. C.: Benign developmental cysts of the mediastinum. Arch. Path. Lab. Med., *101*:136–139, 1977.

626. Sands, W. W., and Clark, W. K.: Diastematomyelia. Amer. J. Roentgen., *72*:64–67, 1954.

627. Sarnat, H. B., Case, M. E., and Graviss, R.: Sacral agenesis. Neurology (Minneap.), *26*:1124–1129, 1976.

628. Sarwar, M., and Kelly, P. J.: Adult diastematomyelia. Spine, *2*:60–64, 1977.

629. Saunders, R. L.: Intramedullary epidermoid cyst

associated with a dermal sinus. Case report. J. Neurosurg., *31*:83–86, 1969.

630. Saunders, R. L. de C. H.: Combined anterior and posterior spina bifida in a living neonatal human female. Anat. Rec., *87*:255–278, 1943.

631. Say, B., Carpenter, N. J., and Coldwell, J. G.: Anterior sacral meningocele (letter). J.A.M.A., *237*:2602, 1977.

632. Sayers, M. P.: The significance of the Arnold-Chiari malformation. *In* McLaurin, R. L., ed.: Myelomeningocele. New York, Grune & Stratton, Inc., 1977, pp. 241–249.

633. Scarcella, G.: Radiologic aspects of Dandy-Walker syndrome. Neurology (Minneap.), *10*:260–266, 1960.

634. Scarff, J. E.: Spastic hemiplegia, produced by a congenital cyst replacing cerebellar vermis. J. Nerv. Ment. Dis., *78*:400, 1933.

635. Scatliff, J. H., Till, K., and Hoare, R. D.: Incomplete false and true diastematomyelia. Radiological evaluation by air myelography and tomography. Radiology, *116*:349–354, 1975.

636. Scherzer, A. L., Kaye, D., and Shinefield, H. R.: Proteus mirabilis meningitis: Report of two cases treated with ampicillin. J. Pediat.,*68*:731–740, 1966.

637. Schey, W. L., and Selker, R. G.: Anterior fontanel meningoencephalocele. Report of a case. Radiology, *104*:79–80, 1972.

638. Schey, W. L., Shkolnik, A., and White, H.: Clinical and radiographic considerations of sacrococcygeal teratomas: An analysis of 26 new cases and review of the literature. Radiology, *125*:189–195, 1977.

639. Schmidt, P. H., and Luyendijk, W.: Intranasal meningoencephalocele. Arch. Otolaryng. (Chicago), *99*:402–405, 1974.

640. Schreiber, M. S., and Reye, R. D. K.: Posterior fossa cysts due to congenital atresia of the foramina of Luschka and Magendie. Med. J. Aust., *2*:743–748, 1954.

641. Schroeder, H. G., and Williams, N. E.: Anaesthesia for meningomyelocele surgery. Anaesthesia, *21*:57–65, 1966.

642. Schut, L., Pizzi, F. J., and Bruce, D. A.: Occult spinal dysraphism. *In* McLaurin, R. L., ed.: Myelomeningocele. New York, Grune & Stratton, Inc., 1977, pp. 349–368.

643. Schwalbe, E., and Gredig, M.: Über Entwicklungsstorungen des Kleinhirns Hirnstamms und Halmarks bei Spina bifida (Arnold'sche und Chiari'sche (Mibbildung). Beitr. Path. Anat., *40*:132–194, 1907.

644. Schwartz, H. G.: Congenital tumors of the spinal cord in infants. Ann. Surg.,*136*:183–192, 1952.

645. Schwidde, J. T.: Spina bifida, survey of 225 encephaloceles, meningoceles and myelomeningoceles. Amer. J. Dis. Child., *84*:35–51, 1952.

646. Scobie, W. G.: Malignant sacrococcygeal teratoma—a problem in diagnosis. Arch. Dis. Child., *46*:216–218, 1971.

647. Scobie, W. G., Eckstein, H. B., and Long, W. J.: Bowel function in myelomeningocele. Develop. Med. Child Neurol., *12*:suppl. 22:150–156, 1970.

648. Scott, F. B.: The management of neurogenic bladder in patients with myelomeningocele: sphincterotomy, bladder flap urethroplasty, and the artificial sphincter. *In* McLaurin, R.

L., ed.: Myelomeningocele. New York, Grune & Stratton, Inc., 1977, pp. 753–772.

649. Scoville, W. B., Manlapaz, J. S., Otis, R. D., and Cabieses, F.: Intraspinal enterogenous cyst. J. Neurosurg., *20*:704–706, 1963.

650. Seagle, J. B.: Congenital dermal sinus complicated by meningitis. Arch. Pediat., *71*:244–251, 1954.

651. Seaman, W. B., and Schwartz, H. G.: Diastematomyelia in adults. Radiology, *70*:692–695, 1958.

652. Sedzimir, C. B., Roberts, J. R., and Occleshaw, J. V.: Massive diastematomyelia without cutaneous dysraphism. Arch. Dis. Child., *48*:400–402, 1973.

653. Sensenig, E. C.: The early development of the human vertebral column. Contrib. Embryol., *34*:21–41, 1949.

654. Shaker, I. J., Lanier, V. C., and Amoury, R. A.: Congenital anal stenosis with anterior sacral meningocele. J. Pediat. Surg., *6*:177, 1971.

655. Shands, A. R., Jr., and Bundens, W. D.: Congenital deformities of the spine: An analysis of the roentgenograms of 700 children. Bull. Hosp. Joint Dis., *17*:110–133, 1956.

656. Shapiro, B., and Tosti, V. G.: Ventricular dilatation in spina bifida. J. Pediat., *16*:318–325, 1940.

657. Shapiro, K., and Shulman, K.: Late complications of the Arnold-Chiari malformation. *In* McLaurin, R. L., ed.: Myelomeningocele. New York, Grune & Stratton, Inc., 1977, pp. 251–262.

658. Sharpe, N.: Spina bifida. An experimental and clinical study. Ann. Surg., *61*:151–165, 1915.

659. Sharpe, W., and Sharpe, N.: Neurosurgery—Principles, Diagnosis and Treatment. Philadelphia, J. B. Lippincott Co., 1928.

660. Sharrard, W. J. W.: The Mechanism of paralytic deformity in spina bifida. Develop. Med. Child Neurol., *4*:310–313, 1962.

661. Sharrard, W. J. W.: Myelomeningocele: Prognosis for immediate operative closure of the sac. Proc. Roy. Soc. Med., *56*:510–512, 1963.

662. Sharrard, W. J. W.: The segmental innervation of the lower limb muscles in man. Ann. Roy. Coll. Surg. Eng., *35*:106–122, 1964.

663. Sharrard, W. J. W.: Spinal osteotomy for congenital kyphosis in myelomeningocele. J. Bone Joint Surg., *50-B*:466–471, 1968.

664. Sharrard, W. J. W.: Neuromotor evaluation of the newborn. *In* American Academy of Orthopaedic Surgeons: Symposium on Myelomeningocele. St. Louis, C. V. Mosby Co., 1972, pp. 26–40.

665. Sharrard, W. J. W.: Assessment of the myelomeningocele. child. *In* McLaurin, R. L., ed.: Myelomeningocele. New York, Grune & Stratton, Inc., 1977, pp. 389–410.

666. Sharrard, W. J. W.: Lordosis and lordo-scoliosis in myelomeningocele. *In* McLaurin, R. L., ed.: Myelomeningocele. New York, Grune & Stratton, Inc., 1977, pp. 591–607.

667. Sharrard, W. J. W.: Muscle balancing procedures in hip deformity in myelomeningocele. *In* McLaurin, R. L., ed.: Myelomeningocele. New York, Grune & Stratton, Inc., 1977, pp. 523–538.

668. Sharrard, W. J. W.: Paralytic convex pes valgus

(paralytic vertical talus). *In* McLaurin, R. L., ed.: Myelomeningocele. New York, Grune & Stratton, Inc., 1977, pp. 461–467.

669. Sharrard, W. J.: Paralytic pes cavus and claw toes. *In* McLaurin, R. L., ed.: Myelomeningocele. New York, Grune & Stratton, Inc., 1977, pp. 469–474.

670. Sharrard, W. J. W., and Drennan, J. C.: Osteotomy-excision of the spine for lumbar kyphosis in older children with myelomeningocele. J. Bone Joint Surg., *54-B*:50–60, 1972.

671. Sharrard, W. J. W., Zachary, R. B., Lorber, J., and Bruce, A. M.: A controlled trial of immediate and delayed closure of spina bifida cystica. Arch. Dis. Child., *38*:18–22, 1963.

672. Shaw, J. F.: Diastematomyelia. Develop. Med. Child Neurol., *17*:361–364, 1975.

673. Shealy, C. N., and LeMay, M.: Intrathoracic meningocele. J. Neurosurg., *21*:880–883, 1964.

674. Shenkin, H. A., Hunt, A. D., Jr., and Horn, R. C., Jr.: Sacrococcygeal sinus (pilonidal sinus) in direct continuity with the central canal of the spinal cord. Surg. Gynec. Obstet., *79*:655–659, 1944.

675. Sheptak, P. E., and Susen, A. F.: Diastematomyelia. Amer. J. Dis. Child., *113*:210–213, 1967.

676. Shidler, F. P., and Richards, V.: Anterior sacral meningocele. Ann. Surg., *118*:913–918, 1943.

677. Shopfner, C. E., Jabour, J. F., and Vallion, R. M.: Craniolacunia. Amer. J. Roentgen., *93*:343–349, 1965.

678. Shorey, W. D.: Diastematomyelia associated with dorsal kyphosis producing paraplegia. J. Neurosurg., *12*:300–305, 1955.

679. Shryock, E. H.: Complete obstruction of the cerebral aqueduct associated with lumbar meningocele. Bull. Los Angeles. Neurol. Soc., *9*:163–166, 1944.

680. Shryock, E. H., and Alexander, H. B.: Congenital malformation of the cerebellar vermis associated with dilatation of the fourth ventricle and cisternal arachnoidal cyst. Bull. Los Angeles Neurol. Soc., *8*:11–17, 1943.

681. Shulman, K., and Ames, M. D.: Intensive treatment of fifty children born with myelomeningocele. New York J. Med., *68*:2656–2659, 1968.

682. Shurtleff, D. B., and Sousa, J. C.: The adolescent with myelodysplasia—development, achievement, sex and deterioration. *In* McLaurin, R. L., ed.: Myelomeningocele. New York, Grune & Stratton, Inc., 1977, pp. 809–835.

683. Shurtleff, D. B., Kronmal, R., and Foltz, E. L.: Follow-up comparison of hydrocephalus with and without myelomeningocele. J. Neurosurg., *42*:61–68, 1975.

684. Shurtleff, D. B., Hayden, P. W., Loeser, J. D., and Kronmal, R. A.: Myelodysplasia: Decision for death or disability. New Eng. J. Med., *291*:1005–1011, 1974.

685. Sieben, R. L., Hamida, M. B., and Shulman, K.: Multiple cranial nerve deficits associated with the Arnold-Chiari malformation. Neurology (Minneap.), *21*:673–681, 1971.

686. Silvernail, W. I., Jr., and Brown, R. B.: Intramedullary enterogenous cyst. Case report. J. Neurosurg., *36*:235–238, 1972.

687. Silvis, R. S., Riddle, L. R., and Clark, G. C.: An-

terior sacral meningocele. Amer. Surg., *22*:554–566, 1956.

688. Siris, I. E.: Spina bifida: Treatment and analysis of 84 cases. Ann. Surg., *103*:97–123, 1936.

689. Small, J. M.: Some disturbances of the neural crest affecting the nervous system. Proc. Roy. Soc. Med., *48*:597–601, 1955.

690. Smith, E. D.: Congenital sacral anomalies in children. Aust. N.Z. J. Surg., *29*:165–176, 1959.

691. Smith, E. D.: Spina Bifida and the Total Care of Spinal Myelomeningocele. Springfield, Ill., Charles C Thomas, 1965.

692. Smith, G. F., and Altman, D. H.: Occipital dermal sinus. Amer. J. Dis. Child., *98*:713–719, 1959.

693. Smith, G. K., and Smith, E. D.: Selection for treatment in spina bifida cystica. Brit. Med. J., *4*:189–197, 1973.

694. Smith, J. R.: Accessory enteric formations. A classification and nomenclature. Arch. Dis. Child., *35*:87–89, 1960.

695. Smith, M. T., and Huntington, H. W.: Inverse cerebellum and occipital encephalocele. Neurology (Minneap.), *27*:246–251, 1977.

696. Smith, T. E.: Anterior or perineal pilonidal cysts. J.A.M.A., *136*:973–975, 1948.

697. Smyth, B. T., Piggot, J., Forsythe, W. I., and Merrett, J. D.: A controlled trial of immediate and delayed closure of myelomeningocele. J. Bone Joint Surg. *56-B*:297–304, 1974.

698. Sokol, G. M., and Schwartz, M. W.: Urinary complication of lipomyelomeningocele. Arch. Dis. Child., *48*:560–562, 1973.

699. Sostrin, R. D., Thompson, J. R., Rouhe, S. A., and Hasso, A. N.: Occult spinal dysraphism in the geriatric patient. Radiology, *125*:165–169, 1977.

700. Spiller, W. G.: Congenital and acquired eneuresis from spinal lesion a) myelodysplasia; b) stretching of the cauda equina. Amer. J. Med. Sci., *151*:469–475, 1916.

701. Stammers, F. A. R.: Spinal epidural suppuration with special reference to osteomyelitis of the vertebrae. Brit. J. Surg., *26*:366–374, 1938.

702. Stark, G.: The pathophysiology of the bladder in myelomeningocele and its correlation with the neurological picture. Develop. Med. Child Neurol. suppl., *16*:76–86, 1968.

703. Stark, G. D.: Neonatal assessment of the child with a myelomeningocele. Arch. Dis. Child., *46*:539–548, 1971.

704. Stark, G. D.: Prediction of urinary continence in myelomeningocele. Develop. Med. Child Neurol., *13*:388–389, 1971.

705. Stark, G. D.: The nature and cause of paraplegia in myelomeningocele. Paraplegia, *9*:219–223, 1972.

706. Stark, G. D.: Myelomeningocele: The changing approach to treatment. *In* Wilkinson, A. W., ed.: Recent Advances in Paediatric Surgery, 3rd Ed. London, Churchill Livingstone, 1975.

707. Stark, G. D.: Spina Bifida. Problems and Management. Oxford, Blackwell Scientific Publications, 1977.

708. Stark, G. D., and Drummond, M.: Neonatal electromyography and nerve conduction studies in myelomeningocele. Neuropädiatrie, *3*:409–420, 1972.

709. Stark, G. D., and Drummond, M.: Results of se-

lective early operation in myelomeningocele. Arch. Dis. Child., *48*:676–683, 1973.

710. Stedman's Medical Dictionary. Baltimore, Williams & Wilkins Co., 1961.

711. Steele, G. H.: The Arnold-Chiari malformation. Brit. J. Surg., *34*:280–282, 1946.

712. Stein, S., Schut, L., and Borns, P.: Lacunar skull deformity (Lückenschädel) and intelligence in myelomeningocele. J. Neurosurg., *41*:10–13, 1974.

713. Stein, S. C., Schut, L., and Ames, M. D.: Selection for early treatment in myelomeningocele: A retrospective analysis of various selection procedures. Pediatrics, *54*:553–557, 1974.

714. Stookey, B.: Intradural spinal lipoma: Report of a case and symptoms for 10 years in a child age 11; review of the literature. Arch. Neurol. Psychiat., *18*:16–43, 1927.

715. Stoyle, T. F.: Prognosis for paralysis in myelomeningocele. Develop. Med. Child Neurol., *8*:755–760, 1966.

716. Strand, R. D.: Spinal dysraphism in certain occult forms examined by air myelography without tomography. Ann. Radiol. (Paris), *12*:393–399, 1969.

717. Strand, R. D., and Eisenberg, H. M.: Anterior sacral meningocele in association with Marfan's syndrome. Radiology, *99*:653–654, 1971.

718. Strandberg, B.: Cephalocele of posterior part of orbit. General survey with report of a case. Arch. Ophthal. (Chicago), *42*:254–265, 1949.

719. Strandgaard, L.: The Dandy-Walker syndrome —a case with a patent foramen of the fourth ventricle demonstrated by encephalography. Brit. J. Radiol., *43*:734–738, 1970.

720. Streeter, G. L.: The development of the venous sinuses of the dura mater in the human embryo. Amer. J. Anat., *18*:145–178, 1915.

721. Streeter, G. L.: Factors involved in the formation of the filum terminale. Amer. J. Anat., *25*:1–12, 1919.

722. Stritch, S. J.: Chiari's cerebellar malformations and the spinal cord. Develop. Med. Child Neurol., *8*:84–85, 1966.

723. Sutherland, C. G.: A roentgenographic study of developmental anomalies of the spine. J. Radiol., *3*:357–364, 1922.

724. Sutow, W. W., and Pryde, A. W.: Incidence of spina bifida occulta in relation to age. J. Dis. Child., *91*:211–217, 1956.

725. Sutton, J. B.: The lateral recesses of the fourth ventricle. Their relation to certain cysts and tumours of the cerebellum and to occipital meningocele. Brain, *9*:352–361, 1887.

726. Suwanwela, C.: Geographical distribution of fronto-ethmoidal encephalomeningocele. Brit. J. Prev. Soc. Med., *26*:193–198, 1972.

727. Suwanwela, C., and Hongsaprabhas, C.: Frontoethmoidal encephalomeningocele. J. Neurosurg., *25*:172–182, 1966.

728. Suwanwela, C., and Suwanwela, N.: A morphological classification of sincipital encephalomeningoceles. J. Neurosurg., *36*:201–211. 1972.

729. Suwanwela, C., and Suwanwela, N.: Air study in infants and children with frontoethmoidal encephalomeningocele. Neuroradiology, *4*:190–194, 1972.

730. Suwanwela, C., Poshyachinda, V., and Poshya-

chinda, M.: Isotope cisternography and ventriculography in frontoethmoidal encephalomeningocele. Acta Radiol. [Diag.] (Stockholm), *14*:5–8, 1973.

731. Suwanwela, C., Sukabote, C., and Suwanwela, N.: Frontoethmoidal encephalomeningocele. Surgery, *69*:617–625, 1971.

732. Swanson, H. S., and Barnett, J. C., Jr.: Intradural lipomas in children. Pediatrics, *29*:911–926, 1962.

733. Swanson, H. S., and Fincher, E. F.: Arnold-Chiari deformity without bony anomalies. J. Neurosurg., *6*:314–319, 1949.

734. Tadmor, R., Davis, K. R., Roberson, G. H., and Chapman, P. H.: The diagnosis of diastematomyelia by computed tomography. Surg. Neurol., *8*:434–436, 1977.

735. Taggart, J. K., Jr., and Walker, A. E.: Congenital atresia of the foramens of Luschka and Magendie. Arch. Neurol. Psychiat., *48*:583–612, 1942.

736. Tan, T. I.: Epidermoids and dermoids of the central nervous system (with two exceptional cases not represented in the literature). Acta. Neurochir. (Wien), *26*:13–24, 1972.

737. Tandon, P. N.: Meningoencephalocoeles. Acta: Neurol. Scand., *46*:369–383, 1970.

738. Tarlov, E.: Sacral perineurial cysts. New observations on diagnosis, relationship to symptoms and treatment. American Association of Neurological Surgeons, Toronto, 1977.

739. Tarlov, I. M.: Perineurial cysts of the spinal nerve roots. Arch. Neurol. Psychiat., *40*:1067–1074, 1938.

740. Tarlov, I. M.: Cysts (perineurial) of the sacral roots, Another cause (removable) of sciatic pain. J.A.M.A., *138*:740–744, 1948.

741. Tarlov, I. M.: Sacral Nerve Root Cysts. Another Cause of the Sciatic or Cauda Equina Syndrome. Springfield, Ill., Charles C Thomas, 1953.

742. Tavafoghi, V., Ghandchi, A., Hambrick, G. W., Jr., and Udverhelyi, G. B.: Cutaneous signs of spinal dysraphism. Report of a patient with a tail-like lipoma and review of 200 cases in the literature. Arch. Derm. (Chicago), *114*:573–577, 1978.

743. Teng, P., and Papatheodorou, C. A.: Arnold-Chiari malformation with normal spine and cranium. Arch. Neurol. (Chicago), *12*:622–624, 1965.

744. Teng, P., and Papatheodorou, C. A.: Dermal sinus and intraspinal dermoid and epidermoid cyst in children. Bull. Los Angeles Neurol. Soc., *35*:153–163, 1970.

745. Thieffry, S., Lepintre, J., Masselin, S., and Fauré, C.: Fistules dermiques congénitales communiquant avec le système nerveux central. Sem. Hop. Paris, *34*:1178–1187, 1958.

746. Thijssen, H. O. M., Walder, H. A. D., Wentges, R. T. R., Slooff, J. L., and Meyer, E.: Acquired basal encephalocele. Neuroradiology, *11*:209–213, 1976.

747. Thomas, J. E., and Miller, R. H.: Lipomatous tumors of the spinal canal. A study of their clinical range. Mayo Clin. Proc., *48*:393–400, 1973.

748. Thompson, M. W., and Rudd, N. L.: The genetics of spinal dysraphism. *In* Morley, T. P., ed.:

Current Controversies in Neurosurgery. Philadelphia, W. B. Saunders Co., 1976, pp. 126–146.

749. Tibbs, P. A., James, H. E., Rorke, L. B., Schut, L., and Bruce, D. A.: Midline hamartomas masquerading as meningomyeloceles or teratomas in the newborn infant. J. Pediat., 89:928–933, 1976.

750. Till, K.: Spinal dysraphism; a study of congenital malformations of the back. Develop. Med. Child Neurol., 10:470–477, 1968.

751. Till, K.: Spinal dysraphism. A study of congenital malformations of the lower back. J. Bone Joint Surg., 51-B:415–422, 1969.

752. Till, K.: Pediatric Neurosurgery for Paediatricians and Neurosurgeons. Oxford, Blackwell Scientific Publications, 1975.

753. Tizard, J. P. M.: Congenital dermal sinus (connexion with intradural dermoid cyst leading to spinal meningitis). Proc. Roy. Soc. Med., 43:247–249, 1950.

754. Toglia, J. U., Netsky, M. G., and Alexander, E., Jr.: Epithelial (epidermoid) tumors of the cranium. Their common nature and pathogenesis. J. Neurosurg., 23:384–393, 1965.

755. Tomlinson, B. E.: Heterotopic, non-functioning masses of nervous tissue in spina bifida cystica. J. Clin. Path., 18:732–736, 1965.

756. Traicoff, D., and Mishkin, F. S.: The diagnosis of Dandy-Walker cyst by brain scanning. Amer. J. Roentgen., 106:344–346, 1969.

757. Tytus, J. S., and Pennybacker, J.: Pearly tumors in relation to the central nervous system. J. Neurol. Neurosurg. Psychiat., 19:241–259, 1956.

758. Udvarhelyi, G. B., and Epstein, M. H.: The so-called Dandy-Walker syndrome: Analysis of 12 operated cases. Child's Brain, 1:158–182, 1975.

759. Vandresse, J. H., and Cornelis, G.: Diastematomyelia: Report of eight observations. Neuroradiology, 10:87–93, 1975.

760. Van Epps, E. F.: Agenesis of the corpus callosum with concomitant malformations, including atresia of the foramens of Luschka and Magendie. Amer. J. Roentgen., 70:47–60, 1953.

761. Van Hoytema, G. J., and van den Berg, R.: Embryological studies of the posterior fossa in connection with Arnold-Chiari malformation. Develop. Med. Child. Neurol. suppl., 11:61–76, 1966.

762. Van Nouhuys, J. M., and Buryn, G. W.: Nasopharyngeal transsphenoidal encephalocele, crater-like hole in the optic disc and agenesis of the corpus callosum. Pneumoencephalographic visualisation in a case. Psychiat. Neurol. Neurochir., 67:243–258, 1964.

763. Variend, S., and Emery, J. L.: The weight of the cerebellum in children with myelomeningocele. Develop. Med. Child Neurol., 15:suppl. 29:77–83, 1973.

764. Variend, S., and Emery, J. L.: The pathology of the central lobes of the cerebellum in children with myelomeningocele. Develop. Med. Child Neurol., 16:suppl. 32:99–106, 1974.

765. Veeneklaas, G. M. H.: Pathogenesis of intrathoracic gastrogenic cysts. Amer. J. Dis. Child., 83:500–507, 1952.

766. Venes, J. L.: Multiple cranial nerve palsies in an infant with Arnold-Chiari malformation. Develop. Med. Child Neurol., 16:817–820, 1974.

767. Venes, J. L.: The use of intravenous fluorescein in the repair of large myelomeningoceles. J. Neurosurg., 47:126–127, 1977.

768. Villarejo, F. J., Blazquez, M. G., and Gutierrez-Diaz, J. A.: Intraspinal lipomas in children. Child's Brain, 2:361–370, 1976.

769. Vogel, E. H.: Anterior sacral meningocele as a gynecologic problem. Report of a case. Obstet. Gynec., 36:766–768, 1970.

770. Von Recklinghausen, F.: Untersuchungen über die Spina bifida. Virchow. Arch. [Path. Anat.], 105:243–373, 1886.

771. Voris, H. C.: Spina bifida and cranium bifidum. J. Int. Coll. Surg., 11:634–639, 1948.

772. Vuia, O., and Pascu, F.: The Dandy-Walker syndrome associated with syringomyelia in a newborn infant. Confin. Neurol., 33:33–40, 1971.

773. Wald, N. J., Brock, D. J. H., and Bonnar, J.: Prenatal diagnosis of spina bifida and anencephaly by maternal serum-alpha-fetoprotein measurement. A controlled study. Lancet, 1:765–767, 1974.

774. Wald, N. J., Cuckle, H., Brock, J. H., et al.: Maternal serum-alpha-fetoprotein measurement in antenatal screening for anencephaly and spina bifida in early pregnancy. (Report of United Kingdom collaborative study on alpha-fetoprotein in relation to neural tube defects.) Lancet, 1:1323–1332, 1977.

775. Walker, A. A., and Moore, C. H.: Tumors of the spinal cord in children; report of a case of teratoid tumor. Amer. J. Dis. Child., 57:900–906, 1939.

776. Walker, A. E.: Dilatation of the vertebral canal associated with congenital anomalies of the spinal cord. Amer. J. Roentgen., 52:571–582, 1944.

777. Walker, A. E.: A case of congenital atresia of the foramina of Luschka and Magendie. J. Neuropath. Exp. Neurol., 3:368–373, 1944.

778. Walker, A. E., and Bucy, P. C.: Congenital dermal sinuses; a source of spinal meningeal infection and subdural abscesses. Brain, 57:401–421, 1934.

779. Walker, E., Moore, W. W., and Simpson, J. R.: Intranasal encephaloceles; survey of problem with recommendations for reducing mortality Arch. Otolaryng. (Chicago), 55:182–187, 1952.

780. Walker, R. M., and Dyke, S. C.: Abscess of the spinal cord. Lancet, 2:1413–1414, 1936.

781. Waring, J. I., and Pratt-Thomas, H. R.: Congenital dermal sinus as a source of meningeal infection. J. Pediat., 27:79–83, 1945.

782. Warkany, J.: Morphogenesis of spina bifida. In McLaurin, R. L., ed.: Myelomeningocele. New York, Grune & Stratton, Inc., 1977, pp. 31–39.

783. Watt, I., and Park, W. M.: The abdominal aorta in spina bifida cystica. Clin. Radiol., 29:63–68, 1978.

784. Wealthall, S. R., Whittaker, G. E., and Greenwood, N.: The relationship of apnoea and stridor in spina bifida to other unexplained infant deaths. Develop. Med. Child Neurol., 16:suppl. 32:107–116, 1974.

785. Weed, L. H.: The establishment of the circula-

tion of cerebrospinal fluid. Anat. Rec., *10*:256–258, 1916.

786. Weed, L. H.: The development of the cerebrospinal spaces in pig and in man. Contrib. Embryol. Carnegie Inst., *4*:1–116, 1917.

787. Weed, L. H.: Meninges and cerebrospinal fluid. J. Anat., *72*:181–215, 1938.

788. Weil, A., and Matthews, W. B.: Duplication of the spinal cord with spina bifida and syringomyelia. Arch. Path. (Chicago), *20*:882–890, 1935.

789. Weinstein, M. A., Rothner, A. D., Dushesneau, P., and Dohn, D. F.: Computed tomography in diastematomyelia. Radiology, *118*:609–611, 1975.

790. Werner, J. L., and Taybi, H.: Presacral masses in childhood. Amer. J. Roentgen., *109*:403–410, 1970.

791. Whatmore, W. J.: Sincipital encephalomeningoceles. Brit. J. Surg., *60*:261–270, 1973.

792. Wheeler, T.: Variability in the spinal column as regards defective neural arches. Contrib. Embryol., *9*:97–106, 1920.

793. Whitten, C. A., Jr., Moyar, J. B., and Wise, B. L.: Hydrocephalus syndrome: Obstruction of the foramina of the fourth ventricle. Amer. J. Dis. Child., *103*:55–60, 1962.

794. Wiese, G. M., Kempe, L. G., and Hammon, W. M.: Transsphenoidal meningohydroencephalocele. Case Report. J. Neurosurg., *37*:475–478, 1972.

795. Williams, D. I., and Nixon, H. H.: Agenesis of the sacrum. Surg. Gynec. Obstet., *105*:84–88, 1957.

796. Williams, R. F.: Colonization of the developing body by bacteria. *In* Davis, J. A., and Dobbing, J., eds.: Scientific Foundations of Paediatrics. London, William Heinemann Medical Books Ltd., 1974.

797. Willis, T. A.: An analysis of vertebral anomalies. Amer. J. Surg., *6*:163–168, 1929.

798. Wilson, D. S.: Value of preoperative electrodiagnosis in assessment of locomotor function of lower limbs in spina bifida cystica. Develop. Med. Child Neurol. suppl., *16*:111–112, 1963.

799. Wilson, E. S., Jr.: Neurenteric cyst of the mediastinum. Amer. J. Roentgen., *107*:641–646, 1969.

800. Winter, R. B., Haven, J. J., Moe, J. H., and Lagaard, S. M.: Diastematomyelia and congenital spine deformities. J. Bone Joint Surg., *56-A*:27–39, 1974.

801. Wise, B. L., and Foster, J. J.: Congenital spinal extradural cyst. Case report and review of the literature. J. Neurosurg., *12*:421–427, 1955.

802. Wolpert, S. M., Haller, J. S., and Rabe, E. F.: The value of angiography in the Dandy-Walker syndrome and posterior fossa extraaxial cysts. Amer. J. Roentgen., *109*:261–272, 1970.

803. Wolpert, S. M., Scott, R. M., and Carter, B. L.: Computed tomography in spinal dysraphism. Surg. Neurol., *8*:199–206, 1977.

804. Woltman, H. W.: Spina bifida: A review of 187 cases including three associated cases of myelodysplasia without demonstrable bony defect. Minn. Med., *4*:244–259, 1921.

805. Wright, R. L.: Congenital dermal sinuses. Progr. Neurol. Surg., *4*:175–192, 1971.

806. Yamada, S.: Personal communication, 1978.

807. Yamashita, J., Maloney, A. F. J., and Harris, P.: Intradural spinal bronchiogenic cyst. Case report. J. Neurosurg., *39*:240–245, 1973.

808. Yashon, D., and Beatty, R. A.: Tethering of the conus medullaris within the sacrum. J. Neurol. Neurosurg. Psychiat., *29*:244–250, 1966.

809. Young, J. R., and Feder, J. M.: Ectopic endometrial tissue occurring in connection with lipoma and spina bifida occulta. Southern Med. J., *32*:1044–1046, 1939.

810. Yu, H. C., and Deck, M. D. F.: The clivus deformity of the Arnold-Chiari malformation. Radiology, *101*:613–615, 1971.

811. Zachary, R. B.: Early neurosurgical approaches to spina bifida (an address to the American Academy of Cerebral Palsy, New York, December 11, 1964). Develop. Med. Child Neurol., *7*:492–496, 1965.

812. Zachary, R. B.: An appraisal of the surgery for meningocele. Clin. Neurosurg., *13*:313–323, 1965.

813. Zachary, R. B.: Recent advances in the management of myelomeningoceles. Progr. Pediat. Surg., *2*:155–169, 1971.

814. Ziter, F. M. H., and Bramwit, D. N.: Nasal encephaloceles and gliomas. Brit. J. Radiol., *43*:136–138, 1970.

815. Zook, E. G., Dzenitis, A. J., and Bennett, J. E.: Repair of large myelomeningoceles. Arch. Surg. (Chicago), *98*:41–43, 1969.

36

HYDROCEPHALUS IN CHILDREN

Hydrocephalus is a dilation of the ventricular system caused by an imbalance in production and absorption of cerebrospinal fluid. Usually the problem is due to impaired absorption of the fluid; in rare cases there may be an overproduction of fluid by a choroid plexus papilloma.

CEREBROSPINAL FLUID CIRCULATION

At 35 days' gestational age, the choroid plexus appears as a mesenchymal invagination of the roof of the fourth, lateral, and third ventricles in that order. At 50 days, normal cerebrospinal fluid circulation begins in conjunction with three important events: (1) perforation of the roof of the fourth ventricle by an active process of differentiation, (2) development of the secretory function of the choroid plexus, and (3) independent formation of the subarachnoid space.[6,23,34,35]

The major fraction of cerebrospinal fluid is formed in the cerebral ventricles at a rate of 0.35 to 0.4 ml per minute, or approximately 500 ml per day.[12] The choroid plexus probably contributes the major portion, although there is evidence that extrachoroidal sites are important.[5,10,26,31,38] The exact mechanism of cerebrospinal fluid formation is unknown, but active transport and serum dialysis are both involved.[54]

The ventricular pulsations are probably the most important mechanism by which the cerebrospinal fluid is propelled along its pathways. This ventricular pulse wave results mostly from cerebral arterial pulse transmission and respiratory variations and less from choroid plexus pulsations.[4,14] The outpouring of newly formed fluid, postural effects, and the ciliary action of the ependymal epithelium are influencing factors of lesser importance.

Most of the cerebrospinal fluid passes out of each lateral ventricle via the foramen of Monro to the third ventricle, and on through the aqueduct of Sylvius, the fourth ventricle, and then into the subarachnoid space through one of three exits. By way of the paired lateral openings of the fourth ventricle, the foramina of Luschka, the fluid flows around the brain stem into the cerebellopontine and prepontine cisterns. This fluid proceeds cephalad by way of two routes: (1) ventrally into the interpeduncular and prechiasmatic cisterns and then to the subarachnoid space over the lateral and frontal areas of the cerebral hemispheres by way of the sylvian fissures and callosal cistern, and (2) dorsomedially up over the medial and posterior areas of the cerebral hemispheres by way of the ambient and quadrigeminal cisterns. The cerebrospinal fluid exiting the fourth ventricle through the midline foramen of Magendi flows through the vallecula into the cisterna magna. From the cisterna magna it passes superiorly over the cerebellar hemispheres, inferiorly into the spinal subarachnoid space, or ventrally into the basilar cisterns to follow the cephalad route.[13,53]

Most absorption of cerebrospinal fluid occurs at the site of the arachnoid villi. The exact mechanism by which it takes place is not known, but hydrostatic pressure differences between cerebrospinal fluid and venous sinuses are important.[55] The capacity for absorption is two to four times as great as the normal rate of cerebrospinal fluid production.[8,11]

M. S. O'BRIEN

PATHOGENESIS OF HYDROCEPHALUS

Any lesion that isolates the major source of cerebrospinal fluid production from the major absorptive site will lead to an excessive volume of fluid. The excess volume of fluid results in progressive dilatation of the ventricular system, recognized clinically as hydrocephalus (Fig. 36–1).[33] Obstruction of the cerebrospinal fluid pathway is the only proved cause of hydrocephalus. There is no firm evidence that hydrocephalus is caused by oversecretion of cerebrospinal fluid, even in the case of oversecretion secondary to choroid plexus papilloma.[37] Nor is there any proof that dural sinus thrombosis causes hydrocephalus by impairing venous absorption.[22]

Hydrocephalus has been variously classified as obstructive or nonobstructive, congenital or acquired, and communicating or noncommunicating.[9,47] These terms have led to some redundancy and confusion. For example, the term "obstructive hydrocephalus" is used by some clinicians to signify noncommunicating hydrocephalus. Actually, the word "noncommunicating" implies only that the ventricles do not communicate with the lumbar subarachnoid space—an observation derived from the old diagnostic study of injecting a dye into the lateral ventricle and subsequently performing a lumbar puncture.

Since all causes of hydrocephalus are obstructive either within the ventricular system or within the subarachnoid space, the terms "obstructive" and "nonobstructive" should be discarded. A much less confusing classification is based on the location of the cerebrospinal fluid pathway block and its pathogenesis in relation to birth. For example, "ventricular obstruction" is substituted for "noncommunicating hydrocephalus" and "subarachnoid obstruction" for "communicating hydrocephalus." The etiological classification would be "prena-

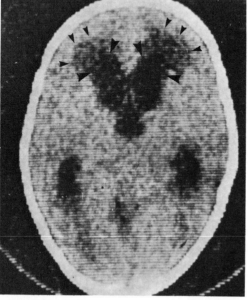

Figure 36–1 Computed tomographic scan demonstrating acute ventricular dilatation (*large arrows*) and paraventricular edema (*small arrows*).

TABLE 36–1 COMMON CAUSES OF HYDROCEPHALUS BY LOCATION OF OBSTRUCTION*

SITE OF BLOCK	CAUSE
Lateral ventricle	Perinatal subependymal and intraventricular hemorrhage
	Intra- or extraventricular tumor (glioma, papilloma)
	Ventriculitis
Foramen of Monro	Ventriculitis
	Glioma of septum, tuberous sclerosis
	Colloid cyst
	Extension of third ventricle or suprasellar masses
Third ventricle	Colloid cyst
	Glioma of optic pathway, hypothalamus, or thalamus
	Suprasellar craniopharyngioma, arachnoid cyst
	Pineal tumor
Aqueduct of Sylvius	Arteriovenous malformation of the galenic system
	Developmental stenosis (gliosis, forking, X-linked)
	Infectious ependymitis (pyogenic, viral)
	Mesencephalic tumor or arteriovenous malformation
	Cerebellar tumor (medulloblastoma, astrocytoma)
Fourth ventricle	Intraventricular tumor (ependymoma, papilloma, dermal cyst)
Fourth ventricular outlets	Cerebellar tumor
	Dandy-Walker malformation
	Arachnoid cyst
	Meningitis (pyogenic, tuberculous)
	Arnold-Chiari malformation
Subarachnoid spaces	Meningitis (pyogenic, tuberculous)
	Subarachnoid hemorrhage (traumatic, spontaneous [arteriovenous malformation, aneurysm], anoxic [prematurity])
	Subdural hematoma

* Modified from Lemire, R. J., Loeser, J. D., Leech, R. W., and Alvord, E. C.: Normal and Abnormal Development of the Human Nervous System. New York, Harper & Row, 1975, p. 100.

tal'' or ''congenital'' and ''postnatal'' or ''acquired.''

ETIOLOGY

The cause of hydrocephalus presenting during the neonatal to late-infancy period (0 to 2 years) is usually a major developmental abnormality. Aqueductal stenosis is the most common of the developmental causes. Intrauterine infection, anoxic or traumatic perinatal hemorrhage, and neonatal bacterial or viral meningoencephalitis are other causes of hydrocephalus presenting in this age group. The remainder are various obstructive masses such as tumors, arachnoid cysts, or arteriovenous malformations of the galenic system.

The most common causes of hydrocephalus in early to late childhood (2 to 10 years) are posterior fossa tumors and aqueductal stenosis.

The common causes of hydrocephalus in relation to the site of obstruction are listed in Table 36–1.

CLINICAL FEATURES OF HYDROCEPHALUS

The clinical features of hydrocephalus are those of increased intracranial pressure. The major factors influencing these features are the time of onset in relation to closure of the cranial sutures and the nature of the obstruction.

Neonatal Period Through Late Infancy (0 to 2 Years)

Prior to 2 years of age, the head enlarges excessively because the cranial sutures are open. This enlargement will almost invariably be the presenting sign and modifies the increased pressure features by its decompressing effect.

An abnormal head shape may suggest the diagnosis. Occipital prominence is seen in the Dandy-Walker malformation; biparietal enlargement may occur with bilateral subdural hematoma; a disproportionately large forehead is common with hydrocephalus caused by aqueductal stenosis. The disproportion of cranial size to facial size may be quite evident.

The anterior fontanel is usually enlarged and full even when the infant is upright and quiet. Normally the anterior fontanel is depressed in a relaxed sitting infant. A soft flat anterior fontanel, however, does not exclude hydrocephalus because of the decompressing effect of open sutures. Palpation of spread sutures may be more helpful in this instance. The percussion note of the infant's skull, normally that of a ''cracked pot,'' comes to resemble that of a ripe watermelon when hydrocephalus is present. This sound is particularly striking when the examiner places his ear against the infant's skull as he percusses.

Auscultation of the head may reveal the presence of a cranial bruit. It is of limited diagnostic importance. Bruits are not uncommon in children with or without increased intracranial pressure and do not necessarily indicate a vascular lesion.[40]

The scalp veins are usually prominent, particularly in a crying infant. The prominence is caused by compression of the basal venous outlets by the increased pressure, which results in shunting of blood through the valveless collateral system into the easily distended scalp veins (Fig. 36–2).

As hydrocephalus progresses, the eyes are displaced downward by pressure on the thinned orbital roofs. The displacement of the eyes causes the sclera to be visible above the iris, the ''setting sun'' sign (Fig. 36–3).

Frequently, cranial nerve abnormalities are found. Optic atrophy is a common finding in advanced hydrocephalus. The atrophy is due to compression of the chiasm and optic nerves by a dilated anterior third ventricle as well as by diffuse increased intracranial pressure. Except in the case of chronic subdural hematoma, papilledema and retinal hemorrhages are rare in the presence of open sutures. Sixth nerve paresis secondary to stretching is common. Random eye movements and nystagmus may be present. Divergent strabismus and impairment of upward gaze (Parinaud's syndrome), a consequence of compression of the mesencephalic tectum by the dilated suprapineal recess of the third ventricle, may be noted.[49] The pulsatile pressure of a dilated third ventricle on the optic chiasm can result in impairment of vision and pupillary reaction. Vision can also be impaired by damage to the occipital cortex by grossly dilated occipital horns. Dysfunction

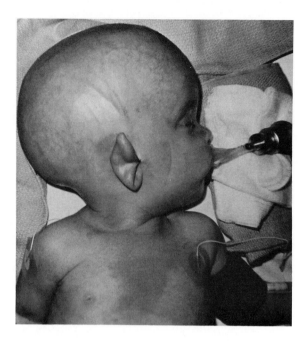

Figure 36–2   Infant with aqueductal stenosis. The cranial vault is greatly enlarged and there is obvious craniofacial disproportion. The anterior fontanel is bulging and the scalp veins prominently distended.

of the lower brain stem secondary to bilateral corticobulbar disruption can be manifested by difficulty in sucking and feeding, which frequently results in vomiting and aspiration. Laryngeal stridor related to vagus nerve traction is not uncommon in patients with the Arnold-Chiari malformation, particularly when it is exacerbated by progressive hydrocephalus.[2] Corticobulbar deficits may account for the characteristic high-pitched cry of the hydrocephalic infant.

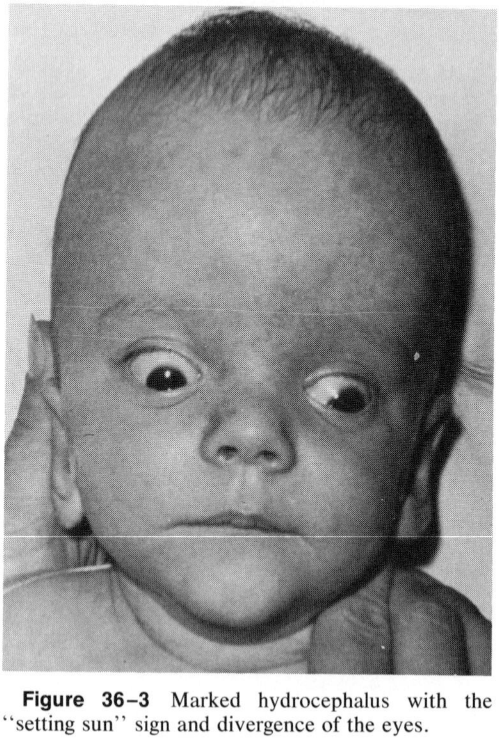

As hydrocephalus progresses, the deep tendon reflexes and tone in the lower extremities are increased. These changes result from disproportionately greater stretching and myelin disruption of the paracentral corticospinal fibers arising from the leg area of the motor cortex by the dilated lateral ventricles.[46,57] Growth failure and delayed neurological development are common. Head and trunk control is particularly affected.

In the later stages of chronic hydrocephalus or with the more rapidly progressive type secondary to bacterial meningitis, there will be increasing irritability, vomiting, lethargy, and seizures. In untreated cases, death usually results from respiratory failure secondary to brain stem compression by transtentorial herniation of the temporal lobes. Transforaminal herniation of the cerebellar tonsils occurs less commonly.

In summary, the clinical features of hydrocephalus in the infant depend largely upon how effectively the expanding head decompresses the intracranial pressure. With slow advancement there may be no other symptoms or signs in an infant with

Figure 36–3   Marked hydrocephalus with the "setting sun" sign and divergence of the eyes.

excessive head growth. On the other hand, when the skull cannot expand rapidly enough, the signs and symptoms of progressively increasing pressure and ventricular dilatation will become manifest.

Early to Late Childhood (2 to 10 Years)

During early to late childhood (2 to 10 years) the patients fall into two groups, differentiated by the presenting clinical features. The first group are those children who have pre-existing (infantile) but unrecognized progressive hydrocephalus that may or may not be marginally compensated. Their neurological development may be normal, borderline, or retarded. Their heads may be only mildly or severely enlarged. Occasionally they carry the misdiagnosis of "arrested hydrocephalus."[48] For some, an incidental head injury may lead to a skull x-ray that reveals spread sutures and demineralization of the dorsum sellae. These patients may have rapid deterioration of neurological function following the head injury. For others, the hydrocephalus may lead to rapid decompensation due to chronically increased intracranial pressure. The decompensation may occur spontaneously or may be associated with a mild illness such as a viral respiratory tract infection. Examination will reveal a head circumference at or above the upper limits of normal. Optic atrophy or papilledema may be present.

Additional features seen in this group include endocrine changes resulting in small stature, obesity, gigantism, delayed or precocious puberty, primary amenorrhea or menstrual irregularities, and diabetes insipidus.[24] The hormonal changes probably are secondary to abnormal hypothalamic function as a consequence of increased intracranial pressure and dilatation of the third ventricle. Spasticity in the lower extremities is not uncommon, and both upper limbs may exhibit mild pyramidal tract signs manifest in fine motor incoordination. Perceptual motor deficits and visual spatial disorganization can result, probably as a consequence of stretched corticospinal fibers of the parietal and occipital cortex. Performance IQ is considerably worse than verbal IQ, and learning problems are common.[39] These children can be quite engaging socially, with bright conversation and relatively good memory. They often, however, are also hyperkinetic, emotionally labile, and unable to conceptualize. As they approach late childhood it may become apparent that they are less competitive than their peers.[19] Occasionally they may lead normal lives until adulthood before symptoms and signs of increased intracranial pressure become manifest. It is not uncommon for hydrocephalus secondary to aqueductal stenosis or the Dandy-Walker malformation to present in this fashion.

When the ventricular system of a patient in this first group is examined, it is usually markedly dilated in contradistinction to that of the child in the next group.

The second group consists of children who develop hydrocephalus after the cranial sutures are closed. In these children neurological symptoms due to increased intracranial pressure or focal deficits referrable to the primary lesion tend to appear prior to any significant change in the head growth pattern. Occult progressive hydrocephalus can be insidious, existing for a long time before head enlargement or decompensation takes place.

When hydrocephalus develops after closure of the sutures, the head circumference usually is within normal limits. The percussion note of the skull may suggest a "cracked pot" (Macewen's sign), indicating split sutures. Papilledema frequently is present. Sixth nerve paresis is a common finding. Knee and ankle jerks may be hyperactive. The child may show regression in motor skills. Morning headaches and vomiting are common. Thus, the clinical features resemble those of any lesion producing increased intracranial pressure. As in the first group, head injury, viral infection, or other factors may cause deterioration in neurological function.

DIAGNOSIS

Differential Diagnosis

The differential diagnosis of excessive head growth with relation to age of presentation is given in Table 36–2.

**TABLE 36–2   DIFFERENTIAL DIAGNOSIS OF EXCESSIVE HEAD
ENLARGEMENT BY AGE OF PRESENTATION**

BIRTH TO SIX MONTHS
Hydrocephalus
  Developmental disorders
    Myelomeningocele, encephalocele, Arnold-Chiari malformation, aqueductal stenosis
  Mass lesions
    Neoplasm, arteriovenous malformation, arachnoid cyst
  Intrauterine infections:
    Bacterial, granulomatous, parasitic
  Perinatal or postnatal hemorrhage
    Anoxia, vascular malformation, trauma
Hydranencephaly
Subdural effusion
  Hemorrhagic, infectious
Normal variant (often familial)

SIX MONTHS TO TWO YEARS
Hydrocephalus
  Mass lesions
    Tumor, cyst, abscess
  Bacterial or granulomatous meningitis
  Developmental disorders
    Dandy-Walker malformation, Arnold-Chiari malformation
  Posthemorrhagic
    Trauma, vascular malformation
Subdural effusion
Increased intracranial pressure syndrome
  Pseudotumor cerebri
    Lead, tetracycline, hypoparathyroidism, steroids, excess or deficiency of vitamin A, cyanotic congenital heart
      disease, anemia
Primary skeletal cranial dysplasias (thickened or enlarged skull)
  Osteogenesis imperfecta, hyperphosphatemia, osteopetrosis, rickets
Megalencephaly (increase in brain substance)
  Metabolic central nervous system disease
    Leukodystrophies (e.g., Canavan's, Alexander's), lipidoses (Tay-Sachs), histiocytosis, mucopolysaccharidoses
  Proliferative neurocutaneous syndromes
    Von Recklinghausen's, tuberous sclerosis, hemangiomatosis
  Cerebral gigantism
    Sotos' syndrome
  Achondroplasia
  Primary megalencephaly
    May be familial and associated or unassociated with abnormalities of cellular architecture

AFTER TWO YEARS
Hydrocephalus
  Mass lesions
  Developmental disorders
    Aqueductal stenosis, Arnold-Chiari malformation
  Postinfectious
  Posthemorrhagic
Megalencephaly
  Proliferative neurocutaneous syndromes
  Familial
Pseudotumor cerebri
Normal variant

Modified from Menkes, J. H.: Textbook of Child Neurology. Philadelphia, Lea & Febiger, 1974, p. 154.

Diagnostic Procedures

Head Circumference

The head size should be measured in a standardized fashion by taking the maximal obtainable circumference with a steel metric tape. Using the maximal circumference on each examination will facilitate accurate comparison of serial measurements, and the metric system is most accurate in denoting small changes. The circumference must be plotted against age on a head growth chart.[42] This procedure is of greatest importance in demonstrating, by serial measurements, an excessive rate of head growth (Fig. 36–4). Serial measurements will demonstrate mild but progressive hydrocephalus in an infant whose head is grossly normal to visual inspection (Fig. 36–5). The growth chart showing continued abnormal head enlargement in an older child thought to have arrested hydrocephalus will prove this

diagnosis to be in error. Progressive hydrocephalus beginning before closure of the cranial sutures will prevent fusion of the sutures and allow continued excessive head enlargement in the older child (Fig. 36–6). On the other hand, a normal head growth curve does not preclude progressive ventricular dilatation in the older child. This fact is of particular importance in following children in whom hydrocephalus is possibly arrested, regardless of whether or not they have had shunts implanted (Fig. 36–7).

Transillumination

If the cortical mantle is thinner than 1 cm, transillumination of the head will be abnormal, measuring more than 1 to 2 cm at the rim of the light source in hydrocephalus. It is also abnormal in prematurity, hydranencephaly, subdural effusion, porencephalic cyst, Dandy-Walker malformation, scalp edema, subgaleal fluid accumulation, and even with normal subarachnoid path-

Text continued on page 1392

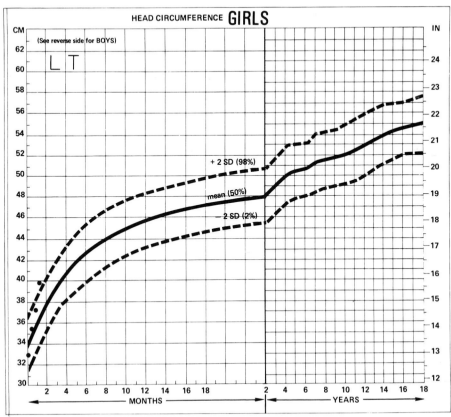

Figure 36–4 Serial measurements demonstrating excessive rate of head growth in a neonate. Note dots at left of graph, denoting head growth from birth to 4 weeks of age.

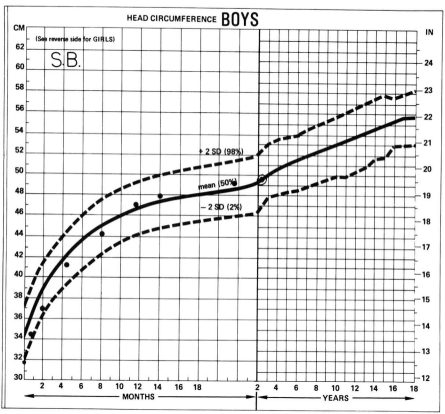

Figure 36–5 Serial measurements demonstrating progressive excessive rate of head growth beginning at age 2 months and terminating at age 12 months following insertion of ventricular shunt.

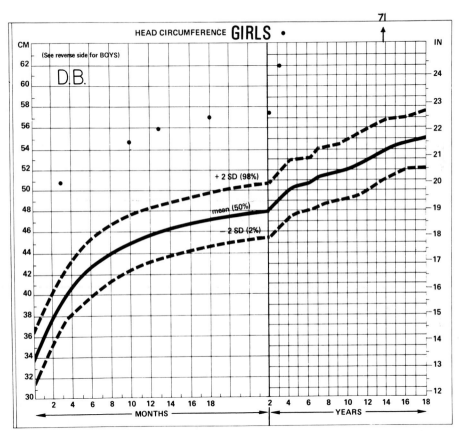

Figure 36–6   Head growth chart of a 14-year-old child whose hydrocephalus was misdiagnosed as "arrested." Note continuation of excessive head expansion throughout childhood, characteristic of progressive hydrocephalus beginning in infancy.

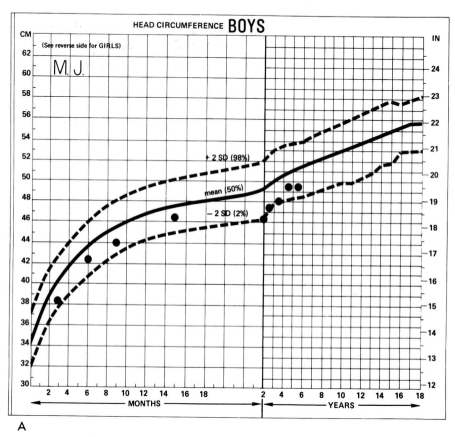

A

Figure 36–7 Child with a ventriculoatrial shunt placed during infancy. Hydrocephalus was misdiagnosed as "arrested" at age 2 years after the child had outgrown the cardiac catheter. At age 4½ years he had rapid alteration of consciousness following a two-week history of headaches and vomiting. *A*. Head size was never excessive.

Illustration continued on opposite page

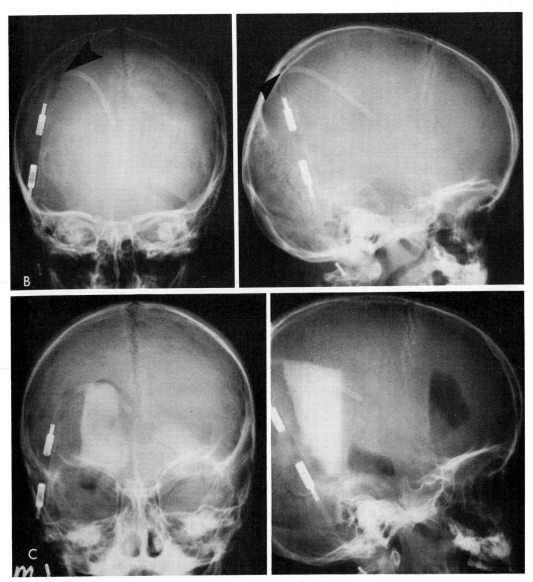

Figure 36-7 (continued) B. Plain x-rays of the skull demonstrate poor placement of the ventricular catheter. The burr hole was placed too high (arrow), and the catheter is directed into the choroid plexus in the body of the lateral ventricle. C. Lack of reservoir necessitated ventricular tap through coronal suture. Opening pressure was 600 ml of water. Air and Conray ventriculograms demonstrate moderate ventricular enlargement.

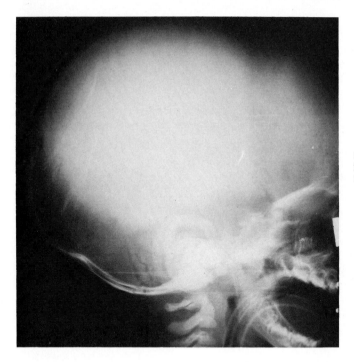

Figure 36–8 Plain skull x-ray showing an enlarged head with craniofacial disproportion and spreading of the coronal and lambdoid sutures.

ways.[27] Thus, while transillumination may suggest a diagnosis, it is not a definitive procedure and further studies are indicated for an accurate diagnosis.

Plain Skull X-Rays

Plain skull x-rays will confirm many of the clinical findings, such as an enlarged head, craniofacial disproportion, spread sutures, and a large anterior fontanel (Fig. 36–8). In addition, they may show the small posterior fossa and the low position of the lambdoid sutures characteristic of aqueductal stenosis, and the prominence of the posterior fossa seen with the Dandy-Walker malformation. In the older child, elongated interdigitations of the suture lines may indicate chronic increased intracranial pressure. Because of the decompressing effect of open sutures, demineralization of the dorsum sellae is usually not present in infants with increased intracranial pressure. Changes in the sella can occur, however, owing to the pulsation of a dilated anterior third ventricle.

Intracranial calcifications may give an indication of the location of the obstruction and its cause. Suprasellar calcifications occur with craniopharyngiomas (Fig. 36–9). In older children, a curvilinear or circular band of calcium can be seen in the wall of a vein of Galen dilated by an arteriovenous malformation of this system. Periventricular calcification suggests cytomegalic inclusion disease, toxoplasmosis, or tuberous sclerosis. In older children there may be evidence of increased convolutional markings (beaten silver skull) and demineralization of the dorsum sellae (Fig. 36–10).

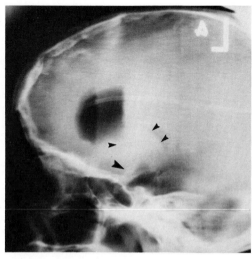

Figure 36–9 Suprasellar calcification (*large arrow*) in a craniopharyngioma obstructing the foramen of Monro and anterior third ventricle (*small arrows*).

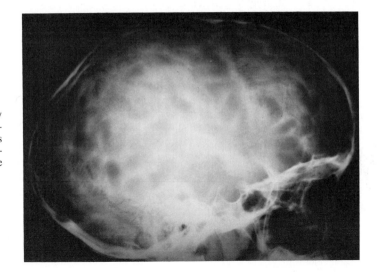

Figure 36–10   Plain skull x-ray of an 8-year-old boy showing increased convolutional markings (beaten silver skull) and demineralization of the dorsum sellae (same case as shown in Figure 36–18).

Electroencephalography

There is no indication for electroencephalography in the evaluation of hydrocephalus except when there is a concomitant seizure disorder.

Radioisotope Brain Scan

The radioisotope brain scan's usefulness in diagnosing subdural hematomas and brain tumors has been all but eclipsed by the computed tomographic scan. It is of essentially no value in the assessment of congenital hydrocephalus. Isotope cisternography has been helpful in tracing cerebrospinal fluid flow patterns, but its usefulness in diagnosis is questionable (Fig. 36–11).

Echoencephalography

With well-trained personnel, sonographic scanning has been fairly accurate in estimating the size of the lateral and third ventricles. This, however, is not a definitive study and has also given way to computed tomography.

Computed Tomography

Computed tomographic scanning has significantly altered the diagnostic approach to the infant or child suspected of having hydrocephalus. The reasons for this are that the scan can demonstrate with a high de-

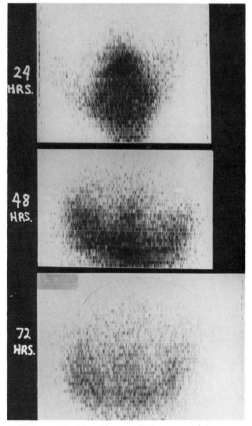

Figure 36–11   Abnormal isotope cisternogram showing persistence of the isotope in the basal cisterns at 72 hours. Child had shunt-independent arrested hydrocephalus documented by a nonfunctioning shunt, an asymptomatic clinical picture, and persistently normal ventricular size on serial CT scans.

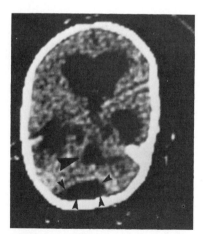

Figure 36–12 Computed tomographic scan demonstrating communicating hydrocephalus. Not only the lateral ventricles but also the fourth ventricle (*large arrow*) and cisterna magna (*small arrows*) are enlarged, indicating a subarachnoid obstruction.

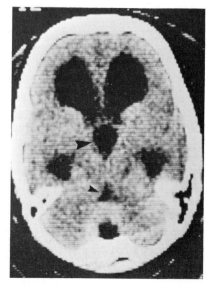

Figure 36–13 Computed tomographic scan demonstrating obstruction at the aqueduct of Sylvius, an enlarged third ventricle (*large arrow*), and a small fourth ventricle (*small arrow*). A small tumor or arteriovenous malformation in the region of the aqueduct can be excluded by the lack of contrast enhancement.

gree of accuracy the size of the ventricular system, the extracerebral spaces, and the site of obstruction; and it has decreased the need for more invasive procedures such as angiography and pneumoencephalography.[41] It is the procedure of choice following physical examination and plain x-rays of the skull. Subarachnoid obstruction (communicating hydrocephalus) can be diagnosed in most instances (Fig. 36–12). When contrast enhancement demonstrates no abnormality, aqueductal stenosis is inferred from the presence of enlarged lateral

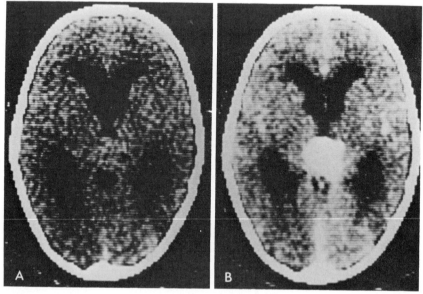

Figure 36–14 *A.* Computed tomographic scan without contrast enhancement shows only ventricular enlargement. *B.* With contrast enhancement, a posterior third ventricle tumor is demonstrated.

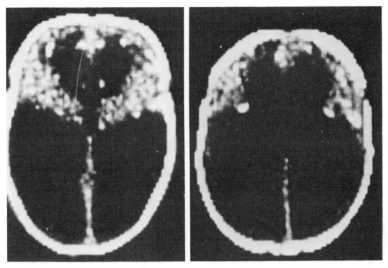

Figure 36–15 Computed tomographic scan showing periventricular calcifications secondary to intrauterine infection by the cytomegalic inclusion virus that has resulted in severe hydrocephalus.

and third ventricles and a normal fourth ventricle (Fig. 36–13). Midline and posterior fossa tumors obstructing the cerebrospinal fluid pathway can easily be identified, provided contrast enhancement is used (Fig. 36–14).[3] Another entity that requires contrast enhancement is the chronic subdural hematoma. The hematoma can easily be missed by computed tomography unless contrast enhancement is used to identify the subdural membrane because the absorption coefficient of the subdural fluid can be the same as that of the brain.

Acute epidural, subdural, intraventricular, and intracerebral hematomas are identified without contrast. Intracranial calcifications, including those too small to be seen on plain x-rays, are easily visualized (Fig. 36–15). Hydranencephaly can usually be distinguished from severe hydrocephalus by the prominence of the basal ganglia and the absence of a cerebral mantle except in the occipital region (Fig. 36–16).

The decision for further diagnostic procedures or operation and the use of computed tomography in the overall management of

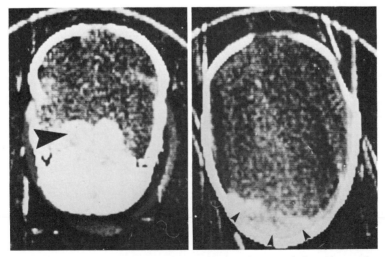

Figure 36–16 Computed tomographic scan demonstrating hydranencephaly with prominent basal ganglia (*large arrow*) and lack of cortical mantle except in the occipital region (*small arrows*).

infants and children with hydrocephalus are discussed subsequently.

Angiography

If computed tomography is not available, cerebral angiography is the procedure of choice for evaluating infants with excessive head growth and older children with signs of increased intracranial pressure. Technical refinements in angiographic procedures, particularly the perfection of the transfemoral catheter method, are currently such that cerebral angiography can be performed in any infant or child regardless of age.[45] Cerebral angiography not only will show the size of the ventricular system but in most cases will determine the level of the cerebrospinal fluid pathway obstruction and its cause. It is of particular importance in defining intracranial mass lesions. Angiography is quite definitive in the diagnosis of vascular tumor, aneurysm, arteriovenous malformation, and subdural hematoma or effusion. Another advantage of the angiogram is that it avoids disturbing cerebrospinal fluid dynamics and possible subsequent decompensation. The angiographic features of hydrocephalus depend, of course, on the degree of ventricular enlargement. As the lateral ventricles increase in size, the lateral arterial phase will show anterior stretching and bowing of the anterior cerebral group of vessels by the frontal horns and elevation of the middle

cerebral group by the temporal horns (Fig. 36–17). In the venous phase the lateral view will show the size of the lateral ventricle by the end points of the terminal branches of the septal and thalamostriate veins. The frontal projection in the arterial phase will demonstrate lateral displacement of the lenticulostriate and middle cerebral arteries, and on the frontal projection in the venous phase, the thalmostriate vein will be rounded and more laterally displaced (Fig. 36–18). It should be noted that with markedly increased pressure, minimal evidence of ventricular enlargement does not preclude mild ventricular dilatation. This situation frequently is seen in the older child with obstruction due to a posterior fossa neoplasm.

Ventriculography

Ventriculography as the initial neuroradiological procedure in evaluating infants with excessive head growth or older children with signs of increased intracranial pressure has been largely replaced by computed tomography and cerebral angiography. Air or water-soluble positive contrast ventriculography is quite accurate in establishing the size of the ventricles and the site of ventricular obstruction (Fig. 36–19). It is not useful in determining the site of a subarachnoid obstruction. It must be pointed out that failure to visualize the recesses of the anterior or posterior third ventricle, the

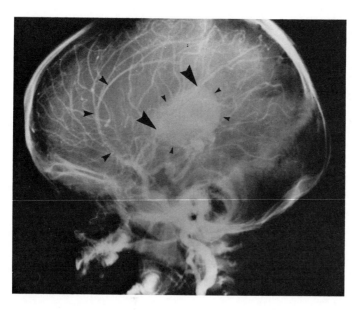

Figure 36–17   Lateral carotid angiogram diagnosing hydrocephalus caused by an arteriovenous malformation of the galenic system. Note dilatation of the lateral ventricle shown by the marked stretching of the pericallosal artery (*medium arrows*). Enlargement of the temporal horn is shown by the elevation of the middle cerebral group (*large arrows*). The arteriovenous malformation, demonstrated by the supplying posterior cerebral arteries and by the enlargement of the vein of Galen, is producing posterior third ventricle and aqueductal obstruction (*small arrows*).

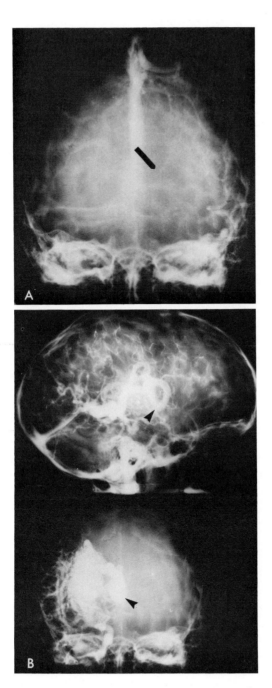

Figure 36–18 *A.* Left anterior venous phase of the angiogram demonstrates lateral displacement and rounding of the thalamostriate vein (*arrow*) by an enlarged lateral ventricle. *B.* Ventricular enlargement was caused by obstruction at the foramen of Monro by an enlarged right thalamostriate vein (*arrows*) draining a deep arteriovenous malformation (same case as shown in Figure 36–10).

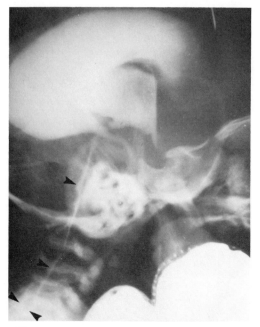

Figure 36–19 Lateral brow-up ventriculogram with water-soluble positive contrast (meglumine iothalamate 60 per cent) demonstrating marked enlargement of the lateral and third ventricle and the Arnold-Chiari type II malformation. Fourth ventricle is elongated with its outlets in the lower cervical canal (*arrows*).

aqueduct of Sylvius, or the fourth ventricle renders the study inadequate, and it must be followed by angiography or pneumoencephalography for an accurate diagnosis.

Complications include disturbance of cerebrospinal fluid dynamics and the development of needle porencephaly (Fig. 36–20).[56]

Ventriculography with Water-Soluble Positive Contrast Agents

Seizures secondary to chemical irritation of the cortex by the water-soluble positive contrast medium can be eliminated by adhering to the following technique: (1) Use a nonrigid needle or catheter for the ventricular tap, thereby preventing enlargement of the needle tract by the movement of a rigid needle, or place the contrast agent through the shunt reservoir. These precautions prevent leakage of the medium back up the needle tract to the cortex (Fig. 36–21). (2) Inject no more than a 2-ml bolus of the contrast agent and do not increase the volume by dilution. (3) Repeat only once, using a total of no more than 4 ml. (4) Use a low-toxicity contrast agent such as meglumine iothalamate 60 per cent (Conray). With this technique there were no complications in 354 consecutive procedures in the author's clinic.

To allow the bolus of contrast to fall into the medial aspect of the frontal horn, the patient's head should be flexed forward and tilted away from the side of injection. Next, the head should be slowly extended but kept tilted until it is finally placed in the straight supine position. This maneuver

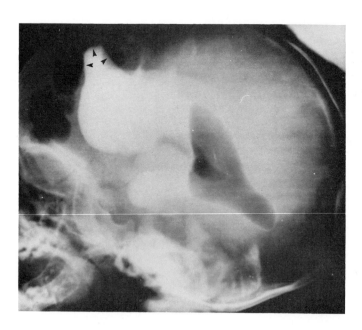

Figure 36–20 Needle porencephaly (*arrows*) produced by percutaneous transcoronal ventricular tap with a rigid needle. Movement of the extracranial portion of the needle causes enlargement of the intracerebral needle tract by the fulcrum effect of the dura (see Fig. 36–21).

causes the bolus of contrast that is medially placed in the frontal horn to flow through the foramen of Monro into the third ventricle, aqueduct of Sylvius, and fourth ventricle. Brow-up lateral, anteroposterior, and Townes views are obtained without further positioning (see Fig. 36–19). The procedure is easily performed in the operating room with a portable x-ray machine. Its advantages are the rapid and complete visualization of the axial ventricular system and minimal movement of the patient.

Pneumoencephalography

Until there is further refinement of computed tomography, pneumoencephalography still provides the most accurate information regarding the subarachnoid space and basal cisterns. It is particularly useful in evaluating suprasellar masses. In combination with positive contrast ventriculography it can definitively delineate aqueductal stenosis (Fig. 36–22). There is a risk in performing this procedure in patients with increased intracranial pressure, and its use has been significantly reduced by computed tomography and cerebral angiography in the initial neuroradiological evaluation of an infant with excessive head growth or the

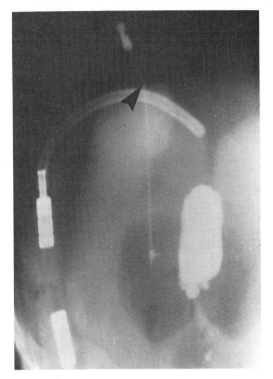

Figure 36–21 Anterior view of percutaneous transcoronal ventricular tap with a flexible needle. Angulation of the nonrigid needle at dural level (*arrow*) is not carried through intracerebrally, preventing enlargement of the needle tract in the brain.

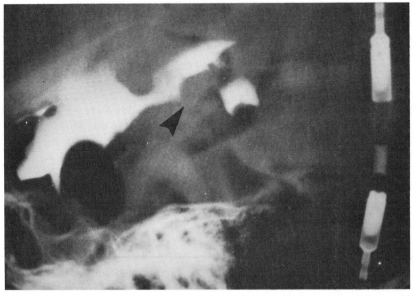

Figure 36–22 Combined pneumoencephalogram and ventriculogram with water-soluble positive contrast agent demonstrating aqueductal stenosis (*arrow*).

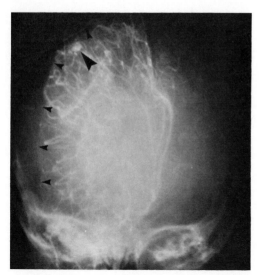

Figure 36–23 A 6-month-old infant with meningitis deteriorated following percutaneous transcoronal subdural tap. Anterior carotid angiogram demonstrates massive subdural hematoma (*small arrows*) secondary to laceration of a cortical artery (*large arrow*) by the subdural needle.

older child with increased intracranial pressure.

Percutaneous Intracranial Tap

As a therapeutic procedure for rapid reduction of the intracranial pressure secondary to hydrocephalus or chronic subdural hematoma, the percutaneous subdural or ventricular tap can be lifesaving in an infant with an open anterior fontanel or an older child with spread coronal sutures.

Ideally, percutaneous subdural and ventricular taps should not be used in the initial diagnostic evaluation of the infant with excessive head enlargement. If available, computed tomography should be performed to assess the status of the intracranial contents. If it is not available, an angiogram will be necessary. It should be noted that, otherwise, these taps are blind procedures and carry the risk of infection and laceration of the vascular structures and cerebral tissue. Further, it is easy to give them a false interpretation, particularly when the physician performing the tap has not had training in neurological surgery (Fig. 36–23).[51]

TREATMENT

Initial Management

If the growth curve of the infant or child's head indicates the possibility of hydrocephalus and the history and physical examination suggest increased intracranial pressure or the possibility of occult progressive hydrocephalus, plain x-rays of the skull and a CT scan should be performed.

In infants and young children, computed tomography is done under general anesthesia. No sedation is necessary in older children who can cooperate. Neuroradiological procedures performed under heavy sedation in the infant or young child with increased intracranial pressure are dangerous, particularly in the absence of monitoring of the vital signs and airway by an anesthesia team.[1] While lighter sedation will allow the infant or young child to sleep through an unenhanced scan, the necessity for intravenous injection of the contrast agent for an enhanced scan will preclude any further cooperation on the part of the patient. General anesthesia avoids both this problem and oversedation, and in addition, maintains constant monitoring by highly competent personnel.

Occasionally the patient will present in a decompensated state requiring immediate reduction of increased intracranial pressure by hyperosmotic diuresis or a subdural or ventricular tap prior to any definitive evaluation. As soon as such a patient's condition is stabilized, computed tomography is performed to determine the size and extent of the subdural hematoma or the configuration of the ventricular system and the cause of its obstruction in the case of hydrocephalus.

How long an excessive growth curve should be watched prior to treatment depends upon its rate of increase, the clinical condition of the patient, the nature of the obstruction, and the size of the ventricles on the initial CT scan. Hydrocephalus secondary to subarachnoid obstruction from perinatal or postnatal trauma or a ruptured vascular anomaly may undergo arrest spontaneously.[50]

An infant with mild ventricular enlargement, a depressed anterior fontanel, and no rapid excessive head enlargement is examined at first daily and then weekly. If there are no signs or symptoms of increased pressure, if the anterior fontanel remains depressed, and if the head circumference follows a normal brain growth curve, computed tomography is repeated in one month. The scan must be repeated under these circumstances because progressive ventricular enlargement can continue in the absence of signs and symptoms of pressure, and with a depressed anterior fontanel and a normal brain growth curve. If the repeat scan shows no change in the minimal enlargement on the original scan, the infant may then be followed at two-week intervals until age 2 months. At 2 to 3 months of age, a third CT scan is performed. If again there is no change, the infant is followed at monthly intervals until six months, when a fourth CT scan is performed. If again there is no further enlargement, the chance of future progressive ventricular dilatation is slight. An infant with this history should be seen at three-month intervals until he is 12 months of age. If his neurological development and his brain growth curve have remained normal, computed tomography is repeated at 12 months. He should then be followed at six-month intervals and another scan should be obtained at about 2 years of age. If his neurological development and brain growth curve remain normal and his CT scan is unchanged, he may be discharged from further neurosurgical follow-up. It should be noted that follow-up scans for ventricular size can be limited to a single rotational plane, thereby significantly reducing the time, cost, and radiation dose.

Unless an adequate initial evaluation of ventricular size is made and the case is followed up closely, progressive hydrocephalus may continue for many years before the situation becomes obvious or neurological decompensation occurs. The diagnosis of spontaneously arrested hydrocephalus should not be made in the presence of delayed neurological development, continued excessive rate of head growth, progressive ventricular enlargement, or, in particular, an inadequate initial neuroradiological procedure (Fig. 36–24). Serial computed tomographic demonstration of the lack of progressive ventricular dilatation is mandatory for the diagnosis of arrested hydrocephalus.

Operative Management

Although drugs such as isosorbide that produce hyperosmotic diuresis and those such as acetazolamide that decrease the secretion of cerebrospinal fluid may temporarily alleviate the clinical situation, their brief action and side effects preclude their use in the definitive control of progressive hydrocephalus.[21,29]

Since the obstruction in the subarachnoid pathways may not be permanent, in some instances hydrocephalus secondary to intracranial hemorrhage may be treated by multiple lumbar punctures. Most cases of hydrocephalus, however, will require an operative procedure for successful control of progressive ventricular dilatation.

While it is desirable to approach the cause of the obstruction with a direct operative procedure, i.e., removal of a posterior fossa tumor or opening of an arachnoid cyst, in most instances subsequent ventricular shunting will be necessary because of persistent cerebrospinal fluid pathway obstruction. This statement applies particularly to hydrocephalus associated with suprasellar or posterior fossa arachnoid cysts and Dandy-Walker malformations.[18]

Posterior fossa decompression for the treatment of hydrocephalus associated with the Arnold-Chiari type II malformation and fenestration or intubation of a stenosed aqueduct of Sylvius have few advocates and have rarely been successful.

Because of subarachnoid obstruction the results of third ventriculostomy, ventriculocisternostomy, and ventriculocervical shunting have been generally poor. These procedures should not be performed unless the subarachnoid space is judged to be competent by pneumoencephalography and isotope cisternography. The number of cases that meet this criterion are few.[33,34,43]

The failure of choroid plexectomy for the treatment of hydrocephalus has been thoroughly documented and is of historical interest only.[32,36]

Wrapping of infants' heads as a means of forcing the cerebrospinal fluid into alternative absorptive pathways has been proposed.[16] This produces increased intracranial pressure and may cause progressive dilatation of the central canal of the spinal cord, resulting in its possible impairment.[20] Head wrapping at the present time must be

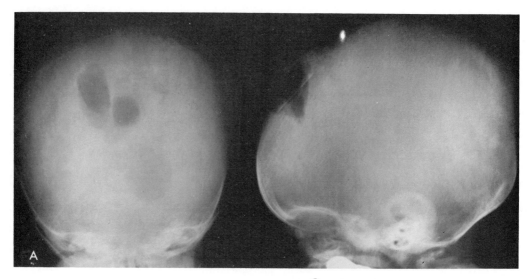

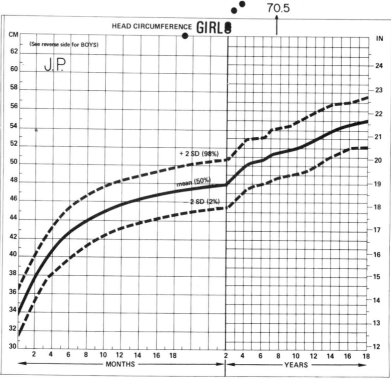

Figure 36-24   A 7-year-old child with an IQ of 115 presented with headaches, vomiting, and a 70.5-cm head circumference. *A*. Original inadequate air study performed by transcoronal tap led to misdiagnosis of hydranencephaly. No further diagnostic studies were performed. *B*. Hydrocephalus was misdiagnosed as "arrested" at age 4 years, and child was discharged from care. Presenting head circumference and those obtained from old chart are shown plotted on head growth curve. This head size demonstrates obvious progressive hydrocephalus since infancy and precludes diagnosis of arrested hydrocephalus.

Illustration continued on opposite page

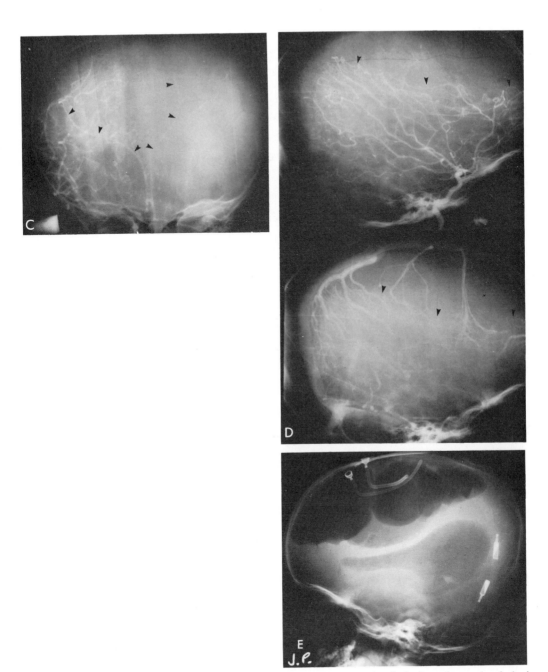

Figure 36–24 (*continued*) *C* and *D*. Angiograms demonstrated interhemispheric and suprahemispheric arachnoid cystic space (*arrows*) and agenesis of the corpus callosum. *E*. Bilateral shunt in arachnoid cyst. Air in cyst and lateral ventricle entered at time of operation, confirming communication between ventricular system and arachnoid cyst. Note tethering of hemisphere by cortical-dural bridging veins. Child had no further enlargement of the head following insertion of the shunt.

considered an experimental and unproved method of treating hydrocephalus.

Extracranial Ventricular Shunt

Shunting the ventricular fluid to a body cavity outside the cranium is the preferred method of treatment of progressive hydrocephalus of whatever cause (congenital, neoplastic, traumatic, infectious, or the like).

The distal end of the shunt should be placed in the peritoneal cavity unless contraindicated by intraperitoneal disease. If peritoneal placement cannot be performed, indirect placement of the shunt in the right atrium by way of the jugular vein and superior vena cava intrapleurally, or direct placement in the atrium by thoracotomy is used in that order of preference.

The advantages of peritoneal over atrial placement of the distal catheter are (1) avoidance of vascular and cardiopulmonary complications, (2) faster and simpler placement of the distal catheter, (3) space to place a longer distal catheter, prolonging the interval before revision, and (4) preservation of the distal tract as the child outgrows the shunt, allowing easy replacement if necessary.

Indications for Extracranial Ventricular Shunt

Progressive ventricular dilatation with or without excessive rate of head growth is the indication for ventricular shunt in the infant. In the presence of open sutures this condition may or may not be associated with symptoms and signs of increased intracranial pressure.

In the older child with closed sutures and increased intracranial pressure, a ventricular shunt is indicated despite the presence of only mild ventricular dilatation because with the more acute hydrocephalus secondary to obstruction by tumors in this age group, decompensation usually occurs prior to significant ventricular enlargement.

Sequence of Radiological Studies and Operative Procedures

When computed tomography reveals congenital hydrocephalus, a ventriculoperi-toneal shunt is indicated, and the procedure may need to be done on an emergency or urgent basis. If by enlargement of the lateral and third ventricles and a normal sized fourth ventricle without evidence of a mass lesion the enhanced CT scan suggests aqueductal stenosis, no further diagnostic tests are performed. If there is doubt regarding an aqueductal obstruction, a ventriculogram with a water-soluble positive contrast agent should be performed in the operating room at the time of the shunt procedure.

If the CT scan shows ventricular dilatation associated with an arachnoid cyst in the suprasellar region or in the posterior fossa, a ventriculogram with water-soluble positive contrast and a pneumoencephalogram should be performed to determine whether the cyst communicates with the ventricular or subarachnoid pathways. If the arachnoid cyst does not communicate, a shunt should be placed in the cyst as well as in the lateral ventricle (Fig. 36–25). If the CT scan reveals hydrocephalus and the Dandy-Walker malformation, a ventriculogram with water-soluble positive contrast should be performed in the operating room immediately prior to the shunt procedure to determine whether the aqueduct is patent. If the aqueduct is patent, a shunt of the Dandy-Walker cyst is indicated (Fig. 36–26). If the aqueduct is stenosed, a shunt of the lateral ventricle and the Dandy-Walker cyst is necessary. Double shunts should be connected to a single valve and distal catheter by means of a T-connector.

If the CT scan reveals hydrocephalus secondary to a mass lesion (intraventricular, suprasellar, or posterior fossa tumor; arteriovenous malformation of the galenic system; or the like), an emergency or urgent insertion of a ventriculoperitoneal shunt may be necessary. After stabilization of the patient's intracranial problem, cerebral angiography should be performed to determine the vascular nature of the mass lesion and its effect on the intracranial contents. Occasionally, it may be necessary to perform ventriculography with water-soluble positive contrast and pneumoencephalography to further delineate the extent of tumors in the third ventricle and suprasellar region before a direct operative approach to the mass. In the case of arteriovenous malformations and posterior fossa tumors, no further diagnostic studies beyond cerebral

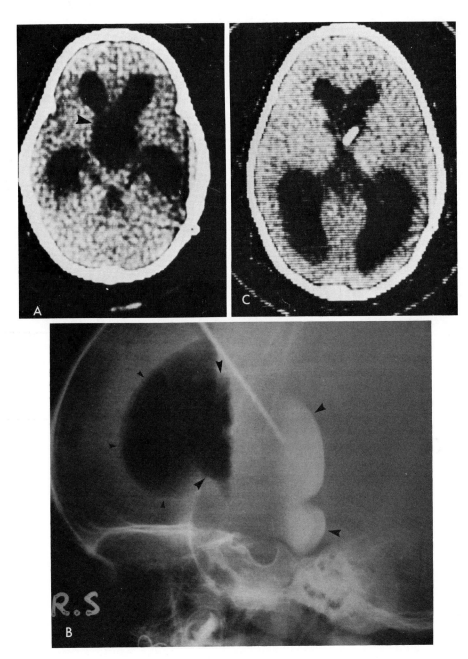

Figure 36–25 *A.* Computed tomographic scan demonstrating hydrocephalus and suprasellar arachnoid cyst (*arrow*). *B.* Brow-up lateral intraoperative ventriculogram showing air in the anterior horns (*small arrows*) and air and water-soluble positive contrast in the arachnoid cyst, clearly delineating its extensions (*large arrows*). Note a catheter in the lateral ventricle as well as in the arachnoid cyst. *C.* Postoperative CT scan showing decompression of the cyst as well as of the ventricular system. Note catheter within the cyst.

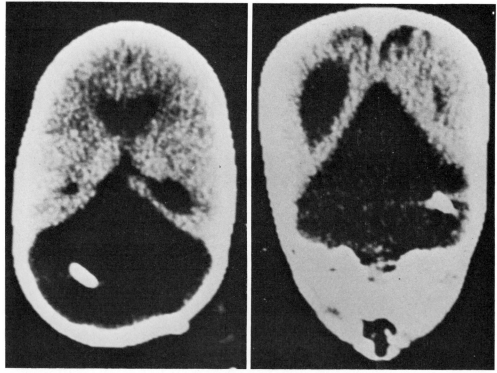

Figure 36–26   Horizontal (*left*) and coronal (*right*) CT scans demonstrating a Dandy-Walker malformation with a posterior fossa shunt.

angiography are done prior to a definitive operation.

Technique of Shunt Placement

The surgeon must pay meticulous attention to every aspect of the operative procedure. This attention, if given, significantly reduces the incidence of shunt malfunction and infection.

VENTRICULOPERITONEAL SHUNT. The skin is shaved in the operating room after the induction of anesthesia. A five-minute povidone-iodine scrub is followed by three applications of providone-iodine solution. After the skin has air dried, one application of tincture of benzoin is applied. The benzoin will increase the adherence of the polyethylene towels and drapes. The incisions may be outlined with a sterile marking pen. For right-sided shunts, a small posterior parietal incision is used and should be in the shape of a semicircle with one limb longer than the other to increase the width of the pedicle. The skin incision is placed so that the burr hole is in direct line with the lateral ventricle. The burr hole site should be at a point several centimeters above the tip of the external ear and several centimeters posterior to the posterior border of the external ear (Fig. 36–27). Obviously the more anteriorly the burr hole is placed, the more chance there is of passing the catheter through the motor cortex. For a right-sided shunt the ventricular catheter can also be placed through a burr hole at the level of the coronal suture and 2.5 cm lateral to the midline. With the sterile marking pen, a transverse right upper quadrant abdominal incision approximately 2 cm in length is then outlined midway between the lower rib and the umbilicus and with its midpoint overlying the rectus abdominus muscle. In older children and more obese patients a longer incision will be necessary. The periphery of the operative field is sealed off with polyethylene towels with adhesive edges (Steri-Drape). Care should be taken to seal off the skin around the ear, which has been sutured forward out of the operative field. A polyethylene drape is then placed over the operative field so that no area of skin is exposed. Sterile sheets complete the draping procedure.

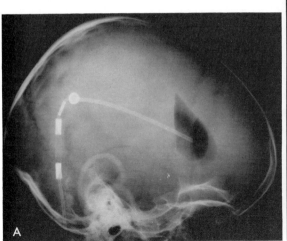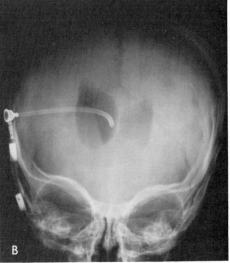

Figure 36-27   Postshunt skull x-rays demonstrating proper placement of the ventricular catheter anterior to the foramen of Monro. Note proper placement of the burr hole (Rickham reservoir site) parallel on a horizontal plane to the lateral ventricle and positioned superior to the tip of the external ear and posterior to the posterior border of the external ear. *A*. Lateral view. *B*. Anterior view.

The scalp is incised down through the galea and the flap is reflected on its base. Bleeding is controlled by bipolar coagulation. It is important to mark the burr hole site by cauterizing the periosteum before placing a self-retaining retractor. Otherwise, the scalp may be displaced by the retractor, which may in turn cause an error in the placement of the burr hole. The periosteum is incised, and a burr hole is made with a small Hudson perforator. The opening is enlarged enough to accommodate a Rickham reservoir. The dura is cauterized and the outer layer is incised. Bipolar cautery is used to penetrate the inner layer of the dura and seal it to the pia and cortex. Sealing the dura to the pia and cortex prevents ventricular fluid from entering the subdural space, which increases the risk of postoperative subdural hematoma. A straight ventricular catheter with multiple perforations is then passed with a stylet into the posterior aspect of the lateral ventricle. As soon as the ventricle is entered, the stylet is removed and the opening pressure is recorded. A length of catheter predetermined by measurement on a preoperative lateral skull x-ray is then advanced without its stylet until its tip passes beyond the foramen of Monro, as shown in Figure 36-27. Care is taken to insure that no more than 1 or 2 ml of ventricular fluid is lost dur-

ing the procedure to prevent cortical collapse and subdural hematoma. If the intraventricular pressure is markedly elevated, it is reduced to approximately 200 mm of water. At this point 5 to 10 cc of air is injected into the catheter, which has been attached to a blunt 16-gauge needle and a stopcock. An intraoperative overhead lateral x-ray of the skull is taken for confirmation of catheter placement.

Next, attention is directed to the abdomen, where a transverse incision is carried down to the anterior rectus sheath. Using a long tube passer to avoid intermediate skin incisions, a distal catheter is passed from the scalp incision to the abdominal incision subcutaneously. In the larger child a small intermediate cervical incision may be necessary. At this point a Rickham reservoir with a side arm cap is attached to the proximal end of the valve with a stainless steel connector and a 2-0 silk ligature. In infants with thin scalps it is important to place the knot on the underside to prevent it from eroding through the skin. The Rickham reservoir is then in turn attached with a 2-0 silk ligature to the ventricular catheter, which has been cut to its proper size. The 2-0 silk is used because a smaller suture or a monofilament suture may cut through the Silastic tubing. The valve mechanism lies in the subgaleal space behind the ear. At this point a 1-cm longitudinal incision is made in the anterior rectus sheath, and the rectus abdominus muscle is split bluntly in the direction of its fibers. The posterior rectus sheath and transversalis fascia are grasped with forceps, and a 1-mm incision is made with tenotomy scissors. The peritoneum is then grasped, and a 1-mm incision is made in it. A trochar is not used for placing the peritoneal catheter because it increases the risk of *Escherichia coli* shunt infections.[7] The peritoneal catheter is then passed into the intraperitoneal space for approximately 15 cm. The wounds are irrigated with bacitracin solution (50,000 units per 100 ml saline). To close the abdominal incision, interrupted 4-0 polypropylene sutures are used for the anterior rectus sheath and subcutaneous and subcuticular layers, and Steri-Strips are used for the skin. The 1-mm incision in the peritoneum is not closed. Methicillin (100 mg) is injected into the ventricle by way of the Rickham reservoir after compression of the valve, and the scalp incision is then closed with interrupted 4-0 polypropylene sutures for the galeal layer and Steri-Strips for the skin. In order to decrease the penetration of bacteria to the deep layers, surface skin sutures are not used.[15] A sterile Telfa dressing is then applied to each incision. Using Telfa prevents adherence of the Steri-Strips to the dressing.

VENTRICULOATRIAL SHUNT. In placing a ventriculoatrial shunt, the steps for preparation of the skin and draping of the head and neck are the same as described for the ventriculoperitoneal shunt. A transverse incision is made in the right anterior cervical region following a skin crease approximately 2 cm below the angle of the jaw and with its midpoint overlying the anterior border of the sternocleidomastoid muscle. This incision is carried down through the platysma muscle. If a large external jugular vein is encountered at this point, an attempt is made to pass the catheter into the right atrium through it. Frequently it is impossible to pass the catheter through the external jugular vein and it is then necessary to dissect out the common facial vein and ligate it about 1 cm distal to its entrance into the internal jugular vein. A small venotomy is made with tenotomy scissors, and a distal Silastic catheter with an open end is passed into the common facial vein and then into the internal jugular vein and advanced into the right atrium. The distance is estimated by preoperative measurements on a chest x-ray. This catheter must be attached to a three-way stopcock and filled with saline prior to entering the vein. A manometer is then placed on the stopcock and the atrial pressure is measured. Next, the catheter is advanced into the right ventricle to identify the intraventricular pressure, after which it

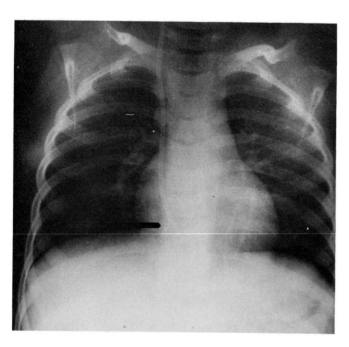

Figure 36–28 Chest x-ray demonstrating proper placement of tip of cardiac catheter just above level of tricuspid valve (*arrow*). This is confirmed by intraoperative cardiac ventricular and atrial pressure recording as well as by chest x-ray.

is slowly withdrawn until the pressure of the ventricular pulsations in the manometer drops to that of atrial pulsations, indicating that the tip of the catheter is above the tricuspid valve. Correct placement of the catheter is confirmed with an intraoperative chest x-ray (Fig. 36–28). The catheter is then connected to the distal end of the valve mechanism in the same manner as the peritoneal catheter with a stainless steel connector and 2-0 silk ligatures. The cervical incision is closed by using interrupted 4-0 polypropylene sutures for the platysma and subcutaneous layers and Steri-Strips for the skin.

Left-sided ventricular shunts should always be placed by way of a coronal burr hole to avoid passing the catheter through the posterior aspect of the dominant hemisphere. This precaution is particularly important when placing the catheter in older children with small ventricles.

Prophylactic Antibiotics

All children are given methicillin (50 mg per kilogram) intravenously during induction of anesthesia and 100 mg of methicillin intraventricularly into the shunt mechanism at the termination of the procedure. Methicillin (50 mg per kilogram) is then administered intravenously every six hours for a total of four doses. Gentamicin is used if there is an allergy to the penicillins.

Selection of Shunt Components

No ventricular catheter design will prevent choroid plexus from entering its perforations and blocking the flow of cerebrospinal fluid. The simple straight catheter with multiple small perforations appears to be the most satisfactory for maintaining patency. It also causes less trauma on removal. Placement of the catheter tip beyond the foramen of Monro will decrease the incidence of choroid plexus obstruction but will not prevent it. The choroid plexus tends to extend toward the perforations of the catheter wherever it is placed.

A reservoir is an essential component of the shunt system. It allows for percutaneous instillation of antibiotics, measurement and reduction of intracranial pressure, and identification of the site of a shunt obstruction. The Rickham reservoir is one of the most satisfactory ones.

A high-pressure Hakim valve (95 to 125 mm of water) is used in most cases except the mildly dilated ventricles under very high pressure secondary to obstruction by posterior fossa tumors. In these latter cases a very-high-pressure Hakim valve (140 to 165 mm of water) is used. It is rarely necessary to use a medium-pressure valve and never necessary to use a low-pressure valve. The author does not use an antisiphon device.

The distal cardiac catheter has a single opening at the end, allowing for intracardiac pressure measurement during placement. The distal peritoneal catheter has a single opening at the end. In the author's experience, shunt mechanisms with slits in the valve or distal catheter malfunction more frequently because slits fail to open when flow is stopped by obstruction elsewhere in the shunt system. Distal intraluminal obstruction by tissue debris or blood clot will occur more readily when the catheter is not open at the end.

POSTOPERATIVE CARE OF THE CHILD WITH A SHUNT

The operative approach to the management of hydrocephalus requires the persistent effort of an interested and dedicated neurosurgeon. The initial placement of the ventricular shunt is only the beginning in the care of the hydrocephalic child. Unless the neurosurgeon is willing to devote the necessary time to the continuing care of the child, he should not initiate operative treatment. Instead, he should refer the child to a surgeon or a medical center that can undertake this responsibility.

Routine clinical follow-up begins two weeks after discharge from the hospital. During the first year of life the infant is evaluated every three months. From age 1 year to 3 years the child is evaluated every 6 months; beyond age 3 years, every 12 months. The history of symptoms of increased intracranial pressure such as irritability, anorexia, vomiting, headache, and changes in personality is obtained. The head circumference is measured and plotted on a head growth chart. Following insertion of the shunt there should be no further increase in the head circumference of the infant for several months. From then on the head growth curve should be that of normal brain growth. In the older child with closed sutures and a head circumference initially significantly above the upper limits of normal there should be no further increase in head size until the head circumference comes within the normal range. From then on the increase in head size should follow a normal brain growth curve. After placement of the shunt the anterior fontanel should be depressed in a quiet sitting infant. It is important to follow infants and children with shunts by means of CT scans for evaluation of ventricular size. In the infant the scan is repeated within the first 6 months of age and again at age 12 months. Following this, computed tomography is

performed yearly. As mentioned before, a single-level scan significantly reduces the time, cost, and radiation dosage.

Elective Shunt Revision

Elective shunt revision of the short distal catheter is not needed if the child meets all the following criteria: (1) no history of increased intracranial pressure secondary to shunt malfunction after 1 year of age, (2) normal brain growth curve, and (3) no evidence of silent ventricular enlargement on follow-up CT scans. If the distal end of a ventriculoperitoneal shunt appears to be out of the peritoneal cavity or above the

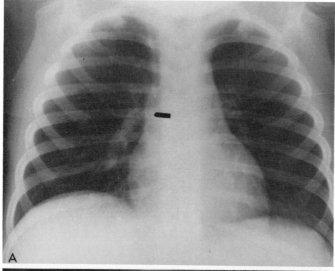

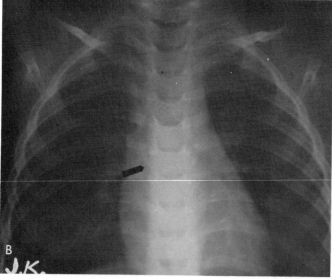

Figure 36–29 Catheter tip (*arrow*) projected against, *A,* T5-T6 vertebral body level by cephalad angulation of x-ray tube and, *B,* T6-T7 vertebral level by caudad angulation of the tube. Actually, interpretation against the cardiac shadow shows the tip of the catheter to be at the superior vena caval–atrial junction on both x-rays.

level of the vena caval–atrial junction with a ventriculoatrial shunt, close re-examination of all these factors is indicated. In determining the level of the cardiac catheter it is important to interpret it against the shadow of the heart rather than against that of the vertebral bodies. The surgeon should familiarize himself with the x-ray shadow of the junction of the superior vena cava and right atrium and the level of the tricuspid valve. Because of the angulation of the x-ray tube, the level of the cardiac catheter can be misinterpreted when it is measured against the vertebral bodies (Fig. 36–29).

Management of Shunt Complications

The following discussion of ventricular shunts is based on 778 consecutive shunt operations performed by or under the direct supervision of the author. Two hundred and forty-five of these operations were initial shunts. Five hundred and thirty-three operations were revisions of both the author's cases and other cases in which the initial shunts had been inserted elsewhere.

Infection

Infection Outside Shunt

Infections that are external to the shunts (i.e., wound infection, cutaneous infection overlying a part of the shunt mechanism or along its entire course, and breakdown of the skin exposing the shunt mechanism) are treated by removal of the entire shunt system and intravenous antibiotic therapy as determined by the appropriate sensitivity studies (Fig. 36–30). If the child becomes symptomatic from increased intracranial pressure after the shunt is removed, external ventricular drainage is instituted. A closed drainage system with a one-way valve is used and antibiotics are instilled intraventricularly daily.

Infection Inside Shunt

An infection inside the shunt produces ventriculitis and colonization of the shunt mechanism that results in bacteremia in the case of a ventriculoatrial shunt or a low-grade peritonitis in the case of a peritoneal shunt. There is no evidence of infection of the skin. There is a marked decrease in the incidence of this type of infection if meticulous attention is given to preparation, draping, and operative technique and to the use of intraoperative antibiotic irrigation and prophylactic intraventricular and intravenous administration of antibiotics.[52]

Of the 778 shunt procedures performed in the author's hospital, 21 were followed by shunt infections (2.7 per cent). The highest incidence of shunt infections occurred in infants less than 1 year of age. Seventy per cent of the infections were detected within one year of the previous shunt procedure.

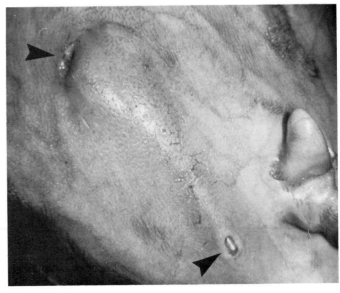

Figure 36–30 External shunt infection caused by breakdown of skin over valve component and wound infection (*arrows*).

There was no significant difference between ventriculoatrial and ventriculoperitoneal shunts with regard to incidence of infection. *Staphylococcus epidermidis* was the organism most commonly identified.

The major clinical manifestation of shunt infection is fever. This usually is intermittent and low-grade. Any infant or child with a ventricular shunt and a history of unexplained intermittent fever, particularly over a period of several weeks, must be considered to be infected, and appropriate cultures must be obtained. Apnea episodes, particularly in premature neonates, anemia, dehydration, hepatosplenomegaly, and stiff neck are other presenting signs. Signs of malfunctioning of the shunt system are frequently the only indication of infection. These signs consist of a bulging anterior fontanel and an excessive rate of head growth. With shunts to the peritoneum, the cerebrospinal fluid may back up along the subcutaneous course of the shunt tubing, which indicates failure of the peritoneum to absorb the infected cerebrospinal fluid. Six of the twenty-one shunt infections were asymptomatic and diagnosed only by routine cultures obtained during shunt revision.

In addition to the 21 infections following the author's own operative procedures, there were 18 patients who were operated on elsewhere and were initially admitted to this clinic for treatment of active infection. The results of treatment of all 39 infections are given in Table 36–3.

Except for the three external infections (wound), which responded to treatment only after removal of the shunt, 26 of 27 infections treated with antibiotics alone or antibiotics and immediate shunt replacement were cured.

Specimens for routine cultures for bacteria should be taken during each shunt revision. If the culture is positive and the patient is asymptomatic, methicillin (200 mg per kilogram per day) or other appropriate antibiotic is given intravenously for 14 days.

For symptomatic gram-positive infections the treatment is immediate removal of

TABLE 36–3   TREATMENT OF VENTRICULAR SHUNT INFECTIONS

TYPE OF TREATMENT	ORGANISM	NO. OF CASES	RESULT	SUBSEQUENT TREATMENT
Intravenous antibiotics	*Staphylococcus epidermidis*	6*	Cured	
Intravenous and intraventricular antibiotics	*Propionibacterium*	2	Cured	
	Klebsiella	1	Cured	
	S. epidermidis	1	Cured	
	Unidentified	1	Cured	
Intravenous and intraventricular antibiotics, immediate shunt replacement	*S. epidermidis*	10	Cured	
	S. epidermidis	1	Recurred	Shunt removed, replacement delayed
	S. epidermidis	2†	Recurred with *Staphylococcus aureus*	Shunt removed, replacement delayed
	Proteus mirabilis	1	Cured	
	Escherichia coli	1	Cured	
	Micrococcus	1	Cured	
	Corynebacterium	1	Cured	
	Unidentified	1	Cured	
	Unidentified	1†	Recurred with *Candida tropicalis* (suspect contaminant)	Shunt removed, replacement delayed (*Candida* cleared without treatment)
Removal of shunt and delayed replacement	*Listeria monocytogenes* and *S. epidermidis*	1	Cured	Delayed replacement
	P. mirabilis	1	Cured	Delayed replacement
	P. mirabilis	1†	Cured	Delayed replacement
	S. epidermidis	3	Cured	Delayed replacement
	S. aureus	1†	Cured	Delayed replacement
	Unidentified	1†	Cured	Delayed replacement
	S. epidermidis (intraperitoneal abscess)	1	Cured	Delayed replacement

* Asymptomatic infections diagnosed by routine cultures during shunt revision.

† Wound infection

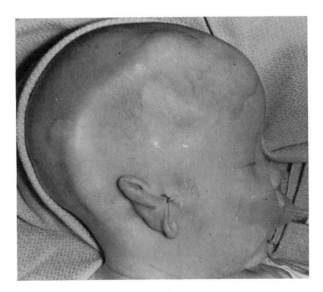

Figure 36–31 Accumulation of cerebrospinal fluid along subgaleal course of coronally placed shunt indicates malfunction. Note ear tied forward for operation.

the shunt system and its replacement in the same site with a new system.[28,44] Fourteen days of methicillin at 100 mg per day intraventricularly and 200 mg per kilogram per day in divided doses intravenously is the antibiotic regimen that should be used. Cultures are obtained and sensitivities determined prior to initiating methicillin therapy, and the appropriate antibiotic is substituted if necessary. Specimens of cerebrospinal fluid are obtained intermittently to assay effective antibiotic levels. Gentamicin is used when there is an allergy to the penicillins.

For gram-negative infections, the shunt is removed and the patient is treated with the appropriate antibiotic both intraventricularly by way of an indwelling ventricular catheter and Rickham reservoir and intravenously for 14 days. External ventricular drainage is used when control of increased intracranial pressure is necessary. Gentamicin has been the most commonly used antibiotic in gram-negative infections.

Shunt Malfunction

The clinical manifestations of shunt malfunction are persistent bulging of the anterior fontanel and excessive rate of head growth in the infant, and signs and symptoms of increased intracranial pressure in either the infant or child. Fluid along the subcutaneous course of the shunt may occur without other signs initially (Fig. 36–31). As stated earlier, silent progressive enlargement of the ventricular system may occur in children without evidence of ex-

cessive rate of head growth or signs and symptoms of increased intracranial pressure. Serial CT scans will diagnose this problem prior to the onset of decompensation.

Site of Obstruction

The most common site of obstruction is within the ventricle at the tip of the catheter (Fig. 36–32). An obstruction of an open-ended catheter within the cardiac atrium has not occurred in the author's series. When the catheter begins to ascend into the superior vena cava because of the child's skeletal growth, however, obstruction of the vascular catheter invariably results (Fig. 36–33). The most common cause of malfunction at the peritoneal end is failure of absorption by the peritoneum or the development of an intraperitoneal pseudocyst by loculation of the area surrounding the catheter (Fig. 36–34). Using an open-ended peritoneal catheter, the author has had no obstruction by omentum entering the lumen of the catheter. This type of obstruction has occurred, however, when slits were present in the peritoneal catheter.

Reliability of the Pumping Mechanism as an Indicator of Shunt Function

When the pumping mechanism is compressed and does not refill, the ventricular end of the system is not draining. When there is undue firmness to compression,

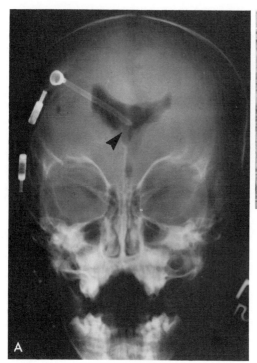

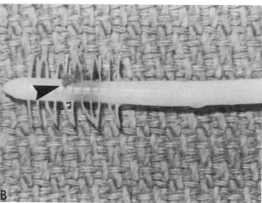

Figure 36–32 *A.* Ventriculogram showing shadow of the choroid plexus attached to the tip of the ventricular catheter (*arrow*). *B.* Extra- and intraluminal obstruction of the ventricular catheter by choroid plexus (*arrow*). No ventricular catheter design will prevent this problem.

Figure 36–33 Chest x-ray demonstrating obstructed cardiac catheter within the superior vena cava (*arrow*) several centimeters above shadow of its entrance into the cardiac atrium.

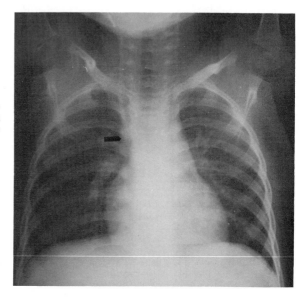

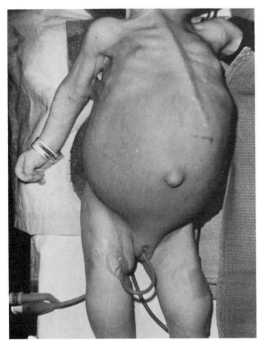

Figure 36–34 Marked abdominal distention due to an intraperitoneal cerebrospinal fluid pseudocyst. Note accumulation of cerebrospinal fluid along the subcutaneous tract of the shunt.

one can suspect an obstruction of the valve or distal catheter. The pumping chamber, however, can be compressed and appear to refill even when the shunt is obstructed. The apparent refilling of the shunt will give a false negative observation for shunt obstruction. Therefore, an apparently normally functioning pumping chamber should not be relied upon as an indication of shunt patency.

Evaluation of Shunt Patency

Proximal and distal flow can be evaluated by percutaneously tapping the reservoir with a short No. 25 Butterfly needle such as those used for scalp vein infusions. After a circular area at least 5 cm in diameter over the reservoir is shaved, the skin is prepared with povidone-iodine, and a short No. 25 Butterfly needle is passed percutaneously into the Rickham reservoir through its cap. If there is no flow of fluid from the ventricular catheter, an obstruction of this catheter can be diagnosed. In this case a manometer is attached to the needle and filled with sterile saline. The distal runoff is then evaluated by observing the drop of the saline column within the manometer. If the fluid column drops rapidly down to the opening pressure of the valve, the valve and distal catheter are open.

If the fluid does not drop unless the valve mechanism of a ventriculoperitoneal shunt is pumped, then an abdominal pseudocyst or failure of the peritoneum to absorb the cerebrospinal fluid can be diagnosed. These same findings with a ventriculoatrial shunt probably would mean that the distal end had been pulled back into the vena cava and was obstructed. If there is no drop in the fluid column when the valve mechanism is pumped, this indicates obstruction within the valve mechanism itself. This technique makes it possible to determine the level of the obstruction of the shunt mechanism prior to operation.

Sometimes it is possible to clear the ventricular catheter obstruction by injecting 2 cc of air or saline through the Rickham reservoir after compressing the valve. If good proximal flow is not obtained by this maneuver, it is unsafe to continue injecting larger volumes of saline into the ventricular system because it will increase the intracranial pressure.

Management of Ventricular Catheter Obstruction in a Child with Slit Ventricles

Children who are dependent on the shunt but who have normal or smaller than normal ventricles can undergo rapid decompensation when obstruction of the shunt mechanism occurs—frequently without ventricular dilatation.

First, the site of the obstruction is determined by the foregoing method of tapping the reservoir. When the ventricular catheter is open, the distal obstruction is revised by operation. If the ventricular catheter is obstructed, emergency preoperative computed tomography is performed to define the largest area of the ventricular system. Many times the scan will show some dilatation of the occipital horns even when the anterior aspects of the ventricular system are small slits. There may be a porencephalic area available for placing the ventricular catheter. This preoperative CT scan will obviate multiple blind passes with a ventricular catheter in attempting to enter the small ventricle. If no dilated areas of the ventricular system are found by the scan,

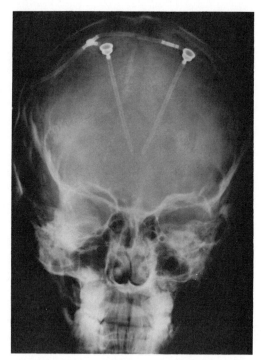

Figure 36–35 X-ray demonstrating bicoronal placement of ventricular catheters into both anterior horns and their attachment to a single valve mechanism by way of a T-connector.

an attempt is made to remove the obstructed catheter and place a new catheter through the same tract without the use of a stylet. Frequently, however, the obstructed catheter will be firmly adherent to the choroid plexus and the risk of intraventricular hemorrhage will preclude its removal. The next step is to place catheters into the anterior horns of both lateral ventricles through bicoronal burr holes. Small ventricles are more easily entered and less vital brain tissue is penetrated via this route. These bilateral ventricular catheters are connected to a single valve mechanism (Fig. 36–35).

Using this technique will make it unnecessary to resort to subtemporal decompression to expand the lateral ventricle in these difficult cases of malfunctioning shunts in very small ventricles.[17] It is possible that bidirectional flow between the two ventricular catheters occurs above the unidirectional valve. This variation of flow may decrease constant one-way flow through the perforations of the ventricular catheter and thus keep the choroid plexus out. In the series reported earlier, five children have been treated by this technique without further recurrence of ventricular catheter obstruction.

Postshunt Subdural Hematoma

The incidence of postshunt subdural hematoma in the author's series is 3 in 245 new shunt procedures (1.2 per cent). No subdural hematomas have occurred following 533 shunt revision procedures. The overall incidence of postshunt subdural hematoma is, therefore, 3 in a total of 778 shunt procedures (0.4 per cent). Several precautions are important in preventing postshunt subdural hematomas: (1) careful intraoperative technique to prevent cerebrospinal fluid from entering the subdural space, i.e., sealing the cortex against the dura at the time of placing the original ventricular catheter; (2) removal of only a small amount of cerebrospinal fluid for laboratory studies prior to connection of the valve; and (3) use of the high-pressure valve.

Postshunt subdural hematoma usually occurs when an initial shunt is placed in a child over 3 years old with a very large head and a markedly dilated ventricular system. The three cases mentioned earlier were successfully treated with a concurrent subdural-peritoneal shunt. Figure 36–36 shows one case of postshunt hematoma occurring in a 7-year-old child with very large ventricles secondary to aqueductal stenosis. A bilateral subdural-peritoneal shunt using a very-low-pressure Hakim valve (5 to 12 mm of water) was placed and the ventricular shunt with the high-pressure valve (95 to 125 mm of water) was left intact. As with other subdural shunts, the parents are instructed to pump the subdural valve frequently (40 times at least 4 to 6 times daily), whereas they are advised never to pump a ventricular valve (cf. Fig. 36–36).

Postshunt Craniosynostosis

In the author's series, there has been no significant cosmetic deformity secondary to craniosynostosis in children who have received shunts and have had normal brain growth. Significantly abnormal skull configurations have occurred only in children with shunts who have had primary failure of brain growth. Of course, with primary failure of brain growth, operative treatment of the craniosynostosis is contraindicated.

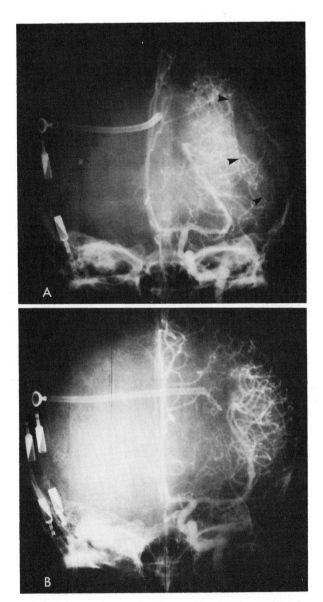

Figure 36–36 *A*. Carotid angiogram demonstrating postshunt subdural hematoma (*arrows*). Note medial displacement of ventricular catheter in the compressed left lateral ventricle. *B*. Repeat angiogram demonstrating resolution of subdural hematoma by a subdural shunt (5- to 12-mm valve) without removal of original ventricular shunt (95- to 125-mm valve). Note return of ventricular catheter.

Infants who have very large heads and markedly dilated ventricles may have an overlap of the cranial bones after a shunting procedure in which a low- or medium-pressure valve is used. In exceptional cases this overlap may persist and it may be necessary to operate to relieve this therapeutically induced craniosynostosis. The use of a high-pressure valve in the initial shunt should preclude this problem.

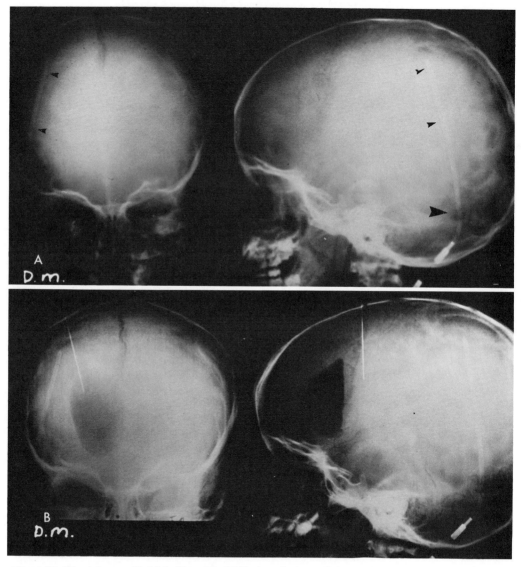

Figure 36–37 A 5-year-old child with an IQ of 145 whose hydrocephalus was diagnosed as shunt-independent arrested at age 3 years, despite the fact that his head had not stopped expanding. *A.* Plain x-rays of the skull show marked enlargement of the cranial vault and poor placement of the shunt. Note the low burr hole below the level of the lambdoid suture (*large arrow*) and the misplacement of the ventricular catheter (*small arrows*). *B.* In the absence of a reservoir, a percutaneous transcoronal ventricular tap was performed. The opening pressure was 250 mm of water. The child did not have symptoms of increased pressure. The ventriculogram, however, demonstrated large ventricles with a frontal cerebral mantle of 3.5 cm.

Illustration continued on opposite page

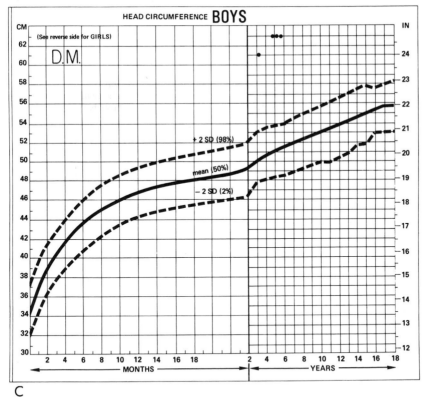

Figure 36–37 (*continued*) *C*. Head growth chart demonstrating the continued rate of excessive growth between ages 3 and 5 years, which is incompatible with the diagnosis of arrested hydrocephalus. Note abatement of growth rate beyond age 5 years following shunt revision.

CRITERIA FOR THE DIAGNOSIS OF ARRESTED HYDROCEPHALUS

Shunt-Independent Arrested Hydrocephalus

When the child has ventricles of normal or nearly normal size and does not require a functioning shunt to maintain this state, he is considered to have shunt-independent arrested hydrocephalus. The criteria for this diagnosis are: (1) there should be no episode of shunt malfunction after 12 months of age, (2) there should be a normal head growth curve, (3) the ventricles should be of normal size or only mildly dilated, (4) there should be no progression of ventricular size as determined by serial CT scans, and (5) the child's shunt should be nonfunctioning. Children with a tentative diagnosis of shunt-independent arrested hydrocephalus should be followed indefinitely. The shunts in these children should not be removed unless there is a problem with infection. Failure to meet any of these criteria is incompatible with a diagnosis of shunt-independent arrested hydrocephalus (Fig. 36–37).

Shunt-Dependent Arrested Hydrocephalus

If the child has ventricles of normal or nearly normal size but requires a function-

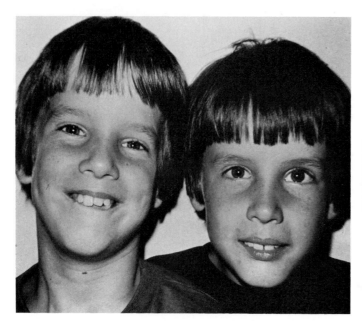

Figure 36–38 The twin on the left has hydrocephalus controlled by a functioning ventricular shunt initially placed during infancy (shunt-dependent arrested hydrocephalus). The twin on the right is normal. Both boys have normal intelligence.

ing shunt to maintain this state and to prevent increased intracranial pressure, he is considered to have shunt-dependent arrested hydrocephalus.

Unless there is an underlying brain impairment, congenital or acquired, there is no reason that the child with hydrocephalus who is treated early and followed closely cannot lead a normal life and have a normal-sized head (Fig. 36–38). These shunt-dependent arrested hydrocephalic children should have: (1) normal- or nearly normal-sized ventricles, (2) normal head growth curves after the ventricles have returned to normal or near-normal size, (3) no progression of ventricular size as determined by serial CT scans, and (4) no symptoms or signs of increased intracranial pressure (Fig. 36–39).

If the child does not meet these criteria, the shunt should be revised because it is not working properly.

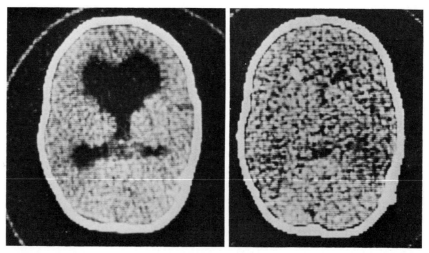

Figure 36–39 Preshunt and postshunt CT scans demonstrate return of ventricular system to normal by a functioning shunt.

REFERENCES

1. Abramowicz, M., ed.: Sedation and analgesia for minor painful procedure. Med. Lett. Drugs Ther., *19*:26, 1977.
2. Adeloye, A., Single, S., and Odeku, E.: Stridor, myelomeningocele, and hydrocephalus in a child. Arch. Neurol., *23*:271, 1970.
3. Berger, P. E., Kirks, D. R., Gilday, D. L., Fitz, C. R., and Harwood-Nash, D. C.: Computed tomography in infants and children: Intracranial neoplasms. Amer. J. Roentgen., *127*:129, 1976.
4. Bering, E. A., Jr.: Circulation of the cerebrospinal fluid. Demonstration of the choroid plexus as the generator of the force for flow of fluid in ventricular enlargement. J. Neurosurg., *19*:405, 1962.
5. Bering, E. A., Jr., and Sato, O.: Hydrocephalus: Changes in formation and absorption of cerebrospinal fluid within the cerebral ventricles. J. Neurosurg., *20*:1050, 1963.
6. Brockelhurst, G.: The development of the human cerebrospinal fluid pathway with particular reference to the roof of the fourth ventricle. J. Anat., *105*:467, 1969.
7. Carmel, P.: Shunt infections. Surg. Neurol., in press.
8. Cutler, R. W. P., Page, L. K., Galicich, J. H., and Waters, G. V.: Formation and absorption of cerebrospinal fluid in man. Brain, *91*:707, 1968.
9. Dandy, W. E., and Blackfan, K. D.: Internal hydrocephalus. An experimental clinical and pathological study, Amer. J. Dis. Child., *8*:406, 1914.
10. Davson, H.: Physiology of the Cerebrospinal Fluid. London, J. & A. Churchill, 1967.
11. Davson, H.: The cerebrospinal fluid pressure. *In* Cumings, J. N., and Dremer, M., eds.: Biochemical Aspects of Neurological Disorders. Oxford, Blackwell Scientific Publications, 1968.
12. Davson, H., and Segal, M. B.: Secretion and drainage of the cerebrospinal fluid. Acta Neurol. Lat. Amer., (Suppl. 1) *17*:99, 1971.
13. Di Chiro, G.: Observations on the circulation of the cerebrospinal fluid. Acta Radiol. [Diagn.] (Stockholm), *5*:988, 1966.
14. Dunbar, H. S., Guthrie, T. C., and Karpell, B.: A study of the cerebrospinal fluid pulse wave. Arch. Neurol., *14*:624, 1966.
15. Edlich, R. F., Rodeheaver, G., Kuphal, J., and deHoll, J. D.: Technique of closure: Contaminated wounds. J. Amer. Coll. Emer. Phys., *3*:375, 1974.
16. Epstein, F., Hochwald, G. M., and Ransohoff, J.: Neonatal hydrocephalus treated by compressive head wrapping. Lancet, *1*:634, 1973.
17. Epstein, F. J., Fleischer, A. S., Hochwald, G. M., and Ransohoff, J.: Subtemporal craniectomy for recurrent shunt obstruction secondary to small ventricles. J. Neurosurg., *41*:29, 1974.
18. Fischer, E. G.: Dandy-Walker syndrome: Evaluation of surgical treatment. J. Neurosurg., *39*:615, 1973.
19. Hagberg, B., and Sjogren, I.: The chronic brain syndrome of infantile hydrocephalus. Amer. J. Dis. Child., *112*:189, 1966.
20. Hall, P. V., Lindseth, R. E., Campbell, R. L., and Kalsbeck, J. E.: Myelodysplasia and developmental scoliosis. A manifestation of syringomyelia. Spine, *1*:48, 1976.
21. Hayden, P. W., Foltz, E. L., and Shurtleff, D. B.: Effect of an oral osmotic agent on ventricular fluid pressure of hydrocephalic children. Pediatrics, *41*:955, 1968.
22. Kalbag, R. M., and Woolf, A. L.: Cerebral Venous Thrombosis. London, Oxford University Press, 1967.
23. Kappers, J. A.: Structural and functional changes in the telencephalic choroid plexus during human ontogenesis. *In* Wolstenholme, G. E., and O'Connor, C. M., eds.: Ciba Foundation Symposium on the Cerebrospinal Fluid. Boston, Little, Brown & Co., 1958, p. 3.
24. Kim, C. S., Bennett, D. R., and Roberts, T. S.: Primary amenorrhea secondary to noncommunicating hydrocephalus. Neurology, *19*:533, 1969.
25. Lemire, R. J., Loeser, J. D., Leech, R. W., and Alvord, E. C.: Normal and Abnormal Development of the Human Nervous System. New York, Harper & Row, 1975, p. 100.
26. Lorenzo, A. V., Page, L. K., and Waters, G. V.: Relationship between cerebrospinal fluid formation, absorption and pressure in human hydrocephalus. Brain, *93*:679, 1970.
27. Mazur, R.: Transillumination of the skull in the diagnosis of intracranial disease in children up to three years. Develop. Med. Child Neurol., *7*:634, 1965.
28. McLaurin, R. L.: Treatment of infected ventricular shunts. *In* O'Brien, M. S., ed.: Pediatric Neurological Surgery. New York, Raven Press, 1978.
29. Mealey, J., Jr., and Barker, D. T.: Failure of oral acetazolamide to avert hydrocephalus in infants with myelomeningocele. J. Pediat., *72*:257, 1968.
30. Menkes, J. H.: Textbook of Child Neurology. Philadelphia, Lea & Febiger, 1974, p. 154.
31. Milhorat, T. H.: Choroid plexus and cerebrospinal fluid production. Science, *166*:1514, 1969.
32. Milhorat, T. H.: Failure of choroid plexectomy as treatment for hydrocephalus. Surg. Gynec. Obstet., *139*:505, 1974.
33. Milhorat, T. H., Clark, R. G., and Hammock, M. K.: Structural, ultrastructural, and permeability changes in the ependyma and surrounding brain favoring equilibration in progressive hydrocephalus. Arch. Neurol., *22*:397, 1970.
34. Milhorat, T. H., Hammock, M. K., and Chandra, R. S.: The subarachnoid space in congenital obstructive hydrocephalus. Part 2. Microscopic findings. J. Neurosurg., *35*:7, 1971.
35. Milhorat, T. H., Hammock, M. K., and Di Chiro, G.: The subarachnoid space in congenital obstructive hydrocephalus. Part 1. Cisternographic findings. J. Neurosurg., *35*:1, 1971.
36. Milhorat, T. H., Hammock, M. K., Chien, T., and Davis, D. A.: Normal rate of cerebrospinal fluid formation five years after bilateral choroid plexectomy. J. Neurosurg., *44*:735, 1976.
37. Milhorat, T. H., Hammock, M. K., Davis, D. A., and Fenstermacher, J. D.: Choroid plexus papilloma. Part 1. Proof of cerebrospinal fluid overproduction. Child's Brain, *2*:273, 1976.
38. Milhorat, T. H., Hammock, M. K., Fenstermacher, J. D., Rall, D. P., and Levin, V. A.:

Cerebrospinal fluid production by the choroid plexus and brain. Science, *173*:330, 1971.

39. Miller, E., and Sethi, L.: The effect of hydrocephalus on preception. Develop. Med. Child. Neurol., Suppl. *25*:77, 1971.

40. Moore, R. Y., Baumann, R. J.: Intracranial bruits in children. Develop. Med. Child. Neurol., *11*:650, 1969.

41. Naidich, T. P., Epstein, F., Lin, J. P., Kricheff, I. I., and Hochwald, G. M.: Evaluation of pediatric hydrocephalus by computed tomography. Radiology, *119*:337, 1976.

42. Nellhaus, G.: Head circumference from birth to eighteen years. Practical composite international and interracial graphs. Pediatrics, *41*:106, 1968.

43. Patterson, R. H., Jr., and Bergland, R. M.: The selection of patients for third ventriculostomy based on experience with thirty-three operations. J. Neurosurg., *29*:252, 1968.

44. Perrin, J. C., and McLaurin, R. L.: Infected ventriculo-atrial shunts. J. Neurosurg., *27*:21, 1967.

45. Ramondi, A. J.: Angiographic diagnosis of hydrocephalus in the newborn. J. Neurosurg., *31*:550, 1969.

46. Rubin, R. C.: The effect of severe hydrocephalus on size and number of brain cells. Develop. Med. Child. Neurol., Suppl. *27*:117, 1972.

47. Russel, D. S.: Observations on the Pathology of Hydrocephalus. (Special Report Series Medical Research Council, No. 265) London, Her Majesty's Stationery Office, 1949.

48. Schick, R. W., and Matson, D. D.: What is arrested hydrocephalus? J. Pediat., *58*:791, 1961.

49. Shallat, R. F., Pawl, R. P., and Jerva, M. J.: Significance of upward gaze palsy (Parinaud's syndrome) in hydrocephalus due to shunt malfunction. J. Neurosurg., *38*:717, 1973.

50. Shulman, K., Martin, B. F., Popoff, N., and Ransohoff, J.: Recognition and treatment of hydrocephalus following spontaneous subarachnoid hemorrhage. J. Neurosurg., *20*:1040, 1963.

51. Tindall, G. T., Payne, N. S., and O'Brien, M. S.: Complications of surgery for subdural hematoma. *In* Keener, E. B., ed.: Clinical Neurosurgery. Baltimore, Williams & Wilkins Co., 1976, p. 465.

52. Venes, J. L.: Control of shunt infection. Report of 150 consecutive cases. J. Neurosurg., *45*:311, 1976.

53. Week, L. H.: The Development of the cerebrospinal fluid spaces in pig and man. Carnegie Inst. Wash., Contribs. Embryol., *5*:1, 1917.

54. Welch, K.: Secretion of cerebrospinal fluid by choroid plexus of the rabbit. Amer. J. Physiol., *205*:617, 1963.

55. Welch, K., and Friedman, V.: The cerebrospinal fluid valves. Brain, *83*:454, 1960.

56. Williams, H. J.: Skull erosion complicating traumatic porencephaly in infancy. Amer. J. Roentgen., *106*:129, 1969.

57. Yakovlevpi, P. I.: Paraplegias of hydrocephalics. Amer. J. Ment. Defic., *51*:561, 1947.

37

HYDROCEPHALUS IN ADULTS

NORMAL-PRESSURE HYDROCEPHALUS

Normal-pressure hydrocephalus has been a well-recognized syndrome since the entity was first described.* Other terms such as "occult hydrocephalus," "low-pressure hydrocephalus," "normotensive hydrocephalus," and "hydrocephalic dementia" have been used, but "normal-pressure hydrocephalus" has emerged as the best descriptive term.

Symptoms include difficulty with gait, impairment of mentation, slowness of thought and action, and at times, incontinence. Change in mental function usually occurs with or after the onset of gait disturbance but may at times be the lone symptom. The cerebrospinal fluid pressure is normal (less than 180 mm of water) and radiographic studies, preferably computed tomography, show enlarged lateral ventricles.

Etiology and Pathology

Mechanisms causing development of this syndrome have not been fully defined. The underlying pathological process appears to be obstruction to the flow of cerebrospinal fluid. This may be due to obliteration of the subarachnoid pathways, usually at the base of the brain, which may follow meningitis or subarachnoid hemorrhage from aneurysm, vascular malformation, cerebral trauma, or intraspinal or intracranial operation (most frequently posterior fossa operation). The syndrome can also be produced by partial intraventricular obstruction due

to tumor or congenital anomaly such as aqueductal stenosis.[20]

The possible pathogenesis has been reviewed.[11] Under normal circumstances the brain acts like a sponge of viscoelastic material with a significant ability to "give" because of the venous capillaries, the extracellular space, and the lipids and proteins in the cerebral white matter. The pressure that controls the degree to which fluid may be displaced and the brain parenchyma compressed is the gradient between the intraventricular cerebrospinal fluid pressure and venous blood—the effective cerebrospinal fluid pressure. The normal effective cerebrospinal fluid pressure is lower than the bioelastic limit of the parenchyma, so it produces only a stress distribution within the cerebral tissue and does not squeeze out any liquid. Hydrocephalus is triggered by an initial increase in intraventricular pressure, raising the effective cerebrospinal fluid pressure, producing additional stress, and shifting fluid out of the cells. It is the periventricular region that receives the greatest stress, and as this area yields, the ventricles enlarge.

A reduction of cerebrospinal fluid pressure follows the reversal of one or more abnormal conditions: The resistance to flow may become reduced as some of the drainage pathways become unblocked or new pathways open up; cerebrospinal fluid production may be decreased; a deficient absorption mechanism may be improved. The inability of the dilated ventricles to return to normal size is due to the continuing increased force exerted on the walls. This force is directly proportional to the ventricular wall area and the intraventricular pressure. Therefore, even with the lowered pressure, the enlarged surface area main-

---

* See references 1, 7, 9, 10, 15, 20–22, 24.

R. G. OJEMANN AND P. M. BLACK

tains an increased force.[10] The continuing symptoms relate to the persistent abnormal stress on the brain parenchyma. In order to change the situation the intraventricular pressure must be further lowered.

Clinical Presentation

The syndrome is progressive, but the tempo of its evolution is highly variable. A history of fluctuating symptoms is not uncommon.[7] In some cases the syndrome may not develop until months or years after the etiological factor has arisen. Cardinal symptoms include disturbance of gait, which may be the first and remain the most prominent symptom. Impaired mentation, which on occasion may be the initial symptom, will more often appear with or follow the disturbance of gait. Some patients show slowness of both motor activity and thought processes. Urinary incontinence is a late symptom. Headache is not present. Abulia, seizures, and Parkinson-like symptoms have been described.[7,20,22,25]

On examination the extraocular movements are full, but nystagmus may be present. There are no focal signs unless there has been brain damage related to the disease process that has caused the hydrocephalus. A gait disturbance is usually found. Tone is usually normal. Limb movements may be slow. Plantar responses vary, and reflexes may be somewhat increased. Sucking and grasping reflexes appear in the late stages. There is no sensory loss.

Disturbance of Gait

Gait disorder, usually the first symptom, may precede the other problems by months or even years.[7] In some patients the changes in gait and mentation occur at about the same time, while occasionally difficulty in walking follows other symptoms.

The gait problem varies from mild imbalance to an inability to walk or even stand.[7,15] There is usually a history of one or more falls. The problem appears to be a matter of balance rather than weakness, spasticity, or sensory loss. There may be a slowness in correcting a potential instability, since progression of the symptom leads to immobility rather than to ataxia.[7]

Examination shows the steps to be shortened, the base widened. Balance is lost when turning. The patient is unable to do tandem walking and sways on the Romberg test. Cerebellar ataxia is not present.

Disturbance of Mentation

The disorder in mentation is often mild.[7,15] It ranges from inability to retain a fact for even a minute to a slight limitation revealed only by detailed testing.[7] The most frequent alteration is impairment of memory. The patient often appears to be slowing up. Spontaneity and initiative are decreased, and interest in conversation, reading, writing, hobbies, and recreational activities declines. The family may report unconcern, apathy, lethargy, or the appearance of being withdrawn. Tests show that tasks are performed more slowly; attention and concentration are impaired. This complex of abnormalities has been termed the "abulic trait" by Fisher.[7]

The Wechsler-Bellevue test will show that in symptomatic hydrocephalus the verbal performance is relatively preserved while nonverbal performance (drawing, copying, arranging blocks, puzzle assembly, digit symbol, and picture story arrangement) is more impaired.[7] Dyscalculia is usually present. As symptoms progress the patient's responses become slower to the point at which there may be no response to questions. Spontaneity is absent. If there is response to a question, it may be brief and only a partial answer. Voluntary movements are slow and delayed. In a few advanced cases, agitation and more complex disturbances in mental function may appear. Only in a small percentage of cases are aberrant behavior, delusions, hallucinations, paranoia, and irrational speech part of the clinical picture.[5,7,20,22]

In an occasional patient, the presenting picture may be that of slowness both of motor activity and thought processes, often with rigidity and tremor and at times profound lethargy that leads to the diagnosis of parkinsonism.[20,22,25]

Incontinence

Urinary incontinence develops in some patients as the illness progresses. In a few patients the incontinence is characterized as an urgency, but in most it is of frontal lobe type in which appropriate concern is diminished or lacking. Incontinence of bowels is rare.

Diagnostic Tests

Computed Tomography

The use of computed tomography (the CT scan) has been a major advance in the evaluation of patients suspected of having normal-pressure hydrocephalus. This test gives an accurate assessment of the ventricular size, the extent of cortical atrophy, and the presence of localized pathologic changes that may account for the hydrocephalic syndrome. The typical computed tomographic scan in normal-pressure hydrocephalus shows marked enlargement of the ventricles but little or no evidence of atrophy (Figs. 37–1A and B, and 37–2A). Postoperatively, ventricular size can be easily measured, as shown in Figure 37–1C and D, and the presence of subdural hematoma or hygroma can be evaluated (Figs. 37–3B and 37–4A and B). The noninvasive nature of this study obviates the worsening of symptoms following pneumoencephalography. It also gives a more accurate assess-

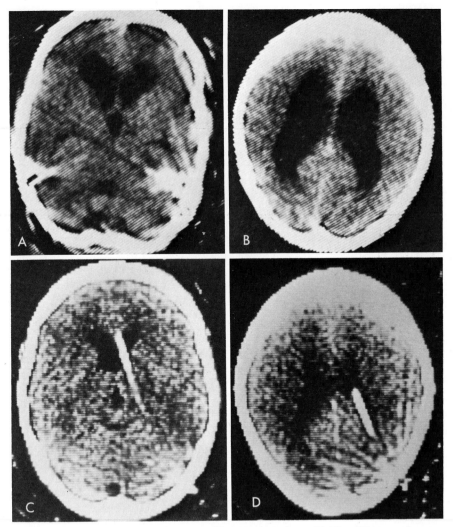

Figure 37–1 A and B. Initial computed tomographic scans in patient with idiopathic normal-pressure hydrocephalus. Gait disorder was the initial and prominent symptom and was associated with mild impairment of memory. The ventricles are large and there is no atrophy. C and D. Postoperative scans showing reduction in ventricular size. Catheter was placed in frontal horn of lateral ventricle from occipital burr hole. Nearly complete recovery from symptoms occurred.

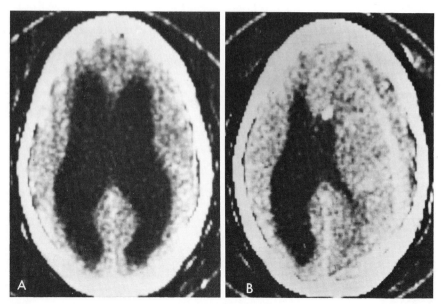

Figure 37–2 *A*. Initial computed tomographic scan in patient with idiopathic normal-pressure hydrocephalus. *B*. Scan done on third postoperative day when drowsiness and mild left hemiparesis were noted. Subdural mass with density similar to brain but with a high-density inner margin was present. Lateral ventricles were shifted and compressed. Subdural hematoma was removed. Shunt reopened one month later with good improvement in symptoms.

ment of the degree of atrophy than the pneumoencephalogram.[13,15]

No firm correlation has been found between the presence or absence of cortical atrophy with large ventricles on computed tomography and the response to operation.[13,15] Reduction in cerebrospinal fluid pressure is not likely to help the patient with cortical atrophy and only moderately enlarged ventricles (Fig. 37–4).

Lumbar Puncture

Careful measurement of the cerebrospinal fluid pressure in the lateral recumbent position reveals a value of less than 180 mm of water. Protein and sugar levels are normal unless altered by the disease process causing the hydrocephalus. Improvement in symptoms after lumbar puncture and removal of cerebrospinal fluid can be striking and is a good prognostic sign.[7,10,24] Failure to improve does not exclude the diagnosis, however, since prolonged sustained reduction in pressure may be required before improvement is seen.

Continuous Pressure Monitoring

Using extradural pressure measurements over a 24-hour period, Symon and Hinz-

peter have been able to separate patients suspected of having normal-pressure hydrocephalus into two groups on the basis of pressure variations during the hours of sleep.[24] In the abnormal group, periods of sustained levels of pressure over 20 mm of mercury with recurrent peak pressures over 53 mm of mercury were seen. In the other group, the intermittent sustained levels of pressure never exceeded 16 mm of mercury and the peak pressures were never over 23 mm of mercury. It was found that two thirds of 30 patients in the abnormal group improved after operation. In another study, none of the seven patients with normal pressure recordings improved with shunting.[4]

Pneumoencephalography

This study is not needed if computed tomography is available. Enlarged lateral ventricles are seen, and the span of the frontal horns is usually greater than 60 mm on the anteroposterior brow-up projection. In typical cases there is complete obstruction of the passage of air through the basal cisterns, but on occasion some air will enter the convexity subarachnoid space.

In idiopathic normal-pressure hydrocephalus cases it has not been possible to

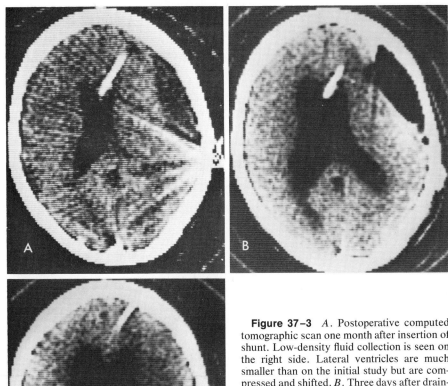

Figure 37–3 *A*. Postoperative computed tomographic scan one month after insertion of shunt. Low-density fluid collection is seen on the right side. Lateral ventricles are much smaller than on the initial study but are compressed and shifted. *B*. Three days after drainage of subdural hygroma and ligation of shunt, the ventricles have enlarged but are still shifted. The density reading in the right subdural space is consistent with air. *C*. One month after scan in *B*. No operative procedure was done in the interim. The brain has re-expanded. The shunt subsequently reopened with no complication.

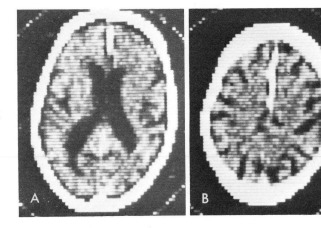

Figure 37–4 Computed tomographic scan in a patient presenting with marked disturbance in mentation but no gait abnormality. Ventricular enlargement is moderate, but marked atrophy is present.

correlate any feature of the pneumoencephalogram with success or failure of the shunt operation.[23] Certain findings, however, may give some indication of the outcome. If the maximum width of the frontal horns is 60 mm or more and little or no air appears in the cerebral sulci, there is more apt to be a good response to treatment, but in some instances, patients with no response may also have these features.[3] Deterioration in neurological symptoms and signs occurs in some patients after pneumoencephalography and it helps to confirm the diagnosis, but an absence of worsening of the patient's condition does not exclude the syndrome.[3,24]

Isotope Cisternography

The most commonly used isotope has been [131]iodine-labeled human serum albumin.[8,17,24] The authors use [111]indium diethyl triamine pentacetic acid (DTPA). A dose of 500 mc is injected into the lumbar subarachnoid space. Scans are made at 4, 24, and 48 hours.

The classification of different flow patterns has been described.[8,24] Clearly abnormal studies with prolonged ventricular retention of the isotope and slight or delayed flow over the cerebral convexity are associated with improvement following shunting in only half to two thirds of the cases with this finding.[3,15] Patients with normal studies, little or no ventricular filling, and flow over the cerebral convexities usually do not respond to operation. Many studies in both the groups of patients who improve with shunts and the groups who do not improve are equivocal.[3,24] The relation of the findings on the scans to the response to shunting is so variable that this test is not of significant help in definitive evaluation of patients with normal-pressure hydrocephalus.[3,23,24]

Other Tests

Skull films are usually normal and show no evidence of chronic increased intracranial pressure.

The cerebrospinal fluid absorption test utilizes a technique in which a constant infusion of saline is given into the lumbar subarachnoid space at a specific rate.[14] The pressure response is recorded. Experience with this test has shown variable correlation with the results of shunting.[3,23,24]

The measurement of transport of radioactive indicators from the cerebrospinal fluid to the plasma as an index of delay in absorption has been reviewed.[24] Definite correlation with the results of shunting has not been studied.

Regional cerebral blood flow measurements have shown that cerebrospinal fluid drainage increased blood flow in patients with hydrocephalus, but the same finding was noted in patients with dementia of other types.[12]

With the use of computed tomography, angiography is no longer needed to determine ventricular size.

Evaluation of the electroencephalogram has shown that there is no type of tracing that is of value in making the diagnosis or predicting the outcome of operation. Little change is seen in studies done on patients who have had good results from operation.[15]

Selection of Patients for Operative Treatment

Idiopathic Hydrocephalus

Numerous studies have attempted to define the criteria, particularly in idiopathic cases, that would indicate which patient would respond to placement of a shunt. In spite of initial enthusiastic reports on a number of tests, no combination of studies has been found to correlate with the results of shunting.[15,23] The clinical presentation remains the most reliable prognostic indicator.[7,24] When enlarged lateral ventricles, demonstrated by computed tomography, are associated with a disturbance in gait alone or in combination with a disturbance in mentation, there is good chance of improvement with a shunt. When impairment of mentation is the initial symptom, the chances of improvement are much less.

Evidence for these conclusions has come from several clinical investigations: Some degree of gait disorder was an early symptom in 15 of 16 patients who improved after a shunting procedure.[7] The only clinical feature in these patients that indicated a favorable prognosis was a predominance of the gait disturbance.[3] The patients with idiopathic hydrocephalus who tended to return to normal function after operation were those in whom the intellectual deterioration was relatively mild and the gait disturbance was a prominent and early sign.[24] The poorest response to shunting occurred in patients who presented with dementia.[15] Of 16 cases that were benefited by shunting, only one showed impairment of mentation prior to the gait disturbance, while in 9 of 11 that did not improve, dementia came first.[7]

The differential diagnosis is primarily concerned with distinction from Alzheimer's or degenerative disease and is based to a great extent on clinical evaluation. The problem usually develops slowly over several years in patients with degenerative disease. The principal symptom is loss of memory, to which are later added defects in speech and thinking. Slowing of mental and physical activity is rarely an early manifestation. The hydrocephalic disturbance of gait is not seen.[7] Computed tomography will show some ventricular enlargement but usually not the massive enlargement seen in the typical case of normal-pressure hydrocephalus. There may be marked widening of the cerebral sulci.

One may encounter patients in whom the diagnosis remains in doubt in spite of the clinical and radiographic studies. Some of these patients seem to have problems with both normal-pressure hydrocephalus and cerebral degenerative disease. They may respond well to shunt for a period of time and then resume a downhill course in spite of smaller ventricles and a lower cerebrospinal fluid pressure shown on repeated studies.[20]

Subarachnoid Hemorrhage

Enlargement of the ventricular system has been reported in 40 to 50 per cent of patients following subarachnoid hemorrhage.[6] Initially there may be a temporary increase in cerebrospinal fluid pressure, but in most cases symptoms of hydrocephalus develop when the pressure has returned to a normal level. Frequently there is delay in the onset of one to several weeks after the hemorrhage. Dementia with severe impairment of memory and slowness of thought and movement may be the most prominent symptom. Gait disorder may not be brought to the examiner's attention, as most patients are confined to bed.[24] Computed tomography shows persistently enlarged ventricles. Not all patients with enlarged ventricles develop related neurological symptoms, and in some who do, spontaneous improvement occurs. If symptoms persist, the response to placement of a shunt is usually good.

Trauma

The natural history of patients who develop large ventricles after head trauma has not been fully studied. In many cases it is difficult to separate the direct effects of the brain injury from those secondary to obstruction of cerebrospinal fluid flow. The mechanism for development of hydrocephalus is thought to be scarring and obstruction of the basal cisterns from subarachnoid hemorrhage. On rare occasion there may be obstruction of a major venous sinus or a block in the third ventricle or the aqueduct. As with spontaneous subarachnoid hemorrhage, symptoms may be associated with mildly elevated or normal cerebrospinal fluid pressure. The onset of disturbance of mentation or a disorder of gait may be delayed for several weeks or even months after the trauma. In these circumstances, improvement after insertion of a shunt can be striking. In cases in which enlarged ventricles are associated with failure to recover fully after a serious head injury, results are variable, probably owing to underlying brain damage.[16,20]

Meningitis

On rare occasions obliteration of the subarachnoid space develops following meningitis. Symptoms of normal-pressure hydrocephalus may be noted early in the illness, but they may not present for several months. A shunt is indicated if spontaneous recovery does not occur.[20]

Intracranial Tumors

Enlarged ventricles associated with partial obstruction of the cerebrospinal fluid pathways by a brain tumor may produce symptoms of normal-pressure hydrocephalus. This phenomenon has been caused by colloid cyst of the third ventricle, craniopharyngioma, pineal region tumor, acoustic neuroma, and other cerebellopontine angle tumors. The cerebrospinal fluid pressure is normal, and often there are no other symptoms of the tumor itself.[20] Preoperative or preradiation insertion of a shunt is indicated in many of these patients.

Several days or weeks after intracranial operation, particularly a posterior fossa exploration, symptoms of normal-pressure hydrocephalus may develop. The CT scan will show enlarged ventricles. If the symptoms do not improve spontaneously over a short period of time, a shunt is indicated.

Aqueduct Stenosis

Symptoms related to hydrocephalus secondary to aqueduct stenosis may not occur until adult life. The majority of patients present with symptoms and signs of increased intracranial pressure, but the syndrome of normal-pressure hydrocephalus may also be seen.[2,20]

Operative Treatment

Either a ventriculovenous or a ventriculoperitoneal shunt may be utilized. In general, the ventriculovenous shunt is preferable. It functions for indefinite periods of time and is relatively free of complication in adults. The type of shunt utilized does not seem to influence the results of operative treatment.[15]

After induction of general anesthesia, the right side of the head and neck, and—when a ventriculoperitoneal shunt is to be inserted—the anterior chest and abdomen are prepared. An adherent drape is utilized so that no skin is directly exposed. The authors usually use a medium-pressure Hakim

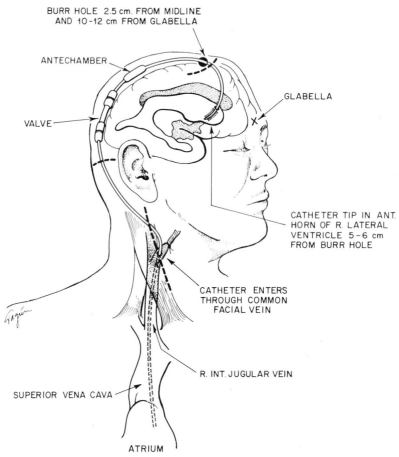

BURR HOLE 2.5 cm. FROM MIDLINE AND 10-12 cm FROM GLABELLA

ANTECHAMBER

GLABELLA

VALVE

CATHETER TIP IN ANT. HORN OF R. LATERAL VENTRICLE 5-6 cm FROM BURR HOLE

CATHETER ENTERS THROUGH COMMON FACIAL VEIN

R. INT. JUGULAR VEIN

SUPERIOR VENA CAVA

ATRIUM

Figure 37–5 Placement of ventriculovenous shunt in the adult via a frontal burr hole. The burr hole is usually on the right side and is placed behind the anterior hairline, 10 to 12 cm from the glabella and 2.5 to 3.0 cm from the midline. The landmarks for insertion are the inner canthus of the eye in the frontal plane and a point just in front of the external auditory meatus in the lateral plane. The catheter should lie at a depth of 5 to 6 cm from the external table of the skull. The neck incision is made in a skin crease and centered over the upper portion of the sternocleidomastoid muscle. Usually the catheter can be inserted through the common facial vein. The position of the distal end of the catheter is checked by x-ray; it should be at the level of the sixth or seventh thoracic vertebra.

valve (60 to 80 mm of water).[19] The Hakim brush ventricular catheter may be inserted through either a frontal or an occipital burr hole. After the burr hole is made, the dura and underlying pia-arachnoid are opened by coagulation. The ventricle is first tapped with a small ventricular needle. If a frontal burr hole is used, it is placed behind the anterior hairline, 10 to 12 cm from the glabella and 2.5 to 3 cm from the midline (Fig. 37–5). The landmarks for insertion are the inner canthus of the eye in the frontal plane and a point just in front of the external auditory meatus in the lateral plane. The catheter should lie at a depth of 5 to 6 cm from the external table of the skull. If an occipital burr hole is utilized, the burr hole is placed approximately 6 cm above and 3 cm to the right of the external occipital protuberance (Fig. 37–6). The ventricular cath-

eter is carefully advanced into the lateral ventricle to the frontal horn while cerebrospinal fluid flow is observed. Insertion of the catheter to a depth of 11 to 12 cm will place the tip in the proper position in the frontal horn. Once the catheter has been inserted, the valve system with reservoir is attached and brought through a subgaleal tunnel to the neck incision.

For a ventriculovenous shunt, an incision is made over the upper portion of the anterior border of the sternocleidomastoid muscle (see Fig. 37–5). The common facial vein is identified and ligated, and the cardiac cathether from the Hakim valve set is inserted through this vein and into the internal jugular vein for a distance of 20 to 25 cm. The catheter is filled with a radiopaque substance, and an x-ray is taken to verify that the tip of the catheter is positioned

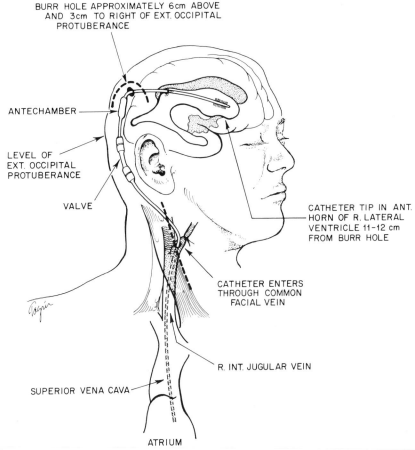

BURR HOLE APPROXIMATELY 6cm ABOVE AND 3cm TO RIGHT OF EXT. OCCIPITAL PROTUBERANCE

ANTECHAMBER

LEVEL OF EXT. OCCIPITAL PROTUBERANCE

VALVE

CATHETER TIP IN ANT. HORN OF R. LATERAL VENTRICLE 11–12 cm FROM BURR HOLE

CATHETER ENTERS THROUGH COMMON FACIAL VEIN

R. INT. JUGULAR VEIN

SUPERIOR VENA CAVA

ATRIUM

Figure 37–6 Placement of ventriculovenous shunt in the adult via an occipital burr hole. The burr hole is usually placed 6 cm above and 3 cm to the right of the external occipital protuberance. The ventricular catheter is advanced into the frontal horn of the lateral ventricle, the glabella being used as a landmark. The tip of the catheter will be 11 to 12 cm from the external table of the skull. Placement of the catheter in the neck is as shown in Figure 37–5.

at about the level of the sixth thoracic vertebra.

For a ventriculoperitoneal shunt, a midline incision is made above the umbilicus (Fig. 37–7). A right rectus muscle–splitting incision may be used. A small opening is carefully made in the peritoneum. The peritoneal catheter is inserted for a distance of at least 18 to 20 cm. The flow in this catheter is checked before final connection of the system. The catheter should be anchored at the peritoneal level and then

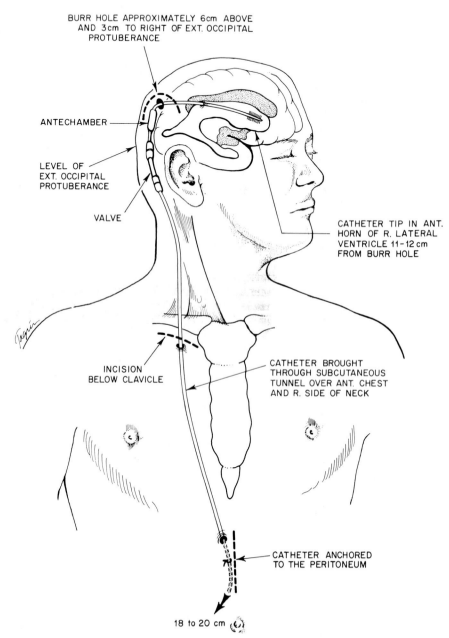

BURR HOLE APPROXIMATELY 6cm ABOVE AND 3cm TO RIGHT OF EXT. OCCIPITAL PROTUBERANCE

ANTECHAMBER

LEVEL OF EXT. OCCIPITAL PROTUBERANCE

VALVE

CATHETER TIP IN ANT. HORN OF R. LATERAL VENTRICLE 11–12 cm FROM BURR HOLE

INCISION BELOW CLAVICLE

CATHETER BROUGHT THROUGH SUBCUTANEOUS TUNNEL OVER ANT. CHEST AND R. SIDE OF NECK

CATHETER ANCHORED TO THE PERITONEUM

18 to 20 cm

Figure 37–7   Placement of ventriculoperitoneal shunt in the adult via an occipital burr hole as depicted in Figure 37–6. Usually a midline incision is made above the umbilicus. The peritoneal catheter is inserted for a distance of at least 18 to 20 cm. It is anchored at the peritoneum and placed in a subcutaneous tunnel over the anterior chest and the right side of the neck.

brought through a subcutaneous tunnel over the anterior chest and right side of the neck. An incision just below the clavicle aids in this placement.

Postoperative Evaluation

Following insertion of a functioning shunt, improvement in both gait and mentation may often be noted almost immediately or within a few days. On occasion a more gradual recovery occurs over several days to weeks. Sustained clinical improvement is the best indication of adequate shunt function. If improvement does not occur or symptoms regress, the function of the shunt is assessed by repeating computed tomography for ventricular size and the lumbar puncture for measurement of pressure. In functioning shunt systems, the cerebrospinal fluid pressure will be less than 80 mm of water, and frequently it will approach zero.[20,24] The CT scan usually will show a decrease in ventricular size (see Fig. 37–1C and D). In patients with conditions known to cause normal-pressure hydrocephalus, the ventricles may appear entirely normal. In idiopathic cases the ventricles are often significantly reduced in size, but they may remain somewhat enlarged. On occasion, no change in ventricular size is seen even when the patient's symptoms have improved and the cerebrospinal fluid pressure is low.[15]

Serious postoperative complications may occur, but the incidence is low. These include infection, shunt malfunction, intracerebral hematoma, subdural hematoma, subdural hygroma, and seizures. Infection remains an inherent problem but fortunately it is infrequent in adults. The authors have not used prophylactic antibiotics. Shunt malfunction is usually manifested by recurrence of symptoms. The onset of a focal neurological deficit or a deteriorating state of consciousness indicates the possibility of a subdural hematoma or hygroma. A CT scan is done (see Figs. 37–3B and 37–4A and B). The lesion must be removed or drained and the shunt temporarily occluded. After four to six weeks a repeat scan is done, and if the ventricles are again enlarged and there is no subdural collection, the shunt is reopened (see Fig. 37–4C). Seizure disorders following insertion of a shunt are infrequent.

HIGH-PRESSURE HYDROCEPHALUS

Etiology and Pathology

High-pressure hydrocephalus in the adult is caused by obstruction of the flow of cerebrospinal fluid through the ventricular system or in the subarachnoid pathways. The lateral ventricles may be selectively obstructed by tumors arising within their cavities, which include choroid plexus papilloma, ependymoma, subependymal giant cell astrocytoma, infiltrating glioma, metastatic tumor, and meningioma.[18]

Obstruction of the third ventricle can be caused by intraventricular tumors (colloid cyst, infiltrating astrocytoma, ependymoma, choroid plexus papilloma, and meningioma); compression of the posterior aspect of the ventricle (pineal region tumor); or compression from inferiorly (craniopharyngioma, pituitary adenoma, ectopic pinealoma, hypothalamic and optic nerve glioma, chordoma, hamartoma, tuberculum sellae meningioma, and metastatic tumor.)[18]

Intrinsic tumors in the aqueduct are rare and are usually ependymoma or astrocytoma. Tumors occurring within the fourth ventricle include ependymoma, medulloblastoma, choroid plexus papilloma, and epidermoid. Extrinsic compression of the fourth ventricle and aqueduct can be found with medulloblastoma, tumor of the cerebellar hemisphere (astrocytoma, hemangioblastoma, metastasis), and lesions of the cerebellopontine angle.[18]

Nonneoplastic masses such as benign cyst, abscess, parasitic cyst, and hematoma may produce obstruction of cerebrospinal fluid flow.

Primary obstruction in the subarachnoid pathways may be seen with any of the tumors occurring outside the ventricular system or following meningitis, subarachnoid hemorrhage, or severe head trauma.

Hydrocephalus due to congenital stricture of the aqueduct of Sylvius may be asymptomatic until adult life. Approximately two thirds of these patients will present with evidence of increased intracranial pressure.[2]

Clinical Presentation

In many patients with the pathologic conditions just noted, the only symptoms will be those of the high-pressure hydrocephalus. They include headache, which tends initially to be bifrontal, is usually worse in the morning, and may be relieved by lying down. As symptoms progress, the headache may awaken the patient at night and become generalized and continuous. Neck pain may develop and is of concern because of the possibility of protrusion of the cerebellar tonsils into the foramen magnum. There may be vomiting, disturbance of vision, incontinence, and impairment in mental and motor performance.[18]

On examination, language ability is usually retained, but recent memory may be impaired and intellectual performance slowed. As the condition progresses, there may be increasing confusion. Papilledema is common and may be accompanied by enlargement of the blind spot, reduction in visual acuity, and constriction of the peripheral visual field. In chronic problems, the optic disc may be pale. Unilateral or bilateral sixth nerve palsy is a common but nonlocalizing sign. Other cranial nerve findings such as paresis of upward gaze and visual field defects may help with localization. Disturbance of gait is common but nonlocalizing and may be due to ataxia or spastic paraparesis. Unilateral cerebellar or motor signs may suggest the location of the disorder. The deep tendon reflex may be generally increased, and the plantar responses are often extensor.

Diagnostic Tests

Skull X-Rays

Nonspecific changes due to increased intracranial pressure may be seen with demineralization or erosion of the dorsum sellae and posterior clinoids. Examination for abnormal calcification, location of the pineal body, and congenital abnormalities of the skull should be done.

Computed Tomography

This has become the most important test in the evaluation of patients with increased intracranial pressure. Not only is the size of the ventricular system evaluated, but with contrast enhancement, the cause of the hydrocephalus may be defined. The use of other radiographic diagnostic tests such as angiography and encephalography is based on the results of the computed tomographic study. In many patients no test other than the CT scan is needed.

The initial clinical presentation of any patient with a disease process causing increased intracranial pressure without hydrocephalus, such as pseudotumor or a mass lesion, may be indistinguishable from that of a patient with hydrocephalus. Computed tomography has provided an effective method for separating these problems.

Treatment

Some patients with focal mass lesions and hydrocephalus with increased intracranial pressure should be treated initially with a shunt procedure. Substantial relief of the increased intracranial pressure may reduce the morbidity and increase the ability to deal with the primary disease at a subsequent operation. Any patient with high-pressure hydrocephalus who is having an operation directly on the primary abnormality should be treated with steroids for at least 48 hours prior to operation.

REFERENCES

1. Adams, R. D., Fisher, C. M., Hakim, S., Ojemann, R. G., and Sweet, W. H.: Symptomatic occult hydrocephalus with "normal" cerebrospinal fluid pressure: A treatable syndrome. New Eng. J. Med., 273:117–126, 1965.
2. Balakrishnan, V., and Dinning, T. A. R.: Nonneoplastic stenosis of the aqueduct presenting in adolescence and adult life. Surg. Neurol., 7:333–338, 1977.
3. Black, P. M., and Sweet, W. H.: Normal pressure hydrocephalus—idiopathic type. Selection of patients for shunt procedures. In Advances in Neurosurgery. Vol. 4. New York, Springer-Verlag, 1977, pp. 106–114.
4. Chawla, J. C., Hulme, A., and Cooper, R.: Intracranial pressure in patients with dementia and communicating hydrocephalus. J. Neurosurg., 40:376–380, 1974.
5. Crowell, R. M., Tew, J. M., Jr., and Mark, V. H.: Aggressive dementia associated with normal

pressure hydrocephalus. Report of two unusual cases. Neurology (Minneap.), *23*:461–464, 1973.

6. Davis, K. R., New, P. F., Ojemann, R. G., Crowell, R. M., and Morawetz, R. B.: Computed tomographic evaluation of hemorrhage secondary to intracranial aneurysm. Amer. J. Roentgen., *127*:143–153, 1976.

7. Fisher, C. M.: The clinical picture in occult hydrocephalus. Clin. Neurosurg., *24*:270–284, 1977.

8. Fleming, I. F. R., Sheppard, R. H., and Turner, V.: CSF scanning in the evaluation of hydrocephalus: A clinical review of 100 patients. *In* Cisternography and Hydrocephalus. A Symposium. Springfield, Ill., Charles C Thomas, 1972, pp. 261–284.

9. Hakim, S.: Algunas observaciones sobre la presion del L. C. R. sindrome hidrocefhlico en al adulto con presion normal del L. C. R. (Prestation de un nuevo sindrome) (Teses de grado). Faculdad de Medicina, Universidad Javeriana. Bogotá, Colombia, 1964.

10. Hakim, S., and Adams, R. D.: The special clinical problem of symptomatic hydrocephalus with normal cerebrospinal fluid pressure: Observations on cerebrospinal fluid hydrodynamics. J. Neurol. Sci., *2*:307–327, 1965.

11. Hakim, S., Venegas, J. A., and Burton, J. D.: The physics of the cranial cavity, hydrocephalus and normal pressure hydrocephalus: Mechanical interpretation and mathematical model. Surg. Neurol., *5*:187–210, 1976.

12. Hartmann, A., Alberti, E., and Lange, D.: Cerebral blood flow and cerebrospinal fluid pressure in patients with communicating hydrocephalus. *In* Advances of Neurosurgery. Volume 4. New York, Springer-Verlag, 1977, pp. 144–155.

13. Jacobs, L., and Kinkel, W.: Computerized axial transverse tomography in normal pressure hydrocephalus. Neurology (Minneap.), *26*:501–507, 1976.

14. Katzman, R., and Hussey, F.: A simple constant-infusion manometric test for measurement of CSF absorption. I. Rationale and method. Neurology (Minneap.), *20*:534–544, 1970.

15. Laws, E., and Mokri, B.: Occult Hydrocephalus: Results of shunting correlated with diagnostic tests. Clin. Neurosurg., *24*:316–333, 1977.

16. Lewin, W.: Preliminary observations on external hydrocephalus after severe head injury. Brit. J. Surg., *55*:747–751, 1969.

17. McCullough, D. C., Harbert, J. D., DiChiro, G., and Ommaya, A. K.: Prognostic criteria for cerebrospinal fluid shunting from isotope cisternography in communicating hydrocephalus. Neurology (Minneap.), *20*:594–598, 1970.

18. Milhorat, T. H.: Hydrocephalus and the cerebrospinal fluid. Baltimore, William & Wilkins Co., 1972, pp. 89–96 and 148–152.

19. Ojemann, R. G.: Initial experience with the Hakim valve for ventriculovenous shunts. Technical note. J. Neurosurg., *28*:283–287, 1968.

20. Ojemann, R. G.: Normal pressure hydrocephalus. Clin. Neurosurg., *18*:337–370, 1972.

21. Ojemann, R. G.: Normal pressure hydrocephalus. *In* Critchley, M., O'Leary, F. L., and Jennett, B., eds.: Scientific Foundation of Neurology. London, W. Heinemann Medical Books Ltd., 1972, pp. 302–308.

22. Ojemann, R. G., Fisher, C. M., Adams, R. D., Sweet, W. H., and New, P. F. J.: Further experience with the syndrome of "normal" pressure hydrocephalus. J. Neurosurg., *31*:279–294, 1969.

23. Stein, S. C., and Langfitt, T. W.: Normal-pressure hydrocephalus. Predicting the results of cerebrospinal fluid shunting. J. Neurosurg., *41*:463–470, 1974.

24. Symon, L., and Hinzpeter, T.: The engima of normal pressure hydrocephalus—tests to select patients for surgery and to predict shunt function. Clin. Neurosurg., *24*:285–315, 1977.

25. Sypert, G. W., Leffman, H., and Ojemann, G. A.: Occult normal pressure hydrocephalus manifested by Parkinsonism-dementia complex. Neurology (Minneap.), *23*:234–238, 1973.

Since this manuscript was written, the following papers of importance in adult hydrocephalus have appeared.

1. Black, P. McL.: Idiopathic normal pressure hydrocephalus: Results of shunting in 62 patients. J. Neurosurg., *52*:371–377, 1980.

2. Borgesen, S. E., Gjerris, F., Sorensen, S. C.: Intracranial pressure and conductance to outflow of cerebrospinal fluid in normal-pressure hydrocephalus. J. Neurosurg., *50*:484–493, 1979.

3. DiRocco, C., DiTrapani, G., Maira, G., Bentoviglio, M., Mocchi, G., and Rossi, G. F.: Anatomico-clinical correlations in normotensive hydrocephalus. J. Neurol. Sci., *33*: 437–452, 1977.

4. Greenberg, J. O., Shenkin, H. A., and Adam, R.: Idiopathic normal-pressure hydrocephalus: A report of 73 patients. J. Neurol. Neurosurg. Psychiat., *40*:336–341, 1977.

5. Hughes, C. P., Siegel, B. A., Coxe, W. S., Gado, M. H., Grubb, R. L., Coleman, R. E., and Berg, L.: Adult idiopathic commuinicating hydrocephalus with and without shunting. J. Neurol. Neurosurg. Psychiat., *41*:961–71, 1978.

6. Jensen, F.: Acquired hydrocephalus. Acta Neurochir. (Wien), *47*:91–104, 1979.

7. Lamas, E., and Lobato, R. D.: Intraventricular pressure and CSF dynamics in chronic adult hydrocephalus, Surg. Neurol., *12*:287–295, 1979.

8. Palma A., Kolberg T., Wüst, R., and Entzian, W.: New aspects of cerebrospinal fluid dynamics in humans investigated by sequential gamma-camera cisternography, with data evaluation by the digital multichannel analyzer. Acta Neurochir. (Wien), *45*:53–88, 1978.

9. Vassilouthis, J., and Richardson, A. E.: Ventricular dilatation and communicating hydrocephalus following spontaneous subarachnoid hemorrhage. J. Neurosurg., *51*:341–351, 1979.

10. Wenig, C., Huber, G., and Emde, H.: Hydrocephalus after subarachnoid bleeding. A correlation of clinical findings, the results of radioisotope cisternography and computer assisted tomography. Eur. Neurol., *18*:1–7, 1979.

38

ARACHNOID CYSTS

Arachnoid cysts are benign cysts that occur throughout the cerebrospinal axis in relation to the arachnoid membrane and the subarachnoid spaces.[44] The synonymous term "leptomeningeal cyst" is not preferred because the word "leptomeninges" refers to both pia and arachnoid; since the pia mater is not involved in the pathogenesis of these cysts, the term "arachnoid cyst" is more specific.

In the current literature, the term "arachnoid cyst" is used when the lesion has no communication with the subarachnoid pathways; when it is in communication with subarachnoid pathways various terms such as "arachnoid diverticulum," "arachnoid hernia," "arachnoid pouch," "internal meningocele," and "arachnoidocele" are used. This terminology is confusing. Simpler—and unifying—terms are "communicating" and "noncommunicating" arachnoid cysts. The distinction between them, however, loses significance in symptomatic cases, because even the communicating arachnoid cysts progressively enlarge and cause compression of the underlying neural tissue. This enlargement occurs because the communication between the cyst and the subarachnoid pathways is almost always small and valvular. The communication is demonstrated by the entry of air, Pantopaque, radioisotope, or other contrast material into the cyst during neurodiagnostic work-up. Arachnoid cysts produce symptoms purely by mechanical compression. Because the majority of them are surface lesions, the compression is felt by both the neural tissue and the bone encasing it. Bony changes may be noticeable on inspection of the calvarium or may be detected by radiological examination of the skull and spine. The cysts are usually filled with clear spinal fluid although occasionally xanthochromic fluid of high protein content may be found, particularly in the noncommunicating cysts. Without exception, all intracranial congenital arachnoid cysts are located intradurally. They are distributed in close association with the subarachnoid cisterns, whereas the majority of spinal arachnoid cysts are located extradurally.

DIFFERENTIATION FROM OTHER BENIGN CYSTS

Porencephaly

This term implies primary loss of brain tissue and its replacement by a fluid-filled cavity, either from congenital failure of development or as a result of acquired conditions like vascular infarction. The cyst communicates freely with the ventricular system or the subarachnoid space.

Ependymal Cysts

Benign epithelial cysts that occur either intracranially or within the spinal canal, ependymal cysts differ in several respects from arachnoid cysts.[9,35] They are rare; fewer than 20 cases of histologically documented supratentorial ependymal cysts have been reported to this date.[18] They occupy the central white matter of the frontal or temporoparietal lobes, causing progressive neurological deficit referable to these lobes along with increased intracranial pressure and seizures. The protein content of the cyst fluid is generally greater than that of spinal fluid. The wall is lined by columnar or cuboidal cells with or without cilia. Blepharoblasts may or may not be identi-

C. E. BRACKETT and S. S. RENGACHARY

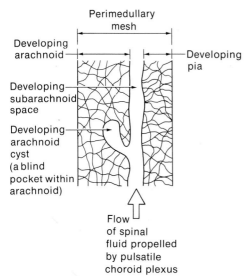

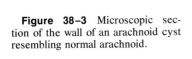

Figure 38–1 Hypothesized development of leptomeninges, the subarachnoid space, and an arachnoid cyst.

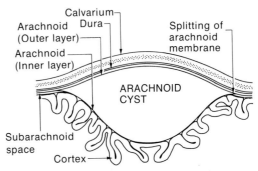

Figure 38–2 Diagrammatic cross section of an arachnoid cyst showing the splitting of the arachnoid membrane at the margin of the cyst.

fiable. These cysts never communicate with the ventricular system, but in rare instances may lie in the subarachnoid space.[24,38] They are believed to arise from sequestration of a small segment of primitive neural tube into the cortical mantle. Treatment consists of drainage of the cyst and excision of the cyst wall.

PATHOGENESIS AND DISTRIBUTION OF ARACHNOID CYSTS

In the developing embryo, the loose mesenchymal tissue around the nervous system known as "perimedullary mesh" differentiates to form the pia and arachnoid.[48] The pulsatile force of the choroid plexus exerts a pumping action on the spinal fluid, which establishes communication between the ventricular system and the subarachnoid pathways.[8] Dissection then occurs in the perimedullary mesh, and the subarachnoid spaces around the brain and spinal cord are thus established. It is postulated that arachnoid cysts develop because of a minor aberration in the flow of cerebrospinal fluid during the earliest stages of embryological development of the arachnoid pathways, resulting in sequestration of an enclosed chamber or diverticulum within the perimedullary mesh (Fig. 38–1).

Detailed pathological study of the cyst in its various parts from autopsy specimens shows that the cysts are intra-arachnoid in location (Fig. 38–2).[19,48] At the margin of the cyst the arachnoid splits into two layers, enclosing the cyst. Both the inner

Figure 38–3 Microscopic section of the wall of an arachnoid cyst resembling normal arachnoid.

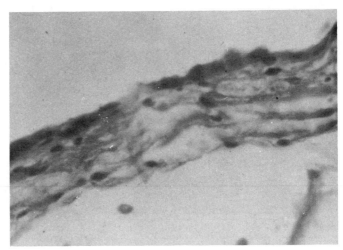

and outer layers histologically resemble normal arachnoid tissue, consisting of a thin layer of connective tissue lined by flattened cells (Fig. 38–3). The inner arachnoid membrane is separated from the pia mater by the subarachnoid space containing leptomeningeal blood vessels. The underlying brain tissue is either normal or shows signs of chronic compression; in no instance has there been valid histological evidence of primary failure of development of underlying neural tissue. Thus, an earlier postulate that arachnoid cysts represent merely a localized enlargement of subarachnoid space due to agenesis of the underlying brain is no longer tenable. In this context, one other observation pertaining to pathogenesis deserves emphasis. In all critically examined cases of spontaneous intracranial or spinal arachnoid cysts (excluding enlarging skull fractures) there has been no histological evidence of inflammation or trauma such as the presence of acute or chronic inflammatory cells or hemosiderin deposits. Thus, the composite of evidence indicates overwhelmingly that arachnoid cysts develop from an aberration of development of the arachnoid membrane and the related subarachnoid space.

Recent observations using scanning electron microscopy show differences between the inner surface of normal arachnoid and the inner surface of an arachnoid cyst. Normal arachnoid shows either a fenestrated surface or a surface embossed by parallel fibers.[6] The inner surface of an arachnoid

TABLE 38–1 DISTRIBUTION OF ARACHNOID CYSTS ALONG THE CEREBROSPINAL AXIS

INTRACRANIAL CYSTS
Supratentorial
  Sylvian fissure (2)
  Cerebral convexity
  Interhemispheric fissure (3)
  Sellar and suprasellar (4)
Optic Nerve
  Intraorbital (1)
  Intracranial
Tentorial
  Quadrigeminal plate cyst (5)
Infratentorial
  Clival (6)
  Cerebellopontine angle
  Posterior midline
  Vermis (7)
  Cisterna magna (8)
INTRASPINAL CYSTS
Intradural (9)
Extradural (10) (includes lateral thoracic meningocele)
Intraforaminal (arachnoid root cysts) (11)

---

* The numbers in parentheses refer to Figure 38–5.

cyst is embossed by arachnoid endothelial cells (Fig. 38–4).[54]

The distribution of arachnoid cysts is given in Table 38–1 and Figure 38–5. Again intracranial arachnoid cysts are always intradural and are intimately related to the arachnoid cisterns.

SYMPTOMS, SIGNS, AND DIFFERENTIAL DIAGNOSIS

Since the symptoms and signs depend greatly on the location of the cyst, each type is discussed individually.

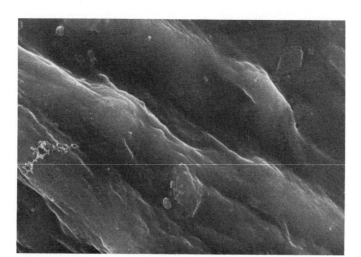

Figure 38–4 Scanning electron microscopic appearance of the inner surface of an arachnoid cyst (Courtesy of Dr. I. Watanabe).

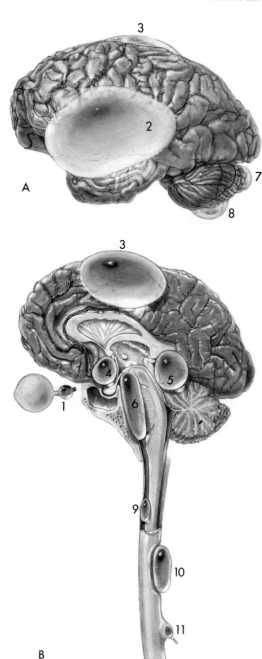

Figure 38–5 The distribution of arachnoid cysts along the cerebrospinal axis. (The numbers shown in the illustration correspond to the numbers in parentheses in Table 38–1).

Intracranial Arachnoid Cysts

Sylvian Fissure Cysts

The sylvian fissure is the most common site for intracranial arachnoid cysts. The cyst slowly expands and opens up the fissure. Depending on the size of the cyst, in late stages the entire insula may be exposed, showing the branches of the middle cerebral artery (Fig. 38–6). The anterior temporal lobe or its anterosuperior part may appear to be deficient (a condition incorrectly termed "temporal lobe agenesis").[43] Similarly, the inferior frontal gyrus may be absent.

The cyst may be manifest clinically at any age but is usually seen in males under 20 years. Headache is the most common symptom. Occasional seizures may occur, which may be focal, grand mal, or psychomotor in nature. A focal bulge in the temporal region or ipsilateral proptosis may be noticeable. Papilledema and mild contralateral hemiparesis are observed in late stages. Visual field defects and dementia are usually absent.

Skull x-rays show evidence of longstanding expansion of the middle cranial fossa as evidenced by elevation of the lesser wing of the sphenoid and thinning and outward bulging of the squamous temporal bone. (Fig. 38–7.)

The most helpful diagnostic test is a computed tomographic scan (Fig. 38–8). It shows an area of decreased density consistent with the density of spinal fluid. There is no contrast enhancement of the cyst wall.

The cerebral angiogram shows evidence of an avascular anterior temporal and sylvian mass. Air studies show shortening of the temporal horn and midline displacement of the ventricular system. The cyst itself may or may not fill with air. A radioisotope brain scan is usually nondiagnostic in uncomplicated cases.

The sylvian fissure cysts may be associated with a unique complication, namely subdural hematoma. The hematoma with its membrane may be located either superficial to the cyst or within the cyst. The plain x-ray and angiographic features are indistinguishable from uncomplicated arachnoid cysts. A radioisotopic scan, however, may be positive, and a computed tomogram may show evidence of subdural hematoma. The entity described by Davidoff and Dyke as "chronic relapsing juvenile subdural hematoma" might be the same as middle fossa arachnoid cyst complicated by subdural hematoma.[14]

The presence of an observable temporal

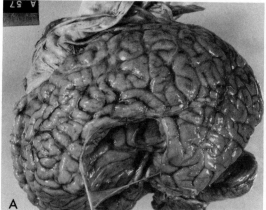

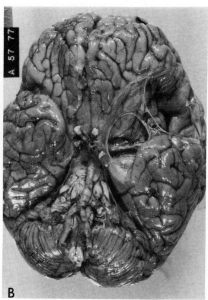

Figure 38–6 Typical sylvian fissure arachnoid cyst after the cyst wall has been partially removed. Note the displacement of the inferior frontal and temporal lobes exposing the insula and branches of the middle cerebral artery. *A*. Lateral aspect. *B*. Superior aspect.

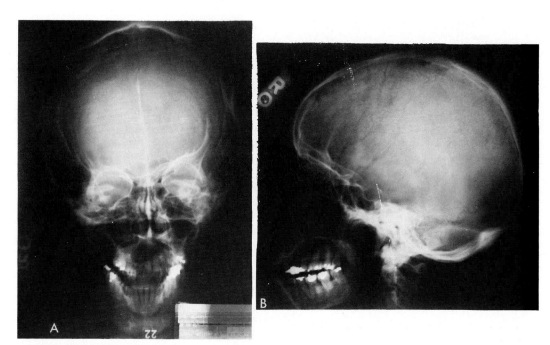

Figure 38–7 Plain x-rays of skull in a patient with sylvian fissure arachnoid cyst. *A*. Note the thinning and outward bulging of the temporal bone and elevation of the sphenoidal ridge. *B*. Lateral view of the skull shows forward displacement of the anterior wall of the middle fossa when compared to the normal side.

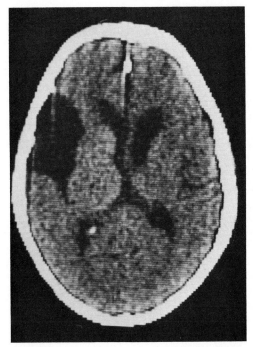

Figure 38–8 Computed tomogram of an arachnoid cyst of the sylvian fissure. The ventricular system is displaced.

bulge and unilateral proptosis is not unique to sylvian fissure arachnoid cysts. It may be seen with neurofibromatosis or low-grade temporal lobe glioma in children and sphenoidal ridge meningioma in adults. It should be easy, however, to differentiate between these conditions from the radiologic data just described.

Cerebral Convexity Cysts

The symptoms and clinical manifestations of cerebral convexity arachnoid cysts depend on the age group in which they are found.

In infants, the lesion is characterized by seizures and progressive but asymmetrical enlargement of the head.[2,15] Transillumination may outline the margin of the cyst. Bilateral cases may simulate hydrocephalus or hydranencephaly. Attempted subdural taps may yield clear spinal fluid. It should be noted that, in infants, large sylvian cysts may extend superiorly and present as convexity cysts. X-rays of the skull show asymmetrical enlargement of the vault with focal thinning of the bone and separation of the sutures. Computed tomograms will help

to differentiate this entity from subdural hematoma and congenital hydrocephalus.

In adults, the lesion presents with focal or grand mal seizures, headaches, papilledema, and progressive contralateral hemiparesis.[45] The skull deformity is not prominent, though radiological examination may show erosion of the inner table of the skull. Cerebral angiography shows an avascular convexity mass closely mimicking a chronic subdural hematoma. Computed tomography will show a biconvex or semicircular area of lucency over the cerebral convexity. A straight inner margin of this lucent area is claimed to be pathognomonic of arachnoid cysts, but to date, a sufficient number of cysts has not been examined by computed tomography to substantiate the validity of this claim.[4]

Interhemispheric Cysts

Cysts in this location do not produce any specific clinical syndrome. About half the reported cases have, however, been associated with agenesis of the corpus callosum.[56] The carotid arteriogram is characteristic in that there is separation and splaying of A_2 segments of the anterior cerebral arteries around the cyst. The density data and morphologic character of the lesion in a computed tomogram will help to differentiate this entity from lipoma of the corpus callosum or interhemispheric dermoid cyst.

Sellar and Suprasellar Cysts

Essentially two types of arachnoid cysts occur in the sellar region: suprasellar cysts, which may be of communicating or noncommunicating types, and intrasellar cysts, the empty sella syndrome (described in Chapter 100).

The suprasellar cysts arise in relation to the chiasmatic cistern and may or may not communicate with it.[5,12,25,42] They are rare and they occur in all age groups. They may be manifest as incidental asymptomatic lesions or as expanding lesions eroding the sella turcica and compressing the pituitary tissue, optic chiasm, anterior third ventricle, and foramen of Monro, resulting in symptoms of hypopituitarism, visual impairment, and obstructive hydrocephalus. Hypothalamic syndromes such as precocious puberty and adipsia have been reported.[10,17] A curious head-nodding motion described as "Bobble-head doll syndrome" has also been observed in association with suprasellar cyst.[39] Noncommunicating suprasellar cysts may be mistaken for other mass lesions in this location, including pituitary adenomas, craniopharyngiomas, meningiomas, and aneurysms of the internal carotid artery.

This is one of the exceptional locations where computed tomograms may not be very helpful in diagnosing intracranial arachnoid cysts, particularly small lesions. The density of the cyst is that of spinal fluid, and since the cyst lies within the cistern, it may be missed. Conventional neurodiagnostic tests including sellar tomography, magnification angiography, and pneumoencephalography with tomography may be necessary to establish the diagnosis.

The intrasellar arachnoid cyst is nothing but an extension of the chiasmatic cistern through an unduly large hiatus in the diaphragma sellae and is better known as the empty sella syndrome.[31] It is described in detail in Chapter 100.

Cysts of the Optic Nerve

Intraorbital Segment

Cysts of the intraorbital segment of the optic nerve may present with unilateral decreased visual acuity, optic disc edema, and prominent opticociliary veins, suggesting retrobulbar mass.[34] The lesion must be distinguished from other retrobulbar masses such as hemangioma, optic nerve glioma, orbital apex meningioma, and orbital pseudotumor. Polytomography of the orbit, orbital sonography, and computed tomography will help to establish the diagnosis.

Intracranial Segment

Two cases of benign cysts involving the intracranial segment of the optic nerve and chiasm have been reported, but without histological verification.[22]

Cysts of the Quadrigeminal Plate Region

Cysts in this location cause early obstruction of the aqueduct of Sylvius with re-sultant hydrocephalus clinically manifesting with progressive headaches, vomiting, and papilledema.[1,13,23,26,28,33] Parinaud's syndrome or its variant is present in less than one fourth of the cases. The cyst may or may not communicate with the quadrigeminal cistern. The clinical features of this entity may be indistinguishable from pseudotumor cerebri, pinealomas, dermoid cysts, tentorial meningiomas, aneurysms of the vein of Galen, or other mass lesions in this location. Computed tomography supplemented by air study or angiography will establish the diagnosis. If an air study is done, one has to be aware that cases of severe obstructive hydrocephalus with resultant rupture of the third or lateral ventricle may simulate communicating arachnoid cysts.[53] Another helpful fact is that the suprapineal recess may be preserved in cases of arachnoid cysts but are obliterated early with pineal masses.

Cysts of the Cerebellopontine Angle

The clinical syndrome may closely mimic that of an acoustic neuroma with sensorineural hearing loss, impaired corneal reflex, and in late stages, cerebellar signs and increased intracranial pressure.[55] Deviations from this pattern have been reported with early onset of complete facial paralysis in one instance and paroxysmal shooting pain in the face in the second or third division of the fifth cranial nerve in the other.[3,50] Tomograms of the internal auditory canal may show a smooth rounded erosion. Increasing numbers of small arachnoid cysts are being reported as use of Pantopaque angle myelography in evaluation of patients with progressive sensorineural hearing loss has become widespread. It may be impossible to distinguish these lesions from epidermoid cysts and acoustic or facial neuromas preoperatively.

Clival Arachnoid Cysts

This location is the rarest for infratentorial arachnoid cysts.[21] The cyst progressively displaces the midbrain and the pons dorsally as other clival masses do. This displacement results in bilateral impairment of corticospinal tracts and the reticular activating system, along with aqueductal obstruction. Quadriparesis and akinetic mutism are the clinical expressions of the upper brain stem distortion. Absence of destructive changes in the bone, and infrequency of involvement of cranial nerves early in the course of the disease distinguish this condition from clival chordoma. Computed tomography, angiography, and air study will help to differentiate it from giant basilar aneurysms, brain stem glioma, and clival meningioma or chordoma.

Other Infratentorial Cysts

Arachnoid cyst may occur in the region of the cerebellar vermis or hemisphere and the region of the cisterna magna (Figs. 38–9 and 38–10).[32] Presenting symptoms include increased intracranial pressure without focal signs or nystagmus, and truncal or extremity ataxia. Cisterna magna arachnoid cysts have to be distinguished from Dandy-Walker syndrome. This is done by demonstration of a compressed fourth ventricle separate from the arachnoid cyst by computed tomography, air study, or posterior fossa angiography.[30] In the Dandy-Walker syndrome the cystic dilatation is in continuity with and is a part of the dorsal aspect of the fourth ventricle.

Spinal Arachnoid Cysts

The spinal arachnoid cysts may manifest themselves at any age but show a peak incidence in the second and fourth decades. The common juvenile or adolescent type occurring in the second decade exhibits a characteristic clinical syndrome. The cysts are located extradurally in the midthoracic

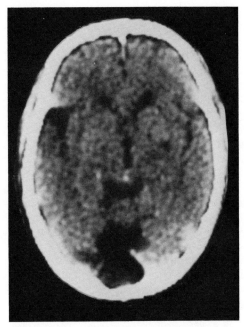

Figure 38–9 Computed tomogram of an arachnoid cyst in the region of the cisterna magna.

region. There is a rounded kyphosis of the thoracic spine. The pathogenesis of juvenile dorsal kyphosis in association with spinal arachnoid cysts remains obscure. There is often interscapular and radiating root pain around the chest. A slowly progressive paraparesis with impairment of all sensory modalities and sphincter disturbances evolves. The motor weakness tends to be worse than the sensory changes. The upper sensory level is usually poorly defined. It is notable that symptoms may fluctuate in time and with change of posture, leading

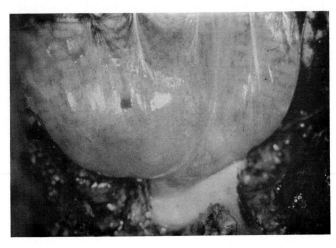

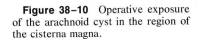

Figure 38–10 Operative exposure of the arachnoid cyst in the region of the cisterna magna.

to a mistaken clinical diagnosis of a demyelinating process or vascular malformation of the cord.*

Plain x-rays show smooth dorsal kyphosis with erosion of the pedicles. During myelography of communicating arachnoid cysts, the contrast material is trapped in the cyst demonstrating a blind lower end with a horizontal fluid level. Noncommunicating arachnoid cysts are indistinguishable from other intraspinal neoplasms (Figs. 38–11 and 38–12).

During myelography the following points should be observed; otherwise the lesion may be missed. A sufficiently large volume of contrast material should be used to visualize the thoracic area adequately. The patient should be examined in the supine and then in the erect position to facilitate filling of the communicating dorsal arachnoid cysts.

In addition to the juvenile type just described, a similar type of cyst may occur in adults. The cervical, lumbar, or sacral region as well as the thoracic region may be involved. The extradural cysts in the thoracic region may extend into the chest cavity, presenting as lateral thoracic meningoceles. Extradural cysts in the lumbar area in adults may present with symptoms of root compression, closely mimicking ruptured intervertebral disc.[20]

Intradural Arachnoid Cysts

Intradural arachnoid cysts are thought to arise from the spaces normally present in the septum posticum, an arachnoid fold that divides the posterior spinal subarachnoid space and extends from the cervical to the lower dorsal region.[40] But this hypothesis does not explain the occurrence of arachnoid cysts entirely ventral to the spinal cord. A carefully designed future study of the arachnoid cyst in its various parts, as found at autopsy, by both gross and histological examination might help to explain the pathogenesis.

Extradural Cysts

Extradural cysts are located in the dorsal midline or dorsolaterally near the dural sleeve of the nerve root. They occur as arachnoid herniations through small dural defects. Such dural defects are known to exist in normal subjects, and are found close to the roots, where arachnoid granu-

---

* See references 7, 11, 16, 27, 29, 36, 37, 41, 46, 49, 52.

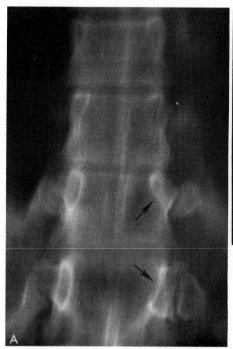

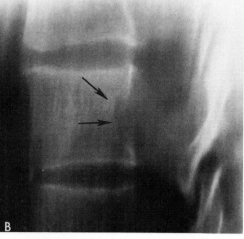

Figure 38–11 *A.* Tomogram of the thoracic spine showing pedicular erosion from a spinal arachnoid cyst. *B.* Lateral tomogram of the thoracic spine showing scalloping of the vertebral body.

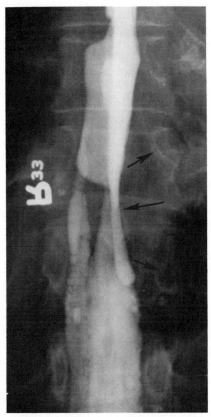

Figure 38–12 Pantopaque myelogram in the lateral decubitus position. A noncommunicating extradural arachnoid cyst displaces the myelographic column away from the eroded pedicles.

lations protrude in a fashion analogous to that of pacchionian bodies. Extradural arachnoid cysts may represent a pathological variant of such normal herniation.

Arachnoid Root Cysts

Arachnoid diverticula are commonly observed along the lower lumbar and sacral roots during lumbar myelography. They are usually clinically insignificant. In rare instances they may produce root symptoms. Plain x-rays may show erosion of sacral foramina.

The fact that they are located in the lumbar and sacral regions, are bilaterally symmetrical in distribution, and may be unobserved on the initial myelographic films but seen on delayed films taken 24 hours later suggest that gravity plays an important part in their pathogenesis and that the communication between the diverticulum and the main subarachnoid space may be very narrow.

Arachnoid root cysts should be distinguished from perineural cysts of Tarlov; the latter contains neural elements.[51]

MANAGEMENT

Since the clinical syndrome of symptomatic arachnoid cysts is produced by mechanical compression by a slowly expansive space-occupying lesion, the treatment is operative excision. The outer layer or dome of the cyst must be removed in its entirety around the margin of the cyst. In addition, the inner layer should be fenestrated to insure communication of the cyst with the subarachnoid space and thus prevent recurrence.

Shunting of the cyst to another space is not required as a primary procedure, but if the cysts recur, shunting may be necessary.

In juvenile extradural spinal arachnoid cysts, the extent of the laminectomy should be limited to prevent progressive worsening of the kyphosis postoperatively.

REFERENCES

1. Alexander, E., Jr.: Benign subtentorial supracollicular cyst as a cause of obstructive hydrocephalus. J. Neurosurg., *10*:317–323, 1953.
2. Aicardi, J., and Bauman, F.: Supratentorial extracerebral cysts in infants and children. J. Neurol. Neurosurg. Psychiat., *38*:57–68, 1975.
3. Bengochea, F. G., and Blanco, F. L.: Arachnoidal cysts of the cerebello-pontine angle. J. Neurosurg., *12*:66–71, 1955.
4. Banna, M.: Arachnoid cysts in the hypophyseal area. Clin. Radiol. 25:323–326, 1974.
5. Banna, M.: Arachnoid cysts on computed tomography. Amer. J. Roentgen., *127*:979–982, 1976.
6. Barrionvevo, P., Dujonvy, M., Kossovysky, N., and Laha, R.: Scanning electron microscopy study of the inner arachnoid surface. Scientific exhibit S-13 at the Annual Meeting of the Association of Neurological Surgeons, Toronto, April 1977.
7. Bergland, R. M.: Congenital intraspinal extradural cysts. Report of three cases in one family. J. Neurosurg., 28:495–499, 1968.
8. Bering, E. A.: Choroid plexus and arterial pulsation of cerebrospinal fluid. Arch. Neurol. Psychiat., 73:165–172, 1955.
9. Bouch, D. C., Mitchell, I., and Maloney, A. F. J.: Ependymal lined paraventricular cerebral cysts; a report of three cases. J. Neurol. Neurosurg. Psychiat., 36:611–617, 1973.
10. Bradley, W. G., and Price, D. L.: Adipsia in association with arachnoid cysts. Neurology (Minneap.), 21:930–936, 1971.
11. Cloward, R. B., and Bucy, P. A.: Spinal extra-

dural cysts and kyphosis dorsalis juvenilis. Amer. J. Roentgen., *38*:681–706, 1937.

12. Danziger, J., and Bloch, S.: Suprasellar arachnoid pouches. Brit. J. Radiol., *47*:448–451, 1974.

13. Danziger, J., and Bloch, S.: Paracollicular arachnoid pouches. Amer. J. Roentgen., *124*:310–314, 1975.

14. Davidoff, L. M., and Dyke, C. G.: Relapsing juvenile chronic subdural hematoma. A clinical and roentgenographic study. Bull. Neurol. Inst. N.Y., *7*:95–111, 1938.

15. Dee, D., Jr., Woesner, M. E., and Sanders, I.: Biloculated intracranial arachnoid cyst in a neonate. Amer. J. Dis. Child., *127*:700–702, 1974.

16. Elsberg, C. A., Dyke, C. G., and Brewer, E. D.: The symptoms and diagnosis of extradural cysts. Bull. Neurol. Inst. N.Y., *3*:395–417, 1934.

17. Faris, A. A., Bale, G. F., and Cannon, B.: Arachnoidal cyst of the third ventricle with precocious puberty. South. Med. J., *64*:1139–1142, 1971.

18. Friede, R. L., and Yasargil, M. G.: Supratentorial intracerebral epithelial (ependymal) cysts: Review. Case reports and fine structure. J. Neurol. Neurosurg. Psychiat., *40*:127–137, 1977.

19. Ghatak, N. R., and Mushrush, G. J.: Supratentorial intracranial cyst. Case report. J. Neurosurg., *35*:477–482, 1971.

20. Glasauer, E. E.: Lumbar extradural cyst. J. Neurosurg., *25*:567–570, 1966.

21. Grollmus, J. M., Wilson, C. B., and Newton, H.: Paramesencephalic arachnoid cysts. Neurology (Minneap.), *26*:128–134, 1976.

22. Holt, H.: Cysts of the intracranial portion of the optic nerve. Amer. J. Ophthal., *61*:1166–1170, 1966.

23. Huckman, M. S., Davis, D. O., and Coxe, W. S.: Arachnoid cyst of the quadrigeminal plate. J. Neurosurg., *32*:367–370, 1970.

24. Jakubiak, P., Dunsmore, R. H., and Beckett, R. S.: Supratentorial brain cysts. J. Neurosurg., *28*:129–136, 1968.

25. Kasdon, D. L., Douglas, E. A., and Brougham, M. F.: Suprasellar arachnoid cyst diagnosed preoperatively by computerized tomographic scanning. Surg. Neurol., *7*:299–303, 1977.

26. Katagiri, A.: Arachnoidal cyst of the cisterna ambiens. Neurology (Minneap.), *10*:783–786, 1960.

27. Kim, J. H., Shucart, W. A., and Haimovici, H.: Symptomatic arachnoid diverticula. Arch. Neurol., *31*:35–37, 1974.

28. Kruyff, E.: Paracollicular plate cysts. Amer. J. Roentgen., *95*:899–916, 1965.

29. Lake, P. A., Minckler, J., and Scanlan, R. L.: Spinal epidural cyst: Theories of pathogenesis. J. Neurosurg., *40*:774–778, 1974.

30. LaTorre, E., Fortuna, A., and Occhipinti, E.: Angiographic differentiation between Dandy Walker cyst and the arachnoid cyst of the posterior fossa in the newborn infants and children. J. Neurosurg., *38*:298–308, 1973.

31. Leclercq, T. A., Hardy, J., Vezina, J. L., and Mercky, F.: Intrasellar arachnoidocele and the so-called empty sella syndrome. Surg. Neurol., *2*:295–299, 1974.

32. Little, J. R., Gomez, M. R., and MacCarty, C. S.: Infratentorial arachnoid cysts. J. Neurosurg., *39*:380–386, 1973.

33. Lourie, H., and Berne, A. S.: Radiological and clinical features of an arachnoid cyst of the quadrigeminal cistern. J. Neurol. Neurosurg. Psychiat., *24*:374–378, 1961.

34. Miller, N. R., and Green, R.: Arachnoid cysts involving a portion of the intraorbital optic nerve. Arch. Ophthal., *93*:1117–1121, 1975.

35. Moore, M. T., and Book, M. H.: Congenital cervical ependymal cyst. J. Neurosurg., *24*:558–561, 1966.

36. Nugent, G. R., Odom, G. L., and Woodhall, B.: Spinal extradural cysts. Neurology (Minneap.), *9*:397–406, 1959.

37. Palmer, J. J.: Spinal arachnoid cysts. J. Neurosurg., *41*:728–735, 1974.

38. Patrick, B. S.: Ependymal cyst of the sylvian fissure. J. Neurosurg., *35*:751–754, 1971.

39. Patriquin, H. B.: The Bobble-head doll syndrome —a curable entity. Radiology, *107*:171–172, 1973.

40. Perrett, G., Green, D., and Keller, J.: Diagnosis and treatment of intradural arachnoid cysts of the thoracic spine. Radiology, *79*:424–429, 1962.

41. Raja, I. A., and Hankinson, J.: Congenital spinal arachnoid cysts. J. Neurol. Neurosurg. Psychiat., *33*:105–110, 1970.

42. Ring, A., and Waddington, M.: Primary arachnoid cysts of the sella turcica. Amer. J. Roentgen., *98*:611–615, 1967.

43. Robinson, R. G.: The temporal lobe agenesis syndrome. Brain, *87*:87–106, 1964.

44. Robinson, R. G.: Congenital cysts of the brain: Arachnoid malformations. Prog. Neurol. Surg., *4*:133–174, 1971.

45. Ryvicker, M., and Leeds, N. E.: Developmental cerebral intraarachnoid cysts. Radiology, *109*:105–108, 1973.

46. Sang, U. K., Baloh, R. W., and Weingarten, S.: Intradural arachnoid cyst presenting with cord compression. Bull. Los Angeles Neurol. Soc., *37*:178–183, 1972.

47. Smith, R. A., and Smith, W. A.: Arachnoid cysts of the middle cranial fossa. Surg. Neurol., *5*:246–252, 1976.

48. Starkman, S. P., Brown, T. C., and Linell, E. A.: Cerebral arachnoid cysts. J. Neuropath. Exp. Neurol., *17*:484–500, 1958.

49. Stewart, D. H., and Red, D. E.: Spinal arachnoid diverticula. J. Neurosurg., *35*:65–70, 1971.

50. Sumner, T. E., Benton, C., and Marshak, G.: Arachnoid cyst of the internal auditory canal producing facial paralysis in a three-year-old child. Radiology, *114*:425–426, 1975.

51. Tarlov, I. M.: Spinal perineurial and meningeal cysts. J. Neurol. Neurosurg. Psychiat., *33*:833–843, 1970.

52. Teng, P., and Paptheodorou, C.: Spinal arachnoid diverticula. Brit. J. Radiol., *39*:249–254, 1966.

53. Torkildsen, A.: Spontaneous rupture of cerebral ventricles. J. Neurosurg., *5*:327–339, 1948.

54. Watanabe I: Personal communication.

55. Wilmer, H. I., and Kashef, R.: Unilateral arachnoid cysts and adhesions involving the eighth nerve. Amer. J. Roentgen., *115*:126–132, 1972.

56. Zingesser, L., Schecter, M., Gonatas, N., et al.: Agenesis of the corpus callosum associated with an inter-hemispheric arachnoid cyst. Brit. J. Radiol., *37*:905–909, 1964.

39

CRANIOSYNOSTOSIS

The term "craniosynostosis" refers to the absence of one or more of the cartilaginous sutures that separate the membranous bones of the skull (Fig. 39–1). The term is usually applied to *primary synostosis,* a spontaneous condition that probably is always present before birth. *Secondary craniosynostosis* is the premature obliteration of one or more cranial sutures due to a cause other than an abnormality of the suture itself. Secondary craniosynostosis occurs, for example, when a markedly hydrocephalic child's shunt is installed in such a fashion that the parietal bones can fall together and actually overlap.[10] Secondary synostosis of the sagittal suture may occur if the overlapping persists. The premature disappearance of all cranial sutures in a microcephalic child might be considered a synostosis secondary to failure of development of the brain.

ETIOLOGY

The etiology of primary craniosynostosis is not known. Interesting theories have been proposed.[9,13] Without question the synostosis can occur in utero. Several cases of sagittal synostosis have been diagnosed on the basis of films made of the mother's pelvis prior to delivery. The presence of the typical deformity has been confirmed at birth. It would appear reasonable that this abnormality probably occurs as the membranous bones of the cranial vault develop.

At birth only a small segment of an involved suture may be abnormal (Fig. 39–2). The tethering of the adjacent bones by this segment of synostosis reduces the stress on the adjacent normal suture, which progressively and prematurely disappears as a result. This is the mechanism by which a normal suture is obliterated after cessation of growth of the brain.

CHARACTERISTIC DEFORMITIES

The deformity produced by craniosynostosis depends upon the suture or sutures involved and upon the site and length of synostosis within each suture. For example, total sagittal synostosis will prevent separation of the parietal bones at the vertex. Breadth can be achieved only by the effects of growth of the brain upon the squamosal sutures. The widest point of the head will be at the squamosal area. The brain can also gain volume by utilizing the patency of the coronal and lambdoid sutures to gain in anteroposterior dimension. The resultant deformity will be an elongation of the head, which is narrowed at the vertex, so-called scaphocephaly ("boat-head") (Fig. 39–3). If only the posterior third of the sagittal suture is fused, the anterior portion of the skull will be quite broad and normal in appearance; only the posterior portion will be narrowed, and the occipital bone will protrude. A ridge usually replaces the missing suture (Fig. 39–4).

Absence of both lambdoid sutures will give a flattened appearance to the back of the head. This may easily be confused with positional molding caused by a child's lying continually on the occipital area. The differential diagnosis may be made radiographically. The absence of one lambdoid suture will cause that side of the back of the skull to be flattened, which again may be

J. SHILLITO, JR.

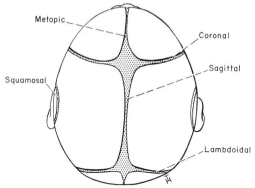

Figure 39–1 Normal sutures, infant's skull. (From Shillito, J., and Matson, D. D.: Pediatrics, *41*:829–853, 1968. Reprinted by permission.)

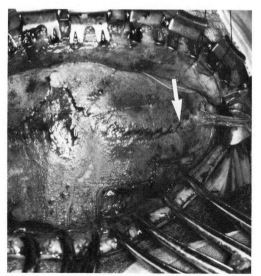

Figure 39–2 Child with complete sagittal and bilateral partial coronal synostosis. Anterior fontanelle is patent. Segment of coronal suture from fontanelle to arrow is not normal. Normal suture appears whiter than surrounding bone, and pericranium is normally adherent to it.

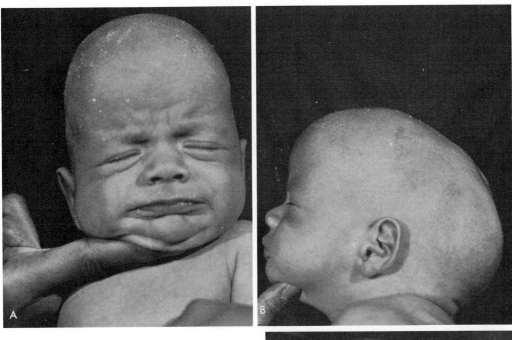

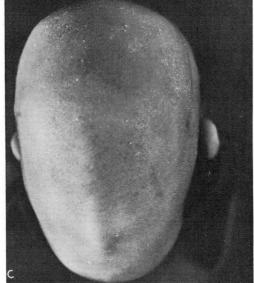

Figure 39–3 Sagittal synostosis. *A*. Except in frontal area, widest portion of skull is at or just above squamosal sutures. *B*. Note elongation of head, particularly noticeable after it has been shaved. *C*. Child is face up; elongation of head is much more noticeable. Note presence of ridge in sagittal region posteriorly where head is also narrowest. In this case, the anterior few centimeters of sagittal suture were patent, as was the anterior fontanelle. (From Shillito, J., and Matson, D. D.: Pediatrics, *41*:829–853, 1968. Reprinted by permission.)

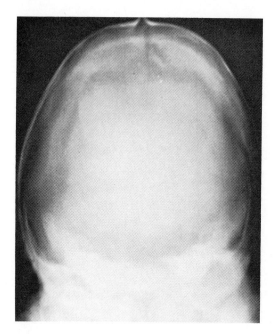

Figure 39–4 Sagittal synostosis. Properly angled anteroposterior view shows synostotic portion of the sagittal suture, which is replaced by a ridge.

confused with positional molding (Fig. 39–5). In the latter case the sutures will appear normal by x-ray.

Bilateral coronal synostosis will present as a flattening of the forehead with absence of the frontal bosses (Figs. 39–6 and 39–7). Unilateral synostosis will appear as a uni-

lateral flattening (Fig. 39–8). With either condition there may be involvement of the orbit to a degree sufficient to produce proptosis. In coronal synostosis, the orbit is usually set obliquely and the sphenoid wing is elevated (cf. Fig. 39–7, Fig. 39–9). The involved orbit will be somewhat shallower

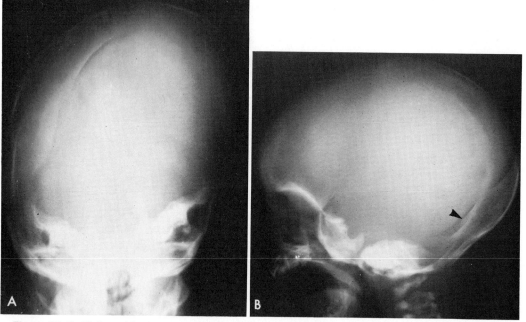

Figure 39–5 Unilateral lambdoid synostosis, right. *A.* Note ridge where the lambdoid suture should be and asymmetry of skull. *B.* In the lateral view one can see only one lambdoid suture and thicker bone in lieu of the other (*arrow*). (From Shillito, J., and Matson, D. D.: Pediatrics, *41*:829–853, 1968. Reprinted by permission.)

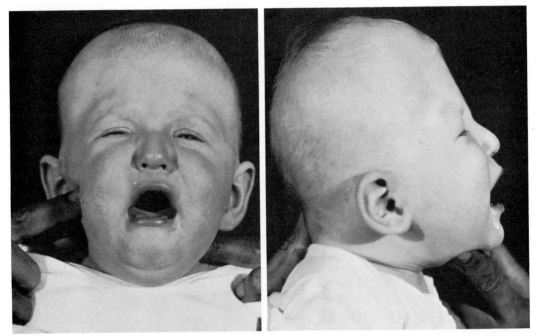

Figure 39–6 Bilateral coronal synostosis, 5-month-old boy. There is flattening of the forehead bilaterally, slightly pinched appearance of the frontal bones, absence of brow ridges. (From Shillito, J., and Matson, D. D.: Pediatrics, *41*:829–853, 1968. Reprinted by permission.)

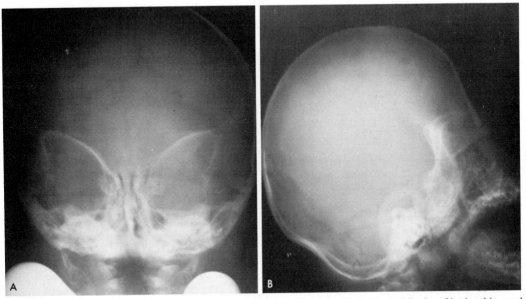

Figure 39–7 Bilateral coronal synostosis, same child as in Figure 39–6. *A.* Note obliquity of both orbits, and normal lambdoid sutures. *B.* Frontal fossa is very small with a steep floor, and no coronal sutures can be seen. (From Shillito, J., and Matson, D. D.: Pediatrics, *41*:829–853, 1968. Reprinted by permission.)

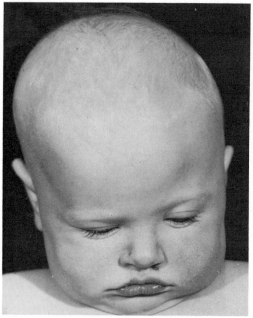

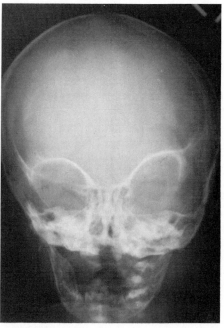

Figure 39–8   Unilateral coronal synostosis, left, 5-month-old girl. There is flattening of left frontal area and relative prominence of right frontal boss. Involvement of left orbit, which is shallower and more oblique, may produce apparent slight proptosis on the involved side, for there is little, if any, overhanging brow ridge. (From Shillito, J., and Matson, D. D.: Pediatrics, *41*:829–853, 1968. Reprinted by permission).

Figure 39–9   Unilateral coronal synostosis, same girl as in Figure 39–8. Note obliquity of left orbital rim on involved side. Normal lambdoid sutures may be seen on this view.

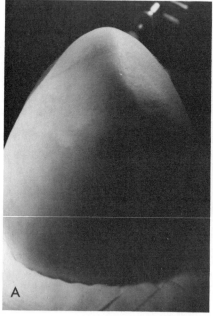

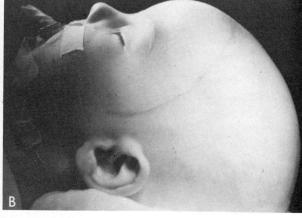

Figure 39–10   *A.* Vertex view of supine child with metopic synostosis. Note the midline ridge extending forward from the anterior fontanelle and the eyebrows, which are just visible bilaterally where the forehead is narrowed. *B.* Side view of same child with intended incision marked on scalp.

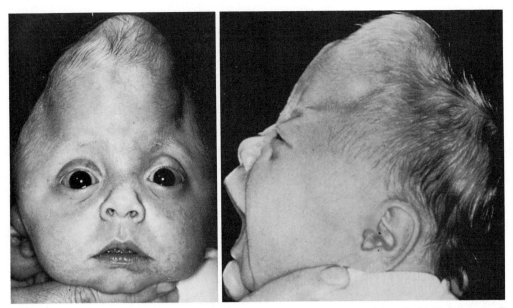

Figure 39–11   Multiple synostosis; sagittal, bilateral coronal, bilateral lambdoid; 1 week old. Brain is protruding through site of anterior fontanelle and also slightly through posterior fontanelle. Widest part of skull is at the squamosal suture level. (From Shillito, J., and Matson, D. D.: Pediatrics, *41*:829–853, 1968. Reprinted by permission.)

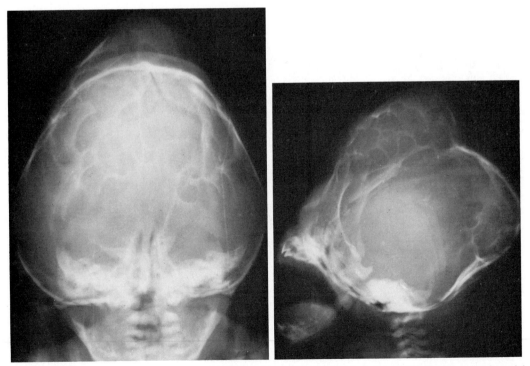

Figure 39–12   Multiple synostosis, same child as in Figure 39-11. The loculations in the skull contained cranial contents, making craniectomy difficult. (From Shillito, J., and Matson, D. D.: Pediatrics, *41*:829–853, 1968. Reprinted by permission.)

than the normal one, and the appearance of a child with unilateral coronal synostosis may suggest an intraorbital tumor on the ipsilateral side or an intracranial cyst on the opposite, normal side.

Metopic synostosis presents as a mid-forehead ridge extending from anterior fontanelle to nasion. The forehead looks as though one had pinched it bilaterally above the orbits, giving the child's head an appearance resembling the bow of an upside-down fisherman's dory (Fig. 39–10).

Multiple suture closures may produce a striking appearance (Fig. 39–11). If some part of a suture or fontanelle is patent, the brain will attempt to grow at this site of less resistance and a grossly misshapen head will result (Figs. 39–11 and 39–12).

In some children, fortunately relatively few, there will be multiple congenital abnormalities involving not only the sutures of the cranial vault but also the sutures of the base of the skull and the face. In children with Crouzon's syndrome (familial craniofacial abnormalities) or Apert's syndrome (craniofacial abnormalities with syndactylism) the characteristic appearance

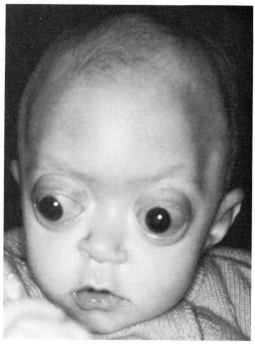

Figure 39–13 Infant with bilateral coronal synostosis and craniofacial abnormalities with marked proptosis. When crying, girl could close lids behind globe.

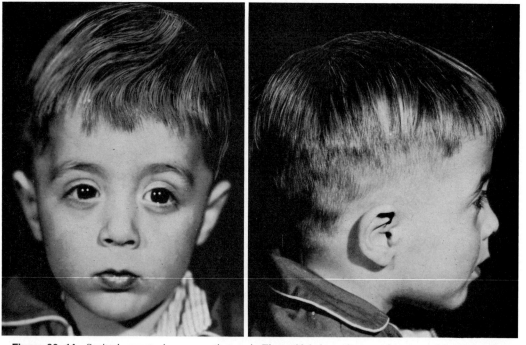

Figure 39–14 Sagittal synostosis, same patient as in Figure 39-3, here shown at 2 years and 3 months of age. Operation was performed at 6 weeks of age. Now over 12 years old, this boy is considered completely normal. (From Shillito, J., and Matson, D. D.: Pediatrics, *41*:829–853, 1968. Reprinted by permission.)

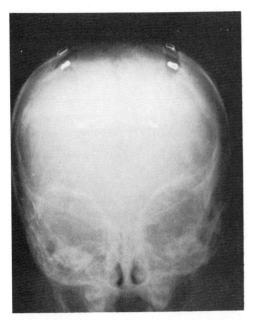

Figure 39–15 Midline craniectomy, initially 1 cm wide, has widened in about 2 years to 5 cm. New bone has filled in craniectomy defect, and a new suture is present in the new bone.

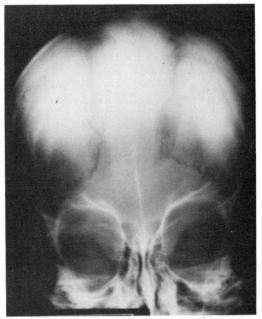

Figure 39–16 Films taken seven months following bilateral parasagittal craniectomies and bilateral coronal craniectomies show what appears to be a normal cranial suture in the center of the new bone formation in each parasagittal craniectomy. Note that the lambdoid suture between these has already disappeared. (From Shillito, J.: Radiology, *107*:83–88, 1973. Reprinted by permission.)

cannot be ameliorated by operative correction of only the abnormal sutures of the cranial vault (Fig. 39–13).[2,4] Methods of dealing with these problems are described in Chapter 40. The purpose of this chapter is to consider some of the factors affecting continued suture patency and to outline simple methods of dealing with craniosynostosis of the sutures of the cranial vault.

DEVELOPMENT OF A SUTURE

Probably there are only two things necessary to permit the development of a fibrous suture between two cranial bones: first, a stress from within that tends to separate them; and second, freedom to move away from one another.

These principles determine the success of simple craniectomies. For example, the ultimate appearance of the child who has had craniectomy for sagittal synostosis usually is excellent (Fig. 39–14). The parietal bone edges migrate away from one another markedly within the first few months after operation. A craniectomy initially 1 cm wide will be 5 cm wide by 2 years of age (Fig. 39–15).

By contrast, a linear craniectomy performed for coronal synostosis will not widen as satisfactorily or as uniformly

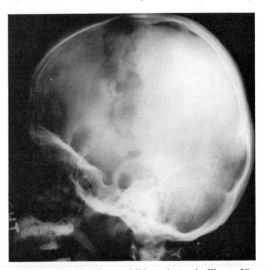

Figure 39–17 Same child as shown in Figure 39–16. New sutures in coronal craniectomy sites have persisted for two years and five months following operation. (From Shillito, J.: Radiology, *107*:83–88, 1973. Reprinted by permission.)

along its length. The width of the craniectomy will become greater at the vertex than in the temporal region. The frontal bone, although freed from the parietal bone, is restricted in its ability to move forward because of its attachment to the base of the skull. If, however, one creates a supraorbital craniectomy extending forward from the coronal craniectomy, the frontal bone is freed from the base of the skull, and will migrate forward and give a more gratifying end result.

About 12 years ago it was first noted in postoperative skull films that a new suture had developed in a craniectomy site in the bone generated by dura.[16] These first iatrogenic sutures were noted in bilateral coronal and bilateral parasagittal craniectomy sites seven months following operation on a boy 2½ years old (Fig. 39–16). Radiograph

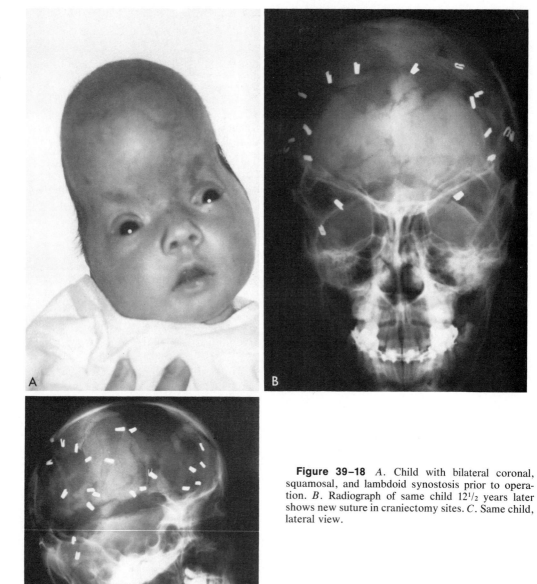

Figure 39–18 *A.* Child with bilateral coronal, squamosal, and lambdoid synostosis prior to operation. *B.* Radiograph of same child 12½ years later shows new suture in craniectomy sites. *C.* Same child, lateral view.

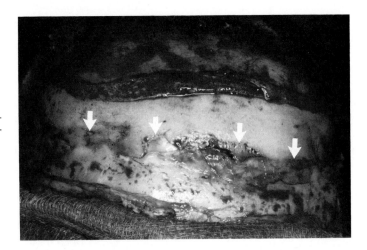

Figure 39-19 New coronal suture 19 years after original craniectomy (*arrows*).

ically the sutures resembled normal sutures. They have persisted (Fig. 39–17). They did not occur at either bone edge, but rather undulated down the midportion of the new bone. Remarkable was the fact that the parasagittal sutures appeared where no natural suture ever exists. The segment of lambdoid suture that lay between the iatrogenic parasagittal sutures disappeared completely (cf. Fig. 39–16). The stress that was formerly applied to that segment of the lambdoid suture was now gone. Many other children have since been noted to have developed these new sutures (Fig. 39–18). Some have persisted for 19 years following operation.

The opportunity came to explore one of these iatrogenic sutures during a corrective craniofacial operation on a 17-year-old girl. Grossly the suture appeared exactly like a natural suture (Fig. 39–19). On its removal, histological examination showed fibrous tissue between membranous bones just as one would expect to find in a naturally occurring suture.

Hanson and co-workers have reported the technique of removal of the entire cranium in an infant with multiple synostosis.[7] New bone generated rapidly from the dura in a more normal configuration. It is interesting to note in postoperative films that sutures developed in this new bone where they would be expected to occur naturally. Although this would tempt one to conclude that there is some organizing factor or stress line in the dura at these positions, this would not appear to be substantiated by the fact that the iatrogenic parasagittal sutures appear and persist at completely unnatural locations.[16]

INDICATIONS FOR OPERATION

Deformities of the skull resulting from craniosynostosis are produced by the skull's inability to respond to the growth of the brain at involved sites. Since its growth is particularly rapid during the first several months of life, early operative intervention will allow the brain to produce optimum improvement in the appearance of the skull.[3] Conversely, if nothing is done, the distortion of the skull can be expected to worsen as the brain enlarges.

If many or all sutures are involved, one could theorize, the brain will be constricted and its function interfered with. Since the author has not allowed a child with multiple synostosis to go without operative correction, he cannot attest to this likelihood. He has, however, seen the results of untreated synostosis of a single suture on more than one occasion. One 8-year-old boy with untreated sagittal synostosis developed symptoms of a duodenal ulcer and had problems keeping up with his work in the second grade. His neurological examination, IQ, electroencephalogram, and intracranial pressure were all normal. He was found to have an emotional problem caused by the taunts of his classmates who referred to him as an "egg head" and a "freak." His uncorrected synostosis had created not only a cosmetic problem but an emotional problem. Rather than wait to see how marked a deformity will be, or whether emotional problems will develop, the best policy is to operate in the first few weeks of life so that the brain's period of rapid growth can be capitalized upon and its expansion allowed to correct the shape of the skull.

SURGICAL PRINCIPLES

If the diagnosis is made at birth, the operation should be deferred until the child is 4 to 6 weeks of age. By that time, the total blood volume has increased significantly and reduces the consequences of blood loss that invariably accompanies the operation. If many sutures are involved and pressure upon the brain seems to be a problem, operation as early as one week of age has been successful.

Linear craniectomies should be done at the normal sites of the missing sutures.[12] The bone edges are lined with polyethylene film in an effort to defer the time at which new bone seals the old bone edges to one another. The film is inert and has caused no late problems.[6] It is thinner than the Silastic material currently available. Scissors or saw cuts in an infant's cranium heal promptly. Wider craniectomies are sealed very soon by new bone regenerating from the dura. Chemical cauterization of the dura is undesirable because it might jeopardize the underlying brain should there be an unseen opening in the dura, and by destroying the osteogenic capacity of the outer layer of the dura it will successfully delay or totally prevent regeneration of bone in the craniectomy.[1] This will leave a defect that might be dangerous to an older, active child. Cranioplasty has been necessary in cases in which a defect has persisted too long.

A craniectomy about 1 cm in width provides adequate room to manipulate the polyethylene film and to control small areas of dural bleeding without difficulty. Wider craniectomies appear unnecessary and involve greater elevation of scalp from the cranium, with attendant bleeding. The craniectomies should be made to extend across the adjacent normal sutures. This makes the operator properly identify the adjacent sutures so that he does not inad-

vertently fall short of his goal. It also allows him to put in a strip of polyethylene film longer than the involved bones at the time of operation. As the child's head grows, the bone edge that has been filmed becomes longer than the film, which will permit premature sealing of the craniectomy at each end. If film of extra length is inserted, this will not occur. The polyethylene film is prepared by wrapping it around the edges of a malleable abdominal retractor, tying it in position, and boiling the assembly for 20 minutes. This procedure molds the film in the folded position for easier application. Then the film and its retractor can be packaged in transparent bags for gas sterilization, after which it may be kept on the shelf for several weeks before use.

To facilitate removal of the film, a shallow groove is put into the abdominal retractor 1 cm from its edges. The scrub nurse can easily pass a knife blade along the four grooves and remove two full strips of film (Fig. 39–20). Commercially available strips of Silastic material now on the market should be equally effective, but they are a little bit thicker and may be more noticeable under an infant's thin scalp. The film may be held to the bone by sutures placed through a hole punched in the bone or by specially made tantalum clips, which speed the application of the film.[5] When the cran-

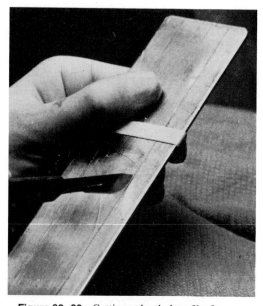

Figure 39–20 Cutting polyethylene film for use on craniectomy margins. Note groove in retractor.

iectomy lies in front of the hairline, it is desirable to use sutures to avoid the small lump produced by the clip, which may be noticeable beneath the infant's thin scalp. The clips do provide useful markers for estimating the width of the craniectomy after new bone has begun to develop, for their progressive separation indicates continued widening of the craniectomy.

Operation may be undertaken with acceptable risks if strict attention is paid to several important principles of surgery in the newborn. Positioning to prevent pressure marks, maintenance of body temperature, and prompt and adequate replacement of blood loss during and after the operation are most important. Since considerable foreign material is left in the wound, meticulous attention to aseptic operative technique is necessary. Postoperative accumulation of blood in the subgaleal space will usually resolve within a week or two. Open drains are not used because of the risk of sepsis. Needle aspiration of the accumulated blood is avoided if possible for the same reason. Some continued subgaleal oozing postoperatively should be anticipated and its amount estimated by hematocrit determinations repeated every six hours for the first day and twice daily for at least two more days. Transfusion is performed as necessary.

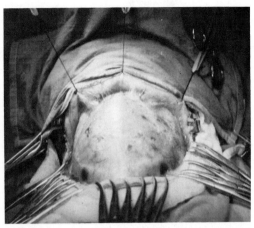

Figure 39–21 Exposed frontal bones of child with metopic synostosis shown in Figure 39–10. Note the midline ridge, patent anterior fontanelle, and normal coronal sutures.

OPERATIVE TECHNIQUES

Metopic Craniectomy

The child is positioned face up, and a coronal incision is made just behind the hairline, extending from one zygoma to the other. The scalp is reflected down to the orbital rim, and the nasion is exposed (Fig. 39–21). Pericranium is stripped from the coronal suture to the nasion over an area 2 cm wider than the ridge. It is also removed from the supraorbital area for a width of about 1 cm. Starting at the anterior fontanelle, if present, or from a small midline burr hole made just anterior to the coronal suture, the midline ridge is removed with various rongeurs down through the nasion. Just above the nasion, there are invariably several small veins running between the sagittal sinus and the bone, and their rupture can cause embarrassing or even dangerous bleeding. Careful hemostasis of

bleeders in both bone and dura must be maintained every centimeter of the way down to this region to prevent excessive blood loss during this short portion of the operation. The width of the craniectomy is determined by the size of the ridge; when it has been completed the thickness of the remaining frontal bone edges should be normal.

Next, a linear cut a few millimeters wide is made from the anterior limit of the metopic craniectomy to the coronal suture on each side. This cut may be made with various instruments; the Stookey rongeur and DeVilbiss rongeur have been useful. It is quite easy, inadvertently, to tear the dura during this maneuver unless it is retracted with a dissector and kept under direct vision while the craniectomy is being made. Any rent must be sutured to prevent persistent cerebrospinal fluid leak and pseudomeningocele formation.

When the frontal bones have been freed except for the attachment at the coronal suture, each is reflected outward, hinged on its coronal suture, and cut free from the skull with a stout pair of scissors. The two frontal bones are removed to the instrument table. There a pair of holes is punched in the medial edge and a pair in the supraorbital edge of each bone. Polyethylene film is sewed to these margins. Two 4-0 silk sutures are used to tie each frontal bone to the other, utilizing the previously placed holes. They should not be tied too securely, but should be slightly moveable to accommo-

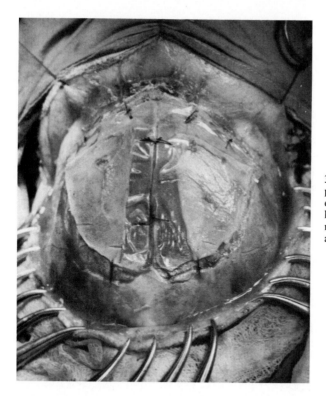

Figure 39–22 Same patient as in Figure 39–21. Frontal bones have been removed, supraorbital and medial margins lined with polyethylene film, and bones sutured together lightly. They have been returned to the cranium with a pair of sutures in the supraorbital and coronal regions tethering them.

date subsequent changes in the shape of the frontal area. The bones are then returned to the cranium. By means of the medial supraorbital holes, they are attached to the pericranium in the supraorbital region. Another suture is passed through the thin edge of each frontal bone, and the bone is sewed to the coronal suture close to the midline. Both bones are, thus, secured to one another and to the skull close to the midline so that their lateral margins may migrate forward to correct the indented appearance of the skull. The midline ridge is gone and there is no unsightly craniectomy defect in its place (Fig. 39–22). One must be careful to trim the lateral inferior corners of the frontal bones appropriately so that they will not protrude in unsightly fashion as the bones migrate forward.

Coronal Craniectomy

Position, preparation, and incision are identical to those for metopic craniectomy. In a unilateral closure, the scalp incision can be stopped above the lateral canthus of the uninvolved eye. A strip of pericranium 3 cm wide, centered over the missing suture site, is removed. The craniectomy is started

from the anterior fontanelle, if present, or a single burr hole. A linear craniectomy 1 cm wide is carried down to a point just in front of the ear, where the squamosal suture can be identified. The middle fossa may be quite deep in this condition, and the squamosal suture is not always easy to find. It must be identified by the adherence of pericranium to it, by the motion of the parietal and temporal bones on one another, and by the adherence of dura to the suture. If the coronal craniectomy is directed too far anteriorly, the squamosal suture may not be encountered at all. The craniectomy is extended 1 cm. beyond the squamosal suture.

Palpating beneath the anterior bone edge thus created, the operator should feel the sphenoid wing. This may present as a deep "keel." Starting just lateral to this keel, a craniectomy about 0.5 cm wide is created, crossing the sphenoid wing just above the lateral margin of the orbit. This margin lies abnormally high because of the synostosis, and care must be taken not to enter the orbit inadvertently. Palpating beneath the frontal bone, the operator can appreciate the position of the orbital roof. The craniectomy should be continued across to the midline just above the orbit. Small rongeurs such as the Stookey or DeVilbiss are used in making this cut. As in metopic synostosis, great care should be used to depress the dura away from the frontal bone lest the dura be torn. If torn, it must be repaired. Polyethylene film is placed on both margins of the coronal craniectomy, but it is difficult to apply and has therefore not been used in the narrow supraorbital craniectomy. The frontal bones can now hinge forward to correct the deformity of the skull. The lateral corner of each frontal bone should be rounded off with rongeurs so that it does not protrude beneath the scalp.

Sagittal Craniectomy

About 10 years ago, the author abandoned the parasagittal craniectomies in favor of the midline sagittal craniectomy. If the operation is performed in infancy, the craniectomy will be filled in with new bone before the child begins to toddle around, at which time he will be more apt to fall and injure himself in this area. If the diagnosis is made later in life and the operation is carried out after a child is ambulatory, one might still consider the use of bilateral parasagittal craniectomies in order to leave some protection over the sagittal sinus.

The single midline craniectomy has several advantages over the parasagittal craniectomy operation. The amount of elevation of the scalp is less, and therefore, bleeding is apt to be less. Adequate scalp elevation can be achieved with the child in the lateral position, which avoids risk of pressure marks on the face. The operation does not require as much time.

Pericranium is stripped from the skull 1.5 cm on either side of the midline, extending from just in front of the coronal sutures to just behind the lambdoid sutures. The outer portion of the fontanelle is removed with this. The epidural space is entered with a knife at the fontanelle or through a burr hole, and a midline strip of bone is removed. The dura adheres only to any normal portions of the suture, and these areas must be elevated with caution lest the sagittal sinus be torn. At other areas where the synostosis is complete, there is no adherence to the dura and the risk of lacerating the sinus is negligible. Ordinarily, a full-length craniectomy is done, removing apparently normal segments of suture. In one or two infants with synostosis involving only a few centimeters of the suture, however, a limited craniectomy, leaving normal suture behind, has corrected the deformity completely. The polyethylene film should cross the lambdoid sutures posteriorly and the coronal sutures anteriorly even though the fontanelle may be large and extend behind the coronal sutures.

Lambdoid Craniectomy

The child is placed in the prone position, and all precautions necessary with a face-down position should be observed. The headrest must be perfectly smooth. Plastic drapes with adhesive edges should be applied to the scalp and cheeks in such a manner that no fluid can reach the headrest at any time during the operation, for it is at these wet points that pressure necrosis is likely to develop. Incision is planned from the posterior end of the sagittal suture to the posterior end of the squamosal suture. This is determined by x-ray or palpation over the involved side or sides. After a strip of pericranium 3 cm wide has been removed, a burr hole is placed parasagittally to avoid entering the sinus. From this point a rongeur usually provides the most expeditious means of making the craniectomy. The sagittal suture must be crossed and the squamosal suture must be identified and crossed. This demands adequate exposure laterally and prompt control of the nearby mastoid emissary vein, which conceivably can be entered in the process of locating the squamosal suture.

Multiple Sutures

Craniectomy techniques as already detailed are used for multiple suture closures. The planning of incisions and the staging of procedures can be summarized as follows: (1) metopic and coronal synostosis—coronal incision, one stage; (2) coronal and sagittal synostosis—coronal and sagittal incisions, two stages; (3) sagittal and lambdoid synostosis—posterior parietal ear-to-ear and sagittal incisions, two stages; and

(4) all sutures—coronal and posterior parietal ear-to-ear incisions, two stages.

In this last situation, anterior halves of sagittal and squamosal craniectomies can be made by using the coronal incision, and the posterior halves completed in the second stage by using the posterior incision. The operations are separated by at least one week.

Other combinations can be dealt with by utilizing these incisions as necessary.

If metopic and bilateral coronal synostoses co-exist, the frontal bones can be removed and repositioned as in the procedure for metopic synostosis.[12]

If the child's cranium is grossly misshapen because of multiple synostosis, the operation described by Hanson and co-workers is certainly attractive and, as has been their experience, probably provides a more satisfactory cosmetic result than multiple linear craniectomies.[7] Whenever a procedure of this magnitude is undertaken in an infant, however, it must be borne in mind that the blood loss is a significant portion of the child's total blood volume and replacement must begin immediately and match the loss continuously. It is mandatory that the operator control bleeding with each step he makes, pausing whenever necessary to allow the child's condition to stabilize.

MORTALITY AND MORBIDITY

In a series of 519 patients treated by operation at the Children's Hospital Medical Center in Boston over a 36-year period up until 1966, there were two deaths, a risk of 0.39 percent.[15] One infant died because of an unsuspected bleeding tendency; the second died in the recovery room of cardiac arrest probably related to inadequate rate of blood replacement. Since that series was reviewed there have been no deaths resulting from any operation for primary craniosynostosis at this center.

Complications have included pressure scars on the forehead resulting from the face-down position.[15] This can be avoided by taking meticulous care in draping so that the headrest remains dry, and by lifting the head and repositioning it slightly every 15 minutes during the operative procedure. Other complications include wound sepsis and hematoma formation requiring reoperation, and cerebrospinal fluid accumulation beneath the scalp requiring reoperation. Tantalum clips when improperly applied have eroded through the scalp in several instances. Only two cranioplasties have been necessary for persistent skull defects. Most of these complications have been prevented by meticulous attention to hemostasis during the operative period, by repairing any

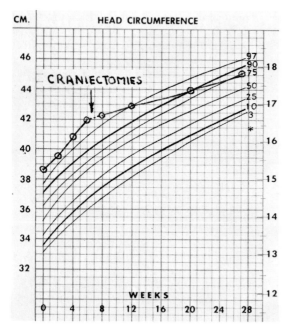

Figure 39–23 Typical growth curve of the head of a child with sagittal synostosis. Several cases in which accurate records were kept by the pediatrician have shown that growth rate is excessive as the head elongates. After craniectomy the head begins to assume a more spherical contour and its growth rate as determined by its circumference becomes less than normal. Theoretically, recurrence of the excessive growth rate should indicate fusion of the operative defect. (From Shillito, J., and Matson, D. D.: Pediatrics, *41*:829–843, 1968. Reprinted by permission.)

tears in the dura, and by using local antibiotic irrigations at the time of the operation.

RESULTS OF OPERATION

The cosmetic improvement can be qualitated but is not easily quantitated. The effect on brain function, however, cannot even be estimated, since by operation on any given child the control study for this child is lost.

The best cosmetic results follow operation performed within the first few weeks after birth. Satisfaction varies with the suture involved, as noted earlier. The results of midsagittal craniectomy have, in general, been excellent. Reoperation has been necessary only when the initial craniectomy was not adequate in length. A useful indicator of continued patency of the craniectomy in sagittal synostosis is the head circumference curve. Before operation, as the head elongates, the circumference increases more rapidly than it would if the head were growing in the shape of the brain. A growth curve not unlike untreated hydrocephalus results (Fig. 39–23). After sagittal craniectomy the growth rate of the skull, as indicated by its circumference, decreases to a rate less than normal until the approximate shape of the brain has been attained. Thereafter, the growth rate should be normal. Theoretically, if the craniectomy fuses prematurely, the head should again begin to elongate and the head growth curve as measured by its circumference should show an abnormally rapid rate. This has, in fact, occurred in one child as the iatrogenic suture was obliterated. Reoperation has not been performed because the cosmetic result is still most acceptable.

INDICATIONS FOR REOPERATION

Reoperation may be necessary when many sutures are involved, since intracranial pressure may increase with sealing of the craniectomies. Follow-up at 6-month intervals by clinical examination and by x-ray after new bone has formed is frequent enough to detect re-fusion. The infant

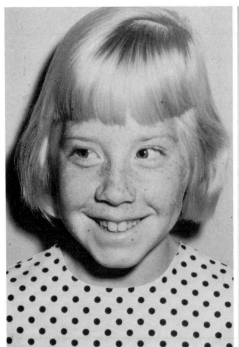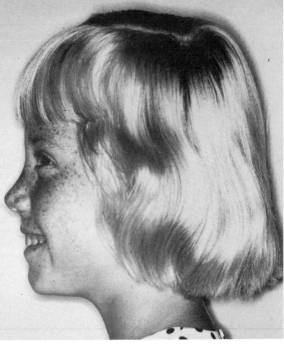

Figure 39–24 Multiple synostosis, postoperative appearance of same girl as in Figures 39–11 and 39–12. She is here 10 years old, has been getting excellent grades in school, and is considered normal. (*Left,* from Matson, D. D.: Neurosurgery of Infancy and Childhood. 2nd Ed. Springfield, Ill., Charles C Thomas, 1969. *Right,* from Shillito, J., and Matson, D. D.: Pediatrics, *41:*829–853, 1968. Reprinted by permission.)

shown in Figure 39–11 underwent a two-stage operation at 1 and 3 weeks of age, and re-fusion dictated reoperation at 18 months of age, when one of the two stages was repeated. The ultimate outcome has been most gratifying (Fig. 39–24).

In any case, if it is certain that the craniectomy is sealed and the child still has considerable brain growth to anticipate, cosmetic improvement will continue if the craniectomy is reopened. In multiple synostosis, if signs of increased intracranial pressure appear, reoperation is indicated even when further cosmetic change can be only slight. For example, a child only 18 months old with a re-fused coronal craniectomy will probably benefit from reoperation. A patient with re-fused coronal, sagittal, and lambdoid sutures at 4 years of age and with signs of increased intracranial pressure, however, also deserves to have further operative treatment considered.

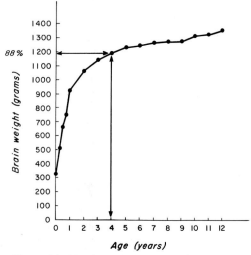

Figure 39–25   Growth curve of brain. By 4 years of age, 88 per cent of the weight of a 12-year-old brain has been achieved. During this period of rapid growth, cosmetic improvement will be most rewarding following craniectomy. Operation carried out during first few weeks of life permits greatest change in appearance. (From Shillito, J., and Matson, D. D.: Pediatrics, 41:829–853, 1968. Reprinted by permission.)

AT WHAT AGE IS OPERATION NOT INDICATED?

Since the linear craniectomy technique relies upon the growth of the brain to effect cosmetic improvement, it is obvious that the later an operation is performed, the less gain there will be. By referring to the growth curve of the brain, one can judge approximately what the returns will be from late operation (Fig. 39–25).[3] In general, craniectomies performed for the first time at an age greater than 2 years will probably have little detectable cosmetic consequence. The author has, on occasion, because of parental pressure, operated even up to the age of 3 years. Serial measurements of the width of the craniectomies showed little widening, and of course, there was no appreciable cosmetic change.

RECENT MODIFICATIONS IN TECHNIQUE

As experience has increased with craniofacial corrective operations, there has been considerable interest in using these techniques to correct the proptosis of Crouzon's and Apert's syndromes during the initial craniectomy (See Chapter 40).

In such cases, the supraorbital craniectomies are modified so that the cuts are made through the orbital roof.[8,14] The frontal bones may then be hinged forward, including the orbital roof, which immediately makes a little more room for the globe. It is hoped that at least part of the major corrective operations later in life may thus be made unnecessary. In cases of bilateral coronal synostosis, if proptosis is not present, it is felt that simpler supraorbital craniectomies combined with coronal craniectomies provide adequate cosmetic improvement (Fig. 39–26).

TOTAL SYNOSTOSIS

In the author's experience, total synostosis is indeed a rare occurrence. A small number of children have been seen at ages up to the late teens for various reasons usually related to head size or appearance of eyegrounds. Films of the skull show absence of all the cranial sutures, marked "beaten silver" appearance of the skull, and usually a head that is quite round and symmetrical (Fig. 39–27). Specifically, there are no areas of protrusion of the brain such as were seen in the child with multiple

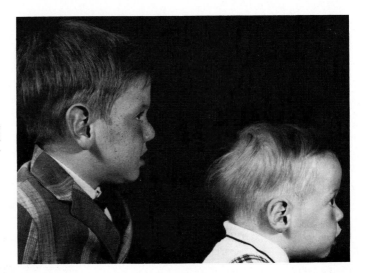

Figure 39–26 Brothers with bilateral coronal synostosis treated with coronal and supraorbital craniectomies in infancy.

synostosis previously described (see Figs. 39–11, 39–12, and 39–24). By careful inspection of the films and direct examination at operation, one may note the remnant of a suture here or there in a normal location. The head size is usually just below normal. There may be evidence of mild increased intracranial pressure. When craniectomies are completed there appears to be a popping apart of adjacent bone edges as the intracranial contents expand slightly.

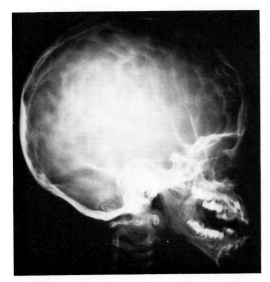

Figure 39–27 Skull films of a child with total synostosis. Note the ''beaten silver'' appearance of the skull and the absence of all sutures. The shape of the skull is perfectly acceptable, and its circumference is at about the third percentile for age. There was no clinical evidence of increased intracranial pressure.

None of these children has had serial preoperative x-rays. One can only guess at what has happened. It would appear, however, that the head has reached its near normal size by some other process than that permitted by suture spread alone. It may be that resorption of bone from within and deposition of bone from without permits gradual expansion of the cranial contents. Certainly there is no disfigurement of the skull, indicating that the process is perfectly uniform.

When deformity has been discovered at a suitable age or when there is evidence of increased intracranial pressure, linear craniectomies have been performed in two stages. Subsequent spread of these craniectomies has indicated that indeed the operation was needed, and a spurt in the growth rate of the skull following operation confirms that these are not cases of microcephaly with premature obliteration of the sutures because of failure of brain growth. This interesting group deserves further attention.

CONCLUSIONS AND RECOMMENDATIONS

Primary craniosynostosis is, by definition, a congenital defect involving the membranous bones of the skull. The defect probably always occurs in utero, where it has been documented radiographically. There is no evidence that abnormality of the underlying brain causes primary synostosis. It can almost always be diagnosed at birth by clinical and radiographic criteria. The synostotic suture may be abnormal over only a *part* of its length. This phenomenon may be one of the factors that delay diagnosis, since the roentgenographic appearance of those portions of the abnormal suture visualized by conventional projections may be falsely reassuring. Since the adjacent membranous bones are effectively tethered where the suture is absent, the remaining normal portions of the suture will be obliterated progressively and prematurely as they would in an adult when the growth of the brain ceases. This phenomenon accounts for the fallacy that primary synostosis develops after birth; it will, however, *progress* after birth.

The anterior fontanelle may be patent when synostosis is present in any one or in some combination of the four adjacent sutures. Therefore, the presence of the patent anterior fontanelle does not *rule out* primary craniosynostosis. Conversely, early disappearance of the fontanelle does not, in itself, *indicate* craniosynostosis. Nevertheless, radiographic investigation may be indicated when a physician feels the fontanelle has closed too soon; this is the only reliable way to rule out craniosynostosis. Rarely an anterior fontanelle bone will further confuse the diagnosis until x-rays are made. Its appearance, like that of a wormian bone in the lambdoid suture, is characteristic.

It has been repeatedly shown that early and proper surgical intervention will remove or significantly lessen cranial deformities due to primary cranial synostosis. The operative risk is justified by the cosmetic result alone and it can be acceptably small if certain principles are respected.

REFERENCES

1. Anderson, F. M., and Geiger, L.: Craniosynostosis: A survey of 204 cases. J. Neurosurg., *22*:229–240, 1965.
2. Apert, E.: De l'acrocéphalosyndactylie. Bull. Soc. Méd. Paris, *23*:1310–1331, 1906.
3. Coppoletta, J. M., and Wolbach, S. B.: Body length and organ weights. Amer. J. Path., *9*:55–70, 1933.
4. Crouzon, Q.: Dysostose cranio-faciale héréditaire. Bull. Soc. Méd. Hôp. Paris, *33*:545–555, 1912.
5. Fowler, F. D., and Matson, D. D.: A new method for applying polyethylene film to the skull in the treatment of craniosynostosis. J. Neurosurg., *14*:584–586, 1957.
6. Ingraham, F. D., Alexander, E., Jr., and Matson, D. D.: Polyethylene, a new synthetic plastic for use in surgery. J.A.M.A., *135*:82–87, 1947.
7. Hanson, J. W., Sayers, M.P., Knopp, L. M., MacDonald, C., and Smith, D. W.: Subtotal neonatal calvariectomy for severe craniosynostosis. J. Pediat., *91*:257–260, 1977.
8. Hoffman, M. J., and Mohr, G.: Lateral canthal advancement of the supraorbital margin. J. Neurosurg., *45*:376–381, 1976.
9. Hoyte, D. A.: A critical analysis of the growth in length of the cranial base. Birth Defects, *11*:255–282, 1975.
10. Kloss, J. L.: Craniosynostosis secondary to ventriculoatrial shunt. Amer. J. Dis. Child., *116*:315–317, 1968.
11. Matson, D. D.: Surgical treatment of congenital anomalies of the coronal and metopic sutures. J. Neurosurg., *17*:413–417, 1960.
12. Matson, D. D.: Neurosurgery of Infancy and Childhood. 2nd Ed. Springfield, Ill., Charles C Thomas, 1969.
13. Moss, M. L.: Functional anatomy of cranial synostosis. Child's Brain, *1*:22–33, 1975.
14. Raimondi, A. J., and Gutierrez, F. A.: A new surgical approach to the treatment of coronal synostosis. J. Neurosurg., *46*:210–214, 1977.
15. Shillito, J., Jr., and Matson, D. D.: Craniosynostosis: A review of 519 surgical patients. Pediatrics, *41*:829–853, 1968.
16. Shillito, J.: A new cranial suture appearing in the site of craniectomy for synostosis. Radiology, *107*:83–88, 1973.

40

CRANIOFACIAL CONGENITAL MALFORMATIONS

HISTORICAL BACKGROUND

Patients with congenital or acquired craniofacial abnormalities have benefited from the collaboration of teams of specialists working in the transitional area of the cranium and face. Early efforts to treat severe malformations commonly consisted of using superficial soft-tissue camouflage techniques in order to make the deformities less conspicuous. Correction of a bifid nose would improve somewhat the overall appearance of a patient with bifid nose and hypertelorism, and would, to some extent, minimize the orbital deformity.

Webster and Deming worked with the nose and surrounding soft tissue in an effort to change the face or to create facial optical illusions that made hypertelorism less conspicuous. Moving the eyebrows closer together and removing the excess tissue from the nasal bridge helped to camouflage the deformity of widely spread orbits. In 1962, Converse and Smith described an extracranial operation for correction of hypertelorism.[3] They removed a medial section of nasal bone and performed osteotomies of the anterior medial orbit so that the medial orbital walls could be more closely approximated. Silicone implants were inserted subperiosteally along the lateral orbital wall to deviate the orbital contents medially.

Lewin and later Longacre and deStefano described their use of onlay rib grafts to augment hypoplastic areas of the face.[14,15] Patients with Crouzon's disease (craniofacial dysostosis) and exophthalmos were treated with grafts only; however, problems with graft resorption made this a less than adequate operation.

In 1951, Gillies and Harrison reported a bold procedure for midface hypoplasia in a patient with Crouzon's disease and laid the groundwork for corrective craniofacial surgery.[11] Using a Le Fort III osteotomy, they advanced the hypoplastic midface region to correct the basic underlying deficiency in bony structure. For years, however, preference was given to camouflage procedures and onlay grafts, and the operation of Gillies and Harrison lay dormant.

In 1966, Murray performed a three-staged operation to correct maxillary hypoplasia and exophthalmos.[18] Utilizing Gillies and Harrison's concept of osteotomies to separate the face from the cranium, Murray advanced the patient's hypoplastic maxilla, produced good dental occlusion, and created deeper orbits.

In 1967, Tessier and co-workers reported a two-staged combined intracranial-extracranial operation to obtain medial displacement of the bony orbits.[20] Their basic technique is still in use today, although it has undergone some modification. In 1970, Converse and his associates noted that, in most patients with hypertelorism, the cribriform plate was not appreciably enlarged.[5] They suggested that Tessier's technique be modified into a one-stage procedure that would preserve the cribriform plate and the sense of smell. The removal of two paramedian segments of bone lateral to the cribriform plate made it possible to displace the orbits medially without disturbing the olfactory apparatus. From these diverse beginnings, craniofacial surgery has, during the last 10 years, developed into a combined specialty capable of managing patients with heretofore untreat-

J. E. MANISCALCO AND M. B. HABAL

able trauma, tumor, and congenital deformities. Centers have developed at major institutions that promote not only therapy but also research to better understand the complexities of many developmental defects.

THE CRANIOFACIAL TEAM

The basic clinical team consists of a plastic surgeon, a neurosurgeon, and an anesthesiologist. These three specialists form the mainstay of the operative team; their performance demands skill and coordinated effort and will greatly influence the success of the unit. Supportive team members who have a vital role during the preoperative and postoperative periods vary among institutions and with the needs of individual patients. These may include a psychologist, ophthalmologist, otorhinolaryngolgist, oral surgeon, and speech pathologist. Each of these specialists makes a unique contribution to the total evaluation and care of the patients, but the success of the clinical team rests on the collaborative efforts of all working together.

DEVELOPMENTAL ANATOMY

The neural tube forms from surface ectoderm and assumes a position below the surface layer. It is separated from the surface ectoderm by a layer of mesenchyme known as the neural crest (Fig. 40–1). While the neural tube undergoes changes and differentiation into the central nervous system, neural crest cells give rise to the autonomic nervous system and sensory ganglia.

The mesenchyme of the cephalic neural crest ultimately gives rise to all the cranial structures except the retina, lenses, epithelial tissue, vascular endothelium, and voluntary skeletal muscles. Influenced by the presence of substrate availability, inducer agents, and environmental factors, the neural crest cells migrate ventrally, giving rise to structures of the face.

As the facial structures take form, several processes or segments can be identified (Fig. 40–2). The frontonasal segment is distinguishable early in development and gives rise to the forehead, glabella, interorbital region, nose, and prolabium. Below the surface, the crista galli, ethmoid, nasal bones, vomer, nasal septum, premaxillary bone, and anterior palate also spring from the frontonasal segment. Other structures identified are the maxillary process and the mandibular and hyoid arches. During early development, the naso-optic furrow separates the nasolateral and maxillary processes. As these sites enlarge, they eventually fuse across the furrow. The nasomedial and maxillary processes also fuse to form the upper lip. The philtrum of the upper lip is formed by the fusion of both nasal medial processes in the midline.

Abnormalities in facial development result when crest cells fail to form, fail to remain viable, or fail to migrate normally. A range of malformations involving both facial structures and brain results. Failure of proper development of the frontonasal process results in a group of medial facial abnormalities associated with a severly abnormal brain and has led to the concept that, "the face predicts the brain."[7] During early development, the prechordal meso-

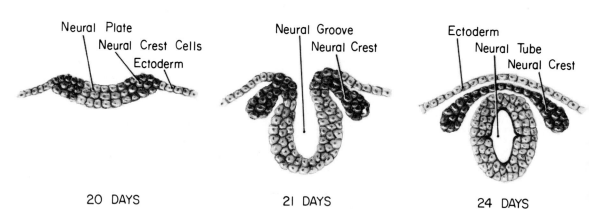

Neural Plate	Neural Groove	Ectoderm
Neural Crest Cells	Neural Crest	Neural Tube
Ectoderm		Neural Crest

20 DAYS   21 DAYS   24 DAYS

Figure 40–1   Development of human neural crest.

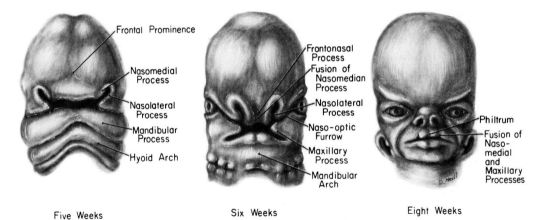

Five Weeks   Six Weeks   Eight Weeks

Figure 40-2   Processes and stages in the development of human facial structures.

derm induces the rostral neural ectoderm, which in turn is responsible for normal cleavage of the prosencephalon into telencephalon and diencephalon.

Midline facial structures developing in this abnormal milieu are affected and have several characteristics. Patients with hypotelorism and in whom midline cranial or facial bones are absent frequently have holoprosencephaly or other severe abnormalities of the central nervous system. An extreme example of this abnormal developmental process is cyclopia. The eyes are fused into one rudimentary optic structure, and the brain is so severely affected that the patient rarely survives the perinatal period. Available evidence suggests that holoprosencephaly and facial dysmorphia may be genetically transmitted as an autosomal recessive trait.[1]

Milder forms of median facial anomalies include hypotelorism and trigonocephaly. With these anomalies, brain development is usually normal. Thus, when hypotelorism is associated with underlying midline facial bony abnormality or with median cleft lip, the incidence of brain malformation is increased.

Hypertelorism, while often occurring as an isolated deformity, is part of a syndrome complex known as median cleft face syndrome (frontonasal dysplasia).[11] Developmentally, this defect is explained as a morphokinetic arrest in orbital migration. As a result of crest cell development, the optic structures remain widely separated in a fetal position while midline structures either fail to fuse or retain clefts. The features of this syndrome are hypertelorism, low or

V-shaped frontal hairline (widow's peak), cranium bifidum occultum, median cleft nose, median cleft upper lip, and median cleft palate. The resulting craniofacial abnormalities are no less severe than those found in the median facial syndrome; however, the most notable difference is the lack of brain involvement in most of these patients.

Although mental retardation and other abnormalities of the central nervous system occur with greater frequency than in the normal population, the incidence of brain involvement is far less than that associated with hypotelorism and the median facial syndrome. According to one authority, when orbital hypertelorism occurs as an isolated facial anomaly and is severe, or if it is accompanied by extracephalic anomalies, the probability of mental retardation is considerably greater than that in the median cleft face syndrome or in the normal population.[6] Occurring most frequently as a sporadic mutation, median cleft face syndrome may be inherited as an autosomal dominant trait.[2]

Crouzon's disease (craniofacial dysostosis) and Apert's syndrome (acrocephalosyndactyly) are developmental abnormalities that share several common clinical traits. Both conditions are characterized by severe midface hypoplasia, resulting in exorbitism or shallow orbits. These anomalies may result from premature fusion or synostosis of the sphenobasilar synchondroses of the cranial base in association with maxillary hypoplasia. The arrest in facial development leads to a compensatory overdevelopment of the greater wings of the sphenoid. The sphenoid wings in turn become translocated anteriorly and depressed inferiorly, the result being enlarged temporal fossae and shallow orbits.

EVALUATION

Evaluation of patients with craniofacial anomalies must be individualized. The craniofacial team composed of many specialists must first, on the basis of their individual examinations, decide what tests and procedures are needed. The neurosurgeon is concerned with the possibility of a malformed brain and chooses the appropriate method of evaluation. For patients who eventually will undergo intracranial exposure, a computed tomogram is the minimal test that should be considered. This examination often will reveal subtle, unexpected abnormalities, such as encephalocele, and will serve as a baseline for comparison with postoperative scans.

Age for Operation

The optimal age for a craniofacial operation has not been agreed on. Ideally, the operation should be performed early enough to keep the child from developing amblyopia. The age at which amblyopia is irreversible is, however, uncertain. Children whose appearances are grotesque should have corrective procedures before they begin school and develop psychological scars from peer criticism. For children with orbital abnormalities, sometime between 3 and 7 years of age seems to be optimal for operation. Patients with midface and alveolar deformities that require interdental fixation should not have the operation until the permanent dentition erupts (after the age of 7 years) to allow for better dental fixation.

Pathological Conditions

Hypertelorism

Hypertelorism is a physical finding characterized by increased interorbital distance. True hypertelorism occurs as a developmental anomaly when medial orbital migration is interrupted during development. The ethmoidal sinuses are widened

anteriorly, while posteriorly the sphenoid sinus and posterior ethmoid sinuses are very nearly their normal size. The optic canals are situated normally (Fig. 40–3). The orbital axis angle normally averages less than 60 degrees in adults. The visual and orbital axes normally form an angle of 22.5 degrees. In hypertelorism, the orbital axis angle is greater than 60 degrees; however, the apex of the projected angle remains in relatively normal position at the posterior sella turcica.[5] The cribriform plates are located on the same plane as the planum sphenoidale in the normal person, and are 1 to 2 cm below the level of the or-

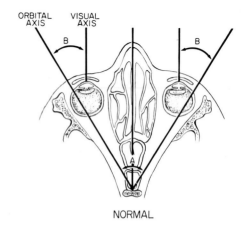

NORMAL

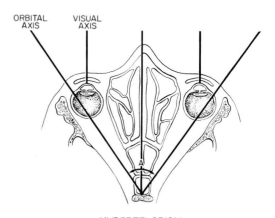

HYPERTELORISM

Figure 40–3 *Top.* Normally situated optic canals. The orbital axis–visual axis angle (B) is normally 22.5 degrees. The orbital axes intersect at the posterior sella turcica and form an angle of up to 60 degrees in normal persons. *Bottom.* Optic canals in hypertelorism. Although the orbital axis angle (A) is larger than 60 degrees, the apex of the angle remains located at the level of the posterior sella turcica.

bital roofs. In patients with hypertelorism, the cribriform plates usually are located below this level; they may be missing entirely in patients with encephaloceles. The understanding of this anatomical pathological change had led to the development of a corrective procedure in which two paramedian wedges of bone and ethmoid are removed and the orbits are rotated medially.

Hypertelorism is not considered a distinct clinical syndrome. It may be present with midline cleft syndrome, encephalocele, or Waardenburg syndrome, or it may be, in rare instances, an isolated finding. It may also be simulated or mimicked by other conditions. To better understand hypertelorism, one should understand the condition known as pseudohypertelorism, that is, epicanthus and telecanthus, as well as other conditions.

Epicanthus is a wide epicanthal fold that extends along the side of the nose over the medial canthus. It may be a normal finding in as many as 30 per cent of infants, and the folds usually recede by the end of the first year. Cursory examination reveals that the folds may impart the illusion of a wide intercanthal distance, simulating hypertelorism.

Increased distance between inner canthi is known as telecanthus. Primary telecanthus is due to excessive soft tissue in the canthal region; however, the interpupillary distance or the interorbital distance is normal. Secondary telecanthus is present whenever the distance between the orbits is increased abnormally. The overgrowth of the canthal region is due to the underlying overgrowth of bone and is seen in all patients with true hypertelorism.

Other conditions such as nasal orbital fractures, flat nasal bridge, widespread eyebrows, and external strabismus may give the illusionary effect of hypertelorism and must be differentiated by careful measurements.

Craniofacial Dysostosis

The craniofacial dysostoses have, as common findings, maxillary hypoplasia, dental malocclusion, relative prognathism, and exophthalmos. In Crouzon's disease, an autosomal dominant inherited trait, there are several abnormalities of the skull.[9] The clivus is oriented more vertically than usual, and the sphenoid plane is angled downward and forward. The floor of the frontal fossa is shorter than normal in the anteroposterior direction, while the transverse diameter of the skull is enlarged. The bones of the skull are thin, with increased digital markings, and multiple suture stenoses are commonly present. Hypertelorism, although frequently an associated finding, is not always present. Because of the maxillary hypoplasia and the foreshortened orbits, these patients have extrusion of the orbital contents and exophthalmos. The patients may have increased intracranial pressure with papilledema and visual loss as well as hydrocephalus, epilepsy, and mental retardation.

Apert's syndrome, inherited as an autosomal recessive trait, has findings very similar to those of Crouzon's disease.[9] Although unusual, both Crouzon's disease and Apert's syndrome have been found in members of the same family. Patients with Apert's syndrome are subject to premature suture stenosis, as are those with Crouzon's disease, the coronal suture seeming to be predominantly the only suture involved. As a result of this closure, the cranium grows vertically rather than laterally, giving the patient's head a turret shape (resembling a fireman's helmet). Clinically, the patients have flat supraorbital ridges with exophthalmos due to shallow orbits. Hypertelorism is a frequent associated finding, along with maxillary hypoplasia and the wide, flat nasal bridge. Features that also distinguish this from Crouzon's disease are syndactyly and polydactyly of the upper and lower extremities. Neurologically, most of these patients are mentally intact; because of the grotesque facial disfigurements, however, they often are institutionalized and treated as mentally defective.

Preoperative evaluation of patients with midface retrusion (hypoplasia) should include cephalometrics. Precise quantitative analysis of abnormalities may be obtained. The plans for operation may be formulated, and reasonable estimates of the required facial advancements, as well as the size of bone grafts that will be needed, may be calculated preoperatively. Cephalometry also provides an objective measure of longitudinal skull growth and facial growth after operation. From the linear and angular mea-

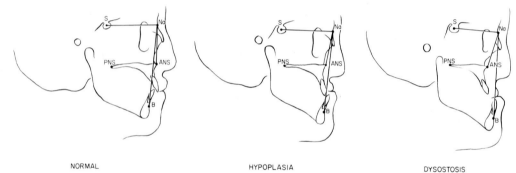

Figure 40–4   Normal cephalometric angles, maxillary hypoplasia, and craniofacial dysostosis. S, sella turcica; Na, nasion; ANS, anterior nasal spine; B, supramentale; PNS, posterior nasal spine.

surements obtained, assessment of the patient's defects may be quantitated and accurately defined. At times, relative prognathism secondary to maxillary hypoplasia is difficult to differentiate from true prognathism; cephalometrics can accurately identify the pathological changes.

Normal and abnormal values are available, but these data serve as guides rather than as absolute criteria for evaluation and operation. Examples of cephalometry in maxillary hypoplasia, craniofacial dysostosis, and normal development are illustrated in Figure 40–4. A few lines and reference points used to perform this evaluation accurately are: the center of the sella turcica (S), the frontonasal suture (nasion, or Na), the anterior nasal spine (ANS), the supramentale (point B), and the posterior nasal spine (PNS).

Midface hypoplasia and an abnormal cranial base develop in patients with craniofacial dysostosis. The distances from sella to nasion (S–Na), from nasion to anterior nasal spine (Na–ANS), and from anterior nasal spine to posterior nasal spine (ANS–PNS) are shorter than normal, indicating the lack of vertical and sagittal facial growth. The angle SNaANS is very acute, while the SNaB angle is greater than normal, reflecting both the maxillary hypoplasia and the relative prognathism. In patients with maxillary hypoplasia who do not have the other associated abnormalities of the cranial base seen in the dysostosis, the distance S–Na is usually normal, and the angle SNB is within a normal range. These differential measurements are the main cephalometric differences between the isolated maxillary hypo-

plasia and the hypoplasia associated with dysostosis. These few measurements are easily traced on the roentgenogram, thus providing not only a simple method for quantitating the underlying skeletal pathological changes but also a means for the accurate planning of the operative corrections. The angles and distances should serve only as a guide for the absolute measurements that the surgeons must make.

Involvement of the superior alveolar ridge may require dental casts to plan for correction of malocclusion. The oral surgeon on the team, in conjunction with a prosthodontist, should provide for this portion of the evaluation as well as for the preoperative placement of interdental bars if operative interdental fixation is anticipated.

Orbital Measurements

Intercanthal Distance

Patients with hypertelorism have intercanthal distances that are greater than 30 mm. This measurement, however, is unreliable as a sole determiner of hypertelorism. In primary telecanthus, patients may have wide epicanthal folds and large intercanthal distances without having true hypertelorism.

Interpupillary Distance

The normal adult interpupillary distance varies between 58 and 71.5 mm. This distance may be difficult to measure accurately in children who are uncooperative. Furthermore, in the presence of ocular strabismus, which many children have, the interpupillary distance is meaningless.

Interorbital Distance

Several methods have been described for the measurement of interorbital distance. Hansman measured the narrowest point be-

tween orbits on a roentgenogram (Waters' view).[13] The normal interorbital distances and ranges for females and males are given in Figure 40–5. This method appears to be simple yet accurate for determining the correct interorbital distance.

Preoperative planning and evaluation of patients with hypertelorism must be indi-

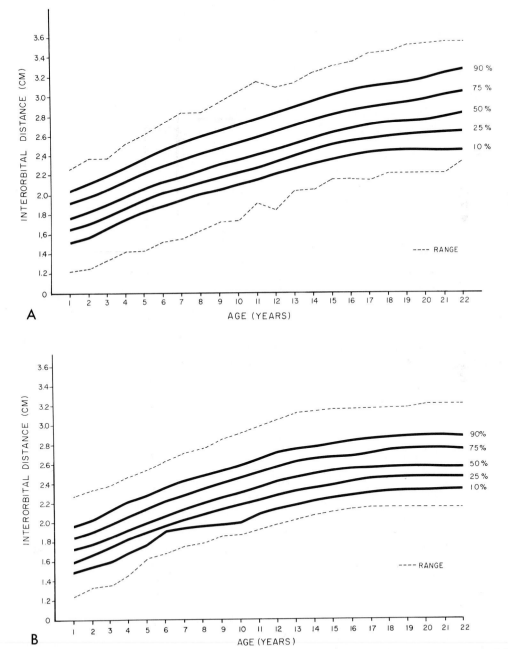

Figure 40–5 Percentile standards for interorbital distance in males, *A*, and females, *B*. (From Hansman, C. F.: Growth of interorbital distance and skull thickness as observed in roentgenographic measurements. Radiology, *86*:87–96, 1966. Reprinted by permission.)

vidualized. Displacement of the orbits may occur in more than one direction, that is, it may be horizontal, sagittal, or vertical.

Tomograms of the skull in anterior, lateral, and basal views provide the means for the proper assessment of interorbital distance, orbital angles, optic canal angle, and location of cribriform plates as well as a survey for missing bones. With tomography, the desired orbital correction can be precisely planned preoperatively. Overcorrection of 2 to 3 mm is desirable to compensate for a certain amount of orbital separation that usually occurs during the first year after operation. This widening, which is seen in approximately 75 per cent of patients, is probably due to bone graft resorption and erosion of the fixation wires.

A careful search for nasal and pharyngeal encephaloceles should be carried out. Absence of bone over these areas may be due to the presence of these abnormalities. Rhinoscopy and pharyngoscopy may be necessary.

Ophthalmological evaluation is vital and should be as complete as the patient will allow. Strabismus, visual fields, exophthalmos, and acuity are evaluated. After operation, strabismus may improve, remain unchanged, or become worse, and often, extraocular muscle procedures are needed.

Auditory acuity is also recorded before operation, and unsuspected hearing losses are often found.

OPERATIVE TECHNIQUES

Basic Principles

Several basic surgical principles apply to craniofacial operations. Loss of blood is a major problem in these procedures. It must be controlled by meticulous technique, and replacement therapy as indicated. Hypotensive anesthesia may be used to reduce the blood loss, but the nature of the operation causes hemorrhage to be expected.

Exposure of the cranial base is obtained by extradural dissection, with gentle retraction on the dura and intradural contents. Drainage of cerebrospinal fluid via the lumbar route facilitates exposure. If needed, mannitol may be used to further enhance the exposure.

Intraoperative monitoring of visual evoked response has been useful in some types of operation around the optic nerves.[8] Although not mandatory for this procedure, the use of intraoperative monitoring enhances its safety.

Autogenous bone grafting is used extensively in craniofacial operations. Grafts are obtained from the chest wall (ribs) and iliac crests to fill gaps created by the osteotomies. When compared with synthetic materials, bone grafts have the physiological advantage of eventually fusing and becoming incorporated into a repair site. Cancellous bone provides a matrix for new bone development (osteoneogenesis) once it becomes revascularized.[15] The ribs are split longitudinally to expose as much cancellous material as possible, and this increases the potential for regeneration. From the iliac crest, cancellous bone is obtained by curetting between the layers of cortical bone. Bone dust is also collected from the sites of the burr holes and is used throughout the reconstruction to fill in small defects and depressions, much as a craftsman uses putty.

In certain unusual situations, alloplastic materials have been used for reconstruction of the craniofacial region. The availability of synthetic substances and the decreased morbidity they cause in chest and hip wounds make them appealing for use. Their main disadvantage, however, is that these materials remain as foreign bodies and never become fully incorporated or fused into the reconstruction sites. Thus, they serve as a nidus for infection, acute and delayed, during the postoperative period.

The Cranial Orbital Region

Hypertelorism

The objectives of the operation are medial rotation of the orbits and contents and preservation of vision and sense of smell.

A bicoronal incision is used to elevate the scalp flap. The pericranium is carefully dissected and taken as a separate layer to be used later for draping over the osteotomized segments of bone. This extra step provides pericranium for direct contact with the bone grafts. The interaction of

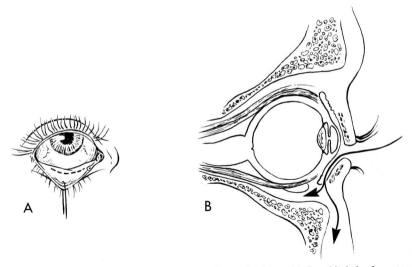

Figure 40–6 *A* and *B*. Transconjunctival approach to floor of orbit and infraorbital rim for osteotomy.

periosteum and bone graft may enhance the revascularization and eventual incorporation of the graft. A subperiosteal dissection is carried out over the orbital rims and into the orbits, exposing the superior, lateral, and medial aspects of both orbits. The nasal bridge is likewise exposed. Soft-tissue dissection is extended to the zygomatic arches to expose the temporal fossa. The intraorbital dissection is gently performed to preserve the integrity of the periorbita and the lacrimal apparatus.

Access to the floor of the orbit is obtained through a separate incision. A transconjunctival incision behind the eyelash line gives excellent exposure of this region, while contact lenses protect the corneas from abrasion and injury.[12,19] The infraorbital neurovascular bundle is identified and preserved by the later performance of an osteotomy just below the level of the infraorbital foramen (Fig. 40–6).

Next, a standard bifrontal craniotomy is performed, leaving a substantial supraorbital rim of bone (frontal bar) for eventual wiring (Fig. 40–7A). An epidural dissection is performed, and both frontal lobes are carefully elevated, leaving the cribriform region attached and undisturbed (Fig. 40–7B and C). Special efforts must be made to avoid penetration of the dura. Frequently, the inner table of the skull is irregular, with spicules of bone projecting into and penetrating the dura, thus making this portion of the operation technically more difficult.

Dural tears should be oversewn immediately with 5-0 silk suture to avoid cerebrospinal fluid leakage after the operation. The dissection is extended posteriorly to the sphenoid ridges bilaterally.

This sequence of operative steps leaves exposure of the brain until last. Doing as much of the facial and soft-tissue dissection as possible before starting the intracranial work exposes the brain less to the potential dangers of trauma or infection. Once the intracranial and extracranial areas have been completely exposed, the osteotomies are performed. On the basis of preoperative measurements, the orbits and frontal bar are marked and cut with an oscillating saw. The roofs of the orbits are cut with tiny, sharp osteotomes from the intracranial approach. In patients with very thin bones, the bony orbit may be as thin as an eggshell and will crack as readily. The precautions of using very sharp osteotomes and avoiding excessive pressure should be taken while these cuts are being made in the orbit. The potential for optic nerve injury is great if fractures occur and extend to the optic canal. A small right-angle oscillating saw blade is used intraorbitally to perform a circumferential osteotomy. This cut must be made no deeper than the posterior ethmoid foramen to avoid injury to the optic nerve. The orbital opening of the optic canal and the posterior ethmoid foramen are separated by approximately 6 mm.[16] The inferior and superior orbital fissures are con-

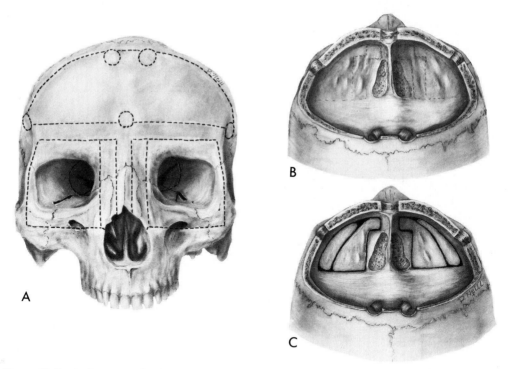

Figure 40–7   *A*. Osteotomy for hypertelorism. Two paramedian nasal segments are measured and outlined prior to performance of the osteotomy. *B*. Outline of osteotomies to be performed on floor of frontal fossa. *C*. Orbits have been rotated medially and bone grafts placed laterally to maintain this position. The cribriform plate is left undisturbed.

nected by the osteotomy, and in order to avoid injury to their contents, dissection and adequate visualization of the fissures must be accomplished before the osteotomies are begun. Throughout this portion of the operation, care is taken to avoid excessive pressure on the osteotomes and inadvertent fracture of the orbit. The orbital contents must be retracted gently to expose the skeleton, and again, care must be taken to avoid injury of the nerves by undue traction.

After the osteotomies are completed and the nasal segments of bone removed, the orbits are medially rotated and wired into place (Fig. 40–8). Blocks of bone graft are used to stabilize the orbits and fill the defects created by the osteotomies. The craniotomy bone plate is replaced, and the burr holes are filled with bone dust.

The medial canthi must be reapproximated in their new position and secured with standard Silastic felt buttons. The lateral canthi are sutured to incline them upward and to avoid the postoperative appearance of the antimongoloid (downward) slant. Closure of the scalp flap is then a rou-

tine procedure, and subgaleal wound drains are placed for 24 hours. Occlusive tarsorrhaphies are performed to avoid conjunctival herniation from edema. A tight compressive dressing is applied to the head and face and is left in place for one week. The subgaleal drains may be removed without disturbing the head dressing if long sutures are sewn through the ends of the drains and allowed to protrude through the dressing. By gently pulling on these sutures, the drains may be easily removed, leaving the dressing relatively undisturbed.

Postoperatively, the spinal subarachnoid drainage is maintained and antibiotics are given prophylactically. Although the pupils are not accessible for postoperative monitoring, the patient's vision may be crudely tested by shining a flashlight below the bandages into the eyes.

Orbital Dystopia

The congenital misplacement of an orbit may occur in any direction. The corrective procedure is similar to that previously described for hypertelorism but involves

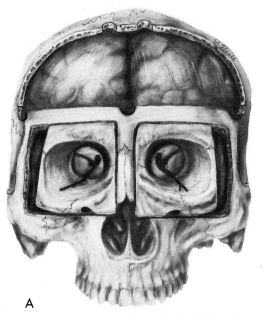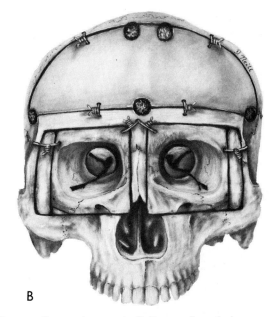

A   B

Figure 40–8 *A*. Orbits rotated medially after removal of paramedian nasal segments. *B*. Bone grafts and wires placed to secure orbital location.

work around one orbit only; the same method is used to move the laterally dystopic orbit medially. Frequently, however, the orbits are deviated in two directions, (that is, laterally and inferiorly), and osteotomies must be planned accordingly. The principles of correction are identical to the ones described earlier.

The Midface Region

Maxillary Hypoplasia

The operative objectives for maxillary hypoplasia are advancement of the hypoplastic midfacial region to produce normal facial contours, deepening of the shallow orbits, and advancement of the superior alveolar ridge for better dental occlusion.

A bicoronal incision is used to expose both temporal fossae and zygomatic arches. A subperiosteal dissection is used to expose the orbital contents and nasal bridge. Burr holes are placed in each frontal fossa, through which cottonoid packs may be introduced carefully to separate the dura from the anterior fossa floor and orbital roofs. While the brain is protected with cottonoid packs, the osteotomies are performed (Fig. 40–9). The osteotomies may

vary slightly according to the specific needs of the patient. For example, if orbital depth is not a problem, a Le Fort II osteotomy is used, and the orbital margins are left undisturbed. The Le Fort III osteotomy shown in Figure 40–9 separates the face from the cranium and provides for orbital volume enlargement as well as alveolar alignment. The osteotomies around the orbits have been performed in different ways, according to the preference of individual surgeons and the needs of the patients. Two variations are shown in Figure 40–10. One type splits the lateral orbital rims and utilizes wedges of bone graft to secure the face in the advanced position (Fig. 40–10*A*). This technique requires a well-developed orbit with wide rims, and therein lies the problem. The patients who need this operation often have thinned bones and narrow rims. The other type—the "spike" osteotomy—allows the locking or fixation of the advanced face by overriding the spikes at the superolateral edges of the orbits (Fig. 40–10*B*). This technique, however, requires onlay grafts to augment the supraciliary ridges.

During the preoperative planning phase and with the aid of cephalometrics, precise measurements are taken to calculate the amount of facial advancement needed.

Generally, these measurements serve only as a guide and are not to be relied on as are the absolute measures that are taken at operation. As with the operation for hypertelorism, overcorrection by several millimeters is done to compensate for the bone absorption that usually occurs in 6 to 18 months after the procedure.

The upper part (orbital region) is advanced farther (tipped forward) than the lower part of the face (alveolar ridge) so that, in effect, the advancement, rather than being a straight line forward, is in a small arc (Fig. 40–11).

The forward and downward movements of the lower orbits increase the volume not only by deepening the orbits but also by widening them. All osteotomy sites are

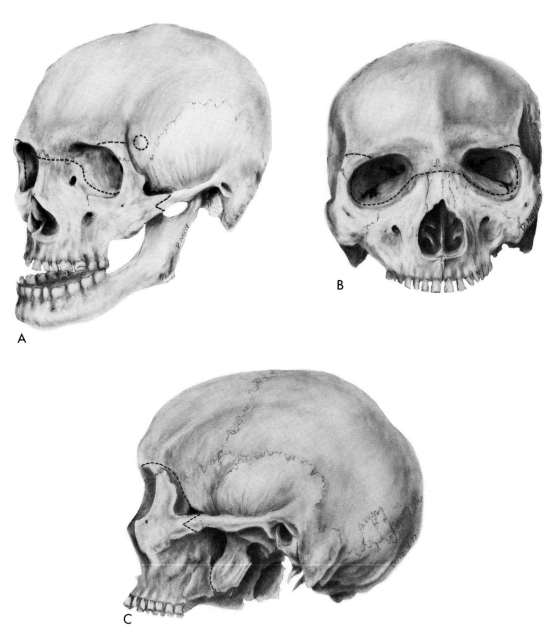

Figure 40–9 Le Fort III osteotomy. *A.* Oblique view. *B.* Anterior view. *C.* Lateral view. Dotted lines indicate the osteotomy used for midface advancement.

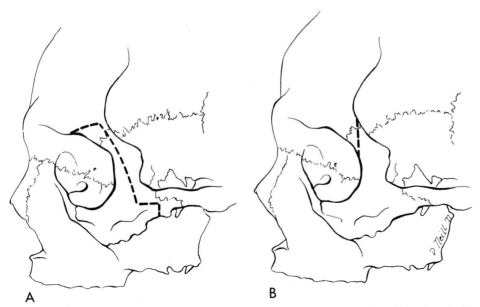

Figure 40–10 Alternative osteotomies for midface advancement. *A*. Osteotomy for well-developed orbits with wide rims splits the lateral orbital rims and uses wedges of bone graft to secure the face in the advanced position. *B*. "Spike" osteotomy locks the advanced face by overriding the spikes at the superolateral edges of the orbits.

Figure 40–11 Le Fort III osteotomy advances midface and orbital rims. A hollowed segment of rib graft is used to encase the zygomatic arches bilaterally. The face is advanced to produce deeper orbits and improved dental occlusion. Bone wedges will be placed to fill all gaps.

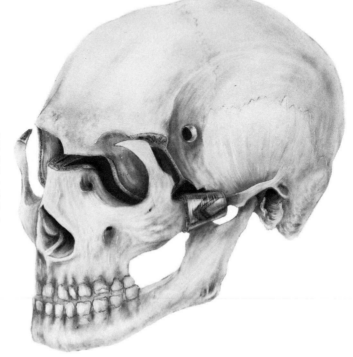

filled with blocks of bone graft. The supra-ciliary ridges are augmented as needed by rib grafts that are wired in place.

POSTOPERATIVE MANAGEMENT

The first 48 to 72 postoperative hours are critical. Cerebral edema usually manifests itself during this time. In an effort to combat this complication, fluids are severely restricted while urinary output and electrolytes are carefully monitored. Dexamethasone is administered in high dosage, and the patient is placed in the semi-Fowler position, with the head of the bed elevated 30 degrees.

Usually there is continuous oozing from the operative sites postoperatively, and blood should be administered as indicated. To avoid fluid overload, patients should receive packed red blood cells rather than whole blood. Occasionally units of fresh whole blood may be needed to replace clotting factors.

The airway is critical and must be maintained until the patient is past the danger of hypoxia or aspiration. The patient should be kept intubated for approximately 24 hours until response to verbal command is brisk and the level of consciousness appears to be normal. Patients with wired teeth are maintained with a tracheostomy for approximately one week until the danger of aspiration is past.

Antibiotics are used prophylactically because of the length of the operation, the number of free bone grafts, and the amount of implanted wire. The penicillins are used prophylactically in combination with an agent such as gentamicin that is effective against gram-negative organisms. The risks of infection are substantial, justifying this aggressive prophylactic use of antibiotics.

Cerebrospinal fluid drainage is maintained via the lumbar subarachnoid catheter for approximately two days after operation to allow dural tears to heal.

There is little indication for the prophylactic use of anticonvulsants unless the brain has been lacerated or cerebral resection has been performed. Hypoxia during the postoperative period may be manifested by generalized convulsions, but the need for anticonvulsants is questionable.

The operative mortality and morbidity rates vary according to the complexity of the case and from one institution to another. Mortality rates have ranged from 0 to 5 per cent.[4,10,17] An operation is fraught with the potential for major complications. Most of the serious ones result from cerebral edema, sepsis, loss of visual function, or intracranial blood clot. These problems are anticipated, and with the slightest indication, a postoperative CT scan should be obtained. The wires used for fixation produce scan artifacts, but enough of the intracranial structures can be seen to make the use of this test worthwhile. An arteriogram may be performed if the scan is not diagnostic.

The face and head dressings are removed for the first time on the seventh postoperative day. Gauze pads moistened in ice-cold saline are applied to the eyes and face to minimize the swelling that will occur. The occlusive tarsorrhaphy sutures are removed if the orbital structures are not excessively swollen or tense. The patients usually have painful photophobia for one or two days.

SUMMARY

The field of craniofacial surgery has developed rapidly over the last 10 years. Congenital malformations heretofore considered hopeless are now being corrected by a team of specialists working together in the craniofacial junction. Experience gained with work in congenital abnormalities has improved the understanding of the anatomical relationships of structures in this region as well as of the behavior of biological tissues. This experience has enhanced the ability to cope with other problems such as tumors and trauma of the craniofacial region.

The effects of operation on facial growth centers remain an unresolved issue. The severe congenital malformations that result from cranial suture stenosis are still poorly understood. Although synchondrosis of the skull base has been proposed as the basis, or underlying cause, for maldevelopment, this entity remains an enigma. Early detection of the maldeveloping face and correction of the underlying problem prior to the formation of grotesque features is a goal we can hope to attain in the future.

REFERENCES

1. Cohen, M. M., Jr., Jirasek, J. E., Guzman, R. T., et al.: Holoprosencephaly and facial dysmorphia: Nosology, etiology and pathogenesis. Birth Defects, 7:125–135, 1971.
2. Cohen, M. M., Jr., Sedano, H. O., Gorlin, R. J., et al.: Frontonasal dysplasia (median cleft face syndrome): Comment on etiology and pathogenesis. Birth Defects, 7:117–119, 1971.
3. Converse, J. M., and Smith, B.: An operation for congenital and traumatic hypertelorism. *In* Troutman, R. C., Converse, J. M., and Smith, B., eds.: Plastic and Reconstructive Surgery of the Eye and Adnexa. Washington, D.C., Butterworth & Co., 1962, pp. 104–110.
4. Converse, J. M., Wood-Smith, D., and McCarthy, J. G.: Report on a series of 50 craniofacial operations. Plast. Reconstr. Surg., 55: 283–293, 1975.
5. Converse, J. M., Ransohoff, J., Matthews, E. S., et al.: Ocular hypertelorism and pseudohypertelorism. Plast. Reconstr. Surg., 45:1–13, 1970.
6. DeMeyer, W.: The median cleft face syndrome. Neurology (Minneap.), 17:961–971, 1967.
7. DeMeyer, W., Zeman, W., and Palmer, C. G.: The face predicts the brain: Diagnostic significance of median facial anomalies for holoprosencephaly (arhinencephaly). Pediatrics, 34:256–263, 1964.
8. Feinsod, M., Selhorst, J. B., Hoyt, W. F., et al.: Monitoring optic nerve junction during craniotomy. J. Neurosurg., 44:29–31, 1976.
9. Francois, J.: Heredity of craniofacial dysostoses. Mod. Probl. Ophthal., 14:5–48, 1975.
10. Freihofer, H. P., Jr.: Results after mid-face osteotomies. J. Maxillofac. Surg. 1:30–36, 1973.
11. Gillies, H., and Harrison, S. H.: Operative correction by osteotomy of recessed malar maxillary compound in a case of oxycephaly. Brit. J. Plast. Surg., 3:123–127, 1951.
12. Habal, M. B.: Experience in the application of the transconjunctival route for surgical exposure in the orbital region. Surgery, 143:437–439, 1976.
13. Hansman, C. F.: Growth of interorbital distance and skull thickness as observed in roentgenographic measurements. Radiology, 86:87–96, 1966.
14. Lewin, M. L.: Facial deformity in acrocephaly and its surgical correction. Arch. Ophthal., 47:321–327, 1952.
15. Longacre, J. J., and deStefano, G. A.: Reconstruction of extensive defects of the skull with split rib grafts. Plast. Reconstr. Surg., 19:186–200, 1957.
16. Maniscalco, J. E., and Habal, M. B.: Microanatomy of the optic canal. J. Neurosurg., 48:402–406, 1978.
17. Matthews, D. N.: Experience in major craniofacial surgery. Plast. Reconstr. Surg., 59:163–174, 1977.
18. Murray, J. E., and Swanson, L. T.: Mid-face osteotomy and advancement for craniosynostosis. Plast. Reconstr. Surg., 41:299–306, 1968.
19. Tessier, P.: The conjunctival approach to the orbital floor and maxilla in congenital malformation and trauma. J. Maxillofac. Surg., 1:3–8, 1973.
20. Tessier, P., Guiot, G., Rougerie, J., et al.: Ostéotomies cranio-naso-orbito-faciales. Hypertélorisme. Ann. Chir. Plast., 12:103–118, 1967.
21. Webster, J. P., and Deming, E. G.: The surgical treatment of the bifid nose. Plast. Reconstr. Surg., 6:1–37, 1950.

41

ANOMALIES OF THE CRANIOVERTEBRAL JUNCTION

The term "craniovertebral junction" refers to an area comprising the inferior portion of the occipital bone surrounding the foramen magnum and the upper two cervical vertebrae. These bones and the ligaments uniting them form a funnel-shaped enclosure within which the spinal cord joins the medulla oblongata and the inferior portion of the cerebellum.

EMBRYOLOGY

It is generally accepted that three or four sclerotomes take part in the formation of the occipital bone, but they are not as clearly individualized as the more caudal spinal sclerotomes.[34,49,56] The latter form the protovertebrae and differentiate into a clear-staining cephalic half and a denser caudal half. These halves are separated by the intervertebral fissure, later to become the intervertebral disc, while the caudal dense portion of a protovertebra joins the clear cephalic portion of the subjacent one to form the definitive vertebra. Each vertebra therefore results from the union of adjacent halves of two protovertebrae (two sclerotomes).

The atlas is an exception to this rule. It is formed, like other vertebrae, by the junction of the caudal dense half of the first spinal sclerotome (proatlantal sclerotome) with the clear cephalic half of the subjacent protovertebra, but the clear cephalic portion of the proatlantal sclerotome also attaches to these two halves and does not unite with the last occipital sclerotomes above, which eventually become the occipital condyles and the margins of the foramen magnum (Fig. 41–1).

The atlas does not develop a vertebral body. Instead, the anlage of this body becomes the main portion of the odontoid process. Since the intervening intervertebral disc fails to develop a nucleus pulposus, the odontoid process unites to the anlage of the body of the axis. An inconstant ossification center for the tip of the odontoid probably originates from the clear uppermost half of the proatlantal sclerotome and may remain separate from the main body of the odontoid. List calls it the "ossiculum terminale."[49] The anterior arch of the atlas does not stem from the anlage of the body of the atlas but from a condensation of mesenchyme in a more ventral portion of the sclerotome, the hypochordal bow, which merges at the sides with the dorsally situated neural arch.

ASYMPTOMATIC ANOMALIES

A variety of anomalies of bony, meningeal, and neural elements can be the result of developmental errors, and others can be produced later, even in adult life, by alterations in the bone structure, meningeal inflammation, and the like. Some of these, although they remain asymptomatic in themselves, are often seen in association with more serious defects.[34,49,54,55,56] Rachischisis (spina bifida) of the anterior or, more commonly, the posterior arch of the atlas, and asymmetries in the occipitoatlantal and altantoaxial joints are seen frequently. The most caudal occipital sclerotomes may fail to fuse completely with the others forming the occiput and can remain as a more or less separate "occipital vertebra" that may be difficult to differentiate

---

G. BERTRAND

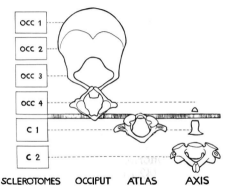

Figure 41–1 Development of the occiput, atlas, and axis according to List. The occipital squama and condyles are viewed from below; atlas and axis are seen from above. The cross-hatched bar represents the craniovertebral border.

from occipitalization of the atlas. In the case of the occipital vertebra, however, the condyles retain their "occipital" characteristics, with their articulating surfaces directed downward and laterally rather than downward and medially like those of the atlas. The posterior arch is usually narrower than the arch of the atlas; it has no groove for the vertebral arteries and the first cervical nerves, which must course beneath the arch. The transverse processes have no foramen for the arteries. On the anterior border of the foramen magnum, a joint or facet-like structure is sometimes found that has been called a "third occipital condyle."[55] It usually does not articulate with the anterior arch of the atlas below it but may be quite close.

SYMPTOMATIC ANOMALIES

Other anomalies may result in serious neurological symptoms. Basilar impression (invagination), occipitalization of the atlas, separate odontoid process or absence of the process, and chronic atlantoaxial dislocation can produce mechanical compression of the spinal-medullary junction. A frequent congenital abnormality of the hindbrain, the Chiari (Arnold-Chiari) malformation, and the less common Dandy-Walker malformation produce a variety of symptoms, chiefly through alterations in the dynamics of cerebrospinal fluid circulation that result in hydrocephalus, hydromyelia, and syringomyelia.

Basilar Impression

Basilar impression is an upward indentation or invagination of the normally convex base of the skull, which looks as though the rigid cervical spine were being pushed up into a softer, more plastic base that yields under the weight of the head. This is indeed the mechanism in disorders such as osteomalacia, osteogenesis imperfecta, cretinism, rickets, and more commonly, Paget's disease that cause softening of the bones and in which the deformity is known to be progressive (Fig. 41–2). The frequent association of basilar impression and congenital fusion of cervical vertebrae to each other or to the occiput indicates that a developmental defect must be at the origin of most cases.

Gardner believes, however, that although the cause is present at birth, the deformity is not truly congenital (since it is never seen in the newborn) but must develop after birth as a result of the upright posture, which causes the relatively heavy head to settle downward on the cervical spine.[36] As in the acquired forms, the bone of the invaginating occiput is compressed radially toward the center of the foramen magnum, whose circumference is reduced.

Since Schüller's first radiological demonstration of basilar impression in 1911, a number of authors have described various

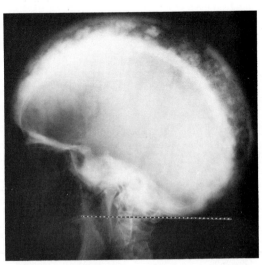

Figure 41–2 Acquired basilar impression in Paget's disease of the skull. Note upward invagination of occipital condyles. Odontoid tip is 23 mm above McGregor's line.

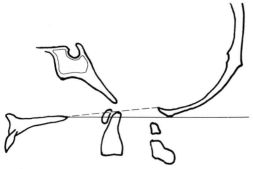

Figure 41–3   Schematic drawing of Chamberlain's line (*dashes*) and McGregor's line (*solid line*) in the normal skull.

roentgenographic measurements of the base that can be used to diagnose or exclude the anomaly.[65] Chamberlain's line, joining the dorsal lip of the foramen magnum to the dorsal margin of the hard palate, should normally lie above the tip of the odontoid process of the axis and pass through the ventral lip of the foramen magnum on a true lateral film of the skull (Fig. 41–3).[15] When invagination is present, the posterior lip of the foramen may be difficult to visualize unless midsagittal tomograms are used. McGregor's line, joining the hard palate to the most caudal portion of the occipital curve, is easier to see.[52] In basilar invagination, the tip of the odontoid can rise far above this line (Figs. 41–4 and 41–5). More than 4.5 mm is considered pathological by McGregor. The anterior margin of the foramen magnum and the occipital condyles that bear the thrust of the spine are also displaced upward. This elevation of the condyles can be appreciated on standard posteroanterior skull films by comparing their location and the level of the odontoid tip with the position of the bimastoid line of Fischgold joining the two mastoid tips (Fig. 41–6).[30] Fischgold's line normally passes through the occipitoatlantal joint and the tip of the dens. These structures are seen well above the bimastoid line in basilar invagination, as the base of the skull becomes concave rather than convex (Fig. 41–7).

Platybasia

The term "platybasia" has been used synonymously with "basilar impression" by some authors.[15,67] It refers, however, only to an abnormally obtuse basal angle—greater than 142 to 147 degrees, depending on how it is measured—joining the plane of the clivus with the plane of the anterior fossa of the skull (Fig. 41–8). It is not a measure of basilar invagination and, although platybasia is often present with basilar impression, it causes no symptom by itself.

Occipitalization of Atlas

Occipitalization, also called assimilation, of the atlas implies a bony union between the skull and the first cervical vertebra. A lack of movement between the two can be suggestive of the malformation but is not diagnostic.[56] This bony fusion occurs most often between the skull and the anterior arch of the atlas. It may also involve the

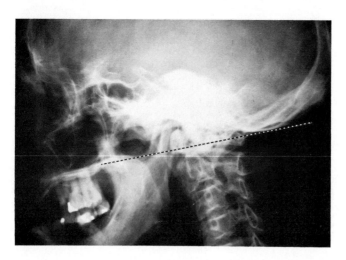

Figure 41–4   Congenital basilar impression, lateral view. Odontoid tip is well above McGregor's line.

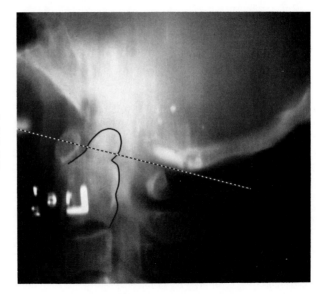

Figure 41–5 Sagittal tomographic view showing odontoid 11.5 mm above McGregor's line. Canal is narrowest between body of axis and posterior arch of atlas (13 mm on films with 20 per cent enlargement). Patient had spastic tetraparesis, posterior column signs.

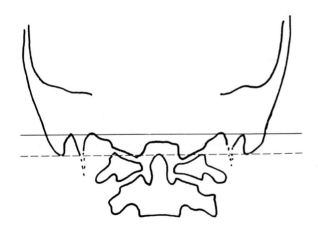

Figure 41–6 Diagrammatic representation of Fischgold's bimastoid line (*dashes*) and Fischgold's and Metzger's digastric line (*solid line*) in the normal skull.

Figure 41–7 Frontal view of case of congenital basilar impression illustrated in Figure 41–4. The upward invagination of the base of the skull projects the odontoid tip far above the bimastoid line and even above the digastric line. Note also the elevated petrosal tips.

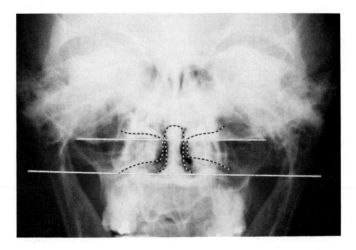

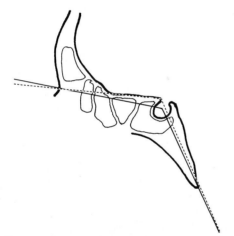

Figure 41–8 Diagrammatic midsagittal view of the base of the skull showing the basal angle according to Boogaard (*solid line,* normal 118 to 147 degrees) and according to McRae (*dashes,* normal 120 to 140 degrees).

posterior arch, the transverse processes, and the lateral masses, causing disappearance of the occipitoatlantal joint space (Figs. 41–9 and 41–10). In some cases, the atlas seems to be so completely assimilated into the skull as to be only a thickened rim around the foramen magnum. In these cases, the vertebral arteries appear to penetrate directly into the base of the skull. Garcin believes that the term "assimilation" should be reserved for these cases in which no vestige of the atlas is recognizable as such above the foramen.[34]

The distance separating the dens from the posterior rim of the assimilated atlas represents the effective anteroposterior diameter of the foramen available to the spinal medullary junction. McRae and Barnum found that, in their series, a reduction of this distance to 19 mm or less usually was associated with neurological signs.[56] They also noted that C2 was fused to C3 in 18 of their 25 cases of occipitalization of the atlas.

Malformation of Axis: Atlantoaxial Dislocation

It is understandable that during flexion and extension of the head on the neck, a congenital fusion of occiput to atlas, particularly if C2 and C3 are also fused, will increase the strain on the ligaments that should normally only allow rotation of atlas on axis. The transverse ligaments that hold the odontoid against the anterior arch of the atlas may be hypoplastic or may become relaxed, allowing the dens to move back into the lumen of the foramen magnum (see Fig. 41–10). In this position, the tip of the displaced dens may press against the ventral aspect of the medulla, compressing it and the cerebellum against the posterior margin of a narrow foramen magnum.[67] Any degree of basilar invagination will intensify the pressure on the medulla by raising the odontoid process even higher and increasing the degree of angulation between the intracranial portion of the medulla and its continuation in the spinal canal. Fortunately, the odontoid itself is often the site of congenital anomalies, being abnormally short, hypoplastic, or tilted ventrally at the tip or to one side. The position of the odontoid in the foramen can be seen on midsagittal tomograms or on axial views of the base. The hyperextended neck posture necessary to obtain these basal projections may be dangerous in symptomatic patients. Computed tomography of the region is much safer, since the neck can be maintained in neutral position.

Relaxation of the transverse odontoid ligaments can result from other causes than congenital malformations. Inflammatory

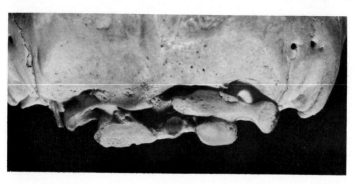

Figure 41–9 Occipitalized atlas. Left transverse process and both halves of left posterior arch are fused to occiput. Right transverse process is not fused. (Courtesy of Dr. D. L. McRae.)

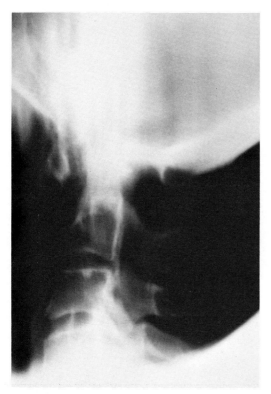

Figure 41–10   Midsagittal tomogram showing occipitalized atlas, posterior arch completely fused to occiput. There is also atlantoaxial dislocation, the odontoid being only 15 mm from the posterior margin of the foramen magnum. Patient had spastic tetraparesis but no sensory symptoms.

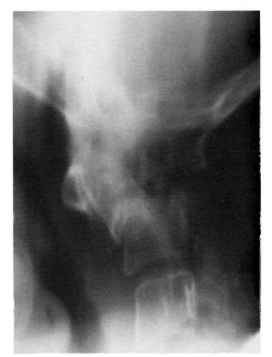

Figure 41–11   Fracture-dislocation of odontoid process, still mobile six months after trauma. Patient had neck pain, but no neurological deficit.

conditions such as rheumatoid arthritis, bacterial or tuberculous osteitis, and neoplasms can lead to atlantoaxial dislocation. In children, the local inflammatory reactions secondary to acute pharyngitis can produce an anteriorly rotated dislocation of one lateral mass of the atlas. The displaced portion may be pushed completely off the corresponding surface of the axis, where it may become locked and produce the characteristic torticollis described by Grisel.[39]

Separate Odontoid Process

In cases of chronic atlantoaxial dislocation, the odontoid process is often found to be separated from the body of C2. This is frequently the result of trauma and merely represents a nonunited fracture of the odontoid. Diagnosis is easy if the films still show the rough irregular edges of the fracture, as illustrated in Figure 41–11, but

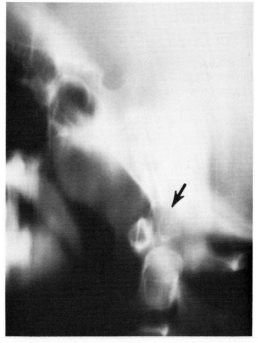

Figure 41–12   Separate odontoid process (*arrow*), probably congenital in origin, in an 8-year-old child. Note smooth, rounded top of body of axis. The patient had transient tetraparesis after a fall on the head.

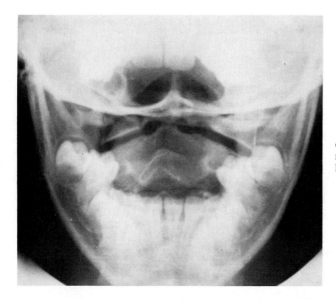

Figure 41–13   Open-mouth view in the case shown in Figure 41–12. Note smooth, rounded top of body of C2, characteristic of long-standing or congenital lesion.

some patients give no history of injury, and the opposing surfaces of the odontoid and the top of axis appear rounded and smooth (Figs. 41–12 and 41–13). Such lesions may be congenital in origin, particularly when associated with other developmental anomalies, but they are undistinguishable from and may be ancient fractures sustained in childhood.[29,32] Cineradiography during flexion and extension of the neck in such cases shows that the atlas glides forward and back on C2, the separate odontoid remaining attached to the anterior arch. Then, as flexion is increased, C1 tilts forward over the anterior rounded edges of the articular pillars of C2. In doing so, the posterior arch, which had come very close to the base of the odontoid during the forward gliding movement, rises, increasing somewhat the "critical distance" separating the arch and the stump of the odontoid (Fig. 41–14).

When the odontoid is separated from C2 and moves with the arch of the atlas, a much greater excursion of C1 on C2 is possible without neurological deficit than when it is intact. Because of the extreme mobility of the bony segments, the inferior component of the cruciform ligament and the membrana tectoria joining the separate odontoid and the rest of C2 become markedly stretched in flexion, but they buckle in extension, narrowing the lumen of the canal even more. These changes were well illustrated in the autopsy reported by Stratford

and explain the patient's respiratory failure, which occurred as the arch of the atlas was being wired to the spine of C2 (Fig. 41–15).[71]

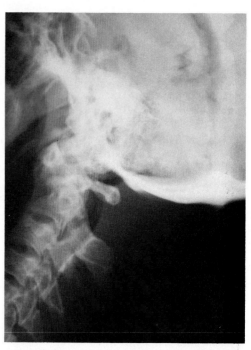

Figure 41–14   Gas myelogram outlining cervical cord compressed between posterior arch of C1 and base of separate odontoid in a case of atlantoaxial dislocation. Critical anteroposterior diameter of canal is reduced to 13 mm. There were spastic tetraparesis and sensory changes.

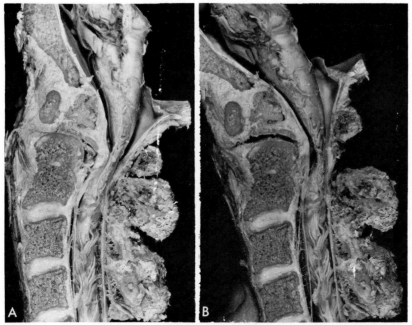

Figure 41–15   Sagittal section of upper cervical cord and clivus at autopsy. Separate odontoid process is dislocated forward with anterior arch of atlas. *A*. Cord is markedly flattened by the thickened ligaments ventral to it, which buckle when posterior arch of atlas is approximated to spinous process of axis. *B*. When C1 is in neutral position and traction is exerted on the skull, the dens and the rest of C2 separate, the ligaments flatten, and compression is relieved. (From Stratford, J.: Myelopathy caused by atlanto-axial dislocation. J. Neurosurg., *14*:97–104, 1957. Reprinted by permission.)

Absence of Odontoid Process

The odontoid process may be completely absent or at least invisible, even on tomographic films, either as a result of a congenital anomaly or possibly following absorption of the distal fragment of a nonunited fracture.[62] In these cases, one sees the same type of dislocation as with a separate odontoid.

Chiari Malformation

In 1881 and 1885, Chiari described an anomaly of the cerebellum and medulla oblongata associated with hydrocephalus. He recognized three types.[16,17]

Type I consisted of lengthening of the cerebellar tonsils, which formed tonguelike prolongations that extended down into the upper cervical canal below the foramen magnum and were closely applied to the medulla oblongata and cord to C1. It was regarded as the adult type (Fig. 41–16; cf. Figs. 41–29 *A* and 41–32 *A*).

In type II, the tonsils extended even farther down, and the lower portion of the narrow, elongated fourth ventricle reached below the foramen magnum. The medulla and upper cord exhibited a curious hump on the dorsal surface and appeared displaced downward. This produced an abnormal course, outward and upward rather than downward, in the upper cervical nerve roots (Fig. 41–17).[63] This type was always associated with myelomeningocele and hydrocephalus and was seen in young children.

In 1894, Arnold reported a single case of type II, also associated with myelomeningocele and many other anomalies.[4] The term "Arnold-Chiari malformation" was coined by two of his pupils, Schwalbe and Gredig, in 1907.[66]

Chiari also described a rare type III in which a large portion of the cerebellum herniates downward through a wide rachischisis of the upper cervical spine and is accompanied by a meningocele.

Intermediate forms of the three types can be found, indicating degrees of hindbrain

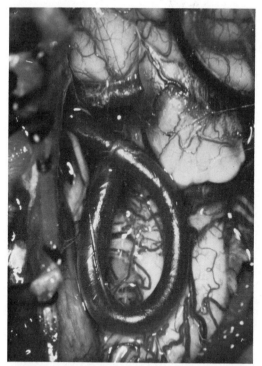

Figure 41–16 Chiari type I malformation. Flattened right cerebellar tonsil with gliosis, lying below margin of foramen magnum and aherent to upper medulla. Note very prominent and low-lying left posterior-inferior cerebellar artery. Right artery is partially hidden under right tonsil. (Operative photograph.)

magnum.[60] But hydrocephalus is not always present with the malformation, and the spinal cord is not always tethered at its lower end. The discovery of other developmental anomalies such as microgyria and craniolacunia suggests that the malformation originates from a basic developmental defect.[44] Simple mechanical factors such as traction from below or pressure from above could not account for all aspects of the pathologic change. Barry, Patten, and Stewart measured the length and volume of various segments of the central nervous system in embryos with the Chiari malformation.[8] Finding each segment examined to be larger than corresponding structures in normal embryos of similar ages, they concluded that the hindbrain herniation was due to an "overgrowth" of these neural elements, including the cerebral hemispheres. They thought that the enlargement of the segments explained why the cerebellum and medulla were forced to herniate out of a relatively small cranium. The "knuckled" appearance of the medulla, seen in various degrees, was also regarded as a result of this overgrowth. Hydrocephalus, they believed, was a secondary phenomenon due to obstruction of the cerebrospinal fluid pathways by the herniated tonsils.

herniation, and type II can be seen in adults without any obvious anomaly lower down. The exact pathogenesis of this malformation is still a matter of debate. Chiari himself believed that the downward displacement was the result of hydrocephalus and noted the frequent occurrence of hydromyelia, a dilatation of the ependyma-lined central canal of the cord, in types I and II.

On the contrary, Russell and Donald believed the malformation, causing obstruction of the foramen magnum, could prevent either the egress of cerebrospinal fluid from the fourth ventricle or its return to the cerebral subarachnoid spaces and was the cause rather than the consequence of the hydrocephalus.[63]

The frequent association of type II with lumbar myelomeningocele suggested to Penfield and Coburn that downward traction by an abnormal attachment of the lower cord in the meningocele might be the mechanism by which the cerebellum and medulla were pulled down into the foramen

Dandy-Walker Malformation

The term "Dandy-Walker malformation" was applied by Benda to a specific

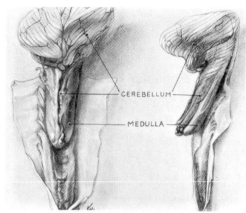

Figure 41–17 Chiari type II (Arnold-Chiari) malformation with low-lying tonsils in cervical canal, redundant "knuckled" dorsal aspect of the medulla, and abnormal upward and lateral course of cervical nerve roots.

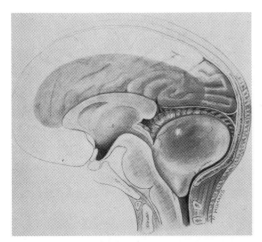

Figure 41–18 Diagrammatic representation of Dandy-Walker malformation. Enormously dilated fourth ventricle occupies most of enlarged posterior fossa. Foramen of Magendie is obstructed by membrane bulging down through foramen magnum. (From Matson, D. D.: Neurosurgery of Infancy and Childhood. Springfield, Ill., Charles C Thomas, 1969. Reprinted by permission.)

type of hydrocephalus due to what Dandy and later Taggart and Walker considered to be atresia of the foramina of Magendie and Luschka.[9,21,22,73] In classic cases, this condition is characterized by a marked enlargement of the fourth ventricle, which becomes cystlike and occupies most of the enlarged posterior fossa (Fig. 41–18). The tentorium, the torcular, and the lateral sinuses are abnormally high, as can be demonstrated by ventriculography or angiography (Fig. 41–19). The cerebellar hemispheres, pushed upward and laterally, are often hypoplastic. The vermis is reduced to a rudimentary bridge or may be absent (Fig. 41–20). The inferior and posterior portion of the fourth ventricle is closed by a membrane, which sometimes bulges down through the foramen magnum. Benda considered this membrane containing arachnoid and ependymal elements to be an abnormally developed medullary velum that had failed to perforate in fetal life. The

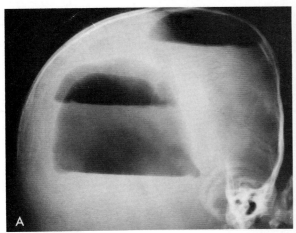

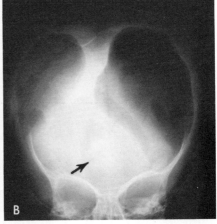

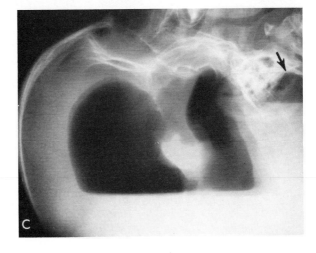

Figure 41–19 Dandy-Walker syndrome. *A.* Brow-down lateral view of ventriculogram showing hydrocephalus of lateral ventricles, enormous fourth ventricle, and greatly enlarged posterior fossa. *B.* Same case, brow-down frontal view. Arrow indicates round shadow of intracranial and extracranial dermoid cyst also present in this patient. *C.* Same case, brow-up lateral view shows dilated lateral and third ventricles. Arrow points to region of foramen of Magendie, obstructed by membrane that prevents escape of gas in cervical canal.

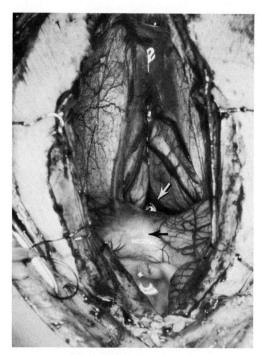

Figure 41–20   Operative photograph of case illustrated in Figure 41–19. Suboccipital craniectomy exposes large fourth ventricle bulging above hypoplastic vermis (*black arrow*) and filling quadrigeminal cistern (*white arrow*) and space between medial temporooccipital regions. Cerebellum is pushed to either side. Membrane occluding foramen of Magendie was removed and hydrocephalus was relieved. Dermoid cyst (*top left*) was also removed.

massive dilatation of the fourth ventricle is also accompanied by hydrocephalus of the third and lateral ventricles, but it produces, in children, a characteristically prominent occiput, as shown in Figure 41–19 *A,* and a dolichocephalic skull, quite different in external appearance from the hydrocephalic skull of aqueductal stenosis in which the posterior fossa is small.

Although it is most common in the young child, the Dandy-Walker malformation has been described later in life.[11,36] In older patients, it is often found in association with syringomyelia. The dilatation of the fourth ventricle is usually not so great in the cases diagnosed in adulthood as in the clearly congenital childhood cases, and the condition may be difficult to differentiate from acquired obstructions of the foramen of Magendie. In these patients the foramen is closed by a thin translucent membrane rather than by matted, feltlike adhesions.

Basal Arachnoiditis

Foster and Hudgson reviewed in detail 18 of their 100 cases of syringomyelia in which arachnoiditis of the upper cervical canal and cisterna magna was responsible for obstruction of the foramen of Magendie and, occasionally, concomitant hydrocephalus.[31] The arachnoid adhesions developed mostly along the dorsal aspect of the cord and the cisterna magna, in the vicinity of the foramen magnum, leaving free passage to the cerebrospinal fluid (and the x-ray contrast medium) along the ventral subarachnoid space and the prepontine cistern. Meningitis was an identifiable cause of the arachnoiditis in three of their cases. Various congenital anomalies such as cerebellar ectopia, basilar impression, and occipitalization of the atlas were also present in one third of the group. No reason was found to explain the unusual amount of adhesions present in these cases in comparison with others of "uncomplicated" tonsillar ectopias. In the author's experience with basal arachnoiditis, obstetrical trauma was clearly responsible for the meningeal adhesions and scarring in two cases with otherwise classic symptoms of syringomyelia.

The experimental evidence derived from kaolin-induced basal arachnoiditis and hydrocephalus shows that hydrosyringomyelia can develop within a few days after the injection of kaolin into the cisterna magna.[25,41,42,53] While the dilatation of the central canal decompresses the ventricles, it produces progressive destruction of the cord.

Syringomyelia

The clinical, pathological, and experimental evidence reviewed recently by Barnett, Foster and Hudgson in their excellent monograph on the subject, and more recent clinical and experimental data indicate clearly that the origin of the syringomyelic cavitation lies in obstruction, partial or complete, of the foramina of the fourth ventricle.[6,11,25,41,42] Congenital lesions affecting the permeability of the rhombic roof, principally cerebellar ectopia, the Chiari malformation, constriction of the foramen magnum in basilar invagination, imperforation of the medullary velum in the Dandy-Walker syndrome, or acquired adhesive arachnoiditis, will produce hydromyelia.

Rupture of the dilated central canal into the substance of the cord, usually at first in the gray matter of the dorsal horns, allows the cerebrospinal fluid to dissect the long syringomyelic cavities that cause the characteristic symptoms. Williams suggested that this pathological entity should be called "communicating syringomyelia."[75] Although they may appear independent from the central canal on some cross sections of the cord, these syringomyelic cysts usually are connected to it somewhere. In contradistinction to tumor cysts, which contain high concentrations of proteins, fluid in the syrinx has the same chemical constituents and appearance as cerebrospinal fluid.

The hydrodynamic mechanisms by which the central canal is forced open have been well studied by Gardner, who summarized them in 1965.[35] He believes that the important factor is obstruction to the pulsatile egress of cerebrospinal fluid that must occur with each systole. Membranes or other mechanical obstructions may be permeable to a slow seepage of fluid but are unable to accommodate the rapid to- and-fro flow that normally occurs with each heartbeat at the only opening of the rigid cranium into the elastic spinal dural tube.

Williams, however, believes that changes in the intracranial venous pressure arising as a result of jugular compression, Valsalva maneuvers, and the like, rather than the systolic pulsations, are the driving force.[75,76] The sudden appearance of symptoms of syringomyelia and syringobulbia following muscular effort or coughing indicate that pressure changes in the intracranial and spinal venous compartments and the resulting pressure gradients that develop between the poorly communicating subarachnoid, ventricular, and eventually intramedullary cerebrospinal fluid compartments play an important role in the process of "hydrodissection" of the nervous tissue substance (Fig. 41–21).[6,11] Whether they are the only driving force, as suggested by Williams, or merely add to the effects of the more con-

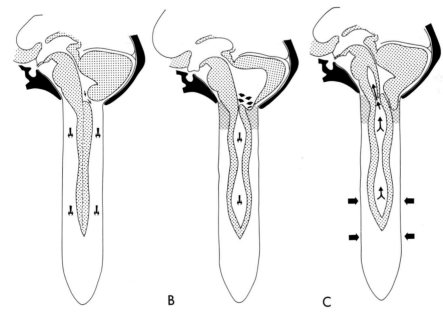

Figure 41–21 Hydrodynamic theory of syringomyelia and syringobulbia. *A.* Normal cerebrospinal fluid dynamics: pulse wave generated by systole and other forces (venous congestion) escapes freely from fourth ventricle. Central canal is closed. *B.* Partial or complete obstruction of foramen of Magendie by adhesions or Chiari anomaly allows fluid wave to reopen and distend central canal, destroying cord substance. *C.* Sudden pressure on dural tube (congestion of spinal epidural veins) forces fluid upward in syrinx, dissecting into substance of medulla if it cannot escape readily through patent central canal: syringobulbia.

stant systolic water-hammer force postulated by Gardner is still a matter of debate.

SYMPTOMS AND SIGNS

In their extensive monograph on craniovertebral anomalies published in 1953, Garcin and Oeconomos reviewed the literature to that date and added 19 observations of their own, for a total of 115 cases.[34] Their paper discussed only cases with bony anomalies, and therefore, the series contains only 15 Chiari malformations. They found isolated basilar impression in 41 instances and isolated occipitalization in 30. All the others were combinations of two or more of the anomalies described in the preceeding paragraphs. There were 15 cases of atlantoaxial dislocation.

Morphological abnormalities of the neck, low hairline, abnormal head posture, limitation of movements, and painful torticollis were present in 63 per cent of the cases reviewed. Occipital headaches and nuchal pain brought on by movements or by coughing or straining, sometimes accompanied by fainting, paresthesias, dizziness, or diplopia, were common, particularly when ectopic cerebellar tissues became impacted in the foramen magnum when the intracranial pressure was abruptly increased.

Like List, Garcin and Oeconomos believed that the different types of anomalies produced two groups of symptoms.[34,49] In the first, occipitalization of the atlas and atlantoaxial dislocations were associated in general with a high cervical cord compression syndrome—spastic tetraparesis affecting the legs at first, posterior column signs, and paresthesias beginning in the upper extremities.[77] In the second group, basilar impression and the Chiari malformation, which impinge on the central nervous system at a higher level, produced a cerebellomedullary syndrome with dizziness and vertigo, nystagmus that was sometimes vertical (downbeat),oscillopsia, and ataxia. There may be involvement of the lower cranial nerves, with fluid regurgitation through the nose, nasal voice, hiccups, atrophy of the tongue, and also sensory problems. The distinction between the two groups of symptoms is not always clear and often they tend to merge. The clinical picture can be complicated further if ectopic cerebellar

tissue or basal arachnoiditis obstructs the cerebrospinal fluid circulation and leads to the development of hydrocephalus and hydrosyringomyelia.[68]

The malformation, although congenital, may remain silent and be discovered fortuitously. In 60 per cent of Garcin and Oeconomos's symptomatic cases, the first symptoms occurred only in the second or third decade of life.[34] This delay in the appearance of neurological impairment has been explained by slow modifications of the bony structure of the foramen, progressive ligamentous relaxation allowing an increasing degree of atlantoaxial dislocation, gradual formation of arachnoid adhesions, and the relentless water-hammer effect of the pulsatile flow of cerebrospinal fluid.

Trauma, often minor, can draw attention to the underlying problem. Particularly in cases of atlantoaxial dislocation, apparently insignificant flexion injuries to the neck produce catastrophic neurological signs that are out of proportion to the forces involved.

When hydrocephalus is present, progressive dementia may occur, and, quite commonly (12 per cent), papilledema and other signs of increased intracranial pressure.[34] In the Dandy-Walker syndrome discovered in childhood, hydrocephalus with the characteristic prominent occiput is often the only clue.[51]

The symptoms of syringomyelia depend on the location and extent of the cord cavitation. Typically, this disorder will produce amyotrophy in the upper extremities, beginning in the interossei and lumbricals, causing the classic "main en griffe," and spreading to upper segments. The deep tendon reflexes are lost in the arms and are hyperactive in the legs. There is a dissociated pain and temperature sensory loss in a cape-like distribution over the neck, shoulders, and arms. Cervicodorsal scoliosis, scars of painless burns and wounds, and a Horner's syndrome are also part of the clinical picture. Paradoxically, the patients often complain of deep aches and pains in areas of the trunk and upper limbs that are totally analgesic. Innumerable variations on this theme are possible. The syndrome may be entirely unilateral, other modalities of sensation may be involved, there may be sensory loss over the face, the amyotrophy may affect the legs with the appearance of a drop foot, reflexes may be preserved and exaggerated everywhere, or the patient may have spastic tetraparesis. Nystagmus and bulbar signs may be prominent.

DIAGNOSIS

With a wide spectrum of clinical signs affecting various structures of the central nervous system in a patchy, apparently unrelated manner and an evolution often marked by temporary exacerbations and remissions of symptoms, it is not surprising that the most common diagnostic error in anomalies of the craniovertebral junction is an erroneous diagnosis of multiple sclerosis. The presence of occipital nuchal headaches, neck pain, and other mechanical factors that produce or modify the symptoms should draw attention to the craniovertebral junction. One must be aware that the Lhermitte sign, the production of electric shock–like sensations in the body on flexion of the neck, a common feature of demyelinating disease, can also be found in chronic atlantoaxial dislocations.[1]

Tumors, particularly meningiomas of the region of the foramen magnum, ependymomas, and astrocytomas of the inferior vermis can produce symptoms of intermittent obstruction and cerebellomedullary compression similar to those caused by the congenital anomalies.

Intramedullary gliomas can form long cystic cavities in the cord substance and produce signs of typical syringomyelia. The fluid aspirated from the cyst at operation or percutaneously under x-ray control will, however, be yellow and proteinacious, quite different from the clear cerebrospinal fluid of communicating syringomyelia (Fig. 41–22).[14,16] Neoplastic cysts usually do not collapse during air myelography. The cord remains large and tense in contrast to its appearance in hydrosyringomyelia, in which it will be quite flat (Fig. 41–23). The ectopic cerebellar tonsils may be visible on the air myelogram (Fig. 41–24). Lack of ventricular filling should make one suspect an obstruction at the foramen of Magendie, but the entry of gas or even oil into the ventricles does not rule out a partial obstruction. Oil myelography should be done in both prone and supine positions in order to demonstrate well the region of the cisterna

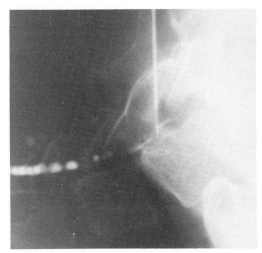

Figure 41–22 Percutaneous aspiration-injection of intramedullary cyst. A 20-gauge needle is used until the dura is penetrated; a 25-gauge one is used to puncture the cord. Clear cerebrospinal fluid–like fluid was obtained; a few drops of Ethiodan outlined the cyst cavity.

magna and the herniated tonsils or adhesions (Figs. 41–25, 41–26, and 41–27).

Computed tomography of the spine will no doubt soon provide reliable visualization

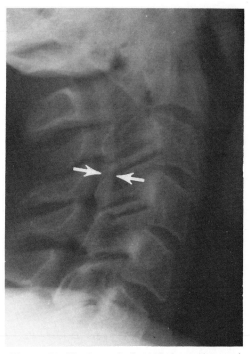

Figure 41–23 Lateral view of air myelogram in syringomyelia. Cord shadow appears flattened to a ribbon (*arrows*).

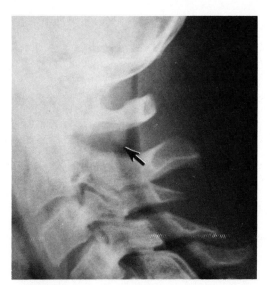

Figure 41–24 Air myelogram showing low-lying cerebellar tonsils in Chiari I malformation (*arrow*).

of spinal cord cysts or herniated tonsils.[2,4] It has proved to be a valuable tool in the detection of hydrocephalus and the study of its evolution. Air myelography and pneumoencephalography are not used as often as in past years in the diagnosis of syringomyelia and anomalies of the craniovertebral junction. Currently, radiographic studies usually consist of (1) plain films of the spine and skull; (2) tomographic studies of the craniovertebral junction, if indicated; (3) Careful flexion-extension films if atlantoaxial dislocation is suspected; (4) computed tomography of the skull for detection of hydrocephalus and a repeat examination with intravenous infusion of diatrizoate (Hypaque) if a tumor is suspected; and (5) iophendylate (Ethiodan) myelography in the prone and supine positions, always done in syringomyelic syndromes but not necessarily in cases of bony anomalies such as chronic atlantoaxial dislocations of which the diagnosis may be clear on plain films and tomograms. Positive contrast and gas ventriculography are very helpful to demonstrate the presence of hydrocephalus due to obstruction of the foramina of the fourth ventricle and to provide proof of the existence of a communication between the ventricular system and the syrinx (Fig. 41–28).[11,74] The advent of computed tomography, however, and the routine use of supine myelography have made this procedure necessary in fewer cases. Vertebral angiography is used if a tumor or a vascular lesion is suspected.

TREATMENT

In the operative management of these anomalies, one should strive to achieve three goals: (1) to decompress nervous structures that are being squeezed and strangled by bony or soft-tissue anomalies, (2) to stabilize joints subjected to abnormal movements that cause secondary neuraxis compression, and (3) to re-establish normal patterns of cerebrospinal fluid circulation.

Posterior Decompression

Posterior decompression by upper cervical laminectomy and occipital craniectomy and opening of the dura is a time-honored procedure. It is the operation of choice whenever posteriorly situated anomalies

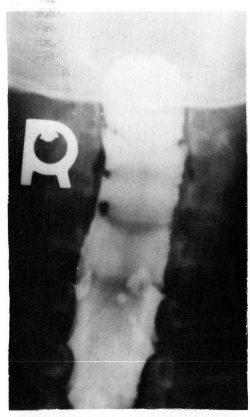

Figure 41–25 Prone iophendylate (Ethiodan) myelogram showing tubular enlargement of cervical cord in syringomyelia.

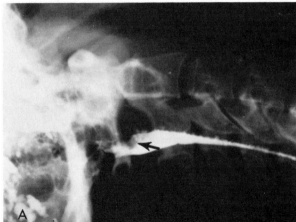

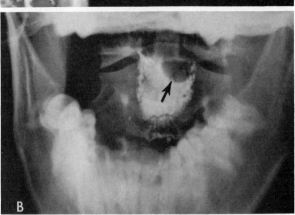

Figure 41–26 Supine iophendylate (Ethiodan) myelogram showing ectopic tonsils outlined below arch of C1 (*arrows*). *A*. Lateral view. Cisterna magna and fourth ventricle do not fill. *B*. Frontal view.

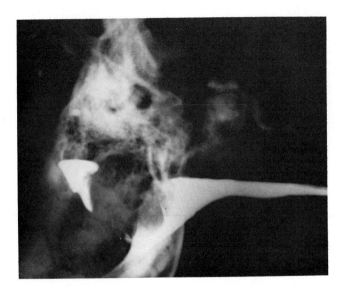

Figure 41–27 Normal supine iophendylate (Ethiodan) myelogram. Large cisterna magna, tonsils well within posterior fossa, oil enters freely into fourth ventricle.

are present, such as the Chiari malformation, with or without syringomyelia, adhesive arachnoiditis, or a narrow foramen with a thick posterior lip impinging on the medulla, as occurs in occipitalization of the atlas or basilar invagination. It may be the simplest treatment also when an anterior dislocation of atlas on axis cannot be reduced by skeletal traction and the posterior arch of the atlas compresses the cord against the stump of a separate odontoid. The author prefers to operate with the pa-

tient prone. The chest should be supported on bolsters to leave the abdomen free, and the shoulders should be elevated to reduce venous congestion. If preoperative studies have shown no dislocation, a Gardner-type pin clamp is used to maintain the head in a neutral or slightly flexed position. If there is evidence of dislocation, skeletal traction with skull tongs is safer. The prone position with the neck horizontal makes the use of the operating microscope easier for the surgeon and his assistant across the table. It

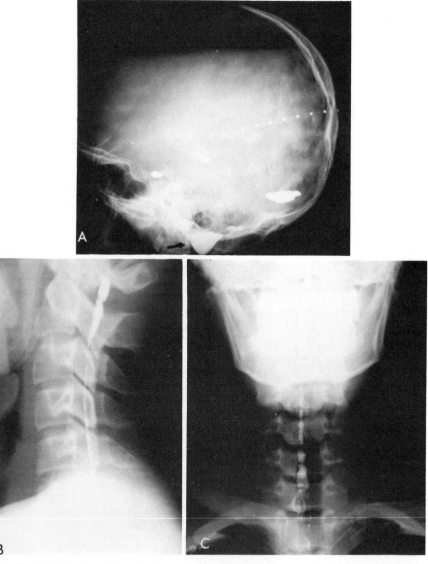

Figure 41–28 *A*. Air-iophendylate (Ethiodan) ventriculogram showing dilated lateral ventricles, rounded lower end of fourth ventricle obstructed by membrane, and beginning of patent central canal (*black arrow*). *B* and *C*. Lateral and frontal views of oil-filled central canal in cervical region with characteristic beaded appearance. Canal extended to T10 vertebra.

requires more rigorous hemostasis during the approach to the lesion, which eliminates many later problems. It also avoids the loss of all the cerebrospinal fluid.

Whenever possible, the long spinous process of C2 should be left intact to prevent flexion deformity of the neck, which may develop later. The upper half of its laminal arch can be resected to gain a few millimeters of exposure for the dura. If visualization lower down is necessary, the laminae can be removed on one side only, leaving all the spinous processes intact. The occipital craniectomy is usually started with a burr hole on either side, and bone is removed from above down toward the foramen. One must remember that in these cases the medulla and cord are already compressed, and there is no room for the jaws of large instruments under the bone. One must also keep in mind the possibility

of anomalies in position of the vertebral arteries, particularly when the atlas is occipitalized.

Removal of the posterior arch of C1 has to be done with the utmost care and without introducing instruments beneath it. The dura is opened in the shape of a Y, beginning in a normal area if possible, above and below, and joining the incisions at the level of the foramen. It is best to keep the arachnoid intact at this stage. The dural sinuses can be coagulated or clipped. When only bony constriction is present, the arachnoid need not be opened. In the presence of cerebellar ectopia, with or without syringomyelia or adhesions, or when the foramen of Magendie is closed by a thin membrane, the arachnoid should be opened and its edges clipped to the dura. The operating microscope is used for the opening of the arachnoid and the dissection of the arach-

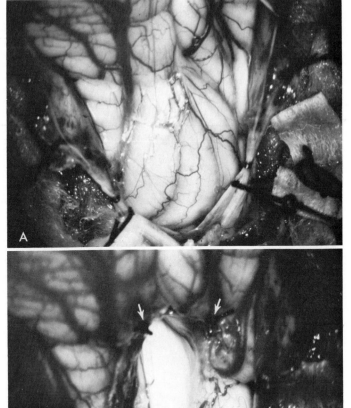

Figure 41–29 *A.* Large cerebellar ectopia extending down to C2, right tonsil much more prominent than left. *B.* Medial portion of tonsils removed, exposing narrow, elongated fourth ventricle now widely open in cisterna magna. Empty tonsillar arachnoid sutured up to keep fourth ventricle open (*white arrows*). A muscle plug has been inserted in open central canal at obex (*black arrow*).

noid adhesions that usually bind the ectopic tonsils over the foramen of Magendie (see Figs. 41–16, 41–29*A*, and 41–32*A* and *B*).[61] Only with the microscope, or at least some magnification, can one avoid damage to fine medullary vessels, which nearly always originate from the abnormally low posterior inferior cerebellar arteries. These arteries are often very prominent, but they may be hidden in dense arachnoiditis. These tough adhesions are best left alone.

The author usually removes the medial and inferior portions of the ectopic tonsils. The small vessels on their dorsal surfaces are coagulated with a bipolar forceps. The pia-arachnoid is incised, and the cerebellar substance is removed from within the arachnoid by gentle suction. Large branches of the posterior inferior cerebellar arteries are left intact as they course to the adjacent cerebellar hemispheres. The empty arachnoid bag can be sutured up and laterally to the cerebellar arachnoid, leaving the lower end of the fourth ventricle open in the cisterna magna (see Figs. 41–29*B* and 41–32*C*). When dense arachnoiditis prevents dissection of the tonsils, the fourth ventricle can still be opened at the lower vermis.

Dural Closure

The foregoing steps provide the necessary posterior decompression of the nervous structures within the foramen and reestablish the normal free communication of the fourth ventricle with the cisterna magna. For this to remain effective, however, every effort must be made to prevent the formation of new and even more dense adhesions. The need for rigorous hemostasis, particularly in the intradural dissection, cannot be overemphasized. The dura should be closed in a watertight manner with a graft to avoid constriction and to prevent bloody exudates and clots from the muscle wound from entering the cerebrospinal fluid. Blood in the subarachnoid space is a well-known cause of meningeal irritation after operation, and it may cause communicating hydrocephalus. Lyophilized dura has, so far, been the most satisfactory material to use for the dural graft. Silastic impregnated Dacron never "heals" and has tended to allow the formation of postoperative meningocele-like cavities in the depth of the incision, which serve as reservoirs of protein-rich bloody fluid (Fig. 41–30). To assure a watertight closure, all clips used on the dural edge should be removed to prevent leakage of cerebrospinal fluid along them. The dural sinuses can be coagulated or closed with a hemstitch. It also is useful to anchor the dorsal arachnoid to the dural suture line to prevent it from flopping down on the underlying cord and closing off the subarachnoid spaces. An epidural suction drain is also used to advantage for the first postoperative day. Using the lyophilized dura and taking these precautions in closing the wound have markedly decreased the postoperative morbidity, and particularly the incidence of aseptic meningitis.

Cyst Aspiration and Drainage, Plugging of Central Canal

When syringomyelia is present, the cavity may be visible along the dorsal root entry zone at C2. When this is the case,

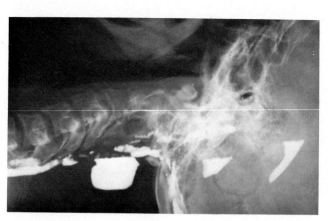

Figure 41–30 Iophendylate (Ethiodan) myelography in supine position outlines "meningocele" left by inadequate closure of dura (Silastic membrane) at previous operation. There was partial obstruction under still intact C1, but oil could enter fourth ventricle. Note flexion deformity that followed extensive laminectomy.

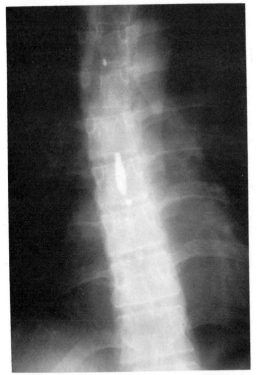

Figure 41–31 Iophendylate (Ethiodan) injected in syrinx at C2 outlines bottom of syrinx at T9–T10 (patient standing).

fluid is aspirated with a 25-gauge needle for analysis and cyst decompression, although the syrinx is usually not under tension. One quarter milliliter of iophendylate (Ethiodan)

can be injected into the cyst to outline its inferior extent (Fig. 41–31). Also, 0.5 ml of a dilute solution of Evans blue (one part Evans blue, nine parts Elliott's solution) may be injected into the syrinx. In approximately half the cases, it will be seen in the fourth ventricle a few minutes later, thus proving the existence of a patent central canal (Fig. 41–32*B* and *C*).

In every case of syringomyelia and in a few cases of Chiari malformation without syringomyelia the author has attempted to close the abnormal opening of the central canal by stuffing small pieces of muscle into it. One of the muscle plugs is marked with a very small clip (for x-ray control later), and a wisp of cotton is added on top of the muscle plug to prevent it from slipping out.[20,35,36] Despite the care taken in doing the procedure, one patient developed unilateral hypoglossal palsy after operation. Undoubtedly this sequel was due to injury to the nucleus. Myelotomy at the dorsal root entry zone and insertion of a Silastic drain were popular in the past but are done less frequently now that the laminectomy is more often restricted to C1 and no effort is made to explore the syrinx.[61]

The more important steps in this operation are: (1) the establishment of an adequate opening at the foramen of Magendie, (2) the maintenance of this opening by a proper dural graft and avoidance of adhe-

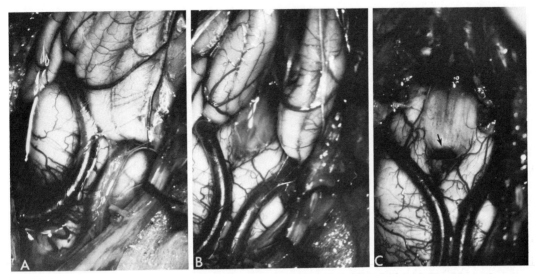

Figure 41–32 *A.* Chiari type I malformation in syringomyelia. Note adherent low tonsils and very low posterior-inferior cerebellar arteries. *B.* Separating tonsils shows bottom part of low-lying fourth ventricle. Dark shadow in ventricle is Evans blue dye injected into cyst exposed at T2 (enlarged thoracic cord was thought to be a tumor after the cisterna magna abnormality was missed on supine myelogram). *C.* Resection of tonsils provides free opening to fourth ventricle. Muscle plug in central canal (*arrow*).

sions, and (3) the closure of the anomalous opening of the central canal. These steps are aimed at re-establishing a normal situation at the foramen magnum. Drainage of the cyst in the cervical region or lower down at the lumbar enlargement, where it tends to widen again, or even at the filum terminale, the so-called "terminal ventriculostomy," also is useful if the cyst extends that far, particularly in those patients in whom procedures at the foramen magnum have failed to arrest the hydrosyringomyelic process.[37] When extremely dense adhesions exist, drainage of the cyst alone or in association with ventricular shunting may be a less hazardous treatment.[31]

Ventricular Drainage

In the author's group of 41 patients who have been operated upon, only 2 have been treated with ventriculoatrial shunting alone. Both had symptomatic hydrocephalus. The syringomyelic symptoms have slightly improved with control of the intracranial pressure. A third patient deteriorated in spite of the shunt until the foramen of Magendie was opened and the central canal was plugged.[11] Two other patients developed hydrocephalus and required shunts after operation. Another patient with hydrocephalus had a shunt inserted after exploration of the foramen magnum.

Anterior Decompression

In basilar impression and particularly in occipitalization of the atlas with atlantoaxial dislocation and an intact odontoid process, posterior decompression alone does not relieve the direct pressure on the ventral aspect of the medulla by abnormal bony elements. In 1951, Scoville and Sherman envisaged the possibility of removing the offending odontoid through a transoral approach, but accounts of this technique did not appear in the literature until Fang and Ong's report in 1962.[4,28,67] Other reports have followed since, describing the technique for removal or fusion of the odontoid through the mouth.[27,38,57,72]

Tracheostomy is performed as a preliminary step, and it is wise to obtain throat cultures before operation in order to establish an adequate pre- and postoperative antibiotic umbrella. At operation, the soft palate is split, and the two halves are retracted laterally. The anterior arch of C1 can be palpated; x-ray may be used to confirm its position if necessary. A midline vertical incision is made over the arch, and the soft tissues are retracted to each side. One must keep in mind the presence of the vertebral arteries on either side of the atlantoaxial joints, as injuries to these vessels have been reported.[28] The anterior arch of the atlas is then drilled out, exposing the odontoid process behind it, and this is drilled out also. The upper part of the body of C2 may have to be removed as well if it is instrumental in the compression of the cord. The pharyngeal and palatal incisions are then closed with absorbable sutures. It is recommended that oral feeding not be allowed for a week after the operation.[38] The risk of infection inherent in this route, two out of six of Fang and Ong's transoral procedures, has led to the development of a retropharyngeal exposure of this area by which one can reach up to the clivus. The technique was first described by Stevenson and his collaborators for the removal of a chordoma of the clivus.[69] It has been used for removal of the odontoid, but most often has been employed for fusion of the skull, atlas, and axis.[3,18,50]

Atlantoaxial Fusion

Chronic atlantoaxial dislocation, whatever the cause, is a serious condition, and death secondary to cord compression and respiratory failure has been described in nearly 10 per cent of the more than 150 cases reported in detail in the literature. Operative mortality rates were particularly high when correction was attempted by posterior decompression only and when operations were performed without traction.[12,23,49,70] In cases of atlantoaxial dislocation, skeletal traction must be applied to the skull until an adequate immobilization apparatus has been installed. Even when the dislocation seems fixed as judged by flexion-extension films, traction with 12 kg overnight will often achieve reduction (Fig. 41–33A and B). The weights must be added slowly and the neurological condition watched carefully during that time (Fig. 41–33C).

When the posterior arch of C1 has been removed or in cases of occipitalization of the atlas with dislocation, the usual practice has been to perform a posterior occipitocervical fusion with bone taken from the iliac crest, the tibia ribs, or the bone bank.[19,43,46,48] A combination of wires and acrylic has also been used, but bone is preferable in cases with a long life expectancy.[58,59] Acrylic never actually fuses to the bone, and the integrity of the "graft" continues to depend only on the wires, which eventually may break.

In cases of separate odontoid with an intact posterior arch of C1 and no occipitalization of the atlas, occipitocervical grafts have also been done. The tendency has been to use shorter grafts to leave the occiput free. Gallie described the wiring of a graft between the posterior arch of the atlas

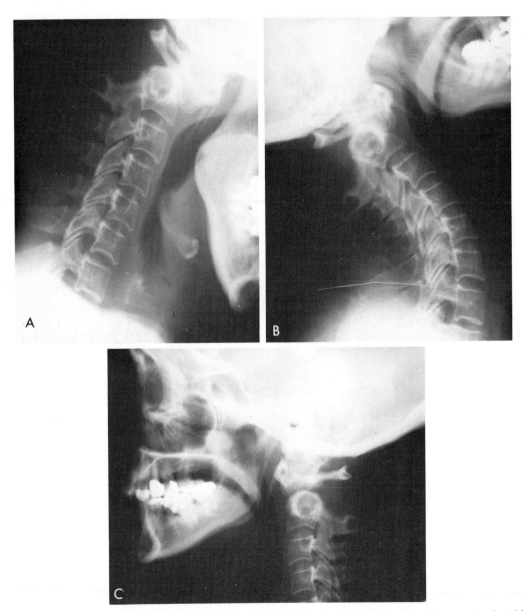

Figure 41–33 *A* and *B*. Lateral view in flexion and extension of atlantoaxial dislocation with separate odontoid process. There is no change in position of C1 or C2. *C*. After overnight traction (12 kg, Cone-Barton tongs) there is almost complete reduction.

and the spinous process of C2.[33] The somewhat longer parallel grafts wired to the laminae of C2 and C3 and to the posterior arch of C1, described by Alexander and his colleagues, provide a more sound immobilization of the dislocation, since they prevent the fore-and-aft gliding movement of C1 on C2 that is not well controlled by the Gallie fusion.[2] A number of other techniques have been devised: simple wiring of C1 to C2, the use of specially prepared skin thongs to tie the atlas to C2 and still preserve some mobility, a metallic clamp to join the arch of C1 to the axis, and acrylic fixation of C1, C2, and C3.[40,45,47,64] These methods may be better suited to recent fractures of the odontoid in which adequate internal immobilization can allow fusion to occur at the fracture site. In chronic dislocations when there is little hope of union of the dens fragment or when it is absent, it probably is safer to use bone for the fusion.

Whatever is done, to prevent the buckling of the ligaments described by Stratford, one should avoid wiring the arch of the atlas tightly to C2 (see Fig. 41–15).[71] The same mechanism was probably responsible for the respiratory difficulties and death in a case described by Bachs and his co-workers.[5]

Traction exerted during the operation serves to maintain the segments in neutral position and keep the ligaments taut. The late William Cone devised a method for

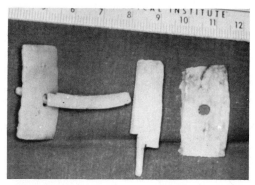

Figure 41–34 Pairs of "paddles" and parallel grafts fashioned from patient's own skull bone. Outer cortex is used for one parallel graft, inner cortex for the other. Paddles are full thickness.

maintaining this relationship after operation by interposing bone blocks between the C1 and C2 joint surfaces. This technique is briefly mentioned in Stratford's paper.[71] A similar technique has been used by the author in 18 cases of chronic atlantoaxial dislocations.[10] After exposure of the occiput, C1, and C2 through a dorsal midline approach, the attenuated ligamentum flavum is removed between atlas and axis. The venous plexus surrounding the C2 roots is dissected and coagulated, the roots are severed close to the dural tube and the ganglia are resected. Before cutting the roots, one must consider the possibly anomalous position of the vertebral arteries. The posterior aspect of the atlantoaxial joint capsules are

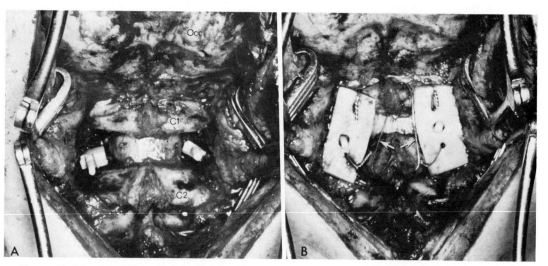

Figure 41–35 *A.* "Paddles" in place in the opened and denuded C1–C2 joint spaces. Joint capsules keep paddles from advancing further, narrow handles engage holes in posterior grafts. *B.* Finished assembly: four No. 20 or No. 18 stainless steel wires are passed around arch of C1 and laminae of C2 and through parallel grafts. In addition, C1 is attached to C2 with a fifth wire (*arrows*).

then coagulated, and a window is cut into them, opening the joint space. The cartilage is carefully removed with an air tool and a small curet, leaving a 4- to 6-mm gap between the bony surfaces. Paddle-shaped bony pegs are then fashioned and are pushed in snugly from back to front into the open joints, keeping their surfaces apart (Figs. 41–34 and 41–35A). The posterior ends of these paddles, protruding beyond the level of the C2 laminal arch, are engaged into suitably placed holes made in two other pieces of bone that form posterior parallel grafts. These are wired to the arch of C1 on either side and to the spinous process of C2 or, better still, around its laminae. A separate wire tightened around the arch of the atlas and the spine of the axis forces the joint surfaces to "bite down" on the bony paddles (Fig. 41–35B). This montage is stable immediately. It allows bony fusion to occur at the joints as well as between the neural arches (Figs. 41–36 and 41–37). Also, it keeps the overstretched ligaments taut and tends to pull down the dens, if it is intact, from its abnormally high position.

Postoperatively, skeletal traction is maintained at about 5 kg until a Minerva jacket or an equivalent brace is in place. Immobilization should be maintained for three months. Human bank bone was used in the first seven cases, and bone was taken

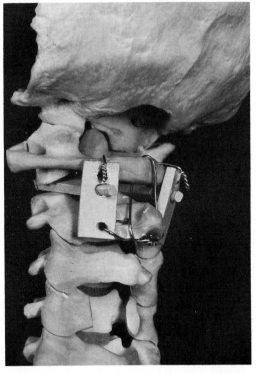

Figure 41–36 Three-quarter view of model spine with grafts in place showing paddles interposed between joint surfaces.

from the patient's own occiput in most of the others. Solid fusion was achieved in all cases except one in which specially pre-

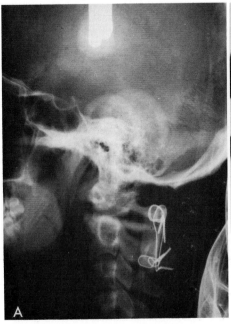

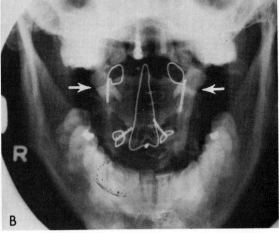

Figure 41–37 Lateral, *A*, and frontal, *B*, views of grafts in position. Arrows indicate position of "paddles" in joints. Patient was still in traction (5 kg) at this stage. After immobilization for three months in Minerva jacket, fusion occurred and reduction was maintained.

pared calf bone ("Boplant," Squibb) had been used. Successful re-fusion was accomplished in this patient with his own skull bone, 18 months later. Obviously, all types of fusion limit neck movements, particularly rotation, and the technique just described leaves some numbness over the occiput as a result of the C2 rhizotomy. Although some neurological deficit has persisted in the more seriously disabled patients, all have shown symptomatic improvement. There was one infection of the acrylic cranioplasty covering the occipital donor site defect.

Following treatment of anomalies affecting the craniovertebral junction, including syringomyelia, one cannot expect complete recovery of all neurological deficits, particularly chronic long-standing ones. There is, however, frequent and gratifying reversal of recently acquired signs. The occipital headaches of the Chiari malformation and those due to atlantoaxial dislocation respond particularly well to posterior decompression and to fusion respectively. The pains of syringomyelia and weakness or numbness of recent onset have improved also following operation, but areflexia and the impairment of pain and temperature sensation have usually remained. Three of the author's 41 patients with syringomyelia deteriorated again after temporary improvement or stabilization, and eventually died in spite of shunting and drainage procedures: one of pneumonia, one of respiratory failure, and the third of acute hydrocephalomyelia that led to complete flaccid tetraplegia and blindness.

Patients treated early in the course of their disease do better than the ones with more advanced lesions. It is recommended that the operative correction be done as soon as the diagnosis is established, particularly if there is evidence of progression of the disease.

REFERENCES

1. Alajouanine, T., Thurel, R., and Papaioanou, C.: La douleur à type de décharge électrique, provoquée par la flexion de la tête et parcourant le corps de haut en bas. Sem. Hôp. Paris, 25:2840–2845, 1949.
2. Alexander, E., Jr., Forsyth, H. F., Davis, C. H., Jr., and Nashold, B. S., Jr.: Dislocation of the atlas on the axis. The value of early fusion of C1,C2 and C3. J. Neurosurg., 15:353–371, 1958.
3. Andrade, J. R. de, and MacNab, I.: Anterior occipito-cervical fusion using an extrapharyngeal exposure. J. Bone Joint Surg., 51A:1621–1626, 1969.
4. Arnold, J.: Myelocyste: Transposition von Gewebskeinem und Sympodie. Beitr. Path. Anat., 16:1–28, 1894.
5. Bachs, A., Barraquer-Bordas, L., Barraquer-Ferré, L., Canadell, G. M., and Modolell, A.: Delayed myelopathy following atlanto-axial dislocation by separated odontoid process. Brain, 78:537–553, 1955.
6. Barnett, H. J. M., Foster, J. B., and Hudgson, P.: Syringomyelia. Philadelphia, W. B. Saunders Co., 1973.
7. Barnett, H. J. M., Botterell, E. H., Jousse, A. T., and Wynn-Jones, M.: Progressive myelopathy as a sequel to traumatic paraplegia. Brain, 89:159–174, 1966.
8. Barry, A., Patten, B. M., and Stewart, B. H.: Possible factors in the development of the Arnold-Chiari malformation. J. Neurosurg., 14:285–301, 1957.
9. Benda, C. E.: Dandy-Walker syndrome or the so-called atresia of the foramen of Magendie. J. Neuropath. Exp. Neurol., 13:14–29, 1954.
10. Bertrand, G.: Chronic atlanto-axial dislocations. A method of reduction and fixation. In Deutsche Gesselschaft fur Neurochirurgie: Proceedings. Freiburg, 1970: Excerpta Medica International Congress Series No. 242. Vol. 2. Cervical Spine Operations, pp. 333–334.
11. Bertrand, G.: Dynamic factors in the evolution of syringomyelia and syringobulbia. Clin. Neurosurg., 20:322–333, 1973.
12. Bharucha, E. P., and Dastur, H. M.: Craniovertebral anomalies (a report on 40 cases). Brain, 87:469–480, 1964.
13. Boogaard, J. A.: Basilar impression. Its causes and consequences. Nederl. T. Geneesk., 2:81–108, 1865.
14. Booth, A. E., and Kendall, D. E.: Percutaneous aspiration of cystic lesions of the spinal cord. J. Neurosurg., 33:140–144, 1970.
15. Chamberlain, W. E.: Basilar impression (platybasia). Yale J. Biol. Med., 11:487–496, 1939.
16. Chiari, H.: Uber Veränderungen des Kleinhirns infolge von Hydrocephalie des Grosshirns, Deutsch. Med. Wschr., 17:1172–1175, 1891.
17. Chiari, H.: Uber die Veränderungen des Kleinhirns, der Pons und der Medulla oblongata infolge von congenitaler Hydrocephalie des Grosshirns. Denkschr. Akad. Wissensch. Wien, 63:71–117, 1895.
18. Cloward, R. B.: Anterior cervical fusion for odontoid fracture. In Hall, R. M., ed.: Air Instrument Surgery. Vol. 1. New York, Springer Verlag, 1970, pp. 152–153.
19. Cone, W., and Turner, W. G.: The treatment of fracture-dislocations of the cervical vertebrae by skeletal traction and fusion. J. Bone Joint Surg., 19:584–602, 1937.
20. Conway, L. W.: Hydrodynamic studies in syringomyelia. J. Neurosurg., 27:501–514, 1967.
21. Dandy, W. E.: Diagnosis and treatment of hydrocephalus due to occlusions of the foramina of Luschka and Magendie. Surg. Gynec. Obstet., 32:112, 1921.
22. Dandy, W. E., and Blackfan, K. D.: Internal hydrocephalus: An experimental, clinical and

pathological study. Amer. J. Dis. Child., *8*:406, 1904.

23. Dastur, D. K., Wadia, N. H., Desai, A. D., and Sinh, G.: Medullospinal compression due to atlanto-axial dislocation and sudden haematomyelia during decompression. Pathology, pathogenesis, and clinical correlations. Brain, *88*: 897–924, 1965.

24. Di Chiro, G., Axelbaum, S. P., Schellinger, D., Twigg, H. L., and Ledley, R. S.: Computerized axial tomography in syringomyelia. New Eng. J. Med., *292*:13–16, 1975.

25. Eisenberg, H. M., McLennan, J. E., and Welch, K.: Ventricular perfusion in cats with kaolin-induced hydrocephalus. J. Neurosurg., *41*:20–28, 1974.

26. Ellertsson, A. B., and Greitz, T.: Myelocystographic and fluorescein studies to demonstrate communication between intramedullary cysts and the cerebro-spinal fluid space. Acta Neurol. Scand., *45*:418–430, 1969.

27. Estridge, M. N., and Smith, R. A.: Transoral fusion of odontoid fracture. J. Neurosurg., *27*:462–465, 1967.

28. Fang, H. S. Y., and Ong, G. B.: Direct anterior approach to the upper cervical spine. J. Bone Joint Surg., *44A*:1588–1604, 1962.

29. Fielding, J. W.: Disappearance of the central portion of the odontoid process. J. Bone Joint Surg., *47A*:1228–1230, 1965.

30. Fishgold, H., and Metzger, J.: Etude radio-tomographique de l'impression basilaire. Rev. Rhum. *3*:261–264, 1952.

31. Foster, J. B., and Hudgson, P.: Basal arachnoiditis. *In* Barnett, H. J. M., Foster, J. B., and Hudgson, P., eds.: Syringomyelia. Philadelphia, W. B. Saunders Co., 1973, pp. 30–49.

32. Freiberger, R. H., Wilson, P. D., and Nicholas, J. A.: Acquired absence of the odontoid process. J. Bone Joint Surg., *47A*:1231–1236, 1965.

33. Gallie, W. E.: Fractures and dislocations of the cervical spine. Amer. J. Surg., *46*:95, 1939.

34. Garcin, R., and Oeconomos, D.: Les aspects neurologiques des malformations congénitales de la charnière cranio-rachidienne. Paris, Masson, 1953.

35. Gardner, W. G.: Hydrodynamic mechanism of syringomyelia. Its relationship to myelocoele. J. Neurol. Neurosurg. Psychiat., *28*:247–259, 1965.

36. Gardner, W. J.: Anomalies of the craniovertebral junction. *In* Youmans, J. R., ed.: Neurological Surgery. Vol. 1. Philadelpha, W. B. Saunders Co., 1973, pp. 628–644.

37. Gardner, W. G., Steinberg, M., and Bell, H.: Terminal ventriculostomy in the treatment of syringomyelia. Presented at the annual meeting of the American Association of Neurological Surgeons. Miami, Florida, April, 1975.

38. Greenberg, A. D., Scoville, W. B., and Davey, L. M.: Transoral decompression of atlanto-axial dislocation due to odontoid hypoplasia. J. Neurosurg., *28*:266–269, 1968.

39. Grisel, P.: Enucléation de l'atlas et torticolis naso-pharyngien. Presse Méd., *38*:50–53, 1930.

40. Guillaume, J., and Lubin, P.: Traitement des luxations de atlas par ostéosynthèse métallique. Presse Méd., *49*:866–867, 1941.

41. Hall, P. V., Kalsbeck, J. E., Wellman, H. N., Campbell, R. L., and Lewis, S.: Radioisotope

42. Hall, P. V., Kalsbeck, J. E., Wellman, H. N., Blanitsky, S., Campbell, R. L., and Lewis, S.: Clinical radioisotope investigation in hydrosyringomyelia and myelodysplasia. J. Neurosurg., *45*:188–194, 1976.

43. Hamblem, D. L.: Occipito-cervical fusion: Indications, technique and results. J. Bone Joint Surg., *49B*:33–45, 1967.

44. Ingraham, F. D., and Scott, H. W., Jr.: Spina bifida and cranium bifidum. The Arnold-Chiari malformation: A study of 20 cases. New Eng. J. Med., *229*:108–114, 1943.

45. Judet, R.: Actualités de chirurgie orthopédique de l'hôpital Raymond-Poincarré. III. Luxation congénitale de la hanche, Fracture du cou-de-pied, Rachis cervical. Paris, Masson, 1964.

46. Kahn, E. A., and Yglesias, L.: Progressive atlanto-axial dislocation. J.A.M.A., *105*:348–352, 1935.

47. Kelly, D. L., Alexander, E., Davis, C. H., and Smith, J. M.: Acrylic fixation of atlanto-axial dislocations. J. Neurosurg., *36*:366–371, 1972.

48. Lipscomb, P. R.: Cervico-occipital fusion for congenital and posttraumatic anomalies of the atlas and axis. J. Bone Joint Surg., *39A*:1289–1301, 1957.

49. List, C. F.: Neurologic syndromes accompanying developmental anomalies of the occipital bone, atlas and axis. A.M.A. Arch. Neurol. Psychiat., *45*:577–616, 1941.

50. Macnab, I.: Anterior occipito-cervical fusion. J. Bone Joint Surg., *49A*:1010–1011, 1967.

51. Matson, D. D.: Neurosurgery of Infancy and Childhood. 2nd ed. Springfield, Ill., Charles C. Thomas, 1969, pp. 259–268.

52. McGregor, M. B.: The significance of certain measurements of the skull in the diagnosis of basilar impression. Brit. J. Radiol. *21*:171–181, 1948.

53. McLauren, R. L., Bailey, P., Schurr, P. H., and Ingraham, F. D.: Myelomalacia and multiple cavitations of the spinal cord secondary to adhesive arachnoiditis. Arch. Path., *57*:138–146, 1954.

54. McRae, D. L.: Bone abnormalities in the region of the foramen magnum: Correlation of the anatomic and neurologic findings. Acta Radiol., *40*:335–354, 1953.

55. McRae, D. L.: The significance of abnormalities of the cervical spine. Amer. J. Roentgen., *84*:3–25, 1960.

56. McRae, D. L., and Barnum, A. S.: Occipitalization of the atlas. Amer. J. Roentgen., *70*:23–45, 1953.

57. Mitsumori, K., Saito, H., Motomiya, M., et al.: Transoral approach for the treatment of atlanto-axial dislocation with the os odontoideum and obstruction of the bilateral vertebral arteries. Neurol. Surg. (Tokyo), *3*:585–591, 1975.

58. Nagashima, C.: Atlanto-axial dislocation due to agenesis of the os odontoideum or odontoid. J. Neurosurg., *33*:270–280, 1970.

59. Nagashima, C.: Surgical treatment of irreducible atlanto-axial dislocation with spinal cord compression. J. Neurosurg., *38*:374–378, 1973.

60. Penfield, W., and Coburn, D. F.: Arnold-Chiari malformation and its operative treatment. A.M.A. Arch. Neurol. Psychiat., *40*:328–336, 1938.

evaluation of experimental hydrosyringomyelia. J. Neurosurg., *45*:181–187, 1976.

61. Rhoton, A. L.: Microsurgery for Arnold-Chiari malformation in adults with and without hydromyelia. J. Neurosurg., *45*:473–483, 1976.
62. Roberts, S. M.: Congenital absence of the odontoid process resulting in dislocation of the atlas on the axis. J. Bone Joint Surg., *15*:988–989, 1933.
63. Russell, D. S., and Donald, C.: The mechanism of internal hydrocephalus in spina bifida. Brain, *58*:203–215, 1935.
64. Schlesinger, E. B., and Taveras, J. M.: Lesions of the odontoid and their management. Amer. J. Surg., *95*:641–650, 1958.
65. Schüller, A.: Zur Roentgen-Diagnose der basalen Impression des Schädels. Wien. Med. Wschr., *61*:2593–2599, 1911.
66. Schwalbe, E., and Gredig, M.: Uber .Entwicklungstörungen des Kleinhirns, Hirnstamms und Halsmarks bei spina bifida (Arnold'sche und Chairi'sche Missbildung). Beitr. Path. Anat., *40*:132–194, 1907.
67. Scoville, W. B., and Sherman, I. J.: Platybasia: Report of ten cases with comments on familial tendency, a special diagnostic sign and the end result of operation. Ann. Surg., *133*:496–502, 1951.
68. Spillane, J. D., Pallis, C., and Jones, A. M.: Developmental abnormalities in the region of the foramen magnum. Brain, *80*:11–48, 1957.
69. Stevenson, G. C., Storey, R. J., Perkins, R. K., and Adams, J. E.: A transcervical transclival approach to the ventral surface of the brain stem for removal of clivus chordoma. J. Neurosurg., *24*:544–551, 1966.
70. Stewart, J. D., Lewis, C. L. H., and Dar, J.: Symptomatic bony craniovertebral anomalies in the Kenyan African. Inst. Neurol. Madras, Proc., *6*:123–129, 1976.
71. Stratford, J.: Myelopathy caused by atlanto-axial dislocation. J. Neurosurg., *14*:97–104, 1957.
72. Sukoff, M. H.: Transoral decompression for myelopathy caused by rheumatoid arthritis of the cervical spine: Case report. J. Neurosurg., *37*:493–497, 1972.
73. Taggart, J. K., Jr., and Walker, A. E.: Congenital atresia of the foramens of Luschka and Magendie. A.M.A. Arch. Neurol. Psychiat., *48*:583–612, 1942.
74. Tjaden, R. J., Ethier, R., and Vézina, J. L.: Iodoventriculography in hydromyelia. J. Canad. Ass. Radiol., *20*:265–268, 1969.
75. Williams, B.: The distending force in the production of communicating syringomyelia. Lancet, *2*:696, 1969.
76. Williams, B.: Combined cisternal and lumbar pressure recordings in the sitting position using differential manometry. J. Neurol. Neurosurg. Psychiat., *35*:142–143, 1972.
77. Wollin, D. G.: The os odontoideum, separate odontoid process. J. Bone Joint Surg., *45A*:1459–1471, 1963.

VII

VASCULAR DISEASE

42

PATHOPHYSIOLOGY AND CLINICAL EVALUATION OF ISCHEMIC VASCULAR DISEASE

In the United States and most developed countries, cerebrovascular disease is the most important cause of chronic disability and the third most frequent cause of death.

The term "cerebrovascular disease" denotes a pathological condition of the central nervous system attributable to a disturbance in its blood supply. Ischemic cerebrovascular disease excludes conditions in which hemorrhage is the primary event and, in common usage, is restricted to those conditions in which the ischemia results in a focal neurological deficit. Both focal and diffuse ischemic events of the cerebral hemispheres, brain stem, and cerebellum are discussed in this chapter. Ischemia of the spinal cord is not discussed.

DEFINITIONS AND CLASSIFICATION

Cerebral ischemic events are classified by their site, vascular mechanism, and time course.

Site

The anatomical localization of a lesion may, in many instances, be deduced from the clinical features. Given the anatomical site and its extent, an attempt must be made to place the lesion with respect to the vascular territory of a single artery, at the border zone or watershed of contiguous arteries, diffusely, or in an area of venous occlusion.

A *single territory infarct* is the lesion most frequently observed in patients presenting with ischemic stroke.[104] Collateral flow can be expected to restrict the volume of the infarct to something less than the region normally perfused by the occluded vessel. Since embolic occlusion and anterograde extension of thrombus from a more proximal occlusion account for most cerebral infarcts, the continuing use of the term "cerebral thrombosis" as a synonym for single territory cerebral infarcts is to be condemned.[65]

If the perfusion pressure is simultaneously reduced in adjacent arteries, the tissue of the *border zone* between the arterial territories will be the site of maximal ischemic damage. Sudden and profound systemic hypotension is the most common cause of *border zone,* or *watershed, infarcts* of the brain.[104]

Diffuse anoxic encephalopathy follows either circulatory arrest or widespread disturbances of the microvascular circulation.

Venous infarction is relatively uncommon, but may develop when cortical veins and their smaller radicles are occluded.

D. D. BURROW AND J. F. TOOLE

Vascular Mechanism

A single territory infarct may follow occlusion of a cerebral vessel by an embolus, by the extension of anterograde thrombus from a more proximal arterial occlusion, or by intrinsic disease of the cerebral vessel. The mechanisms of border zone and venous infarction and diffuse ischemic encephalopathies have already been commented upon. In Tables 42–1 and 42–2, ischemic cerebrovascular events are classified by their initiating mechanisms.

Time Course

The recognition of the significance of transient ischemic attacks is the most important advance in the field of cerebrovascular disease.[41]

Transient ischemic attacks (TIA's) are episodes of temporary and focal cerebral dysfunction of vascular origin commonly lasting from 2 to 15 minutes but occasionally lasting as long as 24 hours.[114]

If the signs or symptoms persist for more than 24 hours but subsequently completely resolve in less than three weeks, the episode is designated a *reversible ischemic neurological deficit* (RIND).

When the neurological deficit has been progressive for six hours or more, cerebral hemorrhage, tumor, and subdural hematoma are diagnostic possibilities. Because of their urgent diagnostic and therapeutic considerations these conditions are designated as *stroke in evolution* or *progressing stroke*.

If the lesion is stable for 18 to 24 hours, further progression is unlikely and it should no longer be categorized as a "progressing stroke." With vertebral-basilar lesions, however, up to 72 hours should elapse before they are designated as "completed stroke."[114]

TABLE 42–1   CAUSES OF FOCAL CEREBRAL ISCHEMIA CLASSIFIED BY SITE OF PRIMARY DISEASE

SITE	CONDITION	MECHANISM
Precardiac	Pulmonary consolidation	Emboli from pulmonary veins
	Deep vein thrombosis and atrial septal defect	Paradoxical embolism
	Clearing a Scribner shunt	Retrograde arterial embolism
Cardiac	Myocardial infarction	Emboli (arrhythmia, hypotension)
	Valvular heart disease (particularly mitral)	Emboli
	Cardiomyopathy	Emboli
	Arrhythmia (particularly chronic and paroxysmal atrial fibrillation	Emboli
	Less common: hypertensive heart disease, infectious endocarditis, marantic endocarditis	Emboli (septic or bland)
Great vessels	Aortic dissection	Extension (thrombosis, emboli)
	Aortitis: Takayasu's, syphilitic, giant cell, rheumatoid, ankylosing spondylitis	Emboli, branch occlusion
Carotid artery	Atherosclerotic plaque (stenotic or ulcerated)	Emboli
	Carotid occlusion	Anterograde thrombosis emboli (hemodynamic)
	Less common: fibromuscuiar hyperplasia, kinking, arteritis	Emboli (hemodynamic)
Vertebral artery	Distal occlusion	Anterograde thrombus, emboli (frequently results in cerebral infarction)
	Proximal occlusion	Emboli (infrequent cause of cerebral infarction)
	Proximal subclavian occlusion	Subclavian steal syndrome
	Neck manipulation	Intimal injury at C2 level
Intracranial (arterial)	Atherosclerosis of major cerebral vessels (particularly vertebral and basilar arteries)	Occlusion
	Arteritis	Occlusion
	Subarachnoid hemorrhage	Spasm and vessel rupture
	Arteriolar sclerosis (hypertension)	Occlusion
	Transtentorial herniation	Compression of posterior cerebral arteries
Intracranial (venous)	Cortical vein thrombosis	Venous infarction
	Occlusion of deep venous system	Venous infarction
Uncertain site	Erythrocytosis (PCV greater than 55%)	Thrombosis (arterial and venous)
	Thrombocytosis	In situ thrombosis, emboli
	Macroglobulinemia (with hyperviscosity)	Sludging
	Oral contraceptives	Thrombosis (arterial or venous)

TABLE 42-2 CAUSES OF DIFFUSE CEREBRAL ISCHEMIA

Circulatory arrest
  Cardiac arrest
Impaired circulation
  Strangulation
  Profound hypotension
  Extensive extracranial vascular disease
Impaired energy substrate supply
  Hypoxemic hypoxia
  Severe anemia
  Hypoglycemia
  Carbon monoxide poisoning
Diffuse small-vessel disease
  Hypertension
  Eclampsia
  Small vessel arteritis, cerebral lupus, polyarteritis nodosa, noninfectious granulomatous angiitis
  Thrombotic thrombocytopenic purpura
Microembolic disease
  Fat embolism
  Disseminated intravascular coagulation
  Cardiopulmonary bypass procedures

EPIDEMIOLOGY OF ISCHEMIC DISEASE

The economic and social importance of ischemic cerebrovascular disease is reflected in the considerable interest in its epidemiology. The diversity of clinical manifestations and the difficulty of determining the pathological changes in and the mechanism of individual cases restricts the usefulness of epidemiological studies; however, we may note that:

1. The incidence of cerebral infarction increases greatly with *age*. In the Mayo Clinic study of the population of Rochester, Minnesota, the incidence increased from 72 per 100,000 population per year among persons 45 to 54 years to 1786 per 100,000 population per year among those of more than 75 years.[110]

2. Most studies have shown the incidence of cerebral infarction to be a little less in women than in men of the same age.[110]

3. The presence of *hypertension* (even an elevation of the systolic pressure taken as a "casual reading") increases the risk of subsequent cerebral hemorrhage or infarction. This risk increases over the whole range of observed pressures, and there is no critical blood pressure above which this risk component commences.[83] The prognosis for an ischemic stroke is a little poorer and the risk of reinfarction is also greater in the hypertensive person.[73]

4. Cardiac disease of all forms is associated with an increased risk of cerebral infarction (usually embolic). Atrial fibrillation increases the risk of cerebral infarction sixfold, and ischemic heart disease increases it fivefold.[41,82]

5. A history of recent transient cerebral ischemia markedly increases the probability of cerebral infarction. Whisnant and coworkers observed 16.5 times the expected incidence of stroke in the first year after a transient ischemic attack.[22,171]

6. Increased serum cholesterol and possibly triglyceride are associated with an increased risk in men before the age of 55 years.[171]

7. In younger persons diabetes mellitus is a risk factor, particularly for discrete small brain stem infarcts.[82]

8. Obesity, cigarette smoking, and decreased physical activity have been suggested as risk factors, but remain unproved.[88,119]

9. Retinopathy, cervical bruit, right-left brachial blood pressure differences, and evidences of peripheral vascular disease are indicators of underlying arterial disease that is related to mechanisms of stroke.

10. The evidence that there are major differences in the incidence of cerebral infarction between geographical boundaries and racial groups is unclear.[91] The belief that the relative frequency of cerebral hemorrhage, compared with cerebral infarction, is greater in Japan is under study.[92]

11. Comparison of the results of observations made upon groups of patients with recent brain infarcts with those of grouped control persons indicate that the viscosity and rheological characteristics of blood, particularly at low flow rates, may influence the size and frequency of cerebral infarcts.[125,130] Circulating platelet aggregates and hypercoagulability are found with greater frequency in stroke patients.[175]

PATHOPHYSIOLOGY OF CEREBRAL ISCHEMIA

When the brain is rendered totally ischemic, electrical activity disappears within 10 to 20 seconds; the sodium-potassium pump fails within 30 seconds; and glucose levels rapidly fall. Water passively follows the influx of sodium, causing intracellular edema within three minutes of the initiation of ischemia. In 5 to 10 minutes intracellular lactate levels have risen fivefold and cellular glucose is exhausted.[102,169] To this point, however, all changes are reversible.

The persistence of ischemia beyond this point causes progressive and ultimately irreversible failure of the cellular organelles. Mitochondrial injury has the most direct influence upon the survival of the cell. For many tissues, ultrastructural changes have been followed through varying durations of total ischemia (except for nervous tissues). It has been possible to compare these changes with cellular viability. The consensus is that the appearance of clumped electron-dense bodies within the mitochondria is a reliable "marker" of cell death.[164] For tissues other than those of the nervous system, 6 to 24 hours of complete ischemia may elapse before cell death occurs. It is interesting to note that the ultramicroscopic criteria of cell death are not observed in the cat brain, even after five hours of *total* ischemia, but will rapidly appear upon reestablishment of circulation.[42] This very important and recently observed phenomenon has its counterpart in myocardial ischemia.[102,164]

What explanations can be offered for this observation? The reperfusion of tissues with their accumulated energy deficit, nonfunctional membrane pumps, and increased cellular permeability allows the cell to be flooded with ions normally excluded (e.g., calcium and sodium ions). The calcium ion, by activating phospholipase enzymes, may initiate further injury to the mitochondrial and cellular membranes.

Although this important observation has not been adequately studied, an exciting possibility has been raised—pharmacological intervention may allow successful reperfusion after prolonged periods of ischemia. It must be cautioned that *total* ischemia is difficult to achieve experimentally and almost never present in focal ischemia of the human brain.

Focal Ischemia

The events that follow obstruction of a cerebral vessel are critical to outcome. Arterial occlusion lowers the perfusion pressure in the vessel's distal vasculature. This pressure drop summons the available collateral flow through channels that rap-idly become maximally dilated by the metabolic effects of ischemia.[154] If the flow into the occluded vasculature is sufficient the patient is spared ischemic injury. Experimental studies indicate that the achieved flow is often close to this "sufficient" or "critical" flow, so for example, clipping the middle cerebral artery of the dog does not cause cerebral infarction unless the dog's blood pressure is simultaneously reduced. It should be noted that flow through the dysautoregulated collateral vasculature is proportional to the perfusion pressure, i.e., the difference between mean arterial and tissue pressures. Cerebral arteriosclerosis, insufficient to initiate an ischemic event, may play a critical role in determining the outcome by limiting the collateral flow.

A cerebral infarct is a rapidly expanding lesion that reaches a maximum volume between the second and fourth days. Swelling is life-threatening in 20 per cent of patients with large cerebral infarcts and 50 per cent of patients with large cerebellar infarcts.[3,131]

Ischemic cerebral swelling is a complex reaction. Vascular dilatation within the zone of ischemia makes a minor contribution to the swelling. Intracellular edema commences within minutes and progresses rapidly, taking water from the extracellular space, which in turn is replenished from the vascular compartment. Perfusion of the ischemic brain causes vasogenic or extracellular edema, particularly when the subsequent breakdown of the blood-brain barrier allows the release of osmotically active substances into the extravascular space. Ischemic cerebral edema is, however, usually maximal before the blood-brain barrier has been significantly disrupted.[122] The early and clinically most significant edema is largely metabolic or cytotoxic in type and intracellular in site, and results directly from ischemic injury of the sodium-potassium cell membrane pump.[123]

Ischemic brain swelling may further compromise the perfusion of ischemic brain by increasing both the local tissue hydrostatic pressure and the overall pressure of its intracranial compartment.[87]

Anastomotic Channels

Effective arterial anastomoses may form at three levels in the vasculature of the brain: extracranially, in the circle of Willis, or in the leptomeninges.

The most common extracranial anastomotic channels are those between the external and the internal carotid arteries. When the internal carotid is obstructed below the origin of the ophthalmic, rich collaterals develop from the maxillary branch of the external carotid to the ophthalmic artery, through which blood flows retrograde to the distal internal carotid and thence to the brain.[48] In certain situations, the ophthalmic artery may carry most of the blood to a hemisphere whose internal carotid artery is occluded. Other anastomoses may develop through the caroticotympanic artery, the artery of the pterygoid canal, or the trigeminal artery.

Congenital variations in the size of the vessels of the circle of Willis are frequently encountered. In more than 50 per cent of normal persons the circle of Willis has one or more hypoplastic vessels, most commonly the posterior cerebrals.[155] These anomalies appear to influence the frequency of cerebral infarctions.[9]

Important anastomotic channels exist between the major cerebral arteries. Because these occur over the surface of the brain, they are commonly described as the leptomeningeal anastomoses. Their potential capacity is less than that of the anastomoses within the circle of Willis, and they are seldom able to protect the brain from infarction when a major cerebral artery is occluded.[165]

Within the substance of the brain there are few if any clinically significant anastomoses. While there are unquestionably capillary and supracapillary anastomoses throughout the brain, the caliber of these is such that they are of little functional importance. Therefore, the penetrating arteries can be considered end-arteries. In certain cases of cerebral infarction, the parenchymal microvascular anastomoses may appear as a "tumor-like" angiographic blush.

Mechanisms of Arterial Occlusion

Embolism

Embolism is the most frequent mechanism of brain infarction.[104] Lhermitte and co-workers concluded that two thirds of middle cerebral artery infarcts were embolic.[99] The heart is the most frequent

TABLE 42–3 FREQUENCY OF CARDIAC LESIONS CAUSING CEREBRAL EMBOLIZATION*

CARDIAC LESION	PER CENT
Myocardial infarction (recent and old)	50
Rheumatic heart disease	26
Congestive cardiomyopathy (and myocardial disease of undetermined causation)	15
Infective endocarditis	7
Thrombotic endocarditis	2
Atrial myxoma	<1

* Data from: Blackwood, W., et al.: Atheromatous disease of the carotid arterial system and embolism from the heart in cerebral infarction: a morbid anatomical study. Brain, 92:897–910, 1969. McCall, A. J., and Fletcher, P. J. H.: *In* Hutchinson, E. C., and Acheson, E. J., eds.: Strokes: Natural History, Pathology and Surgical Treatment. London, W. B. Saunders Co. Ltd., 1975.

source and may account for half of the infarcts within the anterior circulation (Table 42–3).[15] Careful postmortem examination of the brain revealed that of 340 persons dying with heart disease 54 per cent had cerebral infarcts compared with 12 per cent of 100 patients free of heart disease.[87]

Ischemic heart disease is the most frequent cardiac source of cerebral emboli. The risk of embolism is maximal during the first 14 days after an ischemic attack but persists indefinitely. Patients with valvular heart disease, particularly mitral stenosis, are at risk of cerebral embolism, particularly if the valvular disease is complicated by arrhythmia or heart failure. The frequency of both systemic and cerebral embolization in infectious endocarditis is still very marked, but has been reduced by current therapy.[80]

Less frequent cardiac sources of embolism include cardiac myxoma, prolapsing mitral valve, and paroxysmal arrhythmia. Cardiac myxoma is an uncommon benign tumor, usually in the left atrium, that may present at any age with obstruction of the left ventricular inflow tract, peripheral embolism, and constitutional symptoms.[177]

Paradoxical emboli usually enter the systemic circulation through a foramen ovale guarded only by a left atrial flap. The flap is opened by the transient increase in the right atrial pressure that occurs with pulmonary embolism.[157] Embolic occlusion of only 30 per cent of the pulmonary vascular bed is sufficient to produce a reversal of atrial pressures, and 20 per cent of the population have the required atrial septal "defect."[162] As one patient in every five with major pulmonary embolism is at risk, it is not surprising that 4 per cent of all cerebral infarcts are due to paradoxical embolism.[104]

Pulmonary consolidations may initiate phlebothrombosis within the pulmonary veins and generate either septic or sterile emboli.

Emboli of sufficient size to be arrested within a major cerebral artery enter the anterior circulation 10 times as frequently as they enter the posterior and then commonly proceed into the middle cerebral artery. Embolic arrest occurs at bifurcations or major branches because it is at these sites that the arterial cross section takes a stepwise reduction. Microemboli are widely distributed throughout the brain with a frequency of impaction proportional to the blood flow to the region.

The balance between intravascular fibrinolysis and thrombosis will determine the fate of the impacted embolus. Thrombosis of the stagnant vessel distal to the occlusion may be initiated by products from the embolus. This process will occlude the distal vasculature, further reduce the collateral flow, and increase the size of the cerebral infarct. Fibrinolysis may result in dissolution of the embolus and allow reperfusion. Unfortunately, it is unlikely that larger thrombotic emboli will be cleared rapidly enough to avoid irreversible ischemic changes, and indeed reperfusion may both accelerate the ischemic swelling and render the infarct hemorrhagic.[162]

The nature of the embolus will influence this balance. Mature thrombus, particularly if partially organized, is more slowly and incompletely cleared than recent thrombus. Aggregations of platelets are loosely bound by fibrin and therefore may be rapidly and completely cleared from sites of impaction. Such emboli are the most frequent cause of transient ischemic attacks. Many other materials may form occasional emboli: cholesterol, debris from ulcerated atheroma, calcium from cardiac valves, fat, air, dislodged arterial catheters, gun shot, and intravenous cannulae.

Anterograde Extension of Thrombus

Vessel occlusion may be followed by thrombosis and extension of this thrombus distally.[104] Extension becomes significant when it continues past branches bringing significant collateral flow. When the internal carotid artery is occluded at its origin, it is expected that anterograde thrombosis will extend through the unbranched section to a point just short of the ophthalmic artery. In 50 per cent of cerebral infarctions that follow carotid occlusion, thrombus extends beyond the ophthalmic artery, beyond the collateral of the circle of Willis, and into the middle or anterior cerebral arteries or both.[23,162] Similarly, thrombus may extend from the distal vertebral into the basilar artery.[24]

Hemodynamic Infarction

The frequency of asymptomatic carotid and vertebral artery occlusion suggests that the hemodynamic consequences of even complete occlusion of vessels proximal to the circle of Willis is usually insufficient to cause cerebral infarction unless complicated by embolism or anterograde thrombosis.[23,24] It is the opinion of the authors that many cerebral infarcts not associated with demonstrable arterial occlusion are examples of cerebral embolism in which there has been subsequent lysis of the embolus.

Intrinsic Disease of Cerebral Vessels

Severe atherosclerotic stenosis of intracranial vessels is surprisingly infrequent, but may be encountered in the distal portions of the vertebral and internal carotid arteries and in the basilar artery. Battacharji found that only 4 per cent of middle cerebral artery occlusions could be attributed to intrinsic disease.[9] In contrast, the majority of occlusions in penetrating vessels of the hemispheres, pons, and cerebellum are the result of hypertension-related arteriolar sclerosis.

Nonatheromatous arterial pathological conditions are considered later in this chapter.

CLINICAL EVALUATION

History

The clinical interview is conducted to gain adequate historical data to define the neurological symptoms and time course. At a clinical level, the opinion that a patient has ischemic cerebrovascular disease is based almost exclusively upon the temporal profile of the onset and the evolution of symptoms. When the patient is aphasic or comatose, even a fragmentary history of the ictus from a direct witness may be of critical importance and be only as far away as the telephone.

The patient should be asked to begin his story with the first episode rather than with more recent events. This orientation will often cause patients to recount symptoms they considered inconsequential. If multiple episodes have occurred, a description of the first, the most recent, the worst, and any in which the symptoms were substantially different should be reviewed and noted. In each, the symptoms must be adequately reviewed to allow conclusions about the site of ischemia, the time course of events, and whether precipitating factors have been operative.

Although atherosclerosis, ischemic heart disease, and hypertension are the most frequent causes of ischemic cerebrovascular disease, the patient's entire medical and neurological history must be utilized to exclude the many "nonatheromatous" initiating disorders and to assess the coincidental disease.

Neurovascular Examination

The neurovascular examination assesses: (1) cardiac rhythm, (2) pulses of vessels supplying the cerebral circulation, (3) auscultation of the heart and the great vessels, (4) arterial blood pressure recordings, (5) tests of specific precipitants of cerebral ischemia (posture-related hypotension, carotid sinus massage, Valsalva maneuver, head posturing, (6) retinal vasculature, and (7) peripheral vasculature. These techniques are briefly considered, but have been more fully described elsewhere.[161]

Cardiac Rhythm

The opportunity to assess the rhythm occurs during the bimanual radial pulse examination. Dysrhythmia demands electrocardiographic evaluation, and if a paroxysmal rhythm disorder is suspected, prolonged electrocardiographic monitoring is required.[25]

Pulses

The vessels that should be palpated bilaterally simultaneously are: the radial, superficial temporal, facial, common carotid, and subclavian arteries. Diminution, absence, or delay in pulsation may be noted distal to occlusive disease; however, increased pulsation over branches of the external carotid may at times be noted when these vessels supply collaterals to bypass a severe stenosis or occlusion of the ipsilateral internal carotid artery. The technique of palpating the internal carotid pulse by introducing a finger into the oropharynx is difficult and has not received wide acceptance.[30]

Auscultation

The sites worthy of routine auscultation are those that have a propensity for atherosclerosis or are situated over the skull, to which sound is transmitted from such regions. A sequence of examination is illustrated in Figure 42–1. After cardiac auscul-

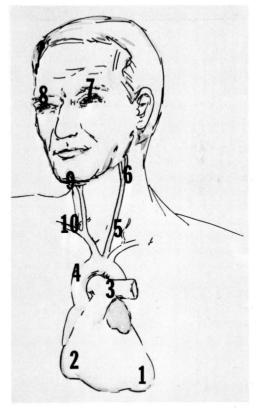

Figure 42–1 A logical sequence for auscultation of the heart, the great vessels in the neck, and the orbits. These are the sites where murmurs are heard most frequently.

tation the aortic outflow tract should be followed to differentiate cervical bruits from those arising proximally. Carotid bifurcation bruits are best heard over the carotid arteries at the level of the upper border of the thyroid cartilage. Because bruits generated at the common carotid bifurcation are seldom transmitted into the cranial cavity, an orbital bruit suggests arterial disease or increased flow through the ipsilateral carotid siphon. A siphon bruit may also be transmitted to the mastoid process.

The significance of arterial murmur can be summarized by the following general rules: (1) Murmurs become audible after the lumen has been reduced about 50 per cent; (2) with increasing stenosis the pitch becomes higher; (3) with increasing stenosis the intensity increases until the lumen is reduced by at least two thirds, at which point the intensity of the murmur decreases until it finally becomes inaudible when occlusion is complete; and (4) as the degree of stenosis increases the duration of murmurs become more prolonged. Murmurs that are continuous into diastole suggest at least 90 per cent reduction in the cross-sectional diameter of the lumen of the vessel. Therefore, the following general points can be made: murmurs of low pitch and of high intensity or volume are generally associated with large orifices through which a large volume of blood is flowing; murmurs of high intensity, of high pitch, and long in duration suggest blood flow high in velocity through a small orifice; and intensity does not correlate well with the severity of the disease that causes it. Consequently, the tightest stenoses are generally accompanied by a high-pitched soft murmur that is accentuated during systole but that continues into diastole.[76]

The finding of a bruit in a patient over 40 years of age indicates arterial disease in three out of four instances; such a bruit would, however, be far less significant if found in a child or young adult. It has been reported that 90 per cent of children under the age of 5 years have bruits and that as many as 30 to 40 per cent of healthy young adults have neck bruits.[61]

Cardiac auscultation incorporates information gathered from inspection of the jugular venous pulse and precordium, and although an important part of the neurovascular examination, is beyond the scope of this text.

Blood Pressure Recordings

It is recommended that the arterial blood pressure be recorded from the right and left arms while the patient is supine and again from the right side after he has been standing for several minutes. The seated, leg-dependent position may be substituted in those unable to stand.

A 20 mm of mercury difference between the systolic pressures recorded in the right and left arms is significant. The diastolic difference is characteristically less. This examination is a valuable screen for the subclavian steal syndrome and is therefore particularly indicated for patients with vertebrobasilar insufficiency.[64]

Tests for Specific Precipitants

Care is required in the application of tests that reproduce symptoms. The patient must be asked to report any symptoms and must be informed of the aim of the specific test. Naturally, the examiner must be prepared to desist at the onset of symptoms.

Carotid Sinus Massage

This test should be reserved for patients having episodes of generalized cerebral ischemia of "syncopal type." A history of attacks being precipitated by forced turning or hyperextension of the neck, wearing a tight collar, shaving the neck, or undertaking violent exercise is often present in patients with carotid sinus syncope.[3] The test is performed both to establish the diagnosis of carotid sinus syncope and to provide information necessary to relieve it by appropriate treatment, and must be preceded by an electrocardiogram because the procedure is contraindicated in the presence of a cardiac conduction disturbance. A further contraindication is a history of a recent carotid transient ischemic attack.

With the patient supine, the bulbous dilation of the carotid sinus is gently massaged on one side for 30 seconds (or less if there is a positive response). If there is no response on one side, the test is repeated on the other side. If massage is tolerated on both sides, it is repeated with the patient seated.

A positive response may take two forms. In the *vagal inhibitory response* there is abrupt cardiac slowing coupled with the possibility of an arrhythmia, heart block, or hypotension. When the patient is lying flat a vagal inhibitory response will be apparent in the pulse and in electrocardiographic recordings. A positive response obviates the need to repeat the test in the seated position.

In the *vasodepressor response* (apparent only when the patient is seated), reflex splanchnic pooling results in decreased venous return and a profound fall in blood pressure. The blood pressure may be restored by having the patient lie back and elevating the legs.

Although complications are rare, cardiac asystole and complete heart block have been reported, and emboli may be displaced from an atheromatous bifurcation.[66]

Other Tests for Precipitants

Placing the patient in postures that he reports have induced symptoms may enable the clinican to evaluate the mechanism involved and test for signs during the symptomatic phase. This is particularly useful if vertigo is a prominent complaint.

Rotation of the neck, particularly when combined with extension, causes compression of the contralateral vertebral artery

upon the anterior border of C2 and may compress the ipsilateral carotid artery.[85] Lord Brain has suggested that the circle of Willis may have evolved as a means of compensating for these imbalances of flow in the four cervical vessels that are the consequences of a mobile neck.

Retinal Vascular Assessment

Although the alterations in the retinal arterioles and venules do not always reflect the condition of their cerebral counterparts, they do provide clues, particularly to embolic events.[140]

Microembolism

Three types of microemboli have been observed in retinal arterioles (Table 42–4). *Platelet-fibrin* emboli are white cylindrical bodies that are highly mobile, rarely produce retinal infarction, and presumably originate from mural thrombi in acute or imminent carotid occlusion. *Cholesterol* emboli appear as bright, highly refractile material and appear larger than the vessel in which they are lodged. Such emboli usually have been cast off from ulcerating

TABLE 42–4 IDENTIFYING FEATURES OF RETINAL MICROEMBOLI*

	TYPES OF EMBOLI		
	Platelet-Fibrin	**Cholesterol-Lipid**	**Calcific or Fibrinoid**
Color	White, nonreflective	Orange-yellow, orange, or bright metallic gold; variable color	Gray-white, dull, nonreflective
Shape	Long, smooth segments with flat discrete ends	Globular, containing bright crystals, indistinct interface with blood Small rectangular flakes alone	Ovoid, discrete, filling arterial lumen
Apparent caliber	Same as blood column	Larger than blood column	Same or slightly larger than proximal blood column
Mobility	Highly mobile; jerks from one bifurcation to the next	Ameboid-gelatinous movement with massage of eye, move or break up over period of days	Fixed
Location in retinal artery	Usually in motion	At bifurcations of medium and small vessels, unless large and mixed with stable fibrin	In unbranched segments of main or medium-sized retinal arterioles
Ischemic changes	Transient slowing of blood flow, no infarction	Dilated vein indicating mild hypoxia, retinal infarction from multiple plaques is variable in density and without clear borders	Usually produce dense, sharply delimited retinal infarct, small ischemic hemorrhages
Vessel change	No damage seen	Gray-white segmental mural opacity at bifurcation; slow appearance	Segmental mural change with narrowing, collateral capillary shunts, or both
Source and significance	Mural or "tail" thrombus in carotid occlusion (acute or imminent)	Eroding atheroma in carotid bifurcation; carotid patent and often without stenosis	Calcific valvular disease (apparent in x-ray of heart); rheumatic heart disease; myocardial disease

* From Hoyt, W. F.: Ocular symptoms and signs. *In* Wylie, E. J., and Ehrenfeld, W. K., eds.: Extracranial Occlusion Cerebrovascular Disease: Diagnosis and Management. Philadelphia, W. B. Saunders Co., 1970. Reprinted by permission.

atheroma at the carotid bifurcation. *Calcific* emboli may be observed in patients with aortic or mitral valvular disease. These bodies are gray, ovoid, stationary, and usually produce dense and sharply limited retinal infarction.[70]

Blood Flow

The mild reduction in retinal blood flow associated with severe stenosis or occlusion of the internal carotid artery seldom produces retinal changes. There are occasional reports of patients in whom the reduced perfusion pressure has protected the eye from severe systemic hypertension and subsequent retinopathy.

A profound decrease in retinal circulation may follow combined occlusions of the common, internal, and external carotid arteries or branches of the aortic arch. Acutely ischemic retinopathy is characterized by a pale fundus, threadlike arterioles, irregularly dilated veins, and a scattered filmy, gray-white exudate within the superficial layer of the retina. This is associated with very low ophthalmic artery pressure as measured with the ophthalmodynamometer. The vision of the ischemic eye is often impaired and fluctuating. A chronic form of ischemic retinopathy produces progressive retinal changes. There are irregular venous dilation, small blossom-shaped hemorrhages, and capillary microaneurysms. Subsequently, visible arteriovenous loops and neovascular formations may appear around the disc and in the midperiphery of the fundus. The appearances are not unlike diabetic retinopathy.[70]

Reduced ocular perfusion pressure often results in lowered intraocular pressure; paradoxically, however, very severe glaucoma may follow occlusion of the anterior chamber angle by rubiosis iridis.[146]

Vessel Changes of Hypertension and Arteriolosclerosis

Only the central retinal artery and its superior and inferior papillary branches are medium-sized arteries (defined as having an internal elastic lamina and a continuous muscular coat). All other arterial channels visible within the fundus are arterioles. Thus, diseases of the arterioles such as arteriolosclerosis may be visualized in the fundus, whereas diseases of the large and medium-sized arteries are not apparent.

Arteriolosclerosis imparts an increased light reflex, sheathing, arteriovenous nipping, tortuosity, or a copper- or silver-like appearance with the development of arteriolosclerosis; when the hypertension is acute and severe, however, the following changes may be noted: segmental and diffuse arteriolar narrowing, widening of the angulation of bifurcations, superficial hemorrhage, retinal infarcts, and papilledema.

Other retinal changes that may be of assistance in the assessment of ischemic cerebrovascular disease include the retinal changes of diabetes, uremia, sickle cell disease, bacterial endocarditis, and systemic lupus erythematosus.

Other Evidence of Arterial Disease

The presence of peripheral vascular disease, ischemic heart disease, heart failure, hypertension, and diabetes mellitus must be noted.

FOCAL CEREBRAL ISCHEMIA

In this section, the ischemic events occurring focally within the area of supply of a cerebral vessel—single territory infarcts or ischemia—are discussed. There may, of course, be cases in which two or more such areas are involved, e.g., anterior and middle cerebral artery occlusion. Ischemia of a more diffuse distribution, such as cardiac arrest and microvascular disease, is discussed later.

Focal ischemic events occurring in the territory of the carotid arteries are considered separately from those of the posterior or vertebrobasilar arteries because the mechanisms, natural history, and treatment differ significantly.[74]

Carotid Territory

Transient Ischemic Attacks

Transient ischemic attacks and cerebral infarction are closely interrelated by mechanism and arterial pathological changes. Since transient ischemia brings to notice degenerative arterial disease before it has been associated with disastrous consequence, the transient ischemic attack has been seen as a gateway to prophylactic treatment of stroke.

Transient ischemic attacks are uncommon before the fifth decade of life but thereafter occur with increasing frequency. The combined incidence of carotid and vertebrobasilar transient ischemic attacks in North American populations has been reported as between 0.3 and 1.3 per 1000 per year.[53,85] Men are at greater risk than women.

Mechanisms

The ultimate mechanism of transient ischemic attacks is a temporary discrepancy between the metabolic needs and the available blood supply of a focal region of the brain.

In the carotid territory the most important cause is fibrin-platelet emboli from the extracranial course of the carotid arteries (Fig. 42–2). Cardiac emboli are less frequently the cause of transient attacks because they are most typically composed of larger pieces of mature clot that cannot undergo dissolution rapidly enough to prevent cerebral infarction. Although vasospasm is important in the genesis of migraine and ischemia after subarachnoid hemorrhage, it is no longer considered of great importance in transient ischemic attacks.

Less frequently, hyperviscosity states, kinking of vessels, disease of the great vessels, focal major cerebral artery stenoses, and hemodynamic factors resulting from severe extracranial and intracranial atheromas may cause transient cerebral oligemia.[27] Unusual arterial pathological conditions are considered separately.

Clinical Features

Common symptoms of transient ischemic attacks of both the carotid and vertebrobasilar territories are listed in Table 42–5. Few symptoms, when taken in isolation, can precisely identify the vascular territory of their origin. Only monocular blindness and dysphasia identify the carotid, and drop attacks and diplopia identify the vertebrobasilar territories.

The visual loss may be partial or complete. When retinal ischemia is caused by a reduction in the perfusion pressure, vision is lost by a rapid constriction in the visual field, whereas embolic retinal ischemia causes sudden loss in sectors corresponding to the anatomy of the retinal circulation. The stepwise progression may be more apparent in the pattern of recovery. Retinal microemboli on other occasions appear as bright sparks of light shooting from the temporal side across the field of vision. Emboli into the supraorbital arteries may produce a

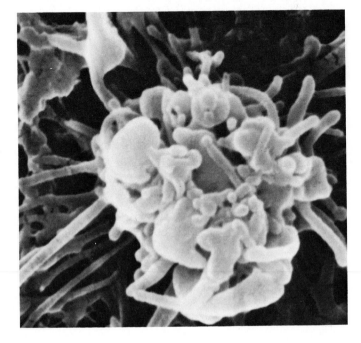

Figure 42–2 Electron microscope picture of aggregation of platelets in areas of traumatized endothelium, which leads to formation of fibrin-platelet thrombin that may become embolic. (Courtesy of B. A. Warren, Department of Pathology, University of Western Ontario, London, Ontario.)

TABLE 42–5 CUMULATIVE INCIDENCE OF SYMPTOMS OF TRANSIENT ISCHEMIC ATTACKS IN 180 PATIENTS*

	ARTERIAL TERRITORY	
SYMPTOM	Carotid	Vertebrobasilar
Dysphasia	20	—
Mono- or hemiparesis	38	12
Hemisensory disturbance	33	9
Confusion	5	1
Visual field disturbances	14	22
Vertigo	12	48
Drop attack	—	16
Diplopia	—	7
Tinnitus	—	1
Dysarthria	3	11
Facial paresthesia	4	22

* Adapted from Marshall, J.: The natural history of transient ischemic cerebrovascular attacks. Quart. J. Med., 33:309–324, 1964.

transient tingling sensation.[70,71] Chronic retinal insufficiency may cause palinopsia (prolonged after-images). Nearly all patients with amaurosis fugax have ipsilateral internal carotid stenosis or occlusion.[111]

Because the sylvian branches of the middle cerebral artery are favored sites of embolic impaction, the most frequent complaints of patients with carotid transient ischemic attacks are of transient motor and sensory deficits. The face and arm are more prominently involved, and remarkable focal deficits of the hand and muscles of articulation are not uncommon.

When a patient transiently displays confused behavior, careful review may reveal the cause to be a specific cortical dysfunction such as anosagnosia, a fluent dysphasia, spatial disorientation, or an unusual dyspraxia. Altered behavior may result when bilateral anterior cerebral artery ischemia follows brief occlusion of a dominant feeder.

Homonymous visual field defects are most commonly an evidence of vertebrobasilar insufficiency. The optic radiations are the only section of the retrochiasmal visual pathways to receive a blood supply from the terminal divisions of the internal carotid. They are nourished by perforating vessels from the parietal and temporal branches of the middle cerebral artery.[40] Quadrantic field defects are common, but may be combined to produce a hemianopsia that often involves one quadrant more intensely than the other.

When the complaint of vertigo occurs in isolation (with a time course suggesting a vascular origin), there should be reservation about accepting it as evidence of a brain stem dysfunction. Vertigo can arise from a hemispheric disturbance with some evidence suggesting a parietal localization.[107]

Approximately 10 per cent of patients will experience pain in the ipsilateral temporal region during and for some time after a carotid transient ischemic attack. The headache may, at times, be severe and have a throbbing quality, features that may cause difficulty in differentiating such an attack from migraine.

More than half the patients presenting with uncomplicated attacks arising in the carotid territory will have experienced only one or two episodes. Unfortunately, the frequency, duration, and symptomatic content of attacks has not been useful in defining a group at greater risk of subsequent stroke.[1] Many neurologists and neurosurgeons, however, have a conviction (not without some foundation) that a recent increase in the frequency of attacks, recurrence of attacks of prolonged duration, and the presence of a bruit of tight stenosis are clinical features of an increased risk of imminent stroke.[160]

Concurrent medical problems are frequently present, as shown in Table 42–6. These must be carefully noted because they have considerable bearing upon the management of the cerebral problem.[112,152]

Differential Diagnosis

The focal neurological symptoms of migraine technically fulfill the definition of transient ischemic attacks; however, there

TABLE 42–6 ASSOCIATED DISEASE IN 178 CONSECUTIVE STROKE PATIENTS*

DISEASE	PER CENT OF PATIENTS
Hypertension	76
Diabetes	31
Myocardial infarction (recent)	10
Ischemic heart disease	51
Hypercholesterolemia	45
Postural hypotension	16
Hyperuricemia	33
Peripheral vascular disease	5
Syphilis	5
Anemia	13
Polycythemia	2

* From Meyer, J. S.: Acute stroke: Biochemical and therapeutic studies. Minn. Med., 47:265–271, 1964. Reprinted by permission.

is seldom any difficulty in differentiating these entities clinically. In migraine, neurological symptoms arise in areas of the cortex other than the occipital lobes in less than 5 per cent of cases. When they do, transient motor, sensory, or dysphasic disturbances are the most common. The rare "Alice in Wonderland" temporal lobe syndromes that have excited considerable interest are typically of migrainous origin. Patients with a long history of vascular headaches occasionally experience their first migraine in association with neurological symptoms after anesthesia, mild head trauma, or menopausal hormonal imbalance. Then, too, the headache may be atypical. The suddennness of onset of transient ischemic attacks is of assistance in separating them from such migrainous phenomena.

Occasionally massive cerebral hemorrhage follows attacks that have appeared to represent transient ischemia, suggesting that small cerebral hemorrhages may infrequently simulate transient ischemic attacks. Hypoglycemia should be considered when focal symptoms are associated with attacks of altered behavior.

Focal epilepsy should be readily distinguished by its tonic or clonic phases and by a characteristic progression. Confusion may arise when the postictal Todd's paresis is prominent and the patient is a poor historian.

The diagnosis of hypertensive encephalopathy should not be made unless there are retinal changes. Occasionally confusion arises because the blood pressure may be transiently elevated during both carotid and vertebrobasilar ischemic attacks.[75]

Investigations

Investigation may be required to confirm the diagnosis, to assess coincidental disease, and to make specific assessments to initiate treatment.

The cost of hospitalization and the relative urgency often make it impossible to assess the results of investigations sequentially, and at least the first two steps will have to proceed concurrently.

As the diagnosis is essentially a clinical one, little or no confirmation may be required; however, it is prudent to exclude a structural cerebral lesion (most particularly a cerebral hemorrhage or infarct) and spe-

cific diagnostic considerations such as hyperviscosity of the blood, cranial arteritis, hypoglycemia, paroxysmal cardiac arrhythmias, valvular heart disease, cardiac myxoma, and neurovascular syphilis. The conditions commonly associated with ischemic cerebrovascular disease have been noted earlier.

Necessary investigations include:

COMPLETE BLOOD COUNT. Polycythemia, thrombocytosis, and the marked leukocytosis that may cause thromboembolic phenomena will be apparent. Anemia may, at times, accentuate the symptoms of cerebral ischemia.

ERYTHROCYTE SEDIMENTATION RATE. Cranial arteritis, hyperviscosity states, hyperglobulinemia, and cardiac myxoma are frequently accompanied by a marked increase in sedimentation rate.

BIOCHEMICAL SCREENS. These include fasting serum glucose, fasting serum lipid, and serum uric acid, creatinine, and urea determinations. A fasting blood sample is required to assess lipid values and screen for diabetes and hypoglycemia. It is convenient to collect all of the required blood from a single venipuncture. Serum uric acid concentrations are elevated in renal failure, hypertension, certain hyperlipidemic states, and by the administration of many diuretics.

ELECTROCARDIOGRAM AND ELECTROCARDIOGRAPHIC MONITORING. The routine electrocardiogram may reveal an arrhythmia or features that increase the probability of paroxysmal arrhythmia; however, it is not uncommon for monitoring during routine activity to show paroxysms of arrhythmia in those in whom the routine tracing was completely normal. The electrocardiogram may also demonstrate features of ischemic and hypertensive heart disease or a conduction disturbance.

SEROLOGICAL TESTS FOR SYPHILIS. Although this test is seldom positive, it is necessary as a public health measure.

BRAIN SCAN. In the dynamic phase of the brain scan, cerebral perfusion may be delayed and reduced on the side of a hemodynamically significant carotid stenosis. The static views should be normal. Brain scans are not a routine study for patients with cardiovascular disease and should be ordered with discretion.

ECHOCARDIOGRAM. This study is the definitive noninvasive method for the detection of atrial myxoma, prolapsing mitral valve, and other cardiac conditions that may result in cerebral embolization.

COMPUTED TOMOGRAPHY. This study is indicated to rule out hemorrhage or other forms of brain disease (see discussion in Management of Cerebral Infarction).

CHEST AND SKULL X-RAYS. The chest x-ray is particularly valuable and should be a routine investigation, as it may reveal unsuspected pulmonary congestion or tumor, or abnormal cardiac configuration. Skull x-ray is of possible value in some cases, but with the advent of the computed tomographic scan, has become decreasingly important.

THYROID FUNCTION TESTS. Hypothyroidism is a sufficiently frequent association to indicate the need for an enlightened clinical awareness.

LUMBAR PUNCTURE. With the advent of computed tomography, this time-honored test is no longer routine for patients with cerebral ischemia but still provides critical information in selected instances (Table 42–7).

NONINVASIVE SCREENING TESTS FOR CAROTID DISEASE. The need for such investigations has called forth ingenuity that has often been in excess of practicality. Instrumentation detects either hemodynamic consequences *distal* to severe internal carotid stenosis or *local* disturbances of flow in the involved segment of the carotid arteries.

Examples of the first type are ophthalmodynamometry, oculoplethysmography, supraorbital thermography, and orbital Doppler ultrasound studies.[15,44,70,158] Doppler evaluation of the direction of flow in the supraorbital and supratrochlear arteries (normally supplied by the internal carotid through the ophthalmic artery) very reliably demonstrates hemodynamically significant internal carotid stenosis but remains of limited clinical value because carotid disease does not have to have progressed to tight stenosis before causing cerebral embolization. Even if these tests were of absolute reliability, they would detect only one third of those patients who have operatively correctable lesions.[15]

Carotid Doppler examination. Scanning of the carotid arteries in the neck with a focused Doppler probe attached to a position-detecting device, develops a map of the carotid flow channels. This map allows a systematic examination of the flow characteristics along the course of these vessels. The focal increase in velocity of flow through stenotic regions causes high-pitched and more continuous Doppler signals, whereas distally, turbulence is noted as a characteristic fluttering signal. In experienced hands, the Doppler examination can detect a stenosis of greater than 50 per cent with reasonable reliability.

ARTERIOGRAPHY. Arteriography is indicated if it is believed very probable that a patient has had carotid territory transient ischemic attacks and if operative treatment will follow the demonstration of an operable lesion. Visualization of all four cervical vessels and their intracranial branches should be obtained. A large proportion of patients will show arteriographic evidence of the focal lesions of the extra- and intracranial vessels.[62]

Treatment

The treatment of extracranial cerebrovascular disease is discussed in Chapter 43.

Prognosis

It is estimated that about one third of those who suffer a transient neurological deficit will continue to have attacks without

TABLE 42–7 ABNORMALITIES IN CEREBROSPINAL FLUID EXAMINATION IN HEMORRHAGIC AND NONHEMORRHAGIC CEREBRAL INFARCTION AND CEREBRAL HEMORRHAGE*

	ISCHEMIC INFARCTION (PER CENT)	HEMORRHAGIC INFARCTION (PER CENT)	CEREBRAL HEMORRHAGE (PER CENT)
Pressure increase	10	15	80
Xanthochromia or blood	0	7	80
Cell count	33	66	(Erythrocyte > 500) 87
Protein increase	Mild 33	Mild 66	Moderate ?90

* From Russell, R. W., ed.: Cerebral Arterial Disease. Edinburgh, Churchill Livingstone, 1976. Reprinted by permission.

developing permanent disability; another third will eventually have cerebral infarction, and in the remaining third the attacks will cease spontaneously.[1,22] There is a close relationship between the site of transient neurological episodes and and the site of subsequent stroke. Following a transient ischemic attack the risk of stroke is maximal in the first two months and disappears within three years.[171] Unfortunately, there is no way to predict the outcome for an individual patient.[1]

The life expectancy of persons under 65 is significantly worsened by the occurrence of a transient ischemic attack but is not demonstrably altered for persons 65 and over.

Cerebral Infarcts of the Carotid Territory

Eighty-five to ninety per cent of brain infarcts occur within the carotid territory.[127]

Although almost all mankind has observed the effects of stroke, knowledge of the etiology is recent and still incomplete. The emphasis of this section is on the mechanisms—to the relative neglect of the many clinical syndromes that have been reported to follow occlusion of particular vessels.

It was noted earlier that the incidence of ischemic stroke increases with age and shows minor sex differences, and that the most important risk factors are previous transient ischemic attack, hypertension, heart disease, and for those under 55 years, diabetes mellitus.

Mechanisms

In discussions of the mechanisms of carotid territory infarcts, a clear distinction must be made between small deeply placed lacunar infarcts within the area supplied by long perforating branches of the middle cerebral artery and infarcts that follow occlusion of the trunk and branches of the middle and anterior cerebral arteries. If a generalization is allowed, the former are the result of local hypertension-related occlusive arterial disease, whereas the latter represent a complication of diseases outside of the skull.

Lacunar infarcts are considered separately in the section on vertebrobasilar insufficiency.

From review of various sources including clinical and postmortem material, it may be concluded that the frequency of mechanisms involved in the development of cerebral infarction within the carotid territory may be as outlined in Table 42–8.

It is likely that stroke patients reaching neurosurgical attention will have been highly selected for carotid artery disease, younger age, and milder neurological deficits or complications requiring operative intervention.

TABLE 42–8 FREQUENCY OF MECHANISMS OF CEREBRAL INFARCTION IN CAROTID TERRITORY*

	CONTRIBUTION OF SUBTYPE TO CLASS (PER CENT)	CONTRIBUTION OF CLASS TO TOTAL (PER CENT)
Precardiac source of embolus		4
Mainly paradoxical embolism		
Cardiac emboli		50
Ischemic heart disease	50	
Valvular heart disease	25	
Cardiomyopathy	15	
Dysrhythmia	5	
Infectious endocarditis	5	
Carotid artery disease		25
Embolism	50	
Anterograde extension of thrombus into cerebral arteries	50	
Hemodynamic effect	Unknown	
Lacunar infarction		15
Atheroma of major branches of carotid		2
Venous infarctions		1
Trauma	Unknown	
Arteritis	Unknown	
Fibromuscular hyperplasia	Unknown	

* Incidence was estimated from numerous clinical and autopsy studies. An attempt was made to correct bias due to referral and interest of authors. Analyses of published data are approximations.

PARADOXICAL EMBOLISM. The mechanisms of paradoxical embolism have been discussed previously. Paradoxical embolism accounts for approximately 4 per cent of cerebral emboli.[104]

CARDIAC EMBOLISM. In all published neuropathological studies the heart has been reported to be the major source of cerebral emboli.[104] Nearly half of carotid infarcts are the result of cerebral emboli.[13] Although the cardiac condition complicated by the greatest frequency of cerebral embolization is subacute bacterial endocarditis, this is a relatively uncommon disorder, and myocardial infarction (both recent and old), valvular heart disease, and congestive cardiomyopathies account for 90 per cent of all cerebral emboli originating in the heart (see Table 42–3).[104] Cardiac myxoma is an uncommon benign curable tumor of the heart most frequently situated in its left atrium.[71] The condition may occur at all ages but is most frequent in the age group of 30 to 60 years. Seventy-five per cent of patients are women. The tumor frequently obstructs the mitral valve, resulting in severe dyspnea from pulmonary venous congestion and edema. More serious valvular obstruction results in syncope in 25 per cent of cases. Cerebral and multiple organ embolization occurs in 50 per cent, and systemic symptoms such as fever, weight loss, and fatigue occur in 90 per cent. Examination frequently reveals murmurs simulating mitral stenosis. Fortunately, echocardiography is a dependable screening test for suspected cases.[177]

EXTRACRANIAL CAROTID ARTERY DISEASE. Perhaps a quarter of cerebral infarcts in the territories of the anterior and middle cerebral arteries result from carotid artery disease, and 40 per cent of these patients will have had preceding transient neurological dysfunction.[104]

Atheroma is the most common arterial disorder, but in young persons trauma accounts for 25 per cent of internal carotid artery occlusions and may result in delayed cerebral infarction.[71] In children, arteritis of the internal carotid may occur in the tonsillar fossa during the course of ear and throat infection.[12]

Fibromuscular hyperplasia of the carotid arteries is noted in 1 per cent of routine carotid arteriograms. This condition is discussed in the section on unusual arterial disorders.

Other uncommon arterial lesions include kinking of the internal carotid in the neck, the Tolosa-Hunt syndrome, and herpes zoster arteritis.[27,47,59]

Atheroma of the carotid arteries most frequently involves the common carotid bifurcation and both the proximal 2 cm and the terminal portions of the internal carotid. Atheroma is seldom completely unilateral. Tight stenosis near the bifurcation on one side is accompanied by at least minor involvement of the opposite side in 9 out of 10 cases. The progression of early lesions cannot be predicted, but when stenosis has reduced the lumen by 50 per cent progression of the stenosis can be expected.

The development of platelet aggregates and thrombus at the site of atheroma is a complex event. Aggregation is enhanced by turbulence, endothelial ulceration, and foci of reduced flow.[149] The platelet aggregate is white, friable, has little interposed fibrin, and is conjectured to be "the embolus of TIA." The activation of thrombosis produces a stable erythrocyte-containing mass that may remain attached as mural thrombus, extend to occlude the lumen completely, or break free and cause embolic cerebral infarction.

Complete internal carotid occlusion may cause cerebral infarction by anterograde extension of thrombus into the cerebral vessels, by embolization from the tail of extending thrombus, or by critically reducing the perfusion of the ipsilateral hemisphere.

It appears that carotid occlusion is often asymptomatic.[31,162] The hemodynamic consequences of internal carotid occlusion can usually be adequately compensated for by collaterals, and cerebral infarction results only when the occlusion is complicated by anterograde extension of or embolization from the tail of the thrombus.[162]

When the proximal internal carotid is occluded, thrombosis commonly extends to the level of the ophthalmic artery, but when collateral flow through the circle of Willis is limited, may extend into the middle or anterior cerebral arteries or both.[23] Of considerable surgical interest is the observation that in as many as 30 per cent there is little thrombosis distal to the occlusion for up to six weeks.[162]

Occlusive disease of the anterior and middle cerebral arteries is uncommon.[104] Small cerebral arteries and arterioles of hypertensive patients, however, frequently show hyaline and fibrinoid hyperplastic changes that are associated with small infarcts deep in the hemispheres. Small infarcts of the cerebral cortex are frequently embolic. With careful examination of the leptomeningeal vessels, Winter and Gyari were able to observe vessel occlusion in 19 of 21 such infarcts, and in six, occlusion was recognized as embolic.[174]

Venous infarction of the brain is discussed in a following section of this chapter.

Pathology

The area of infarction is sharply delineated from the surrounding normal brain and can be identified by its grayish white appearance and soft mushy consistency. Considerable edema accumulates in the infarct and makes an infarct one of the most rapidly expanding cerebral lesions. Swelling is maximal on the third to fourth day and in larger lesions will have a mass effect.

Microscopically, from the second to the fifth day the neurons appear shrunken and stained uniformly pink, glial nuclei are hyperchromatic and blood vessels necrotic, intracellular spaces are accentuated by edema fluid, and polymorphonuclear cells are seen invading the periphery. At this stage, polymorphs may also appear in the cerebrospinal fluid. Subsequently, as necrotic material is engulfed, macrophages become stuffed with foamy material. Gradually the volume of the infarct is resorbed, and cavitation may occur.[104]

Hemorrhagic infarction results when there is early re-establishment of the circulation and is most typical in embolic and venous infarcts and infarction of the occipital poles when the posterior cerebral arteries are intermittently compressed against the edge of the tentorial hiatus. Unlike cerebral hemorrhage, which dissects between nerve fibers and along tracts, hemorrhagic infarction involves all the tissue in the area. When healed, the walls of the hemorrhage are in close opposition; in contrast, those of a hemorrhagic infarct tend to be widely separated. Embolic infarcts frequently are multiple.

Clinical Features

The onset is unheralded and sudden, with the full neurological deficit often apparent within minutes to hours. In occasional cases of major cerebral embolism in younger persons whose cerebral vasculature is undiseased, the onset will appear instantaneous and may be associated with loss of consciousness, probably because of diffuse constriction of the affected vascular tree, that rapidly clears to leave a more limited focal deficit. Typically, cerebral infarction is painless; however, mild to severe headache is reported by up to 25 per cent.[56] Severe constant pain over the carotid artery radiating to the mastoid region has been labeled carotodynia.[34] Carotodynia is an uncommon complaint in stroke, but its presence strongly suggests disease of the extracranial internal carotid.

The neurological deficit is determined by the site of arterial occlusion and the capacity of collaterals to restrict the ischemia.

When the middle cerebral artery is occluded proximal to the lenticulostriate branches, extensive deep hemispheric infarction will include the anterior and posterior limbs of the internal capsule, and a cortical infarct will be centered upon the opercular region. The deficit will therefore include a dense hemiplegia, hemisensory disturbance (of subcortical type), hemianopia, and a cortical deficit appropriate to the hemisphere. The cortical deficits cannot be meaningfully tested but will include a global dysphasia with the possibility of right-left confusion and graphic language disturbances if in the dominant hemisphere; and troublesome dyspraxias, lack of initiative, and a failure to perceive the neurological deficit meaningfully can be expected with nondominant hemisphere involvement.[115]

Involvement of the middle cerebral artery distal to the lenticulostriate vessels results in an infarct of variable extent centered upon the opercular cortex. A faciobrachial motor and sensory disturbance will be the background for inferoparietal and temporal cortical deficits of varying severity. Because the trifurcation of the middle cerebral artery is a frequent point of embolic arrest, recurrent major cerebral embolism, particularly in those patients free of cerebral atherosclerosis, may result in bilateral lesions of the opercular region. In the striking *biopercular syndrome,* paralysis of volitional movements of the tongue, jaw, pharynx, and facial musculature may suddenly be broken by a surprisingly full, emotionally induced movement (e.g., smile or tongue protrusion). As both the upper and lower facial movements are impaired, the lesion could be mistaken for involvement of the lower motor neuron. The jaw, facial, and gag reflexes are characteristically brisk. Emotional continence and limb movements are often spared.[20]

The clinical and angiographic features of branch occlusions of the middle cerebral artery have been studied.[2] Many clinicians believe, however, that the size and shape of cerebral infarcts is not sufficiently consistent for syndrome identification to be useful.

Occlusion of the anterior cerebral artery results in motor and sensory disturbances maximal in the contralateral lower limb. Unilateral lesions rarely cause obvious frontal release signs or behavioral changes. Involvement of Heubner's artery has been said to result in faciobrachial weakness.

Combined occlusions of the anterior and middle cerebral arteries produce a very extensive infarct and have a very poor prognosis.[23]

Jones and Millikan followed the clinical course of 179 patients with carotid territory infarcts, who had been hospitalized less than 48 hours after the ictus.[79] They noted that in 39 per cent of this group, the clinical deficit remained essentially unchanged over the first week. In a further 35 per cent progressive improvement occurred. Nineteen per cent of their patients showed progressive deterioration. In 21 of this latter group of 34 patients, the focal deficit became more severe (often complete), while in the other 13 it was the conscious state that deteriorated. The deterioration began either almost concurrently with the onset or within the first 24 hours. In 4 per cent a late, unexpected, and serious deterioration occurred between the third and seventh day (last day of the study).

Consciousness is impaired in 25 per cent of patients hospitalized with acute carotid system cerebral infarction. Bilateral cerebral infarcts or unrecognized epilepsy may account for the impairment of consciousness observed in some patients but, the authors suspect, not all. Symon's observation that there is a graduation of tissue ischemia that extends into contiguous and unoccluded vascular beds (because they are providing collateral circulation) gives reason to suspect that there may be bilateral diencephalic ischemia with acute embolic occlusion of the proximal middle cerebral artery.[153] This possibility would be enhanced if disease of the contralateral internal carotid or vertebrobasilar systems were to restrict these sources of collateral supply significantly.

Complications

An early study by Shaw and co-workers dealt with the mechanism and time course of fatal complications in patients with large cerebral infarcts resulting from middle cerebral artery occlusion.[145] Fifteen patients met their exacting criteria. Two groups appeared.

In the first group, death occurred between 18 and 108 hours after the ictus. In these patients there was clear evidence of massive hemispheric edema causing compartmental shift. All had been extremely drowsy soon after the onset, and the neurological deficit complete. Such a clinical course was noted by Jones and Millikan in 13 of 179 and terminated fatally in 6 of the 13.[79]

In the second group, death occurred between two weeks and three months after the onset. Evidence of cerebral edema or its complications was no longer present. The cause of death did not directly relate to the pathological state of the brain but to complications initiated by debility such as bronchopneumonia, renal infection, or septicemia. The clinical course suggested that some patients in this group had survived considerable brain swelling. These observations have been confirmed.[118]

Plum and Posner noted that in all of 11 cases of massive hemispheric brain infarction, transtentorial herniation was of the central type. They did not observe uncal herniation with ischemic swellings. These authors have clearly described the clinical features of progressive rostrocaudal brain stem dysfunction from tentorial herniation.[132]

Compartmental shifts are not the only concern that is created by ischemic cerebral edema. Tissue perfusion is compromised by the increased tissue pressure and may therefore cause extension of the zone of critical ischemia and a progressive focal deficit.[108] Because the tissue compliance of white matter is greater than that of gray matter, edema may cause massive white matter swelling, which may be a factor in the development of the rare syndrome of ischemic leukoencephalopathy.[103]

Epilepsy may occur during either the acute (first two weeks) or late course of cerebral infarction. The ictus or early postictal phase is complicated by epilepsy in 3 per cent of patients. Seizures are purely focal in half and generalized in the remainder. Although typically frequent and difficult to control, they abate spontaneously and almost never herald the onset of a chronic seizure disorder.[101]

When epilepsy complicates the late course, the peak of onset occurs between the sixth and twelfth months, but the cumulative incidence continues to rise for at least five years. Seizures are focal in two thirds and generalized in one third. Moskowitz and co-workers reported the frequency as 5 per cent in a period up to two years and 9.5 per cent at five years.[116]

Hemorrhage into an acute infarct is a complication more often feared than seen. With close observation of patients in stroke intensive care units, minor symptomatic changes have been observed during the conversion of a bland to a hemorrhagic infarct.[120] This conversion occurs when the infarct is exposed to normal arterial perfusion pressures. The blood-brain barrier is breeched, vasogenic edema formation is enhanced, and erythrocyte diapedesis occurs. All factors contribute an increase in volume. Despite the drama of these changes, frank hemorrhage is uncommon, but remains a threat. That risk would be enhanced by increases in the perfusion pressure from uncontrolled or induced hypertension or the use of anticoagulants, inhibitors of platelet function, or fibrinolytic therapy. The risks of fibrinolytic therapy have been found intolerable, but the risks of platelet inhibition and anticoagulant therapy have not been adequately investigated to assess their indications in the immediate treatment of cerebral infarction with a risk of recurrent embolism, e.g., cerebral embolism from mitral valve disease.[37]

Electrocardiographic monitoring has demonstrated arrhythmia in half of patients hospitalized for acute stroke.[120] In some, the arrhythmia is the cause of the ischemic event; in others, the arrhythmia is a coincidental expression of arterial disease. Changes in the electrocardiographic complexes or arrhythmia, however, may result from the cerebrovascular lesion. Prolongation of the Q-T interval and an inverted and large T wave may be accompanied by ST segment changes that simulate myocardial ischemia. The induced arrhythmias have been reviewed by Cooper and West.[25] The importance of these arrhythmias is largely undetermined.

Inhalational and bronchopneumonia, decubitus ulceration, and catheter-induced urinary tract infections threaten the debilitated victims of stroke—particularly those of advanced years. As noted, these complications are the major cause of death between the second and twelfth weeks of the course.

Management

The management of brain infarcts within the carotid and vertebrobasilar territories is discussed in the following section, Management of Cerebral Infarction.

Lacunar Infarcts

Although about 10 per cent of brains examined at necropsy will have one or more lacunae, many of these areas of infarction appear to be silent, i.e., there is no record of the patient having sought medical attention for sudden neurological deficit.[104]

Sites of lacunae in order of frequency are: putamen, pons, thalamus, caudate nucleus, internal capsule, corona radiata, white matter of the hemisphere, cerebellum, and corpus callosum. They do not occur in the spinal cord, medulla, mesencephalon, or cortex of either the cerebellum or cerebrum.

Lacunae are most frequent in patients who have had long-sustained arterial hypertension.[43] There may be an ictus consisting of a mild neurological deficit such as hemiparesis, sensory symptoms, ataxia of limbs, and dysarthria. Cortical symptoms such as aphasia are uncommon. The recovery from individual episodes is good, but multiple attacks may lead to the syndrome of pseudobulbar palsy with dysphagia, dysarthria, incontinence, and dementia.

Atherosclerotic Dementia

There is little basis for the widespread belief that atherosclerosis of the aortocranial vessels can cause brain atrophy and neuronal fallout without first producing infarction. There is no clear evidence of a greater incidence of cerebrovascular disease in demented persons than in an age-matched population.

If one adopts the limited concept of dementia as being impairment or loss of any single aspect of intellectual function, it follows that cerebral infarction, particularly if multiple or extensive, can result in "dementia." If one adopts the more usual definition of dementia, cerebrovascular disease is an infrequent cause of dementia.[84]

Except for large bilateral infarcts, the lacunar state is the only atherosclerotic vascular disease that may lead to dementia.[57]

Vertebrobasilar Territory

The pathology, mechanisms, management, and prognosis of ischemic events within the posterior circulation differ markedly from those in the carotid territory. Because of the dangers of vertebral arteriography, the limited possibilities for operative intervention, and the difficulties with postmortem examination of the vertebral arteries, there is less precise information upon which to build an understanding of these events.

Vertebrobasilar Transient Ischemia

The relative frequencies of transient cerebral ischemia of the carotid and vertebrobasilar territories is noted in Table 42–9.

TABLE 42–9 VASCULAR TERRITORY OF TRANSIENT ISCHEMIC ATTACKS

	TERRITORY (PERCENTAGE)		
STUDY	Carotid	Vertebral-Basilar	Mixed
Baker et al.*	53	44	—
Hutchinson and Acheson†	28	71	—
Ziegler and Hassanein‡	17	40	42
Cartlidge, Whisnant, and Elveback§	60	30	10

* Prognosis in patients with transient ischemic attacks. Neurology (Minneap.), *18*:1157–1165, 1968.
† Strokes: Natural History, Pathology and Surgical Treatment. London, W. B. Saunders Co., Ltd., 1975.
‡ Prognosis in patients with transient ischemic attacks. Stroke, *4*:666–673, 1973.
§ Carotid and vertebral-basilar transient cerebral ischemic attacks: a community study, Rochester, Minnesota. Mayo Clin. Proc., *52*:117–120, 1977.

The remarkable differences noted appear to reflect referral bias and differing diagnostic criteria. When a referral bias was excluded by prospective study of a population, it was found that one third of transient ischemic attacks arose within the posterior circulation.[22]

Mechanisms

The relative importance of platelet aggregation–embolization and hemodynamic mechanisms is impossible to define.

Unique features of the vertebrobasilar arterial system have led to the conviction that hemodynamic mechanisms frequently may be involved. Focal high-grade stenoses frequently involve the origins of the subclavian and vertebral arteries, and the intracranial portions of the vertebral and basilar arteries.[142] The severity of stenosis may relate to the size of the vessels. Congenital hypoplasia of a vertebral or posterior communicating artery occurs in more than 70 per cent of the population.[100] When the head is rotated 60 degrees to the side, flow begins to decrease in the contralateral vertebral artery and ceases altogether at about 80 degrees.[159] The circulation time of the vertebrobasilar system is normally considerably slower than that of the carotid system.[100]

When the mechanism of ischemia within the vertebrobasilar system is clearly hemodynamic, as for example, in the subclavian steal syndrome, the symptoms usually lack the focal (or multifocal) nature of more common attacks. There is, also, a reduction in the frequency of attacks when symptomatic patients are treated with drugs that inhibit platelet aggregation.

These mechanisms should not be considered mutually exclusive: it is likely that many attacks of vertebrobasilar ischemia result from the embolization of platelet aggregates formed at sites of hemodynamically significant arterial disease.

Atheroma is by far the most frequently noted arterial disorder, but occasionally fibromuscular hyperplasia, cranial arteritis, traumatic dissection, and fusiform ectasia may be responsible.[148]

Clinical Features

Vertebrobasilar transient ischemic attacks affect men and women with equal frequency. Their duration and frequency, and the associated medical conditions, are the same as those associated with carotid insufficiency. The relative frequency of symptoms is seen in Table 42–4.

The symptoms seldom appear in isolation, but occur in combinations as numerous "as the association of dysfunctions of the brain stem can be. It is the concurrence of different symptoms which is so important in diagnosis, not the exact pattern."[172]

Two patterns are of particular help in diagnosis. The first is the association of symptoms of brain stem dysfunction with visual disturbances, and the second is the occurrence over a period of time of transient or fluctuating symptoms from different regions of the brain stem.[172] The symptomatic content of vertebrobasilar transient ischemic attacks is much more likely to vary from one episode to the next than is that of attacks related to anterior circulation.

Visual changes of some kind occur in two thirds of attacks, but are frequently trivial and may therefore be dismissed by the patient. The most common phenomena are floating black dots that may have a scintillating margin. Visual field defects may be hemianopic, altitudinal, or quadrantic, or may affect any sector that corresponds to the vascular topography of the calcarine cortex. Only the field defects that involve *both* the right and left visual fields can be considered diagnostic in their own right. Visual hallucinations of unformed structure are not uncommon, and occasionally static emotive scenes occur, with the patient maintaining insight into their nature. The latter are considered to arise from ischemia of the anterior temporal lobe.

Vertigo is experienced during nearly 50 per cent of vertebrobasilar ischemic attacks. The examiner should search the history for associated phenomena that are so often overlooked by a patient experiencing severe vertigo. A clear history of associated spots before the eyes "identifies the episode as vascular." As the internal auditory artery is supplied from the basilar system, vertigo may have either a central or peripheral origin. Isolated vertigo is not absolute proof of a brain stem dysfunction.[172]

Drop attacks are particularly frequent in elderly women. While walking or standing, particularly when under some stress, the patient crumples forward without warning, on flexed knees, tending to bruise the knee, chin, and hands. Loss of consciousness is at most momentary. Recurrent drop attacks are believed by most neurologists to be an evidence of vertebrobasilar insufficiency; however, when these attacks occur in isolation, they very seldom carry the same risks for subsequent stroke.[150]

Headache is usually suboccipital, may be severe and throbbing, and may outlast the neurological deficit. When associated with visual scotomas, the headache is difficult to distinguish from migraine.

Hemiplegia and hemisensory disturbances occur in approximately 10 per cent of attacks but, when they do occur, seem to be associated with an enhanced risk of subsequent cerebral infarction. A common, characteristic, and neglected symptom is circumoral anesthesia or tingling. In the absence of acroparesthesia (which would suggest hyperventilation), this symptom is a specific indicator of vertebrobasilar insufficiency.

Examination of the patient should reveal no persisting neurological signs. Bruits over the vertebral arteries are infrequent and indicate increased flow rather than focal stenosis. Patients with vertebral-basilar insufficiency must be specifically examined for features of a subclavian steal mechanism and postural hypotension.

Transient Global Amnesia

There is increasing evidence that this well-defined clinical syndrome is caused by transient ischemia within the distribution of the terminal basilar artery.

Transient global amnesia is the most common cause of attacks of amnesia in persons over 50.[63] A history of previous hysterical illness or epilepsy is notably absent. Because episodes are transient, associated with hypertension and occasionally with visual disturbances, they are thought to be due to vascular insufficiency of the mediobasal temporal lobe structures.[109]

Memory is lost suddenly and without warning, often after a burst of healthy but unaccustomed exercise.[172] During the attack perceptual and personal identity are preserved while amnesia for events of recent days is combined with an inability to lay down new memories. Patients frequently appear agitated about the circumstances they find themselves in. Answers to questions probing their personal whereabouts and that of their family appear to be accepted, but the questions are repeated within minutes as if the answers had been unregistered. As the attack progresses, the retrograde amnesia shrinks until, in the end, it remains only for the attack, and subsequently islands of retention will appear for the events of the attack itself. The duration of an attack is usually between one half and five hours.[39] One third of patients will have recurrent episodes, and clear evidences of a vascular causation are apparent in a third.

The prognosis for full recovery is excellent, and surprisingly few patients have subsequently developed cerebral infarction.

Transient global amnesia is a distinctive disorder. When the clinical features can be fully reviewed there should be no diagnostic uncertainty.[35] Automatism, depersonalization, and abnormal behavior are usually apparent during temporal lobe attacks for which a patient is amnesic. The previous history, brevity, and recurrent nature of epileptic attacks also assist in this distinction. Hysterical fugue states, temporal lobe encephalitis, and a temporal lobe syndrome of migraine are seldom difficult to differentiate.

Differential Diagnosis

Brief attacks of clearly focal dysfunction of regions of the brain stem, cerebellum, and occipital lobes are diagnostic.[172] Unfortunately, some attacks with a clearly hemodynamic mechanism result in nonfocal symptoms. An example is the occurrence of lightheadedness and giddiness (resembling presyncopal sensations) in the subclavian steal syndrome, and another is the recently recognized persistent mental slowness and intermittent giddiness and presyncopal sensations that may be precipitated by changes in position of patients with very advanced extracranial vascular disease.[129] These patients are few, but they do require some liberalization of the definition of transient ischemic attacks.

The history must be searched for precipitants of individual episodes such as rotation and extension of the neck.[159]

Advanced extracranial vascular disease has been noted to result in slowness of all intellectual activity more than in objective intellectual impairment. In these patients, changes in neck and body position may precipitate faintness and instability. All symptoms may resolve with successful cerebral revascularization.[129]

The Steal Syndromes

Because atheromatous plaques have a predilection for the great vessels at their points of origin from the aortic arch, stenosis or occlusion of one of them may occur while the distal arterial tree is still relatively normal. Reduced pressure in the distal segment of the artery results in a variety of shunts or "steals." The most common is the subclavian steal, which may occur when stenosis or occlusion of the subclavian artery (most often the left subclavian) proximal to the origin of the vertebral artery reduces blood pressure in that vessel. The resultant inversion of the pressure gradient between the proximal and distal segments of the vertebral artery causes blood to flow from the cranial portion of the artery, down through the neck, via the subclavian artery, into the arm. Under these circumstances, blood is stolen from the normal vertebral artery and diverted from the cranial to the brachial circulation. Other extra- and intracranial steal syndromes are most infrequent and have been reviewed elsewhere.[64]

Arterial Pathology

Atherosclerosis is the most common cause, but Takayasu's disease, dissecting aneurysm, and congenital anomalies have all been cited.[64] Angiography in patients with cerebrovascular insufficiency has demonstrated asymptomatic subclavian steals in up to 3 per cent of examinations.[33]

Clinical Features

The maximal incidence occurs in the sixth and seventh decades, and men outnumber women in a ratio of 2.5:1. Symptoms may arise from either the posterior circulation or the ischemic upper limb. The neurological symptoms of giddiness, vertigo, headaches, impaired consciousness, and visual disturbances are usually very brief (seconds only) and often lack the clearly focal character of vertebrobasilar insufficiency of other causations. In only 10 per cent of patients are the attacks precipitated by use of the ischemic limb or by neck rotation.[64] Half of symptomatic cases are marked by tingling, coldness, or heaviness in the ischemic arm.

It is the examination that suggests the diagnosis by demonstrating a differential in the brachial blood pressure greater than 20 mm of mercury, a murmur in the region of the subclavian-vertebral junction, and a delayed pulse on the involved side.[126] The diagnosis can be made with certainty only by aortocranial angiography, however, and this is justified only when symptoms are sufficiently disabling and operation is contemplated.[33]

Vertebrobasilar Infarcts

Mechanism

Thrombotic occlusion of a related vessel is found in more than 75 per cent of patients with infarcts in the territory of the vertebrobasilar system and in the majority has occurred at a tight atherosclerotic stenosis of an intracranial segment of the vertebral or basilar arteries.[23] Here the common causes of cerebral infarction found in the carotid territory, namely cardiac emboli and extracranial vascular disease, are relatively infrequent.

Occlusion of the distal and intracranial portion of the vertebral artery is three times as frequent as occlusion of the proximal and intermediate segments.[142] Vertebral artery occlusion is often well tolerated; however, occlusion of the intracranial course may result in local or distal infarcts. The local infarct involves the lateral medulla or inferior cerebellum or both, particularly if the origin of the posterior inferior cerebellar artery is involved.[36] The distal infarcts are caused by either embolization or anterograde propagation of thrombus and are as common as the local infarcts.[24]

Occlusion of the basilar artery is always associated with local infarction and frequently causes embolization of the posterior cerebral arteries. The anterograde extension of thrombosis into the full length of the basilar and into the posterior cerebral arteries is facilitated by disease or hypoplasia of the posterior communicating arteries.

When induced by occlusion at the origin of the vertebral arteries, anterograde thrombosis does not extend further than the midpoint of the extracranial course of this vessel, and the cervical branches to the vertebral usually maintain adequate distal perfusion.[24] The lesion may, however, occasionally initiate embolization.

Vertebrobasilar stroke may follow trauma to the vertebral artery during chiropractic manipulations, congenital atlantoaxial dislocation, and fracture-dislocations of the cervical spine.[112] Temporal arteritis and fibromuscular hyperplasia are occasional causes of vertebral or basilar arterial disease.[148]

Pathology

Discrete, single territory infarcts of the lateral medullary region, paramedian pontine tegmentum, cerebellum, and midline are not infrequent. Their clinical and pathological features have been elaborated.[100,127] More frequently, multiple infarcts are present, often combining a lesion at the site of arterial occlusion with scattered infarcts within the occipital and temporal cortex or diencephalon.

Clinical Features

Over the preceding days, months, or even years, about 25 per cent of patients will have experienced transient neurological warnings.

A sudden onset of the full neurological deficit occurs in 80 per cent; in 20 per cent a subacute and irregular progression occurs with the development of multifocal signs. In contrast to those resulting from infarction of the cerebral hemisphere, many of the deaths occur quickly (12 hours to 3 days) and are the direct result of the neurological deficit. Brain swelling from ischemic edema is seldom life-threatening, because these infarcts are of limited volume; however, when one third or more of a cerebellar hemisphere is infarcted (as may follow occlusion of the trunk of the posterior inferior cerebellar artery), swelling may be critical.[156]

Recent clinical reports have established the syndrome of massive cerebellar infarction.[156] The initial symptom in most patients is the sudden onset of inability to stand or walk because of severe ataxia. Nausea, vomiting, vertigo, and unilateral limb ataxia are frequent complaints. There is an acute but transient loss of consciousness in 15 per cent and more persistent drowsy confusion in nearly half. Examination at this stage reveals evidence of cerebellar dysfunction in nearly all patients, ipsilateral facial weakness and loss of pain and temperature appreciation in half. An ipsilateral gaze palsy is also common.

The clinical features remain stable until between the third and sixth days when nearly half the patients experience a progressive deterioration over 6 to 12 hours because of brain stem compression by the expanding cerebellar infarct. Posterior fossa decompression may be lifesaving and allow the patient to recover with surprisingly mild disability.[97]

The clinical features of the classic brain stem syndrome can be found in neurology texts.[100,127]

Prognosis

The mortality rate, morbidity, and risk of subsequent stroke are marginally better for a patient with a vertebrobasilar stroke than for one with a carotid stroke.[104]

MANAGEMENT OF CEREBRAL INFARCTION

The management of *both carotid* and *vertebrobasilar* territory brain infarcts is as follows.

Emergency Care

Urgent management problems are often found in patients presenting with brain infarction. These include coma, epileptic seizures, acute agitation, and coincidental medical problems, e.g., diabetic complications, electrolyte disturbances, hypertensive crises, drug overdose, cardiac arrhythmia, and myocardial infarction. These must be recognized and treated in a manner appropriate to their urgency.

Coma

The adequacy of airway and ventilation must be assured. Difficulty in maintaining either is an indication for assisted ventilation through an endotracheal tube or face mask and pharyngeal airway. Vital signs including pulse, blood pressure, and the skin color and temperature are then noted, and a neurological examination is performed to establish the cause of coma.[132] An assistant should be seeking available history of the ictus from witnesses or ambulance attendants. When abnormalities of the blood pressure or pulse are noted, the electrocardiogram should be monitored. If the diagnosis is at all uncertain, blood, gastric aspirate, and urine samples should be collected for drug estimations; and blood glucose, electrolytes, and ketone concentrations should be assayed. An intravenous line should be established, and possible hypoglycemia treated by the administration of a bolus of 50 ml of 50 per cent glucose.

Epilepsy may be controlled for the short term with intravenous diazepam, and phenytoin or phenobarbital in loading doses *if* the patient is not already receiving the latter medications. When doubt exists, the loading dose should be withheld until serum levels have been assessed.

The most frequently confused metabolic emergency is hyperosmolar (nonketotic) diabetic "coma." Diagnostic difficulty arises because the patients are often elderly, are not known to be diabetic, and may present with a focal neurological deficit and seizures. Their neurological symptoms may indeed be a manifestation of cortical vein thrombosis and cerebral infarction.

Investigation

A "working diagnosis" of the site and nature of the lesion, the time course (e.g., transient ischemic attack, progressing stroke or the like), and the vascular mechanism should be constructed from the history and examination. The "working diagnosis" and pertinent differential diagnosis may then be tested with laboratory investigation.

Necessary investigations include complete blood count, erythrocyte sedimentation rate, biochemical screens (fasting), lipid screen (fasting for those less than 60 years), chest and skull x-rays, and an electrocardiogram. Since blood for the lipid screen must be taken with the patient fasting and as early in the course as possible, it is often convenient to arrange for all samples of blood to be collected on the first morning.

Commonly indicated investigations include thyroid function tests, and serological tests for syphilis must be considered because it is important not to miss treatable disease.

Electroencephalography

A normal record is obtained in 25 per cent of patients with hemispheric infarcts and many with brain stem infarcts. A slow-wave focus is the most typical evidence of cortical involvement. Because of the frequency of middle cerebral artery infarction, the focus is commonly in the temporal regions. The focus may increase if the infarct is accompanied by edema, and usually resolves in weeks but occasionally persists for months.

Focal spike and sharp waves may appear early in the course of cortical infarction associated with epilepsy. Thalamic lesions may cause synchronous and bilateral bursts of delta and theta activity. Although 90 per cent of chronic subdural hematomas result in abnormal ties in the electroencephalograms, they rarely are specific.[106]

The electroencephalogram has been found useful for confirming the presence of minor lesions away from the motor and sensory strips and for following lesions of uncertain pathology.

Echoencephalography

Midline shifts are noted in only the 10 per cent of patients with hemispheric infarcts that are complicated by massive cerebral edema. When present, the shift is maximal between the second and seventh days.[139] The presence of any shift within hours of the ictus is reasonable evidence that the lesion is *not* an infarct.

Brain Scans

In most series approximately 5 per cent of patients initially considered to have a cerebral infarct are ultimately shown to have a neoplasm.[120] Therefore, it is desirable, at least in most patients, to confirm the nature of the neurological lesion by computed tomography. If this procedure is not available, serial brain scanning is very useful in distinguishing between tumor and infarct. Scans performed within the first two days usually are negative. Over the remainder of the first week only 30 per

cent show abnormal uptake on the static studies. The frequency of abnormal scans increases to 50 per cent during the second week and reaches a maximal incidence of 60 to 80 per cent between the second and fourth weeks.[168]

Delayed scans only marginally increase the yield in the abnormalities that are diagnosed.

Radionuclide dynamic or flow studies are often performed concurrently. An abnormal flow study may be a useful indicator of severe stenosis or occlusion of the carotid artery; however, the very important distinction between these entities is impossible, and less than one third of patients with operatively significant carotid disease can be identified.[15]

Computed Tomography

Computerized axial tomography has revolutionized evaluation of the stroke patient by providing a highly accurate diagnostic examination, which is rapid enough to be utilized in acute emergencies, and safe enough to be utilized for serial follow-up and screening out patients with equivocal findings. At present, CT is the only diagnostic method which will distinguish reliably between the mass effects of cerebral edema and hematoma. For these reasons it has become a major tool for diagnosis of cerebrovascular disease.[117]

The cost of computed tomography is such that it cannot at the present time be advocated as a screening test for all patients who are suspected of having ischemic cerebrovascular disease. If used in this manner, it would often be an elegant but costly display of pathological changes that could be adequately defined clinically.

A CT scan is indicated when the nature of the cerebral lesion is uncertain and the diagnostic considerations include those in which therapeutic intervention is vital. The indications therefore are: uncertain history of onset, headaches, any impairments of consciousness (particularly in hemispheric lesions), atypical cases, as a routine in centers with a research interest in stroke.

Lumbar Puncture

Computed tomography has considerably reduced the need for the "reflection of cerebral events" provided by cerebrospinal fluid examination; however, lumbar puncture is essential when meningeal infection is a possibility and to establish or exclude the presence of neurosyphilis. The reported changes and data concerning their incidence, extracted from several sources, were presented in Table 42–7.[138]

Noninvasive Assessment of Extracranial Vasculature

A number of investigations detect the hemodynamic effects of occlusion or tight stenosis within the internal carotid artery. These include ophthalmodynamometry, oculoplethysmography, orbital Doppler ultrasonic evaluation, and facial thermography.[15,44,95,161] Ophthalmodynamometry is both simple and relatively available. Orbital Doppler studies, also simple and inexpensive, have proved to be more accurate. It must be noted that all these investigations are of limited usefulness because they cannot distinguish high-grade stenosis from occlusion of the internal carotid artery and fail to detect two thirds of the significant lesions of the carotid in the neck that may be treated by operation.[15]

Carotid Doppler angiography and B-scan ultrasound examinations of the carotid arteries in the neck are noninvasive investigations at present under clinical evaluation. Both have the potential of serving as useful noninvasive screens for surgically significant lesions.[16,147]

Angiography

Angiography is seldom required to establish the diagnosis in ischemic cerebrovascular disease, particularly if computed tomography is available. The following groups of patients, however, may need angiography: those in whom the diagnosis remains obscure; those in whom there is a deterioration in consciousness or of a focal neurological deficit; and those in whom recovery from a carotid territory cerebral infarction is excellent and an investigation to exclude an operatively correctable vascular cause is warranted.

The most common angiographic finding in the second group is internal carotid occlusion; however, it is important to insure that a treatable lesion such as a subdural hematoma or swollen cerebellar infarct is not being overlooked.

Treatment

Treatment aims at minimizing the neurological deficit, observing for and attempting to modify complications, and managing coexistent medical problems.

For both ischemic heart and cerebral vascular disease, considerable effort is being directed to minimizing the size of parenchymal infarcts. Induced hypertension, hypothermia, hyperbaric oxygen, barbiturate protection, revascularization procedures (operative and chemical with fibrinolytic therapy), modification of the rheological characteristics of blood, inhibition of released neurotransmitters, and inhibition of calcium ion transport are among the many measures that have been considered. It would be simplistic either to dismiss these attempts as folly or to suggest that currently they can be advocated for routine patient care.[138]

Although no specific active intervention can be recommended, care is required to minimize extension or further damage. Hypoxemia should be corrected by increasing the oxygen saturation of inspired air until the arterial Po_2 is 100 mm of mercury, insuring the adequacy of ventilation, and finally by ruling out pulmonary disease or left ventricular failure.

Improvement in neurological signs has been noted in patients with cerebral infarcts when hypertension is induced; however, increase in the perfusion pressure also accelerates the formation of vasogenic cerebral edema. Hypotension, fluctuations in blood pressure, and uncontrolled hypertension should be avoided. The treatment of hypertension, unless it is of malignant grade, should be unhurried, and care should be taken to avoid fluctuations and rapid falls in pressure.

There is evidence that hypertension will accelerate atherosclerosis and so is an important risk factor for ischemic and hemorrhagic stroke and adversely affects the prognosis, particularly in men, by increasing the incidence of recurrent episodes.[83,104]

In men with cerebral infarction, Carter noted a five-year mortality rate of 75 per cent in hypertensive patients (i.e., systolic pressure > 200 mm or diastolic > 110 mm of mercury) compared with only 8 per cent in normotensive patients.[21] It is therefore important to ensure that hypertension is adequately treated and followed when the acute events of stroke have settled.

Assisted Ventilation

The use of assisted ventilation to maintain patients with extensive cerebral infarction is seldom justified. Lancaster observed that 23 of 25 patients so treated either died or required continuous nursing care.[93] The two who made good recovery presented with pontine infarcts. Because of the remarkable recovery noted in patients with lateral medullary infarcts, they too should have endotracheal intubation or tracheostomy if choking on pharyngeal secretions or food is a problem. The third exception is the rare patient with disordered automatic respiration but preserved voluntary breathing (Ondine's curse).

Anticoagulants*

Completed Stroke

Despite the number of patients at risk, there are no satisfactory trials of the usefulness of anticoagulants in acute cerebral infarction. Of the five available studies, there are three in which treated patients fared the same or worse than controls and two in which the treated patients fared better (Table 42–10).†

---

* See references 45, 69, 113.
† See references 6, 32, 67, 69, 105, 113.

Cerebral or systemic hemorrhage occurred as a complication in 4 to 11 per cent of patients receiving long-term anticoagulants. The risk was proportional to the duration of their use.

Computed tomography has revealed that an element of hemorrhage is much more common in patients in whom infarction has been diagnosed than has hitherto been believed. The cerebrospinal fluid is neither xanthochromic nor blood stained in a significant number of these patients.[86] Exclusion of these previously undetected cases of cerebral hemorrhage could be expected to reduce the risk of massive cerebral hemorrhage as a complication of anticoagulant therapy.

There is, at present, insufficient evidence to recommend the use of anticoagulants in completed infarction unless there is a previous history of pulmonary embolism or deep vein thrombosis.

Stroke in Evolution

Progressive infarction within the vertebrobasilar system is often the result of progressive arterial occlusion, either by the direct extension of thrombus or its embolization. As the extension is often lethal, it is not surprising that anticoagulant therapy does improve the prognosis. Whisnant reported that the mortality rate of patients with progressing brain stem infarction was reduced from 59 per cent to 9 per cent by the use of anticoagulants.[170] The benefit of

---

TABLE 42–10   ANTICOAGULANT THERAPY FOR PATIENTS WITH CEREBRAL INFARCTION (COMPLETED STROKE)

INVESTIGATOR		NO. OF PATIENTS	FOLLOW-UP (MO.)	REINFARCTION (PER CENT)	HEMORRHAGE (PER CENT)
Baker et al.*	Control	60	11	10	0
	Treated	72	11	16	10
Hill et al.†	Control	65	31	29	0
	Treated	66	28	33	6
McDowell and McDevitt‡	Control	99	34	22	2
	Treated	92	42	22	11
Enger and Bøyesen§	Control	49	23	20	0
	Treated	51	23	10	6
Howell et al.‖	Control	92	36	30	0
	Treated	103	16	7	4

* Anticoagulant therapy in cerebral infarction. Report on cooperative study. Neurology (Minneap.), *12*:823–835, 1962.
† Cerebrovascular disease: Trial of long term anticoagulant therapy. Brit. Med. J., *11*:1003–1006, 1962.
‡ Treatment of the completed stroke with long-term anticoagulant: Six and one-half years experience. *In* Millikan, C. H., Sickert, R. S., and Whisnant, J. P., eds.: Cerebral Vascular Disease. New York, Grune & Stratton, Inc., 1965.
§ Long term anticoagulant therapy in patients with cerebral infarction: A controlled clinical study. Acta Med. Scand. (Suppl.), *438*:1–61, 1965.
‖ Observations of anticoagulant therapy in thromboembolic disease of the brain. Canad. Med. Ass. J., *90*:611–614, 1964.

anticoagulants for progressing infarction within the carotid territory is less striking.

The clinical features of major and progressing brain stem infarction should cause little diagnostic confusion, but patients with a progressive neurological deficit of the cerebral hemisphere will require either computed tomography or angiography to exclude the mass effects of cerebral edema or hemorrhage or subdural collections before anticoagulants are initiated.

In these circumstances, anticoagulation should be initiated with heparin, and this should be followed by a short course of oral anticoagulants.[113]

The management of increased intracranial pressure from ischemic edema is discussed in Chapters 24 and 45. Hyperosmolar solutions (urea, mannitol, and glycerol) may effect a transient reduction in the intracranial pressure that is often followed by an augmented rebound. Corticosteroids are considered to have little effect on ischemic cerebral edema.[135] Hyperventilation will also temporarily reduce the intracranial pressure but does not appear to offer sustained benefit. Wide operative decompression of hemispheric infarcts with massive edema has been attempted. Severe residual disability can be expected, however, from cerebral hemisphere infarcts of sufficient size to cause fatal edema. When one third of the cerebellum is infarcted, swelling may cause fatal brain stem compression. Fortunately, decompression is possible and those who recover do well.[156,170]

VENOUS INFARCTION

Thrombosis of the dural venous channels and cortical veins may occur separately or in combination. Cerebral infarction does not follow dural sinus thrombosis, but may develop when the cortical veins and their smaller radicles are extensively occluded.[81] Because of the profusion of venous anastomoses, venous infarction is relatively uncommon and extremely difficult to reproduce experimentally.

Cases of intracranial thrombosis fall into two groups: those associated with intracranial disease and those associated with dehydration or an increased propensity to spontaneous intravascular thrombosis (the so-called "hypercoagulable state").

TABLE 42–11 CAUSES OF INTRACRANIAL VENOUS THROMBOSIS

Trauma	Head injury (penetrating and closed injuries)
Infection	Middle ear, mastoid, and paranasal sinus infection
Endocrine imbalance	Pregnancy
	Puerperium
	Oral contraceptives
Dehydration	Diarrheal illness in children
	Hyperosmolar diabetic coma
	Ulcerative colitis
Hematological disorders	Thrombocytosis
	Sicklemia
	Hemolytic anemia
	Paroxysmal nocturnal hemoglobinuria
	Cryoglobulinemia
Propagation	Spread from an extracranial venous thrombosis following jugular venous canalization
Impaired cerebral circulation	Cerebral arterial occlusion
	Anesthetic in seated position
	Congestive cardiac failure
	Congenital webs in sagittal sinus
Tumor	Compression of intracranial venous channel, particularly parasagittal meningioma

In the first group, infective processes are the most frequent precipitants of intracranial venous thrombosis. Sepsis of the middle ear, mastoid cells, and paranasal air spaces may cause local thrombophlebitis of veins within the cavity's mucosa. Thrombosis may spread to the emissary veins and finally into the sigmoid and lateral sinuses. Thrombosis may remain confined or extend into the sagittal and contralateral lateral sinus. Focal thrombosis of cortical veins is less common but may be initiated by purulent meningitis and subdural empyema.

Fracture across a dural sinus may cause delayed thrombosis of the injured venous canal. Compression or invasion of dural sinuses by tumor is relatively uncommon except with the falx meningioma. Other precipitants of intracranial venous occlusion are listed in Table 42–11.

When an intracranial disease initiates venous occlusion, the features of the primary intracranial process are often predominant. Sinus occlusion may cause a significant increase in the intracranial pressure, and venous infarction may cause focal or generalized seizures.

Patients with Associated Extracranial Diseases

Autopsy studies have suggested that cortical vein and dural sinus thromboses frequently are asymptomatic. Towbin observed intracranial venous occlusion in 9 per cent of consecutive autopsies from a nursing home.[163] Thrombosis usually commences at the midpoint of the sagittal sinus. Extension may occur throughout the sinuses or into cortical veins.

When cortical venous drainage is extensively occluded, intense congestion, edema, and hemorrhagic softening result in the underlying brain. The infarct is confined to the cortex and immediately subjacent white matter by the deep venous system. The venous infarct contrasts sharply with an arterial infarct in shape, color, and the intensity of its edematous swelling. Congested vessels in the zone of infarction may rupture, causing intracerebral or subarachnoid hemorrhage or a subdural hematoma.[46]

Occlusion of the anterior half of the superior sagittal sinus is frequently asymptomatic. More extensive occlusion of the sinus impairs the resorption of cerebrospinal fluid, producing raised intracranial pressure.

Thrombosis usually is confined to the superficial venous drainage, but thrombosis of the vein of Galen may occur in children and causes extensive swelling and hemorrhagic infarction of the basal ganglia, septal regions, and medial and superior portions of the thalamus. Both intracerebral and ventricular hemorrhage may occur. These children present with coma and fever and almost invariably die.

Clinical Features

As previously noted, many cases of dural sinus thrombosis are asymptomatic.[163] Symptoms can be arranged into two syndromes.

Cortical Vein Thrombosis with Venous Infarction of the Brain

The venous infarct is the most potent of epileptogenic lesions known. Convulsions occur in *nearly all* instances. The focal neurological deficit is mild and often localized, most frequently involving the upper limb or face. Fifty per cent of patients have a low-grade fever and headache. Mild drowsiness is common.

Since cortical vein thrombosis is often bilateral, concurrent active epileptic foci may develop in both the right and left cerebral hemispheres. This unusual event is virtually confined to three conditions: herpes simplex encephalitis, anoxic encephalopathy, and cortical venous infarction.

Seizure is the presenting feature in 60 per cent of patients and is characteristically explosive in onset and very difficult to control, but settles within days.

Intracerebral or subdural hemorrhage and occasionally subdural hematoma will complicate the illness in 5 to 10 per cent of untreated patients and is considerably more frequent in those patients "treated" with anticoagulants.[46]

Sinus Occlusion with Intracranial Hypertension

Occlusion of the anterior half of the sagittal sinus and the minor lateral sinus is asymptomatic. When thrombosis extends into the posterior half of the sagittal sinus or involves the lateral sinus draining the sagittal sinus (most frequently on the right), the resorption of cerebrospinal fluid is significantly impaired and the cerebral venous pressure is increased. Both mechanisms result in increased intracranial pressure. This syndrome is so similar to the idiopathic syndrome of *benign intracranial hypertension* or *pseudotumor cerebri* that it is difficult to believe the syndromes are unrelated. Using very complete angiographic investigation, Bresnan and co-workers were able to demonstrate venous sinus occlusion in 10 of 12 children with benign intracranial hypertension.[18] The arterial and early venous phases were considered normal in all of their studies.

Patients with this syndrome complain of severe and generalized headache that is often accompanied by nausea or vomiting and exacerbated by coughing or straining. Transient monocular visual obscurations are common, and persistent visual impairment is present in 10 per cent of patients. A history of episodic drowsiness and diplopia can often be elicited. Examination is remarkable in that it typically reveals florid papilledema in a strikingly alert and otherwise healthy patient. Visual acuity is normal, and the visual fields show only the expected enlargement of the blind spot in all but the 10 per cent with asymmetrical or unilateral field defects. Incomplete sixth nerve palsies are frequently observed.

Investigations will reveal normal or small

cerebral ventricles and chemically normal cerebrospinal fluid, and that the features are not the result of a space-occupying lesion. Cerebrospinal fluid dynamics have been variably reported to show delayed normal or accelerated absorption. The cerebral blood volume is increased.

Chronic venous insufficiency is almost never seen, and in 90 per cent the features resolve spontaneously in less than 12 months, frequently in 3 months or less. Relapse may be expected in 10 per cent.

DIFFUSE CEREBRAL ISCHEMIA

Diffuse ischemic brain damage (anoxic encephalopathy) is a major determinant of the quality of life possible to survivors of overwhelming illness and cardiopulmonary collapse.[176] The advent of intensive care facilities has drastically increased the frequency of these problems and brought to society a new economic and moral dilemma.

Although the details of events during life-threatening emergencies are often complex, careful neuropathological and clinical review has allowed an understanding of the individual roles played by hypoxemia, hypotension, circulatory arrest, microembolism, and venous occlusion.

Impaired Circulation

Cardiac Arrest

Circulatory arrest of more than five to seven minutes' duration causes cerebral injury. The oxygen consumption of the cerebral cortex is 20 times that of skeletal muscle, and after circulatory arrest available tissue stores are soon exhausted. Available glucose or alternative energy sources have been estimated to be adequate for 12 minutes. The ultimate mechanism of brain injury in circulatory arrest is tissue hypoxia. Regions of the brain with greater metabolic activity and oxygen consumption are more vulnerable. This selective vulnerability may cause remarkably "focal" zones of ischemic injury, even though the mechanism is global.

The macroscopic appearance of the brain after cardiac arrest will reflect the extent of neuronal destruction and the duration of survival. Immediately, the brain may appear normal or show only moderate swelling. In time, however, selective areas of gray matter atrophy become apparent. Microscopy reveals more clearly the selective vulnerability of neurons in certain areas.

In the cerebral cortex, ischemic alterations are more severe in the region of the occipital and pre- and postcentral gyri and in the depths of the sulci. The third, fifth, and sixth cortical laminae are the most vulnerable. The hippocampal formations are strikingly involved, particularly in the Sommer section (h_1).

Particularly vulnerable regions of the deep cerebral gray matter are the lateral amygdala, caudate nucleus, putamen, mamillary bodies, and to a lesser extent, the anterior, dorsomedial, and ventrolateral thalamic nuclei. In the cerebellum, the Purkinje cells are the most vulnerable.

The influence of age upon the distribution of ischemic alterations is observed in the brain stem. In adults, damage is commonly minor and restricted to three regions: the substantia nigra, the inferior colliculi, and the olives; in children, however, involvement also includes the third, fifth, and vestibular nuclei, and the gracile, cuneate, and solitary nuclei in the lower medulla.[96]

The severity of brain damage following cardiac arrest will range from immediate death through the already described pattern of widespread softening to foci of gliosis that may present as epilepsy. Many of these lesions are highly epileptogenic.

Clinical Features

Initially, an impairment of consciousness is invariably present. When coma persists for more than 48 hours, complete recovery is unlikely. Seizures may occur during the first four days. Coma is often followed by an organic confusional state with hallucinations. As this clears, an extraordinary variety of intellectual, behavioral, and neurological abnormalities may become apparent.[141] Impaired intellectual function is characterized by a prominent short-term memory deficit, impaired speech and cognitive function, and apraxias. Motor disturbances may include an extrapyramidal syndrome of parkinsonian type, and intention or action myoclonus.[94] Hemiplegia and cranial nerve lesions have been described occasionally.

Profound Hypotension

A constant cerebral blood flow is maintained over a wide range of perfusion pressures by adjustment of the cerebral vascular resistance. As the perfusion pressure falls, cerebral arterioles dilate. When vasodilatation is maximal, autoregulation ceases, and cerebral blood flow falls parallel with the perfusion pressure. It is the boundary zones between major cerebral arteries that are the first regions to experience critical oligemia.[179] In individual cases, developmental anomalies of the cerebral vasculature and stenotic arterial lesions will also influence the pattern of ischemic injury.

The distribution of brain damage caused by prolonged and profound hypotension will be determined by the balance between the selective vulnerability of the region and the blood flow it receives. Lesion distribution conforms to one of three patterns.[19]

Boundary Zone Pattern

Injury is concentrated along the boundary zones of the major cerebral and cerebellar vessels. In the cerebral cortex, damage is most severe in the parietal-temporal-occipital triangle.[179] This region is the junction of the anterior, middle and posterior cerebral arterial territories (Fig. 42–3).

The severity of injury decreases as one approaches the frontal and temporal ends of the anterior-middle, and the middle-posterior arterial border zones. The hippocampal regions are spared. Injury to the cerebellum is restricted to the cortex in the region between the superior and posterior inferior cerebellar arteries. This pattern is seen when there is a *sudden* reduction in blood pressure such as occurs with cardiac arrhythmia or profuse hemorrhage.

Many of the clinical features are similar to those of the anoxic encephalopathy of cardiac arrest; but because of the more restricted cortical defects, apraxias, spatial confusion, and language disturbances are more prominent while short-term memory is spared.

Generalized Pattern

Ischemic lesions are generalized in the cortex of the cerebrum and cerebellum, se-

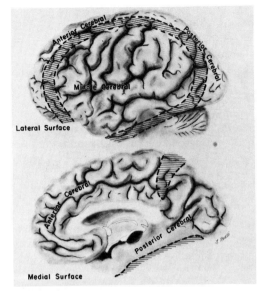

Figure 42–3 Border zone areas of ischemia that may become infarcted in patients with generalized reduction in cerebral perfusion due to hypotension, cardiac dysrhythmia, or the like. (Courtesy of John Moossy, University of Pittsburgh, Pittsburgh, Pa.)

vere in thalamic and cerebellar nuclei, but absent or minor in the hippocampi. This uncommon pattern results when the hypotension is of gradual onset and prolonged duration. Early vasodilatation insures that blood flow to the boundary zone is as adequate as that to other cortical regions. The clinical picture is of symmetrical decerebrate or decorticate coma.

Combined Boundary Zone and Generalized Patterns

Combinations of the foregoing pathological patterns are common. The implications of a sudden onset of hypotension are seen in the boundary zone lesions and those of a more sustained hypotension in the development of generalized lesions.[19] Most typically, this sort of pattern has been observed following brief cardiac arrest followed by prolonged massage or postoperative hypotension. Consciousness is seldom regained.

Impaired Energy Substrate Supply

Hypoxemic Hypoxia

Although it is commonly believed that prolonged hypoxemia can cause brain damage, this contention has not been supported experimentally. Profound hypoxemia, whether achieved by atmospheric decompression or inhalation of gas mixtures depleted of oxygen, causes cardiovascular collapse before it causes detectable brain damage.[19]

When reviewing this subject, Brierley concluded that "hypoxic hypoxia can produce brain damage only through the medium of a secondary depression of the myocardium."[19]

Carbon Monoxide Poisoning

Carbon monoxide both reduces the oxygen carrying capacity of blood and impairs tissue utilization of oxygen. The mechanisms of these actions are similar: by combining strongly with the iron atom of hemoglobin in the first instance and the cytochrome oxidases in the second, carbon monoxide excludes oxygen from its binding site. The lethal dose of carbon monoxide is that which converts 60 per cent of hemoglobin to carboxyhemoglobin; it may be achieved by a 30-minute exposure to 1 per cent carbon monoxide in air.

Pathology

Immediately, there is a marked venous and capillary dilatation, particularly within the deep white matter of the cerebral hemispheres. Petechial hemorrhages are prominent in white matter. The globus pallidus appears ischemic. In severe cases cortical lesions are extensive, more prominently within the third, fifth, and sixth laminae, arterial watersheds, and Somer's sector of the hippocampi. In the cerebellum, the Purkinje cells show coagulation necrosis.

Those who survive develop symmetrical, well-demarcated zones of cortical laminar necrosis and hippocampal atrophy, sometimes with striking areas of circumscribed infarction of the globus pallidus. There may be mild diffuse demyelination secondary to the cortical necrosis. Collections of fat-filled gitter cells must be differentiated from a form of diffuse leukoencephalopathy.

In approximately 5 per cent of cases, a late deterioration occurs. This is related to the development of a remarkable leukoencephalopathy. In its purer form, visible hemorrhages, vascular congestion, edema, and cortical softening are absent. Myelin stains reveal a diffuse or mottled pallor of the cerebral white matter, while subcortical U fibers and the corpus callosum are spared.

Oligodendrocytes in the involved areas are swollen and show nuclear pyknosis. Myelin sheaths are fragmented and vacuolated, with stainable myelin free in the tissue. The continuity of axis cylinders is well preserved, although they may show swelling and tortuosity. In contrast, the nerve cell bodies and demyelinated fibers of the cortex are relatively well preserved. These changes are attributable to a recent diffuse degeneration of oligodendrocytes and myelin sheaths of a shorter duration than the interval since the poisoning.[103]

Mechanism

The immediate and the late ischemic neuronal injury is the result of cardiovascular collapse, severe hypoxemia, and the toxic effects on cellular respiration. The pathological picture is similar to the mixed pattern of hypotension-induced ischemic encephalopathy described earlier. The reason for the prominence of ischemic injury in the globus pallidus remains obscure.

The mechanisms of the leukoencephalopathy are considerably more controversial. Since a similar process has been described in cases in which there has been a hypoxic ischemic insult not related to carbon monoxide poisoning, it is unlikely that carbon monoxide is acting as a specific intoxicant.[133]

Both the infrequency of this condition and the sparing of gray matter suggest that hypoxia is unlikely to be the responsible mechanism. In both experimental and clinical carbon monoxide poisoning the severity of brain damage correlates best with vascular collapse and metabolic acidosis.[50,51] Other suggested, but inadequately documented, factors have included cerebral edema, elevated cerebral and systemic venous pressure, and raised intracranial pressure.

One of the two most likely mechanisms appears to be the combination of inadequate perfusion of the deep cerebral white matter that follows hypotension with the systemic acidosis.[51] The other is specific injury of the glial-myelin unit by agents released by spontaneously occurring intra-

TABLE 42–12 OUTCOME IN 85 CASES OF CARBON MONOXIDE POISONING[*]

	NO.	PERCENTAGE OF TOTAL
Dead on arrival	5	6
Died without recovering consciousness	10	12
Recovery followed by relapse	3	3
Recovery with neurological deficit	6	7
Full recovery	61	72
Total	85	

[*] These 85 consecutive cases of carbon monoxide poisoning were treated at the Toronto General Hospital. (From Richardson, J. C., Chambers, R. A., and Heywood, P. M.: Carbon monoxide poisoning. Arch. Neurol., *1*:178–190, 1959. Reprinted by permission.)

vascular platelet aggregates. It is noted that impaired perfusion, acidosis, venous stagnation, and an increase in circulating catecholamines are all recognized as factors that precipitate intravascular platelet aggregation.

Clinical Features

Carbon monoxide poisoning is accidental in half the cases and of suicidal intent in the remainder. Accidental exposure is much more common in the elderly.

At presentation, nearly all patients are unconscious, many being unresponsive to all stimuli. Most display a generalized increase in tone interrupted by spasms of intense decerebrate posturing and trismus. The face is sweaty and suffused with a characteristic cherry red color. Breathing is rapid and expiration forced. Hyperpnea may be an evidence of developing pulmonary edema, reduced oxygen carrying capacity of the blood, or a central tachypnea with associated respiratory alkalosis. Table 42–12 documents the outcome in 85 consecutive cases from the Toronto General Hospital.[103,137]

Hypoglycemic Brain Damage

Experimental studies in primates have confirmed that the cellular reaction and selective vulnerability of neurons to hypoglycemia are the same as those to anoxia.[19] There is some evidence that the combination of hypoglycemia and anoxia may result in brain damage when neither is sufficiently severe to do so alone.

Prolonged hypoglycemia in man results in diffuse neuronal damage in the third, fifth, and sixth laminae of the cerebral cor-

tex, Sommer's sector of the hippocampus, caudate nucleus, putamen, and isolated thalamic nuclei, while cerebellar damage is moderate.[19] It will be noted that these changes are similar to those of cardiac arrest. Discussion of the clinical features is beyond the scope of this text.

Diffuse Small Vessel Disease

Inflammatory Angiopathies

There is evidence to support the belief that the collagen vascular diseases are autoimmune disorders. Takayasu's disease involves the aortic arch and its primary branches; cranial arteritis, large to medium-sized arteries such as the internal and external carotid arteries; polyarteritis nodosa, the medium-sized and small arteries; and disseminated lupus erythematosus, only the small arteries. Only polyarteritis and lupus are relevant to this section; Takayasu's disease and cranial arteritis are considered in a following one.

Disseminated Lupus Erythematosus

Systemic lupus erythematosus is a disease of small arteries and arterioles, and may involve the vasculature of any organ or tissue; however, its most common presentations are involvement of the skin, joints, kidneys, lungs, and serosal surfaces.[28] Central nervous system involvement is a common late manifestation.

PATHOLOGICAL FINDINGS. The peritoneal, pleural, and pericardial surfaces are usually involved with an inflammatory reaction, adhesions, and effusion. The heart is often enlarged, and the mitral and aortic valves may show verrucous vegetations. When the central nervous system is affected, the brain or spinal cord may be edematous, with thickened meninges. Microscopy reveals that the arterioles, capillaries, and venules of the gray and white matter are diffusely involved with an inflammatory reaction. Many are occluded by thrombus.

CLINICAL FEATURES. In contrast to polyarteritis nodosa, which predominantly affects men, disseminated lupus erythematosus affects women between the ages of 15 and 40 years. The sex ratio is 4 to 1.

The most frequent manifestations of sys-

TABLE 42–13 INCIDENCE OF SYSTEMIC MANIFESTATIONS OF DISSEMINATED LUPUS ERYTHEMATOSUS*

		PER CENT OF 520 PATIENTS
Constitutional	Fever	84
	Weight loss	52
Connective	Arthritis and arthralgia	92
tissue lesions	Pericarditis	31
	Electrocardiographic changes	34
	Hypertension	25
	Pleuritic pain	
	Pleural effusion	30
	Ascites	11
Skin	Skin rash	72
Renal	Albuminuria	46
Hematological	Adenopathy	59
	Anemia (<11 gm)	57
	Leukopenia (<4,500/cm)	43
	LE cell reaction	76

* From Dubois, E. L., and Tuffanelli, D. L.: Clinical manifestations of systemic lupus erythematosus: Computer analysis of 520 cases. J.A.M.A., 190:104–111, 1964. Copyright 1964, American Medical Association. Reprinted by permission.

temic lupus are fever, weight loss, a malar rash, alopecia, arthralgia or arthritis, serositis, lymphadenopathy, renal involvement, pancytopenia, and the presence of circulating antibodies to tissue antigens. The frequency of these manifestations is noted in Table 42–13.

The neurological and psychiatric features are so protean that this condition may have replaced syphilis as the great clinical mimic.

Epilepsy occurs in 20 per cent of patients and is the most common discrete neurological complication. Although a convulsion may be the presenting feature, it is more common for epilepsy to occur during active disease in its later course.[124]

In nearly 50 per cent of patients, a serious psychiatric syndrome occurs. The psychiatric syndrome combines organic symptoms and either affective or schizophreniform syndromes in half of these cases.[11] Even cases without definite organic features are considered by many psychiatrists to be a result of the cerebral lupus itself rather than steroid psychosis or a situational reaction, because episodes are brief (commonly less than six weeks), occur most frequently during activation of the disease, are much more frequently observed in systemic lupus than in other equally debilitating chronic diseases, and may be accompanied by an

abnormal brain scan, low cerebrospinal fluid complement levels, and a response to administration of large doses of adrenocorticosteroids.

Although headache is a common complaint and may be accompanied by mild meningismus, it is usually vague and unexplained, and is not a feature of uncomplicated cerebral lupus. Persisting headache demands consideration of such complications as fungal or tuberculous meningitis and the development of cerebral lymphoma.

Episodes of impaired cranial nerve function most commonly present as disturbances of ocular movement. Of intermediate frequency are involvements of the fifth, seventh, and eighth cranial nerves. The cranial nerves may be affected in their meningeal course or at the level of their nuclei in the brain stem. An associated myasthenic syndrome may also impair ocular movements. A chorea that is similar in course and clinical features to rheumatic chorea may occur.[55] Parkinsonian features have been described.

Focal neurological deficits reflecting cerebral infarcts occur in less than 5 per cent and appear more common in the brain stem.[17,78]

Ophthalmoscopy may reveal superficial fluffy exudates (cytoid bodies) with or without surrounding hemorrhages. The vessels are normal. Such a picture was considered diagnostic of lupus, but its occurrence in polyarteritis, hypertension, leukemia, and retinal tears is now recognized. Papilledema may be present.

Three patterns of peripheral nerve involvement have been recognized. A symmetrical sensory-motor neuropathy is the most frequent, while mononeuritis multiplex is the most specific. A mainly motor neuropathy of Guillain-Barré type may be associated with increased cerebrospinal fluid protein concentration.[52,54]

Other less common neurological manifestations are listed in Table 42–14.

MECHANISM. The widespread arteriolar occlusive disease has appeared sufficient to explain the symptoms of cerebral lupus. Indeed this condition may be seen as a prototype of conditions characterized by diffuse microvascular occlusion; however, it has been noted recently that the cerebrospinal fluid complement and IgG levels fall during

TABLE 42–14 NEUROLOGICAL FEATURES OF SYSTEMIC LUPUS ERYTHEMATOSUS*

	PER CENT TOTAL	PER CENT SUBTOTAL
Emotional disturbances	50	
Convulsions	25	
Dementia		
Cranial nerve involvement	20	
Neuropathy	15	
Symmetrical sensory neuropathy		60
Mononeuritis multiplex		30
Guillain-Barré neuropathy		10
Neuritic pain		
Retinal lesions	10	
Chorea	5	
Cerebral or brain stem infarction	5	
Meningism		
Acute transverse myelitis		
Inappropriate antidiuretic hormone secretion		
Phenothiazine sensitivity causing extrapyramidal syndrome		
Cerebellar ataxia		

* The frequency quoted is a compilation from published series. Data from: Bennahum, D. A., and Messner, R. P.: Recent observations on central nervous system lupus erythematosus. Seminars Arthr. Rheumatol., 4:253–266, 1975. Johnson, R. T., and Richardson, E. P.: The neurological manifestations of systemic lupus erythematosus. A clinical pathological study of 24 cases and review of the literature. Medicine (Balt.), 47:337–369, 1968.

activation of cerebral lupus.[11] This immune reaction may be contributing to the cerebral symptoms.

LABORATORY FINDINGS. Fever, anemia (normochromic, hypochromic, or hemolytic), increased erythrocyte sedimentation rate, a false-positive reaction for syphilis, and at times, isolated thrombocytopenia are nonspecific findings that may suggest the illness. The specific diagnostic test is the presence of high-titer antinuclear-factor antibody.

When the diagnosis is established, a renal biopsy is required to determine the extent of renal involvement (the major prognostic determinant). Examination of the cerebrospinal fluid reveals a pleocytosis that rarely exceeds 200 cells per cubic millimeter. The protein concentration is only slightly increased unless a Guillain-Barré–like neuropathy is present.

Recent observations suggest that decreases in cerebrospinal fluid IgG and complement (C_4) levels may be useful in confirming the suspicion of cerebral lupus.[98]

TREATMENT. The treatment of cerebral lupus is controversial. Most clinicians agree that an acute episode should be treated with increased corticosteroid administration. The frequency of serious complications with high dosages of corticosteroids is a grave concern, however. There is at present no accord as to how much of and for how long these drugs should be administered, and whether the dose can be reduced with the concurrent administration of cyclophosphamide.[11]

Polyarteritis Nodosa*

This disorder is characterized by a widespread arteritis of medium-sized and small arteries that spares the pulmonary circulation.

PATHOLOGY. Of the cases seen at autopsy, 8 to 46 per cent show involvement of the arteries of the brain. Although there has for many years been great interest in this area, the magnitude of the contribution of intracerebral periarteritis to clinically significant cerebral infarction or intracerebral hemorrhage remains unknown.[26] In a recent study, cerebral or brain stem syndromes were reported in 19 of 114 patients. At autopsy of 6 of the 19 symptomatic patients, cerebral infarction was observed in 5 and hemorrhage in the other.[38] Macroscopically involved arteries show visible nodular aneurysms at sites of arterial branching. There are a segmental, necrotizing panarteritis in which the tissues contain fibrin and fibrin products, and a mixed nonspecific cellular response focally. When arterial involvement is widespread, the brain may appear swollen and contains numerous petechial hemorrhages.

CLINICAL FEATURES. This disease is more common in men than in women by a ratio of 4 to 1 and usually has its onset between the ages of 25 and 55. Symptoms and signs secondary to involvement of the central nervous system are seldom the initial manifestation. Myalgia, polymyositis, anemia, and fever almost always precede symptoms of central nervous system involvement by months to years. Hematuria and renal hypertension are frequent initial manifestations. Peripheral nerves are involved in 50 per cent of patients in either a

---

* See reference 26.

generalized symmetrical polyneuropathy or mononeuritis multiplex.

Ill-defined headache, the commonest neurological complaint, is of variable severity, quality, and location.

The more typical evidence of central nervous system involvement is an organic psychosis similar to that described with systemic lupus. Focal or generalized seizures are frequent.

Because major intracranial vessels are very seldom involved, large hemispheric infarcts are uncommon and, when present, are more likely to be related to the associated hypertension.

Cranial nerve palsy occurs in 5 to 10 per cent of cases. More frequently the involvement of either the third or seventh cranial nerve is seen. The third nerve palsy often spares the fibers for pupillary constriction and frequently recovers spontaneously within months. Retinal changes of hypertension are often present. Ischemic optic papillitis or neuritis is occasionally observed.

LABORATORY FINDINGS. Anemia, leukocytosis with eosinophilia, and an elevated erythrocyte sedimentation rate are seen in almost all cases. The urine frequently contains protein, red blood cells, and very characteristically, red blood cell casts. Lumbar puncture usually reveals the pressure to be normal. The spinal fluid often contains increased amounts of protein and abnormal numbers of lymphocytes and polymorphonuclear cells.

Tissue diagnosis is obtained by performing a biopsy of involved tissues such as skeletal muscles, skin, or kidney.

COURSE AND TREATMENT. Polyarteritis nodosa usually has an explosive onset, and the course is often rapidly downhill. About 50 per cent of affected individuals have a remission up to several years in duration, appearing usually in the first year. The prognosis is most closely related to the presence of renal impairment and severe hypertension.

All medications that could possibly precipitate the disorder must be stopped. Among these are hydralazine, the sulfonamides, and certain antibiotics.

Treatment with corticosteroids is effective as a temporary measure and may slow the course of the illness but does not affect the end result.

Noninfectious Granulomatous Angiitis*

In this rare and uniformly fatal central nervous system vasculitis, foci of necrotizing granulomatous and giant cell–containing inflammation involve all coats of the wall of small arteries. Twenty per cent of cases appear to be a response to herpes virus or mycoplasma infection.[135] Segmental saccular aneurysms may be apparent angiographically. Clinically marked by headache and convulsions, rapid mental deterioration with stupor and coma, and multifocal signs, the disease is said to be difficult to distinguish from viral or fungal meningoencephalitis. Because the differentiation is important, brain biopsy is, at times, indicated.

Thrombotic Thrombocytopenic Purpura

This uncommon condition, also known as Moschcowitz's disease, is characterized by hemolytic anemia, thrombocytopenic purpura, fever, and acute renal and cerebral disturbances caused by disseminated microvascular occlusions.[5]

The condition occurs with similar frequency at all ages, attacking females a little more frequently than males. The overall mortality rate is 80 per cent, and many survive less than a week. Frequently the condition appears to be precipitated by an upper respiratory tract infection, vaccination, or drug hypersensitivity.

Exposure to a precipitant, it has been suggested, initiates a reaction in the arteriolar subendothelium that causes fibrin to be deposited and to extend through intercellular spaces into the lumen. Luminal fibrin strands impale circulating red cells, causing hemolysis and fracture of erythrocytes. Thrombocytopenia follows the consumption of platelets and other clotting components. The acute renal and cerebral lesions result from diffuse arteriolar and capillary plugging with fibrin.

The neurological features conform to the pattern of diffuse small-vessel disease that has been described for disseminated lupus erythematosus. Changes in mental function and conscious state tend to mask associated headache, aphasia, seizures, and focal signs. The evolution from headache or

---

* See references 121, 166.

behavior change to coma may take only days.[5]

The differential diagnosis for the most part concerns the viral encephalitides, but subdural hematoma, toxic encephalopathies, septicemia, bacterial endocarditis, and subacute multifocal leukoencephalopathy may need to be considered.

The laboratory investigations are unusually helpful. The blood picture shows both thrombocytopenia and microangiopathic hemolytic anemia at some stage of the illness; elevated direct bilirubin levels and low serum haptoglobin levels confirm the presence of hemolysis. Coagulation studies, microscopic examination of urine, and routine biochemical tests may all show gross abnormalities. Autoantibody titers are normal.

The cerebrospinal fluid usually shows no cells and has normal protein. Neurological investigations seldom reveal structural abnormalities.

Treatment must be commenced before the development of coma if the prognosis is to be altered and consists of administration of aspirin and dipyridamole followed by splenectomy if there is no improvement. Large doses of corticosteroids and heparin have been widely used, although their role is uncertain.[136] These methods of treatment have halved the mortality rate.

Hemolytic Uremic Syndrome

This condition is closely related to thrombotic thrombocytopenic purpura, and as the differences largely relate to its hematological manifestations it is not discussed here.[16]

Hypertensive Encephalopathy

This term was first used by Oppenheimer and Fishburg in 1928 to describe acute and usually transient neurological phenomena occurring in patients with very high blood pressure. They noted the brains of patients who died with this syndrome to be pale, and attributed the abnormality to intense arterial spasm and resultant cerebral edema. Unfortunately, the term has not always been used circumspectly. To avoid further confusion, the diagnosis should be restricted to the rare cases of reversible cerebral features associated with a rapid or marked elevation in systemic blood pressure. Papilledema usually is present.

Etiology

Recent findings challenge the traditional view that hypertensive encephalopathy is caused by uncontrolled vasospasm and resultant ischemic hypoxia. All studies of cerebral blood flow in experimental hypertension indicate that when the limits of autoregulation have been reached a further increase in blood pressure results in an *increase* in cerebral blood flow (see Chapter 23). This increase is greatest in regions where the blood-brain barrier has been damaged. The severe hypertension results in dilatation of the arterioles and rupture of their endothelial cell junctions. This allows fibrin deposition and platelet adhesion, with the release of substances that induce focal edema and necrosis of the arteriolar wall.

Pathology

The brain is usually swollen and pale. Petechiae may be noticed on section and over the surface of the brain. Fibrinoid necrosis involves arterioles diffusely. Areas of abnormal focal dilatation of arterioles have been demonstrated to be the sites of leakage of edema fluid.[77]

Clinical Features

The initial symptoms of hypertensive encephalopathy are headache and emotional lability. The headache is of subacute onset and suboccipital in site, exacerbated by coughing, and most intense on waking. Associated anorexia or vomiting is common. Seizures, an organic confusional state, and transient focal neurological symptoms develop subsequently.

Complaints of visual blurring and transient blindness are associated with hypertensive retinopathy and papilledema. Papilledema is often a reflection of abnormal permeability of the vasculature of the optic nerve head and does not always indicate a marked increase in intracranial pressure.

Examination reveals severe hypertension, retinopathy, and a confusional state, and may show focal twitching, evoked myoclonus, or evidence of focal neurological dysfunction.

Differential Diagnosis

As severe hypertension is often associated with renal disease, the combination of renal failure, encephalopathy, and hypertension has become a common problem in renal units. The nephrologist will have considered a number of metabolic encephalopathies: uremic encephalopathy (underdialysis syndrome), electrolyte disturbances, hypophosphatemia, hypoglycemia, hypocalcemia, hypomagnesemia, and toxic accumulations of heavy metals and aluminum. During or immediately following dialysis, headache, vomiting, confusion, and seizures may indicate development of the cerebral edema of the dysequilibrium syndrome. A rapidly progressive dementia of unknown etiology has become known as dialysis dementia. It may occur at any time after 15 months of dialysis and frequently begins as a confusional state. Specific intoxicants are being sought, but at present no treatment has halted the progression to death in 3 to 15 months. Small-vessel diseases (e.g., disseminated lupus erythematosus) may cause renal disease, headache, and cerebral symptoms, and so should have been considered.

Subdural hematoma may complicate dialysis, particularly if the patient is receiving anticoagulant therapy or has a bleeding disorder. Uremia depresses immunological responsiveness and so predisposes to chronic meningeal infections. There is some evidence that primary cerebral tumors and central nervous system lymphoma are more common in those receiving immunosuppressive therapy for transplantation or immunological renal disease.

Prognosis

The ultimate outlook is dependent on the extent to which the blood pressure can be controlled and on the severity of the accompanying hypertensive cardiac and renal disease.

Management

Patients with hypertensive encephalopathy should be treated in an intensive care unit. The primary treatment is rapid reduction of the blood pressure to a level sufficient to reverse the encephalopathy without precipitating cerebral, myocardial, or renal ischemia. Increased intracranial pressure is reduced when the systemic blood pressure is lowered and does not require specific treatment. Seizures should be controlled with intravenous diazepam; long-term administration of anticonvulsants will not be required.

Once the acute crisis has been controlled, the underlying cause of the patient's hypertension should be sought and when possible treated. Adequate maintenance hypotensive therapy must be initiated.

The Microembolic Syndromes

The impaction of multiple small emboli in the microcirculation is an important mechanism in the development of fat embolism, decompression disease, disseminated intravascular coagulation, post–cardiopulmonary bypass syndromes, and an acute encephalopathy that occasionally complicates carcinoma of the lung. Of these, fat embolism is the most characteristic and possibly the most frequent.

Fat Embolism

Fat embolism is a condition in which fat appears in the blood as droplets of sufficient size (10 to 40 μ) to act as microemboli, temporarily occluding capillaries and arterioles of the pulmonary system and subsequently those of the brain and kidney. It usually arises as a complication of severe trauma with fractures of ribs or long bones.

It is thought that the fat enters the circulation at the site of fracture. With changes in tissue and luminal pressure, torn veins bleed at one moment and then draw free fat into their lumina at another. There is a surge of emboli for some hours, followed by intermittent release with movement of the fracture site. Some pathologists believe the blood and other metabolic pools contribute the fat under the abnormal prevailing metabolic conditions.

Fat embolization is always maximal and earliest in the lung. The mechanisms of impaired lung function are numerous and have been reviewed in Chapters 27 and 77.

Macroscopically, the brain shows a widespread petechial eruption within the white matter of the cerebral and cerebellar hemispheres. Microscopically, fat emboli are widely distributed throughout the central nervous system, being most numerous in gray matter. Their frequency reflects the regional blood flow. Focal lesions of perivascular edema, tissue damage, and hemorrhage, however, predominate in the *white* matter.[144]

As fat globules become coated with platelets, thrombocytopenia develops. Platelet aggregates release powerful proteolytic and inflammatory agents that may contribute to the focal white matter lesions. The susceptibility of the white matter also relates to its paucity of capillary anastomoses.

The result is an encephalopathy with impaired consciousness and confused behavior. Survivors seldom have residua.

Prophylactically, early fracture immobilization and correction of hypoxemia and hypovolemic shock are of proved benefit. Serious cases may benefit from large doses of corticosteroids, positive pressure respiration, and low-dosage heparin therapy.

Neurological Abnormalities After Open Heart Procedures

Neurological disturbances may occur in more than half the patients undergoing open heart procedures. Commonly, there is a delay in postanesthetic recovery, followed by somnolence and irritability after arousal, temporospatial confusion, and diffuse but mild neurological signs. Acute agitation may suddenly appear when the conscious state clears. Half the involved patients will recover within two weeks.[49,90]

The residual neurological deficits are again protean; impaired recent memory and biparietal syndrome are common, however. An interesting study demonstrated that the combination of platelet embolization and hypotension could cause nervous system damage when neither alone was sufficient to do so.

Factors that appear to determine the frequency of subsequent neurological abnormalities are greater age, prolonged cardiopulmonary bypass, hypotension during bypass (mean pressure less than 50 mm of mercury), and fibrin platelet embolism.[4,151,173]

Widespread microembolism and hypotension act in concert to produce the usual clinical picture. Large emboli are occasionally released, causing cerebral infarcts, and intracranial hemorrhage may complicate the use of anticoagulants.

The brain may show scattered petechial hemorrhage and laminar, border zone, and hippocampal cortical necrosis. The frequency and severity of these complications may be halved by the use of filters, ultrasonic monitoring for gas embolism, and modified electroencephalography during bypass.

Prophylactic use of platelet inhibiting drugs may be beneficial. Although no specific therapy is of proved benefit for established lesions, survivors often show remarkable recovery.

UNUSUAL ARTERIAL DISORDERS

Ehlers-Danlos Syndrome

This rare disorder of connective tissue is characterized by hyperelasticity and fragility of the skin, hypermobility of the joints due to increased elasticity in the joint capsule, and a bleeding tendency. It affects the nervous system only secondarily because of the propensity of the arteries to develop aneurysms owing to lack of a normal quantity of elastic fibers in the internal elastic membrane, which leads to herniation of the intima. Subarachnoid hemorrhage and occasionally caroticocavernous fistula may occur.

The disorder tends to run in families as an autosomal dominant trait, and a familial aggregation of aneurysms or caroticocavernous fistulae has been reported.[8]

Thromboangiitis Obliterans

There is controversy concerning whether thromboangiitis obliterans is an inflammatory or an obliterative vascular disease. It affects primarily the arteries of the arms and legs, and rarely the intracranial arteries. Reports of cases emphasize the fact that the disease occurs primarily in young men who smoke heavily. The clinical picture of the disorder is that of cerebral vascular insufficiency and infarction. The diagnosis is made by deduction on the basis of historical information suggesting vascular disease of the legs plus cerebrovascular insufficiency.

Fibromuscular Hyperplasia

This disorder is a nonatherosclerotic, noninflammatory disorder of unknown etiology mainly affecting women. It involves the elastic, muscular, and fibrous elements, and primarily the extracranial portions of the carotid and vertebral systems. Occasionally it affects the major arteries that spring from the circle of Willis.

The first examples of this entity were demonstrated in angiograms of renal arteries, and it is a recognized cause of renovascular hypertension. It has also been reported in the coronary arteries.

Neurologically, the disorder usually presents with a patient's complaint of a sound in the head—an unpleasant pulsing or occasionally whispering or whistling sound—that the patient hears spontaneously in a quiet room or when his ear is placed against a pillow. In time, the sound becomes extremely worrisome to the patient. At times the sound is inaudible to the physician even though quite loud to the patient. In other patients, a murmur in the extracranial arteries is detected during routine physical examination. In such cases angiography is often performed for suspected atherosclerotic disease of the extracranial vasculature, only to reveal the characteristic findings of fibromuscular hyperplasia.

At times, the initial manifestation of fibromuscular hyperplasia is cerebrovascular insufficiency with transient ischemic attacks, and on other occasions an intracranial aneurysm may rupture, causing subarachnoid hemorrhage. There is a known propensity of patients with fibromuscular hyperplasia to have associated intracranial arterial aneurysms. The association first with the aneurysm that may rupture and more recently with the progression of the disorder to secondary cerebral ischemia has led to the conclusion that it is slowly progressive. There is no specific medical treatment, and therefore appropriate operative correction either for the aneurysms or for the progressive stenosis of the extracranial arteries may be necessary.[68]

Moyamoya Disease

This new form of cerebral vascular disease, first described in Japan, is characterized by a combination of cerebral ischemia due to occlusion and small hemorrhages from the secondary rupture of an abnormal network of vessels at the base of the brain. Until recently, the disease was reported only in Japanese, but cases have now been reported in Caucasians and Negroes even though there is a strong predilection to people of Oriental descent. The disease is not considered to be infectious or inflammatory. Some believe the difficulty to be the result of congenital vascular malformation. Others are of the strong opinion that there is primary occlusion of the arteries of the circle of Willis that results in the development of a secondary collateral circulation that gives rise to a network of anastomotic vessels.

As the disease progresses, it produces a focal neurological deficit characteristic of cerebral infarction. There may also develop recurrent headaches, confusion, and convulsions. Subarachnoid hemorrhage may occur spontaneously or with minor trauma.

Arteriography reveals the characteristic neovascularization in the supratentorial vessels. All cases show occlusion of the main branches of the circle of Willis, especially in the region of the carotid bifurcation, with the development of extensive meningeal collateral circulation. The natural history of the disorder is one of recurrent episodes of focal neurological deficit leading to eventual total incapacitation. An intracranial bypass operation has been recommended, but this form of treatment is still under investigation at this time.[134]

Cranial Arteritis

The initial symptoms of this condition, also called temporal arteritis and giant cell arteritis, are usually headache, myalgia, and night sweats in a person older than 50 years. Treatment at this stage may prevent vascular accidents to the eye and brain.

Though it is classified as an autoimmune disorder, the only evidence supporting this classification is the histological appearance of involved arteries, the elevated erythrocyte sedimentation rate, and the dramatic response to corticosteroids.[60]

Pathological Findings

This disorder almost always affects the branches of the external and internal carotid arteries, but it may involve the vertebrobasilar system, the arteries of the upper and lower extremities, the aorta, and rarely the coronary arteries.[89] Probably no part of any large or medium-sized artery is exempt. The arteritis is patchy in distribution, with normal segments of artery lying between severely affected areas.

Histologically, there is a panarteritis with a cellular infiltrate of lymphocytes, plasma cells, macrophages, and giant cells of the foreign body type. Fibroblastic proliferation results in thickening of the wall and narrowing or obliteration of the vessel lumen, and granulomatous panarteritis develops. Damage to the intima may lead to mural thrombosis and arterial occlusion. It should be noted that the histological changes simulate those of polyarteritis and syphilitic arteritis. Care must therefore be taken to consider and exclude these possibilities when a positive temporal artery biopsy is obtained.

Clinical Features

Cranial arteritis affects men and women over the age of 60 equally. Peak incidences occur between 65 and 75 years of age. Almost any segment of a cranial arterial tree may be affected, but headache is most frequently related to involvement of the temporal, ophthalmic, and occipital arteries, one of which is almost always involved.

The most frequent clinical picture is that of an elderly individual with fever, vague myalgia, constitutional symptoms, and a tender temporal artery. He is suffering with a severe headache, is unable to sleep, and is completely incapacitated by the illness. The involved artery, which is exquisitely tender to touch, is thickened like a cord and difficult to compress. The overlying skin is sometimes normal but may be red, hot, and edematous. Ischemia of the skin with resultant areas of necrosis is rare. The head pain is characterized as intense and unremitting, and is localized accurately to the affected artery.

Visual impairment occurs in half the cases of cranial arteritis and is permanent in 20 per cent of these. The most common visual complaint—sudden loss of vision in one eye—is caused by embolic occlusion of the central retinal artery or one of its branches. Emboli have their origin in a proximal vessel, usually the internal carotid or the ophthalmic arteries. Emboli form on the involved segments of the carotid and vertebral arteries and may produce hemispheric or brain stem infarcts. Other ocular manifestations include conjunctival edema, periorbital swelling, photophobia, diplopia, ocular palsy, and homonymous field defects. Funduscopic examination may show the features of a central or branch retinal artery occlusion.

Symptoms such as malaise, lassitude, asthenia, and weight loss are frequent. Some patients have fever (100 to 101°F) and sweats. Polymyalgia rheumatica is closely associated with cranial arteritis and may, in fact, be part of the same disease process. It is characterized by myalgia of a migratory nature, possibly accompanied by severe arthralgia. The patient feels ill and has an elevated erythrocyte sedimentation rate and may have low-grade fever. Neuromuscular examination is normal, as are the electromyogram and the creatinine, phosphokinase, and aldolase levels. Muscle biopsy is normal.

Laboratory Findings

The erythrocyte sedimentation rate is almost invariably elevated, sometimes as much as 100 mm in the first hour. It reaches a peak during the acute inflammatory phase and may continue to be elevated for more than a year. In patients with a normal sedimentation rate the diagnosis of active cranial arteritis is very unlikely.

About 50 per cent of the patients have mild leukocytosis and a normocytic normochromic anemia. Biopsy of the affected artery may show the typical pathological changes. It is important to recognize that segmental distribution of the arteritis may lead to false negative biopsies. Biopsy at times has the benefit of relieving the head pain and is considered essential in atypical cases or in patients who have visual disturbances alone. With a more complete clinical picture, the elevated sedimentation rate and the response to steroids adequately confirm the diagnosis.

Course and Prognosis

If untreated, cranial arteritis usually persists for many months before subsiding. For some patients, the illness is completely debilitating. Untreated, about 50 per cent are left with partial or total blindness and 20 per cent die from cerebral or myocardial infarctions; the remainder, however, regain their former health and vigor.

The course of cranial arteritis is dramatically shortened and the prognosis vastly improved by steroid therapy. Fever may subside within hours, and local pain and constitutional signs resolve completely within one to two days. Appetite returns and along with it the patient's feeling of well-being. When vision has been impaired, the prognosis for its recovery is poor, but it is extremely unusual for visual loss to occur after the initiation of steroid therapy.

Treatment

When cranial arteritis is suspected, it is extremely important to establish the diagnosis adequately and to proceed to steroid therapy. Sixty milligrams of prednisolone or its equivalent in divided oral doses is considered adequate. When symptoms have settled and the patient has been afebrile and without headaches for one week, the daily dose of steroids is gradually reduced and alternate-day steroid therapy is cautiously initiated after two months.[72] Even though the sedimentation rate has been normal for some time, therapy should be continued for at least 12 months.[10]

Takayasu's Disease

This condition, also called pulseless disease and arteritis of young females, bears the name of the Japanese ophthalmologist who so vividly described its ocular changes. Takayasu's disease has a strong predilection for women, but it is not as once was believed restricted to the Orient and has been reported from many parts of the world. Patients are almost always between the age of 15 and 40 years.[58]

Pathological Findings

The disease is often confined to the aortic arch and great vessels but at times involves the entire length of the aorta. There may be involvement of the celiac, superior mesenteric, and renal arteries or the aortic bifurcation. The intracranial vessels are spared.

The vascular lesion is characterized by patchy intimal thickening, longitudinal scarring, and segmental narrowing or aneurysmal dilatation. Luminal thrombosis is common, and evidence of recanalization is often present. Microscopically, there is chronic inflammation in all three coats of the artery, with active lesions showing edema, fragmentation of the elastica, and focal diffuse aggregates of lymphocytes, plasma cells, macrophages, and giant cells.

Clinical Features

Three aortic syndromes occur singly or in combination.

In the *aortic arch* (Takayasu's) *syndrome* involvement of the arch and the great vessels results in a syndrome of cerebral and retinal vascular insufficiency.

The *middle aortic syndrome* involving the celiac, superior mesenteric, and renal arteries results in abdominal angina, malabsorption, and renovascular hypertension.

The *aortic bifurcation* (Leriche's) *syndrome* involving the terminal aorta and the iliac arteries produces intermittent claudication of the hips and lower limbs and male impotence.

Although only the aortic arch syndrome is discussed, the reader should bear in mind that the other two syndromes may coexist.

The classic picture of a young Oriental girl in the head-low position with alopecia, conjunctival injection, and frequent attacks of syncope, vertigo, and visual disturbance is seldom seen. More commonly, the presenting symptoms are those of carotid or subclavian disease manifested as cerebral ischemia or infarction. Some cases present with constitutional symptoms such as fatigue, musculoskeletal pain, and anorexia or weight loss.

Examination may reveal the absence of the subclavian, brachial, and radial pulses, or the brachial blood pressure may be reduced or unrecordable, and pulsations in the carotid arteries may be absent or impaired. The carotid sinuses are often hypersensitive. Pulsations, thrills, and bruits in the collateral circulation of the head, neck, or chest suggest an obstructive lesion of the aortic arch and its major branches, but they are not specific for this syndrome. Trophic changes such as perforation of nasal septum and alopecia are only seen when blood flow to the head has been severely jeopardized. Systemic hypertension and the fundal changes of severe vascular insufficiency are common.

Elevation of the erythrocyte sedimentation rate is almost universal, and 50 per cent of patients show anemia. Chest x-rays may reveal notching of the ribs secondary to collateral circulation. Aortography demonstrates various degrees of stenosis and occlusion of the subclavian, brachiocephalic, carotid, and vertebral arteries. Subclavian steal has been reported. Biopsy of an involved artery may be necessary for definitive diagnosis.

Although there is no specific treatment, corticosteroids have been used in high dosage with good results reported in some instances. Anticoagulant therapy has been of equivocal benefit. Operatively accessible stenotic lesions should be repaired when possible.

This disease is unpredictable in its course, but commonly is relentlessly progressive.

REFERENCES

1. Acheson, J.: Factors affecting the natural history of focal cerebral vascular disease. Quart. J. Med., *40*:25–46, 1971.
2. Adams, R. D., and Victor, M.: Principles of Neurology. New York, McGraw-Hill Book Co., 1977, pp. 501–518.
3. Allsop, J. L.: Carotid sinus syncope. Proc. Aust. Ass. Neurol., *10*:7–12, 1973.
4. Aquilar, M. J., Gerbode, F., and Hill, J. D.: Neuropathologic complications of cardiac surgery. J. Thorac. Cardiovasc. Surg., *61*:676–685, 1971.
5. Aronson, S. M., and Aronson, B. E.: Thrombotic thrombocytopenic purpura: Clinical neuropathological conference. Dis. Nerv. Syst., *30*:493–500, 1969.
6. Baker, R. N.: Anticoagulant therapy in cerebral infarction. Report on cooperative study. Neurology (Minneap.), *12*:823–835, 1962.
7. Baker, R. N., Ramseyer, R. C., and Schwartz, W. S.: Prognosis in patients with transient ischemic attacks. Neurology (Minneap.), *18*:1157–1165, 1968.
8. Bannerman, R. M., Grat, C. J., and Upson, J. F.: Ehlers-Danlos syndrome. Brit. Med. J., *3*:558–559, 1967.
9. Battacharji, S. K., Hutchinson, E. C., and McCall, A. J.: The circle of Willis—the incidence of developmental abnormalities in normal and infarcted brains. Brain, *90*:747–758, 1967.
10. Beevers, D. G., Harpur, J. E., and Turk, A. D.: Giant cell arteritis—the need for prolonged treatment. J. Chron. Dis., *26*:571–584, 1973.
11. Bennahum, D. A., and Messner, R. P.: Recent observations on central nervous system lupus erythematosus. Seminars Arthr. Rheumatol., *4*:253–266, 1975.
12. Bickerstaff, E. R.: Aetiology of acute hemiplegia in childhood. Brit. Med. J., *2*:82, 1964.
13. Blackwood, W., Hallpike, J. F., Kocen, R. F., et al.: Atheromatous disease of the carotid arterial system and embolism from the heart in cerebral infarction: A morbid anatomical study. Brain, *92*:897–910, 1969.
14. Blue, S. K., McKinney, W. M., Barnes, R., et al.: Ultrasonic B-mode scanning for study of extracranial vascular disease. Neurology (Minneap.), *22*:1079–1085, 1972.
15. Bone, G. E., and Barnes, R. W.: Clinical implications of the Doppler cerebrovascular examination: A correlation with angiography. Stroke, *7*:271–274, 1976.
16. Brain, M. C.: The hemolytic uremic syndrome. Seminars Hemat., *6*:162–180, 1969.
17. Brandt, K. D., Lessell, S., and Cohen, A. S.: Cerebral disorders of vision in systemic lupus erythematosus. Ann. Intern. Med., *83*:163–169, 1975.
18. Bresnan, M. J., Strand, R., and Rosenbaum, A.: Jugular venous block associated with benign intracranial hypertension. Neurology (Minneap.), *23*:390, 1973 (abstract).
19. Brierley, J. B.: The neuropathology of brain hypoxia. *In* Critchley, M., O'Leary, J. L., and Jennett, B., eds.: Scientific Foundations of Neurology. Vol. 2. London, William Heinemann Medical Books, Ltd., 1972.
20. Bruyn, G. W., and Gathier, J. C.: The operculum syndrome. *In* Vinken, P. J., and Bruyn, G. W., eds.: Handbook of Clinical Neurology. Vol. 12. Amsterdam, North Holland Publishing Co., 1972, pp. 776–783.
21. Carter, J. B.: Hypertension. Oxford, Permagon Press, 1964, pp. 125–127.
22. Cartlidge, N. E. F., Whisnant, J. P., and Elveback, L. R.: Carotid and vertebral-basilar transient cerebral ischemic attacks: A community study, Rochester, Minnesota. Mayo Clin. Proc., *52*:117–120, 1977.
23. Castaigne, P., Lhermitte, F., Gautier, J. C., et al.: Internal carotid artery occlusion. Brain, *93*:231–258, 1970.
24. Castaigne, P., Lhermitte, F., Gautier, J. C., et al.: Arterial occlusions in the vertebro-basilar system. A study of 44 patients with post-mortem data. Brain, *96*:133–154, 1973.
25. Cooper, E. S., and West, J. W.: Cardiac arrhythmias, cerebral function and stroke. Curr. Conc. Cerebrovasc. Dis., *5*:53–58, 1970.
26. Derby, B. M.: Importance of collagen diseases in the production of strokes. Curr. Conc. Cerebrovasc. Dis., *11*:9–13, 1976.
27. Desai, B., and Toole, J. F.: Kinks, coils and carotids: A review. Stroke, *6*:649–653, 1975.
28. Dubois, E. L., and Tuffanelli, D. L.: Clinical manifestations of systemic lupus erythematosus: Computer analysis of 520 cases. J.A.M.A., *190*:104–111, 1964.
29. Duncan, G. W., Parker, S. W., and Fisher, C.

M.: Acute cerebellar infarction in the PICA territory. Arch. Neurol., 32:364–368, 1975.

30. Dunning, H. S.: Detection of occlusion of the internal carotid by pharyngeal palpation. J.A.M.A., 152:321, 1953.

31. Dyken, M. L., Doepker, J. F., Jr., Kiovsky, R., et al.: Asymptomatic occlusion of an internal carotid artery in a hospital population: Determined by directional Doppler ophthalmosonometry. Stroke, 5:714–718, 1974.

32. Enger, E., and Bøyesen, S.: Long term anticoagulant therapy in patients with cerebral infarction: A controlled clinical study. Acta Med. Scand. (Suppl.), 438:1–61, 1965.

33. Fields, W. S., and Lemak, N. A.: Joint study of extracranial arterial occlusion. VII: Subclavian steal—a review of 168 cases. J.A.M.A., 222:1139–1143, 1972.

34. Fisher, C. M.: Headache in cerebrovascular disease. In Vinken, P. J., and Bruyn, C. W., eds.: Handbook of Clinical Neurology. Vol. 5. North Holland Publishing Co., Amsterdam, 1968.

35. Fisher, C. M., and Adams, R. D.: Transient global amnesia. Acta Neurol. Scand., Suppl. 9, 1964.

36. Fisher, C. M., Karnes, W. E., and Kubik, E. S.: Lateral medullary infarction: The pattern of vascular occlusion. Neuropath. Exp. Neurol., 20:323–379, 1961.

37. Fletcher, A. P., Alkjaersig, N., Lewis, M., et al.: A pilot study of urokinase therapy in cerebral infarction. Stroke, 7:135–142, 1976.

38. Ford, R. G., and Siekert, R. G.: Central nervous system manifestations of periarteritis nodosa. Neurology (Minneap.), 15:114–122, 1965.

39. Fogelholm, R., Kivalo, E., and Bergström, L.: The transient global amnesia syndrome: An analysis of 35 cases. Europ. Neurol., 13:72–84, 1975.

40. Francois, J., Neeten, A., and Collette, J. M.: Vascularization of the optic radiation and the visual cortex. Brit. J. Ophthal., 43:394–407, 1959.

41. Friedman, G. D., Loveland, D. B., and Ehrlich, S. P.: Relationship of stroke to other cardiovascular disease. Circulation, 38:533–541, 1968.

42. Garcia, J. H., et al.: Cerebral ischemia: The early structural changes and correlation of these with known metabolic and dynamic abnormalities. In Scheinberg, P., ed.: Cerebral Vascular Diseases: Transactions of the 10th Princeton Conference. New York, Raven Press, 1975.

43. Gautier, J. C.: Cerebral ischemia in hypertension. In Russell, R. W., ed.: Cerebral Arterial Disease. Edinburgh, Churchill Livingston, 1976.

44. Gee, W., Oller, D. W., and Wylie, E. J.: Noninvasive diagnosis of carotid occlusion by ocular pneumoplethysmography. Stroke, 7:18–21, 1976.

45. Genton, E., Barnett, H. J., Fields, W. S., et al.: Report of the Joint Committee for Stroke Resources. XIV. Cerebral ischemia: The role of thrombosis and of antithrombotic therapy. Stroke, 8:147–175, 1977.

46. Gettelfinger, D. M., and Kokmen, E.: Superior sagittal sinus thrombosis. Arch. Neurol., 34:2–6, 1977.

47. Gilbert, G. J.: Herpes zoster ophthalmicus and delayed contralateral hemiparesis: Relationship of the syndrome to central nervous system granulomatous angiitis. J.A.M.A., 229:302–304, 1974.

48. Gillilan, L. A.: The collateral circulation of the human orbit. Arch. Ophthal., 65:684–694, 1961.

49. Gilman, S.: Cerebral disorders after open-heart operations. New Eng. J. Med., 272:489–498, 1965.

50. Ginsberg, M. D., and Myers, R. E.: Experimental carbon monoxide encephalopathy in the primate. I. Physiologic and metabolic aspects. Arch. Neurol., 30:202–208, 1974.

51. Ginsberg, M. D., Myers, R. E., and McDonagh, B. F.: Experimental carbon monoxide encephalopathy in the primate: II. Clinical aspects, neuropathology and physiologic correlation. Arch. Neurol., 30:209–216, 1974.

52. Goldberg, A. J.: Polyneuritis with albumino-cytologic dissociation in systemic lupus erythematosus. Amer. J. Med., 27:342–350, 1959.

53. Goldner, J. C., Whisnant, J. P., and Taylor, W. F.: Long term prognosis of transient cerebral ischemic attacks. Stroke, 2:160–167, 1971.

54. Granger, D. P.: Transverse myelitis with recovery: The only manifestation of systemic lupus erythematosus. Neurology (Minneap.), 10:325–329, 1960.

55. Greenhouse, A. H.: On chorea, lupus erythematosus and cerebral arteritis. Arch. Int. Med., 117:389–393, 1966.

56. Grindal, A. D., and Toole, J. F.: Headache and transient ischemic attacks. Stroke, 5:603–606, 1976.

57. Hachinski, V. C., Lassen, N. A., and Marshall, J.: Multi-infarct dementia. A cause of mental deterioration in the elderly. Lancet, 2:207–210, 1974.

58. Hachiya, J.: Current concepts of Takayasu's arteritis. Seminars Roentgen., 5:245–259, 1970.

59. Hallpike, J. F.: Superior orbital fissure syndrome: Some clinical and radiological observations. J. Neurol. Neurosurg. Psychiat., 36:486–490, 1973.

60. Hamilton, C. R., Jr., Shelley, W. M., and Tumulty, P. A.: Giant cell arteritis: Including temporal arteritis and polymyalgia rheumatica. Medicine (Balt.), 50:1–27, 1971.

61. Hammond, J. H., and Eisinger, R. P.: Carotid bruits in 1000 normal subjects. Arch. Intern. Med., 109:563–565, 1962.

62. Harrison, M. J. G., and Marshall, J.: Angiographic appearances of carotid bifurction in patients with completed stroke, transient ischemic attacks and cerebral tumour. Brit. Med. J., 1:205–207, 1976.

63. Heathfield, K. W. G., Croft, P. B., and Swash, M.: The syndrome of transient global amnesia. Brain, 96:729–736, 1973.

64. Heidrich, H., and Bayer, O.: Symptomatology of the subclavian steal syndrome. Angiology, 20:406–413, 1969.

65. Hicks, S. P., and Warren, S.: Infarction of the brain without thrombosis. Arch. Path. (Chicago), 52:403–412, 1951.

66. Hilal, H., and Massumi, R.: Fatal ventricular fibrillation after carotid-sinus stimulation. New Eng. J. Med., 275:157–158, 1966.

67. Hill, A. B., Marshall, J., and Shaw, D. A.: Cere-

brovascular disease: Trial of long term anti-coagulant therapy. Brit. Med. J., *11*:1003–1006, 1962.

68. Houser, O. W., Baker, H. L., Sandok, B. A., et al.: Cephalic arterial fibromuscular dysplasia. Radiology, *101*:605–611, 1971.

69. Howell, D. A., Tatlow, W. F. T., and Feldman, S.: Observations of anticoagulant therapy in thromboembolic disease of the brain. Canad. Med. Ass. J., *90*:611–614, 1964.

70. Hoyt, W. F.: Ocular symptoms and signs. *In* Wylie, E. J., and Ehrenfeld, W. K., eds.: Extracranial Occlusive Cerebrovascular Disease: Diagnosis and Management. Philadelphia, W. B. Saunders Co., 1970.

71. Hughes, J. T., and Brownell, B.: Traumatic thrombosis of the carotid artery in the neck. J. Neurol. Neurosurg. Psychiat., *31*:307–314, 1968.

72. Hunder, G. G., Sheps, S. G., Allen, G. L., et al.: Daily and alternate-day corticosteroid regimens in treatment of giant cell arteritis. Comparison in a prospective study. Ann. Intern. Med., *82*:613–618, 1975.

73. Hutchinson, E. C., and Acheson, E. J., eds.: Strokes: Natural History, Pathology and Surgical Treatment, Major Problems in Neurology. Vol. 4. London, W. B. Saunders Co., Ltd., 1975.

74. Hutchinson, E. C., and Acheson, E. J.: Relevance of site of ischemia to prognosis. *In* Strokes: Natural History, Pathology and Surgical Treatment. Major Problems in Neurology, no. 4. London, W. B. Saunders Co., 1975.

75. Ito, A., Omae, T., and Katsuki, S.: Acute changes in blood pressure following vascular diseases in the brain stem. Stroke, *4*:80–84, 1973.

76. Janeway, R.: The art of listening. Curr. Conc. Cerebrovasc. Dis., *4*:17–21, 1971.

77. Johansson, B., Strandgaard, S., and Lassen, N. A.: On the pathogenesis of hypertensive encephalopathy. The hypertensive "breakthrough" of autoregulation of cerebral blood flow with forced vasodilatation, flow increase and blood-brain-barrier damage. Circ. Res., *34*:167–171, 1974.

78. Johnson, R. T., and Richardson, E. P.: The neurological manifestations of systemic lupus erythematosus. A clinical pathological study of 24 cases and review of the literature. Medicine (Balt.), *47*:337–369, 1968.

79. Jones, H. R., and Millikan, C. H.: Temporal profile (clinical course) of acute carotid system cerebral infarction. Stroke, *7*:64–71, 1976.

80. Jones, H. R., Siekert, R. G., and Geraci, J. E.: Neurological manifestations of bacterial endocarditis. Ann. Intern. Med., *71*:21–28, 1969.

81. Kalbag, R. M., and Woolf, A. L.: Cerebral Venous Thrombosis with Special Reference to Primary Aseptic Thrombosis. London, Oxford University Press, 1967.

82. Kannel, W. B.: Current status of the epidemiology of brain infarction associated with occlusive arterial disease. Stroke, *2*:295–318, 1971.

83. Kannel, W. B., Dawber, T. R., Sorlie, P., et al.: Components of blood pressure and risk of atherothrombotic brain infarction: The Framingham study. Stroke, *7*:327–331, 1976.

84. Karp, H. R.: Dementia in cerebrovascular disease and other systemic illnesses. Curr. Conc. Cerebrovasc. Dis., *7*:11–16, 1972.

85. Karp, H. R., Heyman, A., Heyden, S., et al.: Transient cerebral ischemia: Prevalence and prognosis in a biracial rural community. J.A.M.A., *225*:125–128, 1973.

86. Kinkel, W. R., and Jacobs, L.: Computerized axial transverse tomography in cerebrovascular disease. Neurology (Minneap.), *26*:924–930, 1976.

87. Klatzo, I.: Neuropathological aspects of brain edema. (Presidential address.) J. Neuropath. Exp. Neurol., *26*:1–14, 1967.

88. Klaussen, A. V., Loewenson, R. B., and Resch, J. A.: Body weight, cerebral atherosclerosis and cerebral vascular disease: An autopsy study. Stroke, *5*:312–317, 1974.

89. Klein, R. G., Hunder, G. G., Stanson, A. W., et al.: Large artery involvement of giant (temporal) arteritis. Ann. Intern. Med., *83*:806–812, 1975.

90. Kornfeld, D. S., Zimbers, S., and Malm, J. R.: Psychiatric complications of open-heart surgery. New Eng. J. Med., *273*:287–292, 1965.

91. Kurtzke, J. F.: Epidemiology of Cerebrovascular Disease. Berlin-Heidelberg-New York, Springer-Verlag, 1969.

92. Kurtzke, J. F.: Epidemiology of Cerebrovascular Disease. *In* Cerebrovascular Survey Report for Joint Council Subcommittee on Cerebrovascular Disease, National Institute of Neurological and Communicative Disorders and Stroke, National Heart and Lung Institute. Berlin-Heidelberg-New York, Springer-Verlag, revised 1976, pp. 213–242.

93. Lancaster, M. G.: Tracheostomies and strokes. Stroke, *4*:459–460, 1973.

94. Lance, J. W., and Adams, R. D.: The syndrome of intention or action myoclonus as a sequel to hypoxic encephalopathy. Brain, *86*:111–136, 1963.

95. Lance, J. W., and Sommerville, B.: The detection of stenosis or occlusion of the internal carotid artery by facial thermography. Med. J. Aust., *1*:97–100, 1972.

96. Leech, R. W., and Alvord, E. C.: Anoxic-ischemic encephalopathy in the human neonatal period: The significance of brain stem involvement. Arch. Neurol., *34*:109–113, 1977.

97. Lehrich, J. R., Winkler, G. F., and Ojemann, R. G.: Cerebellar infarction with brain stem compression: Diagnosis and surgical treatment. Arch. Neurol. (Chicago), *22*:490–498, 1970.

98. Levin, S. A., et al.: IgG levels in cerebrospinal fluid of patients with central nervous system manifestation of systemic lupus erythematosus. Clin. Immun. Immunopath., *1*:1–5, 1972.

99. Lhermitte, T., Gautier, J. C., and Derousne, C.: Nature of occlusion of the middle cerebral artery. Neurology (Minneap.), *20*:82–88, 1970.

100. Loeb, C., and Meyer, J. S.: Strokes Due to Vertebrobasilar Disease. Springfield, Ill., Charles C Thomas, 1965.

101. Louis, S., and McDowell, F.: Epileptic seizures in nonembolic cerebral infarction. Arch. Neurol. (Chicago), *17*:414–418, 1967.

102. Lowry, O. H., Passonneau, J. V., Hasselberger,

F. X., et al.: Effect of ischemia on known substrates and co-factors of the glycolytic pathway in brain. J. Biol. Chem., *239*:18–30, 1964.

103. Lumsden, C. E.: Pathogenic mechanisms in the leukoencephalopathies in the anoxic ischemic processes in disorders of the blood and in intoxications. *In* Vinken, P. J., and Bruyn, G. W., eds.: Handbook of Clinical Neurology. Vol. 9. Amsterdam, North Holland Publishing Co., 1970, pp. 572–663.

104. McCall, A. J., and Fletcher, P. J. H.: *In* Hutchinson, E. C., and Acheson, E. J., eds.: Strokes: Natural History, Pathology and Surgical Treatment. Major Problems in Neurology. Vol. 4. London, W. B. Saunders Co., Ltd., 1975.

105. McDowell, F., and McDevitt, E.: Treatment of the completed stroke with long-term anticoagulant: Six and one-half years experience. *In* Millikan, C. H., Siekert, R. S., and Whisnant, J. P., eds.: Cerebral Vascular Disease. Transactions of 4th Princeton Conference on Cerebrovascular Disease. New York, Grune & Stratton, Inc., 1965.

106. Marquardsen, J., and Harvald, B.: The electroencephalogram in acute cerebrovascular lesions: A report of 50 cases verified at autopsy. Neurology (Minneap.), *14*:275–282, 1964.

107. Marshall, J.: The natural history of transient ischemic cerebrovascular attacks. Quart. J. Med., *33*:309–324, 1964.

108. Marshall, L. F., Bruce, D. A., Graham, D. I., et al.: Alterations in behavior, brain electrical activity, cerebral blood flow, and intracranial pressure produced by triethyl tin sulfate induced cerebral edema. Stroke, *7*:21–25, 1976.

109. Mathew, N. T., and Meyer, J. S.: Pathogenesis and natural history of transient global amnesia. Stroke, *5*:303–311, 1974.

110. Matsumoto, N., Whisnant, J. P., Kurland, L. T., et al.: Natural history of strokes in Rochester, Minnesota, 1955 through 1969: An extension of a previous study, 1945 through 1954. Stroke, *4*:20–29, 1973.

111. Meyer, J. S.: Acute stroke: Biochemical and therapeutic studies. Minn. Med., *47*:265–271, 1964.

112. Miller, R. G., and Burton, R.: Stroke following chiropractic manipulation of the spine. J.A.M.A., *229*:189–190, 1974.

113. Millikan, C. H.: Reassessment of anticoagulant therapy in various types of occlusive cerebrovascular disease. Stroke, *2*:201–208, 1971.

114. Millikan, C. H., et al.: A classification and outline of cerebrovascular disease II. Ad hoc committee, Advisory Council, National Institute of Neurological and Communicative Disorders and Stroke, National Institutes of Health, Bethesda, Md. Stroke, *6*:565–616, 1975.

115. Mohr, J. P., Fisher, C. M., and Adams, R. D.: Cerebrovascular diseases. *In* Thorn, G. W., et al., eds.: Harrison's Principles of Internal Medicine. 8th Ed. New York, McGraw-Hill Book Co., 1977.

116. Moskowitz, E., Lightbody, F. E. H., and Freitag, N. S.: Long term follow-up of the post-stroke patient. Arch. Phys. Med. Rehab., *53*:167–172, 1972.

117. Naidich, T. P., and Chase, N. E.: Use of computerized axial tomography in evaluation of cerebrovascular disease. Curr. Conc. Cerebrovasc. Dis., *10*:19–24, 1975.

118. Ng, L. K. Y., and Nimmannitya, J.: Massive cerebral infarction with severe brain swelling. A clinical-pathological study. Stroke, *1*:158–163, 1970.

119. Nomura, A., Comstock, G. W., Kuller, L., and Tonascia, J. A.: Cigarette smoking and strokes. Stroke, *5*:483–486, 1974.

120. Norris, J. W., and Hachinski, V. C.: Intensive care management of stroke patients. Stroke, *7*:573–577, 1976.

121. Nurick, S., Blackwood, W., and Mair, W. G. P.: Giant cell granulomatous angiitis of the central nervous system. Brain, *95*:133–142, 1972.

122. O'Brien, M. D., Jordan, M. M., and Waltz, A. C.: Ischemic cerebral edema and the blood brain barrier. Distributions of pertechnetate, albumin, sodium and antipyrine in brains of cats after occlusion of the middle cerebral artery. Arch. Neurol., *30*:461–465, 1974.

123. O'Brien, M. D., Waltz, A. C., and Jordan, M. M.: Ischemic cerebral edema. Distribution of water in brains of cats after occlusion of the middle cerebral artery. Arch. Neurol., *30*:456–460, 1974.

124. O'Connor, J. F., and Musher, D. M.: Central nervous system involvement in systemic lupus erythematosus: A study of 150 cases. Arch. Neurol., *14*:157–164, 1966.

125. Ott, E. O., Lechner, H., and Aranibar, A.: High blood viscosity syndrome in cerebral infarction. Stroke, *5*:330–333, 1976.

126. Patel, A., and Toole, J. F.: Subclavian steal syndrome—reversal of cephalic blood flow. Medicine (Balt.), *44*:289–303, 1965.

127. Paul, B. J.: Brain stem vascular syndromes. Curr. Conc. Cerebrovasc. Dis., *4*:1–6, 1969.

128. Peltier, L. F.: Current concepts: Clinical diagnosis and treatment of fat embolism. J. Kansas Med. Soc., *75*:289–292, 1974.

129. Perry, P. M., Drinkwater, J. E., and Taylor, G. W.: Cerebral function before and after carotid endarterectomy. Brit. Med. J., *4*:215–216, 1975.

130. Phillips, M. L., and Harkness, J.: Plasma and whole blood viscosity. Brit. J. Haemat., *34*:347–352, 1976.

131. Plum, F.: Brain swelling and edema in cerebral vascular disease. Ass. Res. Nerv. Ment. Dis., *41*:318–348, 1961.

132. Plum, F., and Posner, J. B.: The Diagnosis of Stupor and Coma. 2nd Ed. Contemporary Neurology Series, no. 10. Philadelphia, F. A. Davis Co., 1972.

133. Plum, F., Posner, J. B., and Hain, R. F.: Delayed neurological deterioration after anoxia. Arch. Intern. Med., *110*:18–25, 1962.

134. Poór, G., and Góices, G.: The so-called moya-moya disease. J. Neurol. Neurosurg. Psychiat., *37*:370–377, 1974.

135. Reyes, M. G., Fresco, R., Chokroverty, S., et al.: Virus-like particles in granulomatous angiitis of the central nervous system. Neurology (Minneap.), *26*:797–799, 1976.

136. Reynolds, P. M., Jackson, J. M., Brine, J. A., et al.: Thrombotic thrombocytopenic purpura—remission following splenectomy: A report of a case and review of the literature. Amer. J. Med., *61*:439–447, 1976.

137. Richardson, J. C., Chambers, R. A., and Weywood, P. M.: Carbon monoxide poisoning. Arch. Neurol., *1*:178–190, 1959.

138. Russell, R. W., ed.: Cerebral Arterial Disease. Edinburgh, Churchill Livingstone, 1976.

139. Sandok, B. A.: A-mode echoencephalography in the evaluation of cerebrovascular disease. Stroke, *2*:452–455, 1971.

140. Sandok, B. A.: Clinical evaluation of patients with cerebrovascular disease. *In* Seikert, R. G., ed.: Cerebrovascular survey report for Joint Council Subcommittee on Cerebrovascular Disease, National Institute of Neurological and Communicative Disorders and Stroke, and National Heart and Lung Institute. Revised 1976, pp. 96–113.

141. Schneck, S. A.: Cerebral anoxia. *In* Baker, A. B., and Baker, L. H., eds.: Clinical Neurology. Vol. 1, Hagerstown, Md., Harper & Row, 1976.

142. Schwartz, C. J., and Mitchell, J. R. A.: Atheroma of the carotid and vertebral arterial systems. Brit. Med. J., *2*:1057–1063, 1961.

143. Seikert, R. G., ed.: Cerebrovascular Survey Report. Special Task Force of the Joint Council Subcommittee on Cerebrovascular Disease, National Institute of Neurological and Communicative Disorders and Stroke, National Institutes of Health, Revised 1976.

144. Sevitt, S.: Fat embolism: Pathology of fat embolism and its significance. J. Kansas Med. Soc., *75*:299–305, 316, 1974.

145. Shaw, C.-M., Alvord, E. C., and Berry, R. G.: Swelling of the brain following ischemic infarction with arterial occlusion. Arch. Neurol., *1*:161–177, 1959.

146. Smith, J. L.: Unilateral glaucoma in carotid occlusion disease. J.A.M.A., *182*:683–684, 1962.

147. Spencer, M. P., Reid, J. M., Davis, D. L., et al.: Cervical carotid imaging with a continuous-wave Doppler flowmeter. Stroke, *5*:145–154, 1974.

148. Stanley, J. C., Fry, W. J., Seeger, J. F., et al.: Extracranial intercarotid and vertebral artery fibrodysplasia. Arch. Surg. (Chicago), *109*:215–222, 1974.

149. Stein, P. D., and Sabbah, H. N.: Measured turbulence and its effect on thrombus formation. Circ. Res., *35*:608–614, 1974.

150. Stevens, D. L., and Matthew, W. B.: Cryptogenic drop attacks: An affliction of women. Brit. Med. J., *1*:439–442, 1973.

151. Stockard, J. J., et al.: Hypotension-induced changes in cerebral function during cardiac surgery. Stroke, *5*:730–746, 1974.

152. Sundt, T. M., Sandok, B. A., and Whisnant, J. P.: Carotid endarterectomy. Complications and preoperative assessment of risk. Mayo Clin. Proc., *50*:301–306, 1975.

153. Symon, L.: Physiological studies of blood flow in the middle cerebral artery territory. Curr. Conc. Cerebrovasc. Dis., *9*:5–8, 1974.

154. Symon, L., Ishikawa, S., and Meyer, J. S.: Cerebral arterial pressure changes and development of leptomeningeal circulation. Neurology (Minneap.), *13*:237–250, 1963.

155. Symonds, C.: The circle of Willis (Harveian oration). Brit. Med. J., *1*:119–124, 1955.

156. Sypert, G. W., and Alvord, E. C.: Cerebellar infarction: A clinicopathological study. Arch. Neurol., *32*:357–363, 1975.

157. Thompson, T., and Evans, W.: Paradoxical embolism. Quart. J. Med., *23*:135–149, 1930.

158. Toole, J. F.: Ophthalmodynamometry—a simplified method. Arch. Intern. Med., *122*:981–982, 1963.

159. Toole, J. F.: Effects of changes in head, limb and body position on cephalic circulation. New Eng. J. Med., *279*:307–311, 1968.

160. Toole, J. F.: Management of TIA's and acute cerebral infarction. Advances Neurol. *16*:71–80, 1977.

161. Toole, J. F., and Patel, A. N.: Cerebrovascular Disorders. 2nd Ed. New York, McGraw-Hill Book Co., 1974.

162. Torvik, A., and Jörgensen, L.: Thrombotic and embolic occlusion of the carotid arteries in an autopsy material. Prevalence, location and associated diseases. J. Neurol. Sci., *1*:24–39, 1964.

163. Towbin, A.: The syndrome of latent cerebral venous thrombosis: Its frequency and relation to age and congestive heart failure. Stroke, *4*:419–430, 1973.

164. Trump, B. F., Mergner, W. J., Kahng, M. W., et al.: Studies on the subcellular pathophysiology of ischemia. Circulation, *53*:Suppl. 1:17–26, 1976 or Trump, B. F.: Discussion. Ibid., pp. 52–54.

165. Vander Eecken, H. M., and Adams, R. D.: Anatomy and functional significance of the meningeal anastomoses of the human brain. J. Neuropath. Exp. Neurol., *12*:132–157, 1953.

166. Vincent, F. M.: Granulomatous angiitis. New Eng. J. Med., *296*:452, 1977.

167. Vost, A., Wolochow, D. A., and Howell, D. A.: Incidence of infarcts of the brain in heart disease. J. Path. Bact., *88*:463–470, 1964.

168. Welch, D. M., Coleman, R. E., Hardin, W. B., et al.: Brain scanning in cerebral vascular disease: A reappraisal. Stroke, *6*:136–141, 1975.

169. Welch, K. M. A., and Meyer, J. S.: Disordered cerebral metabolism after cerebral ischemia and infarction, therapeutic implications. *In* Meyer, J. S., ed.: Modern Concepts in Cerebrovascular Disease. New York, Spectrum Publications, Inc., 1975, p. 87.

170. Whisnant, J. P.: Discussion. *In* Millikan, C. H., Siekert, R. G., and Whisnant, J. P., eds.: Cerebral Vascular Diseases. Transactions of the Third Princeton Conference on Cerebrovascular Disease. New York, Grune & Stratton, Inc., 1961, pp. 156–157.

171. Whisnant, J. P., Matsumoto, N., and Elveback, L. R.: Transient cerebral ischemic attacks in a community: Rochester, Minnesota 1955 through 1969. Mayo Clin. Proc., *48*:194–198, 1973.

172. Williams, D., and Wilson, T. G.: The diagnosis of

the major and minor syndromes of basilar insufficiency. Brain, *85*:741–774, 1962.

173. Williams, I. M.: Central nervous system dysfunction with open-heart operations. Proc. Aust. Ass. Neurol., *10*:1–6, 1973.

174. Winter, W. J., and Gyari, E.: Pathogenesis of small cerebral infarcts. Arch. Path. (Chicago), *69*:224–234, 1960.

175. Wu, K. K., and Hoak, J. C.: Increased platelet aggregates in patients with transient ischemic attacks. Stroke, *6*:521–523, 1975.

176. Yarnell, P. R.: Neurological outcome of prolonged coma: Survivors of out-of-hospital cardiac arrest. Stroke, *1*:279–282, 1976.

177. Yufe, R., Karpati, S., and Carpenter, S.: Cardiac myxoma: A diagnostic challenge for the neurologist. Neurology (Minneap.), *26*:1060–1065, 1976.

178. Ziegler, D. K., and Hassanein, R. S.: Prognosis in patients with transient ischemic attacks. Stroke, *4*:666–673, 1973.

179. Zülch, K. J., and Behrend, R. C. H.: The pathogenesis and topography of anoxia, hypoxia and ischemia of the brain in man. *In* Bartaut, H., and Meyers, J. S., eds.: Cerebral Anoxia and the Electroencephalogram. Springfield, Ill., Charles C Thomas, 1961, pp. 144–163.

43

EXTRACRANIAL OCCLUSIVE DISEASE OF THE CAROTID ARTERY

HISTORICAL BACKGROUND

Early operations on the cervical carotid artery were mostly ligation procedures for suspected or proved intracranial aneurysms.[11,12] Symptoms of carotid occlusion or insufficiency were recognized in the early twentieth century and publicized by Hunt.[9,30] Fisher, however, is responsible for the modern emphasis on the signs and symptoms associated with carotid occlusion and stenosis.[20,21] In the early 1950's, concomitant with his work, attempts at reconstruction of the carotid artery were reported. Carrea, Molins, and Murphy were the first to reconstruct a stenosed left carotid artery in 1953. They performed an anastomosis between the external carotid artery and the distal internal carotid artery after partial resection of the stenotic segment.[8] The first successful resection of an occluded segment and repair by direct anastomosis between the common and internal carotid arteries was reported by Eastcott, Pickering, and Robb in 1954.[8,16] Thompson gives DeBakey credit for performing the first successful carotid endarterectomy in 1953, but Cooley and coworkers were the first to report success with the procedure in 1956.[10,56] Although Cooley's account was the first to appear in the literature, other surgeons were already practicing the technique of carotid endarterectomy.[25,43] Murphey performed endarterectomies and developed the rationale for operation in patients with carotid atherosclerotic stenotic and ulcerative disease. He and Miller presented a report of 21 cases in 1959 and emphasized operative technique, case selection, and the use of local anesthesia.[43] Murphey had performed the first successful carotid embolectomy in 1949.[41] In 1958, DeBakey and associates described a series of operations for cerebrovascular insufficiency resulting from atherosclerotic disease of the aortic arch.[14] Recently, DeBakey has published a 19-year follow-up of a carotid endarterectomy he performed in 1953.[13]

The Joint Study of Extracranial Arterial Occlusion was begun in 1961, and 24 centers participated.[3,5,10,26] This cooperative study was done by neurologists, neurosurgeons, and other surgeons interested in vascular disease who may be grouped together as "vascular surgeons."[4] It conclusively established the benefits of carotid endarterectomy. Successful operation was followed by significantly fewer transient cerebral ischemic attacks, and when, during follow-up, attacks occurred in the patients who had undergone operation they were usually in the territory of another artery than the one operated on. In addition, occurrence of new strokes in the group who had been operated on was significantly less than in the group who had not. This study and the reports of others contributed greatly in establishing criteria for which patients were best treated by operative or by medical means. The operative morbidity and mortality rates progressively decreased in the decade from 1960

J. T. ROBERTSON AND N. J. AUER

to 1970 until, in good-risk patients, carotid endarterectomy carried an operative mortality rate of under 2 per cent. Additionally, the group reported that deaths during the follow-up of the medically and operatively treated groups were due largely to cardiac disease.

Operative techniques demonstrated the benefits of simple endarterectomy, with and without vein or Dacron patch grafts. In the case of occluded segments or segments destroyed by spontaneous dissection, replacement by vein grafts or various prosthetic materials became routine. Recent operative adjuncts include the use of magnification, close operative monitoring of cerebral blood flow, and electroencephalographic recording.[52]

PATHOPHYSIOLOGY OF OCCLUSIVE AND STENOTIC CAROTID DISEASE

Understanding of the general principles involved in the pathophysiology of ischemic vascular disease of the brain, covered in Chapter 42, is essential to the evaluation of these patients. The most common lesion producing cerebral ischemia for which op-

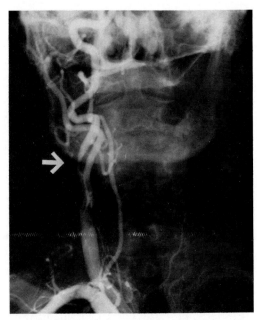

Figure 43–2 A smooth high-grade carotid stenosis.

erative management is readily available is cervical carotid stenosis due to atherosclerosis (Fig. 43–1). The lesion is focal and

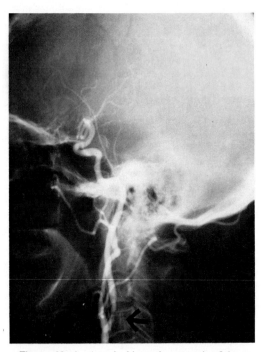

Figure 43–1 A typical irregular stenosis of the carotid artery.

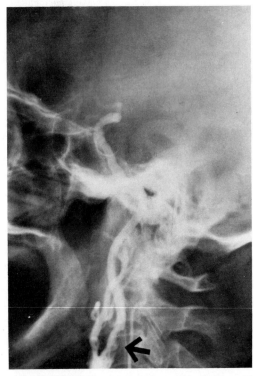

Figure 43–3 An ulcerated carotid plaque with moderate stenosis.

begins in the distal common carotid artery and extends to a variable degree into the external and internal carotid arteries. The atherosclerotic lipid deposition and degeneration is limited to the subendothelial layer of the intima and the inner layer of the media. The process may produce a diffuse smooth stenosis, or more commonly, an ulcerative lesion (Figs. 43–2 and 43–3). The atherosclerotic ulcer may be smooth or filled with platelet aggregates or clot in varying degrees of organization. In addition, frank clot may extend from the ulcer distally into the internal carotid artery, producing partial to complete occlusion (Figs. 43–4 and 43–5). Occasionally, the plaque extends up the posterior wall of the internal carotid artery in a progressively narrowing tongue

toward the skull base.[44] It is rare for it to extend into the carotid canal at the base of the skull. The ulcerative plaque may produce symptoms without significant stenosis by virtue of repeated platelet or atherosclerotic embolization.[37] More commonly, a high degree of stenosis accompanies the symptomatic lesion, which is also ulcerated. Significant impairment of flow in an artery with an isolated stenosis occurs only after the lesion has narrowed the lumen, as seen arteriographically, by 70 per cent or more (2 mm or less in diameter).[44,65] The atheromatous plaque does not inevitably enlarge until the vessel is occluded.[37] It often does, however. The experiences of Thompson and Javid and their co-workers would suggest that, with time, two thirds of plaques

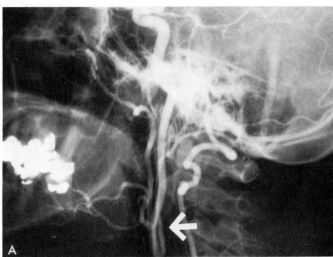

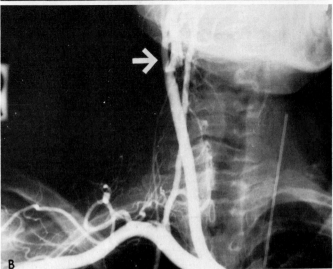

Figure 43–4 Ulcerated carotid lesion with intraluminal clot (*arrows*) capable of causing distal embolization.

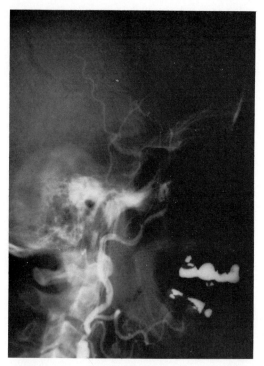

Figure 43–5   External carotid stenosis with internal carotid occlusion. Endarterectomy of external carotid artery may be required.

will show progression of a significant degree, and of those that progress, half will become symptomatic or produce a stroke. The other one third of the plaques will remain relatively stable.[34,58] According to Marshall, the lesion may regress, and recanalization through the plaque may occur.[37] There are, however, no other reports in the literature to support this opinion. Sudden occlusion, secondary to hemorrhage into the wall of the plaque or thrombosis associated with a marked stenosis, is the end result of the process.[33,37,43] With occlusion, approximately three of four patients will have a significant neurological deficit.[20,21,43]

Spontaneous subintimal dissection, a dissecting aneurysm, of the internal and common carotid arteries occurs in 3 to 4 per cent of patients with cervical carotid syndromes.[28] The internal carotid artery is more subject to spontaneous dissection than the common carotid.[1,6,7,29] Usually the cause is unknown, but the dissection probably results from cystic medial necrosis. Conceivably, patients with arteritis or fibromuscular disease could present with

subintimal dissection. Half the reported cases occur in persons under 50 years of age, of whom one third are under 40 years of age.[29] The authors have, however, operated on patients as old as 65 years, and there are older ones on record.[47] This entity may be more common in women than in men; regardless, it is probably more common than heretofore believed. For example, it has been found in 4.4 per cent of a series of 1300 routine necropsies.[28] Trauma is a known cause of dissection. It is considered in Chapter 70. The usual spontaneous variety of dissection begins in an area of cystic medial necrosis just above the origin of the internal carotid artery and may extend well up into the carotid canal. This lesion presents with symptoms of transient ischemic attack or stroke with or without pain in the neck, head, and eye, or may present with a sudden loud bruit. Treatment is directed toward preventing cerebral ischemia or infarction; rupture of the vessel has not been reported.[44]

Other nontraumatic lesions that can produce stenosis leading to cerebral vascular insufficiency or distal embolization include, in certain cases, nonspecific arteritis and fibromuscular hyperplasia of the carotid arteries.[50] Thrombosis with fibromuscular hyperplasia, however, is decidedly unusual.[62]

VASCULAR ANATOMY

The extracranial circulation consists of four cervical arteries: two carotid and two vertebral vessels. The right common carotid artery arises from the right innominate artery. The vertebral arteries arise from the subclavian arteries, and the left common carotid artery takes its origin from the aorta. The common carotids course upward in the neck and bifurcate into the external and internal carotid arteries at the level of the upper thyroid cartilage, the angle of the mandible, or the level of the third or fourth cervical vertebra. The distal portion of the common carotid and the proximal portion of the internal carotid are slightly dilated, forming the carotid bulb. The carotid sinus is at the carotid bifurcation and contains baroreceptors sensitive to changes in blood pressure.[40] In addition, chemoreceptors are contained in the carotid body as well as the aortic body, and impulses from these peripheral chemosensitive cells are carried by the vagus and glossopharyngeal nerves. These impulses may well influence the level of activity of the medullary respiratory neurons. The impulses from the carotid body are carried by the glossopharyngeal nerve.[40]

The first branches of the external carotid artery are the superior thyroid and ascending pharyngeal. Next arise the lingual, external maxillary, and occipital arteries. At its termination, the external carotid bifurcates into the internal maxillary and superficial temporal arteries. The internal carotid normally has no extracranial branches. Rarely, a persistent hypoglossal artery will arise from the internal carotid artery and constitute the sole supply of the vertebrobasilar system. Occasionally, branches of the external carotid, particularly the superior thyroid, will have their origin from the common carotid artery. Rarely, they will arise from the internal carotid artery.[62]

The cervical region most frequently compromised by stenosis is the carotid bifurcation, especially the origin of the internal carotid. Right and left sides develop lesions with equal frequency. The proximal vertebral arteries are the next most frequently stenosed extracranial vessels, the left slightly more frequently than the right (22.3 per cent to 18.4 per cent). The left internal carotid and both vertebrals become occluded with equal frequency. Stenosis of the common carotids occurs with very low frequency, one tenth as often as that of the carotid bifurcation. The portion of the internal carotid just distal to the origin of the ophthalmic artery is the most common location of intracranial stenosis and occlusion.[26] The collateral circulation is discussed in detail in Chapters 23 and 42.

SELECTION OF PATIENTS TO BE TREATED BY OPERATION

Much of carotid operative work is preventive. Operating is indicated to alleviate transient or progressive ischemia, but mainly an operation is performed to prevent further neurological deficit before it results in disability or death.[44,48,53,63]

Transient Ischemic Attacks or Deficit

An operation is indicated in the patient with transient ischemic attacks or reversible ischemic neurological deficits who has a carotid stenosis of 70 per cent or more or a carotid artery with an obvious ulcerated plaque with or without stenosis ipsilateral to the symptoms.[5,44,52,53] The combination of transient attacks and a localized carotid lesion constitutes the best indication for carotid endarterectomy.[42] By conventional definition, transient ischemic attacks can persist up to 24 hours; however, most clinicians would agree that it is very unusual for such an attack to last more than 20 to 30 minutes.[18,20,21] A reversible ischemic neurological deficit (RIND) almost surely is associated with some anatomical lesion but does clear, and this group of patients constitute excellent candidates for operation. The relationship between the number of transient ischemic attacks and when the stroke will occur has been a subject of some controversy. It is generally accepted that transient ischemic attacks are followed by stroke at a rate of 4 to 10 per cent per annum. There is, however, no correlation between the number of ischemic attacks and when the infarction will occur; it must be emphasized that one ischemic attack is just as important as numerous ischemic attacks in demanding immediate therapy.[2] A close correlation of the transient ischemic attack history and the arteriogram is most important. For example, if the arteriogram shows a severe stenosis with greatly reduced distal blood flow or the attack lasted more than an hour or was present on awakening, immediate operation is recommended.[44] Likewise, a progressive or fluctuating neurological deficit constitutes a serious indication for immediate operation.[44,48] In addition, a patient who fails to respond to adequate intravenous heparinization, either by the recurrence of transient ischemic attacks or by the fluctuation of a neurological deficit, should be considered for immediate operation. The patient presenting with a contralateral transient motor or sensory deficit combined with unilateral amaurosis fugax secondary to a lesion in the proximal internal carotid is the best possible operative candidate.[38,63]

Among neurologically intact patients undergoing carotid endarterectomy morbidity ranges from 1 to 2 per cent.[5,44,53,63]

If a patient has symptoms and signs of cerebral ischemia, full evaluation requires adequate three- or four-vessel angiography of the cervical-cranial vessels. This study, therefore, unless otherwise contraindicated, is the definitive procedure that makes the operation possible. Cerebral perfusion may be reduced regionally with isolated severe stenosis. The presence of multiple extracranial or intracranial stenotic or occluded vessels deserves special consideration, because multiple lesions may change the degree of stenosis to be considered for operative correction.[35,57] This patient with multiple lesions must be approached from the standpoint of how disabling the lesions are and, more importantly, where they are located.[62] One study showed that when one carotid artery was completely occluded, a stenosis of only 50 per cent in the opposite carotid artery impaired flow.[5] Another study emphasized that when all four vessels were open in the neck and adequately supplying the brain, it was necessary to constrict the diameter of the carotid artery by 70 per cent or the cross-sectional area by 90 per cent (as measured arteriographically) before a significant reduction in blood flow occurred.[65] On the other hand, after the opposite carotid and both vertebral arteries were occluded, reduction of the diameter of the left carotid artery to 60 per cent produced a significant reduction in blood flow.[57] It is known that constricting the collateral circulation results in an immediate increase in the flow in the patent vessels.[46] A stenosis becomes more significant when the collaterals are occluded because of this increased flow in the patent vessel, which allows the energy lost to turbulence to increase rapidly.[57] Furthermore, there is a tendency to underestimate the degree of stenosis, since the degree of narrowing noted at endarterectomy usually exceeds that estimated from viewing the angiogram.[5]

When there are a proximal carotid lesion and an ipsilateral cerebral artery stenosis, the carotid lesion may be operatively corrected if a source of collateral flow lies between the two, as when the cerebral lesion is in the distribution of the middle cerebral artery. On the other hand, operation on an ipsilateral cervical carotid lesion that is accessible probably is contraindicated when a similar stenotic lesion lies on the inaccessible portion of the carotid artery.[5] This usually means a lesion in the carotid siphon. When this inaccessible lesion compromises the lumen to a greater degree than the proximal lesion, or when the distal lesion compromises the lumen by more than 70 per cent, this tandem situation contraindicates operation on the proximal lesion because the operation would be expected to be of little benefit and, since run-off is interfered with, might even precipitate thrombosis of the vessel.[5,60] When both lesions are accessible, proximal lesions should be operated upon before distal lesions in the same artery or its branches. When concomitant vertebral and carotid lesions exist, the internal carotid lesions should be operated on first because the carotid arteries are capable of supplying a much greater blood flow than the vertebral arteries. Clearly, the continuity of the circle of Willis and the lateral connections between its anterior and posterior portions must be given strong consideration in determining which vessels are operated on in what order. The concept of increasing total cerebral blood flow is valid, particularly if the circle of Willis can be shown to be competent; e.g., patients with transient ischemic attacks ipsilateral to a carotid occlusion with contralateral carotid stenosis of 50 per cent or more should be considered for operation provided cross-circulation occurs through the anterior communicating or anterior cerebral artery. Concomitantly, this lesion that demonstrates 50 per cent narrowing on arteriography may be operated on if the symptoms are ipsilateral. Patients with unilateral stenosis and contralateral occlusion may present with focal symptoms secondary to stenosis or diffuse ischemic symptoms secondary to lack of adequate perfusion. The low-perfusion syndrome can be diagnosed in patients with slowed or impaired mentation, presyncopal or syncopal episodes, transient visual clouding or loss, ataxia, or postural giddiness or vertigo for which no other cause except arterial lesions can be determined.[54] The diagnosis should be made only after careful study. This group carries a higher risk at operation, but the disability of the unaltered disease is also greater, and operation on the stenotic lesion should be considered.[53,54] Bypass procedures available for special circumstances are discussed in Chapter 44. In patients with bilateral carotid stenosis, generally, the symptomatic side is operated on initially. If symmetrical significant stenotic carotid lesions are present and symptoms are not lateralized, the nondominant hemisphere should be operated on first.[44,48,53] Nearly all surgeons stage these operations at least a week apart, and some wait four weeks or more between operations. An attempt to demonstrate patency of the vessel initially operated on prior to operation on the opposite side is recommended. Close scrutiny of arteriographic studies may lead to a decision in cases of bilateral symmetrical carotid lesions; e.g., injection of the left side shows a stenosis similar to that shown by injection of the right side, but, at the time the left side is injected, the anterior communicating artery fills, and this leads to partial filling of the right hemisphere. The arteriogram showing the cross-fill reflects the greater blood flow, and the safest approach would be to operate first upon the opposite side.

In cases of unilateral occlusion and contralateral stenosis, bilateral stenosis, or question about the collateral circulation, it is wise for the average neurosurgeon to use an internal shunt during the endarterectomy.[48,58] A strong argument can be made for the routine use of a shunt unless adequate electroencephalographic monitoring is used.

Neurological Deficit

The patients with extracranial occlusive disease and neurological deficit constitute the group over which an operative versus medical therapy controversy lies. Any form of therapy on these patients will carry a greater risk of morbidity and death than therapy on patients with transient ischemic attacks. Morbidity is greatest and most deaths occur in patients operated on within two weeks of the development of an acute neurological deficit.[5] The risk is always increased in these patients when they are admitted in coma, semicoma, or stupor. Results of operation within the first two weeks following the acute stroke revealed that 34 per cent of patients were improved at discharge, 18 per cent were unchanged, 6 per cent were worse, and 42 per cent had died.

On the other hand, of the medically treated group at the time of discharge, 52 per cent were improved, 22 per cent were the same, 5 per cent were worse, and 20 per cent had died during the hospitalization. The mortality rate, therefore, was twice as great in those treated by early operation. Operation in similar patients after a two-week delay revealed a decrease in mortality rate to 17 per cent. The operative death rate among patients with fixed mild to moderate deficits and unaltered consciousness who were not operated on immediately is about 8 per cent.[5,53] The benefit from operation, when compared with medical treatment, must not ignore or necessarily focus upon operative risks. Patients at high risk are at high risk whether or not they receive medical or operative therapy. Marshall emphasizes that 50 per cent of patients who have had a stroke are dead in four and one half years.[37] It therefore will be necessary to consider operation in the face of significant neurological deficit in the treatment of carotid occlusive disease.[48]

The most controversial issue is that of operation on a patient with neurological deficit and acute carotid occlusion.[5] Granted, operative therapy is hazardous and is not recommended in a patient who has a very minor neurological deficit or simply a transient cerebral ischemic attack. On the other hand, if the occlusion occurs suddenly in hospital, either spontaneously or during or after angiography, or when the patient can be attended by a neurovascular surgeon within one to five hours, for the patient with hemiparesis, hemiplegia, or aphasia, operative therapy is recommended.[48] Support for this position is partly anecdotal; many surgeons can remember cases that were benefited.[48,52] Studies of the microvasculature and progress of experimental infarction resulting from middle cerebral artery occlusion in primates demonstrate advanced ischemic changes after four hours.[61] At 12 hours in areas of marked ischemia, there is beginning necrosis of capillary walls.[22,27] Sundt and co-workers report three dramatic results in 13 patients with only one death related to a hemorrhagic infarction in a patient receiving large doses of heparin for other major vessel occlusion.[53] The patient for whom early operation for an acutely occluded carotid artery is to be done should not be comatose or stuporous but alert, without a visual field defect, and with persistent neurological deficit.[5,48] The arteriograms must be free of evidence of ipsilateral middle cerebral stem or anterior cerebral embolic occlusion. Evidence of collateral flow or filling of the carotid siphon is considered a favorable sign for restoration of flow.[43] A shift of the midline structures and major branch displacement are contraindications to operation. The spinal fluid should be free of blood or xanthochromia. The computed tomogram should reveal no hemorrhage, but it may show areas of decreased density. The operation should be under way within four to six hours of onset of the stroke.[48]

Arterial operative technique is as follows: The initial incision is made in the internal carotid artery, the thrombus is removed, and back flow is established. If this cannot be achieved by simple manipulation or suction, a small Fogarty catheter may be used gently (there is a danger of producing a carotid–cavernous sinus fistula with the Fogarty catheter). If back flow cannot be achieved, then primary ligation of the internal carotid is done. A bypass procedure may then be feasible. If back flow is established, the blood pressure should be temporarily raised 30 to 50 mm of mercury, and the vessel thoroughly flushed while heparin is administered concomitantly. An arteriogram of the distal internal carotid artery is done to reveal its patency, additional clot, or evidence of a middle cerebral or anterior cerebral embolic occlusion.[52] Flow is restored in the internal carotid artery by subsequent routine endarterectomy, provided the carotid artery is patent and branch runoff in the system is demonstrable. Should middle cerebral occlusion be shown, the surgeon should consider an extracranial bypass operation. If additional back bleeding of the carotid does not produce patency in the anterior or middle cerebral arteries, the internal carotid flow should not be restored and the artery should be ligated. Postoperatively, the patient should not be heparinized, and the blood pressure must be controlled to near normotensive levels. The major complication of this operation is hemorrhagic infarction. The routine described should minimize this risk. The true incidence of hemorrhagic infarction in these cases is probably lower than has been reported. Wylie and co-workers reported five of nine patients with recent stroke who were operated on and who developed fresh cerebral hemorrhage within two hours to three days after operation.[63] One hemorrhage was on the side opposite the operation. None of the patients had operative angiography at the time of apparent reopening of the internal carotid arterial flow. Postoperative anticoagulants were not used. Control of blood pressure postoperatively is not mentioned, even though Meyer's experimental work in the production of hemorrhagic infarction emphasized that the administration of anticoagulant drugs or wide fluctuations in blood pressure could produce hemorrhagic infarction.[39]

Some authors advocate only medical therapy for patients with cerebral infarction.[5,31] Most surgeons delay operation on such a patient from two to six weeks to minimize the risk of hemorrhage.[44,48,53,63] In addition, the patients with severe infarcts and whose medical status is poor are excluded within the waiting period.[5] Nevertheless, there are special circumstances in which delayed operation should be performed on a patient with a cerebral infarction. The patients are individually selected on the basis of their capacity to worsen to a hemiplegic or aphasic state.[48] For example, a right-handed person presents with right hemiparesis; speech is not affected. At arteriography, the patient is found to have a significant stenosis of the left internal carotid artery with an embolus partially occluding the left middle cerebral artery. Presumably the embolus originated from the carotid plaque in the neck. This patient has the capacity to worsen, because he could lose the function of speech should another embolus occur or the carotid be occluded.[48] A cerebral infarction is present. This patient is given intravenous heparin, and the rare risk of creating a hemorrhagic infarction is accepted.[39] Only 10 per cent of embolic infarctions are hemorrhagic.[37] Prior to heparin administration, a computed axial tomogram should be obtained to exclude hemorrhage. A spinal puncture should show no blood or xanthochromia. If no hemorrhage is present, heparinization should be continued for 10 days to two weeks. The arteriogram should be repeated and will usually show disappearance of the embolus.[48] Approximately three weeks after the onset, operation for the original insult should be performed by carotid endarterectomy, regardless of the status of the embolus. This approach minimizes the high complication rate seen in operations performed in the presence of a major infarction.[47,48]

Asymptomatic Bruit

There are two special cases in which a patient with an asymptomatic carotid bruit should be considered for angiography and, if significant stenosis is found, should have the stenosis operatively corrected. The operation is acceptable because the risk from the procedure is less than 1 per cent.[44,53] This is lower than the risk of subsequent cerebral infarction.[3] The first case is that of the patient who is otherwise healthy but who on examination has a high-pitched carotid bruit and in whom noninvasive studies show either a decreased ipsilateral cerebral flow or a decreased pressure in the ipsilateral retina. This patient should have an arteriogram, and if the lesion demonstrated is a stenosis of 70 per cent or more, or is ulcerated, operation is recommended.[42] The other case is that of the patient for whom a major operation is being planned for another reason. This is a situation in which operation may be abused. Unless the stenosis is 60 to 70 per cent or certain unusual circumstances exist, for example, a unilateral carotid thrombosis and a contralateral carotid stenosis of 50 per cent or more, then operation to prevent cerebral ischemia during the subsequent operation is difficult to justify. If the plaque shows severe ulceration, however, operation is recommended. Since coronary revascularization procedures have become frequent, some surgeons are doing the carotid endarterectomy at the same time the coronary revascularization is being done.[4] This is justified because of the risk of death from the heart lesions after the endarterectomy and before the coronary operation can be done. Most surgeons stage the procedures.[44]

Common Carotid Stenosis

Common carotid stenosis in the absence of significant internal carotid artery stenosis is unusual; however, the indications for operation are the same in the face of transient cerebral ischemic attacks but different in the face of common carotid occlusion. Serial delayed angiography is mandatory to determine whether the carotid bifurcation is being fed from collaterals through the branches of the external carotid artery. If the bifurcation is found to be open, the obstructed segment can be resected and a vascular prosthesis or vein graft can be interposed between the origin of the common carotid and the internal carotid or the common carotid at the bifurcation. Figures 43–8 through 43–10 illustrate a case of occlusive disease of the common carotid artery. If there is any doubt about the carotid bifurcation being patent, exploration is indicated with or without a concomitant endarterectomy in an effort to reestablish flow from the origin of the common carotid artery into the internal carotid artery. At times, a bypass from the proximal subclavian artery to the internal carotid artery is required. If possible, thoracotomy should be avoided.

External Carotid Stenosis

Operation on the external carotid artery may be considered in a patient with transient ischemic attacks who is shown by angiography to have ipsilateral internal carotid occlusion and significant stenosis of the external carotid artery, provided there is excellent collateral filling of the cerebral hemisphere through the ophthalmic artery (see Fig. 43–5).[5,32,36,62] Additional support for the operation is found in evidence that the circle of Willis cross fills inadequately from posteriorly or from the opposite side. Another indication for operation is a stenosis of the external carotid that must be removed when an extracranial-intracranial bypass of the superficial temporal or occipital arteries is needed. Operation involves the same exposure as carotid endarterectomy. An incision is made in the common cartoid and the plaque is removed by dissection and intussusception. If it does not peel out easily, an incision is made into the external carotid artery to remove the plaque completely and to be certain that the distal intima is left smooth and adherent. Consideration of angioplasty with a Dacron patch or the adjacent internal carotid stump wall is recommended.[32] If the plaque is not ulcerated, angioplasty without endarterectomy can be used.

Fibromuscular Hyperplasia

Although little is known of the natural history of fibromuscular hyperplasia of the carotid and vertebral arteries, it is known that hyperplasia of the renal artery rarely proceeds to total occlusion.[50,62] Operation, therefore, is indicated for the relief of symptoms referable to cerebrovascular insufficiency and not necessarily to prevent occlusion.[62] The disease process often involves a lengthy segment of the internal carotid artery and can extend into the carotid canal and may not be technically approachable for resection (Fig. 43–6). Dilatation of the involved segment has been reported but is not favored in therapy. How frequently this disease produces symptoms other than bruits is unclear. The surgeon should be cautious and have firm arteriographic and clinical grounds before recommending operative intervention. The operation would include, when possible, resection of the involved arterial segment and its replacement by vein graft.

Carotid Dissecting Aneurysms

A patient with a traumatic or spontaneous dissection of the extracranial common or internal carotid artery or both presents with signs of vascular insufficiency or pain or a loud bruit in the neck.* Treatment is indicated to correct acute insufficiency and prevent distal embolization. The traumatic variety usually extends into the carotid canal, and operative therapy is limited to creation of a bypass from the extracranial system. Traumatic lesions are considered in Chapter 70. The spontaneous variety, more common than previously recognized, is demonstrated by adequate biplane angiography.[55] Often seen is a segment of outpouching resembling an aneurysm with a long narrowing proximal to and distal to this dilatation (Fig. 43–7). Close inspection reveals a double lumen at some point in the abnormal segment. At other times there is a long tapering point of dye that may indicate the site of a complete occlusion. If the dissection does not extend into the carotid canal, operative treatment consists of resection of the involved segment and its re-

---

* See references 1, 6, 7, 44, 49, 55.

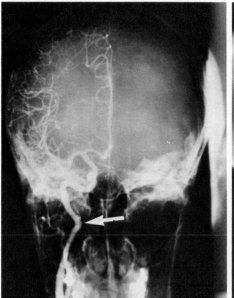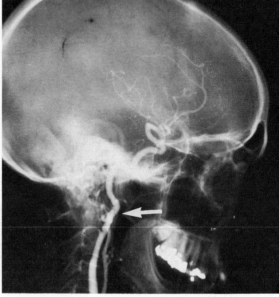

Figure 43–6   A moderate segment of fibromuscular hyperplasia (*arrows*) of the internal carotid artery. The lesion was, and often is, bilateral.

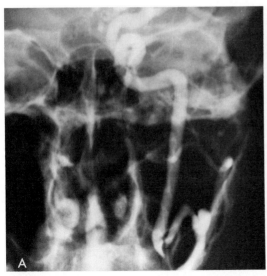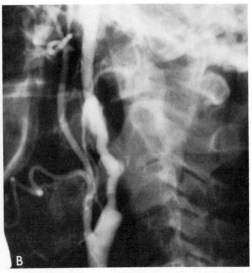

Figure 43–7 Left carotid arteriogram showing dissection beginning just distal to the origin of the internal carotid artery and extending to the level of the C1–C2 vertebral junction. *A*. Anterior arteriogram. *B*. Lateral arteriogram.

placement by a vein or Dacron graft, or an endarterectomy with removal of the intramural clot and involved intima, subsequent tacking down of the distal intima, and primary closure of the vessel with a Dacron or

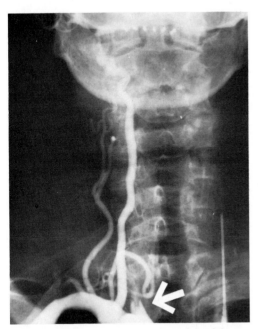

Figure 43–8 The occluded stump of the right common carotid artery and the patent vertebral and thyrocervical trunk arteries are demonstrated. The occlusion resulted from spontaneous dissection of the common carotid artery into a diffuse atherosclerotic plaque. The opposite internal carotid artery was occluded remotely without symptoms.

vein patch graft. When possible, replacement of the involved segment is recommended. Occasionally, the common carotid artery is the site of dissection. Often the dissection is diagnosed at operation. An interesting example of a common carotid occlusion due to dissection leading into atherosclerotic plaque and the operative result is illustrated in Figures 43–8 to 43–10. In dissections that are nonresectable or in lesions in which the vessel is patent that are presenting with transient ischemic symptoms, medical therapy consists of heparin for approximately 10 days to two weeks by a constant intravenous infusion followed by either platelet-inhibiting drugs or warfarin (Coumadin) anticoagulation for an additional one to two weeks and then repeat angiography. At times the artery will heal completely. If healing has not occurred, operative therapy, by either primary resection or carotid ligation after extracranial-intracranial bypass anastomosis, must be considered. The carotid lesions apparently never rupture or enlarge to the point of causing a significant mass. Operation is indicated to avoid distal embolization or subsequent occlusion of the vessel.

CONTRAINDICATIONS TO CAROTID ENDARTERECTOMY

With the exception of patients seen and operated on within 4 to 6 hours of onset, carotid endarterectomy is contraindicated in patients with acute carotid occlusion. Specific contraindicators include (1) the patient with hemiplegia or aphasia or both and with an altered state of consciousness manifested by stupor or coma, (2) the patient with a fixed neurological deficit without an altered state of consciousness whose lesion is estimated to be older than six hours when first examined, and (3) the patient who has had one or more transient ischemic attacks but who is neurologically normal and showing no progressive neurological deficit.

Carotid stenosis accompanied by a fixed neurological deficit should not be operated on immediately but may require delayed operation.

Symptomatic carotid stenosis or ulceration coupled with a limited life expectancy of less than six months from other cerebrovascular, metabolic, infectious, malignant, or degenerative diseases is a contraindication to the procedure. Transient ischemic

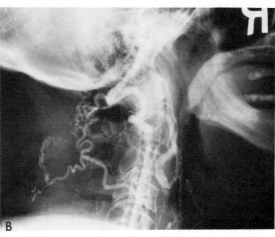

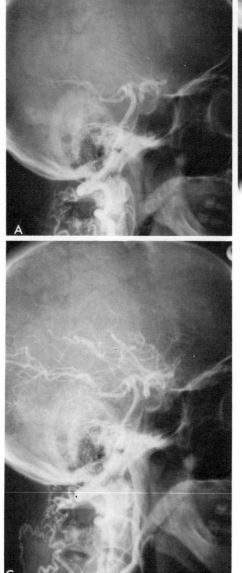

Figure 43–9 Early filling of the vertebrobasilar and intracranial carotid arteries, *A*, is followed by late collateral supply to the carotid bifurcation, *B*, and internal and external carotid arteries distal to the common carotid occlusion, *C*.

attacks in a patient with a myocardial infarction within the previous six months and carotid stenosis with transient ischemic attacks in a patient with severe chronic obstructive pulmonary disease are relative contraindications for operation.

Operation is contraindicated in any patient whose lesions, regardless of etiology, cannot be resected or repaired so as to leave a relatively normal vessel above the lesion.

Carotid endarterectomy should not be performed for an isolated asymptomatic nonulcerated carotid stenosis of less than 60 per cent.[44,52,53]

EVALUATION OF THE PATIENT

History

A good history is invaluable in the evaluation of a patient suspected of having extracranial occlusive disease. The temporal sequence of the patient's symptoms determines the diagnosis. It is important to have several questions answered satisfactorily. Has the patient been having transient ischemic attacks for years or did they begin recently? Are they becoming more frequent? Does the deficit clear completely or do repetitive episodes leave him with a progressive disability? Did the deficit appear suddenly? Is the patient's condition stable? Often, it is helpful to interview a member of the patient's family who has observed the episodes; this is mandatory if the patient is aphasic or has an altered state of consciousness. Risk factors common to patients with atherosclerosis deserve specific attention; e.g., obesity, cigarette smoking, hypertension, diabetes mellitus, and family history of early deaths from cardiovascular disease. Evidence of severe angina pectoris, a myocardial infarction within three to six months, severe chronic obstructive pulmonary disease, and an active malignant disease may be relative or absolute contraindications to operation. A history of hypertension with a sustained dyastolic pressure of 110 mm of mercury should raise the question of intracerebral hemorrhage presenting as a transient ischemic event. The patient's medications should be known, and if possible, long-acting antihypertensive drugs should be discontinued before operation. Reserpine and methyldopa should be stopped up to three weeks before the operation, if feasible. Previously, propranolol hydrocholoride was best discontinued for two or more days before operation. At present, however, unless they are receiving doses of 60 mg or more a day, most patients tolerate operation very well. The use of diuretics should draw the surgeon's attention to the serum potassium level, which should be correct preoperatively.[44]

Physical Examination

The physical examination emphasizes thorough neurological evaluation with particular emphasis on a documented persistent neurological deficit.[20,21] The retina should be examined for signs of increased pressure, significant vascular changes, or emboli. Vital signs, especially the blood pressure and pulse, preferably in both arms, should be determined. The range of motion of the neck should be determined before operative posturing. Occasionally, symptoms will be produced by neck posturing that causes vascular compromise.[50] Auscultation is recommended over palpation to determine the presence of bruits, and if palpation is done, it should be limited to that area of the carotid immediately above the clavicle. Vigorous palpation at the carotid bifurcation has produced distal embolization into the retina and brain.[2,48] If a bruit is located over the lower carotid, it is most likely referred from the heart or aorta. A midcarotid bruit most likely indicates either internal or external carotid stenosis.[62] The higher the pitch of the bruit, the more likely the stenosis is to be significant. Especially important is the presence of a bruit that subsequently disappears, as this is practically diagnostic of a carotid occlusion or severe stenosis.[44] This phenomenon is discussed more fully in Chapter 42.

A cardiac examination including an electrocardiogram should be performed. If there has been a loss of consciousness or there are any cardiac irregularities suggesting a significant arrhythmia, 12- to 24-hour cardiac monitoring is recommended. An echocardiogram should be obtained if an atrial myxoma is suspected.

Additional Studies

Skull x-rays may reveal evidence of trauma or shift of the pineal gland or the presence of intracranial calcification.[37] Chest x-rays determine the presence of cardiomegaly and help to exclude metastatic or primary tumor. Blood examinations should evaluate glucose and serum lipids as well as evidence of hypercoagulability, anemia, or polycythemia.[44]

Certain noninvasive studies of the ca-rotid system should be considered. These include oculoplethysmography, ophthalmo-dynamometry, or, if available, Doppler ultrasonic imaging, as described in Chapter 42. A computed tomogram will exclude a significant intracerebral hemorrhage and may demonstrate an unsuspected cerebral infarction or mass lesion. A spinal puncture supports the impression that there is no bleeding and rules out other disease processes that could present with occlusive disease symptoms; e.g., syphilis. Recent stud-

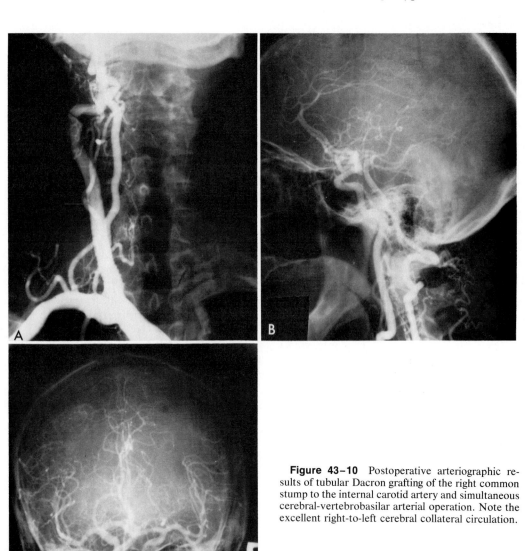

Figure 43–10 Postoperative arteriographic results of tubular Dacron grafting of the right common stump to the internal carotid artery and simultaneous cerebral-vertebrobasilar arterial operation. Note the excellent right-to-left cerebral collateral circulation.

ies suggest acoustically or visually evoked potentials may be helpful in documenting cerebral infarction.[59]

Angiography

The definitive test for cerebral occlusive disease is cerebral angiography. Ideally, the angiogram includes the aortic arch and visualizes all four contributing cerebral vessels. The least acceptable examination should include a percutaneous right brachial and a left carotid injection, which visualizes the vertebral-basilar system as well as both carotid systems. With the advent of readily available femoral catheterization techniques, full arch and cervical vessel–cerebral studies are becoming routine. An adequate study demands visualization of the cervical and cerebral arteries. The carotid bifurcation is best demonstrated by anterior and lateral views; oblique views may be added. This combination insures against overlooking a stenotic or ulcerative lesion.

Magnification views of the cervical vessels may be helpful in identifying ulcerative lesions. An ulcerative lesion is defined as an irregular outpouching or crater deformity seen in either the anteroposterior or lateral view of the carotid artery, which may or may not demonstrate slow dye emptying (Fig. 43–10). Obviously, the angiographic findings and the patient's symptoms must be closely correlated before operative indications become firm.

The risk of angiography in patients with cerebrovascular disease is greater than in the normal population, and the older patient is more likely to have complications than the young.[17,26] The highest incidence of complications occurs in patients above 70 years of age. The risk of angiography is, however, considered to be less than the risk of ignorance.

Preoperative Management

As with any operative procedure, adequate attention to the pre- and postoperative management of patients with extracranial vascular disease reduces complications. Attention to the medications and adjustment of these medications, if practicable,

have been mentioned. Special attention to cardiac reserve is mandatory, because myocardial disease continues to be the leading cause of death after extracranial vascular operations.[18,52,53] Consultation with a specialist in internal medicine may be necessary in these cases, but simple clinical tests like the ability to walk up stairs without angina or unusual dyspnea or severe tachycardia are guides to cardiopulmonary reserve.[44] Patients with chronic obstructive pulmonary disease or who are heavy cigarette smokers are at greater risk.[53] Ideally, cigarette smoking should be discontinued several days before operation. Severe obstructive pulmonary disease remains in the group of relative contraindications to operation.[44,53,62] In less severe cases, vigorous preoperative pulmonary toilet is mandatory. Nutritional status deserves review and correction if time allows. If the patient has been taking a platelet-inhibiting drug, e.g., sulfinpyrazone, aspirin, or dipyridamole, this medication should be discontinued because of increased risk of bleeding. Diabetes should be controlled preoperatively.

OPERATIVE TECHNIQUE

Preoperative medication should be minimized. Heavy doses of narcotics and barbiturates should be avoided to prevent hypotensive and respiratory side effects. A simple regimen of atropine in a dose of 0.4 mg subcutaneously probably is as safe a preoperative medication as any. In addition, as these patients tend to have a relatively diminished blood volume, attention must be given to their intake during the 48 hours prior to operation. If the patient is not in danger of congestive heart failure, the slow administration of a plasma expander prior to the induction of anesthesia is recommended; e.g., 500 ml of 5 per cent human serum albumin.[44] The operation can be performed under local anesthesia, but general endotracheal anesthesia by an informed anesthesiologist is preferred. At present, the anesthesia regimen of choice is halothane, nitrous oxide, and oxygen. The concomitant use of intravenous barbiturates may be indicated for their experimentally proved metabolic brain protection.

Hypercarbia is contraindicated.[51] Meticulous attention to the blood pressure and placing the patient in a supine position are mandatory.[43] The blood pressure should be maintained at the patient's usual level except during the time of carotid occlusion, when it is elevated 30 to 40 mm of mercury until flow is restored.

The patient is placed supine with a sandbag or rolled-up pad beneath the operative shoulder, and the neck is extended comfortably and rotated to the opposite ·side.[44,48,62] After routine skin preparation, which should include the lower part of the ear and the mastoid region, a vertical or horizontal skin incision is made. Generally, the vertical incision, more conventional although not cosmetically pleasing, is used. This incision should extend from just above the clavicle along the anterior medial border of the sternocleidomastoid muscle up to the region of the ear lobe and then posteriorly over the insertion of the sternocleidomastoid muscle. The incision can be varied in length as correlated with the lateral arteriogram. If the horizontal incision is used, it must be of adequate length to allow skin flaps for exposure. Made through the platysma in line with its fibers, the horizontal incision usually preserves the recurrent mandibular branch of the facial nerve.[62] As the vertical incision is made along the anterior medial border of the sternocleidomastoid muscle at the level of the angle of the mandible, it should be curved toward the mastoid process. This maneuver will allow greater exposure at the base of the skull without entering the parotid gland or retracting the lower branches of the facial nerve. The use of magnifying loupes may be helpful.[44]

Sharp dissection throughout the procedure is mandatory.[48] The platysma is divided vertically, usually beginning at the platysma-parotid junction. This exposes the anterior portion of the sternocleidomastoid muscle, which is mobilized and reflected posteriorly and laterally. The internal jugular vein is identified underneath or over the common carotid artery and dissected up to the facial vein, which is carefully isolated, ligated, and divided. The common facial vein usually overlies the carotid bifurcation.[62] The ansa cervicalis, or descending hypoglossal nerve, is identified and followed superiorly to the hypoglossal

nerve, which is carefully freed from the carotid bifurcation or, more commonly, as it crosses the internal and external carotid arteries. The ansa cervicalis can be retracted, but it is usually sectioned. This allows the hypoglossal nerve to be mobilized superiorly. The distal internal carotid artery is carefully exposed by following the plane of the artery. An external carotid branch immediately above the hypoglossal nerve is divided and ligated, which allows the nerve to be dissected superiorly and retracted superiorly and medially easily. This fairly constant artery may be accompanied by a vein and is the sternocleidomastoid artery.[44] The anterior belly of the digastric muscle may be retracted superiorly or divided at its tendon to allow high exposure along the internal carotid artery. The carotid body is blocked with 1 per cent lidocaine hydrochloride. Lymph nodes in the area will occasionally require resection but often can be dissected and reflected laterally. Prior to further carotid bifurcation dissection, the patient is given a bolus of 50 to 75 mg of heparin intravenously. The external carotid artery is dissected medially with particular attention to avoiding the superior laryngeal nerve that lies just medial to the carotid bifurcation. By means of sharp dissection, the internal and external carotid arteries are separated. Meticulous care is taken when dissecting on or about the carotid arteries. Very little trauma is required to dislodge a friable embolus from an ulcerated plaque.

The common carotid artery is mobilized initially, and an umbilical tape is placed around it, fashioning a ramal tourniquet. It is important, as the carotid bifurcation is dissected, to respect the carotid body and to use minimal dissection of its nerve supply, particularly in patients with chronic obstructive pulmonary disease.[62] The surgeon should be familiar with certain anomalies that can occur. For example, the vagus nerve may lie anterior to the carotid. Another umbilical tape is placed around the proximal external carotid, and often the superior thyroid artery is included. The superior thyroid artery can also be temporarily occluded with a separate ligature or with a silver clip. The internal carotid artery is dissected as high as necessary, and an 0 silk ligature is placed around it doubly, while 4-0 silk is placed to serve as a traction suture

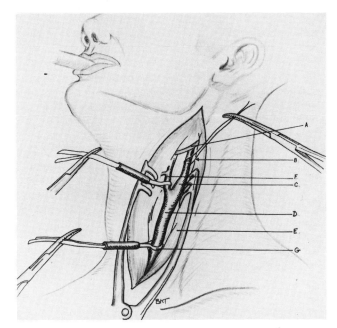

Figure 43–11 Gross anatomy of exposure. A, Twelfth cranial nerve; B, 0-silk ligature around internal carotid artery; C, internal carotid artery; D, common carotid artery; E, sternocleidomastoid muscle (retracted laterally); F, external carotid artery; G, umbilical tape ligature secures common carotid artery.

on the 0 silk. This maneuver avoids placing a clamp or umbilical tape that may slightly but nevertheless critically compromise exposure (Fig. 43–11).

If an angioplastic patch technique is planned, the Dacron patch or vein graft should be obtained and fashioned and preclotted prior to carotid dissection and heparin administration.

If electroencephalographic monitoring is used, the appropriate electroencephalographic leads are secured on the patient's head prior to the induction of anesthesia. If the patient is not so monitored, an internal shunt during carotid endarterectomy is strongly recommended. Chapters 8 and 30 contain further discussion of this matter.

Should the arteriogram demonstrate an apparent clot in the lumen of the artery, the surgeon should give consideration to early occlusion of the external and common carotid arteries or else early occlusion of the internal carotid artery prior to final dissection around the carotid bifurcation. This maneuver minimizes the chance of dislodging an embolus. During occlusion, blood pressure should be elevated 30 to 40 mm of mercury by using a phenylephrine drip or lessening the depth of anesthesia. The vessels are occluded, and the common carotid artery is opened with a No. 11 knife blade. Potts scissors section vertically in the com-

mon carotid artery and through the plaque into the internal carotid artery to normal vessel. A soft Silastic tubing, which has been preselected, is inserted into the internal carotid artery and allowed to fill with

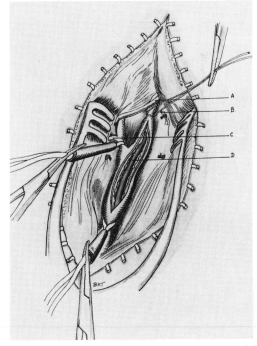

Figure 43–12 Arteriotomy with intra-arterial shunt. A, Twelfth cranial nerve; B, 0-silk ligature; C, superior thyroid artery; D, Silastic intra-arterial shunt.

blood, and air having been excluded from the tube, is inserted in the proximal common carotid artery. The shunt is held in place by the silk above and the ramal tourniquet below (Fig. 43–12). It requires three minutes or less to insert the shunt. Other available shunts include those of Sundt and Javid.[53] Polyethylene tubing is avoided because of its rigidity and occasional sharp edges. If a shunt is not used, electroencephalographic monitoring must be continuous, and the technician must report any change in the electroencephalogram that would indicate hypoxia. At that point, either a shunt can be inserted immediately or the blood pressure can be elevated or both.

A blunt dissector, e.g., a small Penfield dissector, is used to dissect a plane between the plaque and the arterial wall in the common carotid artery (Fig. 43–13). The plaque can be circumferentially dissected by passing a Murphey ball hook between the plane of the plaque and the media of the artery. The plaque is then sectioned sharply proximally in the common carotid artery,

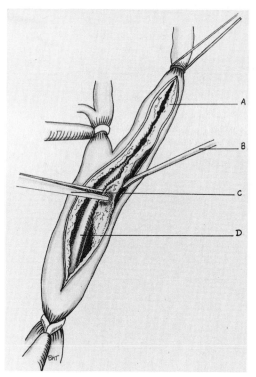

Figure 43–13 Dissection of atherosclerotic plaque. A, Thickest portion of plaque at origin of internal carotid artery; B, Penfield dissector; C, vascular forceps; D, Silastic shunt carrying blood past the arteriotomy site.

lifted gently superiorly and laterally, and dissected to the region of the superior thyroid or the external carotid artery, where it is sectioned sharply at the origin of the thyroid and followed distally into the external carotid artery as necessary to insure that all the plaque is removed from the external carotid. The plaque is peeled free up the internal carotid artery until it can be removed; usually it extends farthest up the posterior wall of the vessel. The surgeon insures that he has adequate exposure of the vessel and that normal intima is seen above the plaque at the time of the original arteriotomy. It is most unusual for the plaque not to peel cleanly without leaving a significant intimal flap in the internal carotid artery. Meticulously, the vessel wall is cleaned of any remaining plaque or debris, and the distal intima is left adhering well to the vessel wall. If an intimal flap is formed and cannot be removed, it is secured by tacking the intima down to the media of the vessel with interrupted 5-0 or 6-0 Prolene sutures. The sutures should be passed from the outer wall through the intima, then out through the muscularis in a vertical or horizontal fashion. The surgeon should make certain that the suture is tied externally.

If an angioplasty with a patch graft is not planned, the arteriotomy can be closed with a running 5-0 or 6-0 Prolene suture; the sutures must be placed close to the edges of the arteriotomy. If a patch is used, it is sutured in place, beginning distally, to the medial wall and subsequently to the lateral wall with a running 5-0 or 6-0 Prolene suture (Fig. 43–14). Just prior to final closure, all vessels are flushed, and the wound is irrigated to remove debris. If a shunt has been placed, it is removed prior to flushing. Final closure is effected after it is certain that air has been flushed out by blood by either forward or back bleeding. After final closure, the external carotid, then the common carotid, and finally the internal carotid arteries are reopened in this sequence (Fig. 43–15). Bleeding is controlled by the application of slight pressure or the use of gelatin foam or hemostatic collagen. The artery is palpated, and if no thrill is present, after a few minutes, the heparin is reversed and the wound is closed. If a thrill is present or pulsation is inadequate, immediate angiography is recommended. If a clot or intimal flap is visualized, it is advisable to reopen

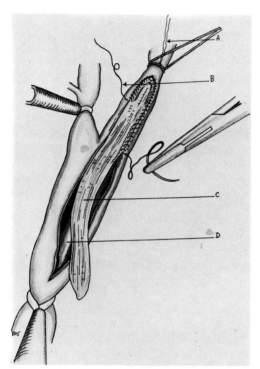

Figure 43-14 Sewing on Dacron patch. A, 4-0 Silk traction ligature facilitates release of 0-silk arterial ligature; B, 5-0 Prolene arterial suture with needles on both ends; C, Dacron patch graft, preclotted; D, intra-arterial shunt.

the wound and remove it. Any time the artery is occluded for more than three to four minutes, heparinization is repeated.

Ojemann and co-workers have described an excellent management routine for extracranial vascular operations.[44] Their technique of endarterectomy differs by using an intussusception method after a graded arteriotomy. This technique is quite satisfactory, but has the disadvantages of possibly dislodging an embolus unless vascular occlusion is done prior to the endarterectomy and, if a shunt is required, requiring that the vessel be opened further before the shunt can be inserted.

POSTOPERATIVE MANAGEMENT

The patient should be observed closely during the first 24 hours after operation. The blood pressure, especially, should be monitored, and if hypotension occurs it should be corrected rapidly. Usually, blood pressure will respond promptly to an intravenous plasma expander. Indeed, intravenous colloid, such as low molecular weight dextran in a dose of 500 ml in 10 per cent invert sugar or 500 ml of 5 per cent serum albumin, may be given postoperatively to avoid hypotension.[44] This hypotension may be due to underactivity of the blocked carotid body. Conversely, hypertension after operation is to be avoided. The systolic pressure should be allowed to rise no higher than 180 mm of mercury, or the diastolic pressure no higher than 110 mm of mercury, in an effort to minimize intracerebral hemorrhage.[44,48] Ideally, if normal, preoperative pressures are maintained. This attention to blood pressure is considered mandatory when the stenosis was of high grade or the patient had cerebral infarction. The blood pressure can be controlled with intravenous propranolol, diazoxide, or a nitroprusside drip. Sometimes hypertension may be due to carotid body malfunction.

Heavy sedation should not be used postoperatively, and it is unusual to require more than 60 mg of codeine hydrochloride intramuscularly every three to four hours for pain. If complications due to hematoma of the neck or obstruction of the artery occur, they usually occur within the first 24 hours. Marked neck swelling should lead to prompt reopening of the wound, evacuation of the hematoma, and control of bleeding.

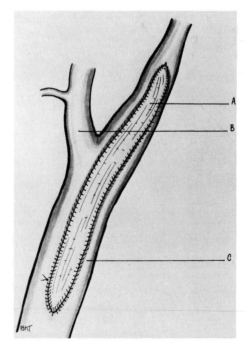

Figure 43-15 Patch angioplasty completed and shunt removed. A, Internal carotid artery; B, external carotid artery; C, common carotid artery.

This problem is manifested by obvious neck swelling with tracheal compression or occasionally with a retropharyngeal hemorrhage. The patient will be unable to speak and will have late respiratory obstruction with the latter. Drains in the wound are not used routinely and do not minimize the degree of hematoma formation. Mild headache is often present in the immediate postoperative period, probably because of increased perfusion in the system. Localized severe headache, however, should raise the question of intracerebral hemorrhage, or in the case of headache localized in and behind the eye and made worse by sitting up, carotid obstruction or dissection should be suspected. If ophthalmodynamometry or oculoplethysmography has been done prior to operation this can be rechecked postoperatively to determine patency.

The patient should receive adequate and continuous oxygen therapy via face mask with careful monitoring of arterial blood gases. Pulmonary toilet must be good, and cardiac monitoring should be continued for 12 to 24 hours.

If the patient awakes with additional neurological deficit or develops a deficit in the postoperative period, aggressive action is required to determine the cause. One routine is to return the patient to the operating suite, reopen the wound under general or local anesthesia, and perform an operative angiogram. The findings dictate subsequent operation or medical therapy.

Postoperatively, intravenously administered heparin minimizes the small risk of embolization or vascular occlusion, but wound hematoma formation may occur.[42,43]

Generally, after three weeks, the vessel is considered healed with regrowth of its endothelial layer. In view of recent evidence, these patients are best given long-term platelet-inhibiting therapy consisting of 5 grains of aspirin four times daily.[19] Additionally, risk factors are minimized whenever possible. Sulfinpyrazone is another platelet-inhibiting drug that may prove beneficial.[23]

COMPLICATIONS OF CAROTID ENDARTERECTOMY

The patients with atherosclerotic disease are usually at risk from widespread atherosclerotic occlusive disease particularly involving the coronary circulation. Recent authors have discussed the complications of this procedure.[15,44,53]

Local Wound Complications

The most serious wound complication in the immediate postoperative period is a hematoma. The hematoma is usually anterolateral to the trachea and causes symptoms by neck distention and tracheal compression. Occasionally, the hematoma will present behind the esophagus and may begin with the patient having difficulty swallowing and being unable to talk. Respiratory embarrassment follows. Cranial nerve paresis may occur, and the most commonly damaged nerve is the hypoglossal nerve as it courses across the carotid bifurcation or just superior to the bifurcation. Occasionally, the vagal nerve can be damaged, and this usually manifests itself with recurrent laryngeal nerve paralysis with hoarseness and vocal cord weakness. The superior laryngeal nerve can be damaged and causes annoying symptoms. This nerve is responsible for sensation in the superior larynx, and when it is sectioned or damaged, the patient has repeated bouts of coughing because he is unable to perceive secretions running into the larynx until they are down into the trachea. The mandibular branch of the facial nerve may be damaged from traction or, occasionally, may be sectioned when high exposure of the carotid artery is necessary. This manifests itself by weakness of the lower face, in particular, the depressor of the lower lip. The arborization of the facial nerve supply usually allows this to disappear spontaneously several months after operation. Occasional patients will have parotidynia, which manifests itself with acute severe pain in the region of the parotid gland when sweet, salty, or sour food is eaten or when the first bite of a meal is taken. This lasts for an indefinite period of time and is thought to be due to retraction of the parotid gland. It usually clears spontaneously. Some patients, usually women, will complain of a drawing or contracting sensation in the mature vertical wound. Occasional patients will have keloid formation significant enough to require a Z-plasty of the vertical scar. This complication could probably be minimized with use of the horizontal incision.

Arterial Complications

Immediate complications revolve around periarterial hemorrhage, vascular occlusion, or occasionally, dissection of the distal intima. These complications can be avoided by meticulous operative technique, and the points regarding them have been made earlier in this chapter. Delayed complications include recurrence of stenosis at the site of the endarterectomy and a false aneurysm that occurs, usually, after the use of an angioplastic technique with Dacron or vein grafting. Ojemann and associates have reported the interval between operation and recurrent symptoms from restenosis in six cases; it was four years in three cases, three years in two, and two years in one.[44] This is an incidence of about 3 per cent. With recurrence, there may be a thickened, fibrous intimal layer or a thin layer of atheroma with adherent thrombus or ulceration. The operative technique described earlier, particularly with the angioplastic technique and meticulous attention to removal of all of the plaque, is followed extremely infrequently by recurrence of stenosis. Recurrent stenosis demands caution and meticulous operative technique. If an atheroma is present, it should be carefully removed, but often considerable scarring and fibrosis or web formation or both constitute the cause of restenosis. In the absence of ulceration or significant plaque formation, a simple angioplasty with a Dacron or vein graft is recommended over endarterectomy.

False aneurysms manifest themselves as sources of emboli or enlarging cervical masses. They require resection of the involved segment and installation of a vein or Dacron graft. They are best avoided by making certain that a generous amount of arterial wall is included in the suturing of the angioplasty at the time of the original endarterectomy. Occasionally, superficial infections, usually due to *Staphylococcus aureus*, will occur. These infections usually respond to appropriate antibiotics and drainage. The infection assumes increasing importance when an angioplastic technique with Dacron or saphenous vein graft has been employed. One author reports treating such an infection with appropriate antibiotics for several weeks, delaying reoperation to remove the foreign graft material until after the arterial wall had regrown.[45] Others insist that use of appropriate antibiotics should be followed by immediate resection of the grafted segment and installation of a fresh saphenous vein graft.

Central Nervous System Complications

The most common complication is the dislodging of an embolus from the atherosclerotic plaque during the dissection of the carotid artery at the time of endarterectomy. Attention to sharp dissection with meticulous gentle technique, as described earlier in this chapter, helps avoid this dreaded complication. Should it occur and should a significant neurological deficit persist, the surgeon should be prepared for immediate superficial temporal or occipital artery to middle cerebral branch bypass. Additional complications include distal embolization with small-vessel occlusion, creation of a hemorrhagic infarction, and local or generalized cerebral ischemia at the time of vessel occlusion. The use of vascular shunting, heparinization, and monitoring minimizes these complications.

Other Complications

These elderly individuals are at considerable risk from cardiovascular complications. In every series, cardiac arrhythmias and myocardial infarction are reported. Congestive heart failure, pulmonary embolism, pneumonia, and complications associated with chronic obstructive pulmonary disease may occur. These complications are best avoided by meticulous attention to postoperative care as described.

CREDENTIALS AND QUALIFICATIONS OF THE NEUROVASCULAR SURGEON

Carotid endarterectomy is one of the procedures that are performed regularly by neurosurgeons and vascular surgeons. It, like disc disease, involves the activities of more than one surgical discipline. The neurosurgeon best understands the pathology and physiology of the brain and its blood supply and should have cervical and cranial vascular operations within his purview. The vascular surgeon, it is to be hoped, after appropriate neurological consultation, approaches cervical revascularization or endarterectomy procedures with technical expertise but perhaps less concern for the sophisticated cerebral pathophysiology. From the beginning, these disciplines have helped to develop the field of neurovascular surgery.

Although operative series have been reported by neurosurgeons and by vascular surgeons, consideration of the operative results of the vascular and neurological surgeons in a large community hospital deserves special attention (Tables 43–1 and 43–2).* During the four-year period from 1973 to 1976, endarterectomies with and without angioplastic technique were performed on 553 arteries in 481 patients on

* See references 5, 8, 10, 13, 14, 16, 36, 42–44, 48, 52, 53, 56–58, 62.

the neurosurgical and vascular surgical services of the Baptist Memorial Hospital in Memphis, Tennessee. Neurosurgeons were

TABLE 43–1 POSTOPERATIVE RESULTS OF CAROTID ENDARTERECTOMY*

	ARTERIES OPERATED ON	PER CENT
Operations	553 (481 patients)	
By neurosurgeons	385	70
By "vascular surgeons"	168	30
Without angioplasty (patch graft)	225	41
With angioplasty	328	59
Dacron graft	249	45
Vein graft	77	14
Teflon graft	2	
Characteristics of Lesions		
Unilateral stenosis—other side normal or with minimal disease	276	
Unilateral stenosis—opposite artery occluded	46	
Acutely occluded artery	18	
Bilateral stenosis, significant	146	
Unilateral operation only	74	
Staged operations, bilateral	72	
Arteriogram not available	6	

* Operations performed by neurosurgeons and "vascular surgeons" at Baptist Memorial Hospital, Memphis, Tennessee, 1973 to 1976.

TABLE 43–2 RESULTS OF CAROTID ENDARTERECTOMY*

RESULTS	ARTERIES OPERATED ON (350)			
	By Two Experienced Neurosurgeons		By "Vascular Surgeons"	
	Number	Per Cent	Number	Per Cent
Total arteries operated on	182		168	
Central nervous system complications (3.7%)				
Cerebral infarction	7 (1 hemorrhagic)	3.8	6	3.6
Local wound neurological complications (2.6%)				
Recurrent laryngeal paresis	1		1	
Superior laryngeal paresis	1			
Hypoglossal nerve paresis	2	2.8		2.4
Partial facial paresis, lower	2			
Facial paresis	1			
Other complications (5.4%)				
Pneumonia	5		1	
Pulmonary embolus	2		0	
Cardiac arrhythmia	2	5.5	2	4.2
Myocardial infarction	2		2	
Congestive heart failure	1		1	
Sepsis	0		1	
Death (3%)				
Cerebral infarction	2		1	
Cardiopulmonary arrest	4	3.8	1	2.3
Gastrointestinal hemorrhage	1			
Liver and/or renal failure	2			

*Selected analysis of operations performed at Baptist Memorial Hospital, Memphis, Tennessee, 1973 to 1976. Neurosurgeons operated on patients at risk, e.g., certain cases of infarction or acutely occluded arteries.

responsible for 70 per cent of the cases, and vascular surgeons responsible for 30 per cent. Fifty-nine per cent of the arteries were repaired by using an angioplastic or patch technique. In about half the arteries there was a simple unilateral carotid stenosis without other significant disease; however, 146 patients had bilateral carotid stenosis, and in 18 cases the carotid arteries were acutely occluded. In patients with acutely occluded arteries and usually in those patients with cerebral infarcts, neurosurgeons were responsible for operation, as shown in Table 43–1.

Table 43–2 contrasts the complications in a retrospective analysis of 350 arteries that were operated on. The experience of two neurosurgeons operating on 182 arteries is contrasted with that of eight vascular surgeons operating on 168 carotid arteries. When it is realized that the neurosurgeons did operate on patients with cerebral infarction and on occasional patients with acutely occluded carotid arteries, while the vascular surgeons did not for the most part, the operative results are remarkably similar. Neurosurgeons tended to record more postoperative specific neck swelling and subtle neurological deficits. Perhaps this is because an active residency program is part of the neurosurgical care, whereas, usually private staff members care for the vascular cases. The neurosurgeons each operated on 91 arteries. One of the neurosurgeons and all the vascular surgeons favored angioplasty with endarterectomy.

An analysis of these data demonstrates that both qualified neurosurgeons and vascular surgeons are capable of achieving acceptable operative results in the wide spectrum of patients presenting with carotid stenosis and varying degrees of transient or permanent cerebral damage. At the time of this retrospective analysis, the data of 16 other neurosurgeons who operated on 203 arteries were analyzed. During this four-year period, the average number of carotid endarterectomies for each of these neurosurgeons was 12.6. This less frequent exposure to and performance of the operation was associated with a considerably higher incidence of central nervous system complications and a higher mortality rate. Clearly, if one is to do this operation, the procedure must be performed frequently enough to maintain competence. How many times per year must one perform the opera-tion to remain competent? This question deserves attention, and obviously, the answer will vary with the technical ability of the surgeon, but one general estimate is that a surgeon should perform not less than 10 to 15 procedures per year to remain competent.

REFERENCES

1. Anderson, R. McD., and Schechter, M. M.: A case of spontaneous dissecting aneurysm of the internal carotid artery. J. Neurol. Neurosurg. Psychiat., 22:195–201, 1959.
2. Barnett, H. J. M.: Platelets, drugs and cerebral ischemia. In Hirsch, J., Cade, J. F., Gallus, A. S., and Schonbaum, E., eds.: Platelets, Drugs and Thrombosis, Proceedings of a Symposium held at McMaster University, Hamilton, Ont., October 1972. Basel, S. Karger, 1975, pp. 233–252.
3. Bauer, R. B., Meyer, J. S., Fields, W. S., Remington, R., Macdonald, M. C., and Collen, P.: Joint study of extranial arterial occlusion. III Progress report of controlled study of long-term survival in patients with and without operation. J.A.M.A., 208:509–518, 1969.
4. Bernard, V. M., et al.: Carotid artery stenosis association with surgery for coronary artery disease. Arch. Surg. (Chicago), 105:837–840, 1972.
5. Blaisdell, W. F., Clauss, R. H., Galbraith, J. G., Imparato, A. M., and Wylie, E. J.: Joint study of extracranial arterial occlusion. IV. A review of surgical considerations. J.A.M.A., 209:1889–1895, 1969.
6. Bostrom, K., and Liliequist, B.: Primary dissecting aneurysm of the extracranial part of the internal carotid and vertebral arteries. Neurology (Minneap.), 17:179–186, 1967.
7. Brice, J. G., and Crompton, M. R.: Spontaneous dissecting aneurysms of the cervical internal carotid artery. Brit. Med. J., 5412:790–792, 1964.
8. Carrea, R., Molins, M., and Murphy, G.: Surgical treatment of spontaneous thrombosis of the internal carotid artery in the neck. Carotid-carotideal anastomosis: Report of a case. Acta Neurol. Latinoamer., 1:71–78, 1955.
9. Chiari, H.: Ueber das Verhalten des Teilungswinkels der Carotid communis bei der Endarteritis chronica deformans. Verh. Deutsch. Path. Ges., 9:326–330, 1905.
10. Cooley, D. A., Al-Naaman, Y. D., and Carton, C. A.: Surgical treatment of arteriosclerotic occlusion of common carotid artery. J. Neurosurg., 13:500–506, 1956.
11. Cooper, A.: Account of the first successful operations, performed on the carotid artery for aneurism, in the year 1808, with the post mortem examination, in 1821. Guy's Hosp. Rep., 1:53, 1836.
12. Cooper, A.: Some experiments and observations on tying the carotid and vertebral arteries, and the pneumo-gastric, phrenic, and sympathetic nerves. Guy. Hosp. Rep., 1:457, 1836.
13. DeBakey, M. E.: Successful carotid endarterectomy for cerebrovascular disease insufficiency. J.A.M.A., 233:1083–1085, 1975.

14. DeBakey, M. E., Morris, G. C., Jr., Jordan, G. L., Jr., and Cooley, D. A.: Segmental thrombo-obliterative disease of branches of aortic arch. J.A.M.A., *166*:988–1003, 1958.

15. Dunsker, B.: Complications of carotid endarterectomy. Clin. Neurosurg., *23*:336–341, 1976.

16. Eastcott, H. H. G., Pickering, G. W., and Rob, C. G.: Reconstruction of internal carotid artery in a patient with intermittent attacks of hemiplegia. Lancet, *2*:994–996, 1954.

17. Feild, J., Robertson, J. T., and DeSaussure, R. L., Jr.: Complications of cerebral angiography in 2,000 consecutive cases. J. Neurosurg., *19*:775–781, 1962.

18. Fields, W. S., Lemak, N. A., Frankowski, R. F., and Hardy, R. J.: Controlled trial of aspirin in cerebral ischemia. Stroke, *8*:301–314, 1977.

19. Fields, W. S., Maslenikow, U., Meyer, J. S., Remington, R. D., and MacDonald, M.: Joint study of extracranial arterial occlusion. V. Progress report of prognosis following surgery or nonsurgical treatment for transient ischemic attacks and cervical carotid lesions. J.A.M.A., *211*:1193–2003, 1970.

20. Fisher, C. M.: Occlusion of the internal carotid artery. Arch. Neurol. Psychiat., *65*:346–377, 1951.

21. Fisher, C. M.: Occlusion of the carotid arteries: Further experiences. Arch. Neurol. Psychiat., *72*:187–204, 1954.

22. Garcia, J. H., Cox, J. V., and Hudgins, W. R.: Ultrastructure of the microvasculature in experimental cerebral infarction. Acta Neuropath. (Berl.), *18*:273–285, 1971.

23. Genton, E., Barnett, H. J. M., Fields, W. S., Gent, M., and Hook, J. C.: XIV. Cerebral ischemia: The role of thrombosis and of antithrombotic therapy. Stroke, *8*:150–175, 1977.

24. Gurdjian, E. S.: Personal communication, February 1978.

25. Gurdjian, E. S., and Webster, J. E.: Thromboendarterectomy of the carotid bifurcation and the internal carotid artery. Surg. Gynec. Ostet., *106*:421–426, 1958.

26. Hass, W. K., Fields, W. S., North, R. R., Kricheff, I. I., Chase, N. E., and Bauer, R. B.: Joint study of extracranial arterial occlusion. II Arteriography techniques, sites, and complications. J.A.M.A., *203*:159–166, 1968.

27. Hudgins, W. R., and Garcia, J. H.: Transorbital approach to the middle cerebral artery of the squirrel monkey: A technique for experimental cerebral infarction applicable to ultrastructural studies. Stroke, V. *1*:107–111, 1970.

28. Hulquist, G. T.: Uber Thrombose und Embolie der Arteria carotis und hierbei vorkommende Gehirnveranderungen. Pathologisch-anatomische Studien. Jena, Germany, Gustav Fischer, 1942, p. 25.

29. Humphrey, J. G., and Newton, T. H.: Internal carotid artery occlusion in young adults. Brain, *83*:565–578, 1960.

30. Hunt, J. R.: The role of the carotid arteries in the causation of vascular lesions of the brain, with remarks on certain special features of symptomatology. Amer. J. Med. Sci., *147*:704–713, 1914.

31. Hutchinson, E. C.: Management of cerebral infarction. *In* Ross-Russell, R. W., ed.: Cerebral Arterial Disease. London, Churchill Livingstone, 1976, pp. 158–180.

32. Jackson, B. G.: The external carotid as a brain collateral. Amer. J. Surg., *113*:375–378, 1967.

33. Jaques, L. G.: Anticoagulant Therapy. Springfield, Ill., Charles C Thomas, 1965.

34. Javid, H., Ostermiller, W. E., Jr., Hengesh, J. W., et al.: Natural history of carotid bifurcation atheroma. Surgery, *67*:80–86, 1970.

35. Kindt, G. W., Youmans, J. R., and Albrand, O.: Factors influencing the autoregulation of the cerebral blood flow during hypotension and hypertension. J. Neurosurg., *26*:299–305, 1967.

36. LePere, R. H., and Hardy, R. C.: Surgical improvement of collateral circulation to the brain. Texas Med. J., *62*:55–58, 1966.

37. Marshall, J.: The Management of Cerebrovascular Disease. 3rd Ed. Oxford, Blackwell Scientific Publications, 1976.

38. Marshall, J., and Meadows, S.: The natural history of amaurosis fugax. Brain, *91*:419–434, 1968.

39. Meyer, J. S.: Importance of ischemic damage to small vessels in experimental cerebral infarction. J. Neuropath. Exp. Neurol., *17*:571–585, 1958.

40. Mountcastle, V. B.: Medical Physiology. Vol. 2. 13th Ed. St. Louis, C. V. Mosby Co. 1974, pp. 1440–1441.

41. Murphey, F.: Presentation at the meeting of the Academy of Neurological Surgery, Bal Harbour, Florida, 1953.

42. Murphey, F., and MacCubbin, D. A.: Carotid endarterectomy. A long-term follow-up study. J. Neurosurg., *23*:156–168, 1965.

43. Murphey, F., and Miller, J. H.: Carotid insufficiency: Diagnosis and surgical treatment. J. Neurosurg., *16*:1–23, 1959.

44. Ojemann, R. G., Crowell, R. M., Roberson, G. H., and Fisher, C. M.: The surgical treatment of extracranial carotid occlusive disease. Clin. Neurosurg., *22*:214–263, 1975.

45. Raskind, R., and Doria, A.: Wound complications following carotid endarterectomy: Report of two cases. Vasc. Surg., *1*:127–135, 1967.

46. Roberts, B., Hardesty, W. H., Holling, H. E., et al.: Studies on extracranial cerebral blood flow. Surgery, *56*:826–833, 1964.

47. Robertson, J. T.: Personal experience in three cases, 1976–1977.

48. Robertson, J. T.: Presidential address: A neurosurgical approach to the therapy of extracranial occlusive disease. Clin. Neurosurg., *23*:1–11, 1976.

49. Roome, N. S., Jr., and Aberfield, D. C.: Spontaneous dissecting aneurysm of the internal carotid artery. Arch. Neurol. (Chicago), *34*:251–252, 1977.

50. Ross-Russell, R. W.: Cerebral Arterial Disease. London, Churchill Livingstone, 1976, pp. 287–316.

51. Smith, A. L.: Barbiturate protection in cerebral hypoxia. Anesthesiology, *47*:285–293, 1977.

52. Sundt, T. M., Jr., Sandok, B. A., and Houser, O. W.: The selection of patients for intracranial and extracranial surgery for cerebrovascular occlusive disease. Clin. Neurosurg., *22*:185–198, 1975.

53. Sundt, T. M., Jr., Sandok, B. A., and Whisnant, J.

P.: Carotid endarterectomy: Complications and preoperative assessment of risk. Mayo Clin. Proc., *50*:301–306, 1975.

54. Tew, J. M., Jr.: Reconstructive intracranial vascular surgery for prevention of stroke. Clin. Neurosurg., *22*:264–280, 1975.

55. Thapedi, I. M., Ashenhurst, E. M., and Rozdilisky, B.: Spontaneous dissecting aneurysm of the internal carotid in the neck: Report of a case and review of the literature. Arch. Neurol. (Chicago), *23*:549–554, 1970.

56. Thompson, J. E.: The development of carotid artery surgery. Arch. Surg. (Chicago), *107*:643–647, 1973.

57. Thompson, J. E., and Patman, R. D.: Endarterectomy for asymptomatic carotid bruits. Heart Bull., *19*:116–120, 1970.

58. Thompson, J. E., Austin, D. J., and Patman, R. D.: Carotid endarterectomy for cerebrovascular insufficiency: Long-term results in 592 patients followed up to 13 years. Ann. Surg., *172*:663–679, 1970.

59. Upton, A.: Personal communication, 1978.

60. Von Ruden, W. J., Blaisdell, F. W., Hall, A. D., et al.: Multiple arterial stenosis: Effect on blood flow. Arch. Surg. (Chicago), *89*:307–315, 1964.

61. Waltz, A. G., and Sundt, T. M.: The microvasculature and microcirculation of the cerebral cortex after arterial occlusion. Brain, *90*:681–696, 1967.

62. Wylie, E. J., and Ehrenfield, W. K.: Extracranial Occlusive Cerebrovascular Disease. Philadelphia, W. B. Saunders Co., 1970.

63. Wylie, E. J., Hein, M. F., and Adams, J. E.: Intracranial hemorrhage following surgical revascularization for treatment of acute strokes. J. Neurosurg., *21*:212–215, 1964.

64. Youmans, J. R., and Kindt, G. W.: Effect of carotid artery impairment on blood flow through a constricted carotid artery. Circulation, *36*:suppl. 2:276, 1967.

65. Youmans, J. R., and Kindt, G. W.: Influence of multiple vessel impairment on carotid blood flow in the monkey. J. Neurosurg., *29*:135–138, 1968.

44

EXTRACRANIAL TO INTRACRANIAL ARTERIAL ANASTOMOSIS

For more than a quarter of a century effort has been directed toward establishing new collateral circulation to the brain by operative means. In 1950 Henschen described an operation by the term "Encephalo-Myo-Synangiose" in which the temporalis muscle was mobilized as a large pedicle flap, passed beneath an osteoplastic craniotomy, and positioned over the surface of the brain in the hope of stimulating ingrowth of new blood vessels into the brain.[81] The patient had a history of seizures and, by arteriography, demonstrated bilateral internal carotid artery stenosis. Following operation the seizures were relieved, but arteriographic proof of function of the graft was never obtained.

In 1951, Fisher acknowledged the potential of applying the newly developing operative techniques to the cerebral circulation. He stated that "It is even conceivable that some day vascular surgery will find a way to by-pass the occluded portion of the artery during the period of ominous fleeting symptoms. Anastomosis of the external carotid artery, or one of its branches, with the internal carotid artery above the area of narrowing should be feasible."[59] In 1963 Woringer and Kunlin reported the placing of a saphenous vein graft between the common carotid artery (end-to-side anastomosis) and the intracranial portion of the internal carotid artery (end-to-end anastomosis) for bypass of an internal carotid artery occlusion.[180] The patient died; however, this type of operation was successfully performed by Lougheed and associates in 1971 and has been developed further by others in a small number of patients.[100,104,117,169,171]

In 1965 Pool and Potts reported having inserted, in 1951, a plastic tube between the superficial temporal artery and the distal portion of the left anterior cerebral artery after trapping an aneurysm at the callosomarginal branch.[125] The patient is known to have been well and employed for at least 12 years, but arteriography performed 10 days after the operation demonstrated that the shunt was not functioning.

Interest in cerebral revascularization had posed two basic questions that seemed beyond a practical solution: (1) Is it possible to identify individuals threatened by stroke and to perform an operation in time to prevent cerebral infarction? (2) In view of the small size of cerebral arteries, their relative inaccessibility, and the requirement of the brain for continuous perfusion, is there a feasible operative technique for cerebral revascularization?

A transient ischemic attack is defined as the sudden onset of focal ischemic neurological deficit that clears in less than 24 hours. Recognition of these attacks as a precursor of a stroke has partially resolved the problem of identifying the individual who is threatened by a stroke and needs to have an operation to prevent a cerebral infarction.[17] Unfortunately, several studies have shown that a majority of stroke patients did not experience premonitory

O. H. REICHMAN

symptoms of a transient ischemic attack and would not have been presumed to be endangered.[107,179] Also, one of those studies reported that 42 of 58 patients (72.4 per cent) had only a single episode of ischemia before the occurrence of cerebral infarction.[107] Nevertheless, numerous studies have developed a more precise definition of a transient ischemic attack, clarified its natural history and the likelihood of a subsequent stroke, identified risk factors, related ischemic episodes to specific arteriographic findings, and summarized experience with various types of therapy.* These studies have been particularly important in identifying stroke-prone individuals and recommending appropriate guidelines for diagnostic evaluation and treatment.[16,148,174]

The second question was resolved by Yaşargil and Donaghy in 1967 by applying micro-operative techniques to creation of an anastomosis between the superficial temporal artery and a cortical branch of the middle cerebral artery.[44,183] The superficial temporal artery is located in an extracranial position closely approximating the intracranial middle cerebral artery territory, the most common site of ischemia resulting from occlusive disease of the internal carotid or middle cerebral artery. It is also accessible to cortical middle cerebral artery branches for anastomosis. It was reasoned that good collateral circulation exists between cortical branches of the middle cerebral artery; hence, temporary interruption of the flow through one of the branches, as required during anastomosis, would not subject the dependent cerebral tissue to ischemia as would the temporary occlusion of the arterial trunk. Furthermore, cortical vessels are readily accessible without manipulation or retraction of the brain and are relatively free of arterial disease.

Micro-operative techniques have facilitated anastomosis between small undiseased vessels with reliable long-term patency.[40,41,54,184] In spite of the small size of the new collateral channel resulting from anastomosis of the superficial temporal to the middle cerebral artery, a significant volume of blood flow can be derived from this source as from other small collateral vessels such as the anterior communicating,

posterior communicating, and ophthalmic arteries.

Early impressions of the superficial temporal to middle cerebral arterial anastomosis were reported as encouraging by several investigators.[12,29,42,72,136] Many investigators now recognize this procedure as a reliable method for establishing a new pathway of collateral circulation to the brain and have reported significant clinical experience.† During the past decade several books have been published that summarize the proceedings of symposia and document, in a comprehensive way, the history and development of microvascular neurological surgery.‡

The patency rate achieved with anastomosis of the superficial temporal artery to the middle cerebral artery is better than 90 per cent. The collateral pathways increase in size with time and provide significant volumes of blood flow for cerebral perfusion. Clinically, the operation is well-tolerated, rarely associated with complications, rarely followed by new ischemic events, and considered clearly beneficial under several well-defined circumstances.

SUPERFICIAL TEMPORAL ARTERY TO MIDDLE CEREBRAL ARTERY ANASTOMOSIS

Operative Technique

The operation is performed in a way that is quite similar to that originally described by Yaşargil. Several options, modifications, and improvements have, however, been developed by subsequent investigators.§ It is important for a neurological surgeon to have extensive laboratory experience to acquire skillful micro-operative techniques before applying them clinically.

An arterial pressure line is inserted for the continuous monitoring of arterial blood pressure, which is maintained at normotensive levels throughout the operation. After the hair is clipped, the patient is placed in

---

* See references 19, 21, 48, 57, 87, 98, 177, 178.

† See references 11, 27, 70, 83, 93, 101, 111, 123, 131, 144, 146, 167, 170, 186.
‡ See references 9, 43, 55, 77, 95, 110, 128, 150, 182.
§ See references 47, 53, 64, 67, 96, 118, 122, 135, 140, 141, 169, 171.

the supine position and endotracheal anesthesia is established. The shoulder on the side of the proposed operation is elevated with a sandbag, and the head is secured in lateral position with three-point cranial fixation. The head should be positioned so that the cortical artery is at the highest point in the operative exposure and subsequently, as the anastomosis is performed, cerebrospinal fluid, blood, and irrigating fluids will drain away rather than obscure vision. Since the largest cortical branches of the middle cerebral artery are located at the posterior end of the sylvian fissure, the

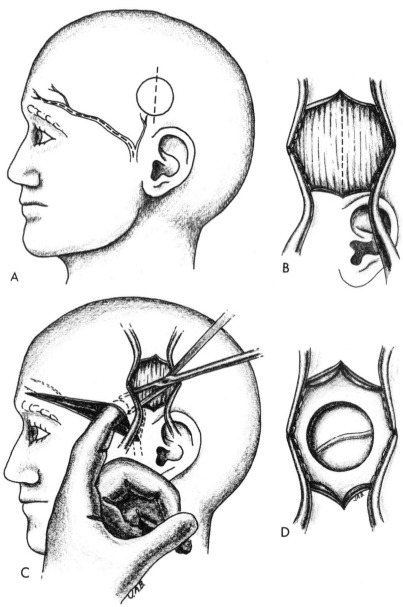

Figure 44–1   Technique for preparing the frontal branch of the superficial temporal artery. *A*. An incision (*broken line*) is placed directly over the artery, which has been localized by preoperative arteriographic films, palpation, and a Doppler ultrasonic probe. A second incision (*broken line*) is placed above the ear so that the center of the craniectomy (*circle*) will be located 6 cm above the external auditory canal. *B*. A retractor exposes the temporalis muscle, which is split (*broken line*) vertically in the direction of its fibers. *C*. A subgaleal tunnel is developed over the temporalis fascia between the two incisions for directing the graft artery to the craniectomy. *D*. Although the angular cortical artery is preferred, the largest branch of the middle cerebral artery is usually selected.

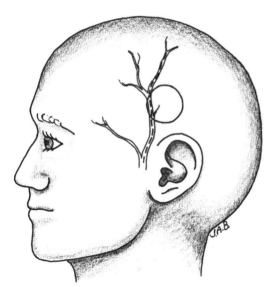

Figure 44-2 Technique for preparing a vertically directed parietal branch of the superficial temporal artery. The incision (*broken line*) is placed directly over the artery. After the artery is dissected from its bed, the same incision will be retracted open for preparation of the craniectomy.

head should be in full lateral position. It may be helpful to rotate the operating table laterally to accomplish this, particularly if the patient has limited neck motion. Usually, however, it is not necessary to place the entire patient in full lateral decubitus position. The scalp is prepared in the usual manner.

The position of the superficial temporal artery and its anatomical configuration are identified by preoperative arteriographic films, palpation, and a Doppler ultrasonic probe. The scalp incision should be planned for optimal use of the donor scalp artery and, in addition, exposure of the posterior end of the sylvian fissure. This can be accomplished in several ways (Figs. 44–1 to 44–5). One is selected that is most favorable for the anatomical arrangement presented by the patient. Usually, it is convenient to expose the donor artery through an incision meticulously placed directly over the artery. When the frontal branch of the superficial temporal artery is selected, a second incision is placed above the ear to expose the posterior sylvian region, and a subgaleal tunnel is developed between the two incisions for passing the free end of the donor artery into proper intracranial position (Fig. 44–1). If the parietal branch of the artery is selected, it may be possible to

expose it and the sylvian fissure through the same incision (Fig. 44–2). This maneuver can be accomplished directly when the parietal branch takes a posterior course, but will require a posterior extension of the incision at its superior extent if the parietal branch is directed anteriorly. In this situation exposure from the undersurface of a scalp flap may be desirable as an alternative method (Fig. 44–3). A scalp flap is generally preferred when both branches of the superficial temporal artery are to be used for anastomosis to two individual cortical arteries (Fig. 44–4).[137] When the superficial temporal artery is not well developed, the occipital artery may be selected as a donor vessel (Figs. 44–5 and 44–6).[157] If a suitable scalp artery does not exist, a free vein or radial artery or, perhaps, a prosthetic graft may serve as a possible alternative.[8,51,163,164] In the event that an intervening graft should be employed, past experience would favor an end-to-side anastomosis at each end (this has less tendency to develop a stricture than does an end-to-end one) (Fig. 44–7).

Under magnification, the donor scalp artery is meticulously dissected from its soft-

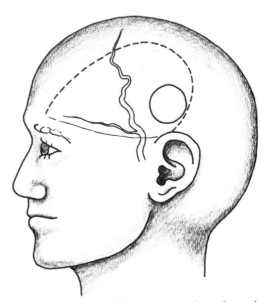

Figure 44-3 Technique for preparing a forward-directed parietal branch of the superficial temporal artery. A scalp flap (*broken line*) is made to include the parietal branch and the craniectomy site. An alternative method is to place an incision directly over the artery, angling it posteriorly from its superior end along the *broken line* for a sufficient distance to expose the craniectomy site.

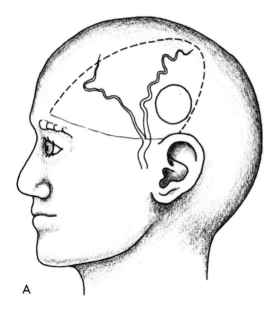

A

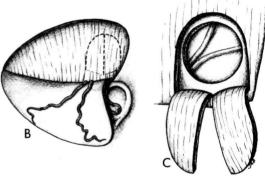

B

C

Figure 44–4 Technique for preparing both frontal and parietal branches of the superficial temporal artery. *A.* A scalp flap (*broken line*) is prepared so that both branches of the artery are included and the craniectomy site is exposed. *B.* After the scalp flap is developed, both arterial branches are dissected from the undersurface. The temporalis muscle is opened (*broken lines*) in the form of two triangular flaps. *C.* When both branches of the artery are used, a larger craniectomy may be required to expose two separate cortical arteries.

tissue bed with small sharp-pointed scissors; bipolar coagulation is used for many tiny branches (under saline irrigation), and ligation for a few larger branches (6-0 silk). The artery is dissected proximally to a level approaching the external auditory canal

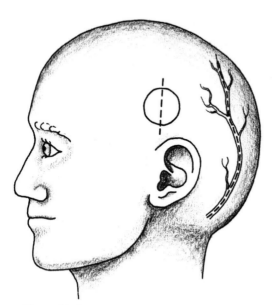

Figure 44–5 Technique for preparing the occipital artery. An incision (*broken line*) is placed directly over the artery and the dissection is carried proximally through dense cervical fascia. The craniectomy is prepared as shown in Figure 44–1, and the occipital artery is directed through a subgaleal tunnel to the craniectomy for anastomosis.

and distally, if its caliber permits, for a length of at least 8 cm. This length will afford flexibility later in routing the donor artery to the branch of the middle cerebral artery to streamline the flow of blood retrograde toward the trifurcation. Sufficient perivascular tissue is retained surrounding the scalp artery to protect it from desiccation, to manipulate it atraumatically, and to insure arterial and venous circulation in the vasa vasorum of the graft artery. The artery is protected in continuity within a moist rubber sleeve, obtained from the finger of a surgical glove, until required for anastomosis.

The temporalis fascia and muscle are opened in a manner that will place the center of a 2.5-cm craniectomy 6 cm above the external auditory canal. The bipolar coagulator is used to occlude meningeal vessels. The dura mater is opened with several radial incisions carried to the margin of the craniectomy, and a suture elevates each triangular flap against the under edge of the bone to secure reliable hemostasis.

With controlled hyperventilation under anesthesia it is unlikely that the intracranial contents will tend to herniate through the craniectomy; but should this occur, the arachnoid is opened quickly, under magnification, for drainage of cerebrospinal fluid and decompression. The cortical surface is examined to identify the largest cortical

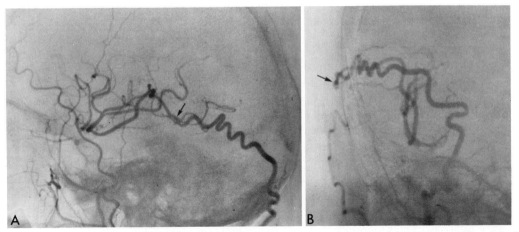

Figure 44–6   Postoperative arteriogram of a patient who had a previous occipital artery to middle cerebral artery anastomosis. *A*. Subtraction version of lateral projection shows the winding course of the hypertrophied occipital artery, which irrigates the entire middle cerebral artery territory through the anastomosis (*arrow*). *B*. Subtraction version of frontal projection shows the occipital artery, which originates medially, coursing upward and laterally to the anastomosis (*arrow*) for irrigation of sylvian vessels.

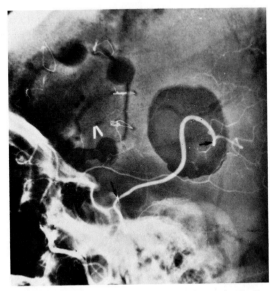

Figure 44–7   Arteriogram (lateral projection) shows free vein graft interposed between superficial temporal artery and cortical branch of middle cerebral artery (*arrows*). The superficial temporal artery was sectioned during a previous craniotomy for coating (with methyl methacrylate) of an infraclinoid aneurysm of the internal carotid artery. A stricture has developed at the proximal end-to-end anastomosis (*vertical arrow*).

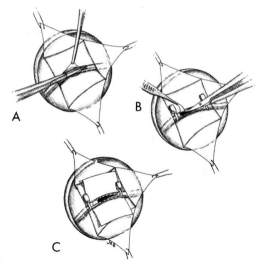

Figure 44–8   Technique for preparing a cortical branch of the middle cerebral artery. The dura has been opened with a series of radial incisions extending to the border of the craniectomy. Each of the resulting triangular flaps has been elevated with a suture to obliterate the epidural space and assure meticulous hemostasis. *A*. The arachnoid is opened under high magnification (25 ×). Drainage of cerebrospinal fluid provides decompression and reduces brain pulsation. A segment of artery is mobilized for anastomosis by dividing the entwining arachnoid fibers. *B*. Atraumatic temporary clips have been applied to isolate the segment of cortical artery. A teardrop-shaped incision is made to streamline the flow of blood proximally toward the middle cerebral artery trifurcation. *C*. An indwelling stent of silicone rubber tubing has been placed inside the lumen to separate the adjacent margins of the opening.

vessel emerging from the sylvian fissure. The angular branch is preferred and usually takes a horizontal course posteriorly from the sylvian fissure.[30,31] Under high magnification (25 ×), the cortical artery is meticulously dissected from a complex array of entangling arachnoid fibers (Fig. 44–8). A segment, relatively free of penetrating branches, is selected. It may be helpful to coagulate a few small cortical veins or to expose the artery for a short distance into the sylvian fissure. Two or three small penetrating branches are frequently coagulated to isolate a segment of cortical artery 1 cm in length. The artery is separated from the surface of the brain by inserting a small moistened triangular strip of rubber (fashioned from a surgical glove). If a rather large penetrating branch arises from an otherwise ideal segment of cortical artery, an incision is made through the strip of rubber to straddle and thereby preserve the branch, which will be temporarily occluded with an additional clip.

An alternative method for selecting a recipient branch of the middle cerebral artery is dissection through the anterior aspect of the sylvian fissure to expose the middle

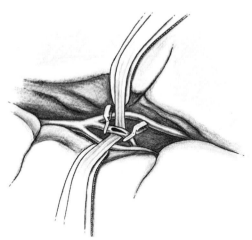

Figure 44–9 Technique for preparing middle cerebral artery branch at the trifurcation. The sylvian fissure has been opened by dividing bridging veins and arachnoid attachments between the frontal and temporal lobes of the brain. The depths of the sylvian fissure have been exposed by retraction, and the middle cerebral artery trifurcation has been identified. The artery that will be used for anastomosis (frequently the angular branch) has been separated from arachnoid attachments and is stabilized by a long thin strip of moistened rubber obtained from a surgical glove. Clips isolate a segment of the artery, and a teardrop-shaped incision has been made.

cerebral artery trifurcation (Fig. 44–9). This is accomplished through a scalp incision placed directly over the frontal branch of the superficial temporal artery and a craniotomy through the pterion as described by Yaşargil and Fox for operations on aneurysm.[185] The sylvian fissure is opened by coagulating and dividing the surface veins, dissecting through arachnoid attachments, and retracting the frontal lobe away from the temporal lobe. The arterial branches follow the lobe to which they have been assigned. The posterior temporal and angular branches and the branch of the ascending frontal complex are exposed at their origin from the trifurcation, and one of these (usually the angular) is freed from its arachnoid investments in preparation for the anastomosis. A long thin strip of rubber is placed beneath this branch, isolating it from adjacent structures. While experience in using it is limited, this method affords an anastomosis at the proximal portion of a middle cerebral artery branch where the lumen is larger and has the potential for greater flow (Fig. 44–10).

Once the recipient branch of the middle cerebral artery has been prepared for anastomosis, attention is returned to the donor superficial temporal artery. A temporary clip is placed across its proximal end, and it is ligated at the distal end. The distal end is sectioned just proximal to the ligature, and the free end of the artery is routed to the recipient middle cerebral artery branch so that flow will ultimately be directed retrograde toward the trifurcation, anticipating irrigation of the entire middle cerebral artery territory. The lumen of the superficial temporal artery is emptied of blood by irrigation with normal saline solution, and any excess length is removed.

Temporary clips are applied to isolate the prepared middle cerebral artery branch (cf. Fig. 44–8). A teardrop-shaped incision is made in the recipient branch, with the largest portion of the opening directed proximally. An indwelling stent of silicone rubber tubing (outside diameter .625 mm) is inserted within the lumen. An incision is made in the free end of the superficial temporal artery on the surface that will lie adjacent to the middle cerebral artery branch. The incision is of such length that the resulting splayed-open end of the superficial temporal artery will match the opening in

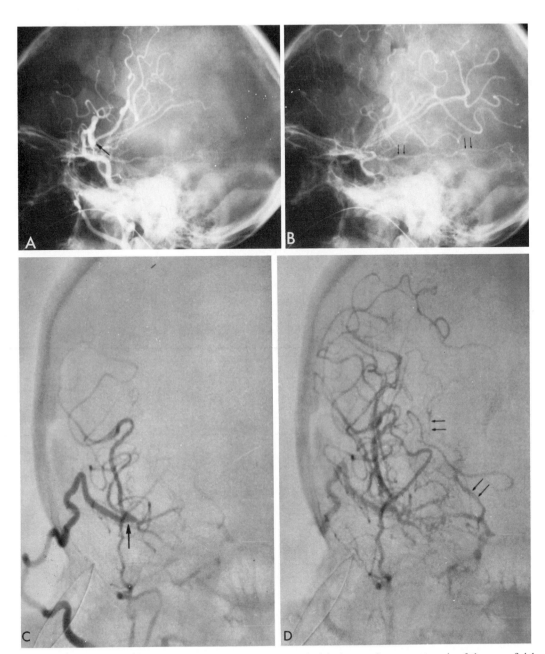

Figure 44–10   Postoperative arteriogram of a patient who had had a previous anastomosis of the superficial temporal artery to the sylvian middle cerebral artery. *A*. Lateral projection. Early phase shows a very large superficial temporal artery irrigating the major branches of the middle cerebral artery through the anastomosis (*arrow*). *B*. Later phase shows perfusion of entire middle cerebral territory with retrograde extension into the distal internal carotid and posterior cerebral arteries (*arrows*). *C*. Subtraction version of frontal projection. Early phase shows a very large superficial temporal artery irrigating branches of the middle cerebral artery through the anastomosis (*arrow*) located deep within the sylvian fissure. *D*. Later phase shows filling of the entire middle cerebral artery territory with retrograde extension into the internal carotid and posterior cerebral arteries (*arrows*).

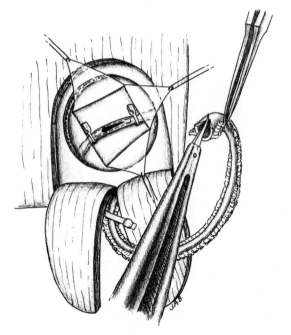

Figure 44–11 Technique for preparing the distal end of the superficial temporal artery. A temporary clip has been placed across its base and the distal end of the artery has been transected perpendicular to its axis. After assessment of the spatial relationships between it and the cortical middle cerebral artery, a surface of the superficial temporal artery has been selected in which to place an incision that will splay open the end of the artery. The length of the incision is made to coincide with the opening in the cortical artery.

the middle cerebral artery branch (Fig. 44–11).

With the openings of both arteries facing the surgeon, a 10-0 monofilament microsuture (25 μ) is placed between the cortical vessel and the superficial temporal artery at each end of the opening (Fig. 44–12). The superficial temporal artery is then rotated over the cortical artery into position and both sutures are tied and cut. A row of interrupted sutures is then placed between the superficial temporal artery and the cortical artery along the side of the anastomosis facing the surgeon. After it has been confirmed by magnified visual inspection that all sutures have been precisely placed (usually 7 to 9 are required), each is tied and cut. The superficial temporal artery is then rotated to expose the other side of the anastomosis, and interrupted sutures are similarly placed along the second side. After visual inspection has confirmed precise placement of sutures, the indwelling stent is withdrawn and the sutures are individually tied and cut.

All temporary clips are removed in rapid sequence. Excellent pulsation confirms patency of the vessels (Fig. 44–13). Any bleeding should cease spontaneously. Wisps of resorbable hemostatic material may be placed along the anastomosis. Papaverine hydrochloride (60 mg) may be applied topically to reduce spasm.

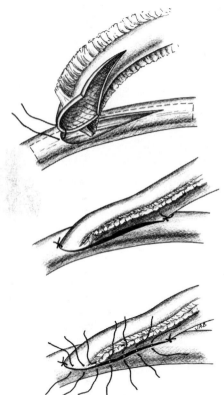

Figure 44–12 Technique for performing the anastomosis. *Top.* With the openings of the cortical artery and the superficial temporal artery facing the surgeon, an anchor suture is placed at each end between the two vessels. *Center.* The superficial temporal artery has been carefully rotated over the cortical artery, and the sutures tightened gently, tied, and cut. *Bottom.* Individual sutures have been placed along the side of the anastomosis facing the surgeon between the superficial temporal artery and the cortical artery. After careful inspection has confirmed perfect placement of all sutures, they are tied and cut in sequence. The arteries are then rotated to expose the opposite side of the anastomosis, where a similar procedure completes the anastomosis.

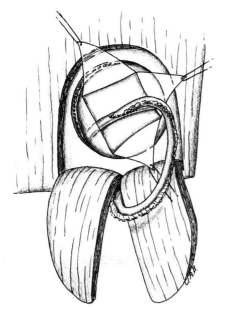

Figure 44–13 Completed anastomosis. All temporary clips have been removed. Distention and pulsation confirm patency. Any bleeding that may occur will usually cease spontaneously.

During closure, the principal consideration is avoiding angulation, twisting, or kinking of the bypass graft. The dura mater may be partially closed but is frequently left open. The temporalis muscle is approximated around the superficial temporal artery in such a way that a watertight closure is obtained without constriction or kinking of the artery (Fig. 44–14). The scalp is closed in layers, and a loose head dressing is applied.

Rationale for Anastomosis

The clinical indication that a person may be endangered by an impending major stroke is the occurrence of a transient ischemic attack or minor reversible stroke. Whisnant and associates reported a 36 per cent incidence of stroke in a series of 198 patients followed for an average duration of 7.5 years after a first episode of a transient ischemic attack.[177,179] Of those experiencing a stroke after the ischemic episode, 21 per cent did so within one month and 51 per cent within the first year. Thereafter, approximately 8 per cent developed a stroke each year.

Baker and co-workers have evaluated the course of patients experiencing an initial transient ischemic attack (average follow-up 41 months) or stroke (average follow-up 44 months) (Table 44–1). While new ischemic events (ischemic attacks and cerebral infarction) occurred more frequently in the group with transient ischemic attacks, the stroke group experienced a higher incidence of new cerebral infarction (26 per cent) than did the group with transient ischemic attacks (22 per cent). Furthermore, the new cerebral infarction was fatal more frequently in the stroke group (35 per cent) than in the transient ischemic attack group (12 per cent).[14,15] These findings suggest that the risk of new cerebral infarction after recovery from a previous one is at least comparable with the risk that has been attributed to transient ischemic attacks.

Fisher reviewed a "more or less unselected" series of cases of middle cerebral

Figure 44–14 Technique for closure. Special care is required to avoid twisting, stretching, kinking, or compressing the superficial temporal artery. A transverse incision through the temporalis muscle or fascia may prove advantageous. *A.* If triangular flaps have been employed, the temporalis fascia is closed around the periphery, and the adjacent flaps are reapproximated by placing sutures between the muscle edges. *B.* If the exposure has been through a simple verticle incision, the temporalis muscle is reapproximated.

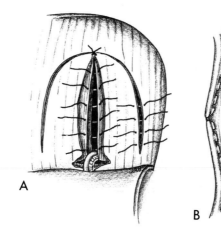

A

B

TABLE 44–1 COMPARISON OF PROGNOSIS AFTER TRANSIENT ISCHEMIC ATTACK AND STROKE*

PATIENTS		NEW ISCHEMIC EVENTS			
			Infarctions		
Group	Number	Transient Ischemic Attacks	New	Fatal	TOTAL
Transient ischemic attack	79	45 (57%)	17 (22%)	2 (12%)	55 (70%)
Stroke	430	85 (20%)	113 (26%)	40 (35%)	164 (38%)

* Average follow-up for transient ischemic attack patients, 41 months; for stroke patients, 45 months. Data from Baker, R. N., Ramseyer, J. C., and Schwartz, W. S.: Prognosis in patients with transient cerebral ischemic attacks. Neurology (Minneap.), *18*:1157–1165, 1968; Baker, R. N., Schwartz, W. S., and Ramseyer, J. C.: Prognosis among survivors of ischemic stroke. Neurology (Minneap.), *18*:933–941, 1968.

artery occlusion (40 patients) and internal carotid artery occlusion (50 patients). These patients were classified into three groups as follows: group I—asymptomatic, group II—slight or nondisabling deficit, group III—moderate to severe deficit (Table 44–2). Of the patients with middle cerebral artery occlusion, there were none assigned to group I, 5 to group II (12.5 per cent), and 35 to group III (87.5 per cent). "These data indicate the grave prospect in individual cases of middle cerebral artery occlusion" and reflect the limited capacity of the leptomeningeal vessels to function as a source of collateral circulation. The patients with internal carotid artery occlusion fared only somewhat better. Eight patients were assigned to group I (16 per cent), thirteen to group II (26 per cent); and twenty-nine to group III (58 per cent).[60-62] The small group of asymptomatic patients with internal carotid artery occlusion, which is observed regularly in clinical practice, has been reported by Dyken and co-workers as 3 per cent of a hospital population, a figure that reflects the extent of collateral circulation derived from the circle of Willis.[49] The observation that 58 per cent of patients with internal carotid artery occlusion have moderate to severe deficit is consistent with reports by Dyken (49 per cent) and McDowell (56 per cent) and their associates, and is reminiscent of the incidence of ischemic neurological complications that follow abrupt internal carotid artery occlusion (59

TABLE 44–2 DISABILITY RESULTING FROM OCCLUSION OF MIDDLE CEREBRAL OR INTERNAL CAROTID ARTERY*

GROUP	OCCLUDED ARTERY	
	Middle Cerebral (40 Patients)	Internal Carotid (50 Patients)
I Asymptomatic	0	8 (16%)
II Transient ischemic attack or "acceptable" nondisabling deficit	5 (12.5%)	13 (26%)
III Moderate to severe deficit	35 (87.5%)	29 (58%)

* Data from Fisher, C. M.: Clinical syndromes in cerebral thrombosis, hypertensive hemorrhage, and ruptured saccular aneurysm. Clin. Neurosurg., *22*:117–147, 1975; The natural history of carotid occlusion. In Austin, G. M., ed.: Microneurosurgical Anastomoses for Cerebral Ischemia. Springfield, Ill., Charles C Thomas, 1976, pp. 194–201; The natural history of middle cerebral artery trunk occlusion. Ibid., pp. 146–154.

TABLE 44–3 MODE OF ONSET OF MODERATE TO SEVERE STROKE*

MODE OF ONSET	OCCLUDED ARTERY	
	Middle Cerebral (Per Cent)	Internal Carotid (Per Cent)
Transient ischemic attacks	65	60
Number before stroke		
1 to 2	50	33
3 to 10	20	33
More than 10	30	33
Duration before stroke		
<2 weeks	27	
3 to 8 weeks	40	
3 to 12 months	33	
1 to 7 days		33
2 to 8 weeks		33
>8 weeks		33
Progressing stroke	13	20
Sudden stroke	22	20

* Data from Fisher, C. M.: Clinical syndromes in cerebral thrombosis, hypertensive hemorrhage, and ruptured saccular aneurysm. Clin. Neurosurg., *22*:117–147, 1975; The natural history of carotid occlusion. In Austin, G. M., ed.: Microneurosurgical Anastomoses for Cerebral Ischemia. Springfield, Ill., Charles C Thomas, 1976, pp. 194–201; The natural history of middle cerebral artery trunk occlusion. Ibid., pp. 146–154.

per cent) reported by the Cooperative Study of Intracranial Aneurysms and Subarachnoid Hemorrhage.[50,109,119] Sixty-five per cent of the patients with middle cerebral artery occlusion and sixty per cent of those with internal carotid artery occlusion had experienced prodromal transient ischemic attacks (Table 44–3).[60–62] However, half the patients with middle cerebral artery occlusion and one third of those with internal carotid artery occlusion had experienced only one or two attacks before cerebral infarction occurred, and the interval between onset of the attacks and infarction was less than two months in two thirds of patients with occlusion of either artery. These data suggest that when a transient ischemic attack occurs, appropriate diagnostic and therapeutic measures should be initiated promptly.

Of 6535 patients registered by the Joint Study of Extracranial Arterial Occlusion (1959 to 1973) 1044 were identified as having an occluded internal carotid artery. From this group 359 with a unilateral internal carotid artery occlusion who were not treated by operation were available for follow-up observation (average 44 months) (Table 44–4). New transient ischemic attacks occurred in 20 per cent and new strokes in 25 per cent. The new events occurred twice as frequently on the occluded side as on the opposite side. Thirty-six patients with bilateral internal carotid artery occlusion were not treated operatively and were available for follow-up observation (average 42 months). New strokes occurred in only four individuals

from this group (11 per cent), but three of the four strokes led to a fatal outcome. Five hundred and fifty-seven patients with occlusion of one internal carotid artery and contralateral stenosis of the other were included in the study. Neurological manifestations at the time of admission were lateralized five and one half times as frequently to the side with the occlusion as to the side with the stenosis (Table 44–5). Two hundred and eleven of these patients were randomly assigned to treatment categories. Of these, 98 were not treated by operation and were available for follow-up observation (average 51 months). New transient ischemic attacks occurred in 12 per cent of patients (referred to the occluded side twice as frequently as to the stenotic side), and new strokes in 33 per cent.[56] These data indicate that occlusion of the internal carotid artery is not necessarily a stable situation.

Since the effectiveness of collateral circulation is thought to play a major role in the clinical outcome of patients with occlusive vascular disease, it is of interest that Alpers and associates found a normal circle of Willis in only 52 per cent of normal brains and 33 per cent of brains harboring cerebral infarction (Table 44–6). The requirement being accepted, as a definition of normal, that each component of the circle has a diameter of 1 mm or more, 23 per cent of the circles from normal brains demonstrated hypoplasia or absence of the posterior communicating artery in comparison with 40 per cent from those with cerebral infarction. Furthermore, an embryonic ori-

TABLE 44–4 "NATURAL HISTORY" OF PATIENTS WITH KNOWN OCCLUSION OF INTERNAL CAROTID ARTERY*

OCCLUSION	LATERALIZATION OF NEW EVENT	NEW TRANSIENT ISCHEMIC ATTACK	NEW STROKES	FATAL STROKES
Unilateral (359 patients)		73 (20%)	89 (25%)	50 (56%)
	Occluded side	30	30	
	Opposite side	16	13	
	Bilateral	3	5	
	Vertebrobasilar—brain stem	24	7	
	Not specified		34	
Unilateral with contralateral stenosis (98 randomly selected patients)		12 (12%)	32 (33%)	16 (50%)
	Occluded side	8		
	Stenotic side	4		
Bilateral (36 patients)		2 (6%)	4 (11%)	3 (75%)

* Average follow-up for patients with unilateral occlusion, 44 months; for patients with occlusion and contralateral stenosis, 51 months; for patients with bilateral occlusion, 42 months. Data from Fields, W. S., and Lemak, N. A.: Joint study of extracranial arterial occlusion: X. Internal carotid artery occlusion. J.A.M.A., 235:2734–2738, 1976.

TABLE 44-5 LATERALIZATION OF CLINICAL MANIFESTATIONS OF OCCLUSION OF INTERNAL CAROTID ARTERY AND STENOSIS OF CONTRALATERAL ARTERY*

	PER CENT
Occluded side	55
Stenotic side	10
Bilateral	16
Asymptomatic	2
Other	17

* Based upon 557 patient studies. Data from Fields, W. S., and Lemak, N. A.: Joint study of extracranial arterial occlusion: X. Internal carotid artery occlusion. J.A.M.A., 235: 2734–2738, 1976.

gin of the posterior cerebral artery (usually associated with hypoplasia of the segment between basilar and posterior communicating arteries) was found in 15 per cent of the circles from normal brains in comparison with 29 per cent of those from brains that demonstrated cerebral infarction. The anterior components were infrequently considered hypoplastic.[1,2] If 1.5 mm or larger were accepted as normal for each component of the circle, however, Perlmutter and Rhoton found the incidence of hypoplasia involving the proximal anterior cerebral artery to increase from 2 to 10 per cent and that for the anterior communicating artery from 16 to 44 per cent (Table 44–7).[124]

TABLE 44-6 ANATOMY OF THE CIRCLE OF WILLIS*

	NORMAL BRAIN (PER CENT)	INFARCTION (PER CENT)
Normal circle[a]	52	33
Anterior cerebral artery		
Hypoplastic	2	5
Fused	1.7	1
Anterior communicating artery hypoplastic	3	4
Posterior communicating artery		
Hypoplastic	22	38
Absent	0.6	1.5
Embryonic posterior cerebral artery	15	29
Accessory vessels	17	19

[a] Normal circle: Closed circuit, fluid may circulate from any entrance point and return, paired anterior cerebral arteries, outside diameter of all component vessels >1 mm.

* Based upon dissection of 350 normal brains and 194 brains with cerebral infarction. Data from Alpers, B. J., and Berry, R. G.: Circle of Willis in cerebral vascular disorders: the anatomical structure. Arch. Neurol. (Chicago), 8:398–402, 1963; Alpers, B. J., Berry, R. G., and Paddison, R. M.: Anatomical studies of the circle of Willis in normal brain. Arch. Neurol. Psychiat., 81:409–418, 1959.

TABLE 44-7 HYPOPLASIA OF THE ANTERIOR COMPONENTS OF THE CIRCLE OF WILLIS*

	HYPOPLASIA DEFINED AS:	
	<1 mm (Per Cent)	<1.5 mm (Per Cent)
Anterior cerebral artery (proximal to anterior communicating artery)	2	10
Anterior communicating artery	16	44

* Based upon a dissection of 50 brains. Data from Perlmutter, D., and Rhoton, A. L., Jr.: Microsurgical anatomy of the anterior cerebral–anterior communicating–recurrent artery complex. J. Neurosurg., 45:259–272, 1976.

The effectiveness of the ophthalmic artery as a source of collateral circulation is not clear. From a small series of patients with occlusion of the internal carotid artery, Krayenbühl and Yaşargil concluded that those patients in whom prominent intracranial filling from retrograde ophthalmic flow could be demonstrated by arteriography fared better than others without this finding.[97] Conversely, Malis has stated that well-developed collateral circulation through the circuitous, high-resistance ophthalmic route reflects a large pressure gradient between the external carotid artery circulation and the intracranial circulation, implies that the brain is existing on marginal sources of circulation, and portends a poor prognosis for the patient.[105]

The lumen diameter of the superficial temporal artery bypass graft averaged 2.0 mm (range 1.3 to 2.8) in a series of 20 patients when measured during arteriography (average 32 weeks after operation) with correction for magnification.[134] Since this is of the same order of magnitude as the component parts of the circle of Willis and since the collateral circulation derived from the latter is considered to be a major factor in determining the clinical course of patients with occlusive cerebral vascular disease, it is logical to conclude that the new source of collateral circulation resulting from superficial temporal artery to cortical middle cerebral artery anastomosis should have equal clinical significance in appropriate cases.

Indications for Operation

The anastomosis is performed most frequently in the treatment of patients with intracranial arterial occlusive disease. Occasionally, it is used to establish a new pathway of collateral circulation in preparation for the deliberate occlusion (abrupt or gradual) of an essential brain artery when required to stop embolization or to treat definitively an exceptional aneurysm, neoplasm, or carotid-cavernous fistula.

Occlusive Cerebral Vascular Disease

The clinical manifestations of occlusive cerebral vascular disease present as a transient ischemic attack (defined as the sudden onset of focal ischemic neurological deficit with complete resolution in less than 24 hours), progressing stroke (evolving over 6 hours or more), or completed stroke (ischemic deficit stabilized for 24 hours or more).[48] A completed stroke with complete resolution within three weeks has been designated as a reversible ischemic neurological deficit.

At the onset of an ischemic event, it is impossible to predict the outcome. Partial or complete resolution may occur promptly or slowly, or the deficit may progress to profound and permanent disability.[127] Furthermore, it is not possible to predict whether a future attack will occur. While some individuals never experience another attack, others experience several attacks that may occur with accelerating frequency and increasing severity as the forewarning of an impending stroke.

Ischemic manifestations relevant to the territories of the internal carotid or the middle cerebral artery are ipsilateral monocular visual loss (amaurosis fugax), dysphasia, contralateral sensory disturbance (face, upper extremity, lower extremity), contralateral weakness (face, upper extremity, lower extremity), and uncommonly, contralateral homonymous visual field disturbance.[65,127] Dysarthria, impairment of memory, and altered behavior may also occur but are not specifically associated with cerebral ischemia and are of little value in localizing the zone of cerebral ischemia or the pathological vascular changes.[123] Deficits that appropriately involve more than one modality may increase the accuracy of diagnosis and improve the localization.[65]

An operation is most appropriately considered for individuals who have become asymptomatic after ischemic events or in whom the residual impairment is minimal or not severely disabling.[101]

While rapidly progressing neurological deficit is not a favorable indication for operation, an occasional patient may present with a slowly developing (hours, days, weeks) partial ischemic deficit or with intervals, alternating between progression and resolution, of abnormal neurological signs. Such patients may benefit from the additional collateral circulation provided by the anastomosis.[131,175] Similarly, an acute major stroke is not generally considered to be a suitable indication for operation. An occasional patient may, however, present with sudden minor partial deficit that may benefit from an early operation.[36,129] This particularly applies to young patients (10 to 20 years of age). Also, an occasional young or older individual whose condition after a minor to moderately severe partial stroke has stabilized and is improving (7 to 21 days after ictus) may demonstrate a striking enhancement of the improvement following operation.[86,131]

A decision to operate is based upon a correlation of clinical manifestations with arteriographic observations.[25,76,106,168] The location and severity of arterial disease

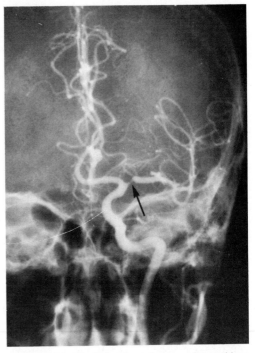

Figure 44–15 Frontal projection of carotid arteriogram demonstrates tight stenosis (*arrow*) of the left middle cerebral artery.

must be consistent with the clinical manifestations.[39] Anastomosis of the superficial temporal artery to the middle cerebral artery should be recommended when recurring transient ischemic events are associated with an appropriate arterial lesion. The lesion may be a stenosis or occlusion of the middle cerebral artery or the intracranial portion of the internal carotid artery, or

an occlusion of the extracranial portion of the internal carotid artery (Figs. 44–15 to 44–18). Arteriographic studies should include a qualitative assessment of the collateral circulation with particular attention directed toward the extent of perfusion derived from anterior communicating artery, posterior communicating artery, and ophthalmic and meningohypophyseal and

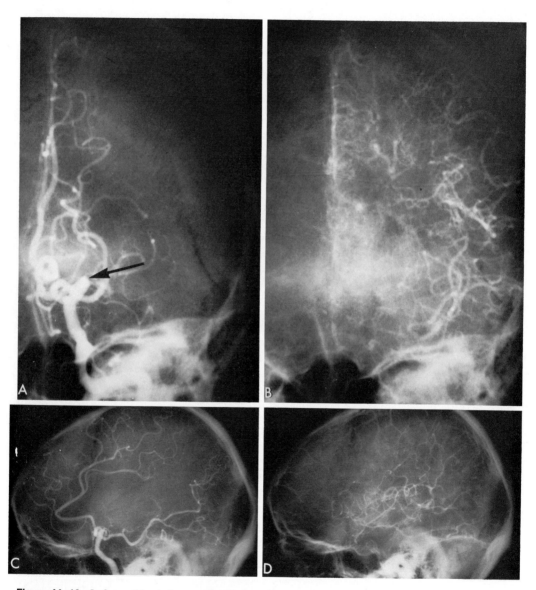

Figure 44–16   Left carotid arteriogram of a 63-year-old man who had experienced three episodes of transient ischemia involving his left cerebral hemisphere. *A.* Frontal projection. Early phase shows prompt filling of the anterior and posterior cerebral arteries with abrupt middle cerebral artery trunk occlusion (*arrow*). *B.* Later phase shows retrograde filling into the vessels of the left sylvian region arising from leptomeningeal collateral circulation. *C.* Lateral projection. Early phase shows prompt filling of anterior and posterior cerebral arteries with absence of sylvian vasculature. *D.* Later phase shows extensive middle cerebral artery filling derived from leptomeningeal sources.

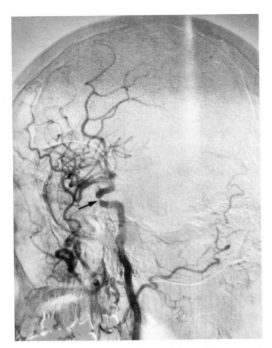

Figure 44–17 Subtraction version of an unusual oblique projection from the carotid arteriogram of a 59-year-old man who had experienced innumerable transient ischemic attacks involving his right cerebral hemisphere. A tight stenosis (*arrow*) involves the cavernous portion of the right internal carotid artery.

leptomeningeal sources (Fig. 44–18).[66] The extent of collateral circulation should be a major factor in determining the need for an anastomosis. The availability of an extensive, intrinsically developed collateral circulation diminishes the need for it.

Determination of regional cerebral blood flow has been advocated as a reliable method for evaluating the effectiveness of the intrinsic collateral circulation. Using intravenous [133]xenon and a frontal and parietal scintillation detector over each cerebral hemisphere, Austin and associates considered a greater than 20 to 25 per cent reduction in gray matter cerebral blood flow as "one good physiologically positive indication" for operation.[12,13] Using intracarotid [133]xenon and 16 scintillation detectors over the ipsilateral hemisphere, Schmiedek and co-workers recommended an operation for patients having "focal cerebral ischemia" alone or superimposed upon a background of moderate general reduction of regional cerebral blood flow (60 to 80 per cent of normal).[151] Because of the diverse techniques used by various investigators, it is not possible to define exact parameters that

are comparable and that can be applied generally to recommend or advise against an operation. As greater experience is acquired, the newer noninvasive methods will be refined further and should serve as an increasingly useful adjunct in patient selection.[121] Additionally, further development and application of positron emission computed tomography in imaging the variables of regional cerebral blood flow and regional cerebral oxygen utilization promise even more precise criteria for patient selection.[73,81]

Although experience is limited, hyperbaric oxygenation promises to be a valuable

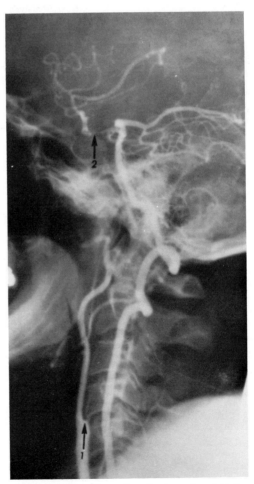

Figure 44–18 Lateral projection of a right brachial arteriogram demonstrates an occlusion, located at the internal carotid artery origin (*arrow 1*). Intracranial filling is derived solely from a thin, irregular posterior communicating artery (*arrow 2*). Other films demonstrated absence of other potential sources of collateral circulation into the right cerebral hemisphere.

method for recognizing viable, but non-functioning, cerebral tissue in the patient with a completed stroke. In a series of 35 patients in the chronic post-stroke stage (average 10 weeks after ictus) and found to have internal carotid artery occlusion, Holbach's group found 15 who improved with hyperbaric oxygenation (1.5 atmospheres for 40 minutes in 10 to 15 daily sessions). The anastomosis was performed in these patients, and 13 in whom a patent anastomosis was demonstrated postoperatively showed further improvement in neurological function. Another patient improved, despite the fact that the anastomosis was not patent. One patient died six days postoperatively because of a subdural hematoma. Five of the twenty patients who did not improve with hyperbaric oxygenation were subjected to an anastomosis, but did not improve following the operation.[83,84] Where available, this modality should be helpful in identifying those patients with stroke who are likely to benefit from an operation.

Atherosclerosis

The most common cause of intracranial arterial occlusive disease is atherosclerosis. Plaques of atherosclerosis may become complicated with calcification, hemorrhage, stenosis, ulceration, and thrombosis.[63,113] While it is generally recognized that these lesions are most common at the origin or cervical portion of the internal carotid artery, Moossy found in an autopsy series of 2650 complete brain dissections that cerebral infarction was most frequently associated with intracranial arterial thrombosis.[112]

Severe arteriosclerosis is a widely disseminated process. Common combinations of lesions include: (1) bilateral internal carotid artery stenosis or occlusion; (2) occlusion of one internal carotid artery and stenosis of the contralateral one; (3) two distinct internal carotid artery stenotic lesions in tandem (cervical and intracranial). Other combinations of lesions occur less frequently.

In the presence of multiple lesions, attention should be directed toward the one that is considered most symptomatic.[114] With tandem lesions, a comparison is made between the relative characteristics of the two lesions in regard to encroachment upon lumen, roughness of arterial surface, and evidence of ulceration. If stenosis of the cervical internal carotid artery is considered to be the more likely cause of the patient's symptoms, and the residual diameter of the lumen at a level of intracranial stenosis is greater than 2 mm, endarterectomy usually is indicated. Superficial temporal to middle cerebral artery anastomosis is indicated if the stenosis in the cervical portion of the internal carotid artery is less than that in the intracranial portion. If the patient has a combined occlusion of the internal carotid artery and stenosis of the contralateral one, the operation should be done on the symptomatic side. For example, superficial temporal artery to middle cerebral artery anastomosis should be done if the ischemic manifestations are compatible with the side of the internal carotid artery occlusion. Conversely, endarterectomy should be performed if the symptoms are relevant to the side with the cervical internal carotid artery stenosis.

Fibromuscular Dysplasia

The histological features of fibromuscular dysplasia include degeneration and disruption of elastic fibers with alternating zones of marked thinning of the media (causing pseudoaneurysm formation) and sharply localized constriction (resulting from hyperplasia of fibrous and fibroelastic tissue, primarily within the media but also involving the intima and adventitia).[149] These alterations cause an arteriographic appearance that resembles a string of pearls. The process may be sharply localized (usually involving the internal carotid artery at the level of the second cervical vertebra) or diffuse, as a tubular narrowing (Fig. 44–19). The vertebral artery is affected less commonly, but the process has also been reported to involve the middle cerebral artery. Intracranial aneurysm is regularly associated with this condition. Ischemic manifestations result from embolization or progression of the stenosis to occlusion.[85] The anastomosis may be utilized to bypass a severely obstructed arterial segment.[162]

Cerebrovascular Moyamoya Disease

This condition is a unique radiological entity, reported most frequently in the Oriental race. The arteriographic features consist of multiple stenoses and occlusions involving the distal intracranial segment of

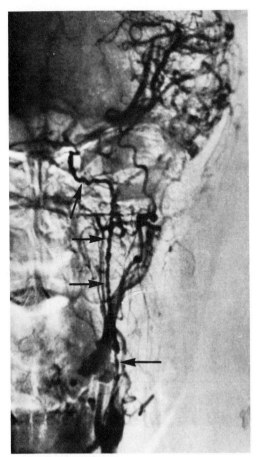

Figure 44–19 Subtraction version of the frontal projection from a carotid arteriogram shows an irregular ("beaded"), diffuse tubular narrowing (*arrows*), characteristic of fibromuscular dysplasia extensively involving the left internal carotid artery.

the internal carotid artery and the trunks of the anterior cerebral and middle cerebral arteries, associated with a dense vascular network in the region of the lenticulostriate and brain stem perforating arteries and a striking telangiectasia of the leptomeningeal arteries (Fig. 44–20). These findings are usually bilateral and exist in children or young adults. Symptoms may result from cerebral ischemia or from intracerebral or subarachnoid hemorrhage.[88] Superficial temporal artery to middle cerebral artery anastomosis has resulted in important clinical improvement in patients with cerebral ischemia, including several who had a long-standing deficit.[3,88,135] The risk of hemorrhage is also thought to be reduced by the anastomosis because the new collateral circulation into the larger conduit arteries of the brain reduces the stimulus for developing new collateral circulation through the small leptomeningeal and lenticulostriate network by the process of telangiectasia.[18,88,93]

Embolization

Many of the patients with middle cerebral artery stenosis or occlusion, who are considered suitable candidates for superficial temporal artery to middle cerebral artery anastomosis, have hypertension or hyperlipoproteinemia and other risk factors suggesting an atherosclerotic cause for the isolated lesion of the middle cerebral artery.[28,82] In other cases the lesion is undoubtedly the result of embolization.[99,156] The two groups of patients may be indistinguishable, even after exhaustive medical evaluation (Fig. 44–21). Candidates from both groups who have recurrent symptoms may be considered appropriate for operation to provide collateral circulation to brain tissue beyond the stenosis or occlusion, even though such a lesion might be expected ultimately to undergo partial or complete resolution.

Craniocerebral Trauma

Superficial temporal artery to middle cerebral artery anastomosis has been performed in a small number of cases of intracranial arterial occlusion associated with trauma.[12,71,159] While these cases have not demonstrated a clear, significant benefit from the operations, the rationale is logical. It is to be expected that in a rare case borderline cerebral ischemia can be corrected by the anastomosis.

Neoplasm

A meningioma of the sphenoid wing, chordoma of the petrous portion of the temporal bone, or other tumor at the base of the skull can cause ischemic manifestations by constricting an enclosed internal carotid artery or middle cerebral artery. Even if the tumor is considered unresectable, a superficial temporal artery to middle cerebral artery anastomosis could prove beneficial in relieving cerebral ischemia.[71]

Deliberate Sacrifice of Essential Brain Vessels

Occlusion of the internal or common carotid artery has been widely employed in the practice of neurological surgery for a

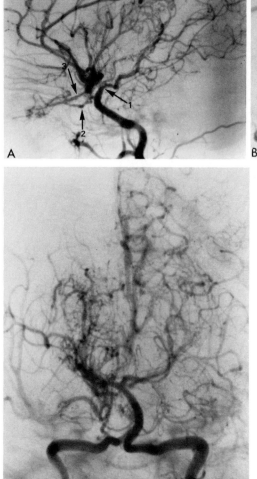

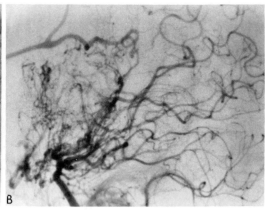

Figure 44–20 Cerebrovascular "moyamoya" disease. *A*. Subtraction version of the lateral projection from a left carotid arteriogram shows occlusion of the internal carotid artery (*arrow 1*) distal to the origin of the posterior communicating artery. The ophthalmic artery (*arrow 2*) irrigates an orbital plexus, from which a prominent posterior ethmoidal artery (*arrow 3*) arises, providing some collateral circulation to the anterior and middle cerebral arteries. Lenticulostriate and posterior pericallosal telangiectasia provides other important sources of collateral circulation. *B*. Subtraction version of lateral projection from a vertebral arteriogram shows telangiectasia forming a complex network of collateral vessels located within the upper brain stem. *C*. Subtraction version of the frontal projection shows the same network from another perspective. This demonstrates even greater involvement on the right and reflects the occlusion of the right internal carotid artery immediately proximal to the origin of its posterior communicating branch. (Courtesy of Arthur E. Rosenbaum, M.D., and Zaid Deeb, M.D.)

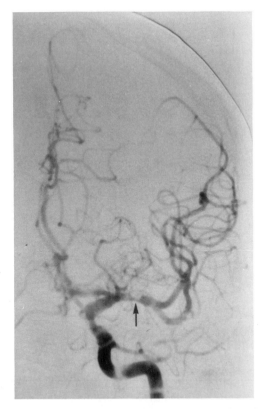

Figure 44-21 Subtraction version of the frontal projection from a carotid arteriogram demonstrates left middle cerebral artery stenosis (*arrow*). On the basis of its arteriographic appearance and the clinical manifestations, it is usually not possible to draw an unqualified conclusion as to whether this lesion is a focal atherosclerotic plaque or partial recanalization of an embolus.

variety of complex vascular abnormalities. The safety of this procedure is unpredictable, however, and depends primarily upon the efficiency of collateral circulation through the circle of Willis.[75,115,119] Several ingenious devices, incorporating external graded control, have been fabricated for partial, gradual, or temporary occlusion.[37,94,153,165] Yet, a high proportion of patients continue to experience grave ischemic complications. Nornes reported 10 patients in whom electromagnetic flow probes were implanted around both internal carotid arteries (distal to a Selverstone clamp on the ipsilateral side) to identify those patients likely to tolerate occlusion of the vessel. Three of the patients demonstrated insufficient collateral circulation, and two others experienced delayed complications (two days, five days), presumed to result from thromboembolism.[120]

Superficial temporal artery to middle cerebral artery anastomosis has substantially increased the safety of deliberately occluding an otherwise essential artery by providing an important pathway of new collateral circulation. While many patients have benefited from this approach, a precisely defined index does not exist for insuring the safety of patients requiring occlusion of major brain arteries. The unpredictable risks must be carefully considered in comparison with the anticipated benefits resulting from a successful operation.

Embolization

A small group of patients has continued to experience ischemic manifestations, subsequent to superficial temporal artery to middle cerebral artery anastomosis for an inaccessible stenosis of the internal carotid artery (atherosclerosis or fibromuscular dysplasia). Sudden or gradual occlusion of the internal carotid artery has been helpful by removing the embolus-generating arterial surface from the circulation.[162] The superficial temporal artery to middle cerebral artery anastomosis is considered appropriate in such cases as a first-stage procedure to increase the safety of deliberately occluding the internal carotid artery as a second-stage procedure.

Intracranial Aneurysm

While microneuro-operative techniques have markedly improved the ability of neurosurgeons to obliterate most intracranial aneurysms directly, some (particularly giant aneurysms) are so related to parent arteries, so large and complex, or so inaccessibly located as to render direct approach excessively dangerous and impractical. The anastomosis may provide collateral circulation to essential vascular territories beyond these lesions so that they can be obliterated more safely, even if it is necessary to deliberately sacrifice a parent artery (Fig. 44-22).[4] Drake has been particularly successful in combining this method with application of a tourniquet device to the parent artery. The stem of the tourniquet has been brought to the surface through a small stab wound. With the patient awake and with concomitant arteriography, the tourniquet has then been tight-

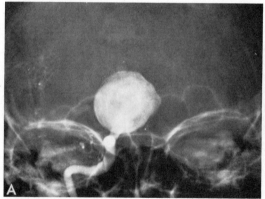
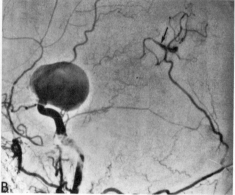

Figure 44–22 Giant aneurysm. *A.* Frontal projection of a right carotid arteriogram demonstrates preferential filling of a giant in-continuity aneurysm of the right internal carotid artery. Note: Contrast material from left carotid injection did not enter the aneurysm. *B.* Subtraction version of the lateral projection from a later right carotid arteriogram (after occipital artery–cortical middle cerebral artery anastomosis had been performed in preparation for gradual internal carotid artery occlusion) shows occipital artery filling vessels in the right parietal region through the anastomosis (*arrow*). [Note] Gradual occlusion of the right internal carotid artery with a Crutchfield clamp was tolerated without event.

ened to test the efficacy and safety of the result without discomfort to the patient. After permanent occlusion, the stem of the tourniquet has been placed beneath the scalp.[46] Spetzler and co-workers have developed a silicone rubber balloon catheter occluder that may be less traumatic and provide better control.[160]

Cerebral Arterial Dolichoectasia

This rare condition is recognized by marked elongation and dilation of major intracranial arteries.[172] The process may appear indistinguishable from a fusiform aneurysm, but it tends to affect multiple arteries and usually exists in the perforator-bearing trunk of the artery rather than arising from a bifurcation (Fig. 44–23). Since the process does not usually encroach upon the arterial lumen, ischemic manifestations presumably result from embolization. It seems unlikely that this condition would often be an appropriate indication for combined superficial temporal–cortical middle cerebral artery anastomosis and arterial occlusion because the resulting extremely slow flow through the cavernous parent artery, indispensable because it irrigates the tiny perforating branches, would add to the already ideal circumstances for thrombus formation. The reduced volume and velocity of flow could, however, conceivably, lessen the frequency of embolization and thereby reduce ischemic manifestations.

Carotid-Cavernous Fistula

Superficial temporal artery to middle cerebral artery anastomosis has been reported as a distinct aid in the successful obliteration of a carotid-cavernous fistula in at least two patients.[74,154]

Intracranial Neoplasm

A rare benign tumor may be so adherent to essential brain vessels that complete removal would require sacrificing them, even though they might seem quite normal in other respects. While actual experience with this approach is very limited, superficial temporal artery to middle cerebral artery anastomosis may provide the required collateral circulation to achieve a safe removal of such an otherwise unresectable tumor.[71]

Diagnostic Evaluation

Since the diagnosis of a transient ischemic attack is made primarily by history, a carefully detailed interview is essential. The date, time, duration, and specific characteristics of the first event should be documented. The frequency and duration of subsequent events should be noted with descriptions of each, in order to determine whether there has been a similar or a variable pattern of involvement. The patient may be able to recall most completely those facts pertaining to the most recent event,

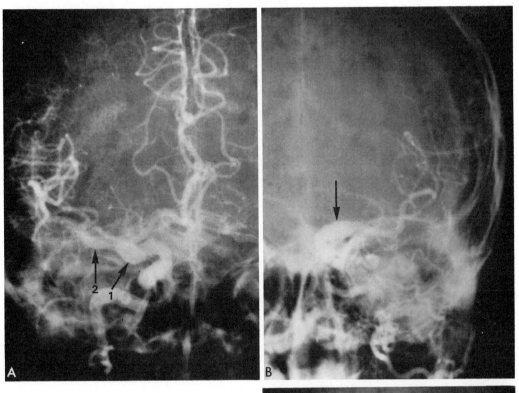

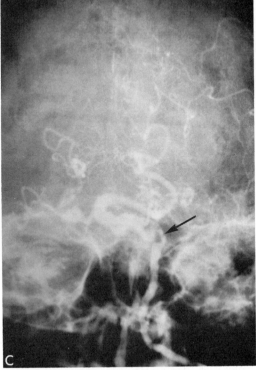

Figure 44–23 Cerebral artery dolichoectasia. *A.* Frontal projection of a right carotid arteriogram shows a dilated segment of the intracranial portion of the internal carotid artery (*arrow 1*) involving the bifurcation and extending into the right middle cerebral artery (*arrow 2*). *B.* Left carotid arteriogram shows involvement of the intracranial internal carotid artery bifurcation and proximal portion of the middle cerebral artery. *C.* The vertebral arteriogram shows an irregularly dilated, tortuous basilar artery beyond a proximal stenosis (*arrow*).

suggesting clues to earlier details that may have been disregarded. This meticulous search for information may greatly help the surgeon to understand the urgency of an ischemic process or to recognize another diagnosis.

The physical examination should disclose that the patient has no abnormal neurological findings or, if abnormalities are present, the extent of involvement. The findings should be clearly and completely documented as a baseline for future comparisons. The physical examination should also include several recordings of blood pressure, a careful determination of the cardiac and peripheral vascular status, and an assessment of other organ systems that could influence the outcome of an operation or preclude it because of an unrecognized grave disease.

Special diagnostic tests have little or no importance in establishing the diagnosis but may be of value (1) to determine possible causes of the transient ischemic attacks, (2) to detect risk factors and associated conditions of importance in the overall prognosis, (3) to rule out alternative diagnoses, and (4) to assess the patient's ability to tolerate various methods of treatment.[68]

Those tests generally considered to be routine include: complete blood count, urinalysis, chest roentgenogram, electrocardiogram, and measurement of blood urea nitrogen, fasting blood sugar, and serum electrolytes. An automated sequential analysis of multiple serum constituents is considered routine in many institutions. Serum triglyceride determination and lipoprotein electrophoresis are important in detecting abnormalities of lipid metabolism.[32,68]

Ophthalmodynamometry, oculoplethysmography, directional Doppler studies, and phonangiography may provide interesting information regarding indications for arteriography.[173]

Since it is cardiac disease that eventually accounts for approximately 50 per cent of the deaths of patients with cerebral vascular disease, formal consultation with a cardiologist is requested regularly. Frequently monitoring of the electrocardiogram during stress or for an extended period of time (24 hours) is included.[24,32] Since cerebral vascular disease may affect various aspects of higher cerebral function, psychological testing is usually recommended pre-operatively to establish a baseline of intellectual and communicative function.[52]

Electroencephalography may provide important information for distinguishing between a minor focal seizure and a transient ischemic attack. The radionuclide brain scan, which reflects the integrity of the blood-brain barrier, can assist in distinguishing between cerebral ischemia and infarction, and in clarifying the extent of cerebral destruction.[68] Computed tomography is particularly informative in assessing the presence or extent of cerebral damage and in excluding other diagnostic possibilities.[152]

Some investigators consider the focal reduction of regional cerebral blood flow to be an appropriate indication for the anastomosis.[12,13,151] Wider experience with these techniques is required, however, to define clearly their usefulness and limitations in the preoperative evaluation of patients considered for the procedure. In patients with stable neurological deficit, hyperbaric oxygenation has been recommended as a useful method for distinguishing those who would likely benefit from an anastomosis.[83,84] Unfortunately the equipment is expensive, special expertise is required, and this capability is not widely available.

Cerebral arteriography is the definitive diagnostic technique for evaluation of cerebral vascular disease.[106,139,155,168] It should include a study of the aortic arch and origins of the great vessels.[39] Both common carotid bifurcations, the vertebrobasilar system, and all other intracranial vasculature should be visualized. Magnification and subtraction techniques can be particularly helpful because many clinically important lesions involve small intracranial vessels, and important collateral pathways may otherwise be obscured by overlying structures of bone. In the interpretation of arteriographic studies, attention should be focused on the location and severity of all abnormalities.[168] A conclusion should be drawn concerning the pathogenesis.[39] Potential sources of collateral circulation should be identified, and a qualitative assessment of its extent considered an important factor in patient selection.[66] Only 3 of 478 patients (0.65 per cent) sustained permanent neurological deficit related to cerebral arteriography, as reported by the Cooperative Study of Hospital Frequency and Character of Transient Ischemic Attacks. A single death occurred in a deeply comatose patient. Transitory neurological complications developed in 25 patients (5.4 per cent), and transitory nonneurological complications in 29 (6.3 per cent).[168]

Differential Diagnosis

Thirteen-hundred, twenty-eight patients considered to have symptoms like those of transient ischemic attacks were registered into the Cooperative Study of Hospital Frequency and Character of Transient Ischemic Attacks.[48] Critical review of the records of these patients disclosed that that diagnosis could be confirmed in only 38 per cent. It was considered to be possible in 31 per cent, and in 30 per cent (395 patients) disorders other than transient ischemic attack were diagnosed. Of the 395 patients without a transient ischemic attack, 95 probably had a minor cerebral infarction, so the distinction seems relatively insignificant. A different diagnosis was suggested in 123 patients, however, and in 177, while the diagnosis of a transient ischemic attack was excluded, there was insufficient information to provide a correct diagnosis. In the group of 123 patients who did not have a transient ischemic attack the following conditions were found: postural hypotension (18), syncope (16), dizziness (14), cardiac arrhythmia and myocardial infarction (9), seizure disorder (18), anxiety (14), migraine headache (5), visual disturbance (4), mental confusion (7), brain tumor (5), and miscellaneous (13).[20]

Neurological disturbances resulting from brain tumor or subdural hematoma can be erroneously attributed to progressive cerebral ischemia. The literature contains at least one report of a case in which an extensive glioblastoma multiforme developed nine months later in the area where superficial temporal artery to middle cerebral artery anastomosis had been performed for symptoms attributed to occlusion of the internal carotid artery.[38]

Contraindications to Operation

An acute stroke—manifest by profound aphasia, hemiplegia, forced deviation of the head and eyes, and altered consciousness —is the result of extensive cerebral destruction and clearly a contraindication to microvascular reconstructive operations. Similarly, patients with a severe degree of stable neurological deficit (completed stroke) are not appropriate candidates for superficial temporal artery to middle cerebral artery anastomosis. Except under unusual circumstances, asymptomatic patients or patients who have been asymptomatic for many months are not encouraged to undergo an operation.

An operation should not be performed in the face of recent myocardial infarction, uncontrollable diabetes, or severe and uncontrolled hypertension. It is unwise to perform this type of operation upon any patient with widespread malignant disease or failure of any major organ system, or in the presence of any other condition expected to result in death within a short time.

Preoperative Management

Preoperative preparation, in addition to precise documentation of the patient's history, physical findings, and laboratory data, consists of meticulous medical management of hypertension, diabetes, cardiac disease, and other coexisting disease processes.[24] Readjustment of antihypertensive medication may be required before operation to avoid hypotension during the procedure and hypertension in the immediate postoperative period.

Platelet-suppressive medication may be prescribed preoperatively.[21,57] If a patient has been treated with anticoagulants, these should be discontinued and platelet-suppressive therapy may be substituted before an operation is performed.

Timing of Operation

It is preferred that a patient be asymptomatic when the anastomosis is performed. In the event of frequent transient ischemic attacks unrelieved by medical measures, however, one might elect to proceed with operation early in an ischemic event in an effort to reverse the ischemic process and minimize the resulting neurological deficit. In patients with mild to moderate grades of completed stroke, early operation (within one to two weeks after onset) seems to be beneficial in some cases and does not seem to threaten the conversion of an anemic infarct into a hemorrhagic infarct, as has been experienced occasionally with carotid endarterectomy. If hypertension has been controlled before operation, this complication does not seem to be a contraindication to the procedure. An operation performed several months after cerebral infarction is of no immediate benefit; it may, however, assist in preventing a future stroke in patients whose collateral circulation is marginal.

A few patients become asymptomatic or nearly so after an ischemic event but demonstrate a small hemorrhagic infarction on computed tomography. With them it is best to defer operation until this finding is no longer present.

Intracranial arterial occlusive disease is commonly associated with ipsilateral, contralateral, or bilateral extracranial carotid or vertebral artery disease.[114] Furthermore, arterial occlusive disease may involve the aorta or coronary, renal, or lower extremity vessels. If multiple operations are required, a decision should be made regarding priority. The operation for the most conspicuous and symptomatic lesion will usually be performed first unless external carotid artery reconstruction is required before the anastomosis.

Postoperative Care

Arterial pressure monitoring is continued during the early postoperative period be-

cause patients with incompletely controlled hypertension may develop labile blood pressure. Hypotension is rarely a problem, but moderate or severe hypertension is not uncommon. Moderate hypertension usually subsides spontaneously, but severe hypertension requires prompt and vigorous treatment (for a few hours in some cases) with intravenous trimethaphan camsylate or sodium nitroprusside. Longer-acting antihypertensive agents are then used for long-term maintenance. Antihypertensive medication must be used cautiously to avoid hypotensive episodes that may dangerously reduce perfusion and cause syncope or other manifestations of cerebral or cardiac ischemia.

Platelet-suppressive medication usually is continued postoperatively when the patient resumes oral intake.[21,57,87] It is continued for an indefinite period. Measures to control cardiac disease and diabetes are carefully followed. Dietary recommendations are made, physical exercise is encouraged, and smoking is proscribed.[24,32,87]

Results After Operation

Arteriographic Studies

Arteriography provides the most precise and complete assessment of the effectiveness of superficial temporal artery to middle cerebral artery anastomosis as a new channel of collateral circulation and its relationship to the preoperative cerebral circulation.[5,8] Selective external carotid injection (frontal and lateral projections should

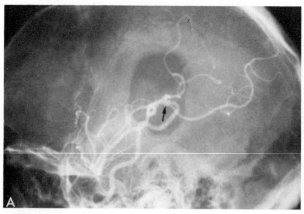
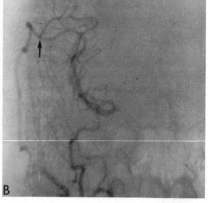

Figure 44–24 Typical postoperative arteriogram. *A.* Lateral projection shows superficial temporal artery irrigating entire middle cerebral artery territory through the anastomosis (*arrow*). *B.* Subtraction version of frontal projection shows superficial temporal artery irrigating sylvian vessels through the anastomosis (*arrow*).

be included) demonstrates patency of the anastomosis, diameter of the new collateral pathway, and extent of perfusion. Perfusion of the entire middle cerebral territory is most frequently demonstrated (Fig. 44–24).

Cinearteriography can be added to the study for estimating the actual volume of flow through the new collateral channel.[134] Selective internal carotid (bilateral, unless occlusion is present) and vertebral injections demonstrate the status of occlusive lesions and the interrelationships of the various sources of perfusion.

A patency rate of better than 90 per cent has been achieved by surgeons who have had extensive laboratory and clinical experience with micro-operative anastomosis. The bypass graft usually remains patent indefinitely, once good flow has been demonstrated by postoperative angiography, because the anastomosis was performed between two vessels rarely subject to atherosclerosis or other occlusive disease (Fig. 44–25). Serial arteriographic studies have shown gradual enlargement of the bypass graft.[5,8] This phenomenon occurs because the bypass graft, which was originally of small caliber, has been redirected into a large low-resistance network.[102,132,136]

Postoperative arteriographic studies have consistently demonstrated that perfusion of the middle cerebral artery territory is derived extensively from the superficial

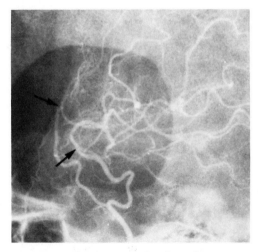

Figure 44–25 Arteriogram performed seven years after operation. Lateral projection demonstrates flow irrigating the entire left middle cerebral territory through two separate anastomoses (*arrows*). This arteriogram is similar to one that was performed six months after the operation.

temporal artery bypass.[5,8] The total perfusion reflects a balanced input from the normal anatomical pathways, other sources of collateral circulation, and flow from the bypass.[132,136] If the normal anatomical pathway was totally obstructed and other sources of collateral circulation were sparse, the superficial temporal artery bypass, enlarging with time, has usually irrigated the entire middle cerebral artery terri-

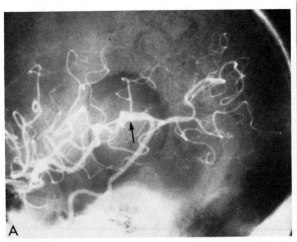
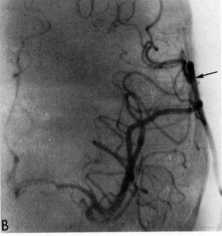

Figure 44–26 Postoperative arteriogram. *A.* Lateral projection demonstrates superficial temporal artery irrigating the entire left middle cerebral artery territory through the anastomosis (*arrow*). *B.* Subtraction version of frontal projection shows luxurious irrigation of the entire sylvian region through anastomosis (*arrow*) with extension across horizontal portion of middle cerebral artery into the anterior cerebral circulation.

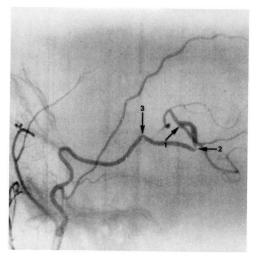

Figure 44–27 Subtraction version of lateral projection from postoperative carotid arteriogram shows sparse filling of middle cerebral artery vessels through anastomosis (*arrow 1*). Constriction has developed at two sites (*arrow 2 and arrow 3*) along the course of the superficial temporal artery bypass graft.

tory plus, frequently, some of the anterior cerebral or posterior communicating artery territories (cf. Figs. 44–10 and 44–26).

While arterial lesions have usually been stable, as demonstrated by serial postoperative arteriography, several have undergone change. Improvement of a lesion has been observed almost as frequently as progression of the occlusive process.[28,131] Rarely, a stenosis has developed in the grafted segment of superficial temporal artery (Fig. 44–27). Autopsy findings in two

cases reported by Steinbok suggest intimal hyperplasia as a probable cause for such a stenosis.[161]

Another rarity observed during postoperative arteriography was an aneurysm adjacent to the anastomosis (Fig. 44–28). The cause may have been failure of the suture to include an adequate amount of the medial layer of the arterial wall.

Electromagnetic flow measurements, performed during operation after completion of the anastomosis, have demonstrated flow rates ranging from 10 to 60 ml per minute.[26,35,158] One would expect these rates to increase postoperatively to correspond with the enlargement of the superficial temporal artery that is demonstrated by serial arteriographic studies. This inference has been strengthened by observations of Reichman, who has devised an arteriographic method for estimating flow through the bypass.[134] The average flow in a series of 20 patients studied 7 to 68 weeks (average 32 weeks) after operation was 90 ml per minute (with a range of 30 to 240 ml per minute). In each instance, the flow value correlated well with the extent of perfusion demonstrated by arteriographic study and with the presence of input from other sources. Postoperative studies of regional cerebral blood flow suggest an increase in blood flow after a superficial temporal artery to middle cerebral artery anastomosis.*

---

* See references 11, 13, 73, 79, 80, 102, 151.

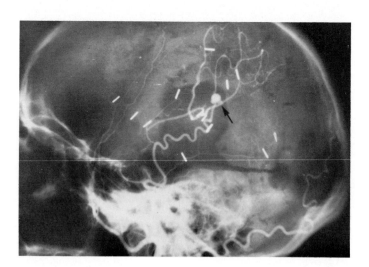

Figure 44–28 Lateral projection of carotid arteriogram shows modest irrigation of middle cerebral artery territory arising from superficial temporal artery with an aneurysm located immediately proximal to anastomosis (*arrow*). (Courtesy of Jae M. Noh, M.D.)

Clinical Outcome

Randomized clinical trials of the efficacy of this procedure are in progress.[108,130,131,138] Clinical follow-up of patients operated upon during the past decade, however, indicates that new ischemic events rarely have involved the hemisphere that was operated on in the presence of a functioning superficial temporal artery bypass.* Contralateral ischemic events also have been uncommon but have been observed in a few instances in which the preoperative arteriographic studies were incomplete.

Many patients with a progressing stroke or mild to moderate completed stroke have demonstrated an abrupt enhancement of improvement after operation.[86,131,175] Patients with long-standing stable deficit have, in general, not benefited from operation. Roski and associates reported a most remarkable exception in a man with a well-documented seven-year-old visual field defect that completely resolved immediately following operation.[142] Exceptions have also occurred in patients with cerebrovascular "moyamoya" disease who, having demonstrated stable deficit for several months, improved significantly following operation.[88,135]

Evans and Austin have reported upon the results of psychological testing performed before and after operation in 14 patients. They found that 12 of the 14 scored better postoperatively.[52]

Complications after superficial temporal to middle cerebral artery anastomosis are uncommon, usually not serious, and decrease with the increasing experience of the surgeon, the operating team, and other supporting personnel. A combination of the following factors probably is responsible: improvement in case selection, better management of risk factors and coexisting diseases, improved surgical skill, and reduced operating time. Transient neurological deficit as the result of this operation is uncommon, and permanent impairment is rare.[27,126,133,145,167] One complication unique to this type of operation is scalp necrosis, which is the result of scalp devascularization. It occurs rarely and can be minimized by designing the scalp flap carefully or placing the incision directly over the scalp artery.

Deaths attributable to superficial temporal to middle cerebral artery anastomosis are uncommon. Diabetes, hypertensive cardiovascular disease, cancer, and many other complex disease processes developing in the population in which this type of operation is performed have, however, caused a few deaths shortly after operation and several later in the follow-up period.[27,126,133,145,167] As could be predicted, an operation that is performed for acute stroke is associated with high rates of neurological impairment and death.

OTHER TECHNIQUES

Cervical Carotid–Intracranial Carotid Venous Bypass Grafts

The first successful operation involving a venous bypass graft between the cervical carotid and the internal carotid arteries was reported in 1971 by Lougheed and co-workers.[104] The procedure has been performed and further developed in small numbers of patients by other surgeons.[100,117,169,171] Although excellent results have been achieved in several instances, this operation has not received wide acceptance for several reasons: (1) the segment of internal carotid artery is very short, (2) endarterectomy of the short internal carotid artery segment is usually required, (3) atheroma may extend into the anterior and middle cerebral arteries, and (4) interruption of the major collateral pathways to the ipsilateral cerebral hemisphere is required during the anastomosis. Regardless of whether the patient improved or not, the results are most difficult to evaluate. In spite of these drawbacks, this procedure has many appealing features and deserves further investigation, specifically in the development of a temporary bypass shunt and in further refinement of methods for performing endarterectomy of the short intracranial internal carotid artery segment.

Posterior Fossa Revascularization

A large number of uncommon clinical syndromes have been observed in conjunc-

---

* See references 10, 11, 27, 69, 70, 101, 111, 131, 145, 147, 167, 186, 187.

tion with occlusive diseases involving the vertebrobasilar system.[6,22,34,91] The many specialized nuclei and tracts of the brain stem, specifically irrigated by small perforating branches, and the numerous possible sites for occlusion with variable collateral circulation lead to innumerable possible combinations of clinical deficit. Some of these conditions carry a dire prognosis, while others have a much more favorable outlook.[58]

Anticipating the possibility of microvascular anastomosis within the vertebrobasilar system, Weinstein considered possible recipient arteries.[176] Requiring that they be located superficially to avoid brain retraction and sufficiently distal to reduce a risk of infarction, and that they be at least 1 mm in diameter, he identified three possibilities: (1) the tonsillohemispheric branch of the posterior inferior cerebellar artery, (2) the lateral hemispheric branch of the superior cerebellar artery, and (3) the calcarine or parieto-occipital branch of the posterior cerebral artery. Rhoton and coworkers have further clarified the surgical anatomy pertaining to posterior fossa circulation.[78,143,188]

Experience with reconstructive procedures for vertebrobasilar arterial disease is limited. Most of the procedures have been performed for transient ischemic attacks associated with appropriate combinations of hypoplasia and occlusive disease (usually atherosclerosis) involving the vertebral arteries.

Vertebrobasilar system transient ischemic attacks are most commonly characterized by various combinations of dizziness, ataxia, diplopia, bilateral blurring of vision, and bilateral or alternating motor or sensory disturbance.[23,65] Dysarthria is common, but not of localizing value. Auditory disturbances, nystagmus, cranial nerve involvement, dysphagia, and gaze disturbances result more commonly from infarction.

As with cervical internal carotid artery stenosis, Lord recommends endarterectomy (transsubclavian) for stenosis involving the orifice of a vertebral artery.[103] Nagashima reports excellent experience with decompression (removal of hypertrophied "uncovertebral" joints) of the intraforaminal portion of vertebral arteries (C2 to C6) for the "ladder effect" related to cervical spondylosis.[113,116] Corkill and associates have reported end-to-side anastomosis between the external carotid artery and a high cervical segment of the vertebral artery (between C1 and C2 in one patient and between C4 and C5 in another).[33]

Ausman and co-workers, Khodadad, and Sundt and Piepgras report favorable and increasing experience with anastomosis between the occipital artery and the posterior inferior cerebellar artery.[7,89,90,166] This operation is more complex than is the superficial temporal to middle cerebral artery anastomosis because of the dense connective tissues surrounding the occipital artery and the deeper, more critical location of the posterior inferior cerebellar artery. The procedure is usually performed with the patient in the sitting position, but the prone position also has been used. Operative morbidity may be greater, and postoperative management may be more complex than in the previously described procedures. Hypotension, dysphagia, respiratory difficulty, and other signs of brain stem dysfunction may occur and require diligent observation and management. These complications are usually temporary, however, and the clinical outcome for these patients has usually been satisfactory.

Anastomosis has been performed between the superficial temporal artery and the superior cerebellar artery to develop new collateral circulation to the upper basilar region.[7,8a,166] While the results were not entirely satisfactory, experience is too limited to draw a firm conclusion, and this method appears to be a feasible solution for some patients with lesions of the basilar artery. The major limiting factor would be the extent to which atherosclerotic disease had involved the orifices of vital perforating branches. An operative approach similar to that recommended by Drake for aneurysms of the basilar artery is used, and the superior cerebellar artery is readily exposed.[45] The "shallow caudal loop" is quite redundant and relatively free of perforators.[78] The artery averages 1.9 mm (range 0.8 to 2.8 mm) in diameter unless it branches proximally. Good collateral circulation is protective against infarction of the vital distal structures during temporary occlusion. Because of the distance between the superficial temporal artery and the superior cerebellar artery, a free graft may be required. The radial artery has been interposed between the other two arteries with an end-to-side anastomosis being performed at each end.[7,8a] This procedure seems quite promising and deserves further evaluation under appropriate circumstances. Anastomosis to the posterior cerebral artery, which Drake has permanently ligated safely in nine patients (a visual field defect resulted in only one), may be even more suitable because its larger diameter averages 2.9 mm (range 1.7 to 3.5 mm).[46]

REFERENCES

1. Alpers, B. J., and Berry, R. G.: Circle of Willis in cerebral vascular disorders: The anatomical structure. Arch. Neurol. (Chicago), 8:398–402, 1963.
2. Alpers, B. J., Berry, R. G., and Paddison, R. M.: Anatomical studies of the circle of Willis in normal brain. Arch. Neurol. Psychiat., 81: 409–418, 1959.
3. Amine, A. R. C., Moody, R. A., and Meeks, W.: Bilateral temporal-middle cerebral artery anastomosis for moyamoya syndrome. Surg. Neurol., 8:3–6, 1977.
4. Ammerman, B. J., and Smith, D. R.: Giant fusiform middle cerebral aneurysm: Successful treatment utilizing microvascular bypass. Surg. Neurol., 7:255–257, 1977.
5. Anderson, R. E., Reichman, O. H., and Davis, D. O.: Radiological evaluation of temporal artery–middle cerebral artery anastomosis. Radiology, 113:73–79, 1974.
6. Archer, C. R., and Horenstein, S.: Basilar artery occlusion: Clinical and radiological correlation. Stroke, 8:383–390, 1977.
7. Ausman, J. I., Nicoloff, D. M., and Chou, S. N.: Posterior fossa revascularization: Anastomosis of vertebral artery to PICA with interposed radial artery graft. Surg. Neurol., 9:281–286, 1978.
8. Ausman, J. I., Latchaw, R. E., Lee, M. C., et al.: Results of multiple angiographic studies on cerebral revascularization patients. In Schmiedek, P., Gratzl, O., and Spetzler, R. F., eds.: Microsurgery for Stroke. New York-Berlin-Heidelberg, Springer-Verlag, 1977, pp. 222–229.
8a. Ausman, J. I., Lee, M. C., Chater, N., et al.: Superficial temporal artery to superior cerebellar artery anastomosis for distal basilar artery stenosis. Surg. Neurol., 12:277–282, 1979.
9. Austin, G. M., ed.: Microneurosurgical Anastomoses for Cerebral Ischemia. Springfield, Ill., Charles C Thomas, 1976.
10. Austin, G., Hayward, W., and Laffin, D.: Modification of cerebral ischemia by microsurgical intracranial anastomosis. In Austin, G. M., ed.: Microneurosurgical Anastomoses for Cerebral Ischemia. Springfield, Ill., Charles C Thomas, 1976, pp. 281–294.
11. Austin, G., Laffin, D., and Hayward, W.: Evaluation and selection of patients for microneurosurgical anastomosis in the treatment of cerebral ischemia. In Morley, T. P., ed.: Current Controversies in Neurosurgery. Philadelphia-London-Toronto, W. B. Saunders Co., 1976, pp. 294–303.
12. Austin, G., Laffin, D., and Hayward, W.: Physiologic factors in the selection of patients for su-

13. Austin, G., Laffin, D., Vasudevan, R., et al.: Cerebral blood flow in stroke-type patients. In Fein, J. M., and Reichman, O. H., eds.: Microvascular Anastomoses for Cerebral Ischemia. New York-Berlin-Heidelberg, Springer-Verlag, 1978, pp. 241–265.
14. Baker, R. N., Ramseyer, J. C., and Schwartz, W. S.: Prognosis in patients with transient cerebral ischemic attacks. Neurology (Minneap.), 18:1157–1165, 1968.
15. Baker, R. N., Schwartz, W. S., and Ramseyer, J. C.: Prognosis among survivors of ischemic stroke. Neurology (Minneap.), 18:933–941, 1968.
16. Barnett, H. J. M.: Clinical evaluation of strokes and threatened strokes. Clin. Neurosurg., 23:540–554, 1976.
17. Barnett, H. J. M.: Pathogenesis of transient ischemic attacks. In Scheinberg, P., ed.: Cerebrovascular Diseases. Tenth Princeton Conference. New York, Raven Press, 1976, pp. 1–21.
18. Boone, S. C., and Sampson, D. S.: Observations on moyamoya disease: A case treated with superficial temporal–middle cerebral artery anastomosis. Surg. Neurol., 9:189–193, 1978.
19. Brust, J. C. M.: Transient ischemic attacks: Natural history and anticoagulation. Neurology (Minneap.) 27:701–707, 1977.
20. Calanchini, P. R., Swanson, P. D., Gotshall, R. A., et al.: Cooperative study of hospital frequency and character of transient ischemic attacks: IV. The reliability of diagnosis. J.A.M.A., 238:2029–2033, 1977.
21. Canadian Cooperative Study Group: A randomized trial of aspirin and sulfinpyrazone in threatened stroke. New Eng. J. Med., 299:53–59, 1978.
22. Caplan, L. R., and Rosenbaum, A. E.: Role of cerebral angiography in vertebrobasilar occlusive disease. J. Neurol. Neurosurg. Psychiat., 38:601–612, 1975.
23. Cartlidge, N. E. F., Whisnant, J. P., and Elveback, L. R.: Carotid and vertebral-basilar transient cerebral ischemic attacks: A community study, Rochester, Minnesota. Mayo Clin. Proc. 52:117–120, 1977.
24. Cassidy, J. E.: Management of risk factors and other diseases in candidates for microneurosurgical anastomosis in cerebral ischemia. In Fein, J. M., and Reichman, O. H., eds.: Microvascular Anastomoses for Cerebral Ischemia. New York-Berlin-Heidelberg, Springer-Verlag, 1978, pp. 105–116.
25. Chater, N.: Patient selection and results of extra to intracranial anastomosis in selected cases of cerebrovascular disease. Clin. Neurosurg., 23:287–309, 1976.
26. Chater, N.: Surgical results and measurements of intraoperative flow in microneurosurgical anastomoses. In Austin, G. M., ed.: Microneurosurgical Anastomoses for Cerebral Ischemia. Springfield, Ill., Charles C Thomas, 1976, pp. 295–304.
27. Chater, N., and Popp, J.: Microsurgical vascular bypass for occlusive cerebrovascular disease: Review of 100 cases. Surg. Neurol., 6:115–118, 1976.
28. Chater, N. L., and Weinstein, P. R.: Progression

perficial temporal artery–to–middle cerebral artery anastomosis. Surgery, 75:861–868, 1974.

of middle cerebral artery stenosis to occlusion without symptoms following superficial temporary artery bypass: Case report. *In* Fein, J. M., and Reichman, O. H., eds.: Microvascular Anastomoses for Cerebral Ischemia. New York-Berlin-Heidelberg, Springer-Verlag, 1978, pp. 269–271.

29. Chater, N., Mani, J., and Tonnemacher, K.: Superficial temporal artery bypass in occlusive cerebral vascular disease. Calif. Med., *119*:9–13, 1973.

30. Chater, N., Spetzler, R., and Tonnemacher, K.: Anatomical localization of optimal middle cerebral branch for anastomosis. *In* Austin, G. M., ed.: Microneurosurgical Anastomoses for Cerebral Ischemia. Springfield, Ill., Charles C Thomas, 1976, pp. 39–51.

31. Chater, N., Spetzler, R., Tonnemacher, K., et al.: Microvascular bypass surgery. Part 1: Anatomical studies. J. Neurosurg., *44*:712–714, 1976.

32. Conneally, P. M., Dyken, M. L., Futty, D. E., et al.: Cooperative study of hospital frequency and character of transient ischemic attacks: VIII. Risk factors. J.A.M.A., *240*:742–746, 1978.

33. Corkill, G., French, B. N., Michas, C., et al.: External carotid–vertebral artery anastomosis for vertebrobasilar insufficiency. Surg. Neurol., *7*:109–115, 1977.

34. Cravioto, H., Rey-Bellet, J., Prose, P. H., et al.: Occlusion of the basilar artery: A clinical and pathological study of 14 autopsied cases. Neurology (Minneap.), *8*:145–152, 1958.

35. Crowell, R. M.: Electromagnetic flow studies of superficial temporal artery to middle cerebral branch artery bypass graft. *In* Austin, G. M., ed.: Microneurosurgical Anastomoses for Cerebral Ischemia. Springfield, Ill., Charles C Thomas, 1976, pp. 116–124.

36. Crowell, R. M.: STA-MCA bypass for acute focal cerebral ischemia. *In* Schmiedek, P., Gratzl, O., and Spetzler, R. F., eds.: Microsurgery for Stroke. New York-Berlin-Heidelberg, Springer-Verlag, 1977, pp. 244–250.

37. Crutchfield, W. G.: Instruments for use in the treatment of certain intracranial vascular lesions. J. Neurosurg., *16*:471–474, 1959.

38. Cusick, J. F., Komacki, S., and Choi, H.: Superficial temporal–middle cerebral artery anastomosis associated with glioblastoma multiforme: Case report. J. Neurosurg., *46*:381–384, 1977.

39. Davis, D. O., and Pressman, B. D.: Angiography of cerebrovascular disease. Clin. Neurosurg., *22*:163–184, 1975.

40. Donaghy, R. M. P.: Status of microangeional surgery in 1971. *In* Fusek, I., and Kunc, Z., eds.: Present Limits of Neurosurgery. Prague, Avicenum, Czechoslovak Medical Press, 1972, pp. 351–355.

41. Donaghy, R. M. P.: What's new in surgery? Neurologic surgery. Surg. Gynec. Obstet., *134*:269–271, 1972.

42. Donaghy, R. M. P.: Evaluation of extracranial-intracranial blood flow diversion. *In* Austin, G. M., ed.: Microneurosurgical Anastomoses for Cerebral Ischemia. Springfield, Ill., Charles C Thomas, 1976, pp. 256–274.

43. Donaghy, R. M. P., and Yasargil, M. G., eds.: Micro-vascular Surgery. St. Louis, C. V. Mosby Co.; Stuttgart, Georg Thieme Verlag, 1967.

44. Donaghy, R. M. P., and Yasargil, M. G.: Extra-intracranial blood flow diversion. Abstract 52. Presentation before the American Association of Neurological Surgeons, Chicago, April 11, 1968.

45. Drake, C. G.: The surgical treatment of aneurysms of the basilar artery. J. Neurosurg., *29*:436–446, 1968.

46. Drake, C. G.: Giant intracranial aneurysms: Experience with surgical treatment in 174 patients. Clin. Neurosurg., *26*:12–95, 1979.

47. Dujovny, M., Osgood, C. P., Barrionuevo, P. J., et al.: SEM evaluation of endothelial damage following temporary middle cerebral artery occlusion in dogs. J. Neurosurg., *48*:42–48, 1978.

48. Dyken, M. L., Conneally, P. M., Haerer, A. F., et al.: Cooperative study of hospital frequency and character of transient ischemic attacks: I. Background, organization, and clinical survey. J.A.M.A., *237*:882–886, 1977.

49. Dyken, M. L., Doepker, J. F., Kiovsky, R., et al.: Asymptomatic occlusion of an internal carotid artery in a hospital population: Determined by directional Doppler ophthalmosonometry. Stroke, *5*:714–718, 1974.

50. Dyken, M. L., Klatte, E., Kolar, O. J., et al.: Complete occlusion of common or internal carotid arteries: Clinical significance. Arch. Neurol. (Chicago), *30*:343–346, 1974.

51. Epstein, M. H.: External carotid–middle cerebral artery bypass using free graft bypass. *In* Fein, J. M., and Reichman, O. H., eds.: Microvascular Anastomoses for Cerebral Ischemia. New York-Berlin-Heidelberg, Springer-Verlag, 1978, pp. 178–180.

52. Evans, R. B., and Austin, G.: Psychological evaluation of patients undergoing microneurosurgical anastomoses for cerebral ischemia. *In* Austin, G. M., ed.: Microneurosurgical Anastomoses for Cerebral Ischemia. Springfield, Ill., Charles C Thomas, 1976, pp. 320–326.

53. Fein, J. M.: Contemporary techniques of cerebral revascularization. *In* Fein, J. M., and Reichman, O. H., eds.: Microvascular Anastomoses for Cerebral Ischemia. New York-Berlin-Heidelberg, Springer-Verlag, 1978, pp. 161–177.

54. Fein, J. M.: Microvascular surgery for stroke. Sci. Amer., *238*:58–67, 1978.

55. Fein, J. M., and Reichman, O. H., eds.: Microvascular Anastomoses for Cerebral Ischemia. New York-Berlin-Heidelberg, Springer-Verlag, 1978.

56. Fields, W. S., and Lemak, N. A.: Joint study of extracranial arterial occlusion: X. Internal carotid artery occlusion. J.A.M.A., *235*:2734–2738, 1976.

57. Fields, W. S., Lemak, N. A., Frankowski, R. F., et al.: Controlled trial of aspirin in cerebral ischemia. Stroke, *8*:301–316, 1977.

58. Fields, W. S., Ratinov, G., Weibel, J., et al.: Survival following basilar artery occlusion. Arch. Neurol. (Chicago), *15*:463–471, 1966.

59. Fisher, C. M.: Occlusion of the internal carotid artery. Arch. Neurol. (Chicago), *65*:346–377, 1951.

60. Fisher, C. M.: Clinical syndromes in cerebral thrombosis, hypertensive hemorrhage, and

ruptured saccular aneurysm. Clin. Neurosurg., *22*:117–147, 1975.

61. Fisher, C. M.: The natural history of carotid occlusion. *In* Austin, G. M., ed.: Microneurosurgical Anastomoses for Cerebral Ischemia. Springfield, Ill., Charles C Thomas, 1976, pp. 194–201.

62. Fisher, C. M.: The natural history of middle cerebral artery trunk occlusion. *In* Austin, G. M., ed.: Microneurosurgical Anastomoses for Cerebral Ischemia. Springfield, Ill., Charles C Thomas, 1976, pp. 146–154.

63. Fisher, C. M., Gore, I., Okabe, N., et al.: Atherosclerosis of the carotid and vertebral arteries—extracranial and intracranial. J. Neuropath. Exp. Neurol., *24*:455–476, 1965.

64. Fox, J. L., Albin, M. S., Bader, D. C. H., et al.: Microsurgical treatment of neurovascular disease. Neurosurgery, *3*:285–337, 1978.

65. Futty, D. E., Conneally, P. M., Dyken, M. L., et al.: Cooperative study of hospital frequency and character of transient ischemic attacks: V. Symptom analysis. J.A.M.A., *238*:2386–2390, 1977.

66. Gado, M., and Marshall, J.: Clinico-radiological study of collateral circulation after internal carotid and middle cerebral occlusion. J. Neurol. Neurosurg. Psychiat., *34*:163–170, 1971.

67. Gertz, S. D., Kurgan, A., Wajnberg, R. S., et al.: Endothelial cell damage and thrombus formation following temporary arterial occlusion. J. Neurosurg., *50*:578–586, 1979.

68. Gotshall, R. A., Price, T. R., Haerer, A. F., et al.: Cooperative study of hospital frequency and character of transient ischemic attacks: VII. Initial diagnostic evaluation. J.A.M.A., *239*:2001–2003, 1978.

69. Gratzl, O., Schmiedek, P., and Olteanu-Nerbe, V.: Long-term clinical results following extraintracranial arterial bypass surgery. *In* Schmiedek, P., Gratzl, O., and Spetzler, R. F., eds.: Microsurgery for Stroke. New York-Berlin-Heidelberg, Springer-Verlag, 1977, pp. 271–275.

70. Gratzl, O., Schmiedek, P., Spetzler, R., et al.: Clinical experience with extra-intracranial arterial anastomosis in 65 cases. J. Neurosurg., *44*:313–324, 1976.

71. Gratzl, O., Schmiedek, P., and Steinhoff, H.: Extra-intracranial arterial bypass in patients with occlusion of cerebral arteries due to trauma and tumor. *In* Handa, H., ed.: Microneurosurgery. Tokyo, Igaku Shoin; Baltimore, University Park Press, 1975, pp. 68–80.

72. Gratzl, O., Steude, U., and Schmiedek, P.: Indications for extra-intracranial anastomosis between the superficial temporal artery and a branch of the middle cerebral artery in man. *In* Fusek, I., and Kunc, Z., eds.: Present Limits of Neurosurgery. Prague, Avicenum, Czechoslovak Medical Press, 1972, pp. 375–379.

73. Grubb, R. L., Jr., Ratcheson, R. A., Raichle, M. E., et al.: Regional cerebral blood flow and oxygen utilization in superficial temporal–middle cerebral artery anastomosis patients: An exploratory definition of clinical problems. J. Neurosurg., *50*:733–741, 1979.

74. Guegan, Y., Javalet, A., Eon, J. Y., et al.: Extraintracranial anastomosis preliminary to treatment of carotid artery–cavernous sinus fistula. Surg. Neurol., *10*:85–88, 1978.

75. Gurdjian, E. S., Lindner, D. W., and Thomas, L. M.: Experiences with ligation of the common carotid artery for treatment of aneurysms of the internal carotid artery. J. Neurosurg., *23*:311–318, 1965.

76. Haerer, A. F., Gotshall, R. A., Conneally, P. M., et al.: Cooperative study of hospital frequency and character of transient ischemic attacks: III. Variations in treatment. J.A.M.A., *238*:142–146, 1977.

77. Handa, H., ed.: Microneurosurgery. Tokyo, Igaku Shoin; Baltimore, University Park Press, 1975.

78. Hardy, D. G., and Rhoton, A. L., Jr.: Microsurgical relationships of the superior cerebellar artery and the trigeminal nerve. J. Neurosurg., *49*:669–678, 1978.

79. Heilbrun, M. P., Reichman, O. H., Anderson, R. E., et al.: Regional cerebral blood flow studies following superficial temporal–middle cerebral anastomosis. J. Neurosurg., *43*:706–716, 1975.

80. Heilbrun, M. P., Reichman, O. H., Anderson, R. E., et al.: Regional cerebral blood flow studies following superficial temporal–middle cerebral artery anastomosis. *In* Fein, J. M., and Reichman, O. H., eds.: Microvascular Anastomoses for Cerebral Ischemia. New York-Berlin-Heidelberg, Springer-Verlag, 1978, pp. 204–209.

81. Henschen, C.: Operative Revaskularisation des zirkulatorisch geschädigten Gehirns durch Auflage gestielter Muskellappen (Encephalo-Myo-Synangiose). Langenbecks Arch. Klin. Chir., *264*:392–401, 1950.

82. Hinton, R. C., Mohr, J. P., Ackerman, R. H., et al.: Symptomatic middle cerebral artery stenosis. Ann. Neurol., *5*:152–157, 1979.

83. Holbach, K. H., Wassmann, H., and Kutzner, M.: Intracranial vascular reconstructive surgery of the brain—indications. *In* Carrea, R., and Vay, D. L., eds.: Neurological Surgery. International Congress Series No. 433. Amsterdam-Oxford, Excerpta Medica, 1978, pp. 223–232.

84. Holbach, K. H., Wassman, H., Hoheluchter, K. L., et al.: Differentiation between reversible and irreversible post-stroke changes in brain tissue: Its relevance for cerebrovascular surgery. Surg. Neurol., *7*:325–331, 1977.

85. Hood, R. S., Heilbrun, M. P., and Millikan, C. H.: Fibromuscular dysplasia as a primary cause of ischemic events. Presentation before the American Association of Neurological Surgeons, New Orleans, April 26, 1978.

86. Jacques, S., and Garner, J. T.: Reversal of aphasia with superficial temporal artery to middle cerebral artery anastomosis. Surg. Neurol., *5*:143–145, 1976.

87. Kannel, W. B.: Current status of the epidemiology of brain infarction associated with occlusive arterial disease. Stroke, *2*:295–318, 1971.

88. Karasawa, J., Kikuchi, H., Furuse, S., et al.: Treatment of moyamoya disease with STA-MCA anastomosis. J. Neurosurg., *49*:679–688, 1978.

89. Khodadad, G.: Occipital artery–posterior inferior cerebellar artery anastomosis. Surg. Neurol., *5*:225–227, 1976.

90. Khodadad, G.: Atherosclerotic occlusive disease of the vertebrobasilar system in young adults and its surgical consideration. Acta Neurochir. (Wien), *45*:147–154, 1978.

91. Khodadad, G., and McLaurin, R. L.: Syndromes of vertebrobasilar insufficiency and their possible surgical treatment. J. Fam. Pract., 6:1185–1190, 1978.

92. Kikuchi, H., and Karasawa, J.: Extra-intracranial arterial anastomosis in ten patients with moyamoya syndrome (occlusion of the circle of Willis). In Schmiedek, P., Gratzl, O., and Spetzler, R. F., eds.: Microsurgery for Stroke. New York-Berlin-Heidelberg, Springer-Verlag, 1977, pp. 260–263.

93. Kikuchi, H., and Karasawa, J.: Clinical experiences with STA-MCA anastomosis in 54 cases. In Fein, J. M., and Reichman, O. H., eds.: Microvascular Anastomoses for Cerebral Ischemia. New York-Berlin-Heidelberg, Springer-Verlag, 1978, pp. 278–283.

94. Kindt, G. W.: Arterial clamp for more gradual blood flow reduction. Technical note. J. Neurosurg., 30:508–510, 1969.

95. Koos, W. T., Böck, F. W., and Spetzler, R. F., eds.: Clinical Microneurosurgery. Stuttgart, Georg Thieme Verlag; New York, Academic Press, 1976.

96. Koos, W. T., Reichman, O. H., Schuster, H., et al.: Surgical technique of extra-intracranial arterial anastomosis. In Koos, W. T., Böck, F. W., and Spetzler, R. F., eds.: Clinical Microneurosurgery. Stuttgart, Georg Thieme Verlag; New York, Academic Press, 1976, pp. 247–251.

97. Krayenbühl, H., and Yasargil, G.: Der cerebrale kollaterale Blutkreislauf im angiographischen Bild. Acta Neurochir. (Wien), 6:30–80, 1958.

98. Kuller, L. H.: The transient ischemic attack. Curr. Conc. Cerebrovasc. Dis. Stroke, 9:23–26, 1974.

99. Lascelles, R. G., and Burrows, E. H.: Occlusion of the middle cerebral artery. Brain, 88:85–96, 1965.

100. Lazar, M. L., and Clark, K.: Microsurgical cerebral revascularization: Concepts and practice. Surg. Neurol., 1:355–359, 1973.

101. Lee, M. C., Ausman, J. I., Geiger, J. D., et al.: Superficial temporal to middle cerebral artery anastomosis: Clinical outcome in patients with ischemia of infarction in internal carotid artery distribution. Arch. Neurol. (Chicago), 36:1–4, 1979.

102. Little, J. R., Yamamoto, Y. L., Feindel, W., et al.: Superficial temporal artery to middle cerebral artery anastomosis: Intraoperative evaluation by fluorescein angiography and xenon-133 clearance. J. Neurosurg., 50:560–569, 1979.

103. Lord, R. S. A.: Vertebrovasilar ischaemia and the extracranial arteries. Med. J. Aust., 2:32–37, 1973.

104. Lougheed, W. M., Marshall, B. M., Hunter, M., et al.: Common carotid to intracranial internal carotid bypass venous graft. Technical note. J. Neurosurg., 34:114–118, 1971.

105. Malis, L. I.: Personal communication, October 1977.

106. Marshall, J.: Angiography in the investigation of ischaemic episodes in the territory of the internal carotid artery. Lancet, 1:719–721, 1971.

107. Marti-Vilalta, J. L., Lopez-Pousa, S., Grau, J. M., et al.: Transient ischemic attacks. Retrospective study of 150 cases of ischemic infarct in the territory of the middle cerebral artery. Stroke, 10:259–262, 1979.

108. McDowell, F. H.: The extracranial/intracranial bypass study. Stroke, 8:545, 1977.

109. McDowell, F. H., Potes, J., and Groch, S.: The natural history of internal carotid and vertebral-basilar artery occlusion. Neurology (Minneap.), 11:153–157, 1961.

110. Mérei, F. T., ed.: Reconstructive Surgery of Brain Arteries. Budapest, Akadémiai Kiadó, 1974.

111. Mérei, F. T., and Bodosi, M.: Microsurgical anastomosis for cerebral ischemia in ninety patients. In Schmiedek, P., Gratzl, O., and Spetzler, R. F., eds.: Microsurgery for Stroke. New York-Berlin-Heidelberg, Springer-Verlag, pp. 264–270, 1977.

112. Moossy, J.: Cerebral infarction and intracranial arterial thrombosis. Arch. Neurol. (Chicago), 14:119–123, 1966.

113. Moossy, J.: Cerebral infarcts and the lesions of intracranial and extracranial atherosclerosis. Arch. Neurol. (Chicago), 14:124–128, 1966.

114. Moran, J. M., Reichman, O. H., and Baker, W. H.: Staged intracranial and extracranial revascularization. Arch. Surg. (Chicago), 112:1424–1428, 1977.

115. Mount, L. A.: Results of treatment of intracranial aneurysms using the Selverstone clamp. J. Neurosurg., 16:611–618, 1959.

116. Nagashima, C.: Surgical treatment of vertebral artery insufficiency caused by cervical spondylosis. J. Neurosurg., 32:512–521, 1970.

117. Neblett, C. R.: Large vessel vein grafts for cerebral ischemia. Presentation before the Congress of Neurological Surgeons, Vancouver, Canada, September 25, 1974.

118. Nishikawa, M., Yasargil, M. G., Yagi, N., et al.: Experimental extracranial-intracranial anastomosis. Surg. Neurol., 8:249–253, 1977.

119. Nishioka, H.: Report on the cooperative study of intracranial aneurysms and subarachnoid hemorrhage. Section VIII, Part 1. Results of the treatment of intracranial aneurysms by occlusion of the carotid artery in the neck. J. Neurosurg., 25:660–682, 1966.

120. Nornes, H.: The role of the circle of Willis in graded occlusion of the internal carotid artery in man. Acta Neurochir. (Wien), 28:165–177, 1973.

121. Obrist, W. D.: Cerebral blood flow and its regulation. Clin. Neurosurg., 22:106–116, 1975.

122. Peerless, S. J.: Techniques of cerebral revascularization. Clin. Neurosurg., 23:258–269, 1976.

123. Peerless, S. J., Chater, N. L., and Ferguson, G. F.: Multiple-vessel occlusions in cerebrovascular disease—a further followup of the effects of microvascular bypass on the quality of life and the incidence of stroke. In Schmiedek, P., Gratzl, O., and Spetzler, R. D., eds.: Microsurgery for Stroke. New York-Berlin-Heidelberg, Springer-Verlag, 1977, pp. 251–259.

124. Perlmutter, D., and Rhoton, A. L., Jr.: Microsurgical anatomy of the anterior cerebral–anterior communicating–recurrent artery complex. J. Neurosurg., 45:259–272, 1976.

125. Pool, J. L., and Potts, D. G., eds.: Aneurysms and Arteriovenous Anomalies of the Brain. New York, Harper & Row, 1965, pp. 221–222.

126. Popp, A. J., and Chater, N.: Extracranial-to-intracranial vascular anastomosis for occlusive cerebrovascular disease: Experience in 110 patients. Surgery, 82:648–654, 1977.

127. Price, T. R., Gotshall, R. A., Poskanzer, D. C., et al.: Cooperative study of hospital frequency and character of transient ischemic attacks: VI. Patients examined during an attack. J.A.M.A., *238*:2512–2515, 1977.

128. Rand, R. W., ed.: Microneurosurgery. St. Louis, C. V. Mosby Co., 1969.

129. Redondo, A., and Le Beau, J.: Traitement des ischémies cérébrales par anastomose artérielle extra-intra-crânienne précoce. Presentation before the Société de Neuro-chirurgie de Langue Française, Paris, France, December 2, 1975.

130. Reichman, O. H.: Extracranial-intracranial arterial anastomosis. *In* Whisnant, J. P., and Sandok, B. A., eds.: Cerebral Vascular Diseases, Ninth Princeton Conference. New York, Grune & Stratton Inc., 1975, pp. 175–185.

131. Reichman, O. H.: Neurosurgical microsurgical anastomosis for cerebral ischemia: Five years' experience. *In* Scheinberg, P., ed.: Cerebral Vascular Diseases, Tenth Princeton Conference. New York, Raven Press, 1976, pp. 311–330.

132. Reichman, O. H.: Arteriographic flow patterns following STA–cortical MCA anastomosis. *In* Austin, G. M., ed.: Microneurosurgical Anastomoses for Cerebral Ischemia. Springfield, Ill., Charles C Thomas, 1976, pp. 339–358.

133. Reichman, O. H.: Complications of cerebral revascularization. Clin. Neurosurg., *23*:318–335, 1976.

134. Reichman, O. H.: Estimation of flow through STA bypass graft. *In* Fein, J. M., and Reichman, O. H., eds.: Microvascular Anastomoses for Cerebral Ischemia. New York-Berlin-Heidelberg, Springer-Verlag, 1978, pp. 220–240.

135. Reichman, O. H., Anderson, R. E., Roberts, T. S., et al.: The treatment of intracranial occlusive cerebrovascular disease by STA–cortical MCA anastomosis. *In* Handa, H., ed.: Microneurosurgery. Tokyo, Igaku Shoin; Baltimore, University Park Press, 1975, pp. 31–46.

136. Reichman, O. H., Davis, D. O., Roberts, T. S., et al.: Anastomosis between STA and cortical branch of MCA for the treatment of occlusive cerebrovascular disease. *In* Mérei, F. T., ed.: Reconstructive Surgery of Brain Arteries. Budapest, Akadémiai Kiadó, 1974, pp. 201–218.

137. Reichman, O. H., Satovick, R. M., Davis, D. O., et al.: Collateral circulation to the middle cerebral territory by anastomosis of superficial temporal and cortical arteries. *In* Fusek, I., and Kunc, Z., eds.: Present Limits of Neurosurgery. Prague, Avicenum, Czechoslovak Medical Press, 1972, pp. 369–373.

138. Reinmuth, O. M.: Intracranial bypass surgery for cerebral arterial disease and the responsibility of the practicing physician. Stroke, *10*:344–347, 1979.

139. Ring, B. A., and Waddington, M. M., eds.: The Neglected Cause of Stroke. St. Louis, W. H. Green, 1969.

140. Robertson, J. H., and Robertson, J. T.: The relationship between suture number and quality of anastomoses in microvascular procedures. Surg. Neurol., *10*:241–245, 1978.

141. Rosenbaum, T. J., and Sundt, T. M., Jr.: Interrelationship of aneurysm clips and vascular tissue. J. Neurosurg., *48*:929–934, 1978.

142. Roski, R., Spetzler, R. F., Owen, M., et al.: Reversal of seven-year-old visual field defect with extracranial-intracranial arterial anastomosis. Surg. Neurol., *10*:267–268, 1978.

143. Saeki, N., and Rhoton, A. L., Jr.: Microsurgical anatomy of the upper basilar artery and the posterior circle of Willis. J. Neurosurg., *46*:563–578, 1977.

144. Salazar, J. L., Amine, A. R. C., and Sugar, O.: Intracranial neurosurgical treatment of occlusive cerebrovascular disease. Stroke, *7*:348–353, 1976.

145. Samson, D. S., and Boone, S.: Extracranial-intracranial (EC-IC) arterial bypass: Past performance and current concepts. Neurosurgery *3*:79–86, 1978.

146. Samson, D. S., Hodosh, R. M., and Clark, W. K.: Microsurgical treatment of transient cerebral ischemia. J.A.M.A., *241*:376–378, 1979.

147. Samson, D., Watts, C., and Clark, K.: Cerebral revascularization for transient ischemic attacks. Neurology (Minneap.), *27*:767–771, 1977.

148. Sandok, B. A., Furlan, A. J., Whisnant, J. P., et al.: Guidelines for the management of transient ischemic attacks. Mayo Clin. Proc., *53*:665–674, 1978.

149. Sandok, B. A., Houser, O. W., Baker, H. L., Jr., et al.: Fibromuscular dysplasia: Neurological disorders associated with disease involving the great vessels in the neck. Arch. Neurol. (Chicago), *24*:462–466, 1971.

150. Schmiedek, P., Gratzl, O., and Spetzler, R. F., eds.: Microsurgery for Stroke. New York-Berlin-Heidelberg, Springer-Verlag, 1977.

151. Schmiedek, P., Gratzl, O., Spetzler, R., et al.: Selection of patients for extra-intracranial arterial bypass surgery based on rCBF measurements. J. Neurosurg., *44*:303–312, 1976.

152. Schmiedek, P., Lanksch, W., Olteanu-Nerbe, V., et al.: Combined use of regional cerebral blood flow measurement and computerized tomography for the diagnosis of cerebral ischemia. *In* Schmiedek, P., Gratzl, O., and Spetzler, R. F., eds.: Microsurgery for Stroke. New York-Berlin-Heidelberg, Springer-Verlag, 1977, pp. 67–78.

153. Selverstone, B., and White, J. C.: A new technique for gradual occlusion of the carotid artery. Arch. Neurol. Psychiat., *66*:246, 1951.

154. Shen, A. L.: Superficial temporal–middle cerebral artery anastomoses in the treatment of a carotid-cavernous fistula. J. Neurosurg., *49*:760–763, 1978.

155. Silverstein, A., and Hollin, S.: Internal carotid vs. middle cerebral artery occlusions: Clinical differences. Arch. Neurol. (Chicago), *12*:468–471, 1965.

156. Sindermann, F., Dichgans, J., and Bergleiter, R.: Occlusion of the middle cerebral artery and its branches: Angiographic and clinical correlates. Brain, *92*:607–620, 1969.

157. Spetzler, R., and Chater, N.: Occipital artery–middle cerebral artery anastomosis for cerebral artery occlusive disease. Surg. Neurol., *2*:235–238, 1974.

158. Spetzler, R., and Chater, N.: Microvascular bypass surgery. Part 2: Physiological studies. J. Neurosurg., *45*:508–513, 1976.

159. Spetzler, R. F., and Owen, M. P.: Extracranial-

intracranial arterial bypass to a single branch of the middle cerebral artery in the management of a traumatic aneurysm. Neurosurgery, 4:334–337, 1979.

160. Spetzler, R. F., Weinstein, P., and Mehdorn, M: New model for chronic reversible cerebral ischemia. Presentation before the American Association of Neurological Surgeons, New Orleans, April 24, 1978.

161. Steinbok, P., Berry, K., and Dolman, C. L.: Superficial temporal artery–middle cerebral artery (STA-MCA) anastomosis: Pathological study of two cases. J. Neurosurg., 50:377–381, 1979.

162. Stephens, H. W., Jr.: Microvascular anastomosis and carotid artery ligation for fibromuscular hyperplasia and carotid artery aneurysm. In Fein, J. M., and Reichman, O. H., eds.: Microvascular Anastomoses for Cerebral Ischemia. New York-Berlin-Heidelberg, Springer-Verlag, 1978, pp. 307–316.

163. Story, J. L., Brown, W. E., Jr., Eidelberg, E., et al.: Cerebral revascularization: Common carotid to distal middle cerebral artery bypass. Neurosurgery, 2:131–135, 1978.

164. Story, J. L., Brown, W. E., Jr., Eidelberg, E., et al.: Cerebral revascularization: Proximal external carotid to distal middle cerebral artery bypass with a synthetic tube graft. Neurosurgery, 3:61–65, 1978.

165. Sugar, O.: (editorial comment) Results of treatment of intracranial aneurysms using Selverstone clamp by L. Mount. In Mackay, R. P., Wortis, S. B., and Sugar, O., eds.: Year Book of Neurology, Psychiatry and Neurosurgery. Chicago, Year Book Medical Publishers, 1960–61, p. 470.

166. Sundt, T. M., Jr., and Piepgras, D. G.: Occipital to posterior inferior cerebellar artery bypass surgery. J. Neurosurg., 48:916–928, 1978.

167. Sundt, T. M., Jr., Siekert, R. G., Piepgras, D. G., et al.: Bypass surgery for vascular disease of the carotid system. Mayo Clin. Proc., 51:677–692, 1976.

168. Swanson, P. D., Calanchini, P. R., Dyken, M. L., et al.: A cooperative study of hospital frequency and character of transient ischemic attacks: II. Performance of angiography among six centers. J.A.M.A., 237:2202–2206, 1977.

169. Tew, J. M., Jr.: Recontructive intracranial vascular surgery for prevention of stroke. Clin. Neurosurg., 22:264–280, 1975.

170. Tew, J. M., Greiner, A. L., and Berger, T. S.: Intracranial reconstructive surgery indications and operative results. Abstract V-44. Stroke, 8:11, 1977.

171. Tew, J. M., Jr., Greiner, A. L., Berger, T. S., et al.: Intracranial vascular bypass: Can it prevent stroke? Mod. Med., 45:58–61, 1977.

172. Thompson, J. R., Weinstein, P. R., and Simmons, C. R.: Cerebral arterial dolichoectasia with seizure: Case report. J. Neurosurg., 44:509–512, 1976.

173. Toole, J. F.: Diagnostic techniques in the medical evaluation and treatment of transient ischemic attacks. Clin. Neurosurg., 22:148–162, 1975.

174. Toole, J. F.: Management of transient ischemic attacks. In Scheinberg, P., ed.: Cerebrovascular Diseases. Tenth Princeton Conference. New York, Raven Press, 1976, pp. 23–30.

175. Weinstein, P. R., and Chater, N. L.: Cerebral revascularization for stroke in evolution. In Schmiedek, P., Gratzl, O., and Spetzler, R. F., eds.: Microsurgery for Stroke. New York-Berlin-Heidelberg, Springer-Verlag, 1977, pp. 240–243.

176. Weinstein, P. R., Chater, N. L., and Lamond, R.: Anatomical studies of the posterior circulation relevant to occipital artery bypass. In Fein, J. M., and Reichman, O. H., eds.: Microvascular Anastomoses for Cerebral Ischemia. New York-Berlin-Heidelberg, Springer-Verlag, 1978, pp. 23–26.

177. Whisnant, J. P.: Epidemiology of stroke: Emphasis on transient cerebral ischemic attacks and hypertension. Stroke, 5:68–70, 1974.

178. Whisnant, J. P., Cartlidge, N. E. F., and Elveback, L. R.: Carotid and vertebral-basilar transient ischemic attacks: Effect of anticoagulants, hypertension, and cardiac disorders on survival and stroke occurrence—a population study. Ann. Neurol., 3:107–115, 1978.

179. Whisnant, J. P., Matsumoto, N., and Elveback, L. R.: Transient cerebral ischemic attacks in a community: Rochester, Minnesota, 1955 through 1969. Mayo Clin. Proc., 48:194–198, 1973.

180. Woringer, E., and Kunlin, J.: Anastomose entre la carotide primitive et la carotide intra-crânienne ou la sylvienne par greffon selon la technique de la suture suspendue. Neurochirurgie, 9:181–188, 1963.

181. Yamamoto, Y. L., Little, J., Meyer, E., et al.: Krypton-77 positron emission tomography for evaluation of medical and surgical treatment in stroke patients. Presentation before the Society of Nuclear Medicine, Anaheim, June 28, 1978.

182. Yasargil, M. G., ed.: Microsurgery Applied to Neurosurgery. Stuttgart, Georg Thieme Verlag; New York and London, Academic Press, 1969.

183. Yasargil, M. G.: Diagnosis and indications for operations in cerebrovascular occlusive disease. In Yasargil, M. G., ed.: Microsurgery Applied to Neurosurgery. Stuttgart, Georg Theime Verlag; New York-London, Academic Press, 1969, pp. 95–119.

184. Yasargil, M. G.: Microsurgical approach to the cerebrovascular diseases. In Fusek, I., and Kunc, Z., eds.: Present Limits of Neurosurgery. Prague, Avicenum, Czechoslovak Medical Press, 1972, pp. 357–361.

185. Yasargil, M. G., and Fox, J. L.: The microsurgical approach to intracranial aneurysms. Surg. Neurol., 3:7–14, 1975.

186. Yasargil, M. G., and Yonekawa, Y.: Results of microsurgical extra-intracranial arterial bypass in the treatment of cerebral ischemia. Neurosurgery, 1:22–24, 1977.

187. Yasargil, M. G., and Yonekawa, Y.: Experiences with the STA–cortical MCA anastomosis in 46 cases. In Fein, J. M., and Reichman, O. H., eds.: Microvascular Anastomoses for Cerebral Ischemia. New York-Berlin-Heidelberg, Springer-Verlag, 1978, pp. 272–277.

188. Zeal, A. A., and Rhoton, A. L., Jr.: Microsurgical anatomy of the posterior cerebral artery. J. Neurosurg., 48:534–559, 1978.

45

OPERATIVE MANAGEMENT OF INTRACRANIAL ARTERIAL OCCLUSIONS AND ACUTE ISCHEMIC STROKE

It has been proverbial that the treatment of stroke lies in its prevention, and that once infarction has occurred and ischemic deficit been produced, recovery or fatal outcome is a function of the natural course of the insult. Prevention is, of course, ideal. The fatalistic approach to acute stroke, however, precludes more aggressive treatment that might be lifesaving or of dramatic benefit to the patient. This chapter addresses these considerations, particularly as they concern the operative re-establishment of blood flow in occluded intracranial arteries and the management of edema related to ischemic central nervous system lesions.

INTRACRANIAL EMBOLECTOMY

In man, total circulatory arrest at normothermia results in irreversible anoxic brain damage within minutes (see Chapter 23). Observations in both clinical and experimental settings indicate, however, that such total circulatory arrest does not occur with occlusion of a major intracranial artery or its branches, the essential difference in this situation being that some collateral flow exists. The principal collateral avenues include the other major channels of the circle of Willis and leptomeningeal anastomoses between cortical branches of the anterior, middle, and posterior cerebral arteries and between the major cerebellar branches.[37,42] In addition, in man as in subhuman primates, collateral anastomoses probably exist through the choroidal plexus and preparenchymal branches of perforating vessels.[39,40]

The adequacy of these collateral channels in the presence of acute occlusion of a major artery determines the degree of ischemia, which along with its duration, determines the development and extent of infarction. The metabolic changes in the cerebral tissue and the resulting ischemic physical effects, as well as the resulting neurological deficits, can be reversed if blood flow is restored immediately. Studies in experimental animals have shown that temporary occlusion of the middle cerebral artery for as long as several hours can be tolerated without infarction.[6,8,9,26,33] This tolerance varies among species as well as among individual animals of the same species, but a major factor in the tolerance to this temporary occlusion is the level of per-

D. G. PIEPGRAS AND T. M. SUNDT, JR.

sistent local cerebral blood flow, a function of collateral circulation. In monkeys, occlusion of the middle cerebral artery producing local cerebral blood flow levels of 12 ml per 100 gm of tissue per minute for two hours or longer consistently resulted in infarction, whereas flows above this "infarction threshold" prevented irreversible damage.[26] Although similar data are not available for humans, studies in anesthetized patients undergoing carotid endarterectomy indicate that the ischemic threshold for deterioration of normal electrical activity is approximately 18 ml per 100 gm per minute, which also corresponds to that noted in subhuman primates.[34] Equally important are experimental studies showing that restoration of flow through an occluded cerebral artery after four to six hours is associated with a high incidence of hemorrhagic infarction and progressive cerebral edema.[6,8,9,33]

Knowing this, the authors believe that, in severe stroke, emergency attempts to enhance flow beyond a site of a major cerebral arterial occlusion or to restore flow through it might be indicated if it could be accomplished within several hours after onset. Emergency carotid endarterectomy in acute occlusion of the internal carotid artery has, in their experience, proved to be beneficial. Less clear are the indications for emergency collateral augmentation operations in acute stroke, namely superficial temporal–to–middle cerebral arterial anastomosis.[5] These considerations are discussed in Chapter 44.

A pertinent consideration, however, is the direct restoration of flow through a site of major cerebral vessel obstruction, specifically by the removal of an embolus at the carotid bifurcation or in the middle cerebral artery. Although this procedure has not been widely practiced or recommended, at least 36 reports in the English literature have discussed intracranial endarterectomy and embolectomy, including some operations involving removal of metallic fragment emboli.* Many cases have been reported in the French literature, and the authors have had experience with 12 cases during the past eight years.[10,20,29] From this experience and from that de-

scribed in the literature, some general conclusions can be drawn.

Most cerebrovascular neurosurgeons agree that endarterectomy of an atherosclerotic plaque in an intracranial vessel to relieve occlusion or stenosis is inadvisable because such lesions do not separate cleanly from the vascular wall, repair of the diseased wall is difficult, and postoperative thrombosis of the site usually occurs. In symptomatic lesions, such as high-grade stenosis in the distal portion of the internal carotid artery or the middle cerebral artery, a bypass procedure, that is, superficial temporal–middle cerebral artery anastomosis, is the operation of choice.

Pathological and angiographic studies of stroke, however, indicate that most strokes involving the middle cerebral artery distribution are due not to local thrombosis at the site of atherosclerotic plaques in one of these major intracranial arteries but rather to propagation of a thrombus or more frequently to embolization from proximal circulatory system disease.[4,22] The authors believe that, in acute occlusion of the middle cerebral artery resulting in severe stroke with obtundation and dense hemispheric deficit, embolectomy should be considered if it can be performed within several hours and if flow can be restored within six to eight hours of the onset. In the evaluation of such patients, a computed tomographic scan of the head should be done initially to rule out the possibility of an intracerebral hematoma, after which angiography should be performed in an attempt to diagnose the occlusive lesion. Because of delays in bringing the patient to the attention of the neurologist and neurosurgeon and time consumed in mandatory evaluation and diagnostic tests, embolectomy is generally not effective or safe. If emergency and nursing personnel, internists, neurologists, and neurosurgeons are alert to the possibilities, however, the occasional patient who has suffered a severe embolic stroke can be quickly recognized, and expeditious evaluation can be completed within a very short time, during which the diagnosis can be confirmed and operative treatment considered.

From the technical standpoint, extraction of an embolus at the carotid bifurcation or the middle cerebral artery is accomplished more simply than endarterectomy

---

* See references 3, 11, 15, 16, 18, 23, 24, 28, 32, 33, 36, 38, 41, 43, 44.

of these vessels. Experience has shown that restoration of patency can be expected in a great many cases when proper micro-operative techniques are used. Whether or not emergency embolectomy can be justified depends on the likelihood of benefit and the risks as compared with the expected course without such treatment. Reported morbidity and mortality rates in acute stroke due to cerebral embolism vary greatly in the literature. Carter reported that the early mortality rate is 33 per cent and that more than half the survivors have late disability.[2] Likewise, Lascelles and Burrows, after studying patients with middle cerebral artery occlusion, noted that nearly one third who had complete occlusion of the middle cerebral artery trunk or branch died and that half the survivors had significant deficits.[19] To the contrary, Allcock reported a death rate of only 5 per cent and a normal or useful life for 72 per cent of patients with occlusion or stenosis of the middle cerebral artery.[1] In that series, however, the inclusion of patients with angiographically diagnosed stenosis skews the final outcome figures favorably because these patients did much better than those with occlusions. Of the latter group, one third had severe deficits. Nevertheless, results in another series were similar, and the challenge to the surgeon considering emergency embolectomy is acknowledged.[17]

Noteworthy in the series of Lascelles and Burrows were features associated with a high incidence of fatal or poor outcome, including apoplectic onset, dense hemiplegia, conjugate deviation of the eyes, and signs of secondary brain stem involvement.[19] The authors have considered emergency embolectomy in only those patients who present with such severe hemispheric clinical signs and angiographic evidence of an occluded middle cerebral artery or rarely an occlusion at the internal carotid artery bifurcation.

Legitimate concern has been expressed that embolectomy will increase the risk of converting an ischemic infarct to a hemorrhagic infarct. As previously stated, experimental studies have found that hemorrhagic infarction is unlikely if flow is restored to the ischemic region within several hours.[6,8,9,33] Edema (related to a reactive hyperemia) may be transiently increased but is reversible.[33] One clinical study found that recanalization of occlusions in the internal carotid and middle cerebral systems, which was demonstrated angiographically within several days after stroke, was associated with a high mortality rate (63 per cent), undoubtedly because of hemorrhagic complications and severe cerebral swelling.[13] With this in mind, it might be proposed that emergency embolectomy in fact might be capable of reducing the risk of hemorrhagic infarction.

In the authors' experience with 12 patients who underwent intracranial artery embolectomy for acute stroke, there were 10 in whom the middle cerebral artery trunk or a primary division thereof was involved and 2 in whom the internal carotid artery bifurcation was occluded and there was propagation of the thrombus into the anterior and middle cerebral arteries. Operation on the latter 2 patients was delayed beyond the limits recommended at present of four to six hours, but of the 10 patients with occlusion of the middle cerebral artery, 8 underwent operation within six hours of the onset of stroke. Of the 10 patients, 6 were in the hospital at the time of their strokes and 4 were at home or at work at the time of onset. Blood flow was re-established in 8 of the 10, and 5 showed definite benefit from the operative restoration of flow. Remarkable recovery occurred in three of the five, all three eventually having only minimal deficit as the residua of a stroke that was catastrophic at its onset. Postoperative patency of the reopened middle cerebral arteries was confirmed by angiography in six patients and by direct inspection at a second operative procedure done several days later in one. Preoperative and postoperative angiograms of a patient with acute occlusion of the middle cerebral artery who underwent embolectomy are shown in Figure 45–1.

In two patients with middle cerebral artery occlusion, flow could not be restored even though operation was performed within six hours of the onset of the strokes. The embolus in each was friable atherosclerotic material from the ascending aorta. One of the patients died of cardiac complications and pneumonia during the immediate postoperative period; the other survived but remained densely aphasic and hemiplegic on the right side until his death one year later.

In this series of 12 patients, both those who died had advanced cardiac disease, and no patient in whom the arterial occlusion was relieved died. In one of the fatal cases, embolectomy did not restore satisfactory flow through the occluded middle cerebral segment because the friable atherosclerotic embolus, originating from the ascending aorta at cardiac catheterization, had broken into many small fragments and had moved into multiple distal middle cerebral branches, preventing the establishment of retrograde flow and, therefore, runoff in these branches. Postmortem microscopic examination of the middle cerebral artery branches confirmed widespread embolic occlusions with atherosclerotic material. In a similar but nonfatal case of atherosclerotic embolization from the aortic arch during coronary angiography, backflow could not be restored in spite of early operation. This experience suggests that cerebral emboli of friable atherosclerotic material are unsuitable for embolectomy because such emboli tend to break up and move into many branches. In contradistinction, large emboli composed of organized platelet-fibrin material, as might originate from a fibrillating cardiac atrium or cardiac mural thrombus, are not likely to fragment and move into more than one cerebral vessel but are likely to remain intact at the site of occlusion. The extraction of such emboli as a single piece is relatively easily accomplished, with satisfactory restoration of flow after embolectomy. Five of the eight

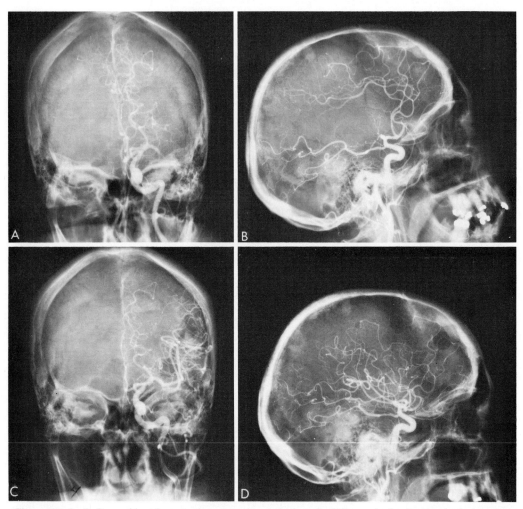

Figure 45–1   Left carotid angiograms demonstrating occlusion of middle cerebral artery trunk. *A*. Anteroposterior view. *B*. Lateral view. Study was done within two hours of onset of stroke, the cause of stroke being an embolus of cardiac origin. *C* and *D*. Study done eight days after middle cerebral embolectomy shows that all major branches of the middle cerebral artery are filling. The absence of mass effect due to cerebral edema is apparent.

patients in the authors' series in whom flow was successfully restored probably had emboli derived from a cardiac source. In two, the site was not determined, although a cardiac source was a definite possibility.

Operative Procedure

For the patient with an acute catastrophic stroke due to embolic occlusion of a major intracranial vessel, in whom emergency embolectomy is being considered, the authors favor administration of barbiturate (pentobarbital 4 mg per kilogram) because of its documented protective effect in cerebral ischemia.[25] Additional doses can be administered during the operation if indicated. Moderate elevation of the blood pressure above normal levels until embolectomy is achieved is likewise proposed to promote collateral circulation.

For the surgeon skilled in microvascular techniques, embolectomy of the middle cerebral artery can be performed expeditiously through a small frontotemporal cra-

niotomy and separated sylvian fissure. The site of the embolic occlusion is readily identifiable as a darkened segment with stasis of blood proximally and distally. After the distal branches have been occluded with temporary microvascular clips, a branch just distal to the occlusion is opened and the embolus is gently milked to the arteriotomy site and extracted (Fig. 45–2). After the proximal vessel has been flushed, a temporary clip is applied proximally, and the distal clips are removed sequentially in order to flush back the propagated clot. The arteriotomy is then repaired with a continuous or interrupted suture of 7-0 to 10-0 monofilament nylon.

OPERATIVE TREATMENT OF BRAIN SWELLING DUE TO INFARCTION

Severe brain infarction may be accompanied in its acute and subacute stages by swelling due to cerebral edema and occasionally to hemorrhagic infarction, which

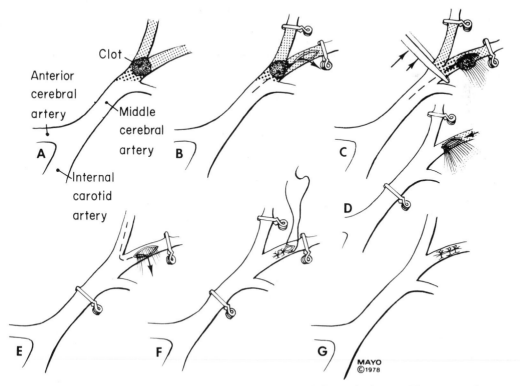

Figure 45–2 *A.* Diagram illustrating embolus at bifurcation of middle cerebral artery. The sequence in restoring blood flow: After temporarily occluding distal branches to prevent displacement of clot, *B*, the embolus is gently milked to the arteriotomy site and extracted, *C.* Retrograde flow washes out propagated clot, *D* and *E*; the arteriotomy is repaired with fine suture, *F*; and flow is restored, *G*.

may be massive and life-threatening in itself. Further, the resulting increased intracranial pressure can be expected to reduce cerebral perfusion pressure and extend infarction into areas of bordering zones that are marginally ischemic. Various studies have estimated that the frequency of severe brain swelling in patients with infarction of a major cerebral hemisphere is 13 to 20 per cent and that such swelling is the primary cause of death in approximately half to three fourths of these patients.[27,30] Massive cerebellar swelling after cerebellar infarction also has been recognized, and in one series it was noted that such swelling occurred with a frequency equal to that of acute spontaneous cerebellar hemorrhage.[35] In a postmortem study, Shaw and co-workers demonstrated that the swelling of the infarcted cerebral hemisphere reaches a maximum on about the fourth or fifth day and may persist for two weeks or longer.[31] Ample evidence indicates that the fatal outcome of massive cerebral or cerebellar infarction within the first week can be directly related to acute brain swelling and to the transtentorial herniation and brain stem compression and hemorrhages that occur secondarily.

Although not widely advocated, emergency decompression by resection of infarcted and necrotic tissue can be lifesaving in certain patients who are rapidly deteriorating because of massive brain swelling secondary to infarction.[12,14,21] Particularly in patients with advanced swelling and brain stem compression due to cerebellar infarction, wide resection of necrotic tissue can be performed and can lead to their eventual recovery to a functional or even near-normal neurological state. In a review of 13 such patients treated operatively, Lehrich and associates found that 4 had died but 9 had recovered sufficiently to be dismissed from the hospital; most of the deficits consisted of ataxia of gait and the ipsilateral limbs. Four patients recovered completely. For a condition that invariably progresses to a fatal outcome, such results are considered good or even excellent.

When cerebral infarction is massive, the stroke always results in a permanent severe deficit (if not death); this is not unexpected because, in all these cases, necrosis involves the entire vascular distribution of the carotid or middle cerebral arteries.[27] If

there is a reasonable possibility that the neurological deficit will be within acceptable limits and medical treatment is failing, emergency operative decompression should be considered for patients who are progressing toward death because of massive cerebral swelling. Most neurosurgeons and neurologists would agree with Greenwood, however, that massive infarction in the dominant hemisphere is a contraindication to such intervention.[12]

In all patients with severe brain swelling due to infarction, medical measures including hyperventilation and dehydrating agents such as urea, mannitol, and steroids should be used before operation is considered. The beneficial effects of steroids in reducing edema secondary to infarction have been debatable, however, and experimental animal studies have shown no benefit.[7] Intracranial pressure monitoring has been advocated in this group of patients and may be beneficial in titrating medical measures and predicting the need for operative decompression.

The clinical condition of the patient is of prime importance. In patients with progressive swelling due to supratentorial infarction, deterioration of the level of consciousness and development of a third-nerve palsy ipsilateral to the side of infarction indicate transtentorial herniation. Probably more common, however, is the "central syndrome," as described by Plum, in which there is deterioration of the level of consciousness, periodic breathing, and bilateral small pupils with preserved light reflex.[30]

In patients with cerebellar swelling, the progression of signs and symptoms is characteristic of an expanding lesion of the posterior fossa, and such a lesion may be difficult to differentiate clinically from an intracerebellar hematoma. Nausea, vomiting, vertigo, and ataxia are typical early manifestations, with ocular palsies, small but reactive pupils, motor dysfunction, and impairment of consciousness occurring as brain stem compression develops.[21,35] In a series of fatal cases of cerebellar infarction, it was found that death usually occurred between the third and the sixth day but only 6 to 30 hours after the onset of obtundation.[35] The admonition to the surgeon is clear—if such patients are to survive or to be spared irreversible brain stem damage, decompression must be done before the end stages are reached. Computed tomography has recently proved to be most valuable in disclosing the underlying disease in such patients and in expediting operative intervention.

For the patient with cerebellar swelling, a standard suboccipital craniectomy is performed, and the necrotic tissue is removed, usually by aspiration. For the patient with swelling of the cerebral hemisphere, a large craniotomy is advised. As advocated by Greenwood, the parietal dura should not be opened until less vital areas have been decompressed by the radical removal of infarcted tissue. Firm areas of the brain that appear viable should not be removed, and speech and motor areas should be preserved unless they are obviously necrotic. Additional decompression can be achieved by resection of the anterior frontal and temporal lobes if necessary. In all patients, the medial temporal lobe should be examined and resected if there is evidence of transtentorial herniation.[12]

REFERENCES

1. Allcock, J. M.: Occlusion of the middle cerebral artery: Serial angiography as a guide to conservative therapy. J. Neurosurg., 27:353–363, 1967.
2. Carter. A. B.: Prognosis of cerebral embolism. Lancet, 2:514–519, 1965.
3. Chou, S. N.: Embolectomy of middle cerebral artery: Report of a case. J. Neurosurg., 20:161–163, 1963.
4. Crawford, T., and Crompton, M. R.: Cited by Lhermitte, F., Gautier, J. C., Derouesné, C., and Guiraud. B., see ref. 22.
5. Crowell, R. M.: Superficial temporal artery–middle cerebral artery bypass for acute focal cerebral ischemia. In Schmiedek, P., Gratzl, O., and Spetzler, R., eds.: Microsurgery for Stroke. New York, Springer-Verlag, 1976, pp. 244–250.
6. Crowell, R. M., Olsson, Y., Klatzo, I., and Ommaya, A.: Temporary occlusion of the middle cerebral artery in the monkey: Clinical and pathological observations. Stroke, 1:439–448, 1970.
7. Donley, R. F., and Sundt, T. M., Jr.: The effect of dexamethasone on the edema of focal cerebral ischemia. Stroke, 4:148–155, 1973.
8. Dujovny, M., Osgood, C. P., Barrionuevo, P. J., Hellstrom, R., and Laha, R. K.: Middle cerebral artery microneurosurgical embolectomy. Surgery, 80:336–339, 1976.
9. Fraser, R. A.: Experimental middle cerebral artery occlusion: Timing of revascularization. Presented at the Fourth Annual Richard Lende Winter Neurosurgery Conference, Snowbird, Utah, February 4 to 9, 1978.
10. Galibert, P., Delcour, J., Grunewald, P., Petit, P., and Rosat, P.: Les oblitérations de l'artère sylvienne: Traitement médical ou chirurgical. Neurochirurgie, 17:165–176, 1971.
11. Garrido, E., and Stein, B. M.: Middle cerebral artery embolectomy: Case report. J. Neurosurg., 44:517–521, 1976.
12. Greenwood, J., Jr.: Acute brain infarctions with high intracranial pressure: Surgical indications. Johns Hopkins Med. J., 122:254–260, 1968.
13. Irino, T., Taneda, M., and Minami, T.: Sanguineous cerebrospinal fluid in recanalized cerebral infarction. Stroke, 8:22–24, 1977.
14. Ivamoto, H. S., Numoto, M., and Donaghy, R. M. P.: Surgical decompression for cerebral and cerebellar infarcts. Stroke, 5:365–370, 1974.
15. Jacobson, J. H., II, Wallman, L. J., Schumacher, G. A., Flanagan, M., Suarez, E. L., and Donaghy, R. M. P.: Microsurgery as an aid to middle cerebral artery endarterectomy. J. Neurosurg., 19:108–114, 1962.
16. Kapp, J. P., Gielchinsky, I., and Jelsma, R.: Metallic fragment embolization to the cerebral circulation. J. Trauma, 13:256–261, 1973.
17. Kaste, M., and Waltimo, O.: Prognosis of patients with middle cerebral artery occlusion. Stroke, 7:482–485, 1976.
18. Khodadad, G.: Middle cerebral artery embolectomy and prolonged widespread vasospasm. Stroke, 4:446–450, 1973.
19. Lascelles, R. G., and Burrows, E. H.: Occlusion of the middle cerebral artery. Brain, 88:85–96, 1965.
20. Lecuire, J., Lapras, C., Dechaume, J. P., Bret, P., Deruty, R., and Yasui, H.: L'embolectomie artérielle intra-cranienne: Données expérimentales et cliniques. Lyon Chir., 69:3–8, 1973.
21. Lehrich, J. R., Winkler, G. F., and Ojemann, R. G.: Cerebellar infarction with brain stem compression: Diagnosis and surgical treatment. Arch. Neurol. (Chicago), 22:490–498, 1970.
22. Lhermitte, F., Gautier, J. C., Derouesné, C., and Guiraud, B.: Ischemic accidents in the middle cerebral artery territory: A study of the causes in 122 cases. Arch. Neurol. (Chicago), 19:248–256, 1968.
23. Lougheed, W. M., Gunton, R. W., and Barnett, H. J. M.: Embolectomy of internal carotid, middle and anterior cerebral arteries: Report of a case. J. Neurosurg., 22:607–609, 1965.
24. Malmros, R.: Cerebral embolectomy (abstract). J. Neurol. Neurosurg. Psychiat., 24:294–295, 1961.
25. Michenfelder, J. D., Milde, J. H., and Sundt, T. M., Jr.: Cerebral protection by barbiturate anesthesia: Use after middle cerebral artery occlusion in Java monkeys. Arch. Neurol. (Chicago), 33:345–350, 1976.
26. Morawetz, R. B., DeGirolami, U., Ojemann, R. G., Marcoux, F. W., and Crowell, R. M.: Cerebral blood flow determined by hydrogen clearance during middle cerebral artery occlusion in unanesthetized monkeys. Stroke, 9:143–149, 1978.
27. Ng, L. K. Y., and Nimmannitya, J.: Massive cerebral infarction with severe brain swelling: A clinicopathological study. Stroke, 1:158–163, 1970.
28. Piazza, G., and Gaist, G.: Occlusion of middle

cerebral artery by foreign body embolus: Report of a case. J. Neurosurg., *17*:172–176, 1960.

29. Piepgras, D. G., Sundt, T. M., Jr., and Yanagihara, T.: Embolectomy for acute middle cerebral artery occlusion. Presented at the Second Joint Meeting on Stroke and Cerebral Circulation, Miami, February 25 to 26, 1977.

30. Plum, F.: Brain swelling and edema in cerebral vascular disease. Res. Publ. Ass. Res. Nerv. Ment. Dis., *41*:318–348, 1966.

31. Shaw, C.-M., Alvord, E. C., Jr., and Berry, R. G.: Swelling of the brain following ischemic infarction with arterial occlusion. Arch. Neurol. (Chicago), *1*:161–177, 1959.

32. Shillito, J., Jr.: Carotid arteritis: A cause of hemiplegia in childhood. J. Neurosurg., *21*:540–551, 1964.

33. Sundt, T. M., Jr., Grant, W. C., and Garcia, J. H.: Restoration of middle cerebral artery flow in experimental infarction. J. Neurosurg., *31*:311–322, 1969.

34. Sundt, T. M., Jr., Sharbrough, F. W., Anderson, R. E., and Michenfelder, J. D.: Cerebral blood flow measurements and electroencephalograms during carotid endarterectomy. J . Neurosurg., *41*:319–320, 1974.

35. Sypert, G. W., and Alvord, E. C., Jr.: Cerebellar infarction: A clinicopathological study. Arch. Neurol. (Chicago), *32*:357–363, 1975.

36. Tew, J. M., Jr.: Reconstructive intracranial vascular surgery. MCV Quart., *10*:139–145, 1974.

37. Vander Eecken, H. M., and Adams, R. D.: The anatomy and functional significance of the meningeal arterial anastomoses of the human brain. J. Neuropath. Exp. Neurol., *12*:132–157, 1953.

38. Van Gilder, J. C., and Coxe, W. S.: Shotgun pellet embolus of the middle cerebral artery: Case report. J. Neurosurg., *32*:711–714, 1970.

39. Watanabe, O., Bremer, A. M., and West, C. R.: Experimental regional cerebral ischemia in the middle cerebral artery territory in primates. Part 1. Angio-anatomy and description of an experimental model with selective embolization of the internal carotid artery bifurcation. Stroke, *8*:61–70, 1977.

40. Watanabe, O., West, C. R., and Bremer, A.: Experimental regional cerebral ischemia in the middle cerebral artery territory in primates. Part 2. Effects on brain water and electrolytes in the early phase of MCA stroke. Stroke, *8*:71–76, 1977.

41. Welch, K.: Excision of occlusive lesions of the middle cerebral artery. J. Neurosurg., *13*:73–80, 1956.

42. Welch, K., Stephens, J., Huber, W., and Ingersoll, C.: The collateral circulation following middle cerebral branch occlusion. J. Neurosurg., *12*:361–368, 1955.

43. Yasargil, M. G., Krayenbuhl, H. A., and Jacobson, J. H., II: Microneurosurgical arterial reconstruction. Surgery, *67*:221–233, 1970.

44. Zlotnik, E. I.: Thrombectomy of the middle cerebral artery: Case report. J. Neurosurg., *42*:723–725, 1975.

46

PATHOPHYSIOLOGY AND CLINICAL EVALUATION OF SUBARACHNOID HEMORRHAGE

Of man's vital organs, the brain stands alone in its propensity to bleed within itself. Almost one fourth of all deaths attributable to disorders of the nervous system are caused by hemorrhage within the intracranial cavity. In the United States, intracranial bleeding produces half of all deaths from stroke.[25,55]

When the bleeding occurs primarily within the subarachnoid space rather than in brain parenchyma, the condition is referred to as subarachnoid hemorrhage. It is more a clinical syndrome than a clear pathological entity. Headache of abrupt onset, meningeal irritation, blood within the cerebrospinal fluid on lumbar puncture, but minimal focal neurological findings describe the condition. It occurs about equally in males and females, although the death rate in females may be slightly higher. For subarachnoid hemorrhage, unlike intraparenchymal brain hemorrhage, no definite seasonal prevalence has been established.[64]

The incidence of subarachnoid hemorrhage varies considerably, depending on the population under study. In Rhodesia, only 3.5 cases per 100,000 population are encountered annually.[36] In Japan, subarachnoid hemorrhage causes 25 deaths per 100,000 population and accounts for 6.6 per cent of all sudden death.[57] In the United States, the death rate from this cause is 16 per 100,000 population.[55] Dietary, hereditary, and socioeconomic factors may have a role in the pathogenesis of this disorder.

Structurally, cerebral arteries differ from their extracranial counterparts. Extracra-

nial organs possess a hilum in which the arterial supply and venous drainage penetrate the internal structure of the organ. Cerebral vessels, on the other hand, after forming a collateral network along the base, enter the organ through its sulci and fissures. Only small vessels penetrate brain substance. The larger arteries are confined to the subarachnoid space and cisterns, where there is little connective tissue to support them. The drainage of blood occurs through thin superficial veins that empty primarily into pericranial sinuses. There are no accompanying cerebral veins (venae comitantes) with the cerebral arteries.[63]

The internal elastic membrane of the intracranial artery is much thicker than that of other arteries. With age, this layer becomes fenestrated and folded.[63] Brain substance may be more susceptible to injury by the pulsation of muscular arteries than other tissues, but the internal elastic membrane serves as a special pressure dampener. Smooth muscle, however, can be stretched by a given force up to 30 times as much as can elastic tissue.[20]

The tunica media of the intracranial artery consists of a spiral network of smooth muscle cells.[63] Compared with that of extracranial vessels, the media contains fewer muscular elements and less elastic tissue. Defects in this muscle layer, commonly referred to as medial gaps, are prominent in all species, including man. They are found most often at arterial bifurcations and are larger in older individuals.[3]

There is relatively little adventitial coating. The elastic tissue in this layer is con-

R. R. SMITH

spicuously decreased. Normally, vasa vasorum are infrequently found on the intracranial arteries of man, although they may be visible on arteries containing arteriosclerotic plaques. The nutrient vessels that supply the muscular layer of normal arteries are yet to be defined.

Nerve bundles can be demonstrated by either electron or special fluorescence microscopy. A rich adrenergic system is present, but nonvaricose cholinergic fibers also accompany the adrenergic fiber. The origin of cholinergic fibers is uncertain. Perhaps, as suggested by Peerless and Kendall, they are derived from the facial nerve or from the oculomotor nerve within the cavernous sinus. The adrenergic fibers apparently originate from the carotid plexus. Once the artery penetrates brain substance, both cholinergic and adrenergic fibers diminish and, perhaps, disappear entirely. At this level the muscular layer of the vessel responds to the metabolic needs of the tissue that it supplies.[51]

The wall of the cerebral artery is exceedingly thin. It is deficient in both muscularis layer and adventitial coating. There are numerous developmental or acquired defects in both the tunica muscularis and the internal elastic layer. The large cerebral artery also lacks external supporting structures provided to muscular arteries elsewhere.

A wide spectrum of clinical manifestations occur with subarachnoid hemorrhage. In three fourths of the patients the symptoms and signs are relatively minor. The most important premonitory clue in the history is the "sentinel headache."[4] The abrupt onset of this headache is usually recognized by the patient as an event unlike anything ever experienced before. If the history is carefully sought, the sentinel headache is found to occur in almost one fourth of all patients who experience subarachnoid hemorrhage, and usually precedes the major catastrophic bleed by about two weeks.[47] Headaches, nausea, vomiting, and transient loss of consciousness are described by two thirds of those who experience subarachnoid hemorrhage. Continued leaking or rebleeding occurs in a significant number of patients. The frequency of rebleeding depends greatly on the underlying pathologic condition in the cerebral vessel. In undifferentiated cases in which the work-up is incomplete, recurrent hemorrhages occur in about one third

within eight weeks.[48] In patients with intracranial aneurysms that are conservatively treated, the mortality rate over a six-year interval reaches 55 per cent. One third of these deaths are caused by proved rebleeding.[44] Bjorkesten noted only three deaths, however, from recurrent hemorrhages over a ten-year interval in 61 patients whose angiograms failed to disclose an aneurysm.[8]

In children and adolescents, subarachnoid hemorrhage is uncommon. When it does occur, an arteriovenous malformation rather than an aneurysm is usually the underlying cause. After about 20 years of age, the reverse is usually true (Fig. 46–1). Of all patients who experience subarachnoid hemorrhage as a result of an intracranial aneurysm, 1.4 per cent have coexisting arteriovenous malformations.[55] Aneurysms appear to develop on major nutrient arteries to arteriovenous fistulae and where there is asymmetry of the circle of Willis. When subarachnoid hemorrhage occurs in a patient with a coexisting aneurysm and vascular anomaly, either lesion may be responsible with about equal frequency.[55] The computed tomogram usually resolves the dilemma (Fig. 46–2).

Subarachnoid hemorrhage, due to both arteriovenous malformations and aneurysms, occurs in association with pregnancy, but aneurysms predominate. In the patient with a malformation, bleeding usually occurs during the sixteenth and twenty-fourth weeks of pregnancy, shortly before labor, during delivery, or in the early puerperium. The patient with an aneurysm

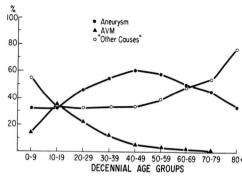

Figure 46–1 Relative probability of major causes of subarachnoid hemorrhage in each decade of life. AVM = arterivenous malformation. (From Sahs, A., Perret, G. E., Locksley, H. B., and Nishioka, H.: Intracranial Aneurysms and Subarachnoid Hemorrhage. Philadelphia, J. B. Lippincott Co, 1969. Reprinted by permission.)

is usually slightly older, and bleeding takes place between the thirtieth and fortieth weeks of gestation, but rarely during delivery. Aneurysms also may be responsible for postpartum subarachnoid hemorrhage. Whether an aneurysm or an arteriovenous malformation is responsible, both fetal and maternal mortality rates are high. In patients with previously demonstrated arteriovenous malformations, there is a ninefold greater risk of hemorrhage during pregnancy. Normal vaginal delivery is acceptable in patients with known aneurysms, but must be considered dangerous in those harboring arteriovenous malformations.[52]

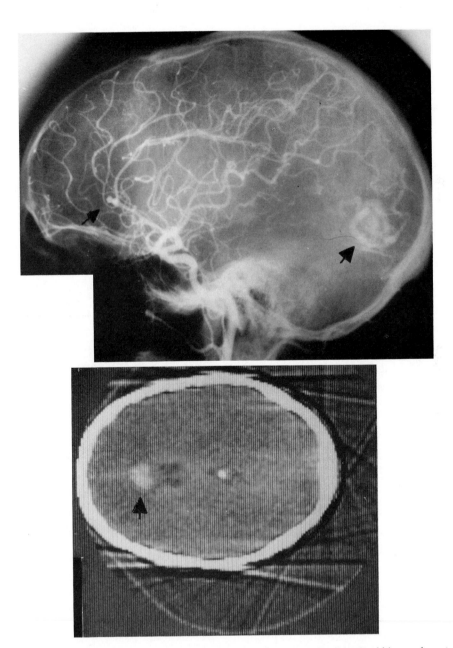

Figure 46–2 In this patient, the computed tomogram clearly relates the subarachnoid hemorrhage to the aneurysm of the anterior cerebral artery (*small arrow*) rather than to the occiptal arteriovenous malformation (*large arrow*).

SUBARACHNOID HEMORRHAGE OF UNKNOWN ETIOLOGY

Spontaneous disruption of an artery or vein of the surface of the cerebrum, cerebellum, or brain stem may be responsible for subarachnoid hemorrhage in some cases.[29] Arteriosclerotic arteries, medial defects in normal vessels, infundibular widenings of communicating arteries, minute aneurysms, and ectatic surface vessels have all been identified as sources of subarachnoid hemorrhage.[26,27] Fatal subarachnoid hemorrhage has been described following use of both intravenous and oral amphetamines. Segmental narrowing and dilatation of the pial vessels, and beading of intracranial arteries characterize the angiographic picture. Definite aneurysm dilatations have also been seen.[38] Granulomatous angiitis of obscure etiology may also result in subarachnoid hemorrhage.[23] Hypertension produces subarachnoid hemorrhage primarily through the formation of intracerebral clots followed by immediate or delayed rupture into the subarachnoid space. Intraventricular bleeding may also lead to a diagnosis of subarachnoid hemorrhage.

After thorough clinical and radiographic study, the cause remains undiscovered in about 20 per cent of cases of spontaneous subarachnoid hemorrhage. The mortality rate in this group of patients is extremely low, on the average less than 3 per cent. In the few necropsy studies performed, half of the deaths have been due to unrecognized ruptured aneurysms.[48] Whether angiography is carried out within 24 hours, seven days, or two weeks, the yield of positive studies changes little. False negative studies are, however, encountered in about 4 per cent of the patients with subarachnoid hemorrhage on the primary radiographic examination.[48] In some cases, aneurysms fail to fill on angiography because of spasm, thrombosis, or their small size. An arteriovenous malformation may likewise be filled by thrombus, or it may be compressed by surrounding hematoma. Repeating the angiogram a week or 10 days later in suspicious cases identifies the lesion in a further one fourth of those studied.[55]

Angiography produces both unexpected complications and benefits in the patient with recent subarachnoid hemorrhage. If all patients whose neurological condition deteriorates within 24 hours following angiogra-

TABLE 46-1 COMPLICATIONS OF ANGIOGRAPHY IN RECENT SUBARACHNOID HEMORRHAGE*

COMPLICATION	PER CENT
Transient hemiparesis	2.0
Permanent deficits	2.5
Deaths	2.6
Aneurysmal rebleedings	1.5
Ischemic deficits worsen	3.0

* From Nibbelink, D. W., Torner, J., and Henderson, W. G.: Intracranial aneurysms and subarachnoid hemorrhage. Stroke, 8:202–218, 1977. Reprinted by permission.

phy are considered, almost 10 per cent develop complications (Table 46–1). This morbidity is often associated with multiple angiographic procedures carried out in acutely ill patients, many of whom are even greater risks than those with ischemic vascular disorders. On the other hand, an intracerebral mass may be delineated in up to 12 per cent of those with subarachnoid bleeding, hydrocephalus may be discovered in an additional 8 per cent, and an extracerebral mass such as a subdural hematoma requiring evacuation will be discovered in almost 5 per cent. The rate of serious complications is increased when angiography is delayed until the second posthemorrhage week.[44] It should preferably be performed soon after the bleeding occurs, prior to the time when ischemic complications and rebleeding are expected.

The computed tomogram is of considerable value in the search for the site and cause of subarachnoid bleeding and may reduce the number of false negative tests. When subarachnoid hemorrhage results from dissection of a primary intraparenchymal hematoma or intraventricular hemorrhage, the accuracy of this method approaches 90 per cent. In predicting the site of aneurysm rupture, it is invaluable. Claims have been made of 100 per cent accuracy in predicting anterior cerebral aneurysms by the location of the associated hematoma. Parasylvian hematomas are pathognomonic of middle cerebral aneurysm rupture, while hematomas implicating the external capsule are characteristic of hypertensive hemorrhage.[28]

CEREBRAL ANEURYSMS

The pathogenesis of the cerebral aneurysm is a subject of continuing debate.

Basically, three schools of thought have developed to explain their presence. One proposes that *congenital weakness* of the muscular layer allows the intima to bulge through, eventually rupturing the elastic membrane by overdistention. The *postnatalists* theorize that degenerative changes within the vessel wall damage the internal elastic membrane, allowing the intima to herniate through the weakness. Followers of a third school insist that aneurysms occur as a result of a *combination* of the two factors, arterial degeneration and developmental deficiency.[55]

Although a consensus as to their hereditary basis is yet lacking, intracranial aneurysms have been described among multiple members of the same family, even twins.[17] At least three familial types have been noted. The first type is associated with known hereditary syndromes such as the Ehlers-Danlos syndrome, coarctation of the aorta, and polycystic kidney disease.[54] As many as 16 per cent of those afflicted with polycystic kidney disease also harbor intracranial aneurysms. In the second group, familial aggregation may be due to possible hereditary factors. Among these, hyperlipemic and hypertensive states carry increased risk factors. Third, fortuitous familial aggregation occurs in 1 to 2 per cent in most reported aneurysm series. If hereditary vascular diseases are excluded, aneurysms probably occur in no more than 1 in 50 of the relatives of patients with ruptured intracranial aneurysms. This number, however, is still somewhat greater than is to be expected from the population at large.[5,31]

Hypertension, if not instrumental in aneurysm development, must promote rupture at an early age. Coarctation of the aorta, polycystic renal disease, and renal artery stenosis all may lead to the development of aneurysms in children and young adults (Fig. 46–3). Certain arterial anomalies of the circle of Willis are also more frequently found in patients harboring aneurysms. Hypoplasia of one or both proximal anterior cerebral arteries is the most commonly encountered anomaly associated with an anterior cerebral aneurysm and probably plays some part in the development of the lesion.[40] Aneurysms occur as well in patients with moyamoya disease.[14] Syphilis, mycotic embolism, and trauma have all, at one time, been suspect, but at present the underlying defect in most cases remains obscure. Arteriosclerosis and ectasia of the vessel wall, commonly seen in elderly individuals, apparently have no relationship to berry aneurysm development.[40]

The wall of the cerebral vessel is thin and consists largely of two layers, the muscular coat and the internal elastic layer, which is as a rule built up in thick lamellae. The muscular coat contains about 25 layers of

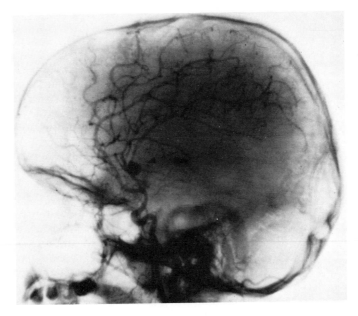

Figure 46–3 This middle cerebral artery aneurysm produced subarachnoid and intracerebral hemorrhage in a 9-year-old child who had hypertension due to renal artery stenosis.

circularly arranged smooth muscle cells with little interspersed elastic tissue.[63] At branches, the muscularis is thin and often absent (medial gaps), and intimal cushions are common.[3,19] These consist of several layers of smooth muscle and intimal connective tissue enveloped by the internal elastic membrane. An internal elastic lamella provides considerable support.[19] Glynn observed that pressures exceeding 600 mm of mercury caused no vessel wall deformity when this layer was intact.[20] Fragmentation of both the muscularis and elastica occurs at the site of the aneurysms, and only scattered smooth muscle cells can be demonstrated in the aneurysm wall.[60]

Using rigid glass models, Forbus demonstrated that the greatest pressure differential occurs at the forks of vessels in line with the flow column (Fig. 46–4).[19] The pressure differential increased as the velocity of flow increased. Employing silicon tubes, Hassler produced pitting at the apex of the bifurcation, once again indicating points of greatest strain on the vessel wall.[27] The location of the pits was similar to that of the intimal cushions observed at points of arterial branching.

At the junction of the aneurysm and parent vessel, the muscular coat rounds off gradually and the elastic layer ends

abruptly.[34] Forbus described similar defects in the muscularis layer at arterial branchings in newborns. He hypothesized that intracranial aneurysms developed from this congenital weakness.[19] In 1960, Stehbens differentiated the congenital medial defects of the newborn from those that develop later, apparently on a degenerative basis. Funnel-shaped dilations, areas of thinning, small evaginations, and changes in the elastic tissue, functionally different from the simple medial defects of the newborn, were described at vessel forks.[60]

Hassler also called attention to minute aneurysms less than 2 mm in diameter that occur either as a progenitor of or in association with major defects or berry aneurysms (Fig. 46–5). None of these were found in 106 arterial preparations from individuals under 31 years of age, but 32 minute aneurysms were present in 27 individuals who were 31 years of age or older. They also occur in half of all those who develop larger berry aneurysms, and are occasionally responsible for the subarachnoid bleeding. Minute aneurysms are morphologically similar to berry aneurysms, consisting primarily of an intima and an adventitial layer.[27] Since microdissection became routine, lesions of this type have been observed on numerous occasions. Thinning of the arterial wall, and small blisters on the vessel surface, not visible angiographically, have been encountered in the dissection of the aneurysm-bearing artery. The development of the berry aneurysm can thus be seen as a continuum, probably beginning with a deficiency in the muscular layer. As the elastic component becomes frayed, minute aneurysms (less than 2 mm) occur and eventually develop into major or berry aneurysms. Once a sac has formed, further distention proceeds at a greater rate. As sac volume increases, lower pressures are required to distend it further. When the wall becomes too thin to support intravascular pressure, rupture and subarachnoid hemorrhage occur. In some instances, minute aneurysms or lesser defects are responsible for the subarachnoid bleeding.[13]

Aneurysms that develop in patients with heart valve vegetations have been known since 1831.[9] Although the incidence of mycotic aneurysms has been reduced, they may yet account for 1 to 2 per cent of all aneurysms. Septic necrosis of the vessel wall, rather than aneurysm formation, some-

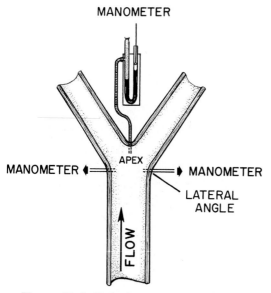

Figure 46–4 Forbus's experiment using glass models indicates that the point of greatest stress placed on the artery wall occurs at the apex of the bifurcation in line with flow channels. Intimal cushions and medial defects also occur at this location.

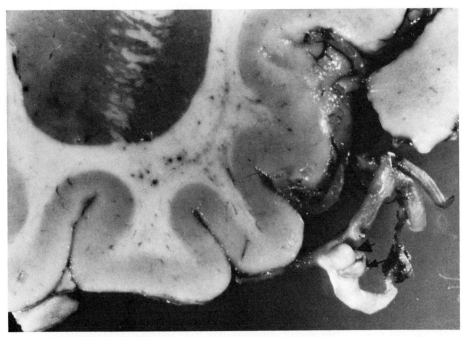

Figure 46–5 Minute aneurysms (less than 2 mm in diameter) are commonly found at the main branching of the middle cerebral artery. They more commonly occur in older individuals and rarely produce subarachnoid hemorrhage. Berry aneurysms take origin from these minor defects. The one depicted here was found incidentally at postmortem examination.

times precedes the hemorrhage.[66] Most mycotic aneurysms, however, are broad-based, saccular, and located on branches of the right middle cerebral artery. Characteristically, parietal lobe hematomas are produced, and they occur about one month or longer after peripheral septic embolization. The embolus passes into penetrating branches, and thus intracerebral, rather than subarachnoid, bleeding is the rule.[30] Frequently, follow-up angiography performed three to four weeks following the original hemorrhage shows resolution of the aneurysm. The rebleeding rate for mycotic aneurysms is unknown, and unless an intracerebral hematoma requires evacuation, a trial of conservative treatment using appropriate antibiotics is probably warranted. Spontaneous resolution has been described at the time of follow-up angiography.[10]

True traumatic aneurysms occur rarely. Aneurysms of meningeal vessels, arteriovenous fistulae, and false aneurysms have also been described following major cranial trauma. With complete disruption of the artery, a hematoma forms around it, producing a false aneurysm. If only the internal elastic lamella is damaged, the intima may bulge through this defect, producing a true aneurysm. Mixed types also occur when true aneurysms rupture and secondary false aneurysms occur.[39] Traumatic aneurysms occur on susceptible vessels: the anterior cerebral artery in relation to the falx, the carotid artery in juxtaposition to the tentorium, or the middle cerebral artery adjacent to a bone flap. Their course is unpredictable, and hemorrhage has resulted in death in 50 per cent of the reported cases.[7] If angiographically demonstrated enlargement occurs, operative obliteration of the sac should be carried out without further delay.

Berry aneurysms usually rupture into the subarachnoid space and cause over half of all cases of subarachnoid hemorrhage (Table 46–2). Hematomas also develop within brain substance, in the ventricles, or in the subdural space.[6,21,42] Internal carotid and middle cerebral artery aneurysms are commonly responsible for intracerebral bleeding.[6]

The peak age for aneurysm rupture is between 55 and 60 years of age in the United States, and 16 deaths per 100,000 population occur each year through aneurysmal

TABLE 46–2 FREQUENCY OF MAJOR CAUSES OF SUBARACHNOID HEMORRHAGE IN THE COOPERATIVE STUDY*

CAUSE	PER CENT
Intracranial aneurysms only	51
Hypertensive and/or arteriosclerotic vascular disease	15
Arteriovenous malformations only	6
Miscellaneous or multiple causes	6
Cause indeterminate (by history plus angiography or autopsy)	22

* From Sahs, A. H., Perret, G. E., Locksley, H. B., and Nishioka, H.: Intracranial Aneurysms and Subarachnoid Hemorrhage. Philadelphia, J. B. Lippincott Co., 1969. Reprinted by permission.

bleeding.[55] Careful examination of routine autopsy material discloses unruptured aneurysms in 1 to 8 per cent.[27,61] Any therapeutic regimen designed for the unruptured aneurysm must take this fact into consideration. McCormick and Rosenfield estimate that these lesions are common and may be found in approximately 4 to 6 per cent of the population by the time they die, and that only one aneurysm out of five ever ruptures.[42] Graf, summarizing the course of 52 patients with incidental unsuspected aneurysms, noted that only two of these subsequently bled and died during the five years after diagnosis was made.[22] Therefore, unless the high-risk unruptured aneurysm can be identified, it is questionable that operative treatment can improve on the natural history of the asymptomatic lesion. Size and location of the aneurysm and age of the patient are all of importance in determining risk factors. Only 2 per cent of all aneurysms less than 5 mm in external diameter ever rupture, while over 40 per cent of those between 6 and 10 mm have already bled when they are found. When the lesion is identified in a patient less than 50 years of age, rupture has already taken place in over 80 per cent of the cases. Sixty per cent of those encountered in individuals less than 60 years of age have previously bled.[22,42] Since they are uncommonly encountered except when associated with subarachnoid hemorrhage, aneurysms of at least 6 mm in size, occurring in individuals 50 years of age or younger, probably fall into this high-risk category and should be operatively obliterated. Symptomatic but unruptured intracranial aneurysms also represent dangerous lesions. The nonoperative mortality

rate over a 12-year period for these aneurysms is about 26 per cent.[22] Aneurysms bearing secondary loculations bleed with twice the frequency of round, smooth-walled lesions.[15] Contrary to popular belief, giant aneurysms (greater than 2 cm in size) may also be responsible for subarachnoid hemorrhage.[43] Calcification of the aneurysm wall appears to provide a modicum of protection.

Certain environmental events seem to promote aneurysm rupture. Among these coitus, lifting, and elimination must be listed. The most common locations for single intracranial aneurysms associated with subarachnoid hemorrhage are listed in Table 46–3. Internal carotid artery aneurysms are slightly more common in females, while anterior communicating artery aneurysms predominate in males (Figs. 46–6 and 46–7). Those that occur on the posterior circulation are most often encountered at the basilar termination, on the basilar trunk, or on the vertebral arteries (Figs. 46–8 and 46–9).[56] Multiple aneurysms are found in about 20 per cent of the patients who experience subarachnoid hemorrhage, the most common being those symmetrically placed on the internal carotid arteries.[55] When more than one aneurysm is seen on the angiogram, identification of the one responsible for the hemorrhage is essential if an operation is contemplated. The largest and most proximal lesion accounts for the rupture in over three fourths of the cases, but spasm, shift, and secondary loculations are all of importance in ascertaining which aneurysm has ruptured.[13] DuBoulay observed that secondary loculation represents a period of instability in the aneurysm wall, and aneurysms that were not

TABLE 46–3 SITE FREQUENCY OF BLEEDING INTRACRANIAL ANEURYSMS*

ARTERIAL SITE	PER CENT
Internal carotid	38
at posterior communicating	25
Anterior cerebral system	36
at anterior communicating	30
Middle cerebral system	21
Vertebral-basilar system	5

* From Sahs, A. H., Perret, G. E., Locksley, H. B., and Nishioka, H.: Intracranial Aneurysms and Subarachnoid Hemorrhage. Philadelphia, J. B. Lippincott Co., 1969. Reprinted by permission.

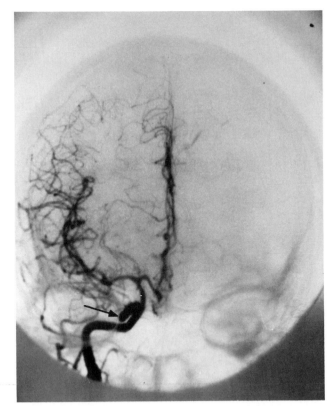

Figure 46–6 The internal carotid artery aneurysm depicted here arises at the posterior communicating branch and projects posterolaterally.

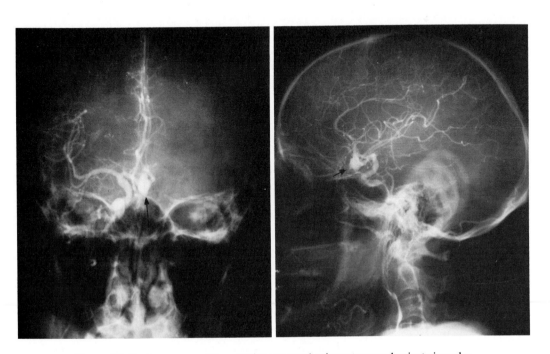

Figure 46–7 Aneurysms of the anterior communicating artery predominate in males.

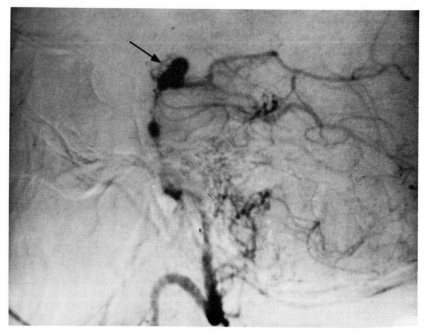

Figure 46–8   Of the aneurysms that occur on the posterior circulation those at the basilar termination (*arrow*) are the most common variety. Severe segmental vasospasm complicates this angiographic picture.

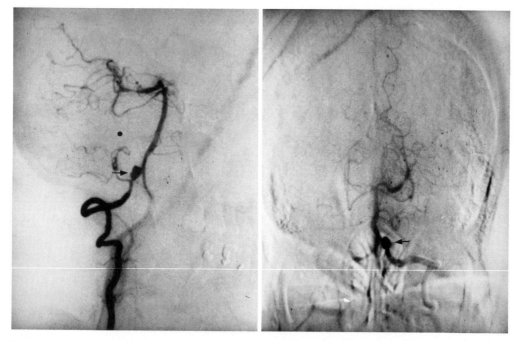

Figure 46–9   Vertebral artery aneurysms arising at the posterior inferior cerebellar artery branch (*arrows*) are the third most common of the posterior circulation aneurysms.

responsible for hemorrhage were rarely loculated in appearance.[15] The mortality rate associated with loculated aneurysms due to hemorrhage is twice that associated with smooth round-wall lesions (31 per cent versus 14 per cent). A widely held notion that vasospasm offers protection against rebleeding has not stood the test of careful analysis.[16]

The greatest incidence of rebleeding from ruptured intracranial aneurysms occurs between the fifth and ninth days after the initial hemorrhage. A mortality rate of about 7 per cent per week until six weeks have passed can be anticipated in conservatively treated cases. Anterior communicating artery aneurysms have a prolonged interval to recurrent hemorrhage in comparison with internal carotid aneurysms and middle cerebral aneurysms, which appear to bleed earlier. One third of all deaths from rebleeding middle cerebral and carotid artery aneurysms occur within two weeks. Two thirds of the deaths from anterior communicating artery aneurysms take place 30 days, or longer, following the hemorrhage. The mortality rate of subarachnoid hemorrhage from intracranial aneurysms continues to rise after completion of a conservative program and after discharge from the hospital. Between 6 and 12 per cent of the survivors die yearly.[44] At all aneurysm sites, the second hemorrhage apparently has greater risk for death than the first (14 per cent versus 42 per cent), but since many patients die suddenly without benefit of complete workup, the true mortality rate for the primary hemorrhage cannot be determined with accuracy.[55]

Thus, after more than a quarter of a century of case studies, no further refinements in Ask-Upmark's assessment of the natural history of subarachnoid hemorrhage can be made.

It may hence be safely stated that if a person has a subarachnoid hemorrhage the chance has hitherto been only one out of five that he will make a good recovery, whilst his chances to become crippled may be judged approximately just as high, and he has three chances out of five to die from his disease sooner or later.[2]

VASCULAR MALFORMATIONS

These vascular anomalies are known by many pseudonyms, including "hamar-toma," "angioma," "hemangioma," and others. Since some malformations slowly increase in size and inflict progressive changes in adjacent brain, they hold a number of features in common with true neoplasms with which they have been confused. Adding to this confusion, certain vascular neoplasms and arteriovenous malformations share similar cellular characteristics. The presence of brain parenchyma between the vessels of an angioma helps to distinguish it from true vascular neoplasms, but this criterion loses its usefulness with large venous angiomas.[40]

The pathology literature contains considerable discussion but little consensus about the classification of vascular malformations. For simplicity, McCormick's outline is used in the following discussion.[40] The term "arteriovenous malformation" is used to describe all vascular malformations as well as the specific subtype containing both arterial and venous structures.

Telangiectasias (capillary angiomas) are congenital malformations that consist of thin-walled capillaries without smooth muscle or elastic tissue and are separated by intervening glial background tissue. They usually occur in the basis pontis and rarely produce subarachnoid hemorrhage. Vascular anomalies of this type accompany Rendu-Osler disease and the Sturge-Weber syndrome. When associated with the latter disorder, they are often accompanied by mental retardation, seizures, and port wine facial nevi (Fig. 46–10).

Varices consist of single or multiple dilated venous channels. The anomalous vessel is usually a thin-walled vein, occasionally with calcification and gliosis surrounding it. The vein of Galen malformation is an example of this type of lesion (Fig. 46–11).

Cavernous angiomas contain thin-walled vessels that are generally not separated by glial tissue (Fig. 46–12). Multilobulation is common. They bleed spontaneously, and hemosiderin is frequently found about them, indicating previous minor hemorrhages.

Arteriovenous malformations constitute the most common and best-known variety. Grossly greatly dilated and thickened venous channels form a pyramidal mass with the apex penetrating the parenchyma and pointing toward the lateral ventricle. At operation it frequently is impossible to differ-

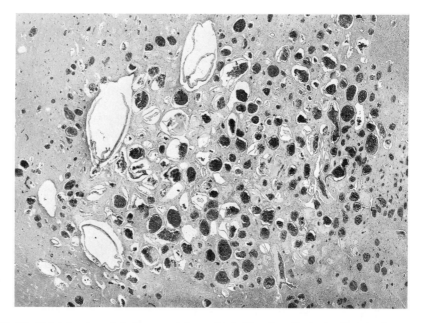

Figure 46–10 This telangiectatic lesion containing multiple dilated capillaries in gliotic background tissue was found incidentally in the subcortical white matter at necropsy examination. (Courtesy of Dr. Jose Bebin, neuropathologist, University of Mississippi.)

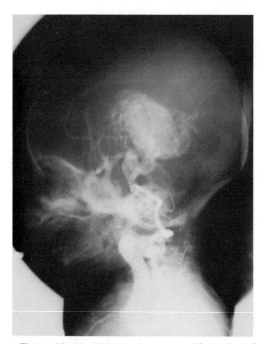

Figure 46–11 This arteriovenous malformation of the vein of Galen contains nutrient vessels from the anterior cerebral artery as well as the posterior choroidal branches. Hydrocephalus, subarachnoid hemorrhage, and congestive heart failure in the newborn may be produced by this anomaly.

entiate arteries from veins. Both are thick-walled and generally filled with oxygenated blood.

Venous angiomas resemble the more common arteriovenous malformations with the exception that arteries are sparse on microscopic examination. Cryptic varieties of the venous angioma occur and may be associated with unexpected massive intracerebral or intracerebellar bleeding.

Although traumatic intracranial varieties exist, arteriovenous malformations apparently develop largely on a congenital basis. The embryological development of the vascular system of the brain begins with common endothelial channels, neither arteries nor veins, which later differentiate through coalescence of these multiple capillary anlagen. The vascular malformation may represent a perpetuation of this primitive arteriovenous communication that normally would be replaced by an intervening capillary network. In the developing vascular system, crossing vessels are often separated by only a double layer of endothelial cells, also providing ample opportunity for fistulous communications.[46] The malformation is wedge-shaped, with the base at the

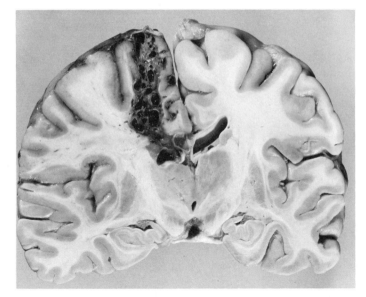

Figure 46–12 The cavernous type of malformation may have no intervening glial tissue between the dilated veins. The one shown was found incidentally. (Courtesy of Dr. Jose Bebin, neuropathologist, University of Mississippi.)

cortex and the apex at the edge of the lateral ventricle, lying for the most part within white matter. Its major blood supply is usually through a dilated arterial branch that would normally supply that region of the brain. Sinusoids and veins become sclerotic with increasing intravascular pressure in much the same manner as renal arteries undergo hypertrophy in hypertension. Venous drainage of malformations takes place through dilated transcerebral veins.[32]

Rarely, intracranial arteriovenous malformations connect and share common blood supply with similar lesions of the scalp (cirsoid aneurysms), cranium, or meninges (Fig. 46–13).[49] The intra-extracranial variety, in addition to producing spontaneous subarachnoid hemorrhage, may also produce spontaneous subdural hematomas. The dense arterial network accompanying moyamoya disease develops primarily as collateral flow channels in response to bilateral carotid artery occlusion. The predilection of these vessels to form aneurysms or to rupture spontaneously and produce subarachnoid hemorrhage is well known.[14]

Arteriovenous malformations rank second to aneurysms among the known vascular lesions that produce subarachnoid hemorrhage, and they are the predominant cause of subarachnoid hemorrhage in childhood.[55] Fewer malformations manifest themselves by epilepsy than by hemor-

rhage. The clinical picture associated with vascular rupture often is indistinguishable from that due to a ruptured aneurysm. When subarachnoid hemorrhage occurs in children or is associated with epilepsy, or when there is a history of repeated bleeding extending over several years, an arteriovenous malformation should be suspected.[55] The natural history of arteriovenous malformations is, if anything, less well understood than that of aneurysms. The events that lead to bleeding from this congenital lesion are also poorly understood. It seems likely that an increase in venous rather than arterial pressure causes the rupture. Activities such as diving, straining, lifting, and playing musical wind instruments carry particular risks for the patient with an intracranial arteriovenous malformation.

Both bleeding and nonbleeding types are more commonly found in the frontal and parietal lobes (Table 46–4). Two thirds of them are larger than 2 cm in diameter, and only 6 per cent are found in the infratentorial space. In this location, the arteriovenous type is the most common variety, and may be responsible for spontaneous intracerebellar hemorrhage. The telangiectatic variety occurs predominantly in the basis pontis or brain stem and rarely produces symptoms.[32]

The microscopic venous malformation that occasionally leads to fatal intracerebral hemorrhage was described by Margolis and

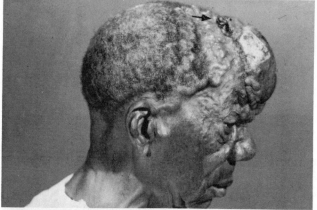

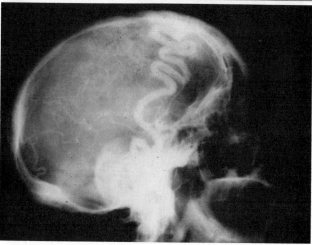

Figure 46–13 This large cirsoid aneurysm of the scalp bled massively on several occasions, producing anemia and heart failure. The site of recent rupture is apparent. Ligation of the greatly dilated superficial temporal arteries under local anesthesia produced softening of the malformation and promoted scalp healing. No recurrent hemorrhages have occurred in four years of follow-up.

associates.[37] This lesion usually is clinically silent. In younger individuals it often produces hemorrhage coincident to minor head trauma. Headaches and delayed loss of consciousness are the earliest clinical findings. The hematoma usually occupies the white matter, and only careful serial studies disclose the thin-walled venous malforma-

TABLE 46–4 LOCATION OF ARTERIOVENOUS MALFORMATIONS*

LOCATION	PER CENT
Parietal lobe	27
Frontal lobe	22
Temporal lobe	18
Intraventricular	18
Occipital lobe	5
Cerebellum	5
Brain stem	2
Other	3

* Data from McCormick, W. F.: The pathology of vascular ("arteriovenous") malformations. J. Neurosurg., *24*: 807–816, 1966.

tion that most often is partly destroyed in the hematoma wall. McCormick and Nofzinger reviewed 48 "cryptic malformations" less than 2 cm in size and found an almost equal distribution between the supratentorial and infratentorial spaces. Epilepsy was infrequent with the cryptic variety, but spontaneous cerebellar hemorrhage was found to coexist with cryptic malformations in one fourth of the cases. The hematomas associated with these lesions are commonly found in the basis pontis and in the frontal and temporal lobes of the cerebrum.[41]

Like aneurysms, vascular malformations are more prevalent among the relatives of those harboring known lesions of similar type. In the case of the capillary hemangioblastoma associated with Von Hippel–Lindau disease, a familial relationship has been found in approximately 20 per cent of cases.[45] Similar hereditary patterns have been established with Rendu-Osler-Weber disease and with Sturge-Weber-Dimitri syndrome.[12,53] In Louis-Bar syndrome (ataxia-telangiectasia), the cerebellar pathologic changes are usually related to neuronal loss and gliosis rather than to vascular malformation.[59] Lindau's syndrome associates angiomatosis of the retina with renal cysts and true neoplasms, hemangioblastomas of the cerebellar hemisphere.[45] Angiomatous lesions of the lungs and other organs are also frequently found in association with intracranial vascular anomalies. With malformations of the arteriovenous type, however, there is no clear familial linkage, although isolated familial cases have been described.[33]

In patients with arteriovenous malformations, subarachnoid hemorrhage occurs in 68 per cent and is by far the most common presenting feature. Seizures occur in 28 per cent, and headaches, syncope, and progressive neurological dysfunction prompt the remainder to seek medical attention. Interestingly, seizures and bleeding may be mutually exclusive. Almost 90 per cent of the patients who hemorrhage from their arteriovenous malformations have no history of convulsive seizures. Conversely, only 18 per cent of those whose arteriovenous malformations causes seizures will have a subarachnoid hemorrhage at a later date. The peak age for hemorrhage occurs between 15 and 20 years of age. Over half of those who bleed will have done so by the age of 30. Recurrent bleeding due to vascular malformations is both less frequent and less life-threatening than bleeding due to aneurysms. More than 25 per cent of these abnormal structures can be expected to rebleed over a 20-year interval, however, with a mortality rate of about 12 per cent.[55]

An unusual malformation involving the vein of Galen occurs in infancy and produces three distinct clinical syndromes, depending upon the age at which the disease is manifested. Neonates present at or shortly after birth with cyanosis and congestive heart failure due to the magnitude of the arteriovenous shunting through the malformation. Infants are often encountered with seizures and hydrocephalus due to obstruction and compression of the cerebral aqueduct by the dilated vein. Older persons may present with multiple subarachnoid hemorrhages. This malformation results when one or more arteries feed directly into the vein of Galen. Most probably it arises in the 20- to 40-mm embryo when arteries and veins are still multiple endothelial tubes.[65]

OTHER CAUSES OF SUBARACHNOID HEMORRHAGE

Hemorrhage into the ventricles of the brain, regardless of the underlying pathologic conditions, may be diagnosed as subarachnoid hemorrhage. In adults, hypertension, blood dyscrasia, vascular anomalies of the basal ganglia or thalamus, and aneurysms are known to cause bleeding within the ventricular cavities (Fig. 46–14).[11,21] Massive hemorrhage is usually accompanied by pinpoint pupils, bilateral rigidity, bilateral Babinski signs, unconsciousness, and ultimately death within 12 hours. Smaller hemorrhages may be accompanied by minimal clinical findings, and spontaneous resolution may occur.

Intraventricular hemorrhage in the newborn strikes almost exclusively in the premature infant.[18] The source of hemorrhage seems to be subependymal blisters that are caused by bleeding from the terminal vein overlying the thalamus. Blood flows from the lateral ventricle caudally, eventually

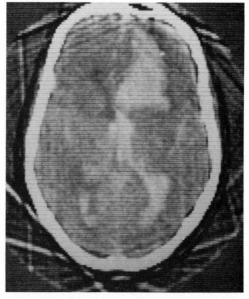

Figure 46–14 CT scan of intracerebral and intraventricular hemorrhage accompanying anterior communicating artery aneurysm rupture.

escaping and accumulating in the cisterna magna.[49] The pathogenesis of the hemorrhage is incompletely understood. Thrombosis of draining veins, fluid overload, deficient clotting mechanisms, and mechanical respirators have all been indicted.[18,35,58] Cyanotic attacks and edema are among the first clinical signs, and death frequently occurs within the first 24 hours following delivery.[18]

Minor hemorrhages quite often occur in intracranial tumors, but by and large, intracerebral rather than subarachnoid bleeding is produced. The exception occurs with pituitary adenomas, intraventricular neoplasms, and hemangioblastomas (Fig. 46–15). Pituitary apoplexy is a well-recognized syndrome that develops in up to 10 per cent of those harboring pituitary adenomas. It may be even more prone to strike the patient who has not been operated on but is receiving radiation therapy. The intrasellar hematoma may erupt through the diaphragm into the subarachnoid space, the hypothalamus, the ventricular system, or the temporal lobe. The optic chiasm and adjacent cranial nerves frequently are affected. Chromophobe adenomas are the histological variety most likely to bleed and undergo spontaneous necrosis. Tumors of this type that occur following adrenalectomy are particularly susceptible to spontaneous hemorrhage. Apparently, spontaneous hemorrhage and necrosis have also resulted in cure of a few cases. Late hemorrhage, spontaneous rupture, and necrosis also occur in craniopharyngiomas.[50] Peculiarly, the lesion may lie dormant for many years, only to produce this complication in the fourth, fifth, or sixth decade of life.

CONCLUSIONS

Only half a century ago the exact diagnosis in cases of spontaneous subarachnoid hemorrhage was rarely established during the patient's lifetime, and only slightly more often after his death. At present, with persistent efforts, the lesions responsible can be identified in the vast majority of cases. Computed tomographic scanning and four-vessel angiography with magnification and subtraction are essential parts of the routine work-up. Cerebral blood flow studies, myelography, spinal angiography, and even ventricular air studies must be part of the diagnostic armamentarium in

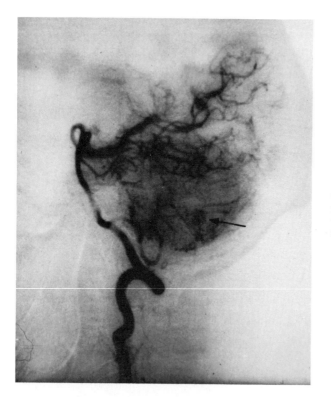

Figure 46–15 This small hemangioblastoma produced several episodes of spontaneous subarachnoid hemorrhage before it was resected. There were no focal neurological disturbances.

difficult cases. Added expense, discomfort, morbidity, and even death sometimes follows these endeavors. No gains are to be made, however, by a passive approach in managing the patient with recent subarachnoid hemorrhage. The severity of this illness, its tendency to recur and produce death and disability, justifies an aggressive attempt by the neurosurgeon to establish a prompt and accurate diagnosis.

REFERENCES

1. Appleton, D. B., Smith, P. J., and Earwaker, W. J. S.: Subarachnoid haemorrhage in children. Proc. Aust. Ass. Neurol., *11*:1–11, 1974.
2. Ask-Upmark, E., and Ingvar, D.: A follow-up examination of 138 cases of subarachnoid hemorrhage. Acta Med. Scand., *138*:15–31, 1950.
3. Baker, A. B.: Structure of the small cerebral arteries and their changes with age. Amer. J. Path., *13*:453–460, 1937.
4. Ball, M. J.: Pathogenesis of the "sentinel headache" preceding berry aneurysm rupture. Can. Med. Ass. J., *112*:78–79, 1975.
5. Bannerman, R. M., Ingall, G. B., and Graf, C. J.: The familial occurrence of intracranial aneurysms. Neurology (Minneap.), *20*:283–292, 1970.
6. Bassett, R. C., and Lammen, L.: Subdural hematoma associated with bleeding intracranial aneurysm. J. Neurosurg. 9:443–450, 1952.
7. Benoit, B. G., Wortzman, G.: Traumatic cerebral aneurysms. J. Neurol. Neurosurg. Psychiat., *36*:127–138, 1973.
8. Bjorkesten, G., and Troupp, H.: Prognosis of subarachnoid hemorrhage. A comparison between patients with verified aneurysms and patients with normal angiograms. J. Neurosurg., *14*:434–441, 1957.
9. Bright, R.: Reports of Medical Cases. Longmau, London, 1831.
10. Cantu, R. C., LeMay, M., and Wilkinson, H. A.: The importance of repeated angiography in the treatment of mycotic-embolic intracranial aneurysms. J. Neurosurg., *25*:189–193, 1966.
11. Caram, P. C., Sharkey, P., and Alvord, E. C.: Thalamic angioma and aneurysm of the anterior choroidal artery with intraventricular hematoma. J. Neurosurg., *17*:347–352, 1960.
12 Courville, C. B.: Encephalic lesions in hereditary hemorrhagic telangiectasis (Rendu-Osler-Weber disease): Report of case with the disclosure of microscopic telangiectasis in the leptomeninges. Bull. Los Angeles Neurol. Soc., *22*:28–35, 1957.
13. Crompton, M. R.: Mechanism of growth and rupture in cerebral berry aneurysm. Brit. Med. J., *1*:1138–1148, 1966.
14. Debrun, G., and Lacour, P.: Case of moya-moya disease associated with several intracavernous aneurysms. Neuroradiology, *7*:277–282, 1974.
15. DuBoulay, G. H.: The significance of loculation of intracranial aneurysms. Bull. Schweiz. Akad. Med. Wiss., *24*:480–485, 1969.

16. DuBoulay, G., and Gado, M.: The protective value of spasm after subarachnoid hemorrhage. Brain, *97*:153–156, 1974.
17. Fairburn, B.: "Twin" intracranial aneurysms causing subarachnoid haemorrhage in identical twins. Brit. Med. J., *27*:210–211, 1973.
18. Fedrick, J., and Butler, N. R.: Certain causes of neonatal death. II Intraventricular hemorrhage. Biol. Neonat., *15*:257–290, 1970.
19. Forbus, W. D.: On the origin of the miliary aneurysms of the superficial cerebral arteries. Bull. Johns Hopk. Hosp., *47*:239–284, 1930.
20. Glynn, L. E.: Medial defects in the circle of Willis and their relation to aneurysm formation. J. Path. Bact., *51*:213–222, 1940.
21. Goldstein, S.: Case reports and technical notes. Ventricular opacification secondary to rupture of intracranial aneurysms during angiography. J. Neurosurg., *27*:265–267, 1967.
22. Graf, C. J.: Prognosis for patients with nonsurgically-treated aneurysms. Analysis of the cooperative study of intracranial aneurysms and subarachnoid hemorrhage. J. Neurosurg., *35*:438–443, 1971.
23. Griffin, J., Price, D. L., Davis, L., and McKhann, G. M.: Granulomatous angiitis of the central nervous system with aneurysms on multiple cerebral arteries. Trans. Amer. Neurol. Ass., *98*:145–148, 1973.
24. Grollmus, J., and Hoff, J.: Multiple aneurysms associated with Osler-Weber-Rendu disease. Surg. Neurol., *1*:91–93, 1973.
25. Haerer, A. F., and Smith, R. R.: Medical and surgical experience in patients of a large Southern stroke center. Southern Med. J., *67*:667–671, 1974.
26. Hamby, W. B.: Spontaneous subarachnoid hemorrhage of aneurysmal origin. J.A.M.A., *136*:522–528, 1948.
27. Hassler, O.: Morphological studies on the large cerebral arteries (with reference to the aetiology of subarachnoid hemorrhage.) Acta Psychiat. Scand. Suppl., *36*:26–58, 1961.
28. Hayward, R. D., and O'Reilly, G. V. A.: Intracerebral hemorrhage. Lancet, *1*:1–5, January 3, 1976.
29. Hochberg, H. H., Fisher, C. M., and Roberson, G. H.: Subarachnoid hemorrhage caused by rupture of a small superficial artery. Neurology (Minneap.) 24:319–321, 1974.
30. Hourihane, J. B.: Ruptured mycotic intracranial aneurysm. Vasc. Surg., *4*:21–29, 1970.
31. Kak, V. K., Gleadhill, C. A., and Bailey, I. C.: The familial incidence of intracranial aneurysms. J. Neurol. Neurosurg. Psychiat., *33*:39–33, 1970.
32. Kaplan, H., Aronson, S. M., and Browder, E. J.: Vascular malformations of the brain. J. Neurosurg., *18*:630–635, 1961.
33. Laing, J. W., and Smith, R. R.: Intracranial arteriovenous malformations in sisters: A case report. J. Mississippi Med. Ass., *15*:203–206, 1974.
34. Lang, E. R., and Kidd, M.: Electron microscopy of human cerebral aneurysms. J. Neurosurg., *22*:554–562, 1965.
35. Larroche, J. C.: Hémorragies cérébrales intraventriculaires chez le prématuré. I. Anatomie et physiopathologie. Biol. Neonat., *7*:26–56, 1964.

36. Levy, L. E., Rachman, L., and Castle, W. M.: Spontaneous primary subarachnoid haemorrhage in Rhodesian African. Afr. J. Med. Sci., 4:77–86, 1973.

37. Margolis, G., Odom, G. L., Woodhall, B., and Bloor, B.: The role of small angiomatous malformations in the production of intracerebral hematomas. J. Neurosurg., 8:564–575, 1951.

38. Margolis, M. T., and Newton, T. H.: Methamphetamine ("speed") arteritis. Neuroradiology, 2:179–182, 1971.

39. Menezes, A. H., and Graf, C. J.: True traumatic aneurysm of anterior cerebral artery. J. Neurosurg., 40;544–548, 1974.

40. McCormick, W. F.: The pathology of vascular ("arteriovenous") malformations. J. Neurosurg., 24:807–816, 1966.

41. McCormick, W. F., and Nofzinger, J. D.: "Cryptic" vascular malformations of the central nervous system. J. Neurosurg., 24:865–875, 1966.

42. McCormick, W. F., and Rosenfield, D. B.: Massive brain hemorrhage. A review of 144 cases and an examination of their causes. Stroke, 4:946–954, 1973.

43. Morley, T. P., and Barr, H. W. K.: Giant intracranial aneurysms: diagnosis, course, and management. Clin. Neurosurg., 16:73–94, 1969.

44. Nibbelink D. W., Torner, J., and Henderson, W. G.: Intracranial aneurysms and subarachnoid hemorrhage. Stroke, 8:202–218, 1977.

45. Nicol, A. A. M.: Lindau's disease in five generations. Ann. Hum. Genet., 22:7–15, 1957.

46. Nystrom, S. H. M.: Development of intracranial aneurysms as revealed by electron microscopy. J. Neurosurg., 20:329–337, 1963.

47. Okawara, S.: Warning signs prior to rupture of an intracranial aneurysm. J. Neurosurg., 38:575–580, 1973.

48. Pakarinen, S.: Incidence, aetiology, and prognosis of primary subarachnoid hemorrhage. Acta. Neurol. Scand. Suppl. 29:1–128, 1967.

49. Pasztor, E., Szabo, G., Slowik, F., and Zoltan, J.: Case report—cavernous hemangioma of the base of the skull. J. Neurosurg., 21:528–585, 1964.

50. Patrick, B. S., Smith, R. R., and Bailey, T. O.: Aseptic meningitis due to spontaneous rupture of craniopharyngioma cyst. J. Neurosurg., 41:387–390, 1974.

51. Peerless, S. J., and Kendall, M. J.: The innervation of the cerebral blood vessels. In Smith, R. R., and Robinson, J. T., eds.: Subarachnoid Hemorrhage and Cerebrovascular Spasm. Springfield, Ill., Charles C Thomas, 1975, pp 38–54.

52. Robinson, J. L., Hall, C. S., and Sedzimir, C. B.: Arteriovenous malformations, aneurysms, and pregnancy. J. Neurosurg., 41:63–70, 1974.

53. Roizin, L., Gold, G., Berman, H. H., and Bonafede, V. I.: Congenital vascular anomalies and syndrome (naevus flammeus with angiomatosis and encephalosis calcificans.). J. Neuropath. Exp. Neurol., 18:75–97, 1959.

54. Rubenstein, M. K., and Cohen, N. H.: Ehlers-Danlos syndrome associated with multiple intracranial aneurysms. Neurology (Minneap.), 14:125, 1964.

55. Sahs, A., Perret, G. E., Locksley, H. B., and Nishioka, H.: Intracranial Aneurysms and Subarachnoid Hemorrhage. Philadelphia, J. B. Lippincott Co., 1969.

56. Sharr, M. M., and Kelvin, F. M.: Vertebrobasilar aneurysms. Experience with 27 cases. Europ. Neurol., 10:129–143, 1973.

57. Shokichi, U., Masumichi, I., Munesuke, S., and Masayoshi, S.: Subarachnoid hemorrhage as a cause of death in Japan. Seitschrift Fur Rechtsmedizin 72:151–160, 1973.

58. Simmons, M. A., Adcoak, E. W., Bard, H., and Battaglia, F. C.: Hypernatremia and intracranial hemorrhage in neonates. New Eng. J. Med., 291:6–10, 1974.

59. Solitare, G. B.: Louis-Bar's syndrome (ataxia-telangiectasia). Neurology (Minneap.), 18:1180–1186, 1968.

60. Stehbens, W. E.: Focal intimal proliferation in the cerebral arteries. Amer. J. Path., 36:289–301, 1960.

61. Stehbens, W. E.: Aneurysms and anatomical variations of cerebral arteries. Arch. Path., 75:45–64, 1963.

62. Stehbens, W. E.: Histopathology of cerebral aneurysms. Arch. Neurol., 8:272–285, 1963.

63. Strong, K. C.: A study of the structure of the media of the distributing arteries by the method of microdissection. Anat. Rec., 72:161, 1938.

64. Talbot, S.: Epidemiological features of subarachnoid and cerebral haemorrhages. Postgrad. Med. J., 49:300–304, 1973.

65. Watson, D. G., Smith, R. R., and Brann, A. W., Jr.: Arteriovenous malformation of the vein of Galen. Amer. J. Dis. Child., 130:520–525, 1976.

66. Yarnell, P. R., and Stears, J.: Intracerebral hemorrhage and occult sepsis. Neurology (Minneap.), 24:870–873, 1974.

47

NONOPERATIVE TREATMENT OF SUBARACHNOID HEMORRHAGE

INTRACRANIAL ANEURYSMS

The management of a patient with a saccular intracranial aneurysm is a problem of considerable complexity, involving such variables as the age, sex, and clinical condition of the patient as well as the specific aneurysm site, the elapsed time since hemorrhage, and the size and configuration of the aneurysm. The experience and enthusiasm of the medical and surgical team and the available facilities deserve equal consideration in selecting the best treatment for a given patient. It is not the purpose of this chapter to decry the value of surgical management of aneurysms but rather to discuss the timing of an operation, to review interim management, and to identify those patients in whom alternative treatment might be just as effective.

Operative treatment of intracranial aneurysms began in modern times. Pioneer work by Ask-Upmark and Hamby called attention to the devastating natural history of these lesions and fostered early attempts to control the recurrent hemorrhages.[4,27] In 1938, Dandy reported the first intracranial cure of a carotid artery aneurysm.[15] During the next quarter century, operative cases accumulated and mortality rates decreased, largely owing to adjuncts of medical and operative treatment and to patient selection. The recent introduction of micro-operative techniques and delayed operative intervention may be the most significant developments in the history of the treatment of aneurysms.[7,70]

The history of nonoperative treatment of cerebral aneurysms is likewise a short one. In 1948, Wechsler said that when treatment was described as conservative, it usually meant that there was no treatment at all.[86] In recent years, regulated bed rest, hypotension, and antifibrinolytic therapy have been added to the medical armamentarium.

Proponents of each type of therapy, operative versus nonoperative, have sponsored comparisons. Until recently, most of these were biased by selection artifacts. When the surgeon withdraws good-risk candidates from the population pool, the mortality rate among the conservatively treated group invariably rises. When a patient assigned for operation suffers rebleeding just before the operation can be performed and is listed as a failure of conservative therapy, further comparisons are impossible. Unfortunately, it is also true that patients who are regarded as poor risks for particular medical measures are excluded from consideration at final statistical analysis. In the past decade, through cooperative arrangements among many centers, it has been possible for the most part to eliminate the bias of selection through random allocation of patients to a treatment protocol. The results of these trials are being evaluated.[53]

R. R. SMITH

The Candidate
for Nonoperative Treatment

Botterell recognized that if comparisons between treatments are to be made, the clinical condition, or grade, at the time therapy is begun is fundamental.[8] Many schemes have been proposed, but in each level of consciousness seems to be the most reliable factor in predicting eventual outcome (Table 47–1). Patients in coma when therapy is begun have the highest mortality rate, and alert patients the lowest. In the group recently randomly assigned to bed rest treatment, the mortality rate among grade I patients was 36.4 per cent, and among grade VI patients, 100 per cent. With each increase in severity, or grade, the mortality rate increases proportionately, regardless of the treatment that is instituted.[53] The quality of survival also correlates closely with clinical grade. Unless an intraparenchymal clot is present, little is to be gained by operative therapy in the high-risk patient. If, however, improvement occurs on a conservative program, definitive operative treatment can be performed later with less risk.

Advanced age must be considered a negative factor in either operatively or medically treated patients. Richardson and co-workers found that three times as many patients over the age of 59 died as did younger patients.[67] Complicating conditions such as hypertension, anemia, and pulmonary disease increase the mortality rate even further. For patients 50 years of age or older in poor neurological condition, Nibbelink and associates record less than a 30 per cent chance of survival after three weeks of regulated bed rest.[53] Although a prior history of hypertension does not necessarily prohibit operative treatment, Walsh found the prognosis of hypertensive patients less favorable than that of normotensive ones (mortality rates of 51 per cent versus 30 per cent).[84] Hypertension following acute subarachnoid hemorrhage may not always accurately reflect antecedent blood pressure alterations, since subarachnoid bleeding through a number of mechanisms, including increased intracranial pressure, may promote a hypertensive response. The presence of elevated cerebrospinal fluid pressure also adversely influences operative survival statistics for patients operated on early as well as for those for whom operation is deferred awaiting improvement in their condition. Klafta found that patients in good condition tended to survive operation regardless of cerebrospinal fluid pressure. In grade III patients, however, the mortality rate was 17 per cent for those with normal pressure, but 41 per cent of those with elevated pressures died at operation or shortly thereafter. In higher-risk patients, fewer died of recurrent hemorrhage than were lost to premature operation, and thus waiting until cerebrospinal fluid pressures are near normal seems justified.[37] Nornes noted that extradural pressures less than 400 mm of mercury favored optimum operative survival figures.[55]

Other factors, notably the patient's sex, the multiplicity of aneurysms, and the number of hemorrhages prior to admission may also influence the survival rate. The number of deaths from subarachnoid hemorrhage among female patients treated nonoperatively is only slightly higher, but the number after operations may be twice as great.[67] There is little difference in mortality rates associated with internal carotid, middle cerebral, and anterior cerebral aneurysms conservatively treated. The presence of more than one aneurysm, however, significantly increases the mortality rates of both operative and medical treatment. There are almost twice as many deaths among patients who sustain more than one episode of subarachnoid hemorrhage before admission to the hospital than among

TABLE 47–1 NEUROLOGICAL GRADING OF SUBARACHNOID HEMORRHAGE (COOPERATIVE STUDY)*

GRADE	DEFINITION
I	Symptom-free
II	Minor symptoms (headache, meningeal irritation, diplopia)
III	Major neurological deficit but fully responsive
IV	Impaired state of alertness but capable of protective or other adaptive responses to noxious stimuli
V	Poorly responsive but with stable vital signs
VI	No response to address or shaking, nonadaptive response to noxious stimuli, and progressive instability of vital signs

* From Nibbelink, D. W., Forner, J. C., and Henderson, W. G.: Intracranial aneurysms and subarachnoid hemorrhage—report on a randomized treatment study. Stroke, 8:202–218, 1977. Reprinted by permission.

those who bleed only once (63 per cent versus 36 per cent).[67]

The size and configuration of the aneurysm as well as the accessibility of its neck are factors to be considered in determining the operability of an aneurysm. Large bulbous aneurysms with significant branches exiting from the fundus are difficult to clip effectively, and wrapping or coating confers less protection than clipping or ligating their necks. Bulbous, up-pointing, anterior communicating aneurysms are more likely to be responsible for death than long, thin, down-pointing lesions.[67]

Micro-operative techniques have added a new dimension to aneurysm therapy, and their benefits in various treatment categories and grades are not yet fully apparent. Statistics for conventional operative treatment, however, indicate that the risk for the patient not fully responsive, the hypertensive patient, and the elderly patient may be prohibitive. Increased risk of death must be weighed against any likely benefit for the patient with a difficult aneurysm, multiple aneurysms, multiple antecedent hemorrhages, or complicating medical illnesses. Any late benefit derived from the prevention of rebleeding by clipping of the aneurysm may be offset by increased risk of immediate death from the operation itself.

The surgeon should not look upon the patient who has not been operated on as a personal defeat. Troupp and Björkesten point out that patients who survive a subarachnoid hemorrhage for six weeks have a good prognosis, and the value of an operation in this group seems questionable. Over an average follow-up of three and one half years, these authors were unable to show a difference in mortality rates or morbidity between patients who had survived the six-week interval who were operated on and those who were not.[82]

Timing of Operation

Of all the factors subject to alteration in a patient with a recently ruptured intracranial aneurysm, the timing of the operation probably influences survival more than any other single factor. In cases operated on later than the seventh day, Saito and associates report a mortality rate of only 3.7 per cent, while almost 18 per cent of those

operated on earlier died.[70] Others have confirmed the great risk of early operation. Graf and Nibbelink noted a 44.5 per cent mortality rate among patients operated on in the first week after subarachnoid hemorrhage.[25] Hunt and others, however, have advocated early operation for grade I and II patients, concluding that the risk of rebleeding and death is higher and the risk of operation lower in these alert patients.[32,33,39] His impressive series lists only 19 deaths among 124 grade I and grade II cases, an 85 per cent survival rate. Widespread popular belief holds that vasospasm and cerebral edema are more often aggravated than relieved by an early intracranial operation.[4,32,33] Progressive decline in neurological function, presumably due to vasospasm, accounts for 8 to 10 per cent of the deaths that follow subarachnoid hemorrhage, and these occur largely within two weeks of the initial hemorrhage.[53] Fifty-seven patients in grade I or II were treated at the University of Mississippi Medical Center with antifibrinolytic agents from 7 to 14 days following their subarachnoid hemorrhages. In this group, there was only one preoperative death attributable to rebleeding of the aneurysm. On the other hand, progressive decline, presumably caused by vasospasm, accounted for four deaths among these conservatively treated patients. The cooperative group described only a 5.8 per cent mortality rate due to rebleeding in all patients during the first 14 days of treatment with antifibrinolytic agents. Although proper management of the grade I or grade II patient is not settled, one point stands out clearly. Unless the surgeon can accomplish his operation in the good-risk patient without occasioning death or morbidity in the first week or 10 days, then delay of the operation is warranted.

In patients in grades III to VI, early operation is difficult to justify. Many patients who are poorly responsive initially improve a grade after 7 to 14 days on a conservative program. Operative deaths decrease sharply as the conscious level rises. The patient in poor-risk status due to complicating medical factors such as diabetes, hypertension, the inappropriate antidiuretic hormone secretion syndrome, or autonomic system dysfunction will frequently improve during a preoperative period of conservative treatment. The last-mentioned condition has usually abated when a drop of 1 per cent epinephrine placed in the conjunctival sac fails to produce a widely dilated pupil.[29] In the patient with more than one aneurysm, an interim period of medical management is frequently helpful in determining which aneurysm has ruptured. Follow-up angiography may reveal spasm or enlargement of the fundus after the intra-aneurysmal clot has lysed.

Intensive Care and Intracranial Pressure Management

There has been an increasing tendency among those dealing with large numbers of acutely ill patients to isolate them in intensive care units. Thus, the concept of the stroke unit for the care of the patient with subarachnoid hemorrhage has evolved. The value of these units has not been clearly established. The stroke unit, when compared with community hospitals where such units are not available, usually has not produced a significant reduction in death rates.

Understanding the problem and anticipating its occurrence has produced a sharp decline in the complications formerly seen in stroke patients. Deep vein thrombosis, pneumonia, pressure sores, and urinary tract infections have been reduced. Approximately 50 per cent of the patients with various kinds of strokes also have cardiac arrhythmias, and these deserve and often require careful monitoring.[26,57]

On postmortem examination, evidence of increased intracranial pressure is an almost universal finding following subarachnoid hemorrhage. Flattening of gyri, herniation, and areas of focal and diffuse edema are found. Focal edema and focally increased pressure may further reduce cerebral perfusion and affect late morbidity. In the acutely ill patient, the measurement of intracranial pressure by means of an intraventricular catheter not only provides the answer to whether pressure is elevated but also permits pressure reduction by removal of ventricular fluid. Epidural, subdural, or subarachnoid devices are likewise helpful, but the cerebrospinal fluid pressure must be reduced by less direct means such as osmotic diuretics.

Nornes has described two types of pressure peaks accompanying subarachnoid hemorrhage.[56] Type 1 pressure peaks are between 900 and 2200 mm of water, last from 8 to 26 minutes, and then fall toward normal levels. Approximately three fourths of the patients who show the type 1 curve survive the subarachnoid hemorrhage. Type 2 peaks occur suddenly, and intracranial pressure may rise from 200 to 2000 mm of water over a very short interval. The elevated pressure is unresponsive to hyperventilation and dehydrating agents. Type 2 curves apparently represent recurrent hemorrhage from the aneurysm and are usually accompanied by deterioration in clinical grade. Fatalities occur in 90 per cent of patients showing type 2 curves. Although type 1 curves are generally not associated with fresh bleeding into the cerebrospinal fluid, they may occur as a prelude to and a warning of the type 2 response.[55] Elevated intracranial pressure following subarachnoid hemorrhage is often resistant to ordinary reduction methods. Minor elevations not associated with peaks can often be reduced by intermittent intravenous administration of mannitol in doses of 20 to 100 gm. Urea, spinal drainage, ventricular drainage, steroids, and hyperventilation may be employed in more resistant cases.

Monitoring intracranial pressure may serve as a guide for the timing of the operation.[56] Lundberg and co-workers advocate ventricular drainage until the fluid pressure is lowered to 200 mm of water and is stabilized there before the operation is performed.[42] In high-risk patients, elevated intracranial pressure remains a significant cause of death. Monitoring and controlling pressures when possible may result in improvement in clinical status, rendering these patients suitable candidates for repair of the aneurysm.

Regulated Bed Rest

Simple bed rest has long been recognized as beneficial in preventing rebleeding from intracranial aneurysms. Since 10 per cent of the rebleedings occur during the third week after the initial hemorrhage, the bed rest program should not be terminated before the fourth week.[53] Beyond the fourth week, rebleeding rates gradually diminish to about 1 per cent per month. At that time, the patient is allowed to sit up in bed and to progress gradually to ambulation in the ensuing weeks. Additional supportive mea-

TABLE 47-2 BED REST THERAPY FOR RUPTURED INTRACRANIAL ANEURYSMS

Hospitalization
Subdued lighting
Elevation of the head no more than 30 degrees
Patient allowed to turn but not sit up or feed himself
Bowel habits regulated with stool softeners
Bedside commode after the first week
Maintenance of airway and oxygenation
Seizure prophylaxis with diphenylhydantoin, 100 mg 3 times daily for 3 weeks
Adequate fluids, 1500 to 2000 ml per 24 hours (by mouth, nasogastric tube, or intravenously)
1000 Calories of nutrition per day
Diazepam, phenobarbital or chloral hydrate for sedation as needed for restlessness
Condom drainage for men, and catheter drainage for women only for incontinence. Otherwise, normal voiding permitted
Analgesic with aspirin, codeine, or meperidine hydrochloride as necessary
Vital sign examination periodically as needed but no more often
Nausea, vomiting, and singultus may be treated with phenothiazines
Steroids or other anti-edema drugs may be used when indicated
Anti-embolic stockings, passive motion of lower limbs several times daily

sures that should be included in the regulated bed rest program are listed in Table 47-2.

In a recent study, 187 patients were randomly allocated to a program similar to the one outlined in Table 47-2 without regard to condition or interval from hemorrhage. The mortality rate was greater with the bed rest program than with either drug-induced hypotension or intracranial operation, (provided that the operation was not performed in the first week after the hemorrhage). After a mean interval of 6.5 years, the overall mortality rate was 55.1 per cent, with proved rebleeding the greatest cause of death. The greatest frequency of rebleeding occurred during the interval from the fifth through the ninth day, and the majority of episodes (65.8 per cent) occurred in the 29 days following the initial bleed. The remainder (34.2 per cent) occurred during the remaining follow-up period.[53]

As expected, the mortality rates for patients allocated to a bed rest program are highest in grade VI and lowest in grade I. The patient's medical condition also influences the mortality and morbidity figures. Patients in poor condition (more than one complication such as myocardial infarction or hypertension) carry mortality risks of over 80 per cent.[53] The complications

directly attributable to bed rest are primarily those accompanying immobilization. Because of age, vascular disease, dehydration, and immobility, the patient with subarachnoid hemorrhage runs a greater risk of thromboembolic disease than the usual patient. Warlow and co-workers described deep vein thrombosis in 60 per cent of their stroke patients with a paralyzed lower extremity.[85] Pulmonary embolism occurs in 7 per cent of all patients with recent stroke.

Hypotensive Therapy

Fundamentally, the proponents of hypotension follow one of two therapeutic plans. The focal point of one method is the lowering of blood pressure to the point of cerebral ischemia by whatever means are required and available. The other method is merely to reduce systolic thrust on the aneurysm wall through a variety of antihypertensive medications.

Slosberg introduced the profound hypotension regimen. It calls for the prompt reduction in arterial blood pressure by both chemical and mechanical means as soon as the diagnosis of aneurysmal subarachnoid hemorrhage is made. The patient is placed on a tilt table and the head is elevated. In the beginning, hydrochlorothiazide and rauwolfia are administered. The desired blood pressure range has been obtained when signs of cerebrovascular insufficiency occur; the pressure must be lowered according to the patient's ability to maintain adequate perfusion of the brain and other vital organs, as judged by careful and frequent assessment. Hypotension is usually maintained by the addition of intramuscular reserpine. An initial dose of 0.625 to 2.5 mg, 0.625 mg every six hours, and oral hydrochlorothiazide, 25 to 50 mg every six hours, are administered. As the risk of rebleeding diminishes, rauwolfia alkaloids and hydrochlorothiazide are given orally. Hydrochlorothiazide is continued at 150 mg per day. Each patient also receives diphenylhydantoin, aspirin as needed for headaches, and potassium supplements as required to maintain normal levels in the serum.[73,74]

Complications of this treatment include decubitus ulcers, septicemia, hypostatic pneumonia, aspiration pneumonia, cardiac arrhythmias, gastrointestinal bleeding, and urinary tract infections. A competent trained nurse is expected to be in attendance at all times, and the therapy is continued until four weeks have elapsed from the day of the initial hemorrhage. The upper acceptable blood pressure limit usually is established at 30 to 40 mm of mercury above the level of cerebral ischemia. When pressure rises above this point, the head of the tilt table is elevated, and if this fails to reduce the pressure, the physician is summoned. If the blood pressure falls below the level previously determined to be safe, the tilt table is lowered until the pressure rises.[73]

At the end of four weeks, the patient becomes ambulatory. Finally, upon discharge, he continues to take hypotensive agents. According to Slosberg, only two deaths occurred among his first 22 consecutive patients treated with hypotensive methods, and late rebleeding was rare. In patients younger than 50 years of age, mortality rates of 5 per cent have been achieved. The therapeutic program is versatile. No patients need be excluded because of age, inaccessibility of the aneurysm, multiple aneurysms, inadequate collateral circulation, reaction to carotid compression, recency of bleeding, or antecedent medical illnesses. A relative contraindication may be a patient's inability to communicate, which restricts the value of clinical assessment.[74]

Profound hypotension, as outlined in the preceding discussion, has never gained a large number of proponents, perhaps more because of its medical complexity than because of disappointment in its results. When profound hypotension is used in the presence of vasospasm, however, cerebral infarction may occur suddenly and unexpectedly.

Moderate hypotension induced by drugs, alone and in combination with other types of therapy, has gained wide support. The international cooperative study allocated 57 patients randomly to a drug-induced hypotension protocol. Diuretics, methyldopa, reserpine, and hydralazine, either alone or in combinations, were administered for a minimum of 7 and not longer than 14 days from the last bleeding episode. Among these patients, 21 (36.8 per cent) died within the 14-day treatment interval, 17 (29.8 per cent) from a proved rebleeding

TABLE 47–3   RANDOMIZED STUDY OF CONSERVATIVE THERAPY

TREATMENT	NO. OF PATIENTS	MORTALITY RATE (PER CENT AT 14 DAYS)
Hypotension	57	29.8
Antifibrinolysis	47	8.5
Combined	53	25.4
Total	157	

episode (Table 47–3). Mechanical means were not used to reduce the blood pressure, and the level of pressure reduction was not comparable to that achieved by using Slosberg's methods. When compared with other forms of therapy (antifibrinolytic and combined), however, hypotension was found to be less effective in preventing rebleeding. On the basis of current information, moderate drug-induced hypotension should be used only when antifibrinolytic therapy is contraindicated, as in pregnancy, or when allergic reaction or thromboembolic complications have intervened.[51]

Antifibrinolytic Therapy

In 1964, Mullen and co-workers noted that the experimentally induced thrombus in the femoral artery of the dog was ordinarily of short duration.[48] When epsilon-aminocaproic acid (EACA) was administered, the duration of the thrombus could be prolonged. Later, lysis of an electrically induced thrombus in an aneurysm was also inhibited by this agent.[47] Epsilon-aminocaproic acid acts principally by competitive inhibition of the activator that converts inactive plasminogen into the active fibrinolytic enzyme plasmin (Fig. 47–1). Active plasmin, normally not present in the circulating blood, is probably the most important

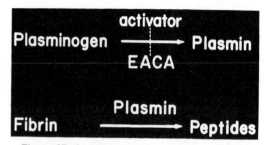

Figure 47–1   The mechanism of action of epsilon-aminocaproic acid (EACA).

factor in fibrin clot dissolution. EACA also plays a role in inhibiting the production of plasminogen. It apparently crosses the blood–cerebrospinal fluid barrier only in very high concentrations, and therefore the effect on the subarachnoid clot and the clot that surrounds the aneurysm is considered minimal. Following subarachnoid bleeding, there is increased natural fibrinolytic activity of both cerebrospinal fluid and blood.[77]

Recognizing that rebleeding from intracranial aneurysms coincided with dissolution of the intravascular blood clot, Mullen administered EACA to 35 patients with recent subarachnoid hemorrhage.[46] Only two patients bled again, and there were no serious complications associated with the therapy. Since this pioneer work was done, antifibrinolytic agents have been tested widely. Epsilon-aminocaproic acid, the most widely used, may be administered intravenously or orally. Since most of the reported rebleedings in patients receiving these agents have occurred before antifibrinolysis was achieved, vigorous intravenous therapy during the first few days following subarachnoid hemorrhage is paramount. During the first several days, 36 to 48 gm per 24 hours is usually required to achieve optimum levels. If the agent is to be administered orally, it must be given at two-hour intervals because it is rapidly excreted in the urine, and three hours following oral administration, fibrinolytic activity of the serum returns toward normal levels (Fig. 47–2). It is quite possible that no single dosage is applicable to all patients. Generally, after two days of treatment the dosage can be reduced to about 24 gm per 24 hours, depending upon the results of fibrin plate studies or analysis of clot lysis time. Some patients require continued high dosage, while in others the optimum level is achieved rapidly.[77] The dosage should be reduced when the streptokinase clot lysis time falls below 12 hours. It should be increased if the lysis time exceeds 24 hours.[24] If fibrin plate studies are used for monitoring serum levels, 155 sq mm of fibrin clot lysis seem to indicate optimum levels.[77]

Tranexamic acid (AMCA), perhaps 10 times as potent as epsilon-aminocaproic acid, effectively crosses the blood-brain barrier and enters the cerebrospinal fluid. Currently it is not available in the United States. After several days of tranexamic acid administration, fibrin breakdown prod-

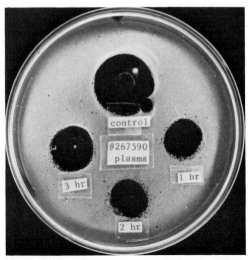

Figure 47–2 The duration of action of epsilon-aminocaproic acid administered orally. Fibrinolytic activity decreases three hours after an oral dose. (From Smith, R. R., and Upchurch, J. J.: Monitoring antifibrinolytic therapy in subarachnoid hemorrhage. J. Neurosurg., *38*:339–344, 1973. Reprinted by permission.)

ucts virtually disappear from the cerebrospinal fluid, and thus hydrocephalus might theoretically complicate prolonged therapy with this agent. Initially, tranexamic acid should be administered intravenously in doses of 1000 mg six times daily for the first week, 1000 mg four times daily during the second week, and 1000 mg three times daily during the third to sixth weeks.[20] Tranexamic acid and epsilon-aminocaproic acid should be discontinued immediately after the aneurysm has been operatively obliterated. Their use is not recommended during pregnancy.

The effectiveness of antifibrinolytic agents in preventing premature rebleeding from aneurysms has now been established. Of 471 patients treated with epsilon-aminocaproic acid by the cooperative group, 12.7 per cent experienced proved rebleeding during the 14-day treatment interval. Most recurrent hemorrhages occurred between the sixth and eleventh days following the initial bleed. Because of the delay in admission, however, 45 per cent of both proved and suspected rebleedings occurred prior to the day proper antifibrinolytic effect would have been achieved.[76] It seems unlikely that an operation could have been performed before bleeding occurred in this group.[52]

The results with tranexamic acid are similarly encouraging. The rebleeding rate in nontreated patients may be as great as nine times that of patients who receive this agent.[20] Table 47–3 compares the mortality rates associated with several treatments during the early posthemorrhage phase.

Since lysis retardation is the primary mechanism of action, antifibrinolytic therapy may simply prolong the interval in which recurrent bleeding is to be expected. Ideally, therefore, this therapy should be combined with operative clipping to forestall late aneurysmal rupture. The effect of these agents on wound healing is a subject about which little is known, however.

Complications associated with antifibrinolytic therapy have been few. Knight and associates have shown that deep vein thrombosis occurs postoperatively in 80 per cent of patients in whose serum fibrinolytic activity is reduced.[38] It is, therefore, not surprising that deep vein thrombosis and pulmonary embolism have been described in patients receiving these agents (Table 47–4).[74] These complications also occur more frequently in all stroke patients than in the general population. Arteriopathic complications of epsilon-aminocaproic acid therapy have now been described in patients with subarachnoid hemorrhage as well as others who have received antifibrinolytic agents.[7] Sonntag and co-workers noted cerebrovascular occlusive disease resembling arteritis in three patients receiving epsilon-aminocaproic acid.[78] An increased incidence of arterial pathological changes may be causally related to these drugs (Fig. 47–3). Dehydration may have contributed to the uremia encountered in six patients in the author's series.[76]

Remarkably, hydrocephalus has not been a frequent complication of antifibrinolytic therapy. Questions have been frequently

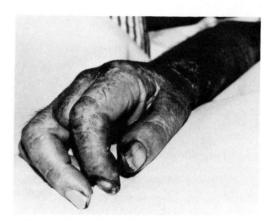

Figure 47–3 This patient developed radial artery occlusion while receiving epsilon-aminocaproic acid therapy. A radial artery catheter had been employed to monitor intraoperative blood pressure. The ischemic changes ultimately resolved spontaneously.

raised as to the effect of these agents on vasospasm. Fodstad and Thulin found vasospasm two weeks after the initial hemorrhage in 80 per cent of patients treated with tranexamic acid as opposed to 25 per cent of the controls who had received no antifibrinolytic drugs. The difference between these two groups was statistically significant. Because small numbers of patients were studied, further confirmation is needed.[20]

Combination Therapy

In Table 47–4 the effectiveness of various treatments currently used in preventing rebleeding are compared. Although the number of patients is small, the trend suggests that hypotensive therapy may erase any benefits derived from antifibrinolytic therapy when the two are used in combination. The group receiving combined therapy contained more of the seriously ill patients, however.[51] Hypotension alone is also apparently less effective than antifibrinolysis. Arterial pressure elevations following subarachnoid hemorrhage may be of the neurogenic type, occurring through ischemic brain centers. Elevated catecholamine levels are observed in both blood and urine. Reduction in systemic arterial pressure under these circumstances may precipitate neurological sequelae. Often, however, the hypertension abates as cerebral edema and increased intracranial pressure subside. Peripheral blood pressure

TABLE 47–4 THROMBOEMBOLIC COMPLICATIONS OF EPSILON-AMINOCAPROIC ACID

	NUMBER OF PATIENTS	PER CENT
At risk	96	
Deep vein thrombosis	3	3
Pulmonary embolism	6	6
Uremia	6	6
Peripheral artery occlusion	2	2
Other	3	3
Myocardial infarction	0	0

reduction through peripheral vasodilators may reduce intracranial pressure, but often at the expense of brain perfusion.

ARTERIOVENOUS MALFORMATIONS

Characteristically, the hemorrhage produced by arteriovenous malformations occurs in younger individuals, causes fewer deaths and less morbidity, and rebleedings occur less frequently than with aneurysms.[62] The mortality rate has been about 10 per cent, but modern therapy may reduce this. Management of the hemorrhagic mass and prevention of recurrent bleeding should be major goals of therapy. When regional intracranial pressure exceeds regional arteriolar pressure, areas of microinfarction occur as a consequence. Although most medical centers do not have the capabilities to measure regional blood flow, monitoring intracranial pressure is now practical on most neurosurgical services and appears worthwhile in acutely and severely ill patients. A reduction in intracranial pressure is often attended by clinical improvement in neurological status, and the beneficial effects in some patients leave little doubt as to the effectiveness of this treatment.

Recurrent hemorrhages from arteriovenous malformations occur less frequently than from aneurysms, and the rebleedings occur randomly over a number of years. Collation of data from several small series reported by a number of investigators indicates that about 30 per cent can be expected to rebleed over a period of about five years of follow-up (Table 47–5). The mortality rate with each hemorrhage is about 12 per cent, and further analysis yields a 2 per cent yearly mortality rate due to rebleeding. Unlike hemorrhage from aneurysms, the frequency of rebleeding is scattered and not grouped about the initial event. Thus, the therapeutic program must cover the long term as well as the short. Of the 105 conservatively treated cases collected by the cooperative study, only two patients rebled and died while in the hospital following the initial event. Four rebled within 2 months, seven between 2 and 12 months; 18 rebleedings occurred between 1 and 5 years, 11 between 5 and 10 years, and 8 others 10 to 20 years following the initial event.[62] Forster concluded that the risk of bleeding in a patient who had never bled was about one chance in four in 15 years. The patient who had rebled once had one chance in four of rebleeding again within four years, and the patient who had rebled twice had one chance in four of rebleeding again within the next year. No correlation was found between the tendency of an arteriovenous malformation to bleed and its site or size, or the age or sex of the patient.[21]

The operative mortality rate with arteriovenous malformations has varied with both the site of the lesion and the age of the patient; overall, it varies between 12 and 15 per cent.[21,45,64] Even after complete excision, rebleedings may occur, and when only coagulation of the vessel or nutrient

TABLE 47–5 RECURRENT BLEEDING FROM ARTERIOVENOUS MALFORMATIONS TREATED NONOPERATIVELY

SERIES	DATE	FOLLOW-UP (YR)	NO. OF CASES	REBLED		DIED	
				PER CENT	NO.	PER CENT	NO.
Perret and Nishioka*	1966	5	103	20	22	5	5
Svien and McRae†	1965	30	47	34	16	6	2
Potter‡	1955	5	44	34	14	9	4
Troupp§	1965	5	60			13	8
Paterson and McKissock‖	1956	5	21	24	5	5	1
Forster et al.¶	1972	12	35	29	10	17	6
Total			220	30	67	12	26

* Report on the cooperative study of intracranial aneurysms and subarachnoid hemorrhage. Section VI. Arteriovenous malformations. J. Neurosurg., 25:467–490, 1966.
† Arteriovenous anomalies of the brain. J. Neurosurg., 23:23–28, 1965.
‡ Angiomatous malformations of the brain: Their nature and prognosis. Ann. Roy. Coll. Surg. Eng., 16:227–243, 1955.
§ Arteriovenous malformations of the brain: Prognosis without operation. Acta Neurol. Scand., 41:39–42, 1965.
‖ A clinical survey of intracranial angiomas with special reference to their mode of progression and surgical treatment A report of 110 cases. Brain, 79:233–266, 1956.
¶ Arteriovenous malformations of the brain. A long-term clinical study. J. Neurosurg., 37:562–570, 1972.

artery ligation is employed, rebleedings occur much more frequently. Recurrent hemorrhages occur in 8 or 9 per cent of those operated on, and in a few even after total excision.[21] Considering all these factors, 10 years or so must pass before any benefit of operative treatment can be appreciated in the patient with bleeding from an arteriovenous malformation. These statistics apply only to patients carefully selected for operative treatment. The small easily accessible malformation located in the frontal, temporal, or occipital pole in young individuals carries lowest risk factors. Deep malformations should be treated nonoperatively. In Moody and Poppen's series, no patients older than 60 survived the operative procedures, and 8 of 14 operative deaths occurred in patients over the age of 40. Eleven of fourteen deaths occurred in patients with large malformations.[45] Spontaneous regression and thrombosis of the malformation have been described after subarachnoid hemorrhage.[40]

In the author's series, a definite correlation has been noted between increased thoracic pressure and the onset of subarachnoid hemorrhage. Hemorrhage has occurred after coughing, diving, straining, and playing musical wind instruments. Apparently, the rupture occurs in thin veins carrying arterial pressures. Increased intrathoracic pressure probably produces engorgement beyond the capacity of these vessels.

The patient should be placed at bed rest until the rent in the vessel wall has had an opportunity to heal by fibrous union. During this interval, anything that might increase venous and arterial pressure is avoided. Excessive hydration and blood volume overload should be avoided. Arterial blood pressure, if it is elevated, should be reduced. Steroids may have some value in reducing cerebral edema, but this has not been established. If pregnancy, with its effect on circulating blood volume, has been a factor in precipitating the hemorrhage, consideration should be given to its termination. The head of the bed should be elevated to approximately 30 degrees to promote venous drainage. Convulsive seizures may be treated prophylactically. Cough, singultus, or vomiting may be ameliorated with codeine, thorazine, or trimethobenzamide respectively. Pulmonary toilet must be maintained, but respirators should be avoided if possible. Increased expiratory pressure is also undesirable.

Antifibrinolytic agents have little place in the management of the patient with a recently ruptured arteriovenous malformation. The low mortality rate with early rebleeding (less than 2 per cent in the first month) would hardly justify their use.[62] The increased incidence of arterial and venous complications and the aggravation of vasospasm or hydrocephalus would balance out any value produced by short-term stabilization of the intravascular thrombus.[20,76]

OTHER SUBARACHNOID HEMORRHAGE

When results of all diagnostic studies are normal following subarachnoid hemorrhage, it must be assumed that the leakage of blood occurred from a minor defect in an artery or vein or from an undisclosed aneurysm. The mortality rates associated with the initial hemorrhage and with recurrence in these cases are probably quite low. Levy described one death among 76 patients with subarachnoid hemorrhage who had normal angiograms.[41] Björkesten and Troupp described prognostic factors in 61 patients with verified subarachnoid hemorrhage who had normal bilateral carotid angiograms. During a follow-up interval of from 1 to 10 years, there were five recurrences. Death resulted in three of these, and one was found to have a ruptured aneurysm.[6] Hook and others reported similar findings.[31] Routinely, approximately half of those who die from recurrent hemorrhages are found to have undisclosed arterial aneurysms. If the autopsy-verified aneurysms are excluded, the mortality rate for the remainder of the patients who have normal bilateral carotid arteriograms is on the average about 3 per cent after five years.[59] If four-vessel angiography and computed tomography are included in the diagnostic regimen, the number of recurrent hemorrhages would probably be further reduced. Hayward and O'Reilly noted that tomography further increases the diagnostic accuracy in subarachnoid hemorrhage. The computed tomogram alone was falsely negative in only 1 of 52 patients harboring cerebral aneurysms and in 4 of 8 with angiomas.[30] Often, a small intracerebral hematoma near the ventricle or subarachnoid space is identified as the source of subarachnoid hemorrhage in these patients. Using four-vessel angiography, Björkesten and Troupp found the source of bleeding in all but 15 per cent of their patients.[6] Repeating the angiogram after a week or 10 days in classic cases often reveals the site of the hemorrhage even when initial studies have been normal.[67] The incidence of rebleeding in cases in which these diagnostic tests are negative must be extremely low. Perhaps arterial windows, medial wall defects, and junctional defects are responsible for hemorrhage in the remainder.

When rebleeding does occur, a scattered, random distribution is found. Pakarinen described hemorrhages during the fourth week, the fifth month, the eighth month, and three years after the initial event.[59] Thus, a conservative therapeutic program in these cases would have to be extremely safe to improve upon the natural history. A prolonged interval of bed rest is probably not justified, since advanced age and generalized vascular disease place these patients in jeopardy for the development of deep vein thrombosis and pulmonary embolism. At best, they should be confined to bed until the rent in the vessel has healed, no longer than two or three weeks. Arterial pressure, if elevated, should be reduced. The use of antifibrinolytic agents seems difficult to justify on the basis of the low natural risk and the complication rates that have been described when these drugs are used.[76–78] It is the author's practice to institute a program of progressive ambulation immediately after repeating the angiogram, usually at the end of the second week.

COMPLICATIONS OF SUBARACHNOID HEMORRHAGE

Cerebral Vasospasm

When a neurosurgeon speaks of vasospasm, he usually refers to a complicated series of clinical and radiographic events that follow subarachnoid hemorrhage from an aneurysm. Lack of understanding of the pathogenesis and the etiological mechanisms has hindered the development of an effective therapeutic plan. No entirely suitable animal experimental model has been developed. While vascular constriction may be produced in a number of animals through a variety of mechanisms, it is usually short-lived, has no recurrent phase, and rarely produces a neurological deficit as a result.

In man, the pathology is not clear. Focal infarction in the territory of the spastic vessel has been shown, but such lesions do not invariably accompany the angiographic vasoconstriction.[13] Cerebral function apparently remains intact until blood flow is reduced to extremely low levels (18 ml per 100 gm of brain tissue per minute). At this level, rapid deterioration follows.[14] The poor correlation between infarction and angiographic spasm may be explained on this basis. Sections of the blood vessel wall sometimes show thickening and granulation tissue in the subintimal layers (Fig. 47–4).[12] The clinical picture of subintimal thickening associated with subarachnoid hemorrhage simulates that often ascribed to vasospasm. Platelet thrombi and emboli may also provoke vessel narrowing.[90]

As a clinical entity, vasospasm rarely occurs before two or three days after the initial hemorrhage. It usually begins toward the end of the first week and persists from one to four weeks. It has also been described as biphasic, occurring during the first few days and again a week or so later.[87] Interestingly, spasm has not been conclusively demonstrated in those angiograms in which rupture complicates the injection.[1] Severe bleeding episodes or multiple hemorrhages favor development of spasm. Elevated catecholamine levels in blood and urine, leukocytosis, and elevated ST segments and Q waves have all correlated positively with the presence of vasospasm.[49,89] The condition occurs in 80 per cent of patients in stupor, in 65 per cent of those with focal neurological deficits, and in 50 per cent of those with only confusion, but in only 14 per cent of the patients who are nearly normal postoperatively.[3] The radiographic and clinical event occurs rarely in conditions other than rupture of intracranial aneurysms. The mere presence of blood in contact with the cerebral vessel apparently does not provoke the clinical response. Perhaps bleeding within the wall of the artery is the prerequisite.

Often the number of adrenergic fibers adjacent to the aneurysm along the vessel wall appears deficient (Fig. 47–5). Catecholamines accumulate in the extraneuronal adventitia layer of the vessel.[22,61] Since the

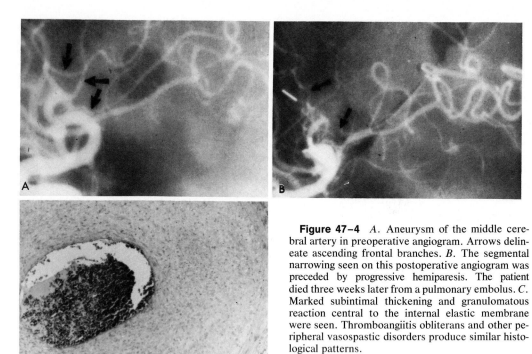

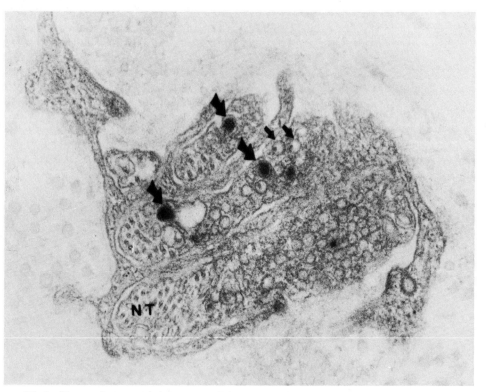

Figure 47–4 *A*. Aneurysm of the middle cerebral artery in preoperative angiogram. Arrows delineate ascending frontal branches. *B*. The segmental narrowing seen on this postoperative angiogram was preceded by progressive hemiparesis. The patient died three weeks later from a pulmonary embolus. *C*. Marked subintimal thickening and granulomatous reaction central to the internal elastic membrane were seen. Thromboangiitis obliterans and other peripheral vasospastic disorders produce similar histological patterns.

Figure 47–5 Biopsy of vasospastic human vessel shows extensive damage of the adrenergic axon with loss of transmitter from the synaptic vesicle (*small arrows*). Large dense core vesicles (*large arrows*) and neurotubulae (NT) are also shown. (Courtesy of Dr. Asa Klein.)

damaged adrenergic axons are unable to take up excess catecholamines, these transmitters may bind the receptor on the smooth muscle cell in a mechanism similar to that originally proposed by Cannon to describe denervation hypersensitivity.[10]

Vasoactive substances have been isolated from both the blood clots surrounding the spastic vessel and from the adjacent cerebrospinal fluid. Serotonin has great spasmogenic potential and it is readily available from platelets found either within the intravascular clot or in the clot of the adjacent subarachnoid space.[35,68] Prostaglandins ($F2_a$ and E2) are spasmogenic and produce prolonged vasoconstriction when injected cisternally. Prostaglandin $F2_a$ is also present in cerebrospinal fluid following subarachnoid hemorrhage.[68] Angiotensin, histamine, and other substances may also act as chemical mediators.[35] Agents from both fresh and aged blood have been shown to provoke constriction of the cerebral artery. Oxyhemoglobin has been identified in mixtures of blood and cerebrospinal fluid as the factor most essential in producing spasm.[91]

Thus, at present, one can only review the various mechanisms that may be responsible for the clinical state and the radiographic findings that occur after aneurysmal subarachnoid hemorrhage. It seems likely that more than one mechanism may be responsible. If a constricted vessel is seen at the time of an operation, vasospasm might be invoked as a causative mechanism. Angiographic narrowing of vessels, on the other hand, may be a result of vasospasm, platelet thrombi or emboli, or subintimal deposits within the artery wall. Perhaps these deposits also alter vascular wall elasticity.

There has been considerable discussion but lack of consensus about the treatment of vasospasm. Zervas and co-workers have noted that pretreatment with reserpine prevents vasospasm in animals subjected to experimental subarachnoid hemorrhage. Kanamycin, a nonabsorbable antibiotic found to be effective in preventing pulmonary arteriospasm, was combined with reserpine in a protocol for treating vasospasm in man.[91] In a controlled trial, this regimen apparently prevented clinical and radiographic spasm in a small number of patients.[90] In the author's experience, serotonin antagonism has not proved to be consistently effective, but it deserves further testing.

A large number of agents that either block the receptor site or act directly on the smooth muscle cell have found use in human vasospasm. Among the former, phenoxybenzamine and phentolamine have been used in human cases.[22] Overall, the results have been disappointing. Sodium nitroprusside, a smooth muscle relaxant, has produced only transient improvement. Sodium nitroprusside, xylocaine, dopamine, and papaverine have all been applied to both the external and internal surfaces of the spastic intracranial artery at the time of operative exposure. Papaverine, in lowest concentrations, produces the greatest dilatation, but even so, the effect is of short duration and not clinically significant.

Recent experimental evidence implicates cyclic AMP in the control of vascular smooth muscle. Either increased synthesis or decreased degradation of this compound produces smooth muscle dilatation. Salbutamol, currently not available in the United States, has been used to relieve experimental vasospasm. The effect is primarily mediated through stimulation of the cyclic AMP system. Flamm and Ransohoff have employed a beta-adrenergic agonist, isoproterenol, and aminophylline in the treatment of human vasospasm.[18] Both these agents are known to increase levels of cyclic AMP. Isoproterenol is infused at 125 mg per hour and aminophylline at 125 mg per hour for a period of up to two weeks. Nine patients improved and three remained unchanged on this regimen.[19] Others have also tested isoproterenol and aminophylline in the treatment of vasospasm and have observed a favorable response in about half of those who were treated.[79] If any benefit is derived from administration of hydrocortisone in large doses, it may be through the stimulation of the cyclic AMP system.[14]

For the present, one must conclude that there is no treatment that will produce uniform success. Although a number of agents are known to dilate the cerebral vessels and improve blood flow on a short-term basis, none has been able to overcome the constrictive force consistently on a long-term basis. In some cases, no doubt, subintimal deposits rather than true spasm of the arterial smooth muscle have produced the arterial narrowing.

Other Complications of Subarachnoid Hemorrhage

Obstructive hydrocephalus as a complication of subarachnoid hemorrhage has been recognized since 1928, when Bagley outlined the pathogenesis of this disorder.[5] The most common symptoms and signs associated with developing ventricular dilatation are headache, mental confusion, and worsening state of consciousness. Occasionally pyramidal tract signs are present, and convulsions have also been described. Signs usually appear within three to four weeks of the hemorrhage, but may be delayed until six months or longer. Bleeding from anterior communicating aneurysms, posterior communicating aneurysms, and basilar artery aneurysms is more likely to be causative. Middle cerebral aneurysms rarely produce the disorder. Multiple episodes of bleeding, rather than the total amount of blood, seems to correlate positively with hydrocephalus.

The mechanism by which blood produces hydrocephalus is yet not clear. Bradford and Sharkey noted that red blood cells block the avenues of escape of saline injected into the subarachnoid space.[9] Fibrous thickening of the leptomeninges and adhesions between the pia mater and arachnoid have also been found.

The diagnosis is easily established in the patient who fails to recover or who deteriorates following subarachnoid hemorrhage. Moderate elevation of cerebrospinal fluid pressure is found on spinal subarachnoid puncture. Pneumoencephalography or computed tomography confirms enlargement of the ventricular system. The condition may be managed by external ventricular drainage alone, repeated lumbar punctures, or shunting procedures. Dramatic improvement in neurological condition frequently follows shunting.

Both electrocardiographic and cardiovascular abnormalities may accompany subarachnoid hemorrhage. By and large, these are changes that accompany massive sympathetic discharge or epinephrine administration. In experimental intracranial hemorrhage, the myocardial necrosis has been averted by pretreatment with reserpine.

Using the enzyme dopamine beta-hydroxylase as a marker for sympathetic activity, Harden and associates found markedly elevated levels of the enzyme during the first week following hemorrhage.[29] Hypertension, glycosuria and intense sweating may also be present. In some patients, a sharp fall in dopamine beta-hydroxylase activity signals both chemical and clinical depletion of sympathetic transmitters. In these patients, during intense vasospasm, a paradoxical reaction of the pupil to cocaine and epinephrine occurs commonly. Normally, a drop or two of 1 per cent epinephrine produces little response when placed in the conjunctival sac. After subarachnoid hemorrhage, and particularly in those patients suffering vasospasm, maximum dilatation of the pupil may be observed, indicating hypersensitivity of the receptors to this transmitter. Management of transmitter depletion calls for minimizing external and internal stress as well as avoiding sympathetic toxins administered in the form of hypotensive therapy. Reduction of elevated intracranial pressure may also be beneficial.

Terson's syndrome (intravitreal hemorrhage), retinal, preretinal, or subhyaloid hemorrhages occur commonly in association with ruptured intracranial aneurysms.[36] Fahmy found 50 patients out of 154 (32.4 per cent) with recent subarachnoid bleeding to have intraocular hemorrhages also. In 21 cases these were bilateral. Few patients experience a complete recovery of vision following massive intravitreal hemorrhage, the scar persisting long after resolution of the blood clot. The mechanism has been a subject of controversy. There is no definite communication between the subarachnoid space and the vitreous cavity of the eye, and thus the hemorrhage must result from rupture of veins secondary to increased venous pressure. It usually occurs immediately or soon after subarachnoid hemorrhage, although delayed onset has also been observed.[17] Again, reduction in intracranial pressure seems to be the only satisfactory solution.

The syndrome of inappropriate antidiuretic hormone secretion (SIADH) has been recognized as a complication of subarachnoid hemorrhage caused principally by anterior communicating artery aneurysm.[34] The criteria for diagnosis of the syndrome are well defined and include: hyponatremia; normal hydration; serum and extracellular fluid hypo-osmolarity; urine osmolarity greater than serum osmolarity; and normal adrenal, renal, and hepatic function.

Expansion of fluid volume may also occur after subarachnoid hemorrhage because of decreased renal blood flow.

The syndrome of inappropriate antidiuretic hormone secretion associated with subarachnoid hemorrhage should be managed primarily through water deprivation. The total water intake from all sources should be limited to approximately 10 ml per kilogram of body weight, or 700 ml per 24 hours. Supplemental sodium is of little benefit. If hyponatremia (sodium less than 100 mEq per liter) threatens, however, more aggressive management prescribes the careful administration of 3 to 5 per cent saline. Solutions containing 200 mEq per liter of sodium may be administered in amounts of 10 ml per kilogram per 24 hours in severely hyponatremic patients. Fluid restriction, of course, must also be used.[34]

CONCLUSION

The ideal treatment of a patient with a recently ruptured aneurysm should be one that carries the lowest immediate risk in its application but one that, at the same time, provides effective long-term protection against rebleeding. An early interval of conservative treatment followed by later clipping of the aneurysm best satisfies these requirements. In the patient over 60 years of age, in the one ill with complicating medical disorders, and in the patient with a difficult or inaccessible aneurysm, nonoperative therapy may be the only reasonable alternative. Pregnancy, specific contraindications to a therapeutic program, and perhaps the patient's peace of mind are likewise factors to be considered in deciding on a nonoperative versus an operative plan. In the patient with hypertension or whose intracranial pressure remains elevated, an interval of nonoperative treatment allows improvement in the clinical condition and increases the opportunity for a successful operative outcome. The proper treatment of the grade I and II patient is less clear. It may be that the risk of interim rebleeding in these patients is higher than the operative mortality risks. An 8 to 10 per cent loss due to postoperative vasospasm must be accepted,

however, and unless the surgeon can carry out his goals with essentially no deaths or morbidity, he should postpone operation for 10 to 14 days following the hemorrhage until a safer interval is reached.

On the basis of present information, a program consisting of bed rest and carefully administered and monitored antifibrinolytic therapy offers the best protection against death from early rebleeding. It is unlikely that antifibrinolytic therapy alone offers any protection against late bleeding, and thus, this program should be combined with operative obliteration of the aneurysm sac. There are yet, however, a number of unanswered questions in relation to antifibrinolytic therapy. Will late vasospasm, hydrocephalus, deep vein thrombosis, or pulmonary embolism erase the benefits derived from preservation of the intra-aneurysmal clot? Do antifibrinolytic agents retard the normal fibrotic healing of the rent in the aneurysm wall? The answer to these questions should be forthcoming as cases accumulate.

When subarachnoid hemorrhage results from an arteriovenous malformation, rebleeding occurs less frequently than with aneurysms. A short interval of bed rest and other supportive measures should be effective in preventing recurrences. In subarachnoid hemorrhage from undefined causes, any treatment program must be extremely safe and effective to improve upon the natural history of the disorder. After completion of the diagnostic work-up, including repeat angiography, discharge arrangements can be safely made in these cases.

The answer to the problem of the diagnosis, pathogenesis, and treatment of vasospasm can be summarized quite simply: there is none. The neurosurgeon speaks of vasospasm as if it were the single entity responsible for all preoperative and postoperative failures, while the pathologist finds no basis for discussion except, sometimes, in the case of distal infarction. Subintimal thickening, thrombi, and emboli are more frequently recognized. When the patient's condition deteriorates following subarachnoid hemorrhage, or when he fares poorly after aneurysmorrhaphy, the surgeon should always look for correctible causes first. Water retention, inappropriate antidiuretic hormone secretion, transmitter depletion, hydrocephalus, cerebral edema, and the hidden clot must be excluded before a less than favorable outcome is accepted on the basis of an indefinite angiographic finding.

REFERENCES

1. Allcock, J. M., and Drake, C. G.: Ruptured I-C aneurysm—the role of arterial spasm. J. Neurosurg., *22*:21–29, 1965.
2. Allen, G. S., Henderson, L. M., Chou, S. N., and French, L. A.: Cerebral arterial spasm. 1. In vitro contractile activity of vasoactive agents on canine basilar and middle cerebral arteries. J. Neurosurg., *40*:433–441, 1974.
3. Antunes, J. L., and Correll, J. W.: Cerebral emboli from intracranial aneurysms. Surg. Neurol., *6*:7–10, 1976.
4. Ask-Upmark, E.: A follow-up examination of 138 cases of subarachnoid hemorrhage. Acta Med. Scand., *138*:15–31, 1950.
5. Bagley, C., Jr.: Blood in the cerebrospinal fluid. Resultant functional and organic alterations in the central nervous system. A. Experimental data. Arch. Surg., *17*:18–38, 1928.
6. Björkesten, G. af, and Troupp, H.: Prognosis of subarachnoid hemorrhage. A comparison between patients with verified aneurysms and patients with normal angiograms. J. Neurosurg., *14*:434–441, 1957.
7. Botterell, E. H., Lougheed, W. M., Morley, T. P., and Vandewater, S. L.: Hypothermia in the surgical treatment of ruptured intracranial aneurysms. J. Neurosurg., *15*:4–18, 1958.
8. Botterell, E. H., Lougheed, W. M., Scott, J. W., and Vandewater, S. L.: Hypothermia, and interruption of carotid, or carotid and vertebral circulation, in the surgical management of intracranial aneurysms. J. Neurosurg., *13*:1–42, 1956.
9. Bradford, F. K., and Sharkey, P. C.: Physiologic effects from the introduction of blood and other substances into the subarachnoid space of dogs. J. Neurosurg., *19*:1017–1022, 1962.
10. Cannon, W. B., and Rosenblith, A.: Autonomic Neuro-Effector System. New York, Macmillan, 1937, p. 229.
11. Ciongoli, A. K., and Poser, C. M.: Pulmonary edema secondary to subarachnoid hemorrhage. Neurology (Minneap.), *22*:867–870, 1972.
12. Conway, L. W., and McDonald, L. W.: Structural changes of the intradural arteries following subarachnoid hemorrhage. J. Neurosurg., *37*:715–723, 1972.
13. Crompton, M. R.: Cerebral infarction following the rupture of cerebral berry aneurysms. Brain, *87*:263–280, 1974.
14. Cruickshank, J. M., Neil-Dwyer, G., and Brice, J.: Electrocardiographic changes and their prognostic significance in subarachnoid hemorrhage. J. Neurol. Neurosurg. Psychiat., *37*:755–759, 1974.
15. Dandy, W. E.: Intracranial aneurysm of the internal carotid artery. Ann. Surg., *107*:654–659, 1938.
16. Estanol, B. V., Loyo, M., Mateos, H., Foyo, E., Cornejo, A., and Guevara, J.: Cardiac arrhythmias in experimental subarachnoid hemorrhage. Stroke, *8*:440–447, 1977.
17. Fahmy, J. A.: Vitreous hemorrhage in subarachnoid hemorrhage–Terson's syndrome. Acta Ophthal., *50*:137, 1972.
18. Flamm, E. S., and Ransohoff, J.: Treatment of cerebral vasospasm by control of cyclic adenosine monophosphate. Surg. Neurol., *6*:223–226, 1976.
19. Fleischer, A. A., Raggio, J. F., and Tindall, G. T.: Aminophylline and isoproterenol in the treatment of cerebral vasospasm. Surg. Neurol., *8*:117–119, 1977.
20. Fodstad, H., and Thulin, C.-A.: Use of tranexamic acid (AMCA) in the preoperative management of patients with ruptured intracranial aneurysms. Unpublished data presented to Sixth International Congress of Neurological Surgery, São Paulo, Brazil, 1977.
21. Forster, D. M. C., Steiner, L., and Håkanson, S.: Arteriovenous malformations of the brain. A long-term clinical study. J. Neurosurg., *37*:562–570, 1972.
22. Fraser, R. A., Stein, B. M., and Barrett, R. E.: Noradrenergic mediation of experimental cerebrovascular spasm. Stroke, *1*:356–362, 1970.
23. Gamble, J. E., and Patton, M. D.: Pulmonary edema and hemorrhage from preoptic lesions in rats. Amer. J. Physiol., *172*:623–631, 1953.
24. Geronemus, R., Herz, D., and Shulman, K.: Streptokinase clot lysis time in patients with ruptured intracranial aneurysms. J. Neurosurg., *40*:499–503, 1974.
25. Graf, C. J., and Nibbelink, D. W.: Cooperative study of intracranial aneurysms and subarachnoid hemorrhage: Report on a randomized treatment and study: III. Intracranial surgery. Stroke, *5*:557–601, 1974.
26. Haerer, A. F., and Smith, R. R.: Medical and surgical experiences in patients of a large southern stroke center. South. Med. J., *67*:667–671, 1974.
27. Hamby, W. B.: Spontaneous subarachnoid hemorrhage of aneurysmal origin. J.A.M.A., *136*:522–528, 1948.
28. Hammer, W. J., Luessenhop, A. J., and Weintraub, A. M.: Observations on the electrocardiographic changes associated with subarachnoid, hemorrhage with special reference to their genesis. Amer. J. Med., *59*:427–433, 1975.
29. Harden, T. K., Klein, R. L., Smith, R. R., Thureson-Klein, A. T., and Lowry, M. W.: Serum dopamine β-hydroxylase activity following subarachnoid hemorrhage in man. Med. Biol., *53*:100–106, 1975.
30. Hayward, R. D., and O'Reilly, G. V. A.: Intracerebral haemorrhage. Accuracy of computerised transverse axial scanning in predicting the underlying aetiology. Lancet, *1*:1–4, 1976.
31. Hook, O.: Subarachnoid haemorrhage. Prognosis when angiography reveals no aneurysm. A report of 138 cases. Acta Med. Scand., *162*:493–503, 1958.
32. Hunt, W. E., and Hess, R. M.: Surgical risk as related to time of intervention in the repair of intracranial aneurysms. J. Neurosurg., *28*:14–20, 1968.
33. Hunt, W. E., and Kosnik, E. J.: Timing and peri-

operative care in intracranial aneurysm surgery. Clin. Neurosurg., *21*:79–89, 1974.

34. Imbeau, S. A., and Rock, W.: Syndrome of inappropriate antidiuretic hormone secretion (SIADH) with subarachnoid hemorrhage. Wisconsin Med. J., *75*:25–28, 1976.

35. Ishii, S., Chigasaki, H., Miyaoka, M., and Nonaka, T.: Experimental and clinical studies on prolonged cerebral vasospasm following SAH. Sixth International Congress of Neurological Surgery, São Paulo, Brazil, 19–25 June, 1977. (R. Carrea, ed., Buenos Aires.)

36. Khan, S. G., and Frenkel, M.: Intravitreal hemorrhage associated with rapid increase in intracranial pressure (Terson's syndrome). Amer. J. Ophthal., *80*:37–43, 1975.

37. Klafta, L. A., Jr.: Intracranial aneurysms factors affecting survival—Part II. Med. Trial Techn. Quart., *17*:392–399, 1971.

38. Knight, M. T. N., Dawson, R., and Melrose, D. G.: Fibrinolytic response to surgery. Labile and stable patterns and their relevance to postoperative deep venous thrombosis. Lancet, *2*:370–373, 1977.

39. Krayenbuhl, H. A., Yasargil, M. G., Flamm, E. S., and Tew, J. M., Jr.: Microsurgical treatment of intracranial saccular aneurysms. J. Neurosurg., *37*:678–686, 1972.

40. Kushner, J., and Alexander, E., Jr.: Partial spontaneous regressive arteriovenous malformation Case report with angiographic evidence. J. Neurosurg., *32*:360–366, 1970.

41. Levy, L. F.: Subarachnoid hemorrhage without arteriographic vascular abnormality. J. Neurosurg., *17*:252–258, 1960.

42. Lundberg, N., Kjallquist, A., Kullberg, G., Ponten, U., and Sungbarg, G.: Non-operative management of intracranial hypertension. *In* Krayenbuhl. H., ed.: Advances and Technical Standards in Neurosurgery, Vol. 1. New York, Springer-Verlag, 1974, pp. 1–193.

43. McKissock, W., Paine, K. W. E., and Walsh, L. S.: An analysis of the results of treatment of ruptured intracranial aneurysms. J. Neurosurg., *17*:762–776, 1960.

44. McNair, J. L., Clower, B. B., and Sanford, R. A.: The effect of reserpine pretreatment on myocardial damage associated with simulated intracranial hemorrhage in mice. Europ. Psychiat., *234*:320–331, 1969, Ch. 16.

45. Moody, R. A., and Poppen, J. L.: Arteriovenous malformations. J. Neurosurg., *32*:503–511, 1970.

46. Mullan, S.: Conservative management of the recently ruptured aneurysm. Surg. Neurol., *3*:27–32, 1975.

47. Mullan, S., and Dawley, J.: Antifibrinolytic therapy for intracranial aneurysms. J. Neurosurg., *28*:21–23, 1968.

48. Mullan, S., Bechman, F., Vailati, G., Karasick, J., and Dobben, G.: An experimental approach to the problem of cerebral aneurysm. J. Neurosurg., *21*:838–845, 1964.

49. Neil-Dwyer, G., and Cruickshank, J.: The blood leukocyte count and its prognostic significance in subarachnoid haemorrhage. Brain, *97*:79–86, 1974.

50. Nibbelink, D. W.: Cooperative aneurysm study: antihypertensive and antifibrinolytic therapy

following subarachnoid hemorrhage from ruptured intracranial aneurysm. Ninth Princeton Conference, January, 1974, Princeton, New Jersey. Reprinted from Whisnant, J. P., and Sandok, B. A., eds.: Cerebral Vascular Diseases. New York, Grune & Stratton, Inc., 1975.

51. Nibbelink, D. W., and Sahs, A. L.: Antifibrinolytic therapy and drug-induced hypotension in treatment of ruptured intracranial aneurysms. Trans. Amer. Neurol. Ass., *97*:145–148, 1972.

52. Nibbelink, D. W., and Torner, J. C.: Intracranial aneurysms and subarachnoid hemorrhage. A cooperative study. Antifibrinolytic therapy in recent onset subarachnoid hemorrhage. Stroke, *6*:622–628, 1975.

53. Nibbelink, D. W., Torner, J. C., and Henderson, W. G.: Intracranial aneurysms and subarachnoid hemorrhage—report on a randomized treatment study. Stroke, *8*:202–218, 1977.

54. Noel, G. L.: How to recognize and treat the inappropriate ADH syndrome. Med. Times, *103*: 119–124, 1975.

55. Nornes, H.: Monitoring of patients with intracranial aneurysms. Clin. Neurosurg., *22*:321–331, 1975.

56. Nornes, H.: The role of intracranial pressure in the arrest of hemorrhage in patients with ruptured intracranial aneurysm. J. Neurosurg., *39*:226–233, 1973.

57. Norris, J. W., and Hachinski, V. C.: Intensive care management of stroke patients. Stroke, *7*:573–577, 1976.

58. Norwood, C. H., Poole, G. J., and Moody, D.: Treatment of delayed cerebral arterial spasm in rhesus monkeys following SAH. Program abstract of the AANS meeting, Miami, 1975, p. 22.

59. Pakarinen, S.: Incidence, aetiology, and prognosis of primary subarachnoid haemorrhage. A study based on 589 cases diagnosed in a defined urban population during a defined period. Acta Neurol. Scand., Suppl. 29: 43, 1967.

60. Paterson, J. H., and McKissock, W.: A clinical survey of intracranial angiomas with special reference to their mode of progression and surgical treatment. A report of 110 cases. Brain, *79*:233–266, 1956.

61. Peerless, S. J., and Kendall, M. J.: Experimental cerebral vasospasm. *In* Whisnant, J. P., and Sandok, B. A., eds.: Cerebral Vascular Disease. Proceedings of the Ninth Princeton Conference, New York, Grune & Stratton, Inc., 1975, pp. 49–58.

62. Perret, G., and Nishioka, H.: Report on the cooperative study of Intracranial aneurysms and subarachnoid hemorrhage. Section VI. Arteriovenous malformations, J. Neurosurg., *25*: 467–490, 1966.

63. Pool, J. L.: Cerebral vasospasm. New Eng. J. Med., *259*:1259–1264, 1958.

64. Pool, J. L.: Excision of cerebral arteriovenous malformations. J. Neurosurg., *29*:312–321, 1968.

65. Potter, J. M.: Angiomatous malformations of the brain: Their nature and prognosis. Ann. Roy. Coll. Surg. Eng., *16*:227–243, 1955.

66. Raimondi, A. J., and Torres, H.: Acute hydrocephalus as a complication of subarachnoid hemorrhage. Surg. Neurol., *1*:23–26, 1973.

67. Richardson, A. E., Jane, J. A., and Payne, P. M.:

Assessment of the natural history of anterior communicating aneurysms. J. Neurosurg., *25*:266–274, 1966.

68. Robertson, E. G.: Cerebral lesions due to intracranial aneurysms. Brain, *72*:100–185, 1949.

69. Sahs, A., Perett, G. E., Lochslen, H. B., and Nishioka, H.: Intracranial Aneurysm and Subarachnoid Hemorrhage. Philadelphia, J. B. Lippincott & Co., 1969.

70. Saito, I., Ueda, Y., and Sano, K.: Treatment of ruptured cerebral aneurysms in the acute stage. Sixth International Congress of Neurological Surgery, São Paulo, Brazil, 19–25 June, 1977. (E. R. Carrea, ed., Buenos Aires.)

71. Shulman, K., Martin, B. F., Popoff, N., and Ransohoff, J.: Recognition and treatment of hydrocephalus following spontaneous subarachnoid hemorrhage. J. Neurosurg., *20*:1040–1049, 1963.

72. Shuster, S.: The electrocardiogram in subarachnoid hemorrhage. Brit. Heart J., *22*:316, 1960.

73. Slosberg, P. S.: Treatment of ruptured aneurysms with induced hypotension. *In* Fields, W. S., and Sahs, A. L., eds.: Intracranial Aneurysms and Subarachnoid Hemorrhage. Springfield, Ill., Charles C Thomas, 1965, pp. 221–236.

74. Slosberg, P. S.: Treatment of ruptured intracranial aneurysms by induced hypotension. J. Mount Sinai Hosp. N.Y., *40*:82–90, 1973.

75. Smith, R. R.: Unpublished data.

76. Smith, R. R.: Unpublished data presented at American Association of Neurological Surgery in San Francisco, Cal., 1975.

77. Smith, R. R., and Upchurch, J. J.: Monitoring antifibrinolytic therapy in subarachnoid hemorrhage. J. Neurosurg., *38*:339–344, 1973.

78. Sonntag, V. K. H., and Stein, B. M.: Arteriopathic complications during treatment of subarachnoid hemorrhage with epsilon-aminocaproic acid. J. Neurosurg., *40*:480–484, 1974.

79. Sundt, T. M., Jr.: Clinical management of cerebral vasospasm. *In* Whisnant, J. P., and Sandok, B. A., eds.: Cerebral Vascular Disease, Proceedings of the Ninth Princeton Conference, 1974. New York, Grune & Stratton, 1975, pp. 77–81.

80. Svien, H., and McRae, J. A. M.: Arteriovenous anomalies of the brain. J. Neurosurg., *23*:23–28, 1965.

81. Troupp, H.: Arteriovenous malformations of the brain: Prognosis without operation. Acta Neurol. Scand., *41*:39–42, 1965.

82. Troupp, H., and Björkesten, G. af: Results of a controlled trial of late surgical versus conservative treatment of intracranial arterial aneurysms. J. Neurosurg., *35*:20–24, 1971.

83. Walsh, L.: Experience in the conservative and surgical treatment of ruptured intracranial aneurysms. Res. Publ. Ass. Res. Nerv. Ment. Dis., *41*:169–179, 1966.

84. Walsh, L. S.: Trials of treatment of intracranial aneurysms. Psychiat. Neurol. Neurochir., *75*:437–440, 1972.

85. Warlow, C., Ogston, D., and Douglas, A. S.: Venous thrombosis following strokes. Lancet, *1*:1305–1306, 1972.

86. Wechsler, I. S.: Discussion of Dr. Wallace B. Hamby's article: Spontaneous subarachnoid hemorrhage of aneurysmal origin. J.A.M.A., *136*:522–528, 1948.

87. Welch, K. M. A., Hashi, K., and Meyer, J. S.: Reconsideration of the role of serotonin in subarachnoid haemorrhage. Proc. Aust. Ass. Neurol., *9*:155–164, 1973.

88. White, R. P., Hagen, A. A., Morgan, H., Dawson, W. N., and Robertson, J. T.: Experimental study on the genesis of cerebral vasospasm. Stroke, *6*:52–57, 1975.

89. Wilkins, R. H.: Aneurysm rupture during angiography: Does acute vasospasm occur? Surg. Neurol., *5*:299–303, 1976.

90. Zervas, N. T.: Prevention of ischemic infarction following rupture of intracranial aneurysms. Trans. Amer. Neurol. Ass., *102*:25–28, 1977.

91. Zervas, N. T., Hori, H., and Rosoff, C. B.: Experimental inhibition of serotonin by antibiotic: Prevention of cerebral vasospasm. J. Neurosurg., *41*:59–62, 1974.

48

MANAGEMENT OF ANEURYSMS OF ANTERIOR CIRCULATION BY INTRACRANIAL PROCEDURES

While both intracranial aneurysms and subarachnoid hemorrhage have been recognized for centuries, it has been only in the last 50 years that cerebral aneurysm has been recognized as the most common cause of spontaneous subarachnoid hemorrhage.[70,108,116] The introduction of cerebral angiography by Moniz in 1927 allowed a diagnosis of cerebral aneurysm to be made in living patients who had sustained subarachnoid hemorrhage.[69] By 1933 Dott could report clinical and angiographic findings in eight patients and operative treatment in two of them.[14] Subsequently, series presented by Krayenbühl in 1941 and Dandy in 1944 showed that aneurysms could be operatively treated, but not without considerable morbidity and mortality at that time.[11,48] By the early 1950's, an increasing number of neurosurgeons had begun to address themselves to the problems of ruptured intracranial aneurysm.[31,64,77,115] Three important concepts emerged during that time: (1) In most cases operation was of value in the prevention of rebleeding and offered little benefit to the course of the initial hemorrhage. (2) Significantly better operative results were obtained if operation was delayed two to three weeks after subarachnoid hemorrhage and the patient was in good preoperative condition. (3) The natural history of ruptured cerebral aneurysm was inadequately delineated, and apparent success of operation might simply represent favorable case selection. The episodic nature of the disease, the extended period of risk, and the multiple variables involved have delayed a final answer to this third problem. In the years it has taken to accrue valid statistical information, however, technical advancements have produced a significant reduction in the morbidity and deaths resulting from operative treatment.

The natural history of ruptured cerebral aneurysm has been most frequently analyzed in terms of gross mortality rates. While many factors enter into this type of mortality figure, a reasonable synthesis of various reports gives a 25 per cent mortality rate at one week, a 50 per cent rate at two months, and a 70 per cent rate at five years.[7,56,80] The clearest conclusion that can be drawn is that the mortality rate is highest in the first week and drops off exponentially over a period of years. Gross mortality figures, however, include both those patients who died as a result of the initial hemorrhage and those who had recurrent hemorrhage. Unless a life-threatening hematoma is present, only those who will sustain recurrent hemorrhage can be expected to benefit from operation. Analyzing the data of the Cooperative Study, Locksley determined a rebleeding rate of 10 per cent the first week, 12 per cent the second week, 7 per cent the third week, 8 per cent the fourth week, and 14 per cent between 5 and 12 weeks.[56] Death from a second hemorrhage occurred in from 41 to 46 per cent depending on the site of the aneurysm. Pakarinen determined the cumulative mortality rate from recurrence of hemorrhage as 24 per cent at one month, 34 per cent at two months, and 38 per cent at one year.[80] While some studies have suggested a very low rate of recurrence after six months, Winn and associates reported a rebleeding rate of 19 to 31 per cent after six months for a group of patients randomly allocated to nonoperative treatment and followed for up to 20 years.[112,117] The differences in the percentages of rebleeding reported in this series depended on the criterion used to determine that the patients had suffered a recurrent hemorrhage. Mortality rates in this group were not stated; only the fact that the main cause of death was a recurrent subarachnoid hemorrhage.

Like the mortality figures, the long-term morbidity of patients sustaining subarachnoid hemorrhage is an important parameter in testing the value of operative treatment. Locksley reported that 74 per cent of patients who were not operated on and who survived one year were able to return to work, 17 per cent were capable of lesser work or at least self care, and 9 per cent were unable to work and required nursing care. Morbidity correlated primarily with the patient's condition at the original hospital admission.[56] Pakarinen found 72 per cent of one-year survivors well, 11 per cent partially disabled, 11 per cent totally disabled, and 6 per cent disabled from unrelated cause.[80]

The foregoing statistics provide a background against which to evaluate the efficacy of operative efforts. This chapter deals with the preoperative evaluation of a patient with subarachnoid hemorrhage as it relates to operative treatment and present operative methods and adjuncts to operation employed in intracranial procedures on aneurysms of the anterior circulation, and evaluates results and complications of intracranial aneurysm operations.

CLINICAL PRESENTATION

Patients who suffer rupture of an intracranial aneurysm present a spectrum of signs and symptoms related to the nature and severity of bleeding. The characteristic presentation is that of subarachnoid hemorrhage: sudden onset of severe headache, temporary clouding of consciousness, nausea and vomiting, meningismus, and transient focal neurological deficits. Oculomotor nerve deficits are common when the aneurysm is in the vicinity of the third cranial nerve. Milder bleeding episodes may be accompanied by only moderate headache and neck stiffness suggesting viral, musculoskeletal, or migrainous headache. A high index of suspicion and readiness of the physician to perform lumbar puncture may allow a patient to receive adequate treatment before subsequent hemorrhage cripples or kills him.[25] At the other end of the spectrum, an initial hemorrhage may result in coma and severe focal neurological deficit such that hypertensive intracerebral hemorrhage or cerebrovascular thrombosis is suspected. When rupture of an aneurysm results in a fall or an accident, the patient's clinical picture may be ascribed to trauma.

In order to establish guidelines for operation and to bring some uniformity to patient analysis it has been customary to grade patients preoperatively. Grading is meant both to describe a patient's clinical condition and to be of prognostic significance. The authors have used the grading system of Botterell as revised by Lougheed and Marshall, which emphasizes the patient's level of consciousness:[10,59]

Grade I—alert and oriented.

Grade II—awake, but with headache, meningismus, or minor neurological deficit.

Grade III—drowsy or confused, with or without neurological deficit.

Grade IV—semicomatose, responding only to pain, with or without focal neurological deficit.

Grade V—comatose, reflex responses, failing vital signs.

Hunt and Hess presented a similar grading system but placed considerable emphasis on headache and nuchal rigidity.[39] Age and associated disease increase both operative and nonoperative risk.

In most cases, a patient's grade will be the result of the injury of the hemorrhage itself, and only supportive measures will be indicated for patients in grades IV and V. Some patients, however, will present in poor condition because of complications of aneurysm rupture, and in these more active intervention may be beneficial. Hydrocephalus may be acute, occurring within hours of subarachnoid hemorrhage, or it may develop over days to weeks while a patient is recovering from the initial ictus.* Shunting or ventriculostomy can produce significant clinical improvement and bring a patient to an acceptable preoperative grade.[51,89] Intracerebral and subdural hematoma when associated with appreciable mass effect are also indications for early operative intervention in poorer grade patients.

RADIOLOGICAL INVESTIGATION

Angiography

Following confirmation of subarachnoid hemorrhage by lumbar puncture, cerebral angiography is necessary to determine the presence and location of an aneurysm. This study is best executed by percutaneous transfemoral catheterization of the carotid and vertebral arteries to allow full visualization of the cerebral circulation. Complete cerebral angiography provides the following information:

(1) *Definition of the aneurysm.* The presence, location, size, and configuration of an aneurysm, and its relationship to adjacent arteries, are evaluated by filming the lesion in at least two views. Stereoscopic views, magnification, subtraction, and angiotomography may be helpful in further delineating the aneurysm. The presence of thrombus within the aneurysm may mislead the surgeon as to the true size and shape of the lesion. Arteriovenous malformation or vascular tumor may be found to be the cause of the subarachnoid hemorrhage.

(2) *Multiple aneurysms.* Multiple aneurysms are reported to be present in from 15 to 33 per cent of cases.† Angiographic evidence that suggests which lesion has bled includes the larger aneurysm, the presence of localized mass effect, the presence of localized spasm, and the presence of secondary loculations on an aneurysm.[5]

(3) *Cerebrovascular degenerative changes.* Atherosclerosis, elongation, tortuosity, and

stenosis of cerebral vessels increase technical difficulty at the time of operation and are associated with greater morbidity and more deaths from cerebral infarction.

(4) *Collateral circulation.* The considerable variability in portions of the circle of Willis has been noted frequently.[49,91] Compression of the opposite carotid artery during angiography provides some indication of the adequacy of the circle of Willis as a collateral channel and the safety of occluding a vessel if this becomes necessary during an operation. This information is especially helpful in deciding the treatment of aneurysms of the anterior communicating and proximal internal carotid arteries. Preoperative vessel occlusion may also be demonstrated.

(5) *Congenital anomalies.* Anomalies of cerebral vasculature are commonly associated with saccular aneurysms and may disorient the operator during the dissection.[90,104] Patterns of anomalies are discussed later when operative technique at specific aneurysm sites is considered.

(6) *Hydrocephalus.* Hydrocephalus may be suspected angiographically when stretching and elevation of the pericallosal arteries, lateral displacement of the middle cerebral and lenticulostriate arteries, and widening of the subependymal veins are seen.

(7) *Cerebrovascular spasm.* Narrowing of the intraluminal diameter of cerebral arteries is seen frequently in association with subarachnoid hemorrhage from ruptured intracranial aneurysms and has been considered to represent spasm of the affected arteries. When Ecker and Riemenschneider described angiographic spasm and its occurrence with a ruptured cerebral aneurysm in 1951, a logical cause for the cerebral infarction and clinical deterioration seen in patients with subarachnoid hemorrhage seemed at hand.[18] Nevertheless, 25 years of intensive research has raised more questions than it has answered concerning the basic problems of etiology, significance, prevention, and treatment of vasospasm.

Many neurosurgeons have believed that spasm is a protective reaction of the vessel. A report of the Cooperative Study of Intracranial Aneurysms and Subarachnoid Hemorrhage has shown, however, that of a group of 242 patients in which 36

* See references 19, 21, 89, 100, 122.
† See references 36, 49, 56, 66, 86.

per cent showed local or diffuse vasospasm and 64 per cent showed no vasospasm, 20 per cent of the group with vasospasm and 11 per cent of the group without vasospasm rebled.[27] Several reports have found some relationship between angiographic vasospasm and cerebral infarction, especially when spasm is severe.[6,93] The Cooperative Study found a consistent correlation between the presence of vasospasm and the neurological condition.[27] However, a report of 198 patients of whom 41 per cent showed vasospasm revealed a slightly higher incidence of neurological abnormalities in those patients who did not demonstrate vasospasm.[68] Significant disparity between angiographic spasm and regional cerebral blood flow has been demonstrated.[8,44,123] Norlén and Olivecrona, Pool and Potts, and Allcock and Drake among others have reported that the presence of angiographic vasospasm increased operative mortality rates.[6,77,84] On the other hand, Graf and Nibbelink give operative mortality rates of 39 per cent for patients without vasospasm, 37 per cent for patients with localized vasospasm, and 29 per cent for patients with diffuse vasospasm.[27] Millikan showed the same mortality rate, 19 to 20 per cent, for cases operated on, with or without vasospasm.[68] It is apparent that the significance of angiographically demonstrated vasospasm has not been determined conclusively, but on the basis of the foregoing evidence and personal experience, it is the opinion of the authors that operative treatment should not be withheld from an alert patient pending disappearance of vasospasm shown by angiography.

It is customary to perform angiography soon after the diagnosis of subarachnoid hemorrhage is made, even in those patients who are in poor condition. The study gives a more definitive diagnosis and helps to determine the presence of a hematoma or hydrocephalus. It has not been believed that angiography contributes adversely to the course of patients with ruptured cerebral aneurysms, although concern about this question still remains.[55,109] Relative contraindications to cerebral angiography include cardiac, pulmonary, or renal insufficiency; allergy; and thrombophlebitis. Computed tomography has somewhat altered the requirement for early angiography in critically ill patients.

Computed Tomography

Computed tomography is useful in many cases of ruptured cerebral aneurysm. It demonstrates hematomas in the subdural and subarachnoid spaces as well as intracerebrally and within the ventricle, shifts of the ventricular system, areas of infarction, and hydrocephalus.[88] Intraventricular hematoma has been shown to be common in cases of ruptured aneurysm. At times an aneurysm will be demonstrated by enhancement of the scan with intravenous contrast medium, and occasionally a significant thrombus within the aneurysm will be shown. In cases of multiple aneurysms, the one that bled may be identified by localized hematoma or infarction.

When computed tomography is available, it is preferable to utilize this modality first with patients who are semicomatose or moribund. If an operable hematoma or hydrocephalus is not found, angiography can be delayed until the patient is in more satisfactory condition. If, on the basis of computed tomography, an operation is contemplated, however, angiography will be required for localization of the aneurysm.

TIMING OF OPERATION

The single most important factor in determining the outcome of an aneurysm operation is the patient's preoperative clinical condition. In general, patients in grades I and II are suitable operative candidates and can undergo operation with acceptable morbidity and mortality risks. Patients in grade III usually are given time to become more alert, although if they are in stable condition or beginning to improve, operation may be deemed advisable, especially if a week or more has elapsed since their hemorrhage. Patients in grades IV and V should usually receive supportive care until they have made some recovery. Operation on these patients carries a high mortality rate, as a damaged brain may sustain further insult at operation. As previously stated, patients who are in poor condition but demonstrate intracranial hematomas with mass effect or hydrocephalus may be operated upon primarily for correction of these problems with treatment of the aneurysm if it can be easily and safely accomplished. Although success is quite limited in these cases, some good results have been obtained, as is discussed later.

For reasons that are as yet unclear, patients undergoing operation within the first week following subarachnoid hemorrhage have been noted by many neurosurgeons to fare worse than those whose operations are delayed one to two weeks.[15,26,77] These surgeons therefore recommend delay of operation in all patients regardless of their grade. Recurrent bleeding has been noted in 11 per cent of cases during this time period, with about half of these recurrent hemorrhages being fatal.[56] The use of epsilon-aminocaproic acid to lower this rate of rebleeding seems, however, to have met with some success.[73,74,76,111] Suzuki has noted that a good outcome can be anticipated in alert patients undergoing operation within two days, but that when operations are performed between two and seven days after hemorrhage, morbidity and mortality rates are increased.[107] While, because of the characteristics of the referral system, a majority of patients seen at the University of Zurich undergo operation after two weeks, a substantial number of cases have been treated within the first week. It is the policy of the senior author that alert patients (grades I and II) undergo operation at the earliest possible time compatible with adequate operating and anesthesia facilities. Nevertheless, the experience of the neurosurgeon and anesthesiologist and the competence of the operating room staff must be considered before one embarks on an operation in a more critical period.

A further problem, as discussed earlier, is that of cerebral vasospasm. While many neurosurgeons recommend delay of operation until vasospasm has cleared, as demonstrated by angiography, it has not been the experience of the senior author that vasospasm correlates well with the patient's clinical status or increases the risk at operation. Meticulous technique and minimal brain retraction are believed to reduce the incidence of postoperative deterioration sometimes attributed to vasospasm.

Finally, a variety of other factors may influence the timing of operation. Elevated cerebrospinal fluid pressure has been used as a contraindication.[33,47] Lability of blood pressure, associated medical problems, and the patient's willingness to have the operation all contribute to the time interval between subarachnoid hemorrhage and operative treatment.

ADJUNCTS TO OPERATION

Anesthesia

Thiopental (Pentothal) anesthesia, generalized paralysis, and topical anesthesia of the vocal cords are used during intubation to allow a smooth induction of general anesthesia without patient excitement and swings in blood pressure and pulse rate. Inhalation anesthesia is most frequently used during the operative procedure. Halothane has the beneficial effect of increasing cerebral blood flow in cases in which adequate regional blood flow may be compromised by the effects of subarachnoid hemorrhage.[63] This increase in blood flow, however, is accompanied by a corresponding increase in intracranial volume and presents some danger when intracranial pressure is increased.[42] Methods for reduction of intracranial volume are discussed later. Controlled ventilation is recommended so that the anesthesiologist can regulate the arterial carbon dioxide tension for cerebral blood volume and the intrathoracic pressure for cerebral venous drainage. An electrocardiograph, radial artery catheter to measure arterial blood pressure, central venous catheter, and urinary catheter are used routinely. A lumbar subarachnoid catheter may be placed for intermittent cerebrospinal fluid drainage.

Reduction of Intracranial Volume

Drainage of spinal fluid by lumbar puncture has been employed for many years as a method of creating operating space. A flexible catheter left in the lumbar subarachnoid space during operation permits the surgeon to drain additional cerebrospinal fluid at his discretion. Significant drainage of cerebrospinal fluid occurs during dissection of the basal subarachnoid cisterns, and for a period of time lumbar puncture was dispensed with to save additional manipulation of the patient and from fear that the subarachnoid cisterns might collapse, hampering precise dissection. More recently lumbar puncture has again been employed to drain 15 to 20 ml of cerebrospinal fluid just prior to beginning the operation. This drainage facilitates epidural retraction of the brain during removal of bone from the sphenoid ridge and does not result in alterations of the basal subarachnoid space. Ventriculostomy is a rarely required option for additional removal of fluid.

Hyperventilation is a safe and effective method for reduction of cerebral blood volume and affects to a considerable degree the increase in blood volume associated with halothane anesthesia.[118] The arterial partial pressure of carbon dioxide should be held at 25 to 30 mm of mercury, as lower values may lead to excessive vasoconstriction.[2]

Dehydrating agents frequently employed include urea, mannitol, and furosemide. Urea readily crosses the blood-brain barrier and may lead to significant "rebound" swelling. Graf and Nibbelink found an increased mortality rate associated with the use of urea as compared with other agents.[27] The relative merits of mannitol versus furosemide are debatable, and both seem to provide a prompt diuresis and reduction in brain size. It is the author's practice to give 20 to 40 gm of mannitol intravenously prior to the skin incision, while some surgeons prefer to give mannitol only in those cases in which the dura is especially tense. Corticosteroids such as dexamethasone and methylprednisolone are almost universally given pre- and postoperatively to prevent cerebral edema, although their beneficial effect in cases of subarachnoid hemorrhage has not been clearly documented.[13,22]

Intraoperative Hypotension

Induced hypotension minimizes the risk of premature rupture of the aneurysm and facilitates dissection and clip placement by reducing the turgor of the lesion. The authors have preferred to keep the systolic pressure at 70 mm of mercury in normotensive patients and at two thirds of the usual systolic pressure in hypertensive patients. Others have reported safely maintaining a mean blood pressure of 40 mm of mercury for short periods.[15] The anesthesiologist begins to lower the blood pressure as the aneurysm becomes visible. For many years

trimethaphan was the agent of choice for controlled hypotension, but nitroprusside is being adopted increasingly, as it allows finer control and more prompt reversal of hypotension.[101,110] Halothane may also be used either alone or in conjunction with other agents to provide hypotension.[43] Continuous monitoring of blood pressure through an intra-arterial cannula adds considerably to the safety of the procedure.

Hypothermia

While theoretically sound, hypothermia as an adjunct to cerebral aneurysm procedures has been disappointing, effecting no improvement in mortality or morbidity levels, and for the most part it has been abandoned. The experience of neurosurgeons who have devoted significant attention to this modality has been published.[1,10,58,114] Recent reports indicate that hypothermia, especially preferential cerebral hypothermia with blood washout, may find a place in the treatment of giant and complex aneurysms not amenable to simple plication or wrapping.[67,96]

GENERAL OPERATIVE TECHNIQUE

Micro-Operative Technique

The introduction of the operating microscope and micro-operative techniques has provided both a new anatomical perspective and enhanced capabilities in the treatment of cerebral aneurysms. A better understanding of the subarachnoid cisterns has allowed them to be used as a natural pathway of dissection to an aneurysm, avoiding brain retraction and damage to nervous tissues. Magnification and improved lighting help the surgeon identify the correct normal and pathological anatomy of the blood vessels giving rise to aneurysms. To make it possible to utilize micro-operative technique fully, new instruments have had to be developed.

It must be emphasized that while the operating microscope and micro-operative technique offer a new perspective and improved capabilities to the operating neurosurgeon, they do not replace sound knowledge of anatomy and familiarity with basic surgical principles. In addition, considerable laboratory practice is required to gain the expertise necessary to utilize these techniques fully.

Subarachnoid Space

It has been recognized that the subarachnoid space and specifically the basal subarachnoid cisterns form a compartmentalized system that retards and perhaps directs the flow of cerebrospinal fluid. Vessels and cranial nerves occupy regular positions in this subarachnoid system and are anchored in the subarachnoid space by variable quantities of connective tissue trabeculae. Following the remarkable work of Key and Retzius in 1875, neuroradiologists have been especially interested in the delineation of this system in connection with pneumoencephalography.[12,46,54] The operating microscope has provided the neurosurgeon with the opportunity to examine this system under nearly physiological conditions and to recognize the areas of trabecular reinforcement that regularly occur at the junction of adjacent cisterns and at the point where a vessel crosses from one cistern to another.[121] Familiarity with this subarachnoid system will help the neurosurgeon maintain his orientation when working under the somewhat altered perspective of the operating microscope.

Subarachnoid cisterns of the anterior and middle fossae that relate to aneurysms arising from the anterior circulation are diagrammed in Figure 48–1. It is seen that a confluens of the several cisterns in the anterior fossa lies just above the bifurcation of the internal carotid artery between the laterobasal frontal lobe and the mediobasal temporal lobe. This confluens of cisterns is a primary landmark for the neurosurgeon to identify following opening of the dura. From it, the carotid cistern containing the internal carotid artery and the origins of its branches runs forward to the anterior clinoid process and shares a common wall with the chiasmatic cistern, a midline structure containing the optic nerves and the pituitary stalk. The olfactory cistern with the olfactory tract indents the inferior surface of the frontal lobe above the carotid cistern. The middle cerebral artery courses into the sylvian cistern, and the anterior cerebral artery and anterior communicating artery are contained in the midline lamina terminalis cistern. The anterior wall of the interpeduncular cistern extends below the diencephalon between the medial aspects of both temporal lobes behind the pituitary stalk. This cisternal wall, "Liliequist's membrane," is well developed and, following subarachnoid hemorrhage, may become quite thickened and tough (Fig. 48–2).[54] The posterior communicating artery passes through this membrane from the carotid to the interpe-

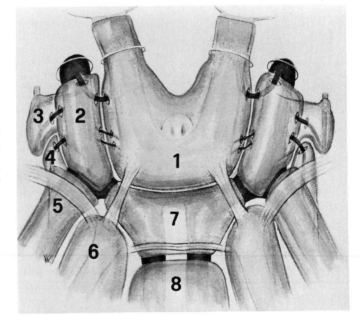

Figure 48–1 Diagrammatic sketch of basal subarachnoid cisterns. 1, Chiasmatic; 2, carotid; 3, interpeduncular; 4, crural; 5, sylvian; 6, olfactory; 7, lamina terminalis; and 8, pericallosal.

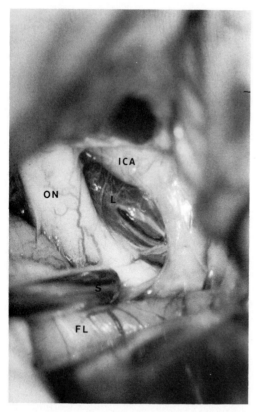

Figure 48–2 Operative photomicrograph showing interpeduncular cistern (Liliequist's membrane, L, between right optic nerve, ON, and internal carotid artery, ICA). FL, frontal lobe; S, suction tip.

duncular cistern, while the oculomotor nerve lies beneath the membrane in the interpeduncular cistern. The anterior choroidal artery does not enter the interpeduncular cistern but rather passes into the crural cistern between the parahippocampal gyrus (uncus) and the cerebral peduncle. Demarcation between the interpeduncular and crural cisterns has been clearly seen under the operating microscope and provides a plane for dissection of the anterior choroidal artery away from aneurysms arising near the posterior communicating artery (Fig. 48–3).

An orderly sequential dissection through the subarachnoid cisterns aids in identification of vital structures, allows for virtually bloodless dissection, contributes to brain relaxation through release of cerebrospinal fluid, and permits freeing of aneurysmal adhesions without undue torsion and traction on the aneurysm fundus.

Vascular Anatomy

The fine anatomy of the cerebral vessels and the relationship of an aneurysm to its parent artery and to adjacent small branches have received considerable attention in recent years. The operating microscope has helped to clarify these anatomical relationships and is of considerable aid

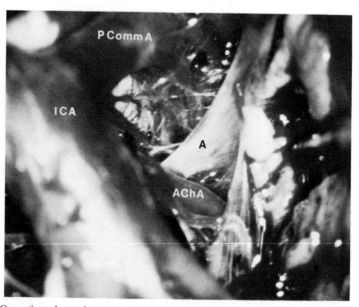

Figure 48–3 Operative photomicrograph showing arachnoid membrane, A, dividing interpeduncular and crural cisterns. ICA, internal carotid artery; PCommA, posterior communicating artery; AChA, anterior choroidal artery.

in identifying important structures and the exact configuration of an aneurysm at the time of operation. Small branches that appear to originate from the aneurysm are most often found to be only apposed to the fundus by arachnoid adhesions. Similarly aneurysms arising at the junction of major vessels such as internal carotid and posterior communicating arteries or the bifurcation of the middle cerebral artery frequently have their necks originating from one vessel with the adjacent vessel adherent to the aneurysm. Small perforating vessels to the brain stem and anomalous configurations of the circle of Willis must be recognized and protected. These perforating arteries and anomalies fall into consistent patterns, as do the relationships of a cerebral aneurysm to its adjacent arteries. These relationships are discussed in detail later when aneurysms in specific locations are considered.

Instrumentation

Newer instrumentation has helped to maximize the usefulness of microsurgical technique.

SKELETAL HEAD IMMOBILIZATION. Microsurgical technique requires complete immobility of the head. A three-point skeletal fixation device such as that devised by Mayfield and Kees provides the most secure stabilization during operation.*

MOBILE OPERATING MICROSCOPE. A significant degree of time loss and inconvenience results from having to make frequent movements and adjustments of the operating microscope. A mobile operating microscope has been developed wherein the microscope head and its accessories are counterbalanced by a weight on the stand.† The microscope is held in place by an electromagnetic braking system and released with a mouth switch. The neurosurgeon's hands are thus free to perform uninterrupted dissection.

BIPOLAR COAGULATION. The development of bipolar coagulation has been a most significant advance in neurosurgery.[28,60]

Small bleeding points may be controlled without heating adjacent structures. In addition, the neck of an aneurysm may be shrunk with bipolar coagulation to accept a clip more readily.[119] Fine bayonet forceps allow dissection and coagulation without need for a change in instruments.

HIGH-SPEED ELECTRIC DRILL. This instrument allows removal of bone with protection of important structures coursing through the bone. It is especially valuable in smoothing the base of the skull along the sphenoid ridge and above the orbits and in removal of the clinoid processes the better to visualize the neck of an aneurysm.

SELF-RETAINING RETRACTORS. Handheld retractors are not satisfactory for micro-operative procedures. A linked socket type of retractor mounted on the operating table allows gentle steady retraction in almost any direction.‡

MICRODISSECTION INSTRUMENTS. A varied selection of hooks, dissectors, ligature passers, scissors, forceps, and clip appliers should be available. General criteria include ease of handling, noninterference with vision (bayonet shape), delicacy, and strength. Micro-operative treatment of aneurysms primarily employs sharp dissection, and the surgeon should avoid pulling or tearing adhesions from the aneurysm with blunt instruments, which may quickly lead to premature rupture.

MICROVASCULAR INSTRUMENTS. With increasing experience, microvascular reconstruction is assuming a more important place in the treatment of intracranial aneurysm. Needleholders and forceps capable of handling 8-0 to 10-0 sutures are necessary.

SURGEON'S STOOL AND ARMREST. To utilize the mobile operating microscope fully, the surgeon must have both mobility and stability for his body and arms. A hydraulically adjustable stool on casters and an armrest that is independent of table or stool allow the required flexibility of position.

Craniotomy

Many operative approaches to cerebral aneurysms have been recommended and in

---

* Mayfield headrest with skull clamp, Codman and Shurtleff, Inc., Randolph, Massachusetts.
† Contraves floor stand, Contraves A.G., Zurich, Switzerland. Zeiss binocular operating microscope mounted on Contraves floor stand, Carl Zeiss Company, New York, New York.

‡ Yaşargil-Leyla brain retractor, Aesculap-Werke AG, Tuttlingen, Germany.

most cases these have varied with the location of the aneurysm.* In addition, different authors have recommended resection of small portions of the frontal or temporal lobes to give better access to the lesion.[20,113] Except for aneurysms on the distal anterior or middle cerebral arteries, most aneurysms of the anterior circulation can be adequately approached through a standard frontotemporosphenoidal (pterional) craniotomy. With bony prominences removed from the base of the skull, this craniotomy provides the most direct access to the circle of Willis, requires little retraction of the brain, and allows most of the procedure to be carried out within the subarachnoid basal cisterns.

The patient is placed supine on the operating table, and the head is immobilized with three-point skeletal fixation. The head is rotated 30 degrees to the side opposite the aneurysm and slightly elevated. The neck is extended so that the vertex of the skull is about 20 degrees down. This will make the malar eminence the superior point in the operating field (Fig. 48–4). For

---

* See references 11, 30, 31, 45, 83, 113.

anterior communicating artery aneurysms, the right-handed surgeon will prefer to operate from the right side unless additional aneurysms or an intracranial hematoma is present on the left. Self-retaining retractors should be draped into the operating field at the same time that the patient is draped.

The skin incision is begun in front of the ear just above the zygoma and continued behind the hairline to the forehead as shown in Figure 48–4). The skin and galea are elevated only enough to allow placement of skin clips on the flap and Dandy hemostats on the skin margin for hemostasis. The incision is then carried through the pericranium and temporalis fascia and muscle in line with the skin incision, and this combined skin and muscle flap is elevated from the skull and retracted inferiorly (Fig. 48–5). The temporalis muscle must be stripped from the zygomatic process of the frontal bone to allow adequate retraction, and it must be reflected deeply enough in the temporal fossa to expose the pterion and greater wing of the sphenoid. Utilizing a combined skin and muscle flap has virtually eliminated frontalis muscle paralysis, which was seen in 30 per cent of cases in

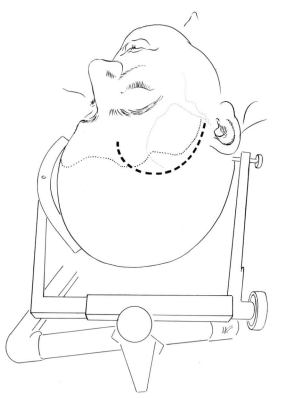

Figure 48–4   Artist's sketch showing skin incision for frontotemporosphenoidal craniotomy. Head is immobilized by skeletal fixation.

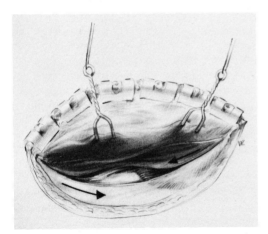

Figure 48–5 Frontotemporosphenoidal craniotomy. Skin and muscle elevated as single flap. Arrows show incisions in the periosteum and temporalis muscle.

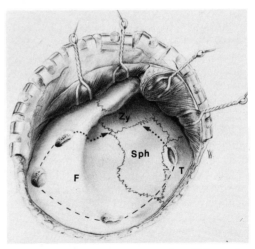

Figure 48–6 Frontotemporosphenoidal craniotomy placement of burr holes. F, frontal bone; Sph, sphenoid bone; T, temporal bone; Zy, zygomatic bone.

which separate skin and muscle flaps were developed.

A diamond-shaped bone flap is outlined with four burr holes. The first burr hole is placed on the posterior edge of the zygomatic process of the frontal bone. The second burr hole is on the superior orbital ridge 2 to 3 cm anterior and superior to the first. The third is 2.5 cm superior and posterior to the first on the anterior temporal line. The fourth is at the pterion posterior to the sphenotemporal suture (Fig. 48–6). The upper limbs of the bone flap are cut with the Gigli saw, while the base is grooved with the electric drill to allow the bone to frac-

ture across the sphenoid bone. The bone flap is removed from the operating field, and under the operating microscope, the sphenoid ridge and projections on the orbital roof are smoothed with the electric drill. Each millimeter removed creates a significant increase in operating space for the surgeon working with the microscope. Removal of the sphenoid ridge is carried medially until the orbitomeningeal artery is visualized and can be coagulated and divided (Fig. 48–7A).

The dural incision extends from the area

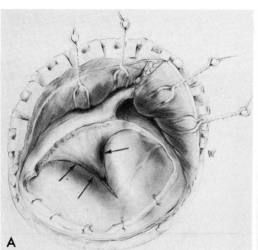

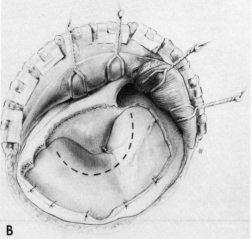

Figure 48–7 *A*. Frontotemporosphenoidal craniotomy. The bone flap has been removed and the dura tacked up to the bone margin. The sphenoid ridge separates the frontal and temporal lobes (*arrows*). *B*. The sphenoid ridge has been drilled away to the level of the orbitomeningeal artery. Dotted line shows dural incision.

of the first or second burr hole in a semicircle across the sylvian fissure to the base of the craniotomy (Fig. 48–7B). The dural flap may be retracted by suturing it to the temporalis muscle and to small drill holes in the bone margin anteriorly. The upper portion of the dura can usually be left closed to protect the brain. The sylvian cistern is opened in its most medial portion on the frontal side of the superficial middle cerebral veins, and the proximal (M_1) segment of the middle cerebral artery is identified. When the frontal and temporal lobes are adherent, judgment must be used as to how much dissection should be performed in the sylvian cistern. Aneurysms on the internal carotid artery usually require exposure of only the first few millimeters of the middle cerebral artery. This artery is followed proximally to the internal carotid artery bifurcation where the already described confluens of basal cisterns is recognized. Thickened fibers are noted over the origins of the middle and anterior cerebral arteries, and these are divided with sharp dissection. Gentle retraction is then applied to the laterobasal aspect of the frontal lobe to expose the carotid cistern and ipsilateral optic and olfactory nerves. A small artery consistently runs from the dorsal surface of the carotid artery to the dura over the anterior clinoid process. This should be coagulated and divided so that it will not tear and retract, giving rise to later bleeding. If adequate brain relaxation has not been achieved, the interpeduncular cistern can be opened through Liliequist's membrane either medial or lateral to the internal carotid artery. This maneuver will allow release of cerebrospinal fluid loculated around the brain stem, usually resulting in significant brain decompression.

Methods of Operative Treatment

Clipping

Ideally the surgeon wishes to eliminate an aneurysm from the circulation while maintaining normal continuity of the parent vessel and to cause no compromise of adjacent vascular or neural structures. Because of pathological changes in the vessel wall and the shape of the aneurysm neck, this ideal frequently cannot be obtained. The most effective method of management at present available is the placement of a clip across the neck of the aneurysm so that no distortion or kinking of the vessel wall results. More often than not, less than ideal placement of the clip must be accepted. In general, however, adequate clip placement is effective in preventing rebleeding and in most cases may be considered a curative procedure.

Early experience with intracranial management of aneurysms was with malleable clips.[63] These clips pose several problems: the aneurysm tends to be pushed forward in the clip, the ends of the clip may tear the aneurysm, in many situations they are difficult to apply, and they are difficult to remove when improperly placed. Subsequently many spring-tension clips have been developed.[35,61,95] Some of them have recently been compared with respect to closing pressure, propensity to slip, width of opening, and vessel wall damage.[106] Each neurosurgeon will develop his own preferences, but these factors should be considered in choosing a clip. Most important is that a great enough variety of sizes and shapes be available at the operating table so that the vagaries of individual aneurysms can be handled adequately. A commonly encountered problem has been that a clip with sufficient closing pressure did not have adequate blade length and opening width. Temporary clips that could open widely were investigated, but it was found that these would not control bleeding from the aneurysm if it ruptured during further dissection. Improved design has produced a clip with longer blades that still provides adequate closing pressure and that most aneurysms will accept primarily.* Only clips with quite low closing pressure should be used as temporary clips on parent vessels. In some situations other methods to reduce the size of the aneurysm neck must be employed, as is discussed later.

In situations in which the neck of the aneurysm is narrow and well defined, the surgeon may proceed directly with application of the clip, making sure that the aneurysm neck is completely enclosed within the blades of the clip, that the parent vessel is not compromised, and that no small perforating arteries or neural structures are

---

* Yaşargil aneurysm clips and appliers, Aesculap-Werke AG, Tuttlingen, Germany.

trapped between the blades of the clip. Following clip application, the aneurysm is opened, the fundus is excised, and a final check is made. Coagulation of cut edges is usually performed.

Frequently, however, difficulty with clip application will be encountered. The following situations have been observed:

Broad-Based Aneurysm

When the neck of the aneurysm is too wide to accept the clip primarily, it may be reduced by one of the four following techniques. Bipolar current may be used, the forceps tips being placed across the neck of the aneurysm, and low-amperage current (2.5 on Malis unit) applied in short bursts. The forceps are gently squeezed and released to check for degree of shrinkage of the tissue until an adequate length of neck has been developed to allow clip placement. A forceps may be employed to compress the neck of the aneurysm while a clip is applied with the other hand, a ligature may be used to reduce the neck, or a wide-opening clip may be applied higher on the fundus to shape the neck for the final clip.

Presence of Atheroma or Thrombus

If a clip can be placed low on the aneurysm neck, the aneurysm may be opened, the thrombus removed or an endarterectomy performed, and the clip moved to a more favorable location while the fundus is held closed with a forceps in the opposite hand. When this maneuver is not possible, the parent vessels may need to be temporarily clipped.

Tightly Distended Aneurysm

At times, despite hypotension, the aneurysm may remain so turgid that clip placement is hampered. Pressure on the fundus, with the sucker over a cottonoid sponge, may help to empty the aneurysm and allow clip placement.

Aneurysm Torn at Base

Temporary clipping of the parent artery and micro-operative repair may allow the parent artery to be saved.

Following clipping of the aneurysm, it is recommended that a small collar of muscle be placed around the base of the clip. This helps to stimulate some fibrosis around the site of aneurysm formation. Not infrequently, a small portion of aneurysm neck will not be amenable to clipping, and this may be protected to some degree by the muscle. The piece of muscle may be held in place by a drop of acrylic bonding agent.

Ligation

Sometimes a ligature passed around the neck of an aneurysm will give a more satisfactory result than clip placement. This is especially true when the aneurysm is located at a major bifurcation such as that of the internal carotid or middle cerebral artery. In general, however, ligature placement is more difficult and somewhat more dangerous than clip placement. When the aneurysm is especially broad-based a ligature tends to kink the parent artery. Ligation may, however, be efficacious in reducing the size of the aneurysm neck to allow subsequent clip placement.

Wrapping and Encasement

Various methods of strengthening the aneurysm wall or providing external support for it have been investigated. Muscle was the first material used and is still employed in many situations. Experimentally, muscle alone has been shown to be inadequate in promoting the necessary fibrosis to protect against aneurysm rupture.[92] Fabrics such as cotton and muslin have been used to promote fibrosis around aneurysms, and some series have shown good results with this method.[24,71,78] The most common alternative to clipping and ligation, however, has been the use of self-hardening plastics: methylmethacrylate and epoxy resins, and more recently cyanoacrylates.[16,17,32,97] It would seem that adequate protection against rebleeding is provided by these agents when the entire aneurysm can be coated, and they retain a place in the management of aneurysms that may not be amenable to clipping or ligation. It is often difficult, however, to achieve the dissection necessary to expose an aneurysm entirely. In addition, one must take care not to allow the material to come in contact with normal neural or vascular structures, as it may cause damage. Strength, adherence, ease of applicability, and safety are among the characteristics to be considered in choosing a compound for aneurysm encasement.

Induced Thrombosis

The finding of thrombus in many aneurysms and the occasional reports of spontaneous cure of an aneurysm by thrombosis have encouraged investigators to seek ways of initiating thrombosis in these lesions. Methods have included injection of animal hair with an air gun, aggregation of iron filings with a magnet, introduction of fine wire into the aneurysm, and application of current to metal needles placed stereotactically.[3,4,23,72,75] More recently, internal occlusion of aneurysms with a radiographically directed Fogarty catheter has been reported.[99] Theoretically the aneurysm could be occluded by the catheter balloon, or an acrylic material could be injected into the aneurysm lumen. Most of these methods remain in an early stage of development.

Additional Technical Considerations

Premature Rupture

An aneurysm may rupture at any time during the operative procedure, and the neurosurgeon must be prepared both technically and psychologically for this event. If rupture occurs early in the course of dissection, the operator can only work quickly toward the aneurysm in hopes of gaining control of the parent arteries. More commonly, however, the aneurysm will rupture during dissection of the parent arteries, when traction may be inadvertently applied to the fundus, or when the aneurysm itself is being freed and attempts are being made to prepare the neck for clipping. Bleeding may frequently be controlled with gentle pressure over a cottonoid sponge with a sucker, and the surgeon should resist the impulse to take a large-bore sucker to clear the field quickly. Forceful suction will generally further damage the aneurysm, leading to increased bleeding, and in addition may injure small perforating arteries and cranial nerves. If bleeding is not controlled, temporary clips are applied to the parent vessels. The anesthesiologist may compress the cervical carotid artery when the aneurysm is proximal on the internal carotid artery and a clip cannot be placed. When dissection has been essentially completed prior to rupture, the aneurysm fundus may be drawn up into the sucker while a clip is applied to the neck with the other hand. When control has been achieved, an attempt is made to rinse the subarachnoid space free of blood prior to further dissection.

Multiple Aneurysms

Fifteen to thirty per cent of patients will have more than one aneurysm. Those aneurysms ipsilateral to the ruptured aneurysm usually can be treated at the same operation, and occasionally contralateral aneurysms on the proximal internal carotid artery and aneurysms of the basilar artery bifurcation are also accessible. The neurosurgeon must exercise judgment as to the condition of the patient, the amount of dissection required, and his own technical ability and experience when deciding whether to attempt treatment of asymptomatic aneurysms. Not infrequently when using the operating microscope the surgeon will encounter "baby" aneurysms and areas of focal thinning on the vessel wall, especially on the anterior cerebral arteries and internal carotid artery bifurcation. Sometimes a neck can be created on these small aneurysms and a clip can be applied. More often it is only possible to place a piece of muscle over the lesion and fix it with a drop of acrylic bonding agent. Whether these lesions would become symptomatic aneurysms is not known.

Mechanical Spasm

Dissection and manipulation of the cerebral arteries can lead to localized spasm of these vessels. Papaverine applied as a 4 per cent solution on a cotton pledget will relieve this type of spasm and is used routinely throughout the operation. Following the application of papaverine, the periadventitial sympathetic plexus of the larger cerebral arteries becomes well delineated and can be stripped from the vessel wall, possibly providing further protection from later spasm.

Repair of Damaged Vessels

Micro-operative techniques applied to vascular operations have made it possible to achieve a good patency rate with anastomosis of vessels less than 1 mm in diameter. If a major branch of the middle cerebral artery or the anterior cerebral artery is lost during dissection of an aneurysm, the surgeon may now consider primary repair of the artery or creation of an extracranial-intracranial anastomosis to provide collateral flow. Degree of back bleeding from the distal arterial segment and local blood flow determinations may help establish indications for such a procedure. Nevertheless, at present, the time required and the lack of effective and practical methods of protecting brain metabolism during the period of ischemia limit its applicability.

INTERNAL CAROTID ARTERY ANEURYSMS

Surgical Anatomy

The internal carotid artery enters the subarachnoid space (carotid cistern) from the cavernous sinus inferior and medial to the anterior clinoid process. The ophthalmic artery arises from its medial aspect, usually after the internal carotid artery has entered the subarachnoid space, although in 8 per cent of cases the origin is intracavernous.[34] Distal to the ophthalmic artery, several small branches arise from the medial aspect of the carotid artery and course into the chiasmatic cistern to supply the optic nerves and chiasm and the pituitary stalk. The largest of these is often called the superior hypophyseal artery and forms an

arcade around the stalk with its opposite mate.[105] The posterior communicating artery takes origin from the lateral aspect of the internal carotid artery a few millimeters distal to the origin of the ophthalmic artery and enters the interpeduncular cistern, where it gives off a group of thalamoperforating arteries before joining the ipsilateral posterior cerebral artery. More distally from the lateral aspect of the internal carotid artery, the anterior choroidal artery passes into the crural cistern between the uncus and cerebral peduncle. Frequently the anterior choroidal artery divides almost immediately, and at times two or even three independent origins will be encountered. The anterior choroidal artery may pass beneath the internal carotid artery bifurcation and be mistaken for a striate vessel. At the internal carotid artery bifurcation, medial striate arteries ascend into the anterior perforated substance. It has been noted that these small vessels never arise directly from the bifurcation but rather a few millimeters distally on the origins of the anterior and middle cerebral arteries.

Internal carotid artery aneurysms constituted 235 of 678, or 35 per cent of, anterior circulation aneurysms in the authors' series. Figure 48–8 shows the frequency of aneurysms at various sites. Intracavernous aneurysms expand the cavernous sinus and often present with cranial nerve deficits rather than subarachnoid hemorrhage.[41] Occasionally they are bilateral. Aneurysms arising from the proximal medial wall of the internal carotid artery (carotid-ophthalmic aneurysms) are intimately related to the

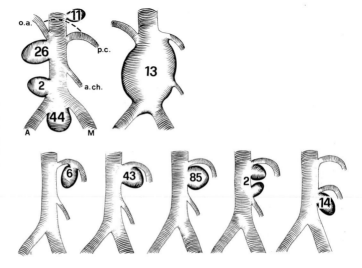

Figure 48–8   Diagram of the locations of 235 supraclinoid and 11 infraclinoid aneurysms of the internal carotid artery. o.a., Ophthalmic artery; p.c., posterior communicating artery; a.ch., anterior choroidal artery; A, anterior cerebral artery; M, middle cerebral artery.

optic nerves and may present above or below the ipsilateral optic nerve. Those presenting below the optic nerve are usually adherent to the dura of the anterior clinoid process and are frequently associated with visual deficit, while those above the optic nerve tend to project back toward the anterior cerebral artery and orbitofrontal lobe (Fig. 48–9). Aneurysms at this location frequently are bilateral (5 of 25 cases). Aneurysms arising more distally from the medial wall of the internal carotid artery are rare. These lesions may involve the anterior cerebral artery, optic chiasm, and pituitary stalk.

By far the most common site of aneurysms on the internal carotid artery is the origin of the posterior communicating artery. These so-called "posterior communicating artery" aneurysms are better termed proximal lateral wall internal carotid artery aneurysms. It must be emphasized that only rarely do aneurysms arise from the posterior communicating artery (see Fig. 48–8). Adhesions between the aneurysm

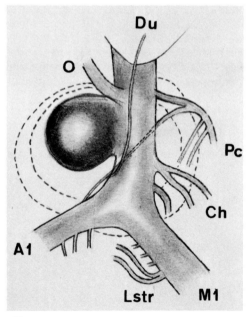

Figure 48–9   Aneurysm arising from medial wall of internal carotid artery (carotid-ophthalmic aneurysm). Dotted lines show how growth of aneurysm may involve adjacent structures. Du, dura over anterior clinoid process receiving small branch from internal carotid artery; O, ophthalmic artery; Pc, posterior communicating artery; Ch, anterior choroidal artery—double origin; A1, anterior cerebral artery with medial striate branches; M1, middle cerebral artery; Lstr, lenticulostriate arteries.

fundus and the posterior communicating artery may create the impression that the aneurysm is arising partially from this artery when, in fact, the neck is based entirely on the internal carotid artery. With growth, aneurysms at this location come to involve the thalamoperforating arteries from the posterior communicating artery, the anterior choroidal artery, and the oculomotor nerve. The neck of the aneurysm and the origin of the posterior communicating artery may lie beneath the anterior clinoid process. The fundus of the aneurysm may be adherent to the mesial temporal lobe. Aneurysms arising from the distal lateral wall of the internal carotid artery (anterior choroidal artery aneurysms) may displace the anterior choroidal artery laterally into the temporal lobe or medially beneath the internal carotid artery bifurcation. The fundus of these aneurysms is frequently buried in the mesial temporal lobe. Two aneurysms arose from the proximal side of the anterior choroidal artery and were associated with proximal lateral wall aneurysms.

In 14 cases internal carotid artery aneurysms took origin from the inferior wall of the internal carotid artery. These aneurysms were large, had poorly defined necks, and may represent a type of atherosclerotic aneurysm. Several of these showed significant thrombosis. In a few of these cases, the aneurysms gave origin to the posterior communicating and anterior choroidal arteries. Aneurysms arising at the internal carotid artery bifurcation tend to be broad-based, rarely involve the major branches at the bifurcation equally, and frequently project into the orbital portion of the frontal lobe in the area of the anterior perforated substance. Although the fundus often is adherent to medial striate arteries, it does not give origin to these arteries. The aneurysm may involve the anterior cerebral artery, recurrent artery of Heubner, medial and lateral striate arteries, anterior choroidal artery, and optic tract.

Operative Technique

Intracavernous Internal Carotid Artery Aneurysms

Aneurysms within the cavernous sinus do not usually lend themselves to direct operative treatment. The operative approach to the cavernous sinus has been described, but the usually benign course of aneurysms in this location has not justified such a radical approach.[81] Cervical common or internal carotid artery ligation remains the treatment of choice. For those patients who cannot tolerate carotid artery occlusion, a superficial temporal artery–middle cerebral artery anastomosis may provide the necessary collateral flow to allow the procedure. Early experience suggests that this procedure may be quite helpful in certain cases.

Medial Wall Internal Carotid Artery Aneurysms

Following frontotemporosphenoidal craniotomy, the thickened arachnoidal fibers over the origins of the anterior and middle cerebral arteries are released to allow gentle retraction of the laterobasal frontal lobe. The carotid cistern is opened superiorly over the carotid artery and the small branch to the dura is coagulated and divided. An attempt is made to gain space on the internal carotid artery below the neck of the aneurysm in case temporary clipping is necessary. With aneurysms originating near the ophthalmic artery, it frequently is not possible to gain enough space to clip the internal carotid artery temporarily, and in this situation, the anesthesiologist is advised that compression of the cervical carotid artery may be necessary. Some surgeons have advocated dissection of the internal carotid artery in the neck at the beginning of the procedure to allow its temporary ligation. In cases in which the aneurysm fundus lies beneath the optic nerve, the anterior cerebral artery should be dissected to facilitate retraction of the frontal lobe. This dissection of the anterior cerebral artery usually is not possible when the fundus of the aneurysm sits above the optic nerves. With the posterior communicating and anterior choroidal arteries identified, adhesions between the aneurysm fundus and internal carotid artery are divided. These arachnoidal adhesions should be divided with sharp cutting instruments. Finally, the surgeon must identify the origin of the ophthalmic artery. In many cases, removal of the anterior clinoid process with a high-speed drill will create the working room needed to separate the aneurysm from the ophthalmic artery. Small branches to the optic nerves and pituitary stalk are dissected from the wall of the aneurysm when possible, and a clip is placed across the neck of the aneurysm. The fundus is resected to decompress the optic nerve. An opposite medial internal carotid artery aneurysm can often be handled at the same procedure. If the neck is to be shrunk with bipolar coagulation, care must be taken not to include the pituitary stalk between the forceps tips, especially when the aneurysm is somewhat distally located.

Lateral Wall Internal Carotid Artery Aneurysms

The initial approach to these aneurysms is the same as that described for medial wall internal carotid artery aneurysms. Following opening of the carotid cistern, the surgeon attempts to find space proximally on the internal carotid artery to place a temporary clip should one be needed. The lamina terminalis cistern is then opened to free the anterior cerebral artery complex. This maneuver will allow for better retraction of the frontal lobe and decrease tension on the fundus of the aneurysm, which may be adherent to the temporal lobe. The anterior choroidal artery must be identified. If it is hidden beneath the aneurysm, it may be found distally in the crural cistern through a small incision in the mesial basal temporal lobe. The aneurysm wall is dissected away from the anterior choroidal artery and the internal carotid artery so that a temporary clip could be placed proximal to the anterior choroidal artery to preserve its collateral flow from the anterior cerebral artery. Finally, a large enough space is created between the posterior communicating artery and the aneurysm neck to allow placement of a clip. No attempt to dissect the fundus of the aneurysm should be made prior to application of a clip. If the origin of the posterior communicating artery is hidden by the aneurysm, the dissection medial to the internal carotid artery frequently will reveal its position. Removal of the anterior clinoid process can provide additional working space. One should try to avoid clipping the posterior communicating artery with the neck of the aneurysm. If the clip should be applied in this manner, a kink may be made in the intima of the internal carotid artery, which compromises its lumen, blood flow may be reduced to thalamoperforating vessels and the ipsilateral posterior cerebral artery, and in some cases retrograde filling of the aneurysm from the posterior communicating artery may occur (Fig. 48–10).

If the aneurysm has arisen distal to the anterior choroidal artery, this artery may be hidden beneath the fundus of the aneurysm. It may be identified beneath the internal carotid artery bifurcation or distally in the crural cistern through a small resection of mesial temporal lobe. The surgeon must consider the early branching of this artery and attempt to separate the neck of the aneurysm from the artery quite near its origin on the internal carotid artery. It is important to identify both the anterior choroidal and the posterior communicating arteries in each case so that the true location and relationships of the aneurysm are appreciated.

Ventral Wall Internal Carotid Artery Aneurysms

The ill-defined necks of aneurysms in this location permitted direct clipping of only 7 of 14 lesions in the authors' series. In the others, cervical carotid artery ligation, muscle wrapping, trapping, and direct ligation were performed. The posterior communicating artery and anterior choroidal artery may be hidden or incorporated into the aneurysm so that a clip cannot be placed. Under the best circumstances a clip may be slipped along the inferior wall of the internal carotid artery to enclose the broad neck. Operative management of aneurysms in this location is not yet satisfactory.

Internal Carotid Artery Bifurcation Aneurysms

After the dura has been opened and retracted, the sylvian cistern must be opened somewhat more distally and the middle cerebral artery exposed. The artery is dissected proximally over a short distance, and the medial and lateral striate arteries are located so that a temporary clip can be placed if needed. The carotid cistern is then opened, and again space is created on the internal carotid artery distal to the anterior choroidal artery to allow placement of a temporary clip if necessary. The lamina terminalis cistern is opened medially over the anterior communicating artery, and the recurrent artery of Heubner is identified. The artery of Heubner and the anterior cerebral artery are dissected toward the bifurcation, and medial striate arteries from the anterior cerebral artery are identified. If a hematoma is present in the orbital frontal lobe, it is evacuated, leaving the pia intact over the fundus of the aneurysm. Removal of the hematoma will create additional working room and minimize the need for retraction. Branches of the anterior choroidal artery may course beneath the internal carotid artery bifurcation and be confused with striate arteries. With all adjacent structures identified, the neck is dissected free and a

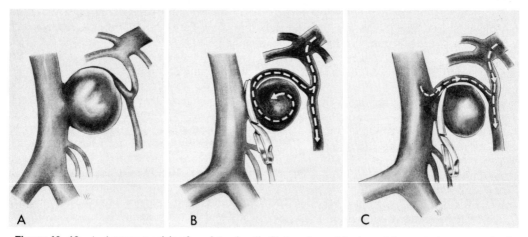

Figure 48–10 *A*. Aneurysm arising from lateral wall of internal carotid artery at the posterior communicating artery. *B*. Clip crossing both neck of aneurysm and posterior communicating artery allows aneurysm to be filled from basilar circulation. *C*. Proper clip placement. The aneurysm is excluded from the circulation and normal flow patterns are maintained.

clip is applied. In this location the neck of the aneurysm frequently is wide and may require bipolar coagulation to shrink it, or ligation or management by another method, as discussed earlier. If the anterior cerebral artery is hypoplastic it may be divided lateral to the striate arteries and included in the clip with the neck of the aneurysm.

MIDDLE CEREBRAL ARTERY ANEURYSMS

Surgical Anatomy

The middle cerebral artery turns laterally from the internal carotid artery and enters the sylvian cistern beneath a band of arachnoid fibers extending from the olfactory area to the mesial temporal lobe. In the sylvian cistern the artery is covered by a variable mesh of arachnoid trabeculations. From this horizontal (M_1) segment, a temporal polar (50 per cent of cases) and an anterior temporal artery course to the temporal lobe. From the medial aspect of the middle cerebral artery arise a few small medial striate arteries within a few millimeters of the internal carotid artery bifurcation. These vessels enter the anterior perforated substance and are joined by the recurrent artery of Heubner. Distal to these vessels, larger lateral striate (lenticulostriate) arteries arise in groups from the medial aspect of the middle cerebral artery. These arteries tend to run proximally (recurrently) in close association with the middle cerebral artery before diverging to enter the anterior perforated substance. These vessels may originate as far distally as the middle cerebral artery bifurcation and are usually found on the medial inferior aspect of the larger main trunk of the bifurcation.

The middle cerebral artery bifurcation occurs as the M_1 segment of the artery curves around the limen insulae. The trunks initially diverge but after 1 to 2 cm reapproximate in the sylvian fissure. Considerable variability of branching patterns is noted. In general, a superior trunk gives branches to the frontal lobe and central sulcus area, while an inferior trunk gives branches to the parietal and temporal lobes. An early temporal or frontal branch may create the impression of a more complex primary division of the middle cerebral artery.

Of 678 anterior circulation aneurysms, 132 (19 per cent) were on the middle cerebral artery (Fig. 48–11). Fourteen of these were on the middle cerebral artery trunk (M_1 segment) at the origins of branches, and six were on the cortical branches, the remainder being found at the middle cerebral artery bifurcation. Aneurysms arising from the trunk of the middle cerebral artery usually were just distal to a small branch, either an anterior temporal or a lenticulostriate artery. Aneurysms arising at the bifurcation of the middle cerebral artery frequently have been described as fusiform dilatations of the middle cerebral artery with the major trunks taking origin from the aneurysm. It has been recommended that these aneurysms be coated rather than clipped. Of the 104 cases just noted, only one showed some ectasia of the middle cerebral trunk at the base of the aneurysm. In all other cases, although arachnoid adhesions created the appearance of a fusiform dilatation, with persistent dissection the branches could be separated from the aneurysm and a clip could be placed across the neck. There is some variability in the

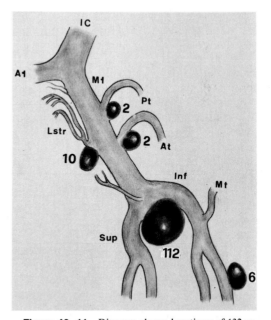

Figure 48–11   Diagram shows locations of 132 aneurysms on the middle cerebral artery. IC, internal carotid artery; AC, anterior cerebral artery; M1, horizontal portion of middle cerebral artery; Pt, temporopolar artery; At, anterior temporal artery; Lstr, lenticulostriate arteries; Inf, inferior trunk at bifurcation; Sup, superior trunk at bifurcation; Mt, middle temporal artery.

course of the horizontal portion of the middle cerebral artery, so on occasion it may be directly beneath the aneurysm from the surgeon's perspective. At the bifurcation the aneurysm will generally be based more on the larger trunk or quite well centered when the trunks are of equal size. Furthermore, in many cases, lenticulostriate arteries originate from the area of the bifurcation just below the neck of the aneurysm to course proximally before turning to enter the anterior perforated substance. Aneurysms arising on the cortical branches of the middle cerebral artery are uncommon and frequently are mycotic or traumatic aneurysms. There was no evidence of inflammation in the six aneurysms in this series, but two of the patients had a history of head trauma.

Operative Technique

Aneurysms of the middle cerebral artery trunk and bifurcation are approached through a standard frontotemporosphenoidal craniotomy. Following retraction of the dura, the carotid cistern is opened first to allow some release of cerebrospinal fluid, and an area is prepared distal to the anterior choroidal artery should temporary clipping be required early in dissection. The sylvian cistern is then entered by dividing the thickened bands over the origin of the middle cerebral artery, and dissection proceeds distally on the M_1 segment as the anterior temporal and lenticulostriate branches are identified. The anterior temporal and temporopolar branches should be mobilized somewhat from the pia so that they are not torn by stretching as the sylvian fissure is opened. Small bridging veins from the superficial middle cerebral veins to the sphenoparietal sinus may require division. The surgeon must free enough of the middle cerebral artery trunk so that a temporary clip can be placed if necessary but does not need to proceed to the aneurysm at this point. When some swelling of the temporal lobe is present, difficulty in identifying the sylvian cistern may be encountered, as the pia of the lobes becomes closely approximated. A cortical branch may be followed proximally to identify the fissure. Aneurysms of the middle cerebral artery trunk may generally be handled directly by freeing the adjacent vessel and applying a clip.

For aneurysms of the middle cerebral artery bifurcation, further dissection of the middle cerebral artery trunk is deferred and attention is turned distally in the sylvian fissure, where the arachnoid is opened on the frontal side of the middle cerebral veins, and the trunks of the middle cerebral artery are identified. A second self-retaining retractor may be necessary to elevate the temporal operculum gently. Dissection is carried proximally along each trunk toward the bifurcation. It is necessary to inspect beneath the temporal operculum, as the inferior trunk may lie hidden and branching of the superior trunk be wrongly assumed to be the primary bifurcation. The distal branches of the middle cerebral artery are especially prone to mechanically induced spasm, and papaverine should be used during dissection. In cases in which a hematoma is present in the superior temporal gyrus, it may be evacuated and the bifurcation approached through the hematoma cavity rather than through the sylvian fissure.

With the major vessels demonstrated, dissection of the neck of the aneurysm may proceed. Adhesions between the trunks and the aneurysm are divided until the neck is adequately defined. Lenticulostriate arteries are generally found beneath the aneurysm neck, arising from the larger trunk or from the middle of the bifurcation if the trunks are equal in size. These are freed from the neck of the aneurysm. With adequate delineation of the neck, a clip may be applied. If thrombectomy or endarterectomy is required, temporary clips should be placed both proximally and distally to the aneurysm to avoid a sump effect on collateral circulation when the aneurysm is opened. The proximal clip should be distal to the largest group of lenticulostriate arteries.

ANTERIOR CEREBRAL–ANTERIOR COMMUNICATING ARTERY ANEURYSMS

Surgical Anatomy

From their origins at the internal carotid artery bifurcation the anterior cerebral arteries enter the lamina terminalis cistern and course medially between the inferior surface of the orbitofrontal lobes and the dorsal surface of the optic nerves and chiasm. They join at the midline through a short arterial segment, the anterior communicating artery. Several groups of perforating arteries arise from the anterior cerebral arteries.[53,82,120] These perforating arteries tend to be somewhat recurrent and course backward along the anterior cerebral artery to enter the anterior perforated substance. Hypothalamic arteries arise from the inferoposterior wall of the anterior communicating artery and enter the septal area and anterior hypothalamus. The recurrent artery of Heubner most often arises at the junction of the anterior cerebral and anterior communicating arteries, although it may take origin distal or proximal to this point.[50] This artery courses laterally, paralleling the anterior cerebral artery and generally lying beneath and posterior to it. It joins the most proximal group of lenticulostriate arteries from the middle cerebral artery. It is contained within the lamina terminalis cistern.

Anomalous configurations of the anterior cerebral–anterior communicating artery complex are common and have an important bearing on the location of aneurysms found in this area. Of 283 cases of aneurysm on the anterior communicating artery, 142 showed the left anterior cerebral artery (A_1 segment) to be larger; 78, the right A_1 segment to be larger; and 63, the two segments to be of equal size. Of those with dominant left A_1 segments, the aneurysm arose from the left corner of the anterior cerebral–anterior communicating artery junction in 138 (49 per cent). Of those with larger right A_1 segments, the aneurysm arose from the right corner in 76, and of those with approximately equal A_1 segments, the aneurysm arose in the middle of the anterior communicating artery in 61. Thus, only 8 of 283 cases had an aneurysm that did not arise from the side of the larger A_1 segment or from the midposition when the two segments were equal. Similarly, the hypothalamic arteries consistently arise from the side of the larger A_1 segment or from the midportion of the anterior communicating artery when these two arteries are of equal caliber. They are therefore found, in almost all cases, to be rather adherent to the posteroinferior wall of the aneurysm. They rarely if ever take origin from the aneurysm, however (Fig. 48–12).

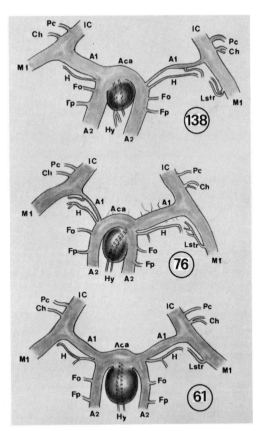

Figure 48–12 Locations of aneurysms and relationship to hypothalamic arteries in 275 of 283 aneurysms of the anterior communicating artery. IC, internal carotid artery; Pc, posterior communicating artery; Ch, anterior choroidal artery; M1, middle cerebral artery; Lstr, lenticulostriate artery; A1, anterior cerebral artery; Aca, anterior communicating artery; H, recurrent artery of Heubner; Fo, fronto-orbital artery; Fp, Frontopolar artery; Hy, hypothalamic arteries; A2, distal anterior cerebral, or pericallosal, artery.

The anterior communicating artery exists in the embryo as a multichanneled network of vessels that coalesce to form the final vessel bridging the two anterior cerebral arteries.[79] Failure of these channels to unite leads to a spectrum of anomalies of the anterior communicating artery ranging from a network of multiple bridges to duplication or triplication of the anterior communicating artery. Although an aneurysm will generally arise from the major communicating artery, cases have been seen wherein the origin of the aneurysm was a small bridge or fenestrated artery. Fenestrations and duplication may also be seen to involve the anterior cerebral arteries (A_1 segments) and the pericallosal (distal anterior cerebral arteries, or A_2 segments). Frequency of these

TABLE 48–1   VARIATIONS OF THE ANTERIOR CEREBRAL–ANTERIOR COMMUNICATING ARTERY COMPLEX*

ARTERY	VARIATION	NO. OF CASES	ARTERY	VARIATION	NO. OF CASES	PER CENT
Proximal anterior cerebral (A₁)	Aplasia		Anterior communicating	Aplasia	0	1.0
	Right	5		Hypoplastia	3	
	Left	4		Duplication		
				Partial	39	
				Full	26	26.5
				Network	10	
					75	
	Inequality		Distal anterior cerebral (A₂)	Single	2	0.7
	Left > right	142		Triple	27	9.5
	Left < right	78				
	Left = right	63				
		283				
	Duplication					
	Right	3				
	Left	2				

SITE OF ANEURYSMS	NO. OF CASES	PER CENT
Left corner	138	48.8
Right corner	76	26.8
Middle	61	21.6
Irregular	8	2.8
	283	

* Variations found in 283 patients with aneurysms of the anterior communicating artery.

anomalies in 283 cases of anterior cerebral–anterior communicating artery aneurysm is summarized in Table 48–1.

The position and size of the recurrent artery of Heubner is also variable and bears some relationship to the other components of the anterior cerebral–anterior communicating arterial complex. Variations of origin of this artery are listed in Table 48–2. It has been noted that when the A₁ segment is small on one side, the recurrent artery of Heubner is also small or aplastic and that a

TABLE 48–2   VARIATIONS IN THE ORIGIN OF THE RECURRENT ARTERY OF HEUBNER*

	No. of Patients	Per Cent	
ORIGIN OF ARTERY			
Bilateral			
ACommA corner	148	52.3	
A₁ corner	6	2.1	
A₂ corner	69	24.4	
Asymmetrical A₁/A₂	47	16.6	
	270		
APLASIA OF ARTERY			
Unilateral			
Right	6	2.1	
Left	3	1.1	
Bilateral	2	0.7	
DUPLICATION OF ARTERY			
Unilateral			
Right	5	1.7	
Left	6	2.1	
Bilateral	3	1.1	

* Variations found in 283 patients with aneurysms of the anterior communicating artery. A₁, proximal anterior cerebral artery; A₂, distal anterior cerebral, or pericallosal, artery; ACommA, anterior communicating artery.

stout medial perforating artery will originate from the midportion of the A_1 segment and pursue a lateral course comparable to that of the normal artery of Heubner.

A small artery originates from the anterior surface of the A_2 segment and runs to the olfactory tract. This artery is almost never adherent to an aneurysm. Fronto-orbital arteries, however, and at times frontopolar arteries may course over the dome of an aneurysm and be densely adherent. The fronto-orbital and frontopolar arteries may show a common origin. In 27 of 283 cases (9.5 per cent) three A_2 segments were present, and in two cases a single A_2 segment was found. In one case there was a fenestration in one of the A_2 segments. The callosomarginal branch runs above the cingulate gyrus. The origin of the callosomarginal artery is the most common site of aneurysms on the distal anterior cerebral (pericallosal) artery. Communications between the distal anterior cerebral arteries distal to the anterior communicating artery have been described.[52]

Operative Technique

Through a frontotemporosphenoidal craniotomy the operator opens the medial aspect of the sylvian fissure to expose the confluens of cisterns over the internal carotid artery bifurcation. It is especially important to divide the reinforcing fibers of arachnoid running from the olfactory area to the optic nerve and mesial temporal lobe in order to allow adequate retraction of the laterobasal frontal lobe without tensing arachnoid bands across the origins of the anterior and middle cerebral arteries. The anterior cerebral artery (A_1 segment) is exposed by opening the lamina terminalis cistern on the anterosuperior aspect of the artery away from the perforating arteries to the basal frontal lobe. Frequently the anterior cerebral artery will be somewhat tortuous and course beneath the frontal lobe. It is not necessary to expose the artery in its entirety, as this may require undue retraction and lead to disruption and spasm of perforating arteries. By following the lamina terminalis cistern medially, the operator will come to the anterior communicating artery complex.

In cases in which the aneurysm projects superiorly into the interhemispheric fissure

(84 per cent), the left anterior cerebral artery is next identified and dissected medially toward the anterior communicating artery by opening the lamina terminalis cistern over it. In those cases in which the aneurysm projects forward over the optic chiasm and may be adherent to the dura of the tuberculum sellae (16 per cent) exposure of the opposite anterior cerebral artery must be postponed. As each anterior cerebral artery is exposed near the anterior communicating artery, the recurrent artery of Heubner on each side can be identified.

Occasionally the configuration of the aneurysm and arteries will be such that the pericallosal arteries (A_2 segments) can be identified with only subarachnoid dissection. More often, however, too much retraction of the basal frontal lobe would be required to expose the interhemispheric fissure and excessive tension would be placed on the aneurysm fundus. Consequently a 0.5- to 1.0-cm subpial resection of the right gyrus rectus is performed to expose these arteries. No attempt is made to dissect the pia from the aneurysm fundus. The A_2 segments are dissected distal to the aneurysm fundus, and the fronto-orbital, olfactory, and frontopolar arteries are identified when they are present. A careful search should be made for a third A_2 segment, as it will usually lie beneath the normal A_2 segments from the surgeon's perspective. The origins of Heubner's arteries are identified. It has commonly been observed that a fronto-orbital artery will be adherent to the fundus of the aneurysm. It has seemed preferable to divide this artery rather than risk tearing the aneurysm fundus. No untoward result of sacrificing these arteries has been noted.

With the major arteries identified and exposed, the final area of dissection is at the neck of the aneurysm. The hypothalamic arteries are freed from the posterior inferior aspect of the aneurysm, and a plane is developed between the optic nerves and the aneurysm and between the pituitary stalk and the aneurysm. In all phases of this dissection arachnoid adhesions should be gently spread with the bipolar coagulation forceps or a blunt dissector and then sharply divided with scissors or a knife. Blunt tearing of adhesions transmits excessive tension to the aneurysm and to normal neural and vascular structures.

The use of bipolar coagulation to shrink the aneurysm neck has been especially advantageous at this location. A small cotton-oid sponge should be placed between the aneurysm and the hypothalamic arteries to protect them from the tips of the coagulating forceps. Temporary clipping of the anterior communicating artery has been used when thrombectomy, endarterectomy, or micro-operative repair has been required, but generally it is not necessary and may lead to psycho-organic sequelae.

Aneurysms located on the proximal portion of the anterior cerebral artery present operative problems similar to those encountered with aneurysms on the anterior communicating artery. An aneurysm at this location arises in conjunction with the origin of a perforating artery, and this should be identified prior to the placement of a clip. Especially important is to avoid excessive retraction on the basal frontal lobe, as the aneurysm is usually adherent to this portion of the lobe and may be avulsed. Otherwise dissection is no different from that required in a standard approach to an aneurysm of the anterior communicating artery.

Clipping of the larger or ipsilateral anterior cerebral artery to treat anterior cerebral and anterior communicating artery aneurysms was advocated by Logue.[57] Pool and Potts and McKissock and associates could not show this method of treatment to be of benefit in their series.[66,84] The Cooperative Study found a high operative mortality rate with this method, but on review of the cases involved, Skultety and Nishioka believed that the procedure had been frequently employed in the face of catastrophe rather than as a primary procedure.[102] More recent series have reported favorable results.[37,94] The authors do not believe that proximal ligation is the optimal treatment for anterior communicating artery aneurysms.

Aneurysms of the distal anterior cerebral artery (pericallosal artery) arise at the origins of the frontopolar or callosomarginal arteries, although more peripherally placed aneurysms occasionally are encountered. The location of these aneurysms is such that they cannot ordinarily be approached satisfactorily through a fronto-temporosphenoidal craniotomy. The patient is placed in the supine position and the head is immobilized brow-up with skeletal fixation. A coronal incision is made behind the hairline, and a rectangular frontal craniot-omy is performed. The medial edge of the craniotomy should be placed over the middle of the superior sagittal sinus so that a rectangular dural flap hinged on the sinus will not compress it when retracted. The mesial frontal lobe is gently retracted a few millimeters to open the interhemispheric fissure. An attempt is made to preserve all bridging veins, although this is often not possible. A cortical artery should be followed proximally to lead the surgeon to the anterior cerebral artery in the corpus callosum cistern. One can easily become disoriented if the callosomarginal artery is mistaken for the pericallosal (distal anterior cerebral) artery. The problem of the surgeon's becoming disoriented is more common when there is some degree of subfalcial herniation of the cingulate gyrus. Following the artery proximally will generally clarify its identity. Because of the limited subarachnoid space, a hematoma often is associated with aneurysms in this location. When a hematoma is present in a cingulate gyrus, dissection may proceed through this gyrus to reach the corpus callosum cistern. Otherwise the often adherent cingulate gyri should be separated by following arterial branches proximally. The subarachnoid cistern measures about 3 to 6 mm in width and height, and contains the paired pericallosal arteries. Special attention must be given to the close relationship of these arteries when the aneurysm neck is being prepared, as the opposite artery may be firmly adherent to the aneurysm and identification of the neck difficult. With adequate isolation of the neck, a clip is applied in the manner described earlier. Papaverine should be used liberally, as these smaller vessels are prone to mechanically induced spasm.

OPERATIVE RESULTS AND COMPLICATIONS

Background

As early as 1953, Norlén and Olivecrona were able to report a mortality rate of less than 4 per cent on 63 patients who were in satisfactory condition and underwent operation at least three weeks after they had sustained a subarachnoid hemorrhage.[77] Eight of fifteen patients on whom the same surgeons operated in the first two weeks after hemorrhage died. Steelman and associates presented a series of 25 patients, treated by operation, in which there were but two deaths.[103] In 1960 Poppen and Fager reported results of 95 intracranial operations for cerebral aneurysm.[87] Seventeen of the patients died following operation (18 per cent), 60 survived in good condition (63 per cent), and 11 survived in fair to poor condition (12 per cent). Six died subsequently, two of recurrent subarachnoid hemorrhage, and one sustained recurrent bleeding but survived. In the same year McKissock and associates reported a series of 599 patients with ruptured intracranial aneurysms, of whom 151 had undergone craniotomy and direct treatment of the aneurysm.[64] Fifty-seven of these patients (38 per cent) died in the rather extended follow-up period. Trying to balance the many variables involved, McKissock came to the conclusion that at that time an intracranial operation could not be shown to provide definite benefit over conservative therapy. Hunt and associates reported their results with intracranial procedures in 55 patients and emphasized the preoperative grade as it related to the mortality rate.[40] There were no deaths among 32 grade I patients, one death among seven grade II patients (14 per cent), two deaths among nine grade III patients (22 per cent), four deaths among five grade IV patients (80 per cent), and both grade V patients died.

The results of these neurosurgeons and others were summarized by Skultety and Nishioka in their report on the Cooperative Study of Intracranial Aneurysms and Subarachnoid Hemorrhage.[102] The Cooperative Study provided for statistical analysis 979 patients who had undergone intracranial operation for treatment of cerebral aneurysm. These patients were derived from 24 participating centers. Analysis of the records, submitted between 1956 and 1964, of patients who had undergone operation for a single aneurysm on the anterior circulation showed mortality rates of 32 per cent for aneurysms on the internal carotid artery, 26 per cent for those on the middle cerebral artery, and 36 per cent for those on the anterior communicating artery. Furthermore, only 46 per cent of the entire group of patients showed a useful functional survival following intracranial operation. Thus, by the end of this study in 1965,

it appeared that while some skilled and experienced neurosurgeons could achieve excellent results in selected cases, the general neurosurgical experience in the treatment of intracerebral aneurysms did not demonstrate a clear advantage for intracranial operation over conservative management.

The past 10 years have seen a significant reduction in the operative mortality rate attending intracranial procedures for aneurysms. Improved neuroradiological capabilities, the use of hypotensive agents and mechanical and pharmaceutical control of intracranial volume, and micro-operative techniques have all contributed toward this decreased mortality rate. In 1970, Bohm and Hugosson published a series of 200 patients with aneurysms, of whom 191 were subjected to intracranial operation.[9] Of 156 grade I and II patients, 3 died (2 per cent). The mortality rate was 5 per cent for 38 patients operated on less than 11 days after hemorrhage, and 0.8 per cent for patients operated on after more than 11 days. Thirty-six per cent of grade III patients in the group operated on under 11 days died, while there were no deaths among nine grade III patients in the group operated on after 11 days. In 1972, Pool reported a 7 per cent mortality rate in 56 patients with anterior communicating artery aneurysms that he had approached through a bifrontal craniotomy in which he used the operating microscope. Sixty-eight per cent of these patients, including 5 of the 15 in grades III or IV, showed excellent results.[83] In 1973, Guidetti presented the results of 98 aneurysm operations that he had performed under the operating microscope, with mortality rates of 2.5 per cent for patients in grades I to III and 55 per cent for patients in grades IV and V.[29] Hollin and Decker have recently reported their series of 70 internal carotid aneurysm operations with micro-operative technique. They had a 9 per cent mortality.[38] Zlotnik and associates reported a series of 137 patients of whom 6 per cent died.[124] Suzuki described his results in over 1000 cases undergoing operation without the microscope. Eight hundred ninety-seven of them had single aneurysms of the anterior circulation. He showed mortality rates of 6 per cent for anterior communicating artery aneurysms, 7 per cent for internal carotid artery aneurysms, and 5 per cent for middle cerebral artery aneurysms.[107] Sengupta and co-workers have described 26 pa-

TABLE 48–3 RESULTS OF OPERATION FOR ANEURYSMS OF THE ANTERIOR CIRCULATION*

| ARTERY AND SITE | NUMBER OF CASES | RESULTS | | | | |
| | | Good | Fair | Poor | Death | |
					Operative	Other Cause
Internal carotid	235					
Ophthalmic artery	26	24	2	—	—	—
Medial wall (distal)	1	1	—	—	—	—
Inferior wall	14	10	1	—	2	1
Lateral wall						
Posterior communicating artery	136	112	10	7	6	1
Anterior choroidal artery	14	11	—	1	2	—
Bifurcation	44	38	4	1	1	—
Middle cerebral	132					
Sphenoid	14					
Bifurcation	112	98	18	6	9	1
Distal	6					
Anterior cerebral	311					
Proximal anterior cerebral artery	8	7	—	—	—	1
Anterior communicating artery	283	246	11	12	7	7
Pericallosal artery	20	17	1	2	—	—
	678	564	47	29	27	11

* Results are for 678 patients with intracranial aneurysms of the anterior circulation who were treated from 1967 through 1976.

tients with anterior communicating artery aneurysms operated on without the use of the microscope with no operative deaths.[98] Many factors and variables go into mortality figures, and these selected series are presented only to give an idea of the present state of operative treatment. While it is unlikely that these results represent an average cross section of neurosurgical practice, the advances that have been made in the field of aneurysm procedures have nevertheless been of value to each neurosurgeon who undertakes an intracranial aneurysm operation.

TABLE 48–4 OPERATIVE RESULTS RELATED TO PREOPERATIVE GRADE

TIME ELAPSED	RESULTS											
	Good						Fair					
	Preoperative Grade						Preoperative Grade					
	I	II	III	IV	V	Total	I	II	III	IV	V	Total
<3 days	4	7	2	2	2	17	—	—	3	1	—	4
3–7 days	18	13	16	8	—	55	—	—	6	6	—	12
7–14 days	32	38	30	8	—	108	—	1	5	3	—	9
2–4 weeks	42	64	53	12	—	171	2	1	6	7	—	16
1–3 months	47	63	52	1	—	163	2	3	—	—	—	5
>3 months	12	8	2	—	—	22	—	—	—	—	—	—
	155	193	155	31	2	536	4	5	20	17	—	46

* Results are for 638 patients with ruptured aneurysms of the anterior circulation. Time elapsed is between the last subarachnoid hemorrhage and operation.

Present Series

Between 1967 and 1976, the senior author has had the opportunity to operate on 678 intracranial aneurysms of the anterior circulation. Forty of these patients had unruptured aneurysms. Table 48–3 summarizes the location of these aneurysms and the results that were obtained in each group of patients. Table 48–4 relates the preoperative grade, postoperative condition, and time elapsed from the day of hemorrhage to the day of operation in the combined group of patients. Postoperative results have been designated as follows:

Good—returned to normal occupation with no or minimal neurological deficit.

Fair—returned to work in a more limited capacity because of residual neurological deficit.

Poor—required supportive care because of serious neurological deficit.

Operative death—died from causes directly related to operation or to cerebral injury.

Death due to other causes—doing well neurologically but died of a medical complication such as pulmonary embolism or myocardial infarction.

The overall operative mortality rate was 4 per cent, with an additional 1.6 per cent of patients subsequently dying of pulmonary embolism or myocardial infarction. The mortality rate for patients in grades I and II was 0.8 per cent; for those in grade III, 4.8 per cent; for those in grade IV, 8 per cent; and for those in grade V, 75 per cent. It is of interest that of patients in grade IV undergoing operation, 64 per cent, usually patients with intracranial hematomas, recovered to a good or fair status. Furthermore, of 72 patients in grades I to III who were operated on within the first week after subarachnoid hemorrhage, only one patient in grade II and two patients in grade III died, while of 32 patients in grade IV, 17 returned to a good or fair status, and 2 patients in grade V made good recoveries.

Tables 48–5, 48–6, and 48–7 list the preoperative grade and postoperative results for aneurysms at the three major locations: supraclinoid internal carotid artery, middle cerebral artery, and anterior cerebral–anterior communicating artery complex. It is seen that the mortality rate for better grade patients does not vary significantly in relation to the location of the aneurysm. Several patients with middle cerebral artery aneurysms underwent operation in terminal condition because of large intracranial hematomas with marked shifts of midline structures. These cases contribute to the relatively higher mortality rate seen in the series of middle cerebral artery aneurysms. Internal carotid artery aneurysms located on the ventral wall of the artery and at the

AND TIME LAPSE BETWEEN HEMORRHAGE AND OPERATION*

					RESULTS							
		Poor						Death				
		Preoperative Grade						Preoperative Grade				
I	II	III	IV	V	Total	I	II	III	IV	V	Total	Summary
—	—	—	3	1	4	—	—	—	4	9	13	38
—	—	—	7	—	7	—	1	2	1	—	4	78
—	1	2	5	—	8	—	—	2	1	—	3	128
—	1	3	5	—	9	—	—	3	—	—	3	199
—	—	—	1	—	1	1	1	2	—	—	4	173
—	—	—	—	—	—	—	—	—	—	—	—	22
—	2	5	21	1	29	1	2	9	6	9	27	638

anterior choroidal artery present technical difficulties, as discussed earlier, that cause these patients to fare less well than other patients with aneurysms. A patient in grade I and a patient in grade II with aneurysms in this location died.

Complications

Intracranial Hematoma

In 2 per cent of cases either epidural, subdural, or intracerebral hematoma devel-oped in the postoperative period. These were evacuated in each case but contributed to increased morbidity and a higher mortality rate.

Hydrocephalus

Between 5 and 10 per cent of patients developed communicating hydrocephalus that was associated with lethargy and focal neurological signs and that required shunting. Evaluation was made by angiography, pneumoencephalography, and isotope cisternography, and more recently by computed tomography.

TABLE 48–5   RESULTS OF OPERATION FOR ANEURYSMS OF THE INTRACRANIAL INTERNAL CAROTID ARTERY*

SITE OF ANEURYSM	PREOPERATIVE GRADE	NO. OF PATIENTS	RESULTS			Death	
			Good	Fair	Poor	Operative	Other Cause
Ophthalmic artery	I	8	8	—	—	—	—
	II	10	9	1	—	—	—
	III	6	5	1	—	—	—
	IV	1	1	—	—	—	—
	V	1	1	—	—	—	—
		26	24	2	—	—	—
Anterior choroidal artery	I	4	3	—	—	1	—
	II	6	6	—	—	—	—
	III	4	2	—	1	1	—
	IV	—	—	—	—	—	—
	V	—	—	—	—	—	—
		14	11	—	1	2	—
Posterior communicating artery	I	27	27	—	—	—	—
	II	72	61	6	4	—	1
	III	21	16	2	1	2	—
	IV	14	8	2	1	3	—
	V	2	—	—	1	1	—
		136	112	10	7	6	1[a]
Carotid bifurcation artery	I	23	23	—	—	—	—
	II	5	5	—	—	—	—
	III	11	10	—	—	1[b]	—
	IV	5	—	4	1	—	—
	V	—	—	—	—	—	—
		44	38	4	—	1	—
Carotid artery (inferior)	I	2	2	—	—	—	—
	II	6	4	1	—	1	—
	III	3	3	—	—	—	—
	IV	1	—	—	—	—	1
	V	1	—	—	—	1	—
		13	9	1	—	2	1

[a] Pulmonary embolism
[b] Rebleeding

* Results for 233 patients with aneurysms of the intracranial internal carotid artery are shown in relation to preoperative grade.

TABLE 48–6 RESULTS OF OPERATION FOR ANEURYSMS OF MIDDLE CEREBRAL ARTERY*

SITE OF ANEURYSM	PREOPERATIVE GRADE	NO. OF PATIENTS	RESULTS				
			Good	Fair	Poor	Death	
						Operative	Other Cause
Middle cerebral	I	44	42	2	—	—	—
artery	II	29	25	2	1	—	1
	III	40	27	10	2	1	—
	IV	11	3	4	3	1	—
	V	8	1	—	—	7	—
		132	98	18	6	9	1[a]

[a] Cardiac infarct

* Results for 132 patients with aneurysms of the middle cerebral artery are shown in relation to preoperative grade.

Epilepsy

A few patients developed seizures in the postoperative period. All patients were treated with diphenylhydantoin in the preoperative and postoperative periods unless there was specific allergy. Postoperative seizures were fairly easily controlled by increasing the dosage of diphenylhydantoin or adding phenobarbital or chloral hydrate.

Infection

Wound infections occurred in about 1 per cent of patients. One patient developed meningitis, and another developed osteomyelitis of the bone flap and subsequently brain abscess. Nonneurosurgical infections included urinary tract infection, pneumonia, and lower extremity and pelvic thrombophlebitis. Most of these latter infections occurred in patients in poorer postoperative condition who were not ambulatory and required supportive care.

Cerebrospinal Fluid Rhinorrhea

Rhinorrhea developed in a few patients and was thought to be due to openings into the frontal sinuses, made either when turn-

TABLE 48–7 RESULTS OF OPERATION FOR ANEURYSMS OF ANTERIOR CEREBRAL–ANTERIOR COMMUNICATING ARTERY COMPLEX*

SITE OF ANEURYSM	PREOPERATIVE GRADE	NO. OF PATIENTS	RESULTS				
			Good	Fair	Poor	Death	
						Operative	Other Cause
Anterior communicating	I	60	57	2	—	—	1
artery	II	71	66	2	—	1	2
	III	105	91	3	4	4 (3)[a]	3
	IV	55	39	4	8	2 (1)[a]	2
	V	—	—	—	—	—	—
		291	253	11	12	7	8[b]

[a] Recurrent subarachnoid hemorrhage
[b] Pulmonary embolism

* Results for 291 patients of the anterior cerebral–anterior communicating artery complex are shown in relation to preoperative grade.

ing the craniotomy flap or while drilling holes for tack-up sutures. Any opening into the sinus should be plugged with muscle and carefully waxed; additionally in this series, a self-hardening bonding agent was used to cover this opening.

Psycho-Organic Syndrome

Many patients, especially those with ruptured anterior communicating artery aneurysms, demonstrated changes in personality, concentration, and mental abilities in the postoperative period. In about 6 per cent of patients this picture appeared in the preoperative period, while in an additional 2 per cent it was first noted after operation. It is probable that injury to the orbitobasal frontal lobes and to the diencephalon contributes to this problem.

General Medical Complications

Pulmonary embolism, gastrointestinal hemorrhage, myocardial infarction, and a variety of other medical problems were encountered.

CONCLUSION

This chapter has presented the basic concepts of preoperative evaluation and planning, intraoperative considerations and techniques, and postoperative results and complications of the treatment of intracranial aneurysms by operative procedures. Differences of opinion exist regarding almost every aspect of operative treatment of aneurysms, and excellent results have been obtained by neurosurgeons employing a variety of methods. It is the belief of the authors that micro-operative techniques and the operating microscope significantly enhance the ability of the neurosurgeon to operate successfully on cerebral aneurysms. Exposure of the well-lighted fine anatomy to binocular vision adds considerable ease and safety to the dissection and control of these lesions. Nevertheless, these technical aids do not replace a thorough understanding of anatomy, nor can they replace judgment and experience in the treatment of the individual patient. Furthermore, considerable laboratory experience is required if the neurosurgeon is to employ these techniques in a useful and meaningful way.

The operative treatment of patients who are in good condition has become quite satisfactory. Much of the future research into cerebral aneurysms will concern methods for improving the patient who is badly injured by the initial hemorrhage, the prevention of rebleeding until a patient is in satisfactory condition, management of very large aneurysms not amenable to clipping or ligation, primary repair of damaged normal vessels, revascularization procedures, and further clarification of the problems of cerebrovascular spasm, cerebral edema, hydrocephalus, and hypothalamic dysfunction that occur with subarachnoid hemorrhage.

REFERENCES

1. Adams, J. E.: Clinical experience with hypothermia. *In* Fields, W. S., and Sahs, A. L.: Intracranial Aneurysms and Subarachnoid Hemorrhage. Springfield, Ill., Charles C Thomas, 1965, pp. 275–294.
2. Alexander, S. C., Cohen, P. J., Wollman, H., Smith, T. C., Reivick, M., and Van der Molen, R. A.: Cerebral carbohydrate metabolism during hypocarbia in man: Studies during nitrous oxide anesthesia. Anesthesiology, 26:624–632, 1965.
3. Alksne, J. F., and Rand, R. W.: Current status of metallic thrombosis of intracranial aneurysms. Progr. Neurol. Surg., 3:212–229, 1969.
4. Alksne, J. F., and Smith, R. W.: Iron-acrylic compound for stereotaxic aneurysm thrombosis. J. Neurosurg., 47:137–141, 1977.
5. Allcock, J. M.: Aneurysms. *In* Newton, T. H., and Potts, D. G.: Radiology of the Skull and Brain. Angiography. Vol II, Book 4. St. Louis, C. V. Mosby Co., 1974, pp. 2472–2473.
6. Allcock, J. M., and Drake, C. G.: Ruptured intracranial aneurysms—the role of arterial spasm. J. Neurosurg., 22:21–29, 1965.
7. Ask-Upmark, E., and Ingvar, D.: A follow-up examination of 138 cases of subarachnoid hemorrhage. Acta Med. Scand., 138:15–31, 1950.
8. Bloor, B. M., Majzoub, H. S., Nugent, G. R., and Carrion, C. A.: Cerebrovascular hemodynamics in intracranial hemorrhage. Excerpta Med. No. 293:46, 1973.
9. Bohm, E., and Hugosson, R.: Results of surgical treatment of 200 consecutive arterial aneurysms. Acta Neurol. Scand., 46:43–52, 1970.
10. Botterell, E. H., Lougheed, W. M., Scott, J. W., and Vanderwater, S. L.: Hypothermia and interruption of carotid, or carotid and vertebral circulation, in the surgical management of intracranial aneurysms. J. Neurosurg., 13:1–42, 1956.
11. Dandy, W. E.: Intracranial Arterial Aneurysms. New York, Hafner Press, 1944, reprinted 1969, pp. 67–90.
12. Davidoff, L. M., and Dyke, C. G.: The Normal

Encephalogram. Philadelphia, Lea & Febiger, 1946.

13. Dick, A. R., McCallum, M. E., Maxwell, J. A., and Nelson, S. R.: Effect of dexamethasone on experimental brain edema in cats. J. Neurosurg., *45*:141–147, 1976.

14. Dott, N. M.: Intracranial aneurysms: Cerebral arterioradiography: Surgical treatment. Trans. Med. Chir. Soc. Edinburgh, *112*:219–240, 1933.

15. Drake, C. G.: Cerebral aneurysm surgery—an update. Princeton Conference, Jan. 1976.

16. Dutton, J.: Intracranial aneurysm. A new method of surgical treatment. Brit. Med. J., *2*:585, 1956.

17. Dutton, J.: Acrylic investment of intracranial aneurysms. A report of 12 years' experience. J. Neurosurg., *31*:652–657, 1969.

18. Ecker, A., and Riemenschneider, P. A.: Arteriographic demonstration of spasm of the intracranial arteries with special reference to saccular arterial aneurysms. J. Neurosurg., *8*:660–667, 1951.

19. Foltz, E. L., and Ward, A. A., Jr.: Communicating hydrocephalus from subarachnoid bleeding. J. Neurosurg., *13*:546–566, 1956.

20. French, L. A., Chou, S. N., and Long, D. M.: The direct approach to intracranial aneurysms. Clin. Neurosurg., *15*:117–128, 1968.

21. Galera, R., and Greitz, T.: Hydrocephalus in the adult secondary to ruptured intracranial arterial aneurysms. J. Neurosurg., *32*:634–641, 1970.

22. Galicich, J. H., French, L. A., and Melby, J. C.: Use of dexamethasone in treatment of cerebral edema associated with brain tumors. J. Lancet, *81*:46–53, 1961.

23. Gallagher, J. P.: Pilojection for intracranial aneurysms. Report of progress. J. Neurosurg., *21*:129–134, 1964.

24. Gillingham, F. J.: The management of ruptured intracranial aneurysm. Ann. Roy. Coll. Surg., *23*:89–117, 1958.

25. Gillingham, F. J.: The management of ruptured intracranial aneurysms. Scot. Med. J., *12*:377–383, 1967.

26. Gillingham, F. J., Barbera, J., Myint, U. M., and Madan, V. S.: Ruptured intracranial aneurysm. Factors influencing prognosis. Pfizer Symposium of "Stroke," Edinburgh, Scotland, 1976.

27. Graf, C. J., and Nibbelink, D. W.: Cooperative Study of Intracranial Aneurysms and Subarachnoid Hemorrhage. Report on a randomized treatment study. Stroke, *5*:559–601, 1974.

28. Greenwood, J., Jr.: Two point coagulation. A new principle and instrument for applying coagulation current in neurosurgery. Amer. J. Surg., *50*:267–270, 1940.

29. Guidetti, B.: Results of 98 intracranial aneurysm operations performed with the aid of an operating microscope. Acta Neurochir., *29*:65–71, 1973.

30. Gurdjian, E. S., and Thomas, L. M.: Operative Neurosurgery. 3rd ed. Baltimore, Williams & Wilkins, 1970, pp. 324–333.

31. Hamby, W. B.: Intracranial Aneurysms. Springfield, Ill., Charles C Thomas, 1952.

32. Handa, H., Ohta, T., and Kamijyo, Y.: Encasement of intracranial aneurysms with plastic compounds. Progr. Neurol. Surg., *3*:149–192, 1969.

33. Hayashi, M., Marukawa, S., Fujii, H., Kitano, T., et al.: Intracranial hypertension in patients with ruptured intracranial aneurysm. J. Neurosurg., *46*:584–590, 1977.

34. Hayreh, S. S.: The ophthalmic artery. *In* Newton, T. H., and Potts, D. G.: Radiology of the Skull and Brain. Angiography, Vol II, Book 2. St. Louis, C. V. Mosby Co., 1974, p. 1334.

35. Heifetz, M. D.: A new intracranial aneurysm clip. J. Neurosurg., *30*:753, 1969.

36. Heiskanen, O.: Multiple intracranial aneurysms. Acta Neurol. Scand., *41*:356–362, 1965.

37. Hockley, A. D.: Proximal occlusion of the anterior cerebral artery for anterior communicating aneurysm. J. Neurosurg., *43*:426–431, 1975.

38. Hollin, S. A., and Decker, R. E.: Microsurgical treatment of internal carotid artery aneurysms. J. Neurosurg., *47*:142–149, 1977.

39. Hunt, W. E., and Hess, R. M.: Surgical risk as related to time of intervention in the repair of intracranial aneurysms. J. Neurosurg., *28*:14–20, 1968.

40. Hunt, W. E., Meagher, J. N., and Barnes, J. E.: The management of intracranial aneurysm. J. Neurosurg., *19*:34–40, 1962.

41. Jefferson, G.: On the saccular aneurysms of the internal carotid artery in the cavernous sinus. Brit. J. Surg., *26*:267–302, 1938.

42. Jennett, N. B., Barker, J., Fitch, W., et al.: Effect of anesthesia on intracranial pressure in patients with space-occupying lesions. Lancet, *1*:61–64, 1969.

43. Keaney, N. P., Pickfrout, V. W., McDowall, D. G., et al.: Cerebral circulatory and metabolic effects of hypotension produced by deep halothane anesthesia. J. Neurol. Neurosurg. Psychiat., *36*:898–905, 1973.

44. Kelly, P. J., Gorten, R. J., Grossman, R. G., and Eisenberg, H. M.: Cerebral perfusion, vascular spasm and outcome in patients with ruptured intracranial aneurysms. J. Neurosurg., *47*:44–49, 1977.

45. Kempe, L. G.: Operative Neurosurgery. Vol 1. Cranial, Cerebral and Intravascular Diseases. Berlin, Heidelberg, New York, Springer-Verlag, 1968, pp. 1–75.

46. Key, A., and Retzius, G.: Studien in der Anatomie des Nervensystems und des Bindegewebes. Stockholm, P. A. Norstad u. Soner, 1875.

47. Klafta, L. A., Jr., and Hamby, W. B.: Significance of cerebrospinal fluid pressure in determining time for repair of intracranial aneurysms. J. Neurosurg., *31*:217–219, 1969.

48. Krayenbühl, H.: Das Hirnaneurysm. Schweiz. Arch. Neurol. Psychiat., *47*:155–236, 1941.

49. Krayenühl, H., and Yasargil, M. G.: Cerebral Angiography. 2nd Ed. Philadelphia, J. B. Lippincott Co., 1968.

50. Kribs, R., and Kleuhues, P.: The recurrent artery of Heubner. *In* Zulch, K. J., ed.: Cerebral Circulation and Stroke. Berlin, Heidelberg, New York, Springer-Verlag, 1971, pp. 40–56.

51. Kusske, J. A., Turner, P. T., Ojemann, G. A., and Harris, A. B.: Ventriculostomy for the

treatment of acute hydrocephalus following subarachnoid hemorrhage. J. Neurosurg., 38:591–595, 1973.

52. Laitinen, L., and Snellman, A.: Aneurysms of the pericallosal artery. A study of 14 cases verified angiographically and treated mainly by direct surgical attack. J. Neurosurg., 17:447–458, 1960.

53. Lazorthes, G.: Vascularisation et Circulation Cérébrales. Paris, Masson & Cie, 1961.

54. Liliequist, B.: The subarachnoid cisterns. An anatomic and roentgenologic study. Acta Radiol. Suppl. 185, 1959, pp. 1–108.

55. Liliequist, B., Lindqvist, M., and Probst, F.: Rupture of intracranial aneurysm during carotid angiography. Neuroradiology, 11:185–190, 1976.

56. Locksley, H. B.: Report on the cooperative study of intracranial aneurysms and subarachnoid hemorrhage. Section V, Part II. Natural history of subarachnoid hemorrhage, intracranial aneurysms and arteriovenous malformations. Based on 6368 cases in the cooperative study. J. Neurosurg., 25:321–368, 1966.

57. Logue, V.: Surgery in spontaneous subarachnoid hemorrhage. Operative treatment of aneurysms on the anterior cerebral and anterior communicating artery. Brit. Med. J., 1:473–479, 1956.

58. Lougheed, W. M., and Marshall, B. M.: The place of hypothermia in the treatment of intracranial aneurysms. Progr. Neurol. Surg., 3:115–148, 1969.

59. Lougheed, W. M., and Marshall, B. M.: Management of aneurysms of the anterior circulation by intracranial procedures. In Youmans, J. R., ed.: Neurological Surgery. Vol. 2. Philadelphia, W. B. Saunders Co., 1973, pp. 731–767.

60. Malis, L. I.: Bipolar coagulation in microsurgery. In Donaghy, R. M. P., and Yasargil, M. G.: Micro-vascular Surgery. Stuttgart, G. Thieme; St. Louis, C. V. Mosby Co., 1967, pp. 126–130.

61. Mayfield, F. H., and Kees, G., Jr.: A brief history of the development of the Mayfield clip. Technical note. J. Neurosurg., 35:97–100, 1971.

62. McDowall, D. G.: The effects of clinical concentrations of halothane on the blood flow and oxygen uptake of the cerebral cortex. Brit. J. Anaesth., 39:186–196, 1967.

63. McKenzie, K. G.: Some minor modifications of Harvey Cushing's silver clip outfit. Surg. Gynec. Obstet., 45:549–550, 1927.

64. McKissock, W., Paine, K. W. E., and Walsh, L.: An analysis of the results of treatment of ruptured intracranial aneurysms. Report of 772 consecutive cases. J. Neurosurg., 17:762–776, 1960.

65. McKissock, W., Richardson, A., and Walsh, L.: Anterior communicating aneurysms. A trial of conservative and surgical treatment. Lancet, 1:873–876, 1965.

66. McKissock, W., Paine, K. W. E., Walsh, L., and Owen, F.: Multiple intracranial aneurysms. Lancet, 1:623–636, 1964.

67. McMurtry, J. G., Housepian, E. M., Bowman, F. O., and Matteo, R. S.: Surgical treatment of basilar artery aneurysms. Elective circulatory arrest with thoracotomy in 12 cases. J. Neurosurg., 40:486–494, 1974.

68. Millikan, C. H.: Cerebral vasospasm and ruptured intracranial aneurysm. Arch. Neurol., 32:433, 1975.

69. Moníz, E.: L'encephalographie arterielle, son importance dans la localisation des tumeurs cérébrales. Rev. Neurol. (Paris), 2:72–90, 1927.

70. Morgagni, J. B.: De sedibus er causis morborum per anatomia indagatis. Venetiis ex typog. Remondiniana. 1791. (Cited in Walton, J. N.: Subarachnoid Haemorrhage. Edinburgh and London, E. & S. Livingstone Ltd., 1956.)

71. Mount, L. A., and Antunes, J. L.: Results of treatment of intracranial aneurysms by wrapping and coating. J. Neurosurg., 42:189–193, 1975.

72. Mullan, S.: Experiences with surgical thrombosis of intracranial berry aneurysms and carotid cavernous fistulas. J. Neurosurg., 41:657–670, 1974.

73. Mullan, S.: Conservative management of the recently ruptured aneurysm. Surg. Neurol., 3:27–32, 1975.

74. Mullan, S., and Dawley, J.: Antifibrinolytic therapy for intracranial aneurysms. J. Neurosurg., 28:21–23, 1968.

75. Mullan, S., Reyes, C., Dawley, J., and Dobben, G.: Stereotactic copper electric thrombosis of intracranial aneurysms. Progr. Neurol. Surg., 3:193–211, 1969.

76. Nibbelink, D. W., Torner, J. C., and Henderson, W. G.: Intracranial aneurysm and subarachnoid hemorrhage. A cooperative study. Antifibrinolytic therapy in recent onset subarachnoid hemorrhage. Stroke, 6:622–629, 1975.

77. Norlén, G., and Olivecrona, H.: The treatment of aneurysms of the circle of Willis. J. Neurosurg., 10:404–415, 1953.

78. Northfield, D. W. C.: Comment on Norlén, G.: The pathology, diagnosis and treatment of intracranial saccular aneurysms. Proc. Roy. Soc. Med., 45:302, 1952.

79. Padget, D. H.: The circle of Willis. Its embryology and anatomy. In Dandy, W. E.: Intracranial Arterial Aneurysms. Reprint of 1944 ed. New York, Hafner Publishing Co., 1969, pp. 67–90.

80. Pakarinen, S.: Incidence, aetiology, and prognosis of primary subarachnoid hemorrhage. Acta Neurol. Scand., Suppl. 29:1–28, 1967.

81. Parkinson, D.: A surgical approach to the cavernous portion of the carotid artery. Anatomical studies and case report. J. Neurosurg., 23:474–483, 1965.

82. Perlmutter, D., and Rhoton, A. L.: Microsurgical anatomy of the anterior cerebral–anterior communicating–recurrent artery complex. J. Neurosurg., 45:259–272, 1976.

83. Pool, J. L.: Bifrontal craniotomy for anterior communicating artery aneurysms. J. Neurosurg., 36:212–220, 1972.

84. Pool, J. L., and Potts, D. G.: Aneurysms and Arteriovenous Anomalies of the Brain. Diagnosis and Treatment. New York, Evanston, London, Harper & Row, 1965.

85. Poppen, J. L.: An Atlas of Neurosurgical Techniques. Philadelphia, W. B. Saunders Co., 1960.

86. Poppen, J. L., and Fager, C.: Multiple intracranial aneurysms. J. Neurosurg., *16*:581–589, 1959.

87. Poppen, J. L., and Fager, C.: Intracranial aneurysms. Results of surgical treatment. J. Neurosurg., *17*:283–296, 1960.

88. Pressman, B. D., Gilbert, G. E., and Davis, D. O.: Computerized transverse tomography of vascular lesions of the brain. Part II. Aneurysms. Amer. J. Roentgen., *124*:215–219, 1975.

89. Raimondi, A. J., and Torres, H.: Acute hydrocephalus as complication of subarachnoid hemorrhage. Surg. Neurol., *1*:23–26, 1973.

90. Riggs, H., and Rupp, C.: Miliary aneurysms; relation of anomalies of the circle of Willis to formation of aneurysms. Arch. Neurol. Psychiat., *49*:615–616, 1943.

91. Riggs. H. E., and Rupp, C.: Variation of form of circle of Willis. Arch. Neurol., *8*:8–14, 1963.

92. Sachs, E., Jr.: The fate of muscle and cotton wrapped about intracranial carotid arteries and aneurysms. A laboratory and clinicopathologic study. Acta Neurochir., *26*:121–137, 1972.

93. Schneck, S. A., and Kricheff, I. I.: Intracranial aneurysm rupture, vasospasm and infarction. Arch. Neurol., *11*:668–680, 1964.

94. Scott, M.: Ligation of an anterior cerebral artery for aneurysms of the anterior communicating artery complex. J. Neurosurg., *38*:481–487, 1973.

95. Scoville, W. B.: Miniature torsion bar spring aneurysm clip. Technical suggestion. J. Neurosurg., *25*:97, 1966.

96. Selker, R. G., Wolfson, S. K., Jr., Maroon, J. C. and Steichen, F. M.: Preferential cerebral hypothermia with elective cardiac arrest: Resection of "giant" aneurysm. Surg. Neurol., *6*:173–179, 1976.

97. Selverstone, B.: Treatment of intracranial aneurysms with adherent plastics. Clin. Neurosurg., *9*:201–213, 1963.

98. Sengupta, R. P., Chiu, J. S. P., and Brierly, H.: Quality of survival following direct surgery for anterior communicating artery aneurysm. J. Neurosurg., *43*:58–64, 1975.

99. Serbinenko, F. A.: Balloon catheterization and occlusion of major cerebral vessels. J. Neurosurg., *41*:125–145, 1974.

100. Shulman, K., Martin, B. F., Popoff, N., and Ransohoff, J.: Recognition and treatment of hydrocephalus following spontaneous subarachnoid hemorrhage. J. Neurosurg., *20*:1040–1047, 1963.

101. Siegel, P., Moraca, P. P., and Green, J. R.: Sodium nitroprusside in the surgical treatment of cerebral aneurysms and arteriovenous malformations. Brit. J. Anaesth., *43*:790–795, 1971.

102. Skultety, F. M., and Nishioka, H.: Report on the cooperative study of intracranial aneurysms and subarachnoid hemorrhage. Section VIII, Part 2. The results of intracranial surgery in the treatment of aneurysms. J. Neurosurg., *25*:683–704, 1966.

103. Steelman, H. F., Hayes, G. J., and Rizzoli, H. V.: Surgical treatment of saccular intracranial aneurysms. J. Neurosurg., *10*:564–570, 1953.

104. Stehbens, W. E.: Aneurysms and anatomical variation of cerebral arteries. Arch. Path., *75*:45–64, 1963.

105. Stephens, R. B., and Stilwell, D. I.: Arteries and Veins of the Human Brain. Springfield, Ill., Charles C Thomas, 1969.

106. Sugita, K., Hirota, T., Iguchi, I., and Mizutani, T.: Comparative study of the pressure of various aneurysm clips. J. Neurosurg., *44*:723–727, 1976.

107. Suzuki, J.: Direct surgery of intracranial aneurysms. Inst. Neurol. Madras Proc., *6*:15–23, 1976.

108. Symonds, C. P.: Spontaneous subarachnoid hemorrhage. Quart. J. Med., *18*:93–122, 1924.

109. Taveras, J. M., and Wood, E. H.: Diagnostic Neuroradiology. Baltimore, Williams & Wilkins, 1964, pp. 17–27.

110. Tinker, J. H., and Michenfelder, J. D.: Sodium nitroprusside: Pharmacology, toxicology and therapeutics. Anesthesiology, *45*:340–354, 1976.

111. Tovi, D.: Studies on fibrinolysis in the central nervous system with special reference to intracranial hemorrhage and to the effect of antifibrinolytic drugs. Umea University Medical Dissertations No. 8. Umea, Sweden, Centraltryckeriet, 1972.

112. Troupp, H., and Björkesten, G. af: Results of a controlled trial of late surgical versus conservative treatment of intracranial aneurysms. J. Neurosurg., *35*:20–24, 1971.

113. Uihlein, A., and Huges, R. A.: The surgical treatment of intracranial vestigial aneurysms. Surg. Clin. N. Amer., *35*:1071–1083, 1955.

114. Uihlein, A., MacCarty, C. S., Michenfelder, J. D., Terry, H. R., and Daw, E. F.: Deep hypothermia and surgical treatment of intracranial aneurysms. A five-year survey. J.A.M.A., *195*:639–641, 1966.

115. Walton, J. N.: Subarachnoid Hemorrhage. Edinburgh and London, E. & S. Livingstone Ltd., 1956.

116. Wilks, S.: Sanguineous meningeal effusion (apoplexy); spontaneous and from injury. Guy's Hosp. Rep., *5*:119–127, 1859. (Cited in Hamby, W. B.: Intracranial Aneurysms. Springfield, Ill., Charles C Thomas, 1952.)

117. Winn, H. R., Richardson, A. E., and Jane, J. A.: Late mortality and morbidity in cerebral aneurysms. A ten-year follow-up of 364 conservatively treated patients with a single cerebral aneurysm. Trans. Amer. Neurol. Ass., *98*:148–150, 1973.

118. Wollman, H., Alexander, S. C., Cohen, P. J., Chose, P. E., Melman, E., and Behar, M. G.: Cerebral circulation of man during halothane anesthesia: Effects of hypocarbia and d-tubocurarine. Anesthesiology, *25*:180–184, 1964.

119. Yasargil, M. G.: Microsurgery Applied to Neurosurgery. New York-London, Academic Press; Stuttgart, Georg Thieme Verlag, 1969.

120. Yasargil, M. G., Fox, J. L., and Ray, M. W.: The operative approach to aneurysms of the anterior communicating artery. *In* Krayenbühl, H.:

Advances and Technical Standards in Neurosurgery. Vol. 2. New York-Wien, Springer-Verlag, 1975, pp. 113–170.

121. Yasargil. M. G., Kasdaglis, K., Jain, K. K., and Weber, H. P.: Anatomical observations of the subarachnoid cisterns of the brain during surgery. J. Neurosurg., *44*:298–302, 1976.

122. Yasargil, M. G., Yonekawa, Y., Zumstein, B., and Stahl, H. J.: Hydrocephalus following subarachnoid hemorrhage. Clinical features and treatment. J. Neurosurg., *39*:474–479, 1973.

123. Zingesser, L. H., Schechter, M. M., Dexter, J., et al.: On the significance of spasm associated with rupture of a cerebral aneurysm: The relationship between spasm as noted angiographically and 71 regional blood flow determinations. Arch. Neurol., *18*:520–528, 1968.

124. Zlotnik, E. I., Oleshkevich, F. V., and Stolkarts, J. Z.: Microsurgical technique in the treatment of intracranial aneurysms. J. Neurosurg., *46*:591–595, 1977.

49

MANAGEMENT OF ANEURYSMS OF ANTERIOR CIRCULATION BY CAROTID ARTERY OCCLUSION

The operative management of intracranial aneurysms has been a source of controversy among neurosurgeons for several decades. McKissock and co-workers, in 1958, questioned whether operative treatment actually decreased the death rate.[45] In 1960, however, following a randomized study, it was found that carotid ligation, as compared with conservative therapy, significantly reduced the mortality rate associated with aneurysms of the internal carotid artery at the junction of the posterior communicating artery.[46] Carotid ligation has subsequently been used for years with a diminished incidence of recurrent subarachnoid hemorrhage and relatively low operative morbidity and mortality rates in the treatment of internal carotid aneurysms and anterior communicating aneurysms associated with a unilateral circulation. The operative technique described in this chapter, if properly used, provides effective treatment for aneurysms in these two locations. Recent advances in microvascular neurosurgical techniques have, however, allowed the direct obliteration of many of these lesions without rebleeding and with lower morbidity and mortality rates than can be obtained with carotid ligation. The role of carotid occlusion in the treatment of intracranial aneurysms must therefore be reassessed.

HISTORICAL BACKGROUND

Abernethy first attempted carotid ligation in 1798 as treatment for a lacerated internal carotid artery.[1-4,29] Although the patient died, carotid ligation attracted interest, and by 1803, both Fleming and Twitchell reported successful control of hemorrhage by carotid ligation.[26,84] In 1805, Cooper ligated the common carotid artery as treatment for an aneurysm of this vessel.[15] His first patient died early in the postoperative course, but four years later Cooper successfully treated a second patient with an extracranial internal carotid aneurysm by this method.[16,17] The patient tolerated the procedure well, and the aneurysm later decreased in size and became nonpulsatile.

No later than 1885, Horsley first used carotid ligation as treatment for an intracranial nonfistulous aneurysm.[9] While operating on a patient for a suspected brain tumor in the middle cranial fossa, he discovered a large pulsating mass arising from the right internal carotid artery. Ligation of the right common carotid artery proved efficacious, and the patient was in good health five years later. Nearly 40 years later, Wilfred Trotter became the first to ligate a carotid artery for a nonfistulous intracranial aneurysm without having first exposed the lesion.[67]

Matas made a noteworthy contribution to carotid ligation by devising a test to determine the efficiency of the collateral circulation to the brain. In patients requiring ligation of one carotid artery, he recommended trial occlusion for a specified time with an aluminum band that could be easily removed if neurological complications occurred. Today the Matas test is sometimes used to determine a patient's tolerance to permanent carotid ligation.

G. T. TINDALL AND A. S. FLEISCHER

No review of this subject would be complete without mention of the outstanding contribution made by Egas Moniz.[47] In 1927, he introduced cerebral arteriography in the diagnosis of intracranial tumors. Not only has this diagnostic procedure proved useful in localizing brain tumors, but it has also contributed invaluably to the field of intracranial vascular operations.

Interest in carotid ligation as a treatment for intracranial aneurysms was further stimulated by the reports of Schorstein in 1940 and Dandy in 1942.[19,67] Schorstein, in an analysis of 60 patients who had had carotid ligation for treatment of intracranial aneurysms, concluded that such an operation was safe in patients with infraclinoid aneurysms but was dangerous in patients with supraclinoid lesions.[67] On the basis of a large clinical experience with patients with intracranial vascular lesions treated by carotid ligation, Dandy recommended ligating the internal carotid artery in two stages: only partly at first, and completely one week later.[19] He contended that this two-stage method reduced the possibility of ischemic neurological complications resulting from carotid ligation.

With the introduction of adjustable clamps for gradual occlusion of the carotid artery, carotid ligation became even more widely practiced in the treatment of patients with intracranial aneurysms. Selverstone and White, Crutchfield, and Poppen and Fager all devised clamps that allow gradual closure of the carotid artery and thus reduce the incidence of ischemic neurological complications.[18,63,69]

Other important contributions toward refining the procedure of carotid ligation include: the use of ophthalmodynamometry or ocular pneumoplethysmography for monitoring indirectly the pressure changes in the internal carotid artery during gradual carotid ligation, the introduction of intravascular pressure measurements at the time of carotid ligation, the monitoring of ligation with cerebral blood flow and electroencephalography, the experimental study of the various physical forces acting on aneurysms, and the use of follow-up carotid angiography to evaluate changes in intracranial aneurysms after carotid ligation.*

The use of carotid ligation in treating intracranial aneurysms has a long and varied history. Numerous authors have discussed the development of this operative procedure, and the reader is referred to their publications for further elaboration of this subject.†

Recently, a long-term follow-up by Richardson and co-workers of the 60 patients in McKissock's 1960 series suggested that carotid ligation did not protect against late rebleeding, as had been reported during the early postoperative period.[65] This report—along with dramatic improvements over the last decade in microsurgical instrumentation and technique, improved magnification and illumination, and associated advances in neuroanesthesiology in which intraoperative hypotension, osmotic dehydrating agents, corticosteroids, and similar agents are used—has resulted in a decline in the popularity of this indirect form of therapy. Direct operative approach to most aneurysms has become the treatment of choice. Carotid ligation, however, does remain an invaluable form of therapy in certain situations.

PHYSIOLOGICAL STUDIES

Intravascular Pressure Measurements

The measurement of intravascular pressure in the carotid vessels has contributed considerably toward an understanding of the physiological changes in the intracranial circulation after carotid occlusion. Sweet and Bennett first measured intravascular pressure in the cervical portion of the internal carotid artery during temporary occlusion and concluded that a substantial reduction in distal intravascular pressure follows proximal carotid occlusion.[77] Their results were later confirmed by other investigators who attributed the success of carotid ligation in treating intracranial aneurysms to this reduction in intravascular pressure in the internal carotid system.[14,50,55,81] The fall in arterial pressure is accompanied by a decrease in the physical forces acting on the aneurysmal wall and a flow reduction in the lesion.[10] Moreover, Ecker and Riemenschneider demonstrated

---

* See references 7, 8, 10, 11, 14, 23, 27, 28, 30, 35, 36, 40, 43–45, 49–51, 53, 56, 64, 71, 76, 77, 81, 92–94.

† See references 29, 61, 66, 67, 86, 88.

arteriographically that extreme slowing of flow or actual stasis—a condition that could lead to intra-aneurysmal thrombosis —occurs in an intracranial aneurysm immediately after carotid occlusion.[23]

After successful measurements of pressure in the neck vessels, some investigators began making similar determinations in intracranial arteries during ipsilateral carotid arterial occlusion.[7,11,92,93] In 17 patients with intracranial vascular lesions, Woodhall and associates measured the pressure in the ipsilateral middle cerebral and internal carotid arteries during occlusion of the carotid vessels in the neck and found that the degree of pressure reduction in these arteries is similar quantitatively to that which occurs in the internal carotid artery in the neck.[92] Bakay and Sweet also recorded intravascular pressure in small intracranial arteries, including branches of the anterior cerebral artery, on the side of the occluded extracranial carotid vessels.[7] They too concluded that the degree of pressure reduction in the extracranial internal carotid artery immediately distal to an occlusion reliably indicates the decrease in arterial pressure that will occur throughout the ipsilateral internal carotid system. Because no one has directly measured the pressure in the ipsilateral anterior and middle cerebral arteries several months or years after ipsilateral carotid ligation, the duration of the pressure reduction in these vessels remains uncertain.

The determination of the pressure changes in the carotid vessels immediately after proximal common carotid occlusion has made it possible to ascertain the direction of flow in the ipsilateral internal-external carotid system.[77,83] Knowing the direction of flow in the system after ipsilateral common carotid occlusion is important in evaluating the adequacy of the intracranial collateral system.[83] Sweet and Bennett measured pressure in the internal carotid artery in eight patients during proximal common carotid occlusion.[77] When the pressure reduction had stabilized, they occluded the ipsilateral external carotid artery and noted the ensuing change in pressure in the internal carotid artery. They reasoned that if there were retrograde flow in the external carotid artery during common carotid occlusion, then the pressure in the internal carotid artery should be higher with the external carotid open than with it closed. In their series of cases, a small rise in pressure in the internal carotid occurred in three, a slight fall in three, and no change in pressure in two patients. In the three patients who showed a fall in internal carotid pressure coincident with external carotid occlusion, Sweet and Bennett correctly predicted that the direction of flow would be from external to internal carotid artery during closure of the common carotid. They postulated that patients who showed flow reversal in the external carotid artery during common carotid occlusion possessed a deficient intracranial collateral circulation. For this group of patients, they predicted, carotid ligation would be potentially hazardous. Later investigators confirmed that patients with a flow reversal in the internal carotid during ipsilateral occlusion of the common carotid artery usually have a well-developed intracranial arterial collateral circulation, whereas those who show flow reversal in the external carotid artery under the same circumstances ordinarily have an inadequate intracranial collateral circulation.[83]

The principal value of measuring internal carotid arterial pressure during proximal carotid occlusion at the time of applying the occlusive clamp to the common carotid artery is that the degree of pressure reduction thus obtained provides a relatively reliable means for predicting whether patients will tolerate carotid ligation.[78] These pressure data also provide an estimate of the number of days required for clamp closure. When the reduction in mean arterial pressure is less than 50 per cent, the clamp can usually be closed within three or four days, whereas when the reduction exceeds 50 per cent, complete closure may require five to seven days. When pressure reduction approaches 75 to 85 per cent, complete ligation may require 10 to 14 days, or may even be impossible. Seldom are pressure measurements at operation misleading. Infrequently a patient whose intravascular pressure falls slightly (30 per cent) may experience a neurological complication during gradual closure of the occlusive clamp after operation.

Retinal Artery Pressure Determination

The change in retinal arterial pressure on the side of carotid occlusion is similar quantitatively to the change in the cervical internal carotid artery after proximal common carotid occlusion.[80] This finding is not surprising, since the ophthalmic artery is the first major branch of the internal carotid and since intravascular pressure changes in the latter vessel are reflected in the ophthalmic artery. One large series of patients had an average reduction of 40 per cent in retinal arterial pressure (systolic), as compared with the opposite or control eye at the time of complete closure of the common carotid artery.[81] More important, a marked reduction in retinal arterial pressure is still demonstrable several months or years after carotid ligation. In a follow-up study of 11 patients in whom carotid ligation had been performed, Heyman and associates observed an average reduction of 23 per cent in retinal arterial pressure 6 to 19 months after carotid ligation.[31] This finding provides indirect evidence that the pressure in the intracranial internal carotid artery remains effectively reduced for many years.

Cerebral Blood Flow and the Electroencephalogram

There was a correlation between the reduction of cerebral blood flow determined by counting the clearance of gamma activity from the frontal and temporal region of patients after the intracarotid bolus injection of [133]xenon and the fall in the internal carotid artery pressure caused by temporary clamping (P < 0.01).[40] This method of monitoring allowed permanent carotid ligation without neurological deficit in 17 of the 20 patients monitored; in the other three patients diminution of blood flow of more than 50 per cent contraindicated ligation. The same study demonstrated that electroencephalographic slowing was usually associated with low cerebral blood flow, but exceptions occurred, making it unreliable as a prognosticating factor. Ligation was safe when, during temporary clamping, cerebral blood flow exceeded 40 ml per 100 gm per minute but was considered unsafe when flow was less than 20 ml per 100 gm per minute. In the range of 20 to 40 ml per 100 gm per minute, consideration of the internal carotid artery pressure permitted more patients to undergo ligation safely than did reliance on cerebral blood flow alone.

CEREBRAL ARTERIOGRAPHY

Cerebral arteriography, which discloses the cause of a spontaneous subarachnoid hemorrhage in most instances, should be done in all patients who have had such a hemorrhage. Aneurysms are a leading cause of subarachnoid hemorrhage, and prompt cerebral arteriography is essential to establish the diagnosis and permit prompt definitive treatment. Because unruptured aneurysms, particularly on the internal carotid artery, often compress the cranial nerves that supply the ocular structures, the diagnosis of an intracranial aneurysm should be suspected in patients with spontaneous onset, gradual or sudden, of paresis of cranial nerves II through VI.[33,34,54] Cerebral arteriography is indicated in these patients to help establish the cause of the cranial nerve involvement.

Four-vessel cerebral angiography via the femoral catheter route is advocated in all patients presenting with spontaneous subarachnoid hemorrhage and in patients with unruptured intracranial aneurysms presenting with clinical signs of mass effect, such as giant aneurysms of the cavernous internal carotid artery and the like. The location, configuration, and number of intracranial aneurysms visualized will determine the form of operative therapy indicated. The authors feel there is no advantage to obtaining cross compression arteriography, since the information obtained will not influence the choice of treatment. This has been confirmed in a recent study by Jawad and associates.[32]

Cerebral arteriography is useful in evaluating the results of operative treatment—either carotid ligation or craniotomy—of intracranial aneurysms. Tindall and his coworkers performed follow-up carotid arteriography in 58 patients who had had carotid ligation for internal carotid aneurysms and found that the aneurysm had become smaller or had undergone thrombosis in 74 per cent.[81] Cerebral arteriography has also shown that after successful obliteration of an intracranial aneurysm by clip ligation, a secondary aneurysm often develops between the clip and the wall of the parent artery. Allcock and Drake found that the aneurysmal sac was still present in 13 of 70 patients with intracranial aneurysms in whom the direct approach was used, although in 6 of these 13 patients, the aneurysmal sac was thought to have been completely obliterated at operation.[5]

In patients with ruptured aneurysms, cerebral arteriography often discloses intracranial vasospasm. When a moderate degree of vasospasm exists, operation is usually deferred. Cerebral arteriography can then be repeated several days later to evaluate the degree of intracranial vasospasm before a decision is made to operate.

As a general rule, cerebral arteriography should not be delayed, since the principal aim of therapy is to prevent recurrent hemorrhage. The earlier an etiological diagnosis is established by arteriography in a patient with subarachnoid hemorrhage, the sooner operation can be performed and the better the chance of avoiding recurrent subarachnoid hemorrhage. In patients who have had a subarachnoid hemorrhage and who show either minimal or no impairment in their level of consciousness and no neurological deficit, carotid arteriography should be done electively shortly following admission to the hospital.

COMPUTED TOMOGRAPHY

Currently, the initial study in the evaluation of patients with subarachnoid hemorrhage is the CT scan, which will disclose the presence of intracerebral hematoma, hydrocephalus, infarction, and possibly the site of ruptured aneurysm. Angiography remains essential to demonstrate cerebral vasospasm, however.

INDICATIONS FOR CAROTID LIGATION

Ruptured Internal Carotid Artery Aneurysms

As evidenced by the probable infrequency of recurrent hemorrhage, gradual ligation of the common or internal carotid artery in the neck has proved successful in treatment of aneurysms of the internal carotid artery. In one reported series, the incidence of recurrent hemorrhage among 136 patients after complete closure of the common carotid artery was only 3.7 per cent.[55] Numerous investigators have shown that carotid ligation significantly decreases the incidence of recurrent hemorrhage, pro-

duces a reduction in pressure in the ipsilateral internal carotid artery, results in a decrease in size or thrombosis of the aneurysm in most patients, and results in clinical improvement, that is, regression or clearing of paralysis of the third cranial nerve.*

For those internal carotid artery aneurysms at the junction of the ophthalmic artery, posterior communicating artery, anterior choroidal artery, or internal carotid bifurcation that have discernible necks and are readily accessible the authors feel that direct clip ligation is currently the treatment of choice, since several recent series have demonstrated no incidence of rebleeding and morbidity and mortality rates lower than those described with carotid ligation. For broad-based or giant aneurysms (greater than 2.5 cm diameter), however, particularly those at the junction of the ophthalmic artery underlying the anterior clinoid, or at the bifurcation of the internal carotid artery, common carotid ligation is felt to be the procedure of choice.

Giant Aneurysms or Inaccessible Aneurysms of the Internal Carotid Artery

Rupture of an aneurysm of the internal carotid artery within the cavernous sinus results in a carotid-cavernous fistula rather than subarachnoid hemorrhage. Carotid-cavernous fistulae are treated effectively in most patients by balloon occlusion of the fistula. If the intracavernous aneurysm has not ruptured and the aneurysm is symptomatic, however, then the gradual ligation of the common or internal carotid artery alone provides satisfactory therapy. Aneurysms of the petrous portion of the internal carotid artery are equally inaccessible, and when presenting with signs of mass effect such as cranial nerve compression or hemorrhage, should be treated with carotid ligation.[48]

Certain Anterior Communicating Artery Aneurysms

A relatively large number of patients who have aneurysms of the anterior communi-

---

* See references 8, 10, 23, 24, 28, 30, 36–38, 44, 45, 49, 51, 53, 56, 63, 68, 70, 71, 74, 81, 88, 94.

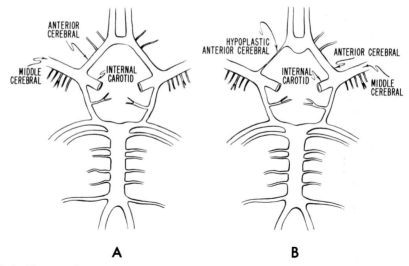

Figure 49-1 Diagram of the circle of Willis, showing a normal pattern, *A*, and severe hypoplasia, *B*, of the proximal portion of one anterior cerebral artery. This developmental anomaly is responsible for the unilateral anterior intracranial circulation in which the blood supply to both frontal lobes is derived from a single internal carotid artery.

cating artery also have associated anomalies of the circle of Willis.[58,73,90] When hypoplasia of the proximal anterior cerebral artery is present in sufficient degree, a unilateral anterior intracranial circulation results (Fig. 49–1). In this common circulatory anomaly, the anterior communicating aneurysm and both anterior cerebral arteries fill from one side only and cannot be filled from the opposite side, even when carotid arteriography is performed with percutaneous contralateral carotid compression.[2] In such patients, ligation of the common carotid artery that fills the aneurysm provides effective treatment. In a series of 40 patients with aneurysms of this type treated by gradual carotid ligation alone, the incidence of recurrent hemorrhage after complete closure of the carotid artery was only 3.1 per cent. Because of the significant morbidity, however, carotid ligation should be reserved for only those broad-based or giant aneurysms that cannot be approached directly without formidable risk to the many small perforating branches in this area.

Middle Cerebral Artery Aneurysms

Although common carotid ligation is considered effective by some, the authors feel that the direct operative approach, craniotomy and either ligation of the aneurysm neck or encasement of the entire aneurysm in acrylic, is the treatment of choice. Common carotid ligation, however, may be of value in the treatment of ruptured aneurysms of the proximal middle cerebral artery.[42]

Inaccessible Traumatic Aneurysms of the Carotid Artery

Those traumatic aneurysms that cannot be repaired directly because of their inaccessible location at the base of the skull frequently may result in life-threatening epistaxis when ruptured. Carotid ligation remains the treatment of choice in this situation.[6]

Mullan has recently advocated the use of subtotal common carotid occlusion to reduce the incidence of rebleeding while awaiting a definitive intracranial procedure.[52] The common carotid artery is completely reopened with removal of the Selverstone clamp following obliteration of the aneurysm.

CONTRAINDICATIONS TO CAROTID LIGATION

In addition to serious systemic disease and location of the aneurysm where it cannot easily be approached directly, the contraindications to carotid ligation include:

Moderate Impairment of Consciousness

The Botterell classification is a practical guide to the advisability of operation in patients with ruptured aneurysms.[12] This classification, based primarily on the patient's level of consciousness, consists of the following five categories:

Grade 1. Conscious patient with or without signs of blood in the subarachnoid space.

Grade 2. Drowsy patient without significant neurological deficit.

Grade 3. Drowsy patient with neurological deficit and probable intracerebral hematoma.

Grade 4. a. Patient with major neurological deficit, deteriorating because of intracerebral hematoma.

b. Elderly patient with less severe neurological deficit but with pre-existing degenerative cerebrovascular disease.

Grade 5. Moribund patient with failing vital centers and extensor rigidity (decerebrate rigidity).

Patients of grades 1 and 2 are candidates for carotid ligation; patients of grades 3 to 5 should not undergo this procedure.

Intracerebral Hematoma

In a patient with an intracerebral hematoma caused by aneurysmal rupture, increased intracranial pressure due to the hematoma exists in addition to the clinical problems associated with subarachnoid hemorrhage. As carotid ligation would only cause a further reduction in an already compromised cerebral blood flow, craniotomy is the recommended operative treatment for evacuating the hematoma and directly obliterating the aneurysm.

Intracranial Vasospasm

Intracranial vasospasm, an unfavorable prognostic finding in patients with ruptured aneurysms, is associated with relatively high mortality and morbidity rates in both those patients who are operated on and those who are not. Impairment in the level of consciousness—probably caused by a reduction in cerebral perfusion, cerebral edema, or both—generally accompanies pronounced vasospasm. In patients with intracranial vasospasm, therefore, carotid ligation should be deferred until a definite improvement in the patient's condition is evident and repeated arteriography shows that the vasospasm has disappeared.

Intolerance to Occlusion

In patients in whom cerebral ischemia develops during gradual closure of the carotid artery, the clamp should be fully opened for two to three days to allow the neurological deficit to regress before the operator reinstitutes clamp closure. If the deficit persists, however, the surgeon should remove the entire clamp and consider the direct approach to treat the aneurysm.

Extracranial Arteriosclerotic Vascular Disease

Carotid ligation is contraindicated in patients with significant stenosis of the contralateral internal carotid artery. In such patients, the major blood supply to the anterior intracranial circulation may be through the carotid artery that is to be ligated. In these patients, the aneurysm should be managed by the direct intracranial approach.

Contralateral Internal Carotid Artery Aneurysm or Junctional Dilation

Common carotid artery occlusion has been demonstrated to cause enlargement and even rupture of a contralateral aneurysm or infundibulum.[75] This is most likely secondary to the increased blood flow through the contralateral circulation that frequently is supplying both hemispheres through the anterior collateral channels.

TIMING OF OPERATION

Provided there are no contraindications to carotid ligation, the procedure can be performed as soon as the diagnosis of aneurysm has been established by carotid arteriography. Operation should, however, be delayed if the interval between onset of subarachnoid hemorrhage and establishment of arteriographic diagnosis is four to six days.[79] This recommendation is based on the observation that the peak incidence of intracranial vasospasm occurs about seven days after the subarachnoid hemorrhage.[89] If craniotomy is done for a direct approach on the fourth to sixth day, postoperative cerebral edema and probably intracranial vasospasm will occur, and the combination of these two adverse factors will reduce the chances for operative success. The principle of delaying operation, however, does not apply to carotid ligation. A gradually occlusive clamp can be applied to the common carotid artery on the fourth to sixth day after subarachnoid hemorrhage, since occlusion of the vessel may require several days. Before completion of carotid ligation, the patient will have passed through the interval of peak incidence of vasospasm.

TECHNIQUE OF CAROTID LIGATION

Choice of Vessel

Previous publications do not indicate a clear preference for the vessel—internal or common carotid—to be ligated in treatment of intracranial aneurysms. Ligation of the common carotid is considered safer from the standpoint of neurological complications, as evidenced by the studies of numerous investigators.* In the Cooperative Study of Intracranial Aneurysms and Subarachnoid Hemorrhage, complications occurred in 41 per cent of 37 patients who had gradual occlusion of the internal carotid artery, but in only 24 per cent of 301 patients who had gradual occlusion of the common carotid artery. Poppen and Fager observed hemiplegia in only 7 of 101 patients in whom they ligated the internal carotid as treatment for intracranial aneurysms.[63] After internal carotid ligation, thrombosis in the isolated segment of the vessel may propagate into the ipsilateral major intracranial arteries and cause cerebral infarction.[41,59,66] In the series reported by Voris, the two patients who had such a compli-

cation died.[85] Recently, the adjunctive use of an extracranial-intracranial bypass procedure has shown promise for markedly reducing morbidity related to internal carotid ligation. For several reasons, gradual ligation of the common carotid artery is preferable in treating intracranial aneurysms. It allows the ipsilateral internal carotid artery to remain patent and thus serve as an important source of collateral circulation to the brain; it provides effective, prolonged reduction of intravascular pressure in the ipsilateral internal carotid artery; and it permits follow-up observations, that is, repeated carotid arteriography and intravascular pressure measurements above the site of ligation.

The Matas Test

Many surgeons recommend a trial period of carotid occlusion before ligation for assessment of the efficacy of the collateral circulation of the brain.[61] This procedure, known as the Matas test, can be performed either percutaneously or on operative exposure of the carotid vessels in the neck. Because the operator can abolish the carotid sinus reflex by applying local anesthesia to the area of the carotid bifurcation, the procedure is considered more reliable when performed at operative exposure of the carotid vessels.

The test is performed by occluding either the internal or common carotid artery for 10 to 30 minutes. During occlusion, the patient is observed for development of neurological signs. If no evidence of cerebral ischemia is found (negative Matas test), then some investigators consider it safe to ligate the vessel completely at that time.[20,22] A serious objection to this method lies in the frequent development of an ischemic neurological complication several hours after carotid ligation despite a negative Matas test.[13,25,57,62,85] In Poppen's series, eight patients had onset of hemiplegia from two hours to eight days after internal carotid ligation.[62] It is principally this delay in onset of ischemic neurological complications beyond the 10- to 30-minute limit of trial occlusion that casts doubt on the value of the Matas test.

Since gradual ligation of the common carotid artery with an adjustable clamp during several days is preferable to abrupt ligation

---

* See references 22, 44, 50, 60, 66, 67, 72, 87.

performed at operation, results of the Matas test have little practical import when the artery is to be occluded gradually.[61] A positive test at operation does not necessarily mean that the patient will not tolerate gradual occlusion of the carotid artery carried out over several days.

Because of the unreliability of the Matas test in identifying patients who will have neurological complications afterward, the test need not be a routine step in the procedure of carotid ligation. It appears that the intravascular pressure measurement in the internal carotid artery at operation is a more reliable index of a patient's tolerance to carotid arterial occlusion than are the results of the Matas test.

Operative Procedure

Although general anesthesia can be used, local anesthesia is usually given to oriented and cooperative patients, whereas general anesthesia is reserved for disoriented, restless, and uncooperative patients.

After making a linear incision along the anterior border of the sternocleidomastoid muscle, the surgeon exposes the distal portion of the common carotid artery and the proximal portions of the internal and external carotid vessels. A Crutchfield clamp is placed around the common carotid about 2 cm below the carotid bifurcation, and the screwdriver portion of the clamp is brought into the operative region through a small stab wound placed behind the incision (Fig. 49–2). With the clamp fully open, a 19-gauge needle is inserted into the proximal internal carotid artery to obtain intravascular pressure recordings with a suitable pressure transducer. After control measurements are obtained, the surgeon occludes the common carotid artery by closing the clamp and records the resulting intravascular pressure reduction. While maintaining the common carotid occlusion, the operator alternately occludes the internal and external carotid arteries and notes the resulting changes in intravascular pressure in the proximal internal carotid artery. From this information, the surgeon can determine the direction of flow in the ipsilateral external-internal carotid arterial system, which, in turn, provides an estimate of the adequacy of the intracranial collateral system.[83] If the pressure in the internal carotid rises when the ipsilateral ex-

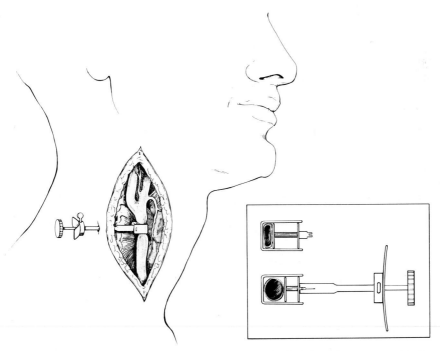

Figure 49–2 Operative sketch showing Crutchfield clamp in position on the common carotid artery. The handle of the clamp is brought out of the operative wound through a small stab incision. Inset shows an enlarged view of the clamp around the vessel.

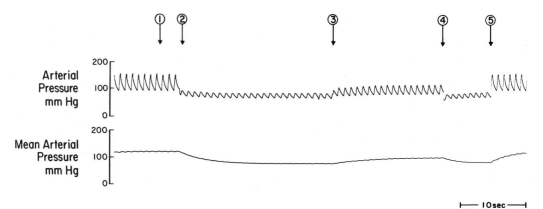

Figure 49–3 Intravascular pressure measurements indicative of reverse flow in the internal carotid artery during occlusion of the ipsilateral common carotid. Arterial pressure measurements were made from the proximal internal carotid artery. Encircled numbers at the top indicate: (1) control values; (2) occluded common carotid; (3) occluded external carotid; (4) released external carotid; and (5) released common carotid occlusion. Note that the pressure in the internal carotid is higher with the external carotid occluded (3) than with this vessel open (2), a finding that indicates that during common carotid occlusion the direction of flow will be from the internal to the external carotid artery.

ternal carotid artery is occluded, the blood flows from internal to external carotid, reflecting an adequate intracranial collateral system (Fig. 49–3). Conversely, if the pressure in the internal carotid falls when the external carotid is occluded, the direction of flow is from external to internal carotid. Such an observation reflects poor or inadequate intracranial collateral vessels, and ischemic neurological complications are more likely to occur during subsequent clamp closure. Finally, the Crutchfield clamp is opened slowly to a position that causes a 10 per cent reduction from control value in systolic or diastolic internal carotid arterial pressure. The clamp is left at this setting, the pressure-recording needle is removed, and the operative wound is closed.

Postoperative Closure of the Occlusive Clamp

The rapidity of postoperative clamp closure depends principally upon the intravascular pressure reduction in the internal carotid artery obtained at operation. When the pressure reduction is less than 50 per cent, the clamp can usually be closed within three to four days, whereas when the reduction exceeds 50 per cent, closure may require five to seven days.[80] In some instances, the clamp cannot be closed completely because of repeated ischemic complications during the closing process.

Postoperatively, the patient is kept at absolute bed rest and under close surveillance until clamp closure is complete. Vital signs are recorded every 30 minutes, and strength in each hand is tested at 5-minute intervals for an eight-hour period after each clamp adjustment. Beginning on the day after operation, the Crutchfield clamp is adjusted daily until the artery is occluded. Retinal arterial pressure is measured in each eye with an ophthalmodynamometer after each half turn of the clamp; when systolic or diastolic ipsilateral retinal arterial pressure has fallen 10 per cent, no further clamp adjustments are made for that day. Before the clamp is turned, a topical anesthetic and a mydriatic are instilled in each eye to facilitate measurement of retinal arterial pressure.

Measuring retinal arterial pressure during postoperative clamp closure is an invaluable technique that provides the only practical means available for monitoring pressure changes in the internal carotid artery on the side of ligation (Fig. 49–4). Flow and pressure reductions in the internal carotid artery do not occur until the lumen of the vessel is seriously compromised.[82] At that point, slight turns (one quarter to one half turn) of the clamp will considerably reduce intravascular pressure and flow above the site of occlusion. For a small pressure reduction (10 per cent) in the internal carotid, therefore, each incremental turn of the clamp must be followed by a measurement of retinal arterial pressure in

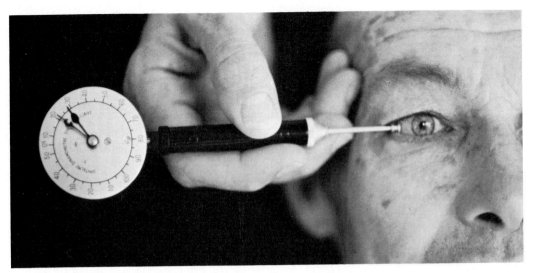

Figure 49–4 Ophthalmodynamometer in position to measure retinal arterial pressure.

the ipsilateral eye. Otherwise, a one- or two-turn clamp closure on any given day may abruptly reduce distal intravascular pressure from normal to fully occluded values. In other words, the latter procedure would be equivalent to carrying out an acute ligation of the carotid artery, and the only reliable guide to preventing this type of clamp closure is careful monitoring of retinal arterial pressure.

When the Crutchfield clamp feels tight around the artery, a roentgenogram of the neck is taken to insure that the clamp is closed. Twenty-four hours later, the detachable screwdriver portion of the clamp is removed. After clamp closure is complete, the patient is allowed to become ambulatory gradually over a two- to three-day period and is then discharged from the hospital.

COMPLICATIONS OF CAROTID LIGATION

Although gradual, as opposed to sudden, ligation of the vessel has materially reduced the incidence of complications by allowing the development of collateral circulation, carotid ligation is not without risks, the most common of which is cerebral ischemia. If ischemia develops while the vessel is being occluded with an adjustable clamp, it can usually be reversed by opening the clamp and allowing more adequate perfusion of the ischemic brain. Among 220 pa-

tients who had gradual ligation of the common carotid artery, Odom and Tindall observed signs of cerebral ischemia in 34 (15.5 per cent).[55] In all patients, the clamp was opened immediately or shortly after onset of the neurological deficit. Twelve of the thirty-four recovered from their neurological deficit completely, 5 remained disabled, 15 died, and in the other 2, follow-up data were not available. Thus, among 220 patients, permanent neurological deficit or death occurred in 20 (9 per cent) during gradual occlusion of the common carotid artery.

Other less frequently encountered complications of gradual carotid ligation include wound infection and erosion of the artery with secondary hemorrhage.[39] In a review of 785 patients undergoing carotid ligation, the Cooperative Study of Intracranial Aneurysms and Subarachnoid Hemorrhage reported ischemic neurological deficits in 233 patients, wound infection in 5, hemorrhage from the neck wound in 1, hypoglossal nerve injury in 1, and a jacksonian seizure during clamp application in 1 patient. On the basis of data accumulated in the Cooperative Study, Nishioka found no evidence that gradual carotid occlusion carries a lower ischemic complication rate than abrupt occlusion, a conclusion that the authors find difficult to accept.[53]

Although it is possible that the long-term effects of carotid ligation may be associated with an increased incidence of ischemic cerebrovascular disease, there is at present no convincing evidence that this potential hazard represents a frequent clinical problem.

Management of Complications of Carotid Ligation

Ischemia

When this complication occurs during gradual closure but before occlusion of the vessel, the adjustable clamp around the artery should be fully opened immediately, and retinal arterial pressure should be measured bilaterally to ascertain if thrombosis of the common or internal carotid artery has occurred. If the retinal arterial pressure is equal bilaterally after the clamp is opened, thrombosis of the carotid vessels has presumably not occurred, and the patient is maintained at absolute bed rest and observed for any change in neurological deficit. If the deficit clears, clamp closure is reinstituted within a few days; if the deficit persists, the clamp is left fully open. Systemic blood pressure should be elevated moderately with a regulated intravenous infusion of metaraminol (Aramine). The raised arterial pressure should be sustained for two to three days. The increased pressure is associated with an increased perfusion of the brain, which lessens the incidence and degree of cerebral ischemia. Marked elevations in arterial pressure should be avoided because of the potential hazard of aneurysm rupture.

When retinal arterial pressure on the side of intended carotid ligation remains significantly decreased after the full opening of the clamp and the patient's condition shows no change, the common or internal carotid artery, or both, are probably thrombosed, a condition demanding immediate operative exploration of the neck vessels. If, however, the carotid artery has been totally occluded for longer than one hour when the ischemic neurological complications arise, the surgeon should reopen the neck incision to insure that there are no clots in the carotid vessels before he opens the clamp.

Wound Infection

Whenever wound infection develops during gradual occlusion of the carotid artery, the surgeon should remove the entire clamp to avoid any danger of vessel erosion.[39]

Fortunately, careful attention to aseptic technique during clamp application and later postoperative closure obviates most wound infections. In 220 patients reported by Odom and Tindall, wound infection occurred in only 11, or 5 per cent.[55] Notably, in only 3 of the 11 patients with wound infection did erosion of the common carotid artery occur with secondary but nonfatal hemorrhage from the vessel. In all three, it was necessary to ligate the common carotid artery proximal to the site of erosion to control the hemorrhage.

RESULTS OF CAROTID LIGATION

Results of many clinical studies indicate the carotid ligation is effective treatment of aneurysms of the internal carotid artery and of the anterior communicating artery associated with a unilateral intracranial circulation. Beneficial results include:

Reduced Incidence of Recurrent Hemorrhage

Internal Carotid Aneurysms

The incidence of recurrent hemorrhage after carotid ligation has varied among the reported series but has usually been less than 8 per cent.[78] From their experience and a review of published reports, Poppen and Fager concluded that carotid ligation has been of undisputed value in preventing recurrent bleeding from internal carotid aneurysms.[63] They found that only 2 of 101 patients had had recurrent hemorrhage during a follow-up period ranging from 1 to 15 years. Equally favorable results have been reported in other large series of patients with internal carotid aneurysms treated by carotid ligation. In the Cooperative Study Program, only 3 per cent of 462 patients treated by carotid ligation had recurrent hemorrhage. In the series reported by Odom and Tindall, the incidence of recurrent hemorrhage after ligation was 3.7 per cent.[53] McKissock, Richardson, and Walsh noted a mortality rate of 36 per cent among 41 patients with internal carotid aneurysms treated conservatively, as compared with only 8 per cent among 37 patients treated by carotid ligation.[46]

In 1974, Richardson and co-workers reported a long-term follow-up of the 60 patients in McKissock's 1960 series and found that carotid ligation did not protect against late rebleeding as well as had been reported during the early postoperative period, seriously challenging the value of the procedure.[65] This is difficult to understand, since significant favorable anatomical changes in aneurysms have been described following carotid ligation.

Mount performed follow-up cerebral arteriography in 13 patients in whom carotid ligation had been carried out and found that the aneurysm was not visualized in 8 patients, was smaller in 4, and was unchanged in 1.[50] In 24 cases of intracranial aneurysm reported by Gibbs, the aneurysm was thrombosed in 4 patients, smaller in 16, and unchanged in size in 4.[28] Tindall and associates performed follow-up carotid arteriography in 66 patients at intervals up to 11 years after carotid ligation and found that the aneurysm was either not visualized or was significantly smaller in 51 patients (77 per cent); in only one patient was the aneurysm larger.[81] Other investigators have described similar findings.[23,30,49,55,71]

Thus, there is ample evidence to show that most internal carotid aneurysms either become smaller or undergo thrombosis after carotid ligation. The aneurysm that becomes smaller rather than becoming thrombosed could remain a potential threat from the standpoint of recurrent hemorrhage. The associated reduction in incidence of recurrent hemorrhage, however, suggests that the aneurysm that has decreased substantially in size after ligation is also less likely to rupture again. Pool and Potts also concluded that carotid ligation can be effective treatment of ruptured aneurysms of the internal carotid–posterior communicating artery even though the aneurysm persists.[61]

Anterior Communicating Aneurysms

In evaluation of the results of carotid ligation in treatment of anterior communicating aneurysms, it is important to distinguish between patients with a unilateral anterior intracranial circulation (discussed in the section on indications for ligation) and those in whom the aneurysm can be visualized during carotid arteriography from either side by appropriate contralateral carotid compression. In the latter situation, carotid ligation alone would be of little or no value in preventing recurrent hemorrhage from the aneurysm of the anterior communicating artery. In a series of patients with a unilateral anterior intracranial circulation reported by Odom and Tindall, the incidence of recurrent hemorrhage from the anterior communicating aneurysm after carotid ligation was 20 per cent.[55] Recurrent hemorrhage usually occurred during clamp closure, the incidence after complete occlusion of the vessel being only 3.1 per cent.

Odom and Tindall performed follow-up cerebral arteriography in 24 patients who had had carotid ligation for anterior communicating aneurysms and found that the aneurysm could not be visualized in 16, was smaller in 3, was unchanged in 3, and was larger in 2 patients. Each of these patients had an associated unilateral intracranial circulation. In the 12 cases reported in the Cooperative Study Program, 5 aneurysms were smaller, 6 were the same size, and 1 was larger on follow-up arteriography.[53]

Middle Cerebral Aneurysms

The Cooperative Study Program reported a total of 36 patients with aneurysms of the middle cerebral artery treated by carotid ligation.[53] Seven of these (19 per cent) experienced recurrent hemorrhage after carotid ligation. In the series reported by Odom and Tindall, postligation hemorrhage occurred in 2 (14.3 per cent) of 14 patients.[55] Lipovšek advocates carotid ligation for proximal middle cerebral artery aneurysms. The incidence of recurrent hemorrhage in this series, however, was 16 per cent.[42]

Although available data suggest that carotid ligation does not afford adequate protection from recurrent hemorrhage of middle cerebral aneurysms, a larger series of cases should be analyzed before this conclusion is accepted.

There have been relatively few reports of repeated carotid arteriography in patients with middle cerebral aneurysms who had had carotid ligation as the only definitive treatment. Of six cases reported by Mount, the aneurysm was not seen in one instance, was smaller in four, and was unchanged in one.[50] Of a total of six cases of middle cerebral aneurysms cited in the Cooperative

Study, two were smaller, two were the same size, and two were larger.[53] In 10 patients reported by Odom and Tindall, the aneurysm was not visualized in 4 patients, was smaller in 3, and was unchanged in 3.[55] Thus, although the number of cases is small, favorable anatomical changes have been observed in middle cerebral aneurysms after carotid ligation.

Reduced Intravascular Pressure in Distal Carotid System

Pressure Measurement at Operation

As previously mentioned, the principal reason for the success of this operation is the reduction in intravascular pressure above the site of ligation. Odom and Tindall measured intravascular pressure in the proximal internal carotid of 214 patients after complete occlusion of the ipsilateral common carotid artery (Table 49–1).[55] During occlusion of the common carotid artery, the reduction in intravascular pressure in the proximal internal carotid was less than 25 per cent in 6 patients, 25 to 40 per cent in 46, 41 to 60 per cent in 109, and greater than 60 per cent in 53 patients. The patients with anterior communicating aneurysms showed greater pressure reductions than did those with either internal or middle cerebral aneurysms. Of the patients with anterior communicating aneurysms, 47 per cent showed pressure reductions greater than 60 per cent, whereas only 14.2 per cent and 30.8 per cent of patients with internal carotid and middle cerebral aneurysms, respectively, showed comparable reductions. That all patients in this series had an associated unilateral intracranial cir-culation contributed to the generally greater pressure reductions in those with anterior communicating aneurysms. Patients with unilateral circulation have greater reduction of pressure than patients with normal intracranial circulation.[21]

Late or Follow-up Pressure Measurements

Carotid ligation should result in a permanent reduction in distal intravascular pressure for lasting benefit in treatment of intracranial aneurysms. Measurement of cervical internal carotid arterial pressure several months or years after carotid ligation indicates that a reduction of about 25 per cent from control mean arterial pressure persists for several years after carotid ligation.[55,56,81,91]

Comparable results have been recorded with ophthalmodynamometry performed in patients several months or years after ligation. In 11 patients studied for 6 to 19 months after carotid ligation, Heyman and associates reported an average reduction of 23 per cent in mean retinal arterial pressure on the side of ligation.[31]

Clinical Improvement After Ligation

The recovery of function in oculomotor nerve paralysis after carotid ligation implies a therapeutically favorable change in the aneurysm responsible for the paralysis. Many authors have noted postligation improvement in extraocular palsies caused by internal carotid aneurysms.*

---

* See references 10, 30, 37, 63, 68, 81, 88.

TABLE 49–1 INTRAVASCULAR PRESSURE REDUCTIONS AT TIME OF APPLICATION OF CRUTCHFIELD CLAMP (214 PATIENTS)

PERCENTAGE PRESSURE REDUCTION	Internal Carotid Patients		Middle Cerebral Patients		Anterior Communicating Patients		TOTAL NO. ANEU-RYSMS
	No.	Per Cent	No.	Per Cent	No.	Per Cent	
Less than 25	6	4.3	0	0	0	0	6
25–40	36	25.7	4	30.8	6	10	46
41–60	78	55.7	5	38.5	26	43	109
More than 60	20	14.2	4	30.8	29	47	53
Total	140		13		61		214

SUMMARY

Carotid ligation is an effective method of treating aneurysms of the internal carotid artery and anterior communicating artery associated with a unilateral circulation. Recent dramatic improvements in microvascular techniques, however, have made the direct obliteration of most of these aneurysms the treatment of choice. Recent series have demonstrated mortality rates of less than 2 per cent associated with clip ligation or acrylic coating of most aneurysms and no occurrence of recurrent hemorrhage.[95] These rates are significantly less than that associated with the potential ischemic complications of carotid ligation, a procedure that does not completely remove the possibility of rebleeding.

Carotid ligation is felt to be indicated in treating those broad-based or giant aneurysms of the internal carotid artery, particularly those at the junction of the ophthalmic artery usually underlying the anterior clinoid, at the bifurcation of the internal carotid artery, or at the anterior communicating artery in the presence of a unilateral circulation. It is also indicated in the treatment of giant aneurysms presenting with signs of cranial nerve compression inaccessible to direct approach, either in the cavernous sinus or in the petrous portion of the internal carotid artery. It remains the treatment of choice for inaccessible traumatic aneurysms of the internal carotid artery. In treatment of these lesions, carotid ligation will decrease the incidence of recurrent hemorrhage, will effectively reduce the intravascular pressure in the carotid system for several years, will decrease the size of or cause thrombosis of the aneurysm in most cases, and will result in clinical improvement, e.g., in third nerve palsy. Carotid ligation is contraindicated if the patient is obtunded, has an intracerebral hematoma, has significant intracranial vasospasm, has severe narrowing of the lumen of the opposite internal carotid artery, or has a contralateral internal carotid artery aneurysm or infundibulum, and obviously if the patient will not tolerate occlusion of the artery.

Gradual ligation of either the internal or common carotid artery with an occlusive clamp is always preferable to abrupt ligation because of the lower incidence of neurological complications with gradual ligation. Because of the unreliability of the Matas test in accurately predicting ischemic neurological complications, its use is not recommended. Intravascular pressure determinations at the time of operation provide an objective and reliable measure of the rate of clamp closure in the postoperative period.

Ophthalmodynamometry is useful in patients undergoing carotid ligation, and the authors recommend that this technique be used in all patients who have gradual closure of the artery.

REFERENCES

1. Abernethy, J.: Surgical Observations. London, Longman & Rees, 1804, p. 193
2. Abernethy, J.: Surgical Observations on Injuries of the Head. Philadelphia, Dobson, 1811, vol. 2, p. 72.
3. Abernethy, J.: Surgical Works, vol. 2. London, Longman, 1815.
4. Abernethy, J.: Surgical and Physiological Works, vol. 2. London, Longman, Rees, Orme, Brown & Green, 1830.
5. Allcock, J. M., and Drake, C. G.: Postoperative angiography in cases of ruptured intracranial aneurysm. J. Neurosurg., 20:752–759, 1963.
6. Araki, C., Handa, H., Handa, J., et al.: Traumatic aneurysm of the intracranial extradural portion of the internal carotid artery. J. Neurosurg. 23:64–67, 1967.
7. Bakay, L., and Sweet, W. J.: Cervical and intracranial intra-arterial pressure with and without vascular occlusion. Surg. Gynec. Obstet., 95:67–75, 1952.
8. Bakay, L., and Sweet, W. H.: Intra-arterial pressure in the neck and brain. Late changes after carotid closure, acute measurements after vertebral closure. J. Neurosurg., 10:353–359, 1953.
9. Beadles, C. F.: Aneurysms of the larger cerebral arteries. Brain, 30:285–336, 1907.
10. Black, S. P. W., and German, W. J.: The treatment of internal carotid artery aneurysm by proximal arterial ligation. J. Neurosurg., 10:590–601, 1953.
11. Bloor, B. M., Odom, G. L., and Woodhall, B.: Direct measurement of intravascular pressure in components of the circle of Willis. Arch. Surg., 63:821–823, 1951.
12. Botterell, W. J., Lougheed, W. M., Scott, J. W., et al.: Hypothermia, and interruption of carotid, or carotid and vertebral circulation, in the surgical management of intracranial aneurysms. J. Neurosurg., 13:1–42, 1956.
13. Brackett, C. E.: The complications of carotid artery ligation in the neck. J. Neurosurg., 10:91–106, 1953.
14. Brackett, C. E., and Mount, L. A.: Some observations on intra-carotid blood pressure made during carotid ligation for intracranial aneurysms. Surg. Forum, 1:344–360, 1950.

15. Cooper, A.: A case of aneurysm of the carotid artery. Med. Chir. Trans., *1*:1–15, 1809.

16. Cooper, A.: Second case of carotid aneurysm. Med. Chir. Trans., *1*:222–233, 1809.

17. Cooper, A.: Account of the first successful operation, performed on the common carotid artery, for aneurysm. Guy's Hosp. Rep., *1*:53–58, 1836.

18. Crutchfield, W. G.: Instruments for use in the treatment of certain intracranial vascular lesions. J. Neurosurg., *16*:471–474, 1959.

19. Dandy, W. E.: Results following ligation of the internal carotid artery. Arch. Surg., *45*:521–533, 1942.

20. Dandy, W. E.: Intracranial Arterial Aneurysms. Ithaca, N.Y., Comstock Publishing Co., 1944.

21. Dukes, H. T., Odom, G. L., and Woodhall, B.: The unilateral anterior cerebral circulation. Its importance in the management of aneurysms of the anterior communicating artery. J. Neurosurg., *22*:40–46, 1965.

22. Echols, D. H., and Rehfeldt, F. C.: Diagnosis and treatment of intracranial aneurysms. South. Surg., *15*:782–788, 1949.

23. Ecker, A., and Riemenschneider, P.: Deliberate thrombosis of intracranial arterial aneurysm by partial occlusion of the carotid artery with arteriographic control. Preliminary report of a case. J. Neurosurg., *8*:348–353, 1951.

24. Editorial Committee: The report on cooperative studies of intracranial aneurysms and subarachnoid hemorrhage. J. Neurosurg., *24*:779–816, 1966.

25. Falconer, M. A.: The surgical treatment of bleeding intracranial aneurysms. J. Neurol. Neurosurg. Psychiat., *14*:153–186, 1951.

26. Fleming, D.: Case of rupture of the carotid artery, and wounds of several of its branches, successfully treated by tying the common trunk of the carotid itself. Med. Chir. J. Rev., *3*:2–4, 1817.

27. Gee, W., Oller, D. W., and Wylie, E.: Non-invasive diagnosis of carotid occlusion by ocular pneumoplethysmography. Stroke, *7*:18–21, 1976.

28. Gibbs, J. R.: Effects of carotid ligation on the size of internal carotid aneurysms. J. Neurol. Neurosurg. Psychiat., *28*:383–394, 1965.

29. Hamby, W. B.: Intracranial Aneurysms. Springfield, Ill., Charles C Thomas, 1952.

30. Harris, R., and Udvarhalyi, G. B.: Aneurysms arising at the internal carotid-posterior communicating artery junction. J. Neurosurg., *14*:180–191, 1957.

31. Heyman, A., Tindall, G. T., Finney, W. H. M., et al.: Measurement of retinal artery and intracarotid pressure following carotid artery occlusion with the Crutchfield clamp. J. Neurosurg., *17*:297–305, 1960.

32. Jawad, K., Miller, J. D., Wyper, D. J., et al.: Measurement of CBF and carotid artery pressure compared with cerebral angiography in assessing collateral blood supply after carotid ligation. J. Neurosurg., *46*:185–196, 1977.

33. Jefferson, G.: On the saccular aneurysms of the internal carotid artery in the cavernous sinus. Brit. J. Surg., *26*:267–302, 1938.

34. Jefferson, G.: Isolated oculomotor palsy caused by intracranial aneurysm. Proc. Roy. Soc. Med., *40*:419–432, 1947.

35. Johnson, H.C.: Cervical intracarotid pressure studies: Their significance in the management of intracranial aneurysms. Surgery, *33*:537–543, 1953.

36. Johnson, R.: Discussion, Norlen, G.: The pathology, diagnosis and treatment of intracranial saccular aneurysms. Proc. Roy. Soc, Med., *45*:301–302, 1952.

37. Krayenbuhl, H.: Immediate and late results of carotid ligature in intracranial aneurysms. Schweiz. Med. Wschr., *76*:908–914, 1946.

38. Krayenbuhl, H., Weber, G., and Yasargil, M. G.: Traitement chirurgical et prognostic. I. La ligature carotidienne. *In* Krayenbuhl, H., ed.: L'Aneurysme de l'Artère Communicante Antérieure. Paris, Masson & Cie, 1959.

39. Lee, J. R., and Tindall, G. T.: Arterial erosion and hemorrhage during graded carotid ligation with the Crutchfield clamp. J. Neurosurg., *27*:52–55, 1967.

40. Leech, P. J., Miller, J. D., Fitch, W., et al.: Cerebral blood flow, internal carotid artery pressure and the EEG as a guide to the safety of carotid ligation. J. Neurol. Neurosurg. Psychiat., *37*:854–862, 1974.

41. Le Fort, L.: Cited by Schorstein, J.: Carotid ligation in saccular intracranial aneurysms. Brit. J. Surg., *28*:50–70, 1940.

42. Lipovšek, M.: Ruptured aneurysms of the proximal middle cerebral artery. J. Neurosurg., *39*:498–502, 1973.

43. Lobstein, A., Phillippsides, D., and Montrieul, B.: La mesure des pressions artérielles reinienne et intracarotidienne au cours de la ligature de la carotide. Rev. Otoneuroophtal., *25*:216–226, 1953.

44. Luessenhop, A. J., Mora, F., and Sweet, W. H.: Subarachnoid hemorrhage, intracranial aneurysms and arterio-venous anomalies; treatment by cervical carotid occlusion. *In* Field, W. S.: Pathogenesis and Treatment of Cerebrovascular Disease. Springfield, Ill., Charles C Thomas, 1961, pp. 516–553.

45. McKissock, W., Paine, K., and Walsh, L. S.: Further observations on subarachnoid hemorrhage. J. Neurol. Neurosurg. Psychiat., *21*:239–248, 1958.

46. McKissock, W., Richardson, A., and Walsh, L.: Posterior communicating aneurysms. A controlled trial of the conservative and surgical treatment of ruptured aneurysms of the internal carotid artery at or near the point of origin of the posterior communicating artery. Lancet, *1*:1203–1208, 1960.

47. Moniz, E.: L'encephalographie artérielle, son importance dans la localisation des tumeurs cérébrales. Rev. Neurol., *2*:72–89, 1927.

48. Moranta, R. A., Kirchiner, F. R., and Kishore, P.: Aneurysms of the petrous portion of the internal carotid artery. Surg. Neurol., *6*:313–318, 1976.

49. Morris, L.: Arteriographic studies in aneurysm of the internal carotid artery treated by carotid occlusion. Acta Radiol. (Stockholm), *1*:367–372, 1963.

50. Mount, L. A.: Results of treatment of intracranial aneurysms using the Selverstone clamp. J. Neurosurg., *16*:611–618, 1959.

51. Mount, L. A., and Taveras, J. M.: The results of surgical treatment of intracranial aneurysms as

demonstrated by progress arteriography. J. Neurosurg., *13*:618–626, 1956.

52. Mullan, S.: Conservative management of the recently ruptured aneurysm. Surg. Neurol., *3*:27–32, 1975.

53. Nishioka, H.: Results of the treatment of intracranial aneurysms by occlusion of the carotid artery in the neck. J. Neurosurg., *25*:660–682, 1966.

54. Odom, G. L.: Ophthalmic involvement in neurological vascular lesions. *In* Smith, J. D.: Neuro-ophthalmology. Springfield, Ill., Charles C Thomas, 1964, pp. 1–96.

55. Odom, G. L., and Tindall, G. T.: Carotid ligation in the treatment of certain intracranial aneurysms. Clin. Neurosurg., *15*:101–116, 1968.

56. Odom, G. L., Woodhall, B., Tindall, G. T., et al.: Changes in distal intravascular pressure and size of intracranial aneurysm following common carotid ligation. J. Neurosurg., *19*:41–50, 1962.

57. Olivecrona, H.: Ligature of the carotid artery in intracranial aneurysms. Acta Chir. Scand., *91*:353–368, 1944.

58. Padget, D. H.: The circle of Willis. Its embryology and anatomy. *In* Dandy, W. E.: Intracranial Arterial Aneurysms. Ithaca, N.Y., Comstock Publishing Co., 1944, pp. 67–90.

59. Perthes, G. C.: Cited by Olivecrona, H.: Ligature of the carotid artery in intracranial aneurysms. Acta Chir. Scand., *91*:353–368, 1944.

60. Pool, J. L.: Diagnosis and recent advance in treatment of subarachnoid hemorrhage. J.A.M.A., *187*:404–409, 1964.

61. Pool, J. L., and Potts, D. G.: Aneurysms and Arteriovenous Anomalies of the Brain. New York, Harper & Row, 1965.

62. Poppen, J. L.: Specific treatment of intracranial aneurysms. Experiences with 143 surgically treated patients. J. Neurosurg., *8*:75–102, 1951.

63. Poppen, J. L., and Fager, C. A.: Intracranial aneurysms. Results of surgical treatment. J. Neurosurg., *17*:283–296, 1960.

64. Rand, R. W.: Retinal arterial pressure studies associated with cervical carotid artery occlusion in the treatment of cerebral aneurysms. Bull. Los Angeles Neurol. Soc., *21*:175–187, 1956.

65. Richardson, A., Winn, R., and Jane, J.: Late results on carotid ligation for posterior communicating aneurysms. Presented at meeting of British Society of Neurosurgeons and American Academy of Neurological Surgery, Bermuda, 1974.

66. Rogers, L.: Ligature of arteries, with particular reference to carotid occlusion and the circle of Willis. Brit. J. Surg., *35*:43–50, 1947.

67. Schorstein, J.: Carotid ligation in saccular intracranial aneurysms. Brit. J. Surg., *28*:50–70, 1940–1941.

68. Scott, M., and Skwarok, E.: The treatment of cerebral aneurysms by ligation of the common carotid artery, Surg. Gynec. Obstet., *113*:54–61, 1961.

69. Selverstone, B., and White, J. C.: A method for gradual occlusion of the internal carotid artery in the treatment of aneurysm. Proc. New Eng. Cardiovasc. Soc., *9*:24, 1952.

70. Shenkin, H. A., Polakoff, P., and Finneson, B. E.: Intracranial internal carotid artery aneurysms. Results of treatment by cervical carotid artery ligation. J. Neurosurg., *15*:183–191, 1958.

71. Somach, F. M., and Shenkin, H. A.: Angiographic end-results of carotid ligation in the treatment of carotid aneurysm. J. Neurosurg., *24*:966–974, 1966.

72. Steelman, J. F., Hayes, G. J., and Rizzoli, H. V.: Surgical treatment of saccular intracranial aneurysms. A report of 56 consecutively treated patients. J. Neurosurg., *10*:564–576, 1953.

73. Stehbens, W. E.: Aneurysms and anatomical variations of cerebral arteries. Arch. Path., *75*:45–63, 1963.

74. Stornelli, S. A., and French, J. D.: Subarachnoid hemorrhage—factors in prognosis and management. J. Neurosurg., *21*:769–780, 1964.

75. Stuntz, T. J., Ojemann, G. A., and Alword, E. C.: Radiographic and histologic demonstration of an aneurysm developing on the infundibulum of the posterior communicating artery. J. Neurosurg., *33*:591–596, 1970.

76. Svien, H. J., and Hollenhorst, R. W.: Pressure in retinal arteries after ligation or occlusion of the carotid artery. Proc. Mayo Clin., *31*:684–692, 1956.

77. Sweet, W. J., and Bennett, H. S.: Changes in internal carotid pressure during carotid and jugular occlusion and their clinical significance. J. Neurosurg., *5*:178–195, 1948.

78. Tindall, G. T., and Odom, G. L.: Treatment of intracranial aneurysms by proximal carotid ligation. *In* Krayenbuhl, H., et al., eds.: Progress in Neurological Surgery. Vol. 3. Chicago, Year Book Medical Publishers, 1969, pp. 66–114.

79. Tindall, G. T., and Odom, G. L.: Saccular Aneurysms of the Brain: Surgical Treatment. Handbook of Clinical Neurology. Vol. 12. Amsterdam, North Holland Publishing Co., 1972, pp. 205–226.

80. Tindall, G. T., Dukes, H. T., Cupp, H. G., Jr., et al.: Simultaneous determination of retinal and carotid artery pressure. Neurology (Minneap.), *10*:623–626, 1960.

81. Tindall, G. T., Goree, J. A., Lee, J. F., et al.: Effect of common carotid ligation on size of internal carotid aneurysms and distal intracarotid and retinal artery pressure. J. Neurosurg., *25*:503–511, 1966.

82. Tindall, G. T., Odom, G. L., Cupp, H. B., Jr., et al.: Studies on carotid artery flow and pressure. Observations in 18 patients during graded occlusion of proximal carotid artery. J. Neurosurg., *19*:917–923, 1962.

83. Tindall, G. T., Odom, G. L., Dillon, M. L., et al.: Direction of blood flow in the internal and external carotid arteries following occlusion of the ipsilateral common carotid artery. J. Neurosurg., *20*:985–994, 1963.

84. Twitchell, A.: Gunshot wound of the face and neck; ligature of the carotid artery. New Eng. Quart. J. Med. Surg., *1*:188–193, 1842–1843.

85. Voris, H. C.: Complications of ligation of the internal carotid artery. J. Neurosurg., *8*:119–131, 1951.

86. Walker, A. E., ed.: A History of Neurological Surgery. Baltimore, Md., Williams & Wilkins Co., 1951, pp. 253–264.

87. Wechsler, I. S., and Gross, S. W.: Cerebral ar-

teriography in subarachnoid hemorrhage. J.A.M.A., *136*:517–521, 1948.

88. Wechsler, I. S., Gross, S. W., and Cohen, I.: Arteriography and carotid artery ligation in intracranial aneurysm and vascular malformation. J. Neurol. Neurosurg. Psychiat., *14*:25–34, 1951.

89. Wilkins, R. H., Alexander, J. A., and Odom, G. L.: Intracranial arterial spasm: A clinical analysis. J. Neurosurg., *29*:121–134, 1968.

90. Wilson, G., Riggs, H. E., and Rupp, C.: The pathologic anatomy of ruptured cerebral aneurysms. J. Neurosurg., *11*:128–134, 1954.

91. Wise, B. L., Boldrey, E., and Aird, R. B.: The value of electroencephalography in studying the effects of ligation of the carotid arteries. Electroenceph. Clin. Neurophysiol., *6*:261–268, 1954.

92. Woodhall, B., Odom, G. L., Bloor, B. M., et al.: Direct measurement of intravascular pressure in components of the circle of Willis. A contribution to the surgery of congenital cerebral aneurysms and vascular anomalies of the brain. Ann. Surg., *135*:911–921, 1952.

93. Woodhall, B., Odom, G. L., Bloor, B. M., et al.: Studies on cerebral intravascular pressure. Further data concerning residual pressure in components of the circle of Willis and in blind arterial segments. J. Neurosurg., *10*:28–34, 1953.

94. Wright, R. L., and Sweet, W. H.: Carotid or vertebral occlusion in the treatment of intracranial aneurysms; value of early and late reading of carotid and retinal pressures. Clin. Neurosurg., *9*:163–192, 1963.

95. Yasargil, M. G., and Fox, J. L.: The microsurgical approach to intracranial aneurysms. Surg. Neurol., *3*:7–14, 1975.

50

MANAGEMENT OF ANEURYSMS OF POSTERIOR CIRCULATION

HISTORICAL BACKGROUND

Direct operative treatment of aneurysms on the vertebral-basilar circulation was slow to develop, not only because routine vertebral angiography was not commonly performed but also because these deadly sacs were hidden in front of and embedded in the brain stem and seemed so inaccessible. A few aneurysms presenting as posterior fossa masses had been explored. In 1937, Dandy shelled out a large aneurysm of the left vertebral artery that he had mistaken for a tumor but failed to relieve extreme pressure in the posterior fossa. He remarked in 1944 that although he knew of no successful outcome from operative attack upon an aneurysm of the posterior cranial fossa, "cures would certainly come in time," especially for those easily exposed on the vertebral and posterior inferior cerebellar arteries.[8] He was unaware that Tönnis, in 1937, had similarly described the inadvertent opening of a large globular aneurysm in the cerebellopontine angle, also explored as a tumor. Tönnis was able to control the bleeding by packing the interior of the sac with muscle, and his patient evidently survived this heroic effort without deficit.[51]

Dandy is also credited with the first vertebral artery ligation for a presumed aneurysm of the left vertebral artery. The vessel was ligated between the axis and the atlas. In another case, in which an atherosclerotic basilar aneurysm was discovered at trigeminal root section, he had been able to ligate the vertebral artery safely "to lessen the strain on the aneurysm." He also described an attempt in 1927 to occlude both vertebral arteries for a huge S-shaped basilar aneurysm. After ligation of the left vertebral artery he temporarily compressed the right with forceps. Death was almost instantaneous: "most rapid death I have ever seen."[8]

Later, Falconer and Poppen used ligation of the vertebral artery in the vertebral triangle, but Logue was the first to describe ligation of the vertebral artery intracranially just proximal to two large fusiform vertebral aneurysms.[23,31,44] The first deliberate occlusion of the basilar artery for aneurysm was done by Mount in 1962.[39]

The first direct attack on an aneurysm in the posterior fossa was described by Schwartz in 1948; remarkably, it was accomplished without previous visualization by an angiogram. The patient presented with a story of repeated headaches and dizziness for three years, then collapsed. The spinal fluid was faintly bloody. At exploration, a small saccular dilatation was found arising from an "abnormal" artery whose exact origin could not be determined. The aneurysm ruptured as it was being freed from an attachment to the pons, so it was trapped with clips and coagulated. The patient remained well thereafter.[46,47]

In the next decade, several surgeons reported their experience with a few cases. In 1961, Drake described four cases of aneurysms in the region of the basilar bifurcation that were treated directly and reviewed the cases reported up to that time (Fig. 50–1).[9]

Fourteen cases had been treated by proximal vertebral artery ligation either in the neck or intracranially with only one death. In 16 of the 33 cases treated directly, the

S. J. PEERLESS AND C. G. DRAKE

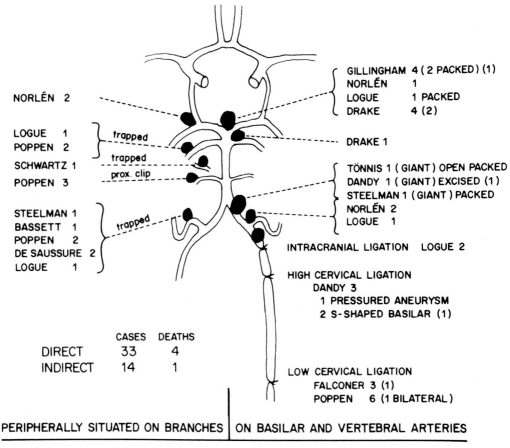

NORLÉN 2

LOGUE 1
POPPEN 2
SCHWARTZ 1
POPPEN 3

STEELMAN 1
BASSETT 1
POPPEN 2
DE SAUSSURE 2
LOGUE 1

trapped
trapped
prox. clip
trapped

GILLINGHAM 4 (2 PACKED) (1)
NORLÉN 1
LOGUE 1 PACKED
DRAKE 4 (2)

DRAKE 1

TÖNNIS 1 (GIANT) OPEN PACKED
DANDY 1 (GIANT) EXCISED (1)
STEELMAN 1 (GIANT) PACKED
NORLÉN 2
LOGUE 1

INTRACRANIAL LIGATION LOGUE 2

HIGH CERVICAL LIGATION
DANDY 3
1 PRESSURED ANEURYSM
2 S-SHAPED BASILAR (1)

LOW CERVICAL LIGATION
FALCONER 3 (1)
POPPEN 6 (1 BILATERAL)

	CASES	DEATHS
DIRECT	33	4
INDIRECT	14	1

PERIPHERALLY SITUATED ON BRANCHES | ON BASILAR AND VERTEBRAL ARTERIES

Figure 50–1 Early operative treatment of aneurysms of the posterior circulation. Sites of vertebrobasilar aneurysms operated upon before 1960. Numbers of deaths are given in parentheses. (Modified from Drake, C. G.: Bleeding aneurysms of the basilar artery. Direct surgical management in four cases. J. Neurosurg., *18*:230–238, 1961.)

aneurysms were situated peripherally on a branch of the basilar or vertebral artery and were therefore more readily accessible. Except for Drake's cases, only six aneurysms arising from the basilar artery had been explored. All were at the basilar bifurcation and three had to be packed. Nevertheless, it was encouraging that for the 33 aneurysms treated directly, there were only four postoperative deaths. Jamieson, however, was discouraged about his results in 19 patients with aneurysms on the vertebral basilar system: 10 died, and only 4 of the survivors were employable.[30] Logue and Hook and co-workers reported their experience and noted the same poor results with aneurysms at the basilar bifurcation.[29,32]

In 1965, Drake was more optimistic about aneurysms along the basilar trunk, as four of his five patients had done well.[10] He recognized that these aneurysms were

more readily obliterated because they were more easily visualized and were not so intimately associated with perforating arteries. The results of direct attack on aneurysms at the basilar bifurcation remained gloomy, however, for of the first seven patients, only two did well while one remained in poor condition and four died. A review of these cases and the anatomy of the region of the basilar bifurcation suggested that the placing of a clip or ligature blindly behind the necks of these aneurysms injured or occluded some of the many perforating vessels that arise from the adjacent posterior cerebral arteries at or near their origin and resulted in midbrain infarction. The tiny, but vital, vessels irrigating the midbrain, pons, and hypothalamus are often numerous and are plastered to the posterior and lateral walls of the aneurysm hidden in the interpeduncular fossa. Once the anatomy of these minute structures was appreciated and precautions taken to preserve their integrity, the operative results immediately improved. Three years later Drake reported 12 additional cases with no operative deaths and good results in all except two patients who were in poor condition at the time of operation. These improved results with basilar bifurcation aneurysms and the continued good results with truncal aneurysms prompted description and illustration of the operative techniques.[11,12]

In the past decade, the remarkable advantages afforded to the surgeon by the operating microscope, fine instruments for dissection, a variety of precisely engineered clips, vastly improved anesthetic techniques, and even more sophisticated neuroradiology have made the operative treatment of all aneurysms of the posterior circulation as safe as procedures on those of the anterior circulation.

MORBID ANATOMY

The incidence of aneurysms on the vertebrobasilar tree has been estimated from angiographic and autopsy studies by several authors (Table 50–1).

These figures, including data from reviews of the literature, suggest an incidence of vertebral-basilar aneurysms of between 5 and 10 per cent of all aneurysms. The most common saccular aneurysms of the posterior circulation are those at the basilar bifurcation, followed in order by those along

TABLE 50–1 INCIDENCE OF VERTEBROBASILAR ANEURYSMS

SOURCE	NO. OF CASES	PER CENT OF ALL ANEURYSMS
Bull*	1769	3.6
McCormick and Nofzinger†		
Adults	7650	5.8
Review of literature		9.6
Cooperative Study‡		
Single aneurysms	2349	5.5
Including multiple aneurysms		7.5

* Contribution of radiology to the study of intracranial aneurysms. Brit. Med. J., 2:1701–1708, 1962.
† Saccular aneurysms: An autopsy study. J. Neurosurg., 22:155, 1965.
‡ Sahs, A. L., et al.: Intracranial Aneurysms and Subarachnoid Hemorrhage. A Cooperative Study. Philadelphia, J. B. Lippincott Co., 1969.

the basilar trunk and on the vertebral artery at the posterior inferior cerebellar artery.

Hamby described three varieties of aneurysms on the vertebral and basilar arteries and their branches: (1) large tortuous, dilated, S-shaped arteriosclerotic vertebral or basilar aneurysms; (2) large spherical vertebral or basilar aneurysms; and (3) smaller saccular aneurysms with subarachnoid hemorrhage.[28]

This classification remains useful with a few qualifications. Hamby considered that the first two groups presented only with signs of focal brain stem or cranial nerve dysfunction, but it is now known that both types may also rupture spontaneously. Although Hamby tended to dismiss the operative importance of these large aneurysms, the authors' experience has shown that much may be accomplished in treating the large spherical aneurysms and even the occasional S-shaped aneurysm as well. Since the problems of operative treatment are proportional to the size and shape of the aneurysms, especially when modified by the relation of the size of the neck to the parent artery, the degree of atheroma at the neck, and the extent of mural thrombosis in the sac, it is more important to classify these lesions according to their dimensions.[18] Although it would be ideal if all aneurysms could be subdivided in accordance with their size and configuration and the complexities of their necks, it was realized that the only readily available measurements are the overall dimensions. It has been proposed, therefore, that aneurysms be classified as small (less than 12.5 mm), large (12.5 to 25 mm), and giant (over 2.5 cm).[4] Hence, Hamby's smaller aneurysms could be subdivided into small and large, while the large globular aneurysms would be of the "giant" variety. Pathologists and radiologists have divided the smaller variety further, but it is believed that the technical problems are much the same for all those under 12 mm.[34]

Saccular aneurysms, in common with those on the anterior circulation, always arise at the distal crotch of a vessel and are conventionally named according to the branch, e.g.: (1) posterior cerebral, first and second segments (P_1 and P_2); (2) basilar bifurcation; (3) basilar–superior cerebellar artery; (4) basilar–anterior inferior cerebellar artery; (5) vertebral-basilar junction; and (6) vertebral–posterior inferior cerebellar artery. A few arise at the carina of origin of small unnamed vessels from the vertebral or basilar arteries and should be labeled according to the nearest named branch. For example, a few have arisen on the basilar artery between the superior cerebellar artery and the anterior inferior cerebellar artery from what may be the site of termination of the primitive trigeminal artery. Another small group arise peripherally at more distal branchings of the named branches themselves. In common with those of the anterior circulation and except in the rare instance of a small fusiform dilatation, the smaller saccular posterior aneurysms do not have branches arising from the sac itself.

Like aneurysms of the anterior circulation, those in the posterior circulation reach their critical size for rupture at 5 to 6 mm. Sacs smaller than 5 mm rupture much less frequently.[14] Although massive intracerebral bleeding is common with aneurysms of the anterior circulation, it is rarely seen with basilar and vertebral aneurysms, which in most cases bleed into the subarachnoid spaces, including the many large cisterns enveloping the brain stem. Like the backward-projecting carotid-communicating aneurysms, posterior circulation aneurysms tend to lie free in the subarachnoid cisterns, and the tougher pial envelope of the brain stem may be more resistant to penetration and even provide strength to the adherent portion of the sac. Only one temporal lobe clot has been seen, from rupture of a large basilar bifurcation aneurysm. Large subdural hematomas are infrequent, although thin collections under a temporal lobe or over a cerebellar hemisphere are not uncommon. Intratemporal and occipital hemorrhage may occur from distally situated posterior cerebral aneurysms, as may cerebellar clots from the rare, peripherally situated aneurysms on the cerebellar arteries. Only one small hematoma has been evacuated from the brain stem in a patient surviving rupture of a high-placed vertebral aneurysm.

Intraventricular hemorrhage is not an infrequent terminal event, however, particularly from recurrent rupture of the dome of a basilar bifurcation aneurysm through the floor of the third ventricle.

The association of aneurysms of the posterior circulation with cerebellar or occipital arteriovenous malformations has been seen in 23 patients. In each instance, the aneurysm arose at the crotch of a branch on a major feeder to the arteriovenous malformation, presumably in response to the high rate of flow. In the authors' experience, subarachnoid hemorrhage in a patient harboring both an arteriovenous malformation and an aneurysm always is from rupture of the aneurysm.

The unusual number of large and giant aneurysms in the authors' series is undoubtedly related to the patterns of referral. The number reaching the borderline between small and large (12.5 mm), however, seems inordinately large, particularly for those at the basilar bifurcation.

Although large fusiform S-shaped aneurysms probably arise on an atherosclerotic basis, the large bulbous and giant globular aneurysms almost certainly result from enlargement of small saccular aneurysms (e.g., vertebrobasilar aneurysms). Many have considered that rupture of giant aneurysms is uncommon, but a surprising proportion in this series have ruptured. Of 198 cases, including aneurysms on both anterior and posterior circulations, rupture of a giant aneurysm was a presenting feature or occurred subsequently in 87 patients (44 per cent). Another 11 patients had a history of subarachnoid hemorrhage some time before, often many years earlier, when presumably the aneurysm was smaller. There was no significant difference between lesions of the anterior and posterior circulations. Massive mural thrombosis in a giant sac did not confer protection, either, for although 60 of the 87 aneurysms were predominantly open sacs, 27 were largely occluded with thrombosis except near the neck. In some of these it is possible that the thrombosis occurred after the rupture, but in many the appearance of the thrombus at operation suggested that it was well organized and old. Most giant sacs along the brain stem are associated with signs of compression of neighborhood structures and often mimic tumors.

NATURAL HISTORY

At one time, aneurysms of the vertebrobasilar system were thought to be more benign than those of the carotid system and its branches; however, there is increasing evidence that they are equally dangerous. Uihlein and Hughes explored 14 posterior aneurysms without definite treatment, and eight of the patients subsequently died of aneurysmal rupture.[53] Gillingham noted that of 26 patients treated nonoperatively in Edinburgh, all died of recurrent hemorrhage within three years; "they seem particularly nasty lesions to have."[27] In a follow-up of 25 cases of ruptured basilar bifurcation aneurysms, Troupp found that there were 13 deaths from rebleeding up to 52 months after diagnosis. He felt that "the future of the patients with this type of aneurysm is actually worse than that of patients with anterior aneurysms."[52]

CLINICAL FEATURES

In spite of a more intimate relation to cranial nerves and brain stem, most small vertebrobasilar aneurysms remain cryptic until their rupture. The authors believe that, like the anterior circulation aneurysms, the vertebrobasilar aneurysms rupture as a result of the emotional and physical stresses in life, including rapid eye movement sleep, that suddenly raise blood pressure beyond the tolerances of luminal volume and wall thickness. Initial minor "warning leaks" seem to be as common, too, as is vicious recurrent bleeding.

While earlier reports suggested features peculiar to their rupture, the ictus does not seem to differ significantly as far as localization of the headache or the incidence of coma is concerned.[8,29] Transient paresis of upward gaze has been seen after rupture of basilar bifurcation aneurysms. A history of respiratory arrest and pulmonary edema seems to be more common with brisk hemorrhage from aneurysms arising in front of the medulla. Abducens nerve palsy as a false localizing sign is common but no more frequent than with other causes of sudden increase in intracranial pressure. Oculomotor nerve palsy must be as common with the laterally projecting basilar–superior cerebellar artery aneurysm as with carotid aneurysms and should always suggest a basilar artery aneurysm, especially when the carotid study is negative. Sixth nerve palsy may occur from rupture of basilar–anterior inferior cerebellar artery an-

eurysms, but the laxity of this nerve spares it most times. It is remarkable how seldom dysfunction of the lower cranial nerves occurs with rupture of vertebral or vertebral junction aneurysms, in spite of their close proximity. The data in the Cooperative Study "support the widely held impression that neither . . . or the site of the aneurysm can be differentiated clinically except when an aneurysm is sufficiently large to produce cranial nerve or other neighbourhood signs."[45]

The phenomena associated with cerebrovascular "spasm" also seem in no way different except that brain stem ischemic syndromes are more commonly featured. Further, in the carotid circulation, the arterial narrowing may occur remotely and be associated with severe cerebral hemisphere ischemia and infarction.

As posterior aneurysms enlarge, however, their location becomes more apparent. With lesions of less than giant proportions, palsies of the cranial nerves predominate—of the third for lesions at the superior cerebellar artery and of the sixth for those lower on the basilar artery. Ninth and tenth nerve palsies are rare except with aneurysms of huge dimensions. Once the aneurysms reach "giant" size, tumor syndromes appear. Medullary signs occur with vertebral aneurysms and, if the mass is laterally placed, will mimic a cerebellopontine angle tumor. Pontine syndromes appear with huge basilar trunk aneurysms, while with those arising at the superior cerebellar artery, Weber's syndrome with third nerve palsy and contralateral hemiplegia is typically produced. Giant aneurysms at the basilar bifurcation cause a variety of syndromes, depending on their projection. Those pointing forward commonly mimic pituitary tumors with compression of the optic apparatus; those directed vertically are associated with amnestic syndromes with bilateral oculomotor palsies and bulbar and quadriparesis; and those aimed posteriorly, with midbrain-pontine syndromes, occasionally with pathological laughter.

Tortuous arteriosclerotic S-shaped aneurysms may compress the cranial nerves in either angle and are said occasionally to produce alternating hemiplegia.[25] All of Dandy's 11 cases were found at posterior fossa operations for tic douloureux (10) or

Menière's disease (1) with a presumed causative relationship.[8]

RADIOLOGICAL DIAGNOSIS

Angiography for investigation of subarachnoid hemorrhage in the posterior fossa follows the same principles as that for hemorrhage elsewhere in the head, but it is made more complex by the increased density of overlying bone and by the overlapping and lack of symmetry of the vessels on each side, particularly in older people. Like any angiogram, it must demonstrate the size and shape of the aneurysmal sac or sacs and the relation of the neck to the parent and adjacent vessels as well as evidence of spasm, and displacement of surrounding vessels to suggest thrombosis in a sac larger than is filled with the contrast agent, or surrounding hematoma.

In the majority of cases subtraction films are necessary to remove the bony shadows. Stereoscopic views may be helpful also. Angiotomography in various planes, where the facilities are available, has often been found to be of most value, as it blurs out the bony shadows and overlying vessels. Because of the large amount of contrast within the sac, however, it is of little help in a patient with a huge aneurysm.

Routine views include a lateral and a Townes projection, the latter needing a tilt of 30 to 35 degrees to show the region of the foramen magnum more clearly. Oblique Townes views are sometimes needed, but the head should usually be turned only 10 to 15 degrees from the midline to avoid overlapping and distortion of vessels. A true anteroposterior view is often helpful to show an aneurysm and also to give a better view of the true relationship of the vessels to each other and to the sac. Basal views may also be needed.

All studies should include demonstration of both carotid and both vertebral systems. Good reflux down one vertebral artery may, when contrast is injected into the other, show the origin of the posterior inferior cerebellar artery in the anteroposterior view, but in the lateral view the two vertebrals may overlap so that the area is obscured. If there is any doubt, the agent must be injected into each vertebral separately.

Both carotid systems must be shown, not only to demonstrate any aneurysms that may be present on that circulation but also, in older people, to detect atheroma in the neck, which may have bearing on the operative treatment.

All injections must be selective, nowadays usually by catheter rather than by direct puncture. Right retrograde brachial injections lead to overlapping of the anterior and posterior circulations. In a number of cases, aneurysms have been missed or mistakenly identified because of this.

With aneurysms arising from the vertebral and basilar arteries, the relationship of the sac to the upper or lower margin of the clivus must be clearly demonstrated to decide the operative approach. If operative occlusion of the basilar artery is contemplated, patency of the first segment of each posterior cerebral artery and of the posterior communicating arteries must be tested. Patency of these vessels may be visualized with routine injections, but if it is not, repeat views with injection into the vertebral and compression of each common carotid artery in turn are needed. These maneuvers will show not only whether the first segment of the posterior cerebral artery is present but also whether there is continuity of flow through it, the posterior communicating artery, and the siphon to provide collateral circulation if needed. The patency of the anterior communicating artery should also be checked by carotid injection, with cross-compression views when necessary. Both vertebral arteries should be demonstrated throughout their length to exclude congenital anomalies or atheroma proximally—this is particularly necessary when distal occlusion of a vertebral artery may be contemplated. Streaming in the basilar artery is quite common, owing to flow of blood from the non-opacified vertebral artery, particularly if this is the larger one. Usually this artifact is obvious, as some opacification of the other side of the basilar artery occurs, but it must not be mistaken for spasm. Sometimes the streaming is so marked that the branches of the basilar artery on the poorly opacified side do not fill with contrast and may appear to be occluded. When there is doubt in this respect, the injection must be made into the other vertebral artery, and sometimes into both at once.

Often the sac is considerably larger than is demonstrated by the portion filled with contrast, owing to the presence of mural thrombus. This may often be suspected by greater displacement of adjacent vessels than would be expected from the size of the sac shown and by the shape of the aneurysm, which may have an irregular or concave rather than convex border. Occasionally, air studies have been done to show the size of the sac, but today computed tomography should solve most of these problems. It is also helpful in cases of multiple aneurysms, demonstrating intracerebral and subarachnoid hematoma, edema, or infarction in the region of the ruptured sac. The CT scan does not, however, obviate the need for careful and full angiography in all cases, in view of the likelihood that aneurysms on vessels close to one another may cause similar appearances on the scan. The scanner can also be used to follow the changes in the brain produced by spasm and infarction and to assess the degree of hydrocephalus.

If it is accepted that unruptured sacs should be treated operatively, it is not enough to show the arteries in only the region implicated by the CT scan; all vessels should be demonstrated. It has also been found that in quite a large number of cases of subarachnoid hemorrhage, no convincing abnormality is seen on the scan.

Sometimes the basilar artery is very tortuous and in the lateral view appears displaced away from the clivus. This might suggest a hematoma, and if there is any doubt, computed tomography should help to resolve the question.

Postoperative angiography should always be performed even if the patient is doing well, partly to insure complete obliteration of the sac, obviously the main object of the operation, and as well to document the presence of spasm or occlusion of a branch vessel. If the aneurysmal sac has been aspirated and collapsed at the time of operation, postoperative angiography may seem redundant, but there will still be occasions when the surgeon will be unpleasantly surprised when, in the postoperative angiogram, he notes imperfect clipping of the aneurysm.

In conclusion, it is of great importance to give meticulous attention to the quality of the radiographs and the positioning of the head in the investigation of the posterior circulation; otherwise aneurysms will be missed, or loops or overlapping branches mistaken for sacs. One must be particularly cautious in older people in whom the vessels are often tortuous and asymmetrical. Precise visualization of the sac in two planes is essential before the diagnosis can be made.

If no source of bleeding has been shown by careful angiography following a hemorrhage, the examination should usually be repeated in a week to 10 days. This occasionally reveals an aneurysm that was not seen previously. The initial failure is more often than not due to human error, faulty positioning, bad injections of contrast, or overlapping vessels. Because these failures of technique are more likely to occur in examinations of the posterior circulation than of the anterior, repeat angiograms are more likely to be productive.

OPERATIVE TECHNIQUE AND RESULTS

This review is based on the experience with 616 patients with aneurysms on the vertebrobasilar circulation treated by operation at the University of Western Ontario. The overall results are given in Table 50–2. The cases are divided into three groups according to the size of the aneurysm, which is the most important factor in determining the outcome of operative treatment.

The success or failure of repair of aneurysms, whether on the posterior or the anterior circulation, is dependent on two general factors: first, the condition of the patient as he enters the operating room, and second, but obviously of equal importance, the techniques by which the aneurysm is exposed and precisely isolated from the cerebral circulation. The authors usually prefer to operate on a patient who is in good clinical condition, has no signs of impaired cerebral perfusion, and is well hydrated 7 to 10 days following the last subarachnoid hemorrhage. Obviously, when one is planning a prophylactic procedure to prevent recurrent hemorrhage, it is ideal to operate as soon as possible after the initial bleed to seal the rent in the cerebral artery. Early operation is at best controversial, however, and rarely proves to be a straightforward matter. Frequently, the swelling of the brain soon after the hemorrhage limits the exposure. The aneurysm is more fragile, since it is sealed with a clot of jellylike con-

TABLE 50-2   RESULTS OF OPERATIVE TREATMENT OF ANEURYSMS OF THE POSTERIOR CIRCULATION*

SIZE OF ANEURYSM	NO. OF CASES	RESULTS							
		Excellent No.	Excellent Per Cent	Good No.	Good Per Cent	Poor No.	Poor Per Cent	Dead No.	Dead Per Cent
Small (<1.2 cm)	411	308	75 (87%)	48	12	33	8 (13%)	22	5
Large (1.2–2.5 cm)	87	52	60 (75%)	13	15	15	17 (25%)	7	8
Giant (>2.5 cm)	118	39	33 (58%)	30	25	31	26 (42%)	18	14
Total	616	399	65 (80%)	91	15	79	13 (20%)	47	8

* All sites and grades are included.

sistency and will burst with the slightest manipulation. Furthermore, the problem of cerebral vasospasm may well be aggravated if not precipitated by early operation. In the authors' unit, it is most uncommon to operate in the first week even on a simple aneurysm in a patient who is completely well. Similarly, it is equally rare to delay beyond two weeks except in patients with persistent high intracranial pressure, cerebral infarction, or vasospasm. Of course, the presence of an intracerebral hematoma in an individual in whom failure of vital centers cannot be controlled by medical measures demands an emergency decompression.

With use of the measures to inhibit fibrinolysis and control blood pressure, the incidence of recurrent hemorrhage is less than 6 per cent. When the operation is delayed for a week or more after the hemorrhage, the brain is slack, Retraction of the brain, and exposure and clipping of the aneurysm can be accomplished with safety and ease. Having the brain slack is particularly important when deep hypotension is used during dissection and clipping of the sac, since retraction pressures exceeding 40 mm of mercury will result in cessation of flow beneath the retractor blade and almost certainly cause ischemia or hemorrhagic infarction. The authors are so convinced of the necessity of having a slack brain during the exposure of the aneurysm that occasionally they will discontinue the procedure when a tight, swollen, and injected brain is encountered upon opening the dura. Reoperation is done 5 to 10 days later after administration of appropriate drugs to reduce intracranial tension.[42]

Preoperative and Anesthetic Considerations

Most patients should be operated upon under general endotracheal anesthesia, and assisted or controlled ventilation should be used. Occasionally when intentional occlusion of a major vessel is contemplated and the patient is cooperative, operation under local anesthesia is indicated. Similarly, when a possible disturbance of medullary flow is anticipated during the dissection, exposure, and obliteration of an aneurysm, it may be preferable to have the patient under general anesthesia but breathing spontaneously, thereby allowing the normal function of respiratory centers to serve as a guide to the adequacy of flow to the brain stem. In all cases, the anesthesia is light and care is taken not to overventilate the patient, keeping the carbon dioxide level in the range of 40 to 45 mm of mercury and the oxygen tension close to 100 mm of mercury. Halothane, nitrous oxide, and narcotic anesthetic techniques may be selected by the neuroanesthetist, depending on the patient's clinical condition.[1]

Almost all aneurysms of the posterior circulation are approached with the patient in the right lateral decubitus, or "park-bench," position. In this position, the patient is lying on the left side with padding under the upper part of the chest and the hip to provide a comfortable position for the left shoulder and neck. For procedures on aneurysms arising between the vertebral junction and the basilar bifurcation, the head is held in a straight lateral position and fixed with the pin headrest (Fig. 50–2). The sagittal plane of the head is then precisely parallel to the floor with the coronal axis either perpendicular to the floor or angled no more than 10 to 15 degrees in the cephalad direction to provide slightly greater access to the base of the brain. The right arm is taped to the right side of the trunk or held on an armboard. The back is supported with well-padded rests that are attached firmly to the table. Pillows are placed between the knees, and all weight-bearing surfaces are adequately padded.

For operations on aneurysms arising from the vertebral arteries, the face is angled 20 to 30 degrees toward the floor and the upper shoulder is taped caudally to open the exposure of the suboccipital region (cf. Fig. 50–13). With both positions, care is taken not to occlude vascular structures of the neck.

Accurate, continuous monitoring of the mean arterial pressure, heart rate, electrocardiogram, blood gases, fluid balance, temperature, and occasionally electroencephalogram is essential during the procedure.

Perhaps the most important monitoring technique is measurement of the systemic arterial blood pressure. This is accomplished by inserting a polyethylene cannula into a radial or dorsalis pedis artery and connecting it directly to an aneroid manometer or to a pressure transducer and then to an electronic pressure recording device. It is important that the artery from which the systemic pressure is measured be at the level of the brain or slightly above so that an accurate estimate of the cerebral arterial blood pressure can be obtained and measured continuously. The electrocardiogram and arterial pressure are monitored continuously on a console beside the anesthesiologist. The bladder is catheterized, and fluid balance is measured continuously. A heating-cooling blanket is placed over the patient to maintain normal body temperature.

With a Tuohy needle, a lumbar subarachnoid catheter (PE 100) is inserted into the lumbar subarachnoid space and attached to a closed drainage bag. This tubing is clamped until the dura is opened, when cerebrospinal fluid drainage is commenced to assist intracranial relaxation.

Adequate intracranial relaxation is essential for the success of the procedure. In the authors' experience, a slack brain is best achieved by administering furosemide (Lasix), 1 mg per kilogram, shortly after induction and mannitol, 1 gm per kilogram intravenously, with the skin incision. Cerebrospinal fluid drainage is commenced with the dural incision, and the removal of 60 to 120 ml of fluid will provide further relaxation of the intracranial contents and also remove the pooled cerebrospinal fluid in the basal cisterns, which tends to obscure the operative field. There are some hazards associated with too vigorous attempts to reduce the intracranial pressure, for example, torsional stresses on the brain stem and even rupture of bridging cerebral veins, which produces acute subdural hematoma. One should be aware of these uncommon complications and aim for only sufficient

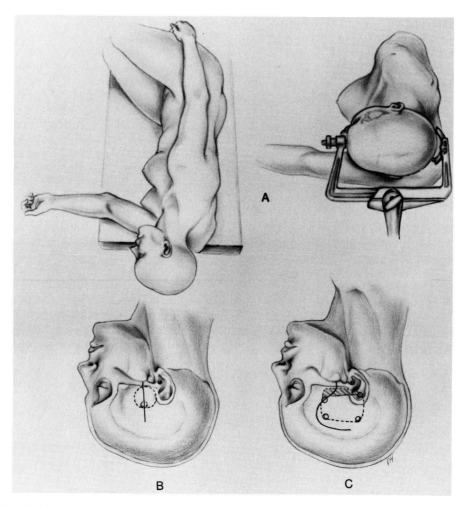

Figure 50–2 Subtemporal approach to region of basilar bifurcation. *A*. Lateral park bench position with head slightly flexed downward. *B*. Subtemporal "tic" craniectomy showing usual extent of bony opening. *C*. Half horseshoe incision, conventional bone flap, and removal of squamous temporal bone to level of zygomatic root and floor of middle fossa.

relaxation to expose the base of the brain without excessive retractor pressure.

If sufficient relaxation for easy exposure of the tentorial incisura has not been achieved, the retractor should be removed, the brain surface should be gently irrigated and covered, and the surgeon should wait while checking the cerebrospinal fluid drainage, the adequacy of ventilation, and the diuretic effect. It is hazardous to hyperventilate the patient in an attempt to reduce the intracranial bulk. To drive the carbon dioxide tension below 35 mm of mercury is to run a significant risk of causing sufficient vasoconstriction to impair cerebral perfusion, particularly during periods of profound hypotension. Gently packing the anterior and posterior margin of the exposed temporal lobe with strips of Gelfoam, carefully wrapping the vein of Labbé and the veins traversing the anterior temporal fossa, raising the head of the table, and exercising patience often achieve sufficient relaxation to allow the surgeon to proceed. If, however, adequate exposure is still not attained by these various maneuvers and the use of gentle retraction, it is best to abandon the procedure until a later time. Cerebral edema is the most likely cause of the brain's tightness, and it cannot be adequately reversed during the operative procedure. Cerebral edema and swelling will also certainly be aggravated by heavy retraction pressures combined with prolonged hypotension and will compromise the outcome of the operation.

Most of the craniectomy and initial exposure of the aneurysm is carried out under normal arterial blood pressure. When the surgeon begins to approach the aneurysm, however, hypotension is induced to reduce pressure in the sac below the bursting point. The preferred hypotensive agents in the authors' unit are sodium nitroprusside (Nipride) and trimethaphan camsylate (Arfonad). Initially, the mean arterial pressure is brought down to approximately 60 mm of mercury during the approach to the aneurysm; when one begins separating perforating arteries or intentionally displacing the sac to gain exposure of the neck, the pressure is further reduced to a mean of 40 mm of mercury. Mean arterial pressures of 40 mm of mercury are safe for more than an hour in otherwise healthy individuals without a history of long-standing hypertensive disease. If the dissection is more prolonged, the pressure can be raised intermittently to 60 or 70 mm of mercury mean to permit reperfusion.[42,48]

The dissection of the aneurysm has been facilitated by the use of magnification of vision, first with loupes and more recently with the microscope. With excellent coaxial illumination, even the finest details of the origin of the sac are revealed and great accuracy attained in freeing the neck from fibrin, clot, arterial branches, and nerves. Coupled with this are delicate new instruments with which to do these intricate dissections. Bipolar coagulation deserves special mention, for with it the neck of an aneurysm can be shrunk and rendered firm to reveal hidden connections and facilitate its dissection and clipping. "Baby" aneurysms, often no more than blisters and too small to be seen in an angiogram, are not infrequently discovered nearby and can be coagulated down to a thickened stump for packing.

The value of these technical adjuncts to the procedure is enhanced by the fact that most saccular aneurysms arise at the distal carina or "crotch" of the branching of a major artery along the base of the brain. At every site, there are important vessels arising from or near this crotch that must be identified and preserved. They may be only the branches forming the crotch, but at most sites there are a few, if not a host of, tiny perforating vessels whose integrity is so important to the outcome of the procedure. Ideally the dissection should be carried to the very neck of the sac. Under magnification and deep hypotension, even sharp dissection may be used on the fragile wall to clear it from adjacent vital structures. The clip or ligature must be placed flush with the origin of the neck so that the normal arterial wall will heal firmly. Since aneurysms grow from the neck, even a small portion of the neck remaining proximal to a clip has the potential of blowing out or forming another aneurysm.[21] If the surgeon is not satisfied with the placement of a clip or is concerned that other structures may be caught in the blades, it should be removed and replaced as many times as necessary to obtain an ideal position. Admittedly, there are circumstances in which a portion of the neck must be left to prevent kinking or narrowing of a major vessel or to avoid injury to an adherent arterial branch or hard atherosclerotic plaque. In these cases, the remaining aneurysm should be packed with gauze or coated with plastic. If there is any doubt that the aneurysm is completely obliterated, or if the sac has not been aspirated and collapsed to verify its obliteration, then postoperative angiography is necessary to enable the surgeon to assure the patient that the aneurysm is no longer a hazard.

The extent and firmness of atheromatous involvement of the neck and parent branching is important. Ordinarily "soft" atheroma in the neck will conform to a clip or ligature, but "hard" atheroma is dangerous in that it may prevent the clip blades from closing in an ideal position. The clip may then migrate to leave the aneurysm exposed or, more tragically, to occlude the parent vessel. It is equally dangerous if the manipulations of a clip fracture the atheroma, resulting in thrombosis of the parent trunk.

Surgical ingenuity has known no bounds in the search for other methods of obliteration of aneurysms, e.g., plastic coating, insertion of thrombogenic hair, wire, or iron filings, but the clip or ligature remains most effective for most aneurysms.[3,24,40,49] These alternate methods may be indicated in cases in which the dissection of an aneurysm would formerly have been left incomplete for fear of rupture or because branches arose from the sac. Now it is known that the latter does not occur in saccular aneurysms except when the aneurysm enlarges to the point that the parent branching becomes ectatic and forms the base of the aneurysm. Further, it is now routinely possible to clear the necks of most aneurysms safely for accurate and permanent occlusion.

Clips Used

Any good spring clip can be used for posterior aneurysms with a neck in clear view. The authors prefer the Scoville clip, which has a well-machined, thin, but strong, blade to work into the narrow confines under perforating vessels and across the neck. Its

major fault is that it tends to rotate easily in the somewhat short applier. Grooving the handle of the clip might solve the rotation problem. The Heifetz clip can be held rigidly in the applier, but the blades are wider and longer, and the longer blades tend to float and slip on the necks of the broad aneurysms. The many varieties and forms of the Sugita clip are strong and close ideally, and the bayonet handle of the applier allows better visualization of the blades and neck. Because of the special problem of the large bulbous bifurcation aneurysms, a new, strong clip was designed with an aperture in its base to accommodate the P_1 segment (Fig. 50–3). This clip is available in lengths up to 24 mm for giant aneurysms. It is important that the blade length selected be exactly the width of the compressed aneurysmal neck so that the P_1 segment, the perforators, and the opposite third nerve are not caught in the tips. The blade can be trimmed and filed, if necessary, to fit the anatomy accurately. This fenestrated clip has been found to be useful to enclose structures other than P_1, such as nearby perforating vessels or even the third nerve. Because of its strength, the Drake-Kees clip is usually satisfactory for very large-necked aneurysms, although caution must be used so that none of the near side of the neck lies free in the aperture. Often a neck can be shrunk down and firmed with coagulation so that a much smaller clip can be used to obliterate the aneurysm precisely.

The Subtemporal Approach

Aneurysms in the region of the basilar bifurcation, including those arising at the superior cerebellar artery, are exposed quite satisfactorily by an anterior subtemporal approach across the floor of the middle fossa and the tentorial edge into the mouth of the incisura in front of the midbrain. Ordinarily the right side is used unless the projection or complexity of the aneurysm or a left oculomotor palsy or right hemiparesis demands an approach under the dominant temporal lobe.

For this approach with the patient in the lateral decubitus position, a small temporal bone flap has been used above and in front of the ear. It is important to remove the temporal squama down to the floor of the middle fossa for a better line of sight with

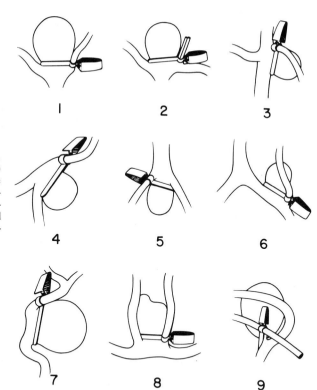

Figure 50–3 The fenestrated drake clip. Structures shown in the aperture include (1) the P_1 segment, (2) perforating arteries, (3) the anterior inferior cerebellar artery (4) the basilar artery, (5) the vertebral artery, (6) the posterior inferior cerebellar artery, (7) the carotid artery, (8) the A_2 segment of the anterior cerebral artery, and (9) the oculomotor nerve.

the least temporal retraction. For the experienced surgeon, a small subtemporal craniectomy through a linear incision like that for the Frazier-Spiller operation for tic douloureux is quite sufficient, and it is now routine on the authors' unit for most ordinary aneurysms in the region of the basilar bifurcation (see Fig. 50–2 *B* and *C*). Ordinarily, a week or more after bleeding, the brain will be slack following administration of mannitol and furosemide and lumbar drainage of spinal fluid prior to and during the opening of the dura. Very little brain retractor pressure will be needed to elevate the anterior temporal lobe out of the floor of the middle fossa. It has never been necessary to resect any portion of the temporal lobe. A sheet of compressed moist Gelfoam is used to cover the brain, for if irrigated, it does not adhere to the brain even after several hours of retraction.

The microscope may now be moved into position. Most of the dissection can be done at 10× or 16×, but higher powers may be advisable for critical sharp dissection. As the edge of the tentorium comes into view, the uncus will be seen disengaging from its position inside the edge of the tentorium. It marks the ideal position for

the tip of the retractor, as it lies just in front of the crus at the entrance to the interpeduncular cistern (Figs. 50–4 and 50–5). The oculomotor nerve is almost universally attached by arachnoidal bands to the tip of the uncus so that, as the uncus is raised with the tip of the retractor, this nerve is elevated with it out of the opening and can be spared from manipulation. It is usually possible to work underneath the nerve to clip the aneurysm except in the case of a high basilar bifurcation aneurysm or a giant sac, when it may be necessary to separate it from the uncus. The lessening of third nerve manipulation by this simple expedient has resulted in fewer postoperative third nerve palsies and earlier and more complete recoveries in those that do occur.

To enlarge the opening into the interpeduncular cistern, a silk suture is placed in the edge of the tent just in front of but free of the insertion of the fourth nerve. After being passed through the dura of the floor of the middle fossa, the suture can be tied tightly, thus drawing the edge of the tentorium laterally, often for a centimeter or more. The fourth nerve is then tucked below the tentorial edge for safety. This simple but effective maneuver to open the

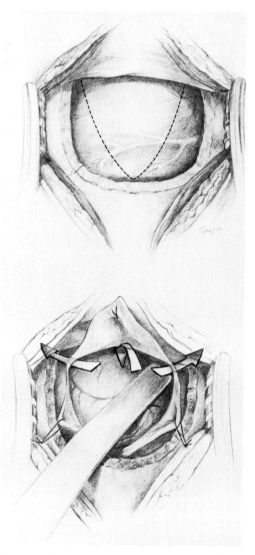

Figure 50-4 Detail of temporal craniectomy and dural opening to show initial exploration of undersurface of temporal lobe to identify and protect the draining veins.

municating artery. Indeed, this vessel should be carefully preserved in case some injury to P_1 occurs or it is necessary to include P_1 in the clip (rarely). Further, this communicating artery gives rise to important diencephalic branches (anterior thalamo-perforating arteries) whose integrity might be compromised by its occlusion.

At this stage, the blood pressure is lowered to mean arterial levels of 35 to 40 mm of mercury by administering intravenous sodium nitroprusside. It is important to be certain the systemic intra-arterial pressure measurements are made with the transducer or manometer at head level if the patient is tilted so that mean *intracranial* arterial pressure is being recorded. This deep hypotension, by reducing the pressure in the sac, permits the careful, complete removal of clot and fibrin from

entrance into the interpeduncular region has obviated the necessity for dividing the tentorium to approach aneurysms at the basilar bifurcation or as low as at the superior cerebellar artery (Fig. 50-6).

Opening the double layer of arachnoid in front of the crus and below the third nerve exposes the interpeduncular cistern. To avoid heavier retractor pressure to visualize the posterior cerebral artery, it is convenient to follow the superior cerebellar artery back to the basilar, where it arises just below the origin of the P_1 segment, which curves upward from its origin. It has never been necessary to divide the posterior com-

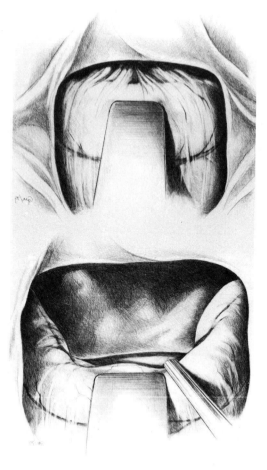

Figure 50-5 Initial view of tentorial incisura with elevation of temporal lobe.

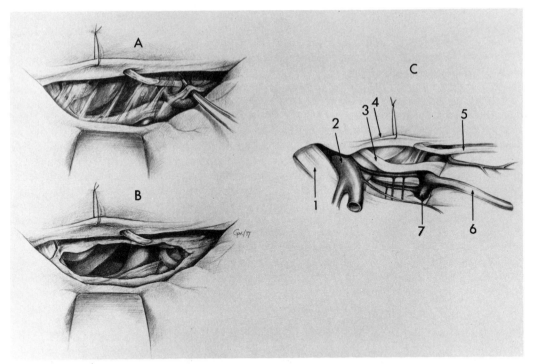

Figure 50–6 Exposure and anatomy of interpeduncular fossa. *A*. Tentorial edge sutured laterally into middle fossa, entry of trochlear nerve into free edge, and hook opening arachnoid between third and fourth cranial nerves. *B*. Extent of arachnoid opening exposing interpeduncular fossa. *C*. Anatomy of region. 1, optic nerve; 2, carotid artery; 3, oculomotor nerve; 4, free edge of tent; 5, trochlear nerve; 6, posterior cerebral artery; 7, aneurysm arising from basilar bifurcation.

the interpeduncular cistern and exposure of the neck of the aneurysm and associated branches. A clear understanding of the anatomical detail is essential before proceeding with any clip application.

Saccular Aneurysms at the Basilar Bifurcation

These aneurysms arise in the crotch of the bifurcation and most commonly project *upward* in line with the curve of the basilar artery. The next most common projection is *posteriorly* into the interpeduncular space. Least common are those aneurysms that project *anteriorly* with the dome above the dorsum sellae or adherent to its posterior surface. Rarely they project laterally from a bifurcation that may be rotated nearly 90 degrees in the coronal plane.

The host of perforating vessels seen in the angiogram in this region are often interpreted as arising from the aneurysm. This is fallacious, since smaller saccular aneurysms cannot be the origin of perforators because they themselves originate as "blow outs" of the elastica and intima through openings in the media at the distal carina of the branching. These small vessels are named according to their distribution, interpeduncular, circumflex, mesencephalic, and posterior thalamic perforating arteries. They arise most often from or very near the origin of the P_1 segment and are usually applied to the sides of the sac posterolaterally. A few interpeduncular vessels may arise from the back of the basilar bifurcation and be applied to the posterior aspects of the sac.

A characteristic feature of these aneurysms is the associated ballooning of the basilar bifurcation, which seems to become ectatic almost routinely as the aneurysm enlarges, so that when viewed from the side the P_1 segments at first appear to emerge from the sac itself.

The *height* of the basilar bifurcation is also very important and varies considerably. Ordinarily, the crotch is at or just above the dorsum sellae. It may be much higher, however, at the apex of the interpeduncular space behind the mammillary bodies. Rarely, it may be even higher if the basilar artery is elongated and tortuous with atheroma, when it may even indent the floor of the hypothalamus and third ventricle. The greater the height above the dorsum sellae, the more the temporal lobe will need to be retracted. As the neck of the sac reaches the apex of the interpeduncular space, it and the perforating arteries are more completely hidden by the mammillary bodies in front and the peduncles behind. With only one smaller aneurysm, however, was it necessary to abandon clipping for gauze packing because of this obscuration by height. Gentle retraction of the mammillary bodies or crus has not produced any known persistent deficit.

On the other hand, the bifurcation may be quite low, at the base of the dorsum sellae or even lower. This position of the neck is confining to the surgeon because the edge of the insertion of the tentorium cannot be reflected downward as much by the "tenting" suture and tends to hide the base of the sac, which is wedged between the pontomesencephalic junction and the clivus. Division of the tentorium does not add much advantage because the fifth nerve as well as the fourth now obscures the region. Even so, with a little more retraction applied laterally under the temporal lobe to increase the angle of vision over the depressed tentorial edge, it is possible to do most of the lowest basilar bifurcation aneurysms without dividing the tentorium. In one case, however, in which the neck was below the level of the sellar floor, the sac tore in the region of the neck on simple removal of an improperly placed clip. Control of bleeding was not possible. Despite division of the tentorium and the fourth nerve and temporary basilar artery occlusion, another clip could not be applied accurately in this confined region. The posterior communicating arteries were tiny, so permanent P_1 occlusion could not be used. The patient became exsanguinated and succumbed before packing of the area stopped the flow. In one other case of a very low bifurcation aneurysm, attempts to clip a small sac wedged into the inferior apex of the interpeduncular fossa failed on two separate occasions because of an inability to gain visual access or room to maneuver the clip in this deep recess. Although the dome of the aneurysm was clearly visible, the origins of

P_1 and associated perforating branches could not be seen and spared; thus, attempts to clip the aneurysm were discontinued and the sac was reinforced with chopped gauze.

A frequent error in interpreting the angiogram has to do with the apparent position of the P_1 segments clear of the aneurysmal neck in the Townes view. It must be remembered that P_1 takes a compound curve forward and outward to cross above the third nerve before turning around the edge of the peduncle hidden under the hippocampal gyrus. The first curve and position of P_1 are therefore not seen in the Townes view, so it seems to come out straighter from the side of the neck. Further, even when the neck seems to be clear for a few millimeters at its origin, as seen in the angiogram, it must be understood that P_1 may well be adherent because the unseen walls of the aneurysm and the artery are usually apposed. Therefore, at operation, P_1 with its perforatoring branches will usually be found applied to the side of the neck. In larger, bulbous sacs it will seem to be arising from the base of the sac itself, although it really originates from the very common ectatic widening of the bifurcation.

Upward-Projecting Aneurysms

Following the superior cerebellar artery to its origin will reveal the basilar artery and the origin of the P_1 segment immediately above with the fibers of the third nerve crossing underneath. This nerve will usually be elevated far enough upward by the arachnoid bands attached to the uncus. This allows sufficient exposure of the P_1 origin and the neck of the sac to allow completion of the dissection and placement of the clip below. It is best to start the dissection across the front of the neck, as there are never perforating vessels in this area. By this maneuver, it is usually simple to see across the front of the aneurysm to the origin of the opposite P_1 segment and even its perforating branches, and to get an estimation of the width of the neck, although the sac may have to be gently depressed posteriorly with a dissector (Fig. 50-7).

The hazards to clipping of this aneurysm lie behind its sac. Rarely it will stand free in the interpeduncular space; more usually it will be buried in the space hidden by the crus. Gentle retraction of the crus is well

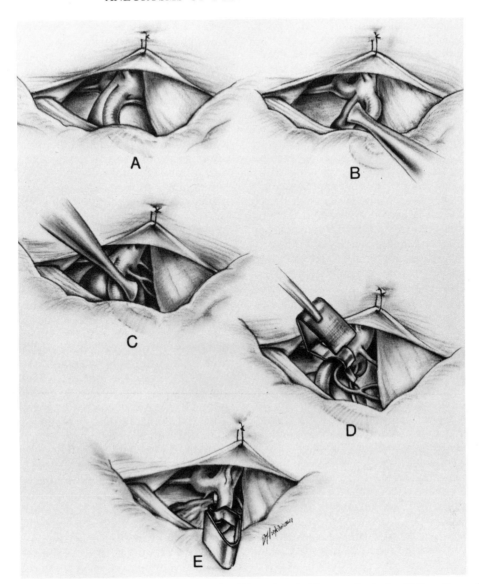

Figure 50–7   Typical bulbous aneurysm at basilar bifurcation. *A*. Note usual ectasia of bifurcation and thalamo-perforating vessel arising from P_1 segment of posterior cerebral artery. *B*. Compression of waist of sac posteriorly to see opposite P_1 segment and posterior communicating artery. *C*. Anterior displacement of sac to reveal interpeduncular fossa to see and separate perforating branches. *D*. Drake clip applied and then rotated to show P_1 and one perforating artery clear in the aperture but a previously unseen perforator caught under the blade. The clip must be removed, the perforator separated from the sac, and the clip properly reapplied. *E*. After application of the clip, the aneurysm has been punctured and collapsed. Blades properly cross only the neck, just missing the thalamo-perforating vessel from the opposite P_1 segment.

tolerated and will expose the posterolateral aspect and the perforating arteries, which can be carefully separated with a tiny dissector. To see the posterior aspect of the neck and waist, usually it is necessary to indent and displace the waist of the sac anteriorly with the dissector or small sucker tip and to retract the crus somewhat with the other instrument. This maneuver will reveal the whole of the interpeduncular space, the exit of the opposite third nerve, the origin of the opposite P_1 segment and the perforating branches arising from it, and the basilar artery. All these perforating vessels must be freed sufficiently to permit a clip blade to slide underneath. A general widening or ballooning ectasia of the basilar bifurcation is common and must be distinguished from the aneurysm. This distinction is frequently obscured by atheromatous change extending from the artery into the base of the aneurysm.

As noted, the P_1 segment arises nearly vertically from its origin beside and gently adherent to the base of the sac before crossing laterally over the third nerve. To apply an ordinary spring clip in this circumstance, P_1 with its perforators must be freed carefully from this adherence so that one blade can be slipped underneath it, either from in front or from behind, to cross the neck. This is quite reasonable where P_1 ascends toward either the front or the back of the sac. When it is placed midway on the side of a more bulbous sac, however, it can be awkward and dangerous to try to free a firm adherence or to try to slide one blade underneath P_1 nearly at right angles to the surgeon. In this case, the Drake-Kees or Sugita aperture clip with the aperture at the base of the blades is very satisfactory. With these clips it is not even necessary to separate P_1, and perforating vessels may also be included safely in the aperture. A common error to be avoided is to choose a clip with blades longer than necessary. The necks of most basilar bifurcation aneurysms in the coronal plane are usually narrower than is apparent on the anteroposterior angiogram and will usually measure between 3 and 5 mm. It is most important to select or trim the blades (with wire cutting pliers and file) so that they fall only across the neck and do not impinge on P_1 or perforating arteries on *either* side.

As the posterior blade of the clip is passed behind the neck, it must be certain that it is inside the perforators. As the blades are allowed to close and narrow the neck, the opposite P_1 segment will come into view, so accurate final alignment of the blades flush with the neck at the upper origin of P_1 on each side is certain before final closure. The posterior blade must not be put too far across, for the root of the opposite third nerve courses up behind the opposite P_1 segment and can be brushed or actually injured by this blade. As for any aneurysm, immediately after first placement, the position of the clip should be assessed by rotating it forward and backward to see the position of each blade. Not infrequently, the first time the clip is placed, the blades will be too high or too low on the opposite side and a perforating artery may be inadvertently caught. As noted earlier, a common error is to use blades longer than

necessary and to place them across the far P_1 segment or up on the waist of the aneurysm. In spite of its apparent width, the neck is often narrower at its very origin, and much shorter blades can be used. It is important to remove, modify, and replace the clip as many times as is necessary until a perfect position is insured. Ordinarily this is no problem with deep hypotension. Moving quickly, the surgeon may take advantage of a malpositioned clip to separate adherent perforators, P_1 from the slack sac, or if necessary, even the sac itself from higher reaches of the interpeduncular fossa. After final positioning of the clip, the aneurysm should be punctured and collapsed. This will provide an even better view of the position of the clip. If it is imperfect still, a little pressure and waiting will always stop the bleeding from a needle hole so that a dry field will be available for repositioning.

Should the slope of the basilar bifurcation in the coronal plane be to one side, the neck of the aneurysm will not be in a direct line away from the operator. Not infrequently this obliquity of the neck is considerable, and if it slants down and away from the surgeon, the clip application is awkward, since not enough temporal retraction can be obtained safely to get a line of sight along the angle of the neck. Even so, except in the rare circumstance in which the basilar bifurcation is directed laterally this is usually not enough of a problem to warrant an approach under the dominant temporal lobe. Usually it is possible to rotate the clip in its applier or to retract P_1 downward enough to level the neck to get accurate placement. Deep levels of hypotension are necessary for these extensive though gentle manipulations.

Rarely, as the neck is closed by a clip, the dome of the sac is dragged inferiorly away from an attachment to the hypothalamic floor or clivus and hemorrhage will begin. If the clip has to be removed and replaced, usually the dome will stop bleeding as it re-expands and is tamponaded against the area where it was formerly adherent, especially if the rent is not too large.

When can a perforating artery be safely occluded? Ideally, never, but it has been possible to include one or two tiny very adherent ones on the back of a very thin neck without evident deficit. Most of these vessels can be freed with a tiny dissector, but if one or more of large size could not be freed, then it would be best to abandon clipping and resort to reinforcement of the sac. Sometimes, thickening the wall of the sac with bipolar coagulation underneath a perforator will make it possible to dissect it free more safely without rupturing the aneurysm. With this lateral subtemporal approach, this vertical aneurysm is perhaps the only one on the basilar circulation whose neck cannot easily be shrunk and firmed up with coagulation, since usually P_1 is squarely in the way of closing the forceps blades.

Frankly ruptured, these aneurysms can be handled in the same manner as any other aneurysm, primarily without panic and on the principle that the dissection must always be completed before the clip is applied. Frantic, imperfect application of clips leads only to disaster. Small rents will stop spontaneously with a little pressure. When the bleeding from larger rents is directed into the sucker, often the aneurysm will collapse, exposing its origin nicely for completion of the dissection. Although a rent at or near the neck may require exquisite placement of clip blades, it would be wise to take a P_1 segment only if a generous posterior communicating artery were present.

In critical situations or in dealing with giant aneurysms, it has been found that the P_1 segment may be occluded at its origin in certain circumstances. The presence of a good posterior communicating artery is prerequisite to deliberate occlusion, and no perforating vessel should be included in the clip. Clip application must therefore be very accurate to leave the small vessels originating from the distal stump to be irrigated retrogradely by the communicating vessel. The decision for this action should not be taken lightly, however, and would depend on the situation and the risk.

Recently, the *sylvian approach* to the basilar bifurcation has been suggested because of the excellent exposure of the region, as seen in removal of supra- and retrosellar tumors.[57] After the inner end of the sylvian fissure has been split, the approach is on one or the other side of the carotid artery, between it and the chiasm medially or the third nerve laterally, to gain maximum visibility and access. The authors have used this approach from time to time over the years, but it can be narrow and confining. It is most suitable for aneurysms with

small necks lying in ideal position just above the dorsum sellae and pointing forward or upward. The level of the bifurcation varies greatly, however, and the neck of the aneurysm may be just out of sight above or hidden below behind the dorsum, for the cisterns are usually much smaller than when ballooned by a tumor. Further, this approach does not allow nearly the same visualization in that important region of the perforating arteries behind the aneurysm or below it when the sac projects posteriorly. Also, the neck of a bifurcation aneurysm is usually more completely obliterated if the clip is placed in parallel with the bifurcation, and there is less risk of kinking. When placed at right angles, a "dog ear" may remain as the sides of the neck are approximated and the bifurcation is crimped. The approach is ideal though to see the opposite P_1 segment and its perforating vessels and to shrink the neck of the aneurysm by coagulation, for P_1 is not in the way, which offsets some of its disadvantages. Also, there is less third nerve manipulation. It has been useful also in the case of multiple aneurysms in this region, e.g., to deal with an intact bifurcation aneurysm after clipping an anterior communicating or an intact basilar–superior cerebellar artery aneurysm projecting to the left after the ruptured basilar bifurcation aneurysm has been clipped from the nondominant side. The neck of a basilar–superior cerebellar artery aneurysm is difficult to see and obliterate from a subtemporal approach from the opposite side across the clivus, although it can be done. The two approaches have been used frequently in a complementary fashion, for the sylvian approach can be quickly modified to be subtemporal merely by displacing posteriorly or elevating the temporal pole if the anterior temporal squama has been removed. Further, a "half and half" combination of the two approaches is useful where the sylvian exposure does not allow visualization of the back of the neck of a larger aneurysm or where the neck has a more horizontal takeoff posteriorly. The mobile temporal pole may be elevated or displaced backward enough to allow the surgeon to dissect on either side of the third nerve. Behind it, the posterior aspect of the neck can be seen and cleared of perforators, after which the clip is applied from in front of the nerve over the dorsum sellae with all the vessels

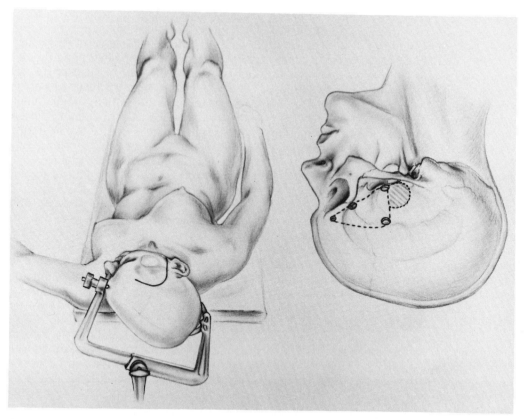

Figure 50–8 Head position and craniotomy for combined approach to anterior circle of Willis and basilar bifurcation region. Initial classic frontotemporal bone flap. Additional subtemporal craniectomy to be done for temporal lobe displacement when the sylvian exposure to the region of basilar bifurcation is unsatisfactory.

in view. Much of the merit of any exposure is a matter of continued use and familiarity with the anatomy (Figs. 50–8, 50–9, and 50–10).

Posteriorly Projecting Aneurysms

Early, it was considered that these aneurysms would be difficult and dangerous. They have, however, proved to be a good group for operative treatment. Once the neck is exposed, the perforating arteries are either free or can easily be freed from the sac, although there may be one or two above the neck as well as on both sides and below.

The same subtemporal approach is used, but the third nerve is more in the way because of its slope from above and behind P_1 to cross down and below it, often across the neck. Only a glimpse of the neck is seen from in front, although the opposite P_1 is clearly visible. Because of the rise of P_1 from its origin, it is necessary to work behind and below it and either above or below the

third nerve, depending on its position and the easiest method of displacing it. As the crus is retracted, the neck will come into view, although the dome, buried in the interpeduncular space, usually is not seen. Occasionally there are perforating branches on the back of the neck, but the usual leash will be present on either side of and below the belly of the neck. They seem to separate as the crus is retracted or the neck is teased into view by pulling gently outward on P_1 with the sucker tip. As the blades of a spring clip are allowed to close slowly, the gradual narrowing of the neck will reveal its opposite side, the perforating vessels on the opposite P_1 segments, and the opposite third nerve. The opposite P_1 segment will not ordinarily be in the way of the blades, and as long as the blades close only across the far side of the neck, it is unlikely that any unseen perforator will be caught. Situations have been seen in which one or two small perforators were free between the tips of the blades, which were held just far

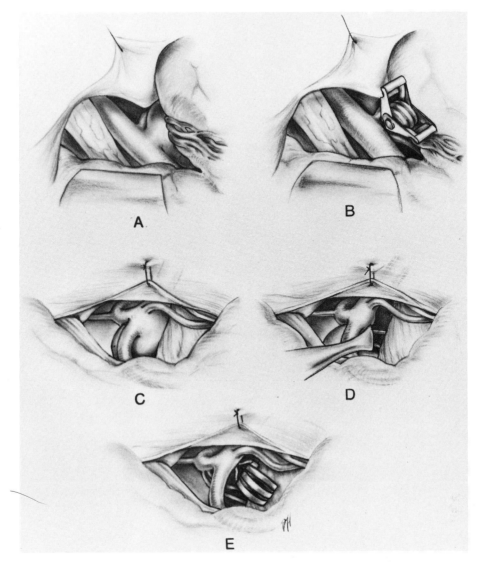

Figure 50–9 Two aneurysms, carotid–communicating artery and basilar bifurcation, ruptured sac unknown. *A*. Carotid–communicating artery aneurysm exposed by usual subfrontal approach. *B*. Aneurysm clipped, sparing posterior communicating and anterior choroidal arteries. Paracarotid approach to the basilar bifurcation was too narrow and dangerous. (Carotid aneurysms can be clipped via a pure subtemporal exposure). *C*. After additional squamous temporal craniectomy and subtemporal exposure of backward-projecting basilar bifurcation aneurysm. *D*. Displacement to see and separate perforating arteries. *E*. Clip is free of perforators from opposite P_1 segment.

enough apart by the bulk of the neck to accommodate them; however, it is not a circumstance on which to rely. Aspiration and collapse of the sac will reveal how accurately the clip has been placed. Caution should be exercised when what appears to be a backward-projecting sac is actually a saccule or tit coming off posteriorly from what is really a neck that has an initial upward projection. This configuration should be viewed and dissected in the same way as an upward-projecting neck.

Anteriorly Projecting Aneurysms

Unfortunately, these are the least common type, for they are the easiest and most straightforward to repair. They project forward and upward from the line of the basilar artery, usually above the dorsum sellae and free in the interpeduncular space, and are free of perforating branches, since none arise from the anterior aspect of the basilar artery. In low-placed basilar bifurcations, caution is needed, for the dome is often ad-

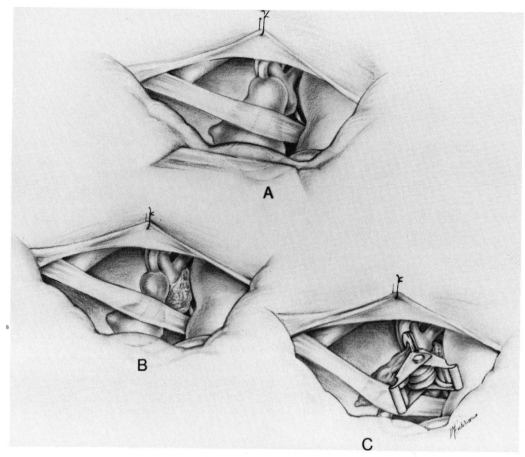

Figure 50–10 Typical basilar–superior cerebellar aneurysm. *A*. Mildly compressing the third nerve, which was not adherent to the uncus, a small intact "beehive" aneurysm at basilar bifurcation is just seen medially and posteriorly. *B*. Neck of the aneurysm has been shrunk with coagulation to reveal all of the bifurcation sac, which is coated in gauze prior to clip placement. *C*. Curved clip is applied to follow the natural contour of the neck between origins of P_1 and the superior cerebellar artery. Aneurysm has collapsed after needle aspiration.

herent to the dorsum sellae or clivus and may be torn loose while access to the neck is being gained. One other hazard is to be avoided: one must be sure that the clip blades do not encroach on the opposite P_1 segment but remain flush with the origin of the neck.

Bilocular Aneurysms

Bilocular aneurysms are not uncommon at the basilar bifurcation. The problem with them is the width of the angle forming the neck of the sac, which may approach 180 degrees. The neck, however, which may be broad in only the sagittal plane, can be "gathered" with the clip as the blades are forced gently upward from an original positioning at the top of the basilar artery. If the saccules are too large, then each can be

clipped separately, for the first clip narrows the other sac nicely for the second clip.

Large (or Bulbous) Basilar Bifurcation Aneurysms

Most of these project vertically and have bulbous necks to whose size the difficulties of exposure and clipping are directly proportional. The major problem is that the basilar bifurcation is almost certainly widely ballooned, forming a funnel that seems to be a part of the neck. As a consequence, the P_1 segment also appears to arise from the side of the aneurysmal neck and project vertically with its perforating arteries in close application to the sac. Enough experience has been gained, however, over many years of follow-up, to suggest that this ectatic bifurcation is composed of atherosclerotic but otherwise normal arterial wall and has not "blown out" to form another aneurysm. Nevertheless, the sheer bulk of the neck makes it more difficult to see either in front of or behind the aneurysm to the other side. The origin and neck of this aneurysm are even more likely to be yellow and firm with atheroma.

Once exposed, the waist of the sac should be indented firmly anteriorly so that the surgeon is able to look across for a glimpse of the origin of the opposite P_1 segment and perhaps its perforating branches. It is critical to identify the opposite segment accurately and not mistake the superior cerebellar artery for it. In one of the authors' cases, death from occlusion of the terminal basilar and posterior cerebral arteries resulted from this error in defining the anatomy (cf. Fig. 50–3). The opposite P_1 segment may be identified either by confirming that the opposite third nerve (usually clearly seen) courses beneath it or that the opposite posterior communicating artery can be seen entering it. Behind, these large aneurysms tend to bulge far back into the interpeduncular space, and fairly firm retraction of the peduncle is necessary even to expose part of the back of the neck. One can often get a "feel" of the curve and extent of the neck by gently, although blindly, working a small curved dissector backward beside the neck inside the medial aspect of the peduncle. It is remarkable how gentle, intermittent retraction of the peduncle is tolerated without any resulting deficit. Finally, it is necessary to work either the sucker tip or a dissector held in the left hand gradually behind the aneurysm, displacing the waist forward, and to separate perforators with a fine dissector held in the right hand until the apex of the curve is reached, when more bold forward displacement of the sac will tilt the waist of the sac toward the clivus to disclose the contents of the interpeduncular fossa, the opposite perforating vessels, and usually the opposite P_1 segment. As this is done, the top of the origin of the opposite P_1 segment should be noted to get a line of sight for the clip blades.

The aperture clip designed for this aneurysm should be used unless P_1 has an unusual course upward on the anterior and posterior portion of the neck, when an ordinary spring clip blade can be worked underneath it. During the foregoing inspection, an estimate of the width of the neck between the P_1 origins should be made. This cannot be exact, for as the neck is closed by the blades, it tends to widen slightly. It must be stressed, however, that the final length of the blades should exactly match that of the closed neck.

Because of the breadth of the aneurysmal neck, it will probably be necessary to use the sucker tip to indent the waist of the sac again from behind to expose the base of the neck and the perforating arteries in the interpeduncular fossa in order to initiate clip application. If it is not too broad, the blades can be gradually worked across the neck with a rocking motion inside the perforators and slowly allowed to close. The application of any clip and particularly the aperture clip is a bit awkward, as the handle and the tips of the applier obscure the anatomical details so that it is sometimes difficult to be sure that P_1 is free in the aperture. Narrowing the handle or offsetting or angling the blades would solve this problem.

If there are no significant perforators behind, the blades can be started low on either side of the basilar bifurcation and then gently worked up on the neck by rocking and sliding just high enough to clear each P_1 segment before closing. As the blades close, the opposite P_1 segment will be seen and adjustments of their angle can be made. The opposite third nerve is more in jeopardy during application of a clip on these aneurysms, for it is thinned and flattened on the far side and is likely to be brushed or even torn by the widely opened posterior blade.

The authors have experienced significant difficulty in the presence of atherosclerotic firmness of the base that caused a clip, initially in good position, to slide down to occlude the bifurcation as it closed. Sometimes the anterior blade can be held up on the far side of the neck with the sucker tip as the blades are allowed to close. Repeated trials seem to "soften up" the neck so the blades will stay, but often it requires drastic narrowing of the waist of the sac with forceps or the sucker tip to produce a slope on which they will close and remain in position. It may be necessary to place the blades up on the waist deliberately and then try to get another set of blades across below or, failing that, to pack the remaining base in gauze. A "hob-nailed" clip blade might be a solution to this dilemma. If there is a good posterior communicating artery, then the ipsilateral P_1 segment can be cautiously taken in the clip, provided there is no alternative and no perforators are included. The sheer bulk of these necks is often such that the tips of the blades are held open a few millimeters on the far side, permitting persistent flow into the aneurysm, for it will bleed when punctured. If the blades are in good position, however, they should be left, for a strong clip will finally occlude the neck. Sometimes rotation of the clip about its long axis will complete the occlusion; it can then be maintained, if necessary, by suturing the rotated handle to nearby dura.

There is still another abnormality seen occasionally with bulbous sacs. This results from ectasia of the bifurcation such that the P_1 segments emerge vertically *downward* from the base of the sac. Here it is almost impossible to prevent the blades of a clip from stenosing both P_1 orifices, and consideration must be given to basilar artery occlusion with the microtourniquet after the patient wakens from the anesthesia, as described later.

Results

The results of operative treatment of small and large (bulbous) bifurcation aneurysms are summarized in Table 50–3. In this table they have been divided into appropriate categories in regard to size and projection. Giant aneurysms, because of their special problems, are discussed separately.

The results have been quite good with small aneurysms at the basilar bifurcation when the projection was forward or backward. Two deaths of patients in this group were due to factors other than the operative obliteration of the aneurysm: in one case rupture of a second, previously intact, aneurysm and in the other meningitis. Similarly, two of the four poor results in good-risk patients were due to cardiopulmonary complications. The other poor results in good-risk patients were from delayed postoperative deterioration associated with arterial spasm.

The bulk of the morbidity encountered with small aneurysms was associated with those projecting upward from the bifurcation. Over half of this morbidity occurred early in the series before the significance of

injury to the perforating vessels in the interpeduncular fossa was recognized. In spite of great care taken in the past 15 years, however, a few more midbrain syndromes, four with bilateral third nerve paresis, have occurred. Three of them are permanently disabling. In two recent patients, a tear into the back of a fragile aneurysm neck occurred at operation, resulting in bleeding that could barely be controlled even with temporary basilar clipping. Both patients died. The remaining morbidity was due to postoperative deterioration with "arterial spasm," postoperative clots, and sepsis.[42]

The large bulbous aneurysms embedded more deeply in the interpeduncular fossa are a greater problem. In two early cases they were explored and ineffectually packed with gauze. Both patients died several months later from recurrent hemorrhage. With the use of the new fenestrated clip, the results have become acceptable. There was only one operative death when inadvertently the clip blades occluded the basilar bifurcation and the opposite P_1 segment, and six of the eleven poor results were in poor-grade patients already severely disabled by the initial hemorrhage.

Posterior Cerebral Aneurysms

These aneurysms arise principally at two places, the posterior cerebral artery's junction with the posterior communicating artery and its first major branching on the side of the midbrain.[19] A few aneurysms appear, however, to arise at the origin of large perforating branches from P_1 and more rarely peripherally in the occipital lobe.

Those arising from P_1 are approached in the same fashion as those at the basilar bifurcation and have much the same intimate involvement with perforating vessels.

The posterior cerebral artery is hidden under the hippocampal gyrus and a distinct layer of arachnoid as it winds around the side of the midbrain, and this arachnoid must be divided and the gyrus elevated with the tip of the retractor in order to expose aneurysms arising at its first major branching. It even may be necessary to remove a small amount of the overlying hippocampal gyrus in order to expose a high-placed or complex aneurysm where it lies on the midbrain in the choroidal fissure. The same care is needed in the dissection of the neck

TABLE 50-3 BASILAR BIFURCATION ANEURYSMS—RESULTS OF OPERATIVE TREATMENT

ANEURYSMS		GRADE (BOTTERELL)	NO. OF CASES	RESULTS			
Size	Projection			Excellent	Good	Poor	Dead
Less than 12 mm	Vertical	1	87	68	6	7	6
		2	28	18	5	5	
		3	12	3	4	3	2
			127*	89	15	15	8
	Posterior	1	34	26	5	2	1
		2	9	3	4	1	1
		3	1		1		
			44*	29	10	3	2
	Forward	1	15	13	1	1	
		2	9	6	2		1
		3	2		1	1	
			26	19	4	2	1†
Total 12 mm			197	137	29	20	11
Large bulbous (12 to 25 mm)		1	40	30‡	4	3	3§
		2	15	9	4	2	
		3	9	1	2	6	
			64	40	10	11	3

* Another patient rebled under anesthesia induction and died—no operation.
† Died from rupture of intact middle cerebral aneurysm.
‡ One patient underwent exploration only.
§ One patient well: unexpected death from coronary thrombosis.

to preserve the branches, although perforating vessels are not ordinarily a problem here. For aneurysms lying more distally, the posterior cerebral artery may be followed to the midline behind the midbrain by the subtemporal approach. Beyond this, an occipital flap should be used so that the mobile occipital pole can be retracted laterally and upward from the dural surface of the falx-tentorial junction.

It has been found that the posterior cerebral artery has a surprisingly good collateral supply—such that its inadvertent (and more recently, deliberate) occlusion has been followed by occipital infarction in only two of eight cases. Advantage may be taken of this observation in dealing with a critical situation such as a tear at the neck of a sac. A clue to the adequacy of the collateral circulation may be had if, with a temporary clip on the posterior cerebral artery just proximal to the aneurysm, the aneurysm still bleeds well after needle puncture or rupture. The P_1 segment can be taken if a good posterior communicating artery is present, and a small segment can even be trapped if it is bare of perforating branches. For large or giant aneurysms, deliberate occlusion of P_1 or P_2 would best be done with the tourniquet while the patient is awake.

Results

Posterior cerebral aneurysms included only small and giant sizes. The results with the small aneurysms have been good, presumably because of their easier exposure, although perforating vessels have been a concern with those arising on the P_1 segment (Table 50–4). One death resulted from massive pulmonary embolism, and the poor result was in a patient already severely hemiparetic who failed to impove.

Basilar–Superior Cerebellar Artery Aneurysms

These aneurysms arise at the distal crotch of origin of the superior cerebellar artery, and as they enlarge, the neck comes to involve most or all of the lateral portion of the basilar artery between the superior cerebellar artery and the P_1 segment. These aneurysms usually project laterally, rarely forward, lying in a shallow bed in the peduncle. There is always an intimate relation to the third nerve, which will course either over or below the sac or be flattened by the dome. Very rarely, the aneurysm arises inferior to the superior cerebellar artery.

The subtemporal approach is used, usually on the side of the fundus of the aneurysm. This aneurysm can also be approached from the opposite side to expose the neck first, but this approach may prove awkward, requiring the surgeon to work across in front of the basilar artery in the narrow space behind the clivus unless the basilar artery is displaced away from the dome toward the opposite side. Frequently it is necessary to dissect behind the basilar artery to free perforating branches that not infrequently arise near the origin of the superior cerebellar artery, are adherent to and displaced by the sac, and cannot be seen as well from the neck side. These disadvantages of the ''opposite side'' approach usually outweigh those of an exposure directly on the dome of the aneurysm. There is a risk, of course, of inadvertent rupture of the aneurysm and, in those projecting to the left, of retraction damage of the temporal lobe. Because of the lower position of these aneurysms, the retraction necessary is somewhat less than for bifurcation aneurysms, and injury to the temporal lobe is less frequent.

The suture tying the edge of the tentorium laterally will suffice for exposure without dividing the tent except for very large aneurysms. Indeed, no further injury to the trochlear nerve has occurred since division of the tentorium was found to be unnecessary for aneurysms in the region of the basilar bifurcation. This thin strand was a nuisance as it crossed the opening created by the tentorial cut and was injured or torn inadvertently in three early cases. The fragile dome with its adherent clot can be avoided by working down the sides of the aneurysm, first in front. If necessary, depressing the sac against the peduncle will

TABLE 50–4 POSTERIOR CEREBRAL ANEURYSMS ($<$12 MM)—RESULTS OF OPERATIVE TREATMENT

ANEURYSM	GRADE	NO. OF CASES	RESULTS			
			Excellent	*Good*	*Poor*	*Dead*
	1	15	14	1		
	2	1	1			
	3	6	1	1	1	3*
		22	16	2	1	3*

* One patient was recovering; died unexpectedly from pulmonary embolus; one patient bled from an associated arteriovenous malformation.

reveal the neck emerging from the basilar artery, and the superior cerebellar artery below it. The P_1 segment may be readily visible too, depending upon its course, but if the sac is of any size, the artery is often hidden above and behind. Then, working behind it, the surgeon can gently dissect and tease the aneurysm out of its bed in the peduncle, using a fine spatula to lift it to show the plane of cleavage. In the same way, the waist and neck are freed from the P_1 segment and the superior cerebellar artery, although the latter is usually not as adherent. With the aneurysm freed and displaced forward, the neck is seen clearly with any nearby perforating branches. During these manipulations, great care is taken not to injure the third nerve, which frequently winds around the neck itself. If this nerve makes application of a clip awkward, a ligature can be gently slipped around the neck inside it and tied firmly, or the neck can be shrunk with coagulation. Not infrequently, the superior cerebellar artery emerges from the side of the neck below, so care is taken not to kink it with the ligature or clip. Often a clip curved in the long axis of the basilar artery fits well across the curve of a larger neck created by the slopes of origin of P_1 and the superior cerebellar artery. Aspiration and collapse of this aneurysm is important to relieve third nerve compression if present.

This aneurysm can also be operated on from the sylvian approach on the side to which it projects (or opposite if necessary).

Rarely this aneurysm projects forward toward or is adherent to the dorsum sellae. Its obliteration is quite straightforward, for there are no perforating branches involved. Care must be taken not to injure the opposite third nerve as the clip is applied and closed.

The bulk of *large bulbous aneurysms* obscures the field more, but they too can be approached on the dome and dissected free in the same way to expose the neck, although more forceful retraction of the sac will be necessary to free it from its bed to see the neck behind. These very large aneurysms tend to distort the parent basilar artery toward the opposite side and are therefore the most suitable type to consider for exposure directly on the neck. Often P_1 is very adherent above and may have to be dissected free with a knife. Coagulation of a thin neck will not only shrink it but also

firm it up for freeing of a very adherent vessel. The third nerve is always displaced and flattened by these large sacs and is more prone to injury.

Aneurysms lying distally on the superior cerebellar artery on the upper surface of the cerebellum are rare. They may be approached subtemporally through the tentorium, but the more distal ones are easily seen by a suboccipital-subtentorial exposure with the patient in either the sitting or park bench position.

Results

Obliteration of ordinary basilar–superior cerebellar artery aneurysms has been very satisfactory, there being no deaths and only four poor results in good-risk patients from dysphasia after an approach under the dominant left temporal lobe (Table 50–5). The morbidity was greater with the large bulbous sacs that obscured their broad necks and necessitated displacement of the dome out of the bed in the peduncle. This maneuver resulted in rupture at the neck in two cases. In one, in which the aneurysm was mycotic, the basilar artery was irreparably torn and the patient did not survive its occlusion. The other patient suffered permanent hemiplegia.

Basilar–Anterior Inferior Cerebellar Artery Aneurysms

These aneurysms arise in the crotch of origin of the anterior inferior cerebellar artery (aica) over the middle third of the clivus, usually nearer its junction with the lower third. They tend to project laterally but are sometimes directed forward against the clivus or even posteriorly into the pons. There is always a near or intimate relation to the abducens nerve (Fig. 50–11).

Aneurysms in this location may be exposed in either of two ways. The whole of the basilar artery and even the upper vertebral arteries may be visualized through the subtemporal transtentorial approach. From behind and below through the standard lateral suboccipital exposure, however, the whole of the vertebral artery and the basilar at least as far as the anterior inferior cerebellar artery can also be exposed. The choice of approaches depends upon the height of the aneurysm on the clivus, its size and projection, and certain other disad-

TABLE 50–5   BASILAR TRUNK ANEURYSMS AT SUPERIOR CEREBELLAR ARTERY— RESULTS OF OPERATIVE TREATMENT

| ANEURYSMS | | | | RESULTS | | | |
Size	Projection	GRADE	NO. OF CASES	Excellent	Good	Poor	Dead
<12 mm	Forward	1	1	1			
		2	2		1*	1	
		3	2 / 5̲	1 / 2̲	1 / 2̲	1 / 1̲	
	Lateral	1	50	49		1	
		2	13	9	2	2	
		3	6 / 69̲	2 / 60̲	2 / 4̲	2 / 5̲	
Totals <12 mm			74	62	6	6	
Bulbous (12 to 25 mm)		1	7	2	1	2	2
		2	2 / 9̲	1 / 3̲	1 / 2̲	2̲	2̲

* Three distal superior cerebellar artery aneurysms and a cerebellar arteriovenous malformation.

vantages of each approach. The latter are: (1) from above—the possibility of injury to the fifth, sixth, seventh, and eighth cranial nerves and the potential need to approach under a dominant temporal lobe; and (2) from below—the chance of injury to the tenth and eleventh nerves. Originally Drake favored the route through the tent because the final exposure in front of the pons is a little larger and unilateral deafness or temporary facial or abducens nerve paresis is far less distressing and dangerous than vagal palsy. Even so, with experience, it is possible to work at the vertebral artery junction and above through the posterior fossa underneath the medulla, between the pharyngeal filaments of the eleventh nerve and the vagal fibers, with little or no injury. The choice would also be predicated on a consideration of the size and projection of the aneurysm and which exposure would best expose the neck and the anterior infer-

ior cerebellar artery and avoid the dome. Generally those over the lower third of the clivus are done from below and those above through the tentorium. The transoral transclival approach has been abandoned for aneurysm as confining, dangerous, and now unnecessary, as described later (Fig. 50–12).

The subtemporal transtentorial approach requires a more posteriorly placed temporal bone flap to avoid restricting the angle of the retractor and permit a line of sight down the posterior slope of the petrous bone. It is most important to preserve the integrity of the vein of Labbé during temporal lobe retraction, since in one case when it was torn, a fatal venous infarction occurred postoperatively.[56] The mid temporal lobe is elevated to display the edge of the tentorium beside the crus cerebri. This edge is picked up 1 or 2 cm *behind* the insertion of the fourth nerve, is clipped or coagulated (or both)

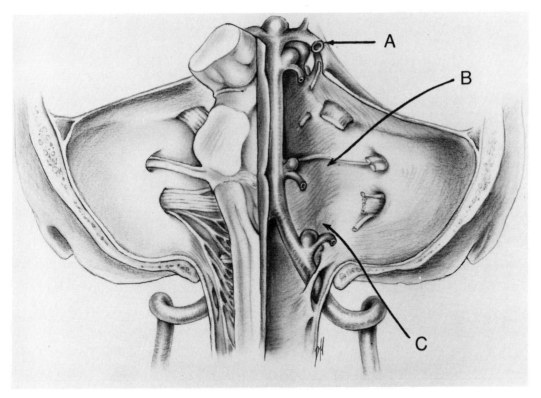

Figure 50–11   Orientation drawing for operative exposure of basilar and vertebral aneurysms. A. Basilar bifurcation and basilar–superior cerebellar aneurysms via the subtentorial approach; B. lower basilar, vertebrobasilar junction, and upper vertebral aneurysms approached through divided tentorium (subtentorial approach); C. vertebral, vertebrobasilar junction, and lower basilar aneurysms exposed via the suboccipital approach.

and divided, and then the tentorium is incised on a line 1 or 2 cm behind the petrous ridge, far laterally to near the lateral sinus. The anterior leaflet can then be folded forward on its attachment to the ridge and tied firmly to the floor of the middle fossa, usually with 3-0 silk sutures. This exposes the fourth and fifth nerves medially under the arachnoid, and midway the petrosal vein (there may be one or several) bridging from the petrosal sinus to the anterior cerebellum. The petrosal vein or veins may be divided after careful coagulation, and after the arachnoid is opened, the cerebrospinal fluid may be evacuated. With a slack brain, very little retraction of the temporal lobe is required as the tip of the same retractor is worked down along the anterior edge of the cerebellum just lateral to the fifth nerve. As the tip gently retracts the pons from the petrous bone and clivus, the bundle of the seventh and eighth nerves will come into view laterally. The final exposure will be in the opening between the fifth nerve medially and the seventh and eighth

nerves laterally. At first, the space may seem too confined, but with suction and further gentle retraction, it opens up considerably to reveal first the sixth nerve, then the basilar artery above the aneurysm. The arachnoid sheet in front of this space may be a nuisance in the sucker and should be sharply divided. If there is much old clot in the cistern, it is best to tease and suck it away, beginning at a distance from the presumed position of the dome of the aneurysm. The sixth nerve is slack enough that it can be laid up against the clivus or gently held on the pons with the retractor tip. Often it has to be separated from an adherence to the aneurysm. Handled gently, the sixth nerve, like the third nerve, has a remarkable capacity for complete recovery of function.

The aneurysm will be disclosed, depending on its position and size, as the basilar artery is followed down from above. Forward-projecting sacs are commonly adherent to the clivus, and those projecting laterally or posteriorly are shallowly em-

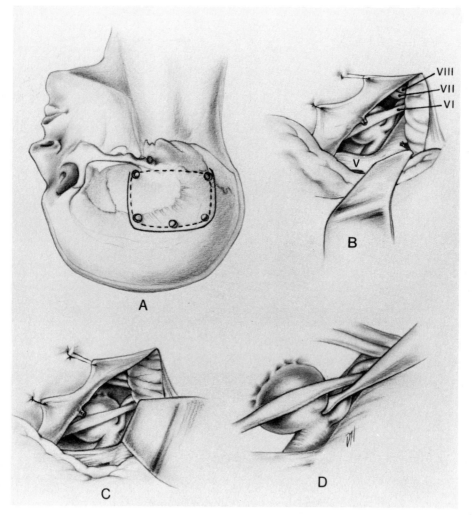

Figure 50–12 Subtemporal transtentorial exposure of lower basilar artery and vertebrobasilar junction. *A*. Bone flap placed posteriorly to allow posterior temporal retraction for line of sight down posterior slope of petrous bone. *B*. Tentorium divided 1 to 2 cm behind petrous ridge to near lateral sinus. Anterior leaflet of tentorium is tied firmly forward to floor of middle fossa. Petrosal vein is coagulated and divided. *C*. Basilar–anterior inferior cerebellar artery aneurysm exposed with sixth nerve flattened over dome, which is adherent to clivus. *D*. Careful separation of the anterior inferior cerebellar artery from the neck of the aneurysm before clipping.

bedded in the pons. Occasionally, the neck will stand out in clear view with the anterior inferior cerebellar artery below, but usually it is necessary to dissect the artery free to its origin and confirm the relationship of this vital vessel to the neck of the aneurysm, the basilar trunk, and other small branches. The fundus often can be held forward against the clivus to facilitate this exposure. For the backward-projecting sac, it is quite possible to work *behind* the basilar artery to free the neck and perforating branches. Rupture of the sac is frustrating because of the narrow confines, but is handled no differently. Clip application can be

awkward in this region, largely because the tips of the applier and the handles are large and difficult to maneuver in the right direction out of line of sight in between the nerves. It may even be necessary to guide the applier in laterally to the seventh and eighth nerves.

A few aneurysms have been seen whose origin from the trunk of the basilar artery is clearly midway between those of the anterior inferior cerebellar and superior cerebellar arteries, probably at the sight of an unnamed vessel or possibly at the origin of the primitive trigeminal artery. This can be an awkward segment of the basilar to see even though the tent is widely divided, for the broad fifth nerve crosses the field and the surgeon must work above and below it. It has not, however, been necessary to divide either the fourth or the fifth nerve.

Bilateral aneurysms arising from the basilar artery at the anterior inferior cerebellar artery have been seen on four occasions ("butterfly" aneurysms). In each case, it has been possible to clip both aneurysms, although it has meant working beneath the basilar artery in two cases to expose the neck of the posteriorly projecting sac. Both anterior inferior cerebellar arteries must be cleared to their origins before clipping. It is prudent to place the first clip so that neither the blades nor the handle interfere with the placement of the second.

Most large bulbous aneurysms at the anterior inferior cerebellar artery have been approached through the tentorium. Coming down on a large, upward-projecting aneurysm may be precarious because the dome will obscure the neck or may be torn. Because of this in two cases the necks were approached through a tentorial opening on the opposite side and dissection was carried across the midline either over or underneath the basilar artery. While this was feasible in both cases, the visualization of the neck was not as clear, so more recent cases have been approached on the same side regardless of the projection of the aneurysm. It is a matter of working down the sides of the sac and displacing the waist of the aneurysm with a spatula or narrow retractor in order to visualize and clear its connections at the base for clipping. The anterior inferior cerebellar artery may be difficult to see below the neck of a large sac, and considerable displacement may be required to see and be sure this vital vessel is freed. The results of operative treatment of basilar–anterior inferior cerebellar artery aneurysms are discussed after the section on vertebral-basilar aneurysms.

Vertebral–Basilar Junction Aneurysms

Because saccular aneurysms always seem to arise at the *distal* carina of a bifurcation on which the axial flow impinges, it would seem unlikely that the crotch of union of the vertebral arteries could be the site of aneurysm formation. Aneurysms

have, however, been seen arising at least in the neighborhood of this junction. Three have occurred in cases in which the opposite vertebral artery ended in the posterior inferior cerebellar artery and did not join its fellow in giving rise to the aneurysm. Three have been associated with fenestrations of the proximal basilar artery, giving further support to the notion that a distal carina is almost always the site of origin.

The vertebral union usually overlies the junction of the lower and middle thirds of the clivus. This region too can be approached from above or below as in the case of basilar–anterior inferior cerebellar artery aneurysms, and the same considerations prevail.

Excepting the giant aneurysms, 10 of the 14 have been approached through the tentorium, although most of these operations were done earlier in the series when it was thought that the midline over the lower third of the clivus was difficult to visualize from behind. Since it has been learned that this is not the case, the more recent procedures have been done through the posterior fossa unilaterally (the approach for vertebral aneurysms is discussed in the following section).

Results

In Table 50–6, the results with small and large aneurysms of the basilar trunk have been grouped together because of their small numbers.

The subtemporal transtentorial exposure of aneurysms lower on the basilar trunk at the anterior inferior cerebellar artery, or even at its origin at the union of the vertebral arteries, has also been satisfactory.

One death occurred in a patient operated on in 1963 under deep hypothermia with cardiopulmonary bypass. The basilar–anterior inferior cerebellar artery aneurysm was clipped uneventfully, but the surface of an associated pontine arteriovenous malformation was merely packed. The patient was well for five hours, when massive pontine hemorrhage from the vascular anomaly occurred, possibly related to the heparinization. There have been three instances of permanent unilateral deafness from apparently gentle retraction of the very tender eighth nerve.

Two early poor results followed a postoperative extradural hematoma and postop-

TABLE 50–6   BASILAR TRUNK ANEURYSMS AT ANTERIOR INFERIOR CEREBELLAR ARTERY—RESULTS OF OPERATIVE TREATMENT

ANEURYSMS	GRADE	NO. OF CASES	RESULTS			
			Excellent	*Good*	*Poor*	*Dead*
12 mm	1	21	14*	2	4*	1†
	2	6	4*	1		1
	3	$\frac{4}{31}$	$\frac{1^*}{19}$	$\frac{1}{4}$	$\frac{2}{6}$	$\frac{}{2}$
Region of union of vertebral arteries	1	21	20‡	1		
	2	$\frac{6}{27}$	$\frac{3}{23}$	$\frac{1}{1}$		$\frac{3}{3}$

* Indicates one large bulbous aneurysm (12 to 25 mm) in each group.
† Midbasilar dissecting aneurysm.
‡ Includes nine large bulbous aneurysms (12 to 25 mm). Three cases of unilateral deafness only.

erative spasm subsequent to early operation one day after the hemorrhage. More recently, however, two were the result of brain stem syndromes that seemed inexplicable, although small unseen vessels may have been injured.

Vertebral Aneurysms

Although their principal origin is at the distal crotch of origin of the posterior inferior cerebellar artery (pica), the notorious tortuosity and wandering of the vertebral artery and the varying level of origin of the posterior inferior cerebellar artery have placed these aneurysms from near the intracranial entry of the vertebral artery under the first dentate ligament to near the vertebrobasilar junction, from the lip of the foramen magnum to the middle third of the clivus, and in both angles. A right vertebral aneurysm has been seen lying to the left of the midline. Most project upward, lying shallowly in the medulla, either on its side or in front. A few project posteriorly into the medulla or forward with the dome adherent to the clivus. Commonly with this aneurysm, the posterior inferior cerebellar artery arises from the side of the neck. A few of the aneurysms arise distinct from the posterior inferior cerebellar artery, probably at the site of origin of the anterior spinal artery or possibly of smaller unnamed branches. Most have an intimate relation to the hypoglossal nerve, which usually lies on the upper distal side of the neck but may be split by the aneurysm or lie in a groove between loculi.

Originally, from an operative point of view, these aneurysms were divided into groups depending on their nearness to the midline, since it was thought that the transoral transclival approach would be best for those at or near the midline over the lower third of the clivus.[15] This low midline region was thought to be a surgical "no man's land." There is no question that a midline vertebral aneurysm can be approached by this transclival route. The authors' first case went uneventfully, but in the second, fatal meningitis occurred. In this case the small aneurysm was just off the midline, not seen clearly, and was packed in gauze. The patient was well for three days and then, although no known cerebrospinal fluid leak into the pharynx existed, he rapidly became comatose and died in six hours from pneumococcal meningitis. This confirmed that, in addition to being confining, the transclival opening was also dangerous. Since then it has been learned that all aneurysms overlying the lower third of the clivus, even in the midline, can be exposed through the posterior fossa via a unilateral suboccipital opening (Fig. 50–13). The "park bench" position is very useful for vertebral and lower trunk aneurysms, allowing the surgeon to sit, while giving a nice angle for dissection up the side of and under the brain stem. This position eliminates most risk of air embolism and allows, if necessary, a combined subtemporal and transtentorial exposure. A midline 7-shaped or paramedian curvilinear incision is used, sparing the occipital nerves to preserve sensation in the scalp above. The major problem facing the surgeon is that most of these aneurysms lie tucked under the medulla so that it is necessary to work under or around the filaments of vagal nerve. More lateral approaches serve no useful purpose and many impede vision because of the muscle mass medially, especially in heavy individuals (Fig. 50–14).

The posterior fossa is slackened by opening the cistern and gently retracting the cerebellum off the medulla with a narrow retractor blade placed on the base of the tonsil. This stratagem exposes the elev-

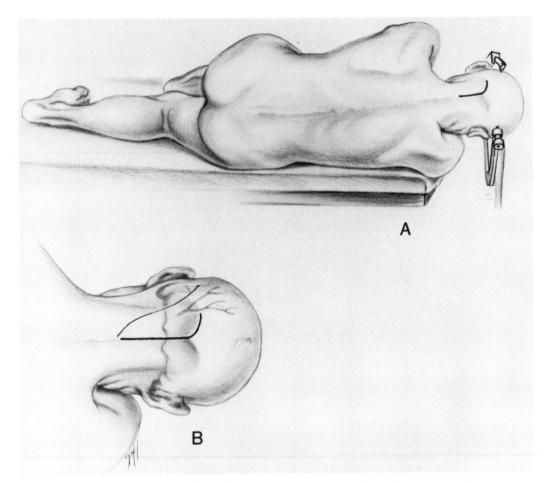

Figure 50–13 *A*. Park bench position with preferred hockey stick incision just short of occipital nerves. Face is cocked a few degrees to floor for comfortable access to premedullary and pontine regions. *B*. Alternate paramedian curvilinear incision may enhance exposure of aneurysms of high midline vertebral and basilar origin.

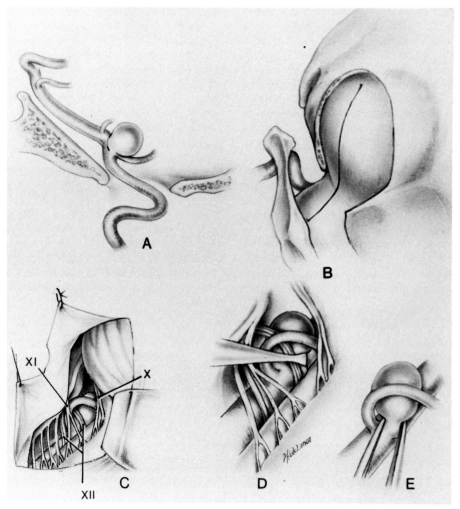

Figure 50–14 *A*. Vertebral aneurysm with posterior inferior cerebellar artery typically originating from base of sac. *B*. Unilateral suboccipital craniectomy through foramen magnum and dural incision. *C*. Elevation of cerebellum to expose dome of aneurysm between lower filaments of vagus nerve and pharyngeal filaments of accessory nerve. Hypoglossal nerve is divided into two bundles, one below and the other above the neck of the aneurysm under the posterior inferior cerebellar artery. *D*. Defintion of vertebral artery distal to the aneurysm. *E*. Neck held with forceps for coagulation or determination of ideal position for clip.

enth nerve with its medullary pharyngeal filaments, the tenth and ninth nerves, the caudal loop of the posterior inferior cerebellar artery, and the vertebral artery as it emerges from under the first dentate ligament. Lower aneurysms will be seen immediately at this stage. The more unusual aneurysms lying up on the side of the medulla above the ninth and tenth nerves will require the microscope to be tilted upward, but only slightly.

Usually it is convenient to begin the dissection proximally and follow the vertebral artery upward toward the assumed site of the neck of the aneurysm. Fortunately in

this regard, the origin of the posterior inferior cerebellar artery is ordinarily just proximal to the neck, so it will be seen first as a landmark to denote the presence of the neck just beyond, even though it may be under the midline of the medulla. Generally, the route is between the pharyngeal filaments of the eleventh nerve and the lower filaments of the vagus, of which great care must be taken, for dysphagia and hoarseness are not only terribly distressing but also dangerous. As the vertebral artery courses upward and medially, the medulla must be gently retracted to follow it. Spontaneous breathing is used as a guide to retractor pressure. At first, as in the case of pontine retraction from above, it will seem that there is just not enough room, but with further gentle retraction and suction the exposure enlarges to satisfactory limits for midline aneurysms over the lower and middle thirds of the clivus to be visualized. Even a left vertebral aneurysm has been operated on inadvertently from the right side. As the neck of the aneurysm is glimpsed, it may be best to work on either side of the posterior inferior cerebellar artery, up the sides of the vertebral artery to the neck, and then underneath the vertebral to follow this large vessel beyond the neck. The vertebral artery beyond the neck must be seen and its direction appreciated to permit proper clip alignment. It may be quite difficult to get a good view of this segment, but visualization will be aided by holding the aneurysm closed with forceps or by allowing the blades of the clip to close slowly to collapse the neck so that they can then be realigned and positioned correctly just before the final closure. The twelfth nerve will usually be seen on the far side of the neck and is gently freed so that it will not be injured by the clip.

The fact that the posterior inferior cerebellar artery emerges from the near side of the neck often makes clipping awkward, for the angle of the neck will be oblique to the exposure and the clip often tends to slip down to occlude the artery. Coagulation to shrink the neck just above this artery is often useful to provide a bed for the clip. The clip should be strong and so placed that the tips lie under the perforating arteries and the twelfth nerve and flush with the far side of the neck. A ligature can be very satisfactory for this aneurysm, although care must be taken that the artery is not kinked. The Drake-Kees clip may also be used and the posterior inferior cerebellar artery placed in the aperture, or an angled Sugita aperture clip may be used to enclose the vertebral artery.

Results

The vertebral aneurysms, too, were either small or giant, there being none between 12.5 and 25 mm. They have been a satisfactory group for operative treatment (Table 50–7). The only two deaths in good-risk patients occurred from pneumococcal meningitis, the result of a transoral transclival approach, and from fatal recurrent hemorrhage after a clip slipped some time before the patient's scheduled discharge. The other two deaths were in poor-grade patients taken to the operating room with medullary infarction secondary to the original bleed who succumbed to cardiorespiratory complications.

Giant Aneurysms of the Posterior Circulation

Giant intracranial aneurysms have been defined as those over 2.5 cm (1 inch) in diameter.[6] It would appear that they reach and exceed this size as a result of nonlinear enlargement of smaller saccular aneurysms that may or may not have ruptured during the course of their development. The elon-

TABLE 50–7   VERTEBRAL ARTERY ANEURYSMS—RESULTS OF OPERATIVE TREATMENT

| ANEURYSM | GRADE | NO. OF CASES | RESULTS | | | |
			Excellent	Good	Poor	Dead
	1	58	51	5		2
	2	11	8	3		
	3	3	1		1	1
	4	2			1	1
		74	60	8	2	4

gated fusiform serpentine variety most commonly seen on the vertebral and basilar arteries probably arise from atherosclerotic weakening of the wall.

Usually, as a saccular aneurysm enlarges, the neck involves more and more of the parent artery, reaching and then exceeding its caliber. The neck becomes splayed out spherically, forming a bulbous origin that is often wider than the parent vessel or its bifurcation, even incorporating the wall of the artery in its base. The neck commonly becomes yellow with atheroma and, rarely, may be calcified. As aneurysms enlarge to "giant" proportions, more and more of the parent artery is splayed out into the neck, even to the point of entering and leaving it separately, in which case no occlusion of the neck can be contemplated.

For the most part, treatment of these masses has been restricted to those on the carotid artery in both its intracavernous and extracavernous segments by hunterian ligature of that vessel in the neck, which has remained the mainstay of their operative treatment. That the hunterian principle is effective also for giant aneurysms on the posterior circulation was shown by Drake's initial experience with vertebral and basilar artery occlusion.[17]

Since reported experience with *direct* operative treatment of giant aneurysms was limited to a few cases, a preliminary communication in 1975 discussed the methods and results in 41 cases, in 26 of which the lesions were on the posterior circulation.[16] Now 195 of these aneurysms have been operated upon on the authors' unit by means of some form of indirect or direct operative procedure. Of these, 76 were on the anterior circulation and 119 were on the vertebrobasilar system. Indirect methods for the posterior aneurysms have utilized the hunterian principle: ligation of the vertebral artery remotely in the vertebral triangle or intracranially near the aneurysm as well as ligation of the upper or lower basilar artery and the superior cerebellar and posterior cerebral arteries. Direct operative methods have utilized the same techniques used for the smaller aneurysms: clipping, trapping, intraluminal thrombosis, and rarely, reinforcement by wrapping in gauze or plastic coating (Table 50–8).

In 12 cases, all in poor-grade patients, only an exploration was done, the sac being considered to be impossible to deal with at the time. Simple exploration is not without hazard, for one patient, critically ill after rupture of a huge vertebrobasilar aneurysm, suffered cardiac arrest and died as the tentorium was being opened, and another patient with a basilar bifurcation sac inexplicably was rendered mute and quadriplegic. The future for such patients seems bleak. Three other survivors have since rebled and died, and three remain totally disabled. Only one has remained reasonably well with only a third nerve palsy; after having largely recovered from a right hemiparesis six years earlier, he deteriorated rapidly with brain stem compression and ischemia, which was the reason for the second heroic attempt to decompress the mass. In the light of present knowledge, it is probable that several of the earlier cases could now be treated reasonably safely. In two, however, temporary occlusion of the basilar and a large vertebral artery, respectively, produced profound cardiorespiratory alterations under anesthesia, and the procedure had to be abandoned.

Hunterian Ligation

Hunterian ligation of the parent artery was the most common method used, in 50 per cent of the cases if the trapping procedures are included. Initially, the vertebral artery was occluded at a distance from the aneurysm in the vertebral triangle in the neck with a Selverstone clamp, and this seemed to be effective for aneurysms filling solely or chiefly from one artery. It was, however, learned that the vertebral artery has an extensive collateral supply from deep cervical branches in its traverse through the cervical spine, which may make its lower occlusion ultimately ineffective. Now it is considered best to clip the vertebral artery intracranially just proximal to the aneurysm above the collateral inflow as long as the other vertebral artery is known to exist and the two join to form the basilar artery. Unfortunately, in vertebral aneurysms, the posterior inferior cerebellar artery usually arises at or from the side of the neck below, so the occlusion usually must be just proximal to this vessel. It is, nevertheless, remarkable how the posterior inferior cerebellar artery will continue to be filled retrogradely from the other vertebral through the stump of the occluded artery beneath a completely thrombosed aneurysm or from superior cerebellar artery collateral channels.

When there is no doubt that the aneurysm is inoperable by direct approach, the vertebral artery may be occluded as effectively by an extracranial exposure in the sulcus arteriosus of the atlas just before it enters the dural sac, thus avoiding an intracranial procedure while excluding the cervical collateral inflow. This was done in two cases, and large fusiform vertebral aneurysms were thrombosed completely in a 14-year-old boy and a 17-year-old boy respectively, as described later in the discussion of bilateral vertebral artery ligations.

As in the case of the basilar artery, trial occlusion of the vertebral artery with forceps or a temporary clip may, from respiratory or cardiac changes, give a clue to the patient's tolerance. Their absence, however, may not mean it is safe, although brain stem infarction has not occurred from single vertebral occlusion per se. Infarction occurred only when massive thrombosis taking place in the aneurysm involved the basilar artery as well. When any doubt exists about intracranial occlusion, it may be best to use the tourniquet, as described later, so that the vessel may be occluded while the patient is awake, especially if only one vertebral artery contributes to the basilar artery.

Unilateral vertebral artery ligation in the neck by a Selverstone clamp was done three times, and bilateral ligation was attempted in three patients. The three single occlusions were well tolerated, and massive thrombosis occurred in the two aneurysms filling solely from that artery. Both patients are well after spectacular recoveries from brain stem compression. There was no lasting benefit in the case of the vertebral aneurysm filling bilaterally, which subsequently re-enlarged and ultimately ruptured fatally one and one half years later. Bilateral cervical vertebral artery ligation was attempted three times but tolerated in only one boy 14 years of age whose vertebrobasilar aneurysm, after initially becoming smaller, enlarged again after five years as a remarkable deep cervical collateral supply developed. The aneurysm was thrombosed completely only when both vertebral arteries were occluded in the sulcus arteriosus above the collateral vessel. (One patient with a basilar bifurcation aneurysm was treated by single vertebral artery occlusion when he could not tolerate bilateral occlusion in the lower portion of the neck. Since he died from rupture of the aneurysm one and one half years later, it is probable that single vertebral occlusion is ineffective for these lesions on the upper part of the basilar artery.) The only death in this group occurred subsequent to massive thrombosis in a huge truncal aneurysm after attempted bilateral ligation, even though the second artery had been reopened when ischemic signs developed 24 hours earlier.

Primary intracranial vertebral occlusion just proximal to the aneurysm was done 13 times. The thrombotic occlusion of the aneurysm was complete in nine and partial in three, and none occurred in one. There were two deaths, both occurring late, at one and two weeks respectively. The first, in a young man already requiring a respirator, was from massive thrombosis in a huge vertebrobasilar aneurysm that spread to involve the basilar artery. The other was in a patient with a similar aneurysm. After clipping of the dominant left vertebral artery, a tourniquet had been placed on the opposite right vertebral intracranially and left open but buried in the back of the neck subcutaneously in case an attempt at bilateral vertebral ligation was necessary. She had renal fibromuscular hyperplasia and was severely hypertensive. Her course was punctuated by three episodes of brain stem failure that seemed to recover completely when she was allowed to remain hypertensive. After one week, she suffered cardiac arrest when her pressure inadvertently was allowed to drop to a systolic value of 80 with nitroprusside. At autopsy, the left vertebral artery was found to be severely stenosed by a dissecting aneurysm at the site of the tourniquet, probably induced by the practice occlusions of the tourniquet in the operating room. Nine survivors have done well, including one in whom the large aneurysm compressing the medulla could be trapped and collapsed. In one, however, temporary spinal hemiparesis resulted on the third day from retrograde thrombosis of the vertebral artery down to the sixth cervical segment. The other poor result is persistent hemianesthesia that was present before vertebral occlusion.

Unilateral ligation of the vertebral artery for large aneurysms of the vertebral artery or at the vertebrobasilar junction appears to

TABLE 50-8 "GIANT" ANEURYSMS (>25 MM)—METHODS AND RESULTS OF OPERATIVE TREATMENT

REGION*	GRADE†	NO. OF CASES	EXPLORATION ONLY				HUNTERIAN LIGATURE Remote‡ 1 Vertebral				Remote‡ 2 Vertebrals				Nearby§ Vertebral				Nearby§ Basilar (or Branch)				TRAPPING				NECK OCCLUSION				INTRALUMINAL THROMBOSIS				WRAPPING OR COATING			
			E	G	P	D‖	E	G	P	D	E	G	P	D	E	G	P	D	E	G	P	D	E	G	P	D	E	G	P	D	E	G	P	D	E	G	P	D
Basilar bifurcation	Good	23	1	1															5	2	2	1					5	2	2	1	1	1		1				
	Poor	24				6							1						2	2	3				1		4	3	3			1						
Basilar trunk at superior cerebellar artery	Good	9																	1				2				2	1	1	2								
	Poor	14				1															1	1			1		2	4	4								1
Below superior cerebellar artery	Good	7																	3				1	1			1											
	Poor	6			1	1	1				1	1				1				1	1	1		1	1	1										1		
Vertebrobasilar junction	Good	5					1								1	1												1	1										
	Poor	8		1								1			2	1	1						1																
Vertebral	Good	8			1	1									3		1						2				1	1											
	Poor	1																																					
Posterior cerebral	Good	11		2			1												5 (pca)				1 (pca)				3			1						1		
	Poor	3																	1	2							2											
		119	1	2	7	2	2		1		1				7	2	2		17	4	6	3	4	3	1	1	12	12	11	10	1	1		2		1		1

* Region used because often difficult to know exact origin of aneurysm.
† Good grade, grade 1 or 2 from hemorrhage and no major deficit from intact aneurysm. Poor grade, grade 3 or 4 from hemorrhage or major deficit from intact aneurysm or both.
‡ Remote indicates vertebral ligation in neck.
§ Nearby indicates vertebral or basilar occlusion intracranially just proximal to aneurysm, superior cerebellar artery, or posterior cerebral artery (pca) in aneurysms on these branches.
‖ E, excellent; G, good; P, poor; D, dead.

be very effective provided the aneurysm fills principally or entirely through one vertebral artery and that the other artery exists, unites with its fellow, and seems large enough to supply the basilar arterial system. The best result is undoubtedly achieved when ligation is done intracranially just proximal to the aneurysm to eliminate the effect of deep cervical collateral supply to the artery.

Bilateral cervical ligation of the vertebral artery was successful in only two of the five cases in which it was tried, and then only when the arteries were secondarily occluded as they entered the skull above the collateral vessel in one and after trapping the aneurysm in another. The three remaining patients died; one from rebleeding two years later, one from vertebral arterial dissection and inadvertent iatrogenic hypotension, and one from massive thrombosis that included the basilar artery. Tolerance of this procedure appears to be less than that of basilar occlusion, possibly because of the extra flow needed through the posterior communicating arteries via the basilar to irrigate the intracranial segments of the vertebral arteries and their branches. It may be worthwhile to attempt this in selected cases, the initial occlusion being staged and done low in the neck to take advantage of the vertebral collateral supply. If occlusion of flow is not well tolerated in this situation, the outlook is gloomy.

Basilar artery occlusion has been done 21 times, 16 at the upper basilar just below the superior cerebellar arteries, 1 between the P_1 segment and the superior cerebellar artery for huge terminal aneurysms, and 4 near its origin for truncal aneurysms (one truncal aneurysm was trapped).*

Initial experience with basilar artery occlusion in seven cases was poor, for two patients were worsened and two died, both when significant sections of the artery were trapped.[17]† What was needed was a means to determine beforehand the patient's tolerance to basilar occlusion, which depends solely on the amount of collateral flow through the posterior communicating arteries. Sometimes these vessels are demonstrated in routine carotid and vertebral angiography, but more often are not. As noted

before, Allcock's simple expedient of carotid compression during vertebral angiography will reveal the size and potential of the communicating artery collateral supply through varying degrees of filling of the carotid siphon and its branches.[3a]

Less collateral flow would be needed if the basilar artery could be occluded between the origins of the superior cerebellar arteries and the P_1 segments, but this segment is usually nonexistent with giant sacs, and one or the other vessel would be compromised. Only in one case in which these origins were separated by the expansion of a large bulbous aneurysm was this possible.

With radiographic knowledge of the collateral potential, there was a need to test and reverse the occlusion in the awake patient. The successful, though harrowing, trial of basilar occlusion under local anesthesia in one patient led to the development and use of a simple tourniquet by which the artery could be occluded after the patient is awake (Fig. 50–15). The tourniquet is made of 3-0 Prolene suture, which slides easily through No. 190 polyethylene tubing whose tip is marked by a small Weck clip to mark its subsequent position radiographically. The Prolene suture is applied around the artery to be occluded at initial exploration of the aneurysm, and the suture in the tubing is left protruding from the head through a small stab wound. Tightening of the tourniquet should be practiced in the operating room to get the "feel" of the device. Then, after the patient has recovered from the anesthetic, the tourniquet can be tightened by hand and, with concomitant angiography through a femoral catheter, the occlusion and its effects can be tested both clinically and radiographically. It has been remarkable how even one posterior communicating artery will successfully perfuse the upper and even the lower basilar system. To leave the artery occluded for several hours or a day or two, the surgeon can pinch the tubing against the suture threads with a Weck clip, and if ischemic signs develop, a nurse can open it almost instantly by cutting the tubing just inside the clip. When tolerance of the occlusion of the basilar artery is evident by the following day, the occlusion can be made permanent by burying the tourniquet after enlarging the stab wound under local anesthesia. Another Weck clip is firmly applied to the tubing flush with the muscle or skull, and the

---

* One patient died of rebleeding before the tourniquet was closed.

† Two patients did not have "giant" aneurysms.

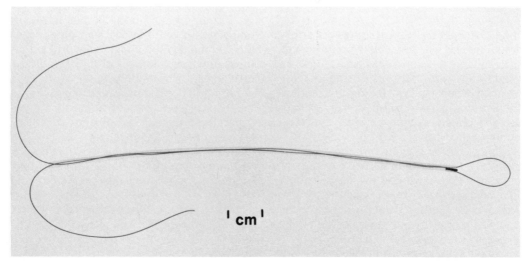

Figure 50–15 Micro-Drake tourniquet. Polyethylene tubing (PE 190) encloses looped Prolene (3.0) suture. Metal clip on the end of the tubing is for radiographic orientation.

tourniquet is cut off just beyond so that the skin can be closed over it.

The tourniquet can also be used to produce significant stenosis in an artery, even in stages, to promote development of collateral circulation when complete occlusion is not tolerated. This has been done on the middle cerebral artery in four cases of giant aneurysms at its trifurcation. In each instance, a superficial temporal–middle cerebral artery anastomosis would not initially support complete occlusion of the artery without resulting aphasia and hemiparesis. Production of severe stenosis with the tourniquet was used to promote the collateral flow through the bypasses. One patient could tolerate only a 75 per cent stenosis at first, but after three months, could tolerate a 90 per cent stenosis following further closure of the tourniquet, which had been left intact under the scalp. Sometime in the next three months, the artery spontaneously became completely occluded at the site of the induced severe stenosis. In another case in which a double anastomosis was done (superficial temporal and occipital arteries to supra- and infrasylvian middle cerebral branches respectively), a 90 per cent stenosis maintained for 24 hours allowed complete occlusion of the artery on the next day. In all cases, the middle cerebral occlusions caused complete thrombosis of the aneurysms without any neurological deficit.

A "bypass" anastomosis to improve collateral circulation to major branches of the posterior circulation would undoubtedly further its propensity to develop, and would add to the safety of their occlusion. Unfortunately, the readily accessible branches of the basilar artery, with the exception of the posterior inferior cerebellar artery, are probably too small for anastomosis with the occipital artery. An anastomosis with the posterior inferior cerebellar artery has, however, been used in vertebral-basilar insufficiency, and this might have a place in the treatment of certain vertebral aneurysms.[43,50]

On 12 occasions, the tourniquet has been used to occlude the basilar artery for giant aneurysms arising from it.* Of the nine attempts on the upper artery (just below the superior cerebellar arteries), one resulted in the death of the patient from rupture of the aneurysm on the evening of the tourniquet's application but *before* it was tightened. Two patients were worsened by the exploration and showed no worthwhile recovery even though the tourniquet subsequently and uneventfully occluded the basilar artery and massive thrombosis was produced in the aneurysm. Another, operated upon in grade 4 condition due to

---

* The tourniquet has been used also to occlude the carotid, vertebral, anterior cerebral, posterior cerebral, and middle cerebral arteries for giant aneurysms, the last named vessel after the superior temporal artery–middle cerebral artery anastomosis.

midbrain and pontine compression, has improved slightly with the aneurysm completely thrombosed but remains an invalid. In the five successful cases, huge bifurcation aneurysms were totally occluded by thrombosis in two and nearly so in the third. One patient showed dramatic recovery from completely disabling partial bilateral oculomotor palsies and quadriparesis and is now working. In another, dementia, thought to be due to the huge inter- and suprapeduncular mass, has receded dramatically. The third patient, with the partially thrombosed aneurysm, has been free of his formerly recurrent subarachnoid hemorrhages for two years. Two others, functional before operation, have remained entirely well with complete thrombosis of the aneurysm.

In addition, since the original report, two other patients have had sudden occlusion of the upper basilar artery during exploration of the aneurysm, although both were known to have good posterior communicating arteries. In the first, the occlusion was deliberate, but in the other, the artery had to be occluded when a tear at its entrance into the aneurysm occurred during attempted placement of the tourniquet. Neither patient suffered ill effects, and in both cases massive thrombosis in the sac occurred, as shown in postoperative angiograms, leaving only a tiny portion of the neck filling from posterior communicating arteries and also giving rise to the origins of both P_1 segments and superior cerebellar arteries.

Among the seven cases of lower basilar occlusion for giant truncal aneurysms, there was one death in the original series when, naively, an attempt was made to trap a giant sac on the basilar artery.[17] In two more recent cases, the lower basilar artery was occluded with the tourniquet, which had to be left protruding from the back of the neck after suboccipital exploration. The first patient, a 4-year-old girl, was quite well several hours after the application when, during angiography preliminary to tightening the loop, it was discovered that even though the tourniquet was open, the basilar artery was occluded and the aneurysm thrombosed, presumably from manipulation of the artery that had produced a dissecting aneurysm, as occurred in the vertebral artery described earlier. Fifteen minutes after what was probably unnecessary closure of the tourniquet, a fatal massive hemorrhage occurred, perhaps because the artery was torn. Unfortunately no autopsy could be obtained to give a definite answer. In the other patient, a girl of 13, the aneurysm was totally thrombosed and the sixth nerve palsy that had prompted the investigation also recovered completely. In another patient, in poor condition from massive brain stem compression, thrombosis of the aneurysm occurred without tightening of the tourniquet, but there has been no subsequent improvement. The remaining four patients have had total thrombosis of their aneurysms and complete recovery of function.

Basilar artery occlusion may seem a radical measure, but when tolerated, it appears to be very effective. The four truncal aneurysms were completely obliterated by thrombosis, but two patients died, both because of surgical misjudgment, from a trapping procedure and a tourniquet injury. Among the 13 completed occlusions for basilar bifurcation aneurysms, thrombosis appeared to be complete in four. In all but one of the others, there was massive thrombosis virtually obliterating the sac except for a few millimeters of the neck through which the basilar bifurcation and the superior cerebellar arteries were being irrigated retrogradely, usually from only one P_1 segment. No patients died but four were worsened, two apparently because of the operative manipulation rather than ischemia. Preliminary angiographic visualization of the collateral potential of the posterior communicating arteries and the use of the tourniquet may in the future make this a safe and effective procedure. Practice occlusion of the tourniquet at operation is not without risk, however. It has resulted in dissection of the vertebral artery in one case and probable dissection of the basilar artery in another. It must be used with great care and gentleness.

The superior cerebellar artery has been occluded deliberately at its origin on five occasions for large sacs at or near its origin, and all sacs were occluded. Three patients did well, one recovering from preoperative hemiparesis after trapping and collapse of the huge aneurysm embedded in the peduncle. That no infarction occurred probably was because the artery was huge and supplied a large cerebellar arteriovenous malformation. One patient died with cerebral infarction from unexplained occlusion of the posterior cerebral artery just above the clip after coming around well initially without evident cerebellar deficit although he had a preoperative hemiplegia. The dilated origin of the cerebellar artery was torn, however, during 6.5 minutes of temporary basilar occlusion at 28° C during the dissection, and it had to be included in the clip. In the third case, isolation of a long fusiform ruptured superior cerebellar aneurysm, by trapping over 1 inch of the artery around the peduncle, resulted in a devastating cerebellar syndrome that fortunately has resolved considerably over many months. It would seem that, when possible, the tourniquet should be used to test the efficiency of the collateral supply to this artery, for it does not appear to be extensive.

Previous experience suggested that the posterior cerebral artery has excellent collateral following its ligation, and this premise has been maintained.[19] In each of the nine giant P_1 (seven) and P_2 (two) aneurysms the artery was occluded, yet only one patient developed a field defect; there were no other deficits produced. Some idea of the collateral flow can be gained by putting a needle hole in the aneurysm after applying a temporary proximal clip. A good pulsating stream suggests that the sac can be trapped, as was done in the first two cases. In huge fusiform aneurysms of P_1, a tiny segment of P_1 at its origin could just be occluded by a small silver clip. At the first attempt, however, the postoperative angiogram showed that P_1 was not completely closed and a tiny stream of dye still entered the sac, but the posterior communicating artery, previously unfilled, now joined with P_2 as it emerged from the sac. At reoperation, after tightening of the McKenzie clip, a Sundt clip could be placed over the union of the posterior cerebral and communicating arteries as they emerged from the sac so that the aneurysm could be collapsed while the posterior cerebral artery was perfused through the clip by the posterior communicating artery. The patient made a useful recovery from a complete Weber's syndrome. This availability of a tiny segment of the P_1 origin before it balloons into a giant fusiform aneurysm is not unique, for in a recent case, the right P_1 segment also could just be occluded by a narrow clip. The huge sac became completely thrombosed in a boy of 17 whose only deficit was a temporary postoperative left third nerve palsy caused by a left sided approach. In this case the aneurysm was so large that the basilar bifurcation was displaced to the lateral edge of the left cerebral peduncle. As in another giant fusiform P_1 aneurysm in a boy of 15, however, it would be best to use the tourniquet when possible. About 1 cm of the P_1 segment was available and the tourniquet was applied to the artery just proximal to the aneurysm. After the artery had been left occluded for 24 hours without deficit, it was permanently occluded and the tourniquet was buried under the scalp. This aneurysm too was thrombosed completely.

Trapping of giant posterior aneurysms has been included in the discussion of hunterian ligatures because the same principle pertains, the occlusion of the artery giving rise to the aneurysm. It is the second "trapping" occlusion of the vessel just beyond the aneurysm that makes this procedure so effective, for the aneurysm usually is isolated from any significant collateral flow. The segment of artery so isolated must obviously not give rise to important branches that do not in turn have their own sufficient collateral supply except when the risk of a deficit is deemed acceptable, e.g., a blind eye or a field defect.

All 11 large aneurysms trapped in this series were done intracranially, on either side of the aneurysm. There was one death from pontine thrombosis following the attempt to trap a huge basilar trunk aneurysm when, too late, it was discovered that both the anterior inferior cerebellar arteries arose from the sac itself. All three patients with trapped posterior cerebral aneurysms did well, presumably because of the excellent collateral circulation to this vessel, and the only one who developed a right field defect had no disturbance of speech. The superior cerebellar artery was trapped twice at its origin. One patient, in whom the aneurysm arose from a huge vessel that was supplying an arteriovenous malformation, suffered no ill effect, but the other, in whom over an inch of vessel was isolated, developed a severe cerebellar deficit. In the only vertebral aneurysm trapped, a ligature could be closed just inside the origin of the posterior inferior cerebellar artery to spare that vessel, which peculiarly arose just distal to the aneurysm.

Trapping of an aneurysm is a very effective procedure, but it must be done with great caution, for two collateral systems are involved, that of the parent vessel and that of any vessel arising from the trapped segment.

The use of the hunterian principle in these 57 cases of giant aneurysms on the posterior circulation suggests that it will be just as effective as for those on the carotid circulation. There were 7 deaths (12 per cent) and 10 poor results (17 per cent). In consideration of the dreadful state and outlook for these patients, however, this trial of operative treatment seems reasonable. Since two of the deaths were due to massive thrombosis in the aneurysm that included the basilar artery, in patients who tolerated the initial arterial occlusion, some thought must be given to anticoagulation in certain situations so that the thrombosis may occur more gradually as the patient is weaned from the drug. The use of the simple tourniquet will now allow maximum safety in making the decision to occlude any intracranial artery for aneurysm, since that decision can be based the patient's actual tolerance of the occlusion while awake and for a day or more if necessary.

It has subsequently been learned that the tourniquet principle has been used intracranially before. Gibbs discussed his experience with occlusion of the anterior cerebral artery to improve the efficiency of carotid ligation for aneurysms on its tree before the British Society of Neurological Surgeons in 1972.[26] He used a tube tourniquet in most cases but also tried torsion of the artery with a hook. Unfortunately, carotid occlusion in isolation from the opposite side was not tolerated, and the technique was abandoned.

Direct Operative Treatment

Direct operative treatment has been used for 50 giant aneurysms on the posterior circulation: coating of the aneurysms for 2, intraluminal thrombosis of the aneurysm with injection of wire or hair for 3, and occlusion of the vertebral artery in the neck for 45.

The opportunity to reinforce a giant posterior aneurysm is rare, since it is unusual to be able to dissect the whole of the sac safely from the brain stem. This was attempted in two cases. In one only the open base of a large partially thrombosed basilar–superior cerebellar artery aneurysm could

be encased in gauze and plastic; the patient has, however, remained relatively well. The other was a fusiform basilar trunk aneurysm in a girl of 14 who also had a huge cavernous carotid aneurysm as well. In spite of apparent complete encasement in plastic, a posterior "blow out" saccule developed after six months, presumably through an incompletely covered area. Fortunately, it and the carotid aneurysm spontaneously became completely and mysteriously thrombosed before a planned second operation.

Three large sacs at the bifurcation were treated by injection of horse hair in two and copper wire in the other. In all three, massive thrombosis occurred except at the neck of the aneurysm. In all three, the remaining portion of the neck "blew out" in three months, one year, and seven years respectively. Two of these lesions reruptured, one with fatal results, and the aneurysm treated with injection of wire took the life of the patient by further massive enlargement.

It would appear that as long as a portion of the aneurysmal neck still fills directly from the pounding axial stream of the parent artery, even massive thrombosis will not prevent further enlargement and even rupture. After the injection, ligation of the parent artery just below the aneurysm to remove the axial stream might be more effective in preventing subsequent enlargement of the neck.

Direct treatment aimed at obliteration of the neck of a giant aneurysm so that it can be opened and evacuated has received little attention in the literature except for sporadic case reports almost entirely restricted to those on the anterior circulation. Aside from being the most effective method for treating any saccular aneurysm, and one in which the major parent artery is spared for the patient's future, there are several situations in which it must be considered: (1) when serious brain compression has occurred and radical decompression is needed; (2) when hunterian ligature is not possible or has failed to halt the growth or rupture of the mass; (3) for bilateral aneurysms on the carotid circulation; and (4) when, from the angiogram or actual inspection, the neck of the aneurysm is known to be small enough.

From an operative point of view, there are distinctive features to these aneurysms related to the bulk of the sac, the degree to which the parent artery and its branching are involved in the neck, and the extent of mural thrombosis and atheroma (Fig. 50–16).

With the gradual inclusion of the parent artery into the neck of an aneurysm reaching giant size and the invasion with atheroma, safe obliteration becomes more treacherous, for the occlusion of a large neck may kink and stenose or even occlude the artery or its branches.

It is surprising, however, how often the neck of a giant aneurysm is smaller than was evident on the angiogram or can easily be made smaller for clipping. For this reason alone, many deserve exploration, for even though clipping is not possible, the tourniquet can be applied for subsequent arterial occlusion. It is remarkable how often even the largest neck that is *free* of adherent thrombus will wrinkle and collapse with a ligature, perhaps not completely, but enough for a smaller clip to be applied accurately—or for a longer clip to be worked across and then out a little on the neck so that when it is closed arterial

continuity is maintained with a little neck proximal to the blades. Occasionally, a "mosquito" arterial snap can be used to close the neck for a ligature or make a site for a long clip. Rarely, a neck is thick enough or access is suitable for end-aneurysmorrhaphy.

The aneurysm and its neck must be soft enough and the pressure sufficiently reduced so that it does not fracture with these manipulations or allow the clip or ligature to slip down the sharply sloping sides to kink or occlude the parent vessels. The development of "hob-nailed" blades may be useful in this regard to prevent the common clip blade from "skiing" off the slope. When the neck is free of thrombus, deep hypotension (mean arterial pressure 40 mm of mercury) will suffice. Occasionally transient very deep hypotension (mean arterial pressure 20 mm of mercury or below) under moderate hypothermia, or the very careful use of a temporary clip on the proximal vessel, is necessary to soften the neck. On very broad necks, clip blades, which may need to be 20 mm long or more (the Drake-Kees clip), often will stay open on

BASILAR BIFURCATION

BASILAR TRUNK AT SCA

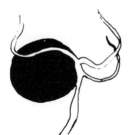

BASILAR TRUNK BELOW SCA

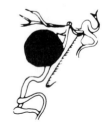

VERTEBRAL-BASILAR JUNCTION

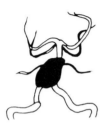

VERTEBRAL

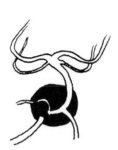

POSTERIOR CEREBRAL

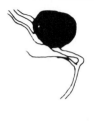

Figure 50–16 Tracings of typical "giant" aneurysms (larger than 25 mm) arising from the posterior circulation. Note the contrast-filled portion of the sac often is much smaller than the actual size of the aneurysm because of the presence of mural thrombus. SCA, superior cerebellar artery.

the far side because the thickness of the neck does not allow them to close in parallel. The aneurysm will still pulsate and bleed when punctured with a needle. Sometimes a few degrees of rotation of the clip handle will finish the occlusion, and the handle can be sutured in the rotated position to nearby dura, or another clip can be applied over the blade ends of the first to give more strength to their closure. If left, however, the blades of this strong clip will, in a few hours or days, finally close off the residual neck so that, if decompression is necessary, the aneurysm can be opened and evacuated at a second operation.

The other major problem with direct operative treatment of giant aneurysms is the extent to which the sac and its neck are occluded with mural thrombus. This thickens and stiffens the neck so that it will not collapse unless the aneurysm is opened and the thrombus removed, a difficult and dangerous proposition. This would be more feasible if the thrombus were soft and suckable, but it is not. It is firm, tough, even fibrous, and very adherent, and must be removed with grasping forceps after cautious separation from its adherence to the wall lest the neck be torn. Once the cavity of the aneurysm is entered, bleeding tends to obscure the field and preclude careful dissection, necessitating temporary proximal occlusion. The major concern is the time factor. Normothermia will permit two to three minutes of occlusion, moderate hypothermia only six to eight minutes. This is usually not sufficient, for even after the neck is freed of thrombus, it still has to be dissected from its adherence to major branches and perforating arteries and then accurately defined and narrowed for clipping. The wall of the neck in large aneurysms usually is thickened and capable of withstanding manipulation, but the junction of the aneurysm to branches is vulnerable and likely to tear. Occasionally, where the thrombus is principally on one side of the waist and the neck, it is possible to remove much of this without getting into the cavity so that the neck will collapse enough for clipping. In some moderate-sized aneurysms in which the neck is reasonably clear of thrombus, it will be sufficient to open the sac, accept the bleeding, and keep the field reasonably clear with suction while freeing the neck. Once a giant aneurysm is opened, the surgeon is committed to a satisfactory occlusion of the neck, but a near certainty of doing so must be assured by preliminary inspection.

Forty-five giant aneurysms were treated directly by neck occlusion, and 10 of the patients died. This high mortality rate seemed to be clearly related to the degree to which the aneurysm was thrombosed and the method used to free the neck. There was no major difference in the size of the aneurysm between the survivors and the fatalities, but the patients with massively thrombosed aneurysms did less well.

Most of the deaths and morbidity occurred in patients with massively thrombosed aneurysms and were directly related to the technical difficulties with these lesions.

Of the five patients operated on under deep hypothermia ($\pm$ 15°C) with cardiac arrest and cardiopulmonary bypass, three died. Two deaths resulted from massive temporal lobe bleeding, presumably heparin-induced, into brain rendered ischemic by retractor pressure. In these cases the repair of the aneurysms was done without undue difficulty. The other patient recovered well after the pump bypass procedure, only to die several hours later from a pinhole-sized rupture in the base of the posterior cerebral artery just proximal to the clip. Since this area was not ruptured at operation, the new hemorrhage apparently occurred in a deteriorated portion of the artery.[21,22,41,54]

There is no question about the usefulness of circulatory arrest in the treatment of these lesions. While the patient is at 15° C, the area of the lesion should be exsanguinated and ample time allowed to empty the neck and sac of the aneurysm to make an area for clipping. Since these aneurysms are deeply embedded in seriously compressed brain stem, only enough of the neck should be exposed to provide room for the clip and its application. The arterial branches, large and small, are often very adherent, but fortunately these necks are thick enough for reasonably bold dissection to free branches to be used.

The problem after cardiac arrest and cardiopulmonary bypass has been bleeding during the rewarming period and neutralization of heparin. The effects of retractor pressure are just being realized, for it appears that ischemic changes begin underneath with forces just over 20 mm of mercury, and frank hemorrhage into the white matter begins with pressures approaching 40 mm of mercury.[2] Any degree of induced hypotension will aggravate this problem. Temporal lobe hematomas occurred in three of the five cases during or after closure, even though the brain appeared to be free of hemorrhage. It appears that retractor pressure produced enough ischemia to result in hemorrhagic infarction, for the clots all developed in the temporal lobe underneath the retractor site. The two patients who did not recover were in extremis with intraventricular hematoma within an hour or so of recovering from the anesthesia. In the other, who had the largest aneurysm, temporal swelling was recognized during dural closure and the clot was evacuated. In spite of this injury to the left temporal lobe, she has had a dramatic recovery from her pre-existing hemiplegia and has no speech defect.

Methods of circulatory arrest under deep hypothermia without heparin probably will emerge and undoubtably will expand our capabilities for dealing directly with giant sacs that have potentially clippable necks. Until then, when conventional cardiopulmonary bypass is used, great care must be taken with brain retraction to prevent the calamity of retractor-induced hemorrhagic infarction. In retrospect, several of these cases could probably have been treated with basilar artery occlusion, which probably would have arrested the course of the brain stem compression. Further, from experience with hunterian ligation of the artery for giant aneurysms, a remarkable but paradoxical improvement has been noted in several cases that is probably related in part to the reduction of pulsatile pressure but also to some shrinkage of the mass as the thrombus is organized.

Multiple Aneurysms

The principles underlying the management of multiple aneurysms elsewhere apply equally well to those of the posterior circulation, viz., the intact sacs are not benign and should be obliterated too. If the operation on the ruptured aneurysm has gone well and the other is nearby and known to be reasonable as far as size and position are concerned, then it can be obliterated at the same time; if more remote, it can be left for another procedure. In a series of 163 cases of subarachnoid hemorrhage and multiple aneurysms, including those on the posterior circulation, there was only one death clearly attributable to the procedures on 174 of the intact aneurysms, a mortality rate far less than to be expected from their natural course.

Intact Aneurysms

Intact aneurysms revealed during the course of angiographic study of other disorders are infrequent but pose the same question as the intact ones of multiple aneurysms. On the authors' unit, 32 patients have been operated on (excluding those with giant aneurysms) with good results in all but one case.[18] All five patients with intact basilar aneurysms had excellent results.

Older Patients

From earlier experience with this age group (over 60), it was concluded that these patients tolerated intracranial aneurysm procedures well and had a gratifying rate of successful outcome.[4] Half of the morbidity, however, occurred unexpectedly from other disease in the postoperative period when the patients had been well. In a more recent review of these patients, the results from operations alone remained good for procedures on the anterior circulation but less so for those on the posterior circulation.[18] A number of technical errors occurred during the earlier years while methods of dealing with posterior aneurysms were being learned, and three of that series were giant aneurysms. Now, since the technical problems for most posterior as well as anterior aneurysms are largely solved, it seems reasonable to consider the older patient carefully, for many are physiologically younger than their years, are active, and deserve the opportunity to have their future made secure.

CURRENT EXPERIENCE

From many personal communications, it is known that many surgeons have operated on one or a few patients with aneurysms on

TABLE 50-9 REVIEW OF RECENT LITERATURE IN THE OPERATIVE TREATMENT OF ANEURYSMS IN REGION OF BASILAR BIFURCATION

		RESULTS		
SOURCE	NO. OF CASES (ALL GRADES AND SIZES)	Good	Poor	Dead
McMurtry et al.*	12	9	2	1
McMurtry†	14	10	2	2
Wilson and Hoi Sang‡	15	11	4	
Sundt§	23	15	6	2
Chou‖	20	8	6	6
Yaşargil¶	38	23	12	3
Totals	122	76	32	14

Note: "Fair" results have been grouped with poor since patients are presumed not to have resumed normal work and life.

* Surgical treatment of basilar artery aneurysms. Elective circulatory arrest with thoracotomy in 12 cases. J. Neurosurg., 40:486–494, 1974.
† Letter to the Editor. J. Neurosurg., 45:361, 1976; personal communication, 1976.
‡ Surgical treatment for aneurysms of the upper basilar artery. J. Neurosurg., 44:537–543, 1976.
§ Personal communication, 1979.
‖ Personal communication, 1976.
¶ Microsurgical pterional approach to aneurysms of the basilar bifurcation. Surg. Neurol., 6:83–91, 1976.

the vertebral-basilar tree. Success has been varied, although the higher incidence of operative problems probably reflects many other surgeons' disinclination to report on successful outcomes in a few cases.

Only five series have been reported in recent years, all tending to put emphasis on aneurysms in the region of the basilar bifurcation (Table 50–9).[37,50,56,57] It is evident, however, that in the hands of experienced surgeons, the techniques evolved in the past decade have, with some variation, resulted in satisfying operative results for patients harboring the smaller aneurysms. Already much has been accomplished for the patient with the larger and giant aneurysms, but some technical problems remain.

THE FUTURE

The techniques for safe obliteration of most small and large aneurysms in good-grade patients in good-risk periods are now available.

A major advance in the management of all aneurysms would be the nearly universal recognition of the minor "warning" hemorrhage. If this state of emergency were recognized, patients could be protected from the catastrophic recurrent hemorrhage or progressive enlargement of the sac to giant proportions. It is probable that the widespread use of computed tomography for faint neurological symptoms or signs may permit early recognition of the sac before "giant" proportions are reached and may thereby reduce the major problems still encountered with these massive lesions.

Techniques for deep hypothermia without heparin for cardiopulmonary bypass may emerge and will vastly improve the means of direct operative treatment of certain giant aneurysms when collapse of the sac is essential for brain stem decompression. In the meantime, application of the hunterian principle will remain effective in promoting massive thrombosis to prevent rebleeding and stay growth of the aneurysm, and even somewhat paradoxically result in improved brain stem function.

REFERENCES

1. Aitken, R. R., and Drake, C. G.: Experience with profound hypotension in intracranial aneurysms. Presented at Harvey Cushing Society Meeting, Washington, D.C., 1971.
2. Albin, M. S., Bunegin, L., Dujovny, M., Bennett, M. H., Janetta, P. J., and Wisotzkey, H. M.: Brain retraction pressure during intracranial procedures. Surg. Forum, 26:499–500, 1975.
3. Alksne, J. F., and Rand, R. W.: Current status of metallic thrombosis of intracranial aneurysms. In Krayenbühl, H., Maspes, P. E., and Sweet, W. H., eds.: Progress in Neurological Surgery. Vol. 3. Chicago, Year Book Medical Publishers, 1969, pp. 212–229.
3a. Allcock, J. M.: Personal communication, 1972.
4. Amacher, A. L., and Drake, C. G.: Aneurysm surgery in the seventh decade. In Fusek, I., and Kunc, Z., eds.: Present Limits of Neurosurgery. Proceedings, Fourth European Congress of Neurosurgery. Prague, Avicenum (Czech. Medical Press), 1972, pp. 263–266.
5. Bull, J. W.: Contribution of radiology to the study of intracranial aneurysms. Brit. Med. J., 2: 1701–1708, 1962.
6. Bull, J. W.: Massive aneurysms at the base of the brain. Brain, 92:535–579, 1969.
7. Chou, S.: Personal communication, 1976.
8. Dandy, W. E.: Intracranial Arterial Aneurysms. Ithaca, N.Y., Comstock Publishing Co., 1944.
9. Drake, C. G.: Bleeding aneurysms of the basilar artery. Direct surgical management in four cases. J. Neurosurg., 18:230–238, 1961.
10. Drake, C. G.: Surgical treatment of ruptured aneurysms of the basilar artery. Experience with 14 cases. J. Neurosurg., 23:457–473, 1965.
11. Drake, C. G.: Further experience with surgical treatment of aneurysms of the basilar artery. J. Neurosurg., 29:372–392, 1968.

12. Drake, C. G.: The surgical treatment of aneurysms of the basilar artery. J. Neurosurg., 29:436–446, 1968.

13. Drake, C. G.: The surgical treatment of vertebral basilar aneurysms. Clin. Neurosurg., 16:114–169, 1969.

14. Drake, C. G.: Formal discussion. In Cerebral Vascular Disease Seventh Conference. Whisnant, J. P., & Sandok, B. A.: New York, Grune & Stratton Inc., 1971, pp. 241–244.

15. Drake, C. G.: Management of aneurysms of posterior circulation. In Youmans, J. R., ed.: Neurological Surgery, Vol. 2. Philadephia, W. B. Saunders Co., 1973, pp. 787–806.

16. Drake, C. G.: Direct surgical treatment of "giant" intracranial aneurysms. Presented at meeting of American Association of Neurological Surgeons, April, 1975.

17. Drake, C. G.: Ligation of the vertebral (unilateral or bilateral) or basilar artery in the treatment of large intracranial aneurysms. J. Neurosurg., 43:255–274, 1975.

18. Drake, C. G.: Cerebral aneurysm surgery—an update. In Cerebral Vascular Diseases, Eleventh Conference. New York, Raven Press, 1976.

19. Drake, C. G., and Amacher, A. L.: Aneurysms of the posterior cerebral artery. J. Neurosurg., 30:468–474, 1969.

20. Drake, C. G., and Girvin, J. P.: The surgical treatment of subarachnoid hemorrhage with multiple aneurysms. In Morley, T. P., ed.: Controversies in Neurosurgery. Philadelphia, W. B. Saunders Co., 1976.

21. Drake, C. G., and Vanderlinden, R. G.: The late consequences of incomplete surgical treatment of cerebral aneurysms. J. Neurosurg., 27:226–238, 1967.

22. Drake, C. G., Barr, H. W. K., Coles, J. C., and Gergely, N. F.: The use of extracorporeal circulation and profound hypothermia in the treatment of ruptured intracranial aneurysms. J. Neurosurg., 21:575–581, 1964.

23. Falconer, M. A.: Surgical treatment of spontaneous intracranial hemorrhage. Brit. Med. J., 1:790–792, 1958.

24. Gallagher, J. P.: Pilojection for intracranial aneurysms. Report of progress. J. Neurosurg., 21:129, 1964.

25. Garvey, P. H.: Aneurysms of the circle of Willis. Arch. Ophthal. (Chicago), 11:1032–1054, 1934.

26. Gibbs, H. R.: Attempts at reversible closure of intracranial arteries for more difficult aneurysms. J. Neurol. Neurosurg. Psychiat., 35:921, 1972.

27. Gillingham, F. J.: Personal communication, 1977.

28. Hamby, W. B.: Intracranial Aneurysms. Springfield, Ill., Charles C Thomas, 1952.

29. Hook, O., Norlén, G., and Guzman, J.: Saccular aneurysms of the vertebral-basilar arterial system. A report of 28 cases. Acta Psychiat. Scand., 39:271, 1963.

30. Jamieson, K. G.: Aneurysms of the vertebrobasilar system. Surgical intervention in 19 cases. J. Neurosurg., 21:781–797, 1964.

31. Logue, V.: The surgical treatment of aneurysms in the posterior fossa. J. Neurol. Neurosurg. Psychiat., 21:66, 1958.

32. Logue, V.: Posterior fossa aneurysms. Clin. Neurosurg. 11:183–207, 1963.

33. MacCarty, C. S., Michenfelder, J. D., and Uihlein, A.: Treatment of intracranial vascular disorders with the aid of profound hypothermia and total circulatory arrest: three years' experience. J. Neurosurg., 21:372–377, 1964.

34. McCormick, W. F., and Acosta-Rua, G. J.: The size of intracranial saccular aneurysms. An autopsy study. J. Neurosurg., 33:422, 1970.

35. McCormick, W. F., and Nofzinger, J. D.: Saccular aneurysms: An autopsy study. J. Neurosurg., 22:155, 1965.

36. McMurtry, J. G. III: Letter to the Editor. J. Neurosurg., 45:361, 1976.

37. McMurtry, J. G. III: Personal communication, 1976.

38. McMurtry, J. G. III, Housepian, E. M., Bowman, F. O., Jr., and Matteo, R. S.: Surgical treatment of basilar artery aneurysms. Elective circulatory arrest with thoracotomy in 12 cases. J. Neurosurg., 40:486–494, 1974.

39. Mount, L. A., and Taveras, J. M.: Ligation of basilar artery in treatment of an aneurysm at the basilar artery bifurcation. J. Neurosurg., 19:167–170, 1962.

40. Mullan, S., Reyes, C., Dawley, J., and Dobben, G.: Stereotactic copper electric thrombosis of intracranial aneurysms. In Krayenbühl, H., Maspes, P. E., and Sweet, W. H., eds.: Progress in Neurological Surgery. Vol. 3. Chicago, Year Book Medical Publishers, 1969, pp. 212–229.

41. Patterson, R. H., Jr., and Ray, B. S.: Profound hypothermia for intracranial surgery: Laboratory and clinical experience with extracorporeal circulation by peripheral cannulation. Ann. Surg., 156:377–391, 1962.

42. Peerless, S. J.: Pre- and post-operative management of cerebral aneurysms. Clin. Neurosurg., 26:209–223, 1979.

43. Peerless, S. J.: Personal observation, 1978.

44. Poppen, J. L.: Vascular surgery of the posterior fossa. Clin. Neurosurg., 6:198–209, 1958.

45. Sahs, A. L., Perret, G. E., Locksley, H. B., and Nishioka, H.: Intracranial Aneurysms and Subarachnoid Hemorrhage. A Cooperative Study. Philadelphia, J. B. Lippincott Co., 1969.

46. Schwartz, H. G.: Arterial aneurysms of the posterior fossa. J. Neurosurg., 5:312–316, 1948.

47. Schwartz, H. G.: Personal communication, 1962.

48. Sellery, G. R., Aitken, R. R., and Drake, C. G.: Anaesthesia for intracranial aneurysms with hypotension and spontaneous respiration. Canad. Anaesth. Soc. J., 20:468–478, 1973.

49. Selverstone, B., and Ronis, N.: Coating and reinforcement of intracranial aneurysms with synthetic resin. Bull. Tufts-New Eng. Med. Cent., 4:8–12, 1958.

50. Sundt, T. M., Jr.: Personal communication, 1979.

51. Tönnis, W.: Zur Behandlung intrakranieller Aneurysmen. Arch. Klin. Chir., 189:474–476, 1937.

52. Troupp, H.: The natural history of aneurysms of the basilar bifurcation. Acta Neurol. Scand., 47:350–356, 1971.

53. Uihlein, A., and Hughes, R. A.: The surgical treatment of intracranial vestigial aneurysms. Surg. Clin. N. Amer., 35:1071–1083, 1955.

54. Uihlein, A., Theye, R. A., Dawson, B., et al.: The

use of profound hypothermia, extracorporeal circulation and total circulatory arrest for an intracranial aneurysm: Preliminary report with reports of cases. Proc. Staff Meet. Mayo. Clin., *35*:567–576, 1960.

55. Warren, K. G., Drake, C. G., Kaufmann, J. C. E., and Seldon, D.: Dissecting aneurysms of the basilar artery. J. Neurosurg., In press.

56. Wilson, C. B., and Hoi Sang, U.: Surgical treatment for aneurysms of the upper basilar artery. J. Neurosurg., *44*:537–543, 1976.

57. Yasargil, M. G., Antic, J., Laciga, R., Jain, K. K., Hodosh, R. M. and Smith, R. D.: Microsurgical pterional approach to aneurysms of the basilar bifurcation. Surg. Neurol., *6*:83–91, 1976.

51

ANEURYSMS AND ARTERIOVENOUS FISTULAE OF THE INTRACAVERNOUS CAROTID ARTERY AND ITS BRANCHES

REGIONAL ANATOMY

Arterial Relationships

The intracavernous segment of the carotid artery begins at the foramen lacerum as the vessel emerges from the carotid canal. The artery ascends briefly toward the posterior clinoid process, then turns abruptly forward in its horizontal portion for a distance of approximately 2 cm. The segment terminates by passing upward on the medial aspect of the anterior clinoid process, where it perforates the dural roof of the cavernous sinus to become the supraclinoid portion of the carotid artery.

Several small branches arise from this segment of the carotid artery (Fig. 51–1).[37,85] The largest and most proximal intracavernous branch is the meningohypophyseal trunk, present in 100 per cent of dissected specimens. This artery arises at the level of the dorsum sellae just before the apex of the first curve of the carotid artery as it begins its horizontal portion. Shortly after its origin, this vessel typically divides into three branches: (1) the tentorial artery (artery of Bernasconi-Cassinari), which courses laterally to the tentorium; (2)

the inferior hypophyseal artery, which travels medially to supply the posterior pituitary capsule; and (3) the dorsal meningeal artery, which perforates the dura of the posterior cavernous sinus wall to supply the clival area and sixth nerve.

The second major intracavernous branch is the artery of the inferior cavernous sinus. This vessel usually arises laterally from the horizontal portion of the intracavernous carotid artery 5 to 8 mm distal to the origin of the meningohypophyseal trunk. It arises directly from the carotid artery in 84 per cent of specimens and from the meningohypophyseal artery in another 6 per cent. It supplies the dura of the inferior lateral cavernous sinus wall and the area of the foramina ovale and spinosum.

The third commonly encountered intracavernous carotid arterial branch is McConnell's capsular artery, identified in 28 per cent of specimens. It arises from the medial side of the carotid artery approximately 5 mm distal to the artery of the inferior cavernous sinus. This vessel supplies the anterior and inferior pituitary capsule.

The ophthalmic artery arises from this segment of the carotid artery in 8 per cent of cases, and the dorsal meningeal artery is

A. L. DAY and A. L. RHOTON, JR.

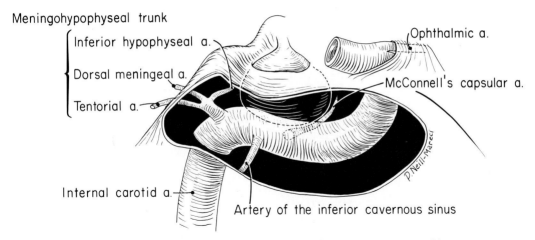

Meningohypophyseal trunk

Inferior hypophyseal a.

Dorsal meningeal a.

Tentorial a.

Ophthalmic a.

McConnell's capsular a.

Internal carotid a.

Artery of the inferior cavernous sinus

Figure 51–1   Arterial branches of the cavernous portion of the internal carotid artery.

a direct intracavernous carotid branch in 6 per cent of specimens. The persistent trigeminal artery may also pass through the cavernous sinus. This vessel arises from the intracavernous carotid artery proximal to the meningohypophyseal trunk and joins the basilar artery between the superior and anterior inferior cerebellar arteries.[89]

The bifurcations formed by the origin of these small arteries from the parent carotid artery frequently mark the site of aneurysm or fistula development. These small arteries

form an extensive network of intradural anastomoses with arteries of the opposite side. They provide important collateral channels following occlusion of the internal carotid artery below the level of the cavernous sinus. These arteries are often visualized angiographically in stenotic carotid lesions, intracranial (parasellar) tumors, and carotid-cavernous fistulae. While their presence is not necessarily pathological, a careful search of the skull base and tentorium should follow their identification.

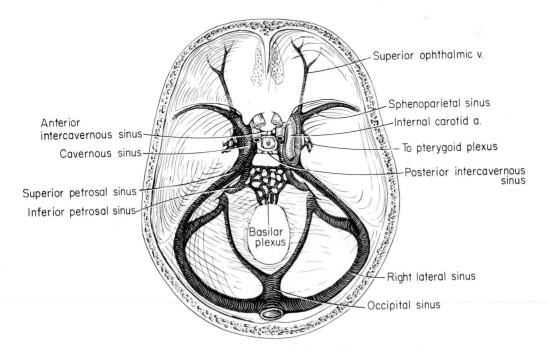

Superior ophthalmic v.

Sphenoparietal sinus

Internal carotid a.

Anterior intercavernous sinus

Cavernous sinus

To pterygoid plexus

Posterior intercavernous sinus

Superior petrosal sinus

Inferior petrosal sinus

Basilar plexus

Right lateral sinus

Occipital sinus

Figure 51–2   Venous tributaries and drainage of the cavernous sinus.

Venous Relationships

The paired cavernous sinuses are located on each side of the sphenoid sinus, sella, and pituitary gland, extending from the superior orbital fissure to the apex of the petrous bone. Each cavernous sinus is connected to the orbit by the superior and inferior ophthalmic veins, to the cerebral hemisphere through the middle and inferior cerebral veins, to the retina by the central retinal vein, to the dura by tributaries of the middle meningeal veins, to the transverse sinus by the superior petrosal sinus, to the jugular bulb by the inferior petrosal sinus, to the pterygoid venous plexus by the emissary vein passing through the cranial base, and to the facial veins through the ophthalmic veins. The cavernous sinus thus has intimate venous connections with the cerebrum, cerebellum, brain stem, face, eye, orbit, nasopharynx, mastoid, and middle ear (Fig. 51–2).[37]

Dural venous pathways that connect both cavernous sinuses are termed intercavernous sinuses. Those connections within the sella turcica are usually named according to their relationship to the pituitary gland; the anterior intercavernous sinus passes anterior to the pituitary gland,

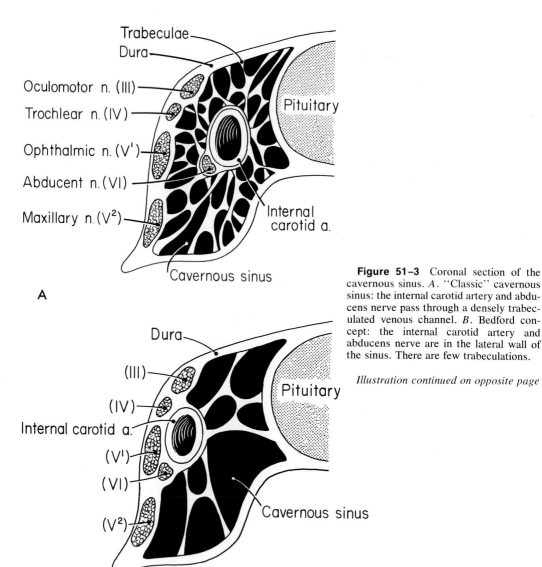

Figure 51–3 Coronal section of the cavernous sinus. *A*. "Classic" cavernous sinus: the internal carotid artery and abducens nerve pass through a densely trabeculated venous channel. *B*. Bedford concept: the internal carotid artery and abducens nerve are in the lateral wall of the sinus. There are few trabeculations.

Illustration continued on opposite page

and the posterior intercavernous sinus passes behind the gland. Intercavernous venous connections posterior to the clivus are called the basilar sinus. The existence of these connections explains the often paradoxical presentation of symptoms contralateral to a fistula in this region.[48,95]

The cavernous sinus is classically described as a large unbroken trabeculated venous channel that surrounds a portion of the carotid artery and abducens nerve. The trabeculated lumen of this "classic" sinus bears close resemblance to the corpora cavernosa of the penis (Fig. 51–3A).[119] The detailed anatomy of this venous structure,

however, has been elucidated by several recent reports. Bedford places the carotid artery and abducens nerve within the lateral dural wall (Fig. 51–3B).[7] Harris and Rhoton describe an intimate association between the artery and nerve laterally within the intraluminal space (Fig. 51–3C).[37] Both reports describe the sinus as a single continuous venous structure containing a small number of trabeculations.

Taptas and Parkinson dispute the concept that the cavernous sinus is a large unbroken venous cavern. They conclude that the cavernous sinus is an intricate plexus of various sized veins that divide and coalesce

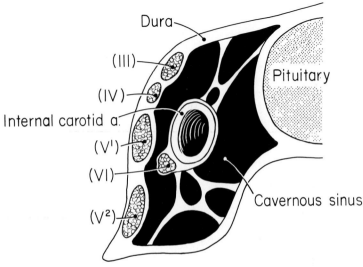

Figure 51–3 (*continued*) *C*. Harris and Rhoton concept: the internal carotid artery and abducens nerve are situated laterally within the venous lumen. There are few trabeculations. *D*. Taptas and Parkinson concept: an outer dural layer surrounds an extensive venous plexus that incompletely envelops the carotid artery and abducens nerve.

C

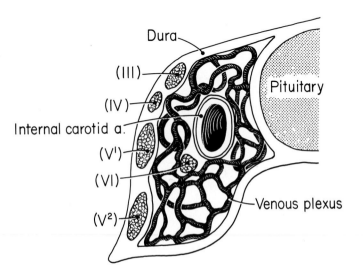

D

to incompletely surround the carotid artery (Fig. 51–3D).[87,109] Bonnet thought that the trabeculations represent cut cross sections of these veins.[11] This "venous plexus" concept allows theoretical exposure of the intracavernous carotid artery without entering the venous lumen, as reported by Parkinson.[86]

Neural Relationships

The cranial nerves that mediate ocular motion and facial sensation pass through the cavernous sinus region. The oculomotor, the trochlear, and the upper divisions of the trigeminal nerve lie within the dura of the lateral sinus wall. The abducens nerve courses within the sinus, adhering to the carotid artery medially and to the lateral sinus wall laterally.[37] As the sinus is viewed from a lateral projection, the oculomotor nerve is located superiorly, followed inferiorly by the trochlear, abducens, and trigeminal nerves (Fig. 51–4).

The ocular sympathetic fibers traverse the cavernous sinus as a grossly visible plexus on the surface of the carotid artery. Some of these fibers jump to the abducens nerve before joining the first division of the trigeminal nerve. These fibers ultimately control the pupillodilator and superior tarsal muscles. The remainder of the plexus continues upward around the carotid artery as it enters the subarachnoid space.[37]

CLASSIFICATION OF VASCULAR LESIONS

Vascular lesions of the intracavernous carotid artery may be divided into two groups: (1) nonfistulous arterial aneurysms and (2) carotid-cavernous fistulae.

NONFISTULOUS ARTERIAL ANEURYSMS

Approximately 3 per cent of all angiographically identified aneurysms originate from the intracavernous carotid artery.[52,61] Aneurysms at this site constitute 14 per cent of all aneurysms arising from the internal carotid artery.[99] Intracavernous an-

eurysms may be divided into three groups: congenital (saccular), arteriosclerotic (fusiform), and traumatic (false).

Congenital and Arteriosclerotic Aneurysms

Clinical Features

The many similarities between arteriosclerotic and saccular intracavernous aneurysms allow their discussion as a single clinical entity. Most intracavernous carotid aneurysms are saccular and are thought to arise from congenital defects in the vessel wall at the site of actual or vestigial branches. Arteriosclerosis and hypertension may also contribute to their development. Saccular and arteriosclerotic aneurysms have been reported to be six times as common in women as in men.[99] Symptoms tend to occur in the fifth and sixth decades, with saccular aneurysms presenting earlier and arteriosclerotic lesions later within this range.

Small arterial aneurysms of the cavernous sinus may be identified either when they rupture to establish fistulous communications or when they are incidentally discovered during a work-up for unrelated symptoms. The confining dural walls of the sinus otherwise allow many of these aneurysms to remain asymptomatic until a certain critical size (approximately 1 cm) is attained. At this point, clinically significant dural and neural compression begins. Intracavernous aneurysms larger than 1 cm make up 15 per cent of all symptomatic unruptured aneurysms.[52,99] The cavernous carotid artery is also a very common site of giant aneurysms (exceeding 2.5 cm in diameter), accounting for 11 of 28 such lesions (39 per cent) in Morley and Barr's series.[75] As the aneurysm expands, it may present as a large mass stretching from the superior orbital fissure to the petrous portion of the temporal bone.

Symptoms are caused by local mass effect against adjacent structures. Onset may be explosive, stuttering, or insidiously progressive. Worsening of symptoms is usually associated with acute enlargement of the aneurysm. A partial third nerve deficit is often the earliest detectable oculomotor abnormality. As symptoms progress, this nerve is almost always involved. The

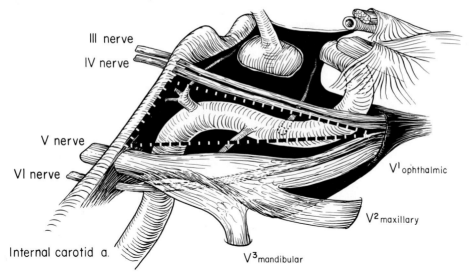

Figure 51–4 Cranial nerve relationships within the cavernous sinus. The dotted line represents Parkinson's triangle, indicating the space for incision to expose the two largest cavernous branches of the internal carotid artery. The boundaries of this triangle are the oculomotor and trochlear nerves superiorly, the trigeminal and abducens nerves inferiorly, and the plane of the clivus posteriorly.

trochlear, the abducens, and the sympathetic nerves may also be affected, regardless of aneurysmal position in the sinus. Associated loss of taste due to compression of the greater superficial petrosal nerve at the petrous ridge has been reported.[116] Pain is generally retro-orbital and is caused by dural and trigeminal nerve compression. Painful symptoms may be episodic, leaving residual facial numbness that is often isolated to the ophthalmic division.

An unruptured saccular or arteriosclerotic intercavernous aneurysm is identified in 20 to 25 per cent of patients with the "cavernous sinus," or "parasellar," syndrome.[110] Pain, usually in the ophthalmic or maxillary trigeminal distributions, is accompanied in this syndrome by deficits of one or more cranial nerves supplying the extraocular muscles. Jefferson attempted to designate specific anatomical locations for such aneurysms within the sinus on the basis of which divisions of the trigeminal nerve were compressed.[46] A large aneurysm, however, may occupy the entire sinus without trigeminal involvement.[47] Nasopharyngeal or metastatic neoplasms also cause this syndrome with equal frequency. The pathological cause of this clinical syndrome cannot be accurately predicted from the mode of onset, frequency of remission, rate of progression, presence or absence of pain, pattern of neurological deficit, or response to steroid therapy.[110]

Mild visual loss is usually caused by the accommodative disturbances that accompany the oculomotor nerve paresis. Occasionally, the aneurysm may bulge upward above the level of the anterior clinoid process and compress the optic nerve or chiasm. The resultant visual loss is usually monocular, but junctional or bitemporal patterns may occur. Anterior extension through the superior orbital fissure may produce exophthalmos.

Subarachnoid hemorrhage from intracavernous aneurysms occurs in less than 10 per cent of cases.[18] When hemorrhage does occur, intracavernous aneurysms must be distinguished from "paraclinoid" aneurysms. The paraclinoid aneurysm arises from the internal carotid artery opposite and slightly distal to the origin of the ophthalmic artery. This type of aneurysm originates at least in part within the subarachnoid space and projects secondarily into the cavernous sinus. Paraclinoid aneurysms have a much higher bleeding rate than intracavernous aneurysms, and their operative management may be different.[82]

Epistaxis following enlargement into the sphenoid sinus is fortunately rare with this type of aneurysm. Once it occurs, however, the potential for morbidity and death is high. Catastrophic results following transnasal biopsy of an unsuspected aneurysm have been reported.

Roentgenographic Features

Plain film abnormalities are present in many cases of symptomatic arteriosclerotic and saccular intracavernous aneurysms. Characteristic changes include elevation and erosion or destruction of the ipsilateral anterior clinoid process.[62] The dorsum sellae, posterior clinoid process, or sellar floor may also be eroded. Expansion into the sella may stimulate a pituitary adenoma. One to three per cent of enlarged sellae are due to aneurysms, most of which arise from the intracavernous carotid artery.[118] Enlargement of the superior orbital fissure may accompany anterior expansion of the aneurysm. This finding, when combined with inferior optic canal erosion, is almost pathognomonic of intracavernous aneurysm. Calcification may be found in one third of patients, and is usually curvilinear and dense. Tomography may be useful in defining subtle osseous changes.

Computed tomography may demonstrate round masses, enhanced by contrast, confined to the cavernous sinus.[111] The definitive diagnosis, however, must be established by arteriography. Mural thrombosis often occurs as the lesion enlarges, causing the aneurysm to appear smaller than its actual size. Bilaterality can be identified in 10 per cent of patients.

Prognosis and Treatment

The symptoms of nontraumatic symptomatic intracavernous aneurysms are usually confined to oculomotor or trigeminal dysfunction. With mild symptoms in this distribution, operative intervention is generally not advisable, as many patients will have a benign clinical course. The presence of visual loss (secondary to optic nerve or chiasmal compression) or severe intractable facial pain should be considered as a relative indication for operation. Subarachnoid hemorrhage and epistaxis should be treated aggressively.

When an operation is indicated for symptoms of oculomotor or trigeminal dysfunction, most surgeons perform common carotid ligation with a gradually occluding device.[28,79] By correlating cerebral blood flow and internal carotid artery pressures, the incidence of prolonged ischemic deficits following common carotid ligation has been significantly reduced.[72] Although several series report stabilization or improvement of symptoms with this treatment, it is not always effective. Oculomotor recovery is rarely complete.[47,62,75]

If visual loss or hemorrhage occurs, internal carotid artery ligation should be considered. Krayenbühl and Yasargil favor cervical internal carotid ligation if the patient has angiographically demonstrated open intracranial collateral channels and meets certain clinical and electroencephalographic criteria.[53] Intracranial carotid ligation is then performed if the aneurysm is visualized on postoperative angiography. Dandy recommended intracranial and cervical internal carotid ligation because in four of his cases the aneurysm ruptured into the intracranial cavity. He reported good results in 9 of 10 cases treated in this fashion.[18] Trapping is the treatment of choice once epistaxis develops.[112]

Ischemic complications will occur in some patients regardless of the choice or sequence of vessels ligated. Since ischemic symptoms may be delayed for hours or days after the ligation, a well-tolerated Matas test or trial carotid occlusion under local anesthesia does not eliminate the potential for hemiplegia. Blood pressure should be carefully monitored during and after ligation. Controlled hypertension may increase collateral flow, and has been successful in reversing some postocclusion deficits. Preliminary extracranial-intracranial bypass procedures may be useful in patients whose collateral circulation does not allow major vessel ligation.

A direct approach using stereotaxically injected iron filings or highly thrombogenic copper-beryllium wires has been reported by several authors.[77,106] These techniques require special skills and devices not readily available to most surgeons, and their effectiveness is not well established.

Traumatic Nonfistulous (False) Aneurysms

Clinical Features

Closed head trauma may injure the internal carotid artery at several sites: the supraclinoid segment, the intracavernous segment, the intrapetrous segment, and the upper cervical segment. Traumatic aneurysm formation, however, occurs predominantly in the intracavernous portion. Such lesions may become symptomatic following expansion in several directions: supraclinoid extension (rare) with potential massive intracranial hemorrhage, intracavernous rupture with resultant fistula formation, and sphenoid sinus extension with subsequent rupture and epistaxis.

The typical patient harboring a traumatic nonfistulous intracavernous aneurysm is a young man who has sustained a severe closed head injury. Skull films frequently demonstrate a fracture across the anterior cranial fossa. As the patient awakens, blindness (usually unilateral) is noted and is due to direct optic nerve injury. Anosmia, extraocular palsies, or trigeminal nerve impairment may accompany the initial injury. The aneurysm itself is not initially symptomatic. It will enlarge silently, extending medially and downward into the sphenoid sinus. Massive epistaxis appears one to three months after the injury. While the initial bleed is rarely fatal, recurrence is expected. Almost 50 per cent of patients die before diagnosis or adequate operative treatment is undertaken.[35]

Traumatic nonfistulous aneurysms may develop following penetrating injuries to the orbit or brain when the wall of the cavernous carotid artery is traumatized. This aneurysm may also be encountered by the otologist who performs operations on the head and neck.[98] Unexplained arterial bleeding following parasphenoidal procedures may be due to disruption of the carotid artery or one of its branches. Epistaxis may develop immediately when packing is removed, or it may be delayed as in the variety that follows head trauma.

Roentgenographic Features

Plain skull films usually demonstrate direct or indirect evidence of a basilar skull fracture. An initial angiogram performed to evaluate the patient's altered mental status may disclose an irregularity or dilatation of the intracavernous carotid artery. This finding reflects a severe injury to the arterial wall, and a repeat arteriogram performed several weeks later may reveal a large false aneurysm extending into the sphenoid sinus, arising exactly from the previously demonstrated abnormal arterial segment.

Prognosis and Treatment

The triad of unilateral blindness, orbital fracture, and massive epistaxis should alert the clinician to the possibility of a traumatic intracavernous aneurysm with sphenoid extension. Once the lesion is suspected, arteriography should be performed as soon as the patient's condition can be stabilized. Aggressive operative therapy should be instituted following angiographic identification, as the death rate attendant on the untreated lesion is high. Cervical internal carotid ligation is usually not sufficient to eliminate rebleeding risks. In their review of 31 cases, Shirai and associates reported that 7 of 13 patients treated with cervical carotid ligation alone experienced recurrent hemorrhage. Trapping (intracranial and cervical carotid ligation) produced excellent results in most patients.[105] Both sites should be ligated simultaneously to accelerate thrombosis and lessen the chances of collateral circulation development.

CAROTID-CAVERNOUS FISTULA

The true pathological nature of an arteriovenous fistula was first recognized by William Hunter in 1757.[42] He noticed that fistulae develop when both an artery and vein are injured simultaneously. This abnormal communication between the two channels produces a localized pulsatile mass that tends to expand as more blood is diverted through less resistant venous channels.

Fistulae in the cavernous sinus area, however, may be pathologically different from those arising elsewhere. The traditional concept of the cavernous sinus allows the carotid artery to rupture directly into the surrounding venous lumen without concomitant venous injury (Fig. 51–5). In contrast, Parkinson and Taptas visualize the cavernous sinus as an extensive plexus of veins.[87,109] According to this concept, a carotid-cavernous fistula would require simultaneous arterial and venous injury, and would conform pathologically with fistulae at other sites.

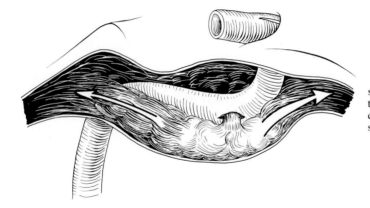

Figure 51–5 "Classic" representation of a carotid-cavernous fistula: the carotid artery empties directly into a large unbroken venous sinus.

Carotid-cavernous fistulae are more common than symptomatic intracavernous aneurysms but are considerably less common than subarachnoid saccular aneurysms. Hamby reported 42 carotid-cavernous fistulae among 550 cases of aneurysms and aneurysm-like lesions, an incidence of 8.6 per cent. Of his remaining 508 cases, 31 (6.1 per cent) were intact subclinoid aneurysms.[33] These fistulae accounted for 39 of the 545 cerebral vascular malformations reported by the National Cooperative Study.[99]

The presence or absence of head injury temporally related to the onset of the fistula allows division of carotid-cavernous fistulae into two groups: post-traumatic and spontaneous.

Post-Traumatic Fistulae

The post-traumatic carotid-cavernous fistula is three times as common as the spontaneous variety.[60] Onset occurs most often near the end of the third decade. Men, with their greater social and occupational susceptibility to head trauma, are afflicted more often than women. The lesion usually follows a head injury violent enough to produce unconsciousness. It is frequently associated with a basilar skull fracture, but may occasionally follow penetrating injuries. Isolated cases following retrogasserian rhizotomy, Fogarty catheter usage during endarterectomy, and blind sphenoid sinus biopsies have been reported.[58,63,76,116]

The head injury directly damages the carotid artery or one of its intracavernous arterial branches. Parkinson reports that post-traumatic fistulae are usually located anteriorly within the sinus, and he divides them into two groups. In type I fistulae, the carotid artery wall is torn, and one fistulous source results. In type II lesions, a branch of the carotid artery is disrupted. The extensive dural arterial anastomoses produce two fistulous sources, making this type of fistula more difficult to obliterate (Fig. 51–6).[85,86]

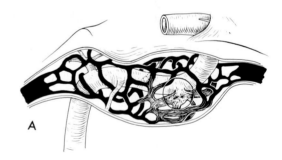

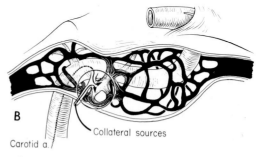

Figure 51–6 Parkinson's representation of a carotid-cavernous fistula. *A*. Type I. A tear in the carotid artery wall allows blood to flow directly into an adjacent and simultaneously injured vein. There is a single fistulous source. *B*. Type II. A cavernous branch of the internal carotid artery has been injured concomitantly with an adjacent vein. The fistula has two potential feeding sources: the main trunk of the carotid artery, and the anastomoses from adjacent dural collaterals.

Clinical Features

Signs and Symptoms

Clinical abnormalities usually arise from the redirection, overfilling, and resultant mass effect of hypertrophied orbital arteriovenous channels. The fistulous diversion of arterial flow away from the eye and brain may produce ischemia and hypoxia of these structures. Subtle signs and symptoms are evident in most patients when consciousness is regained. Some patients complain merely of a vague ocular discomfort or a faint intracranial sound synchronous with the pulse. Uncommonly, the entire symptom complex may be noticed immediately.

Clinical signs of this disorder include exophthalmos, orbital or cephalic bruit or both, ocular pulsations, headache, chemosis, extraocular palsies, and visual failure.[66,101] The frequency of these abnormalities, as collected by Martin and Mabon, is listed in Table 51–1.[66]

Exophthalmos is usually severe, and may prevent the eyelids from completely covering the globes. It is caused by the retrograde flow of blood from the cavernous sinus into the ophthalmic veins. Stimulated by arterial blood pressure, these veins dilate tremendously. The resultant mass of distended orbital veins, usually located superiorly in the orbit, may displace the globe downward and laterally.[101]

The bruit is perhaps the most disturbing symptom to the patient. It becomes louder when the patient is reclining, or when the environment is quiet, and makes sleep difficult. It may be audible over the orbit, temporal region, frontal area, or great vessels of the neck, and can occasionally be heard with the unaided ear. Present in most cases,

it is the most common initial symptom of this disease.[33]

Ocular pulsations may be difficult to visualize unless the eye is carefully observed in lateral profile. The pulsations are usually palpable, and may be accompanied by a thrill. Ocular tonography may aid recognition of this sign.

Headache is usually localized around or behind the affected eye, and is initially sharp in quality. It may be due to acute dural or vessel wall distention, or may be secondary to direct trigeminal nerve compression. The headache may subside as the vessels become adjusted to the engorgement, or it may be replaced by paresthesia and numbness, usually in the upper trigeminal division.

Chemosis results from the dilatation and arterialization of the small veins of the conjunctiva and sclera. In severe cases, the cornea lies depressed in the center of a swollen, angry-red mass of conjunctival tissue that herniates beyond the eyelids. Exposure to the air leads to drying, irritation, and increased risks of superinfection. Panophthalmitis may necessitate removal of the affected eye. The nasal mucosal veins may undergo similar changes, providing a potential source of severe nasal hemorrhages.

Diplopia may result from mechanical restriction of ocular motion as the increased orbital mass stretches and weakens the ocular musculature. More often, however, diplopia is secondary to cranial nerve palsy. The abducens nerve is affected twice as often as the oculomotor and trochlear nerves combined, probably because of its closer relationship to the carotid artery within the sinus.[101] The sympathetic plexus surrounding the cavernous carotid may also be impaired. While these deficits may develop immediately as a consequence of direct nerve injury, they usually are delayed until fistulous enlargement promotes vascular compression of these structures. Deficits of cranial nerves I, VII, and VIII are not directly caused by the fistula, but may accompany the initial injury.

Visual failure is frequently associated with carotid-cavernous fistula. De Schweinitz and Holloway reported impaired vision in 89 per cent of cases.[21] Sattler found visual diminution in 73 per cent of patients, most of whom had less than 10 per cent of vision remaining.[101] The

TABLE 51–1 SYMPTOMS IN ORDER OF FREQUENCY AS SHOWN IN CASES IN LITERATURE SINCE LOCKE'S REVIEW*

SYMPTOM	NUMBER
Bruit	191
Pulsation	178
Chemosis	159
Diplopia	76
Headache	71
Visual disturbance	66

*Symptoms reported in 224 cases of carotid-cavernous fistula. (From Martin, J. D., Jr., and Mabon, R. F.: Pulsating exophthalmos: Review of all reported cases. J.A.M.A., *121*: 330–334, 1943. Copyright 1943, American Medical Association. Reprinted by permission.)

causes of this visual loss are direct optic nerve injury from the initial trauma, corneal ulceration leading to secondary infection and panophthalmitis, and vascular insults to the various ocular components.

Increased ocular venous pressure may lead to intraorbital and retinal hemorrhages. The retina may become detached and the vitreous and anterior chamber filled with blood. Enlarged limbic veins may compress the canal of Schlemm and elevate intraocular tension, causing glaucoma that may be refractory to medications.[38] Cataracts or corneal neovascularity may develop in chronic cases. Papilledema and optic atrophy may develop from direct optic nerve pressure or stretching by the exophthalmos.

The major pathophysiological threat to vision, however, may be hypoxia.[100] The lowered arterial pressure and elevated venous pressure lead to embarrassment of ocular circulation by reducing the ocular perfusion pressure. This hypoxic damage may be irreversible, and visual loss may progress despite intervening control of the fistula.

Clinical Variants

Signs and symptoms of carotid-cavernous fistula are largely dependent on venous drainage patterns. The multiple venous outflow channels from the cavernous sinus allows the clinical features to vary considerably, regardless of the site of the arterial injury. A patient with a unilateral carotid-cavernous fistula may present with ipsilateral, contralateral, or bilateral ocular manifestations or even their absence (Fig. 51–7).

Most post-traumatic carotid-cavernous fistulae drain directly into the ipsilateral ophthalmic veins and present with ipsilateral ocular signs. If these veins are obstructed by thrombosis, traumatic rupture, anomalous course, or the dilated carotid artery, contralateral venous outflow through intercavernous connections may occur. Under these circumstances, ocular signs will appear contralateral to the fistula. Unusually large intercavernous connections may allow a unilateral fistula to present with bilateral ocular signs. True bilateral fistulae, however, are rare. They are more often post-traumatic than spontaneous.[16] The bilaterality may not be appreciated until the more symptomatic side has undergone treatment.

The venous drainage of the atypical carotid-cavernous fistula proceeds mainly through distended cortical vessels rather than orbital channels. This type of fistula is uncommon and may not demonstrate the usual orbital symptoms.[1] The progressive cerebral arterial insufficiency and cortical venous hypertension increase the risk of hemispheric neurological deterioration in these patients. Rarely, major venous outflow through the petrosal sinuses produces signs suggesting disease in the posterior fossa.[6]

Differential Diagnosis

The clinical diagnosis of post-traumatic carotid-cavernous fistula is usually straightforward: a history of trauma followed by the development of exophthalmos, ocular pulsations, and orbital bruit.[19] Occasionally, however, an unusual presentation may resemble that of other clinical entities. Endocrine exophthalmos, orbital pseudotumor, and most retro-orbital tumors should cause little confusion, since they exhibit no pulsations or bruit. Cavernous sinus thrombosis may produce similar ocular changes, but the absence of ocular pulsations and the presence of systemic intoxication usually secure this diagnosis. Congenital, traumatic, or neoplastic defects in the orbital roof or sphenoid ridge may cause pulsatile exophthalmos, particularly when associated with intracranial hypertension. Some intraorbital vascular tumors or malformations may be clinically indistinguishable from a fistula without the use of radiographic aids.[39]

Roentgenographic Features

Plain skull x-rays may demonstrate evidence of the initial inciting skull trauma. Pressure erosion of the sphenoidal fissure or lateral part of the sella turcica may develop as the lesion enlarges and becomes chronically established.[49] Computed tomography may demonstrate a dilated cavernous sinus, but in small fistulae this study will be normal. Computed tomography and plain skull x-rays are most useful in assessing the extent of the initial intracranial injury.

Angiography is the definitive diagnostic

procedure. Characteristic angiographic features include: early dense opacification of the enlarged cavernous sinus, early filling of the ophthalmic or other veins usually draining into the cavernous sinus, and poorer than expected opacification of the cerebral arterial system secondary to the arteriovenous shunt.[92]

Most post-traumatic fistulae are high-flow, high-pressure shunts. The cavernous sinus fills rapidly, making the exact point of fistulous communication more difficult to demonstrate than with spontaneous fistulae.[22] Vertebral artery injection and ipsilateral carotid compression may slow the fistulous flow sufficiently to allow more accurate localization, especially if rapid-sequence filming is used.[41] Although most post-traumatic fistulae appear angiographically to originate directly from one internal carotid artery, bilateral selective external and internal carotid injections and one vertebral injection should be performed, as some fistulae will have unusual arterial feeding patterns or atypical venous drainage. Complete arteriography is necessary to plan the operative approach as well as to explain the failure of previous treatments. Associated congenital anastomotic vessels such as primitive trigeminal or hypoglossal trunks have been reported.[27,29] An ablative procedure that did not spare these congenital arteries could cause brain stem ischemia.

Prognosis and Treatment

Catastrophic complications are uncommon in untreated post-traumatic carotid-cavernous fistulae. Life-threatening intracranial hemorrhage occurs in 3 per cent of patients.[101] Epistaxis and severe orbital bleeding are rare.[56] Impaired cerebral function is usually directly related to the severity of the initial head injury. Spontaneous remission may occur in 5 to 10 per cent of patients.

Indications for operative intervention include patient intolerance to the bruit, delayed visual loss, and hemorrhage. Visual loss is the most threatening problem, and it may not be improved by fistula obliteration. Multiple vessel ligations may further reduce ocular perfusion pressure, and ocular hypoxia may worsen. Ten of sixteen patients in the Sanders and Hoyt series had visual deterioration immediately after the

procedure or within several months thereafter.[100] Most patients seek operative correction because the bruit and cosmetic disfiguration become unbearable.[74]

Subcutaneous gelatin injections, sympathectomy, venous injections of sclerosing solutions, orbital vein ligation, carotid-jugular anastomosis, and digital carotid compression have been previously recommended for this condition.[25] Such forms of therapy have subsequently been discarded as inadequate.

Some surgeons perform preoperative digital carotid compression (Matas test) to evaluate a patient's tolerance to a planned carotid ablative procedure. This test, however, is not always a reliable predictor of the adequacy of collateral circulation.[67,107] Cerebral symptoms may develop because manual arterial compression promotes fistulous shunting of blood from other sources. The surgeon may then erroneously assume that the patient cannot tolerate carotid ligation.

The goals of therapy include preservation of vision, elimination of the bruit, and restoration of the orbit and its contents to normal while avoiding cerebral ischemic complications. The ideal treatment should obliterate the fistula while maintaining patency of the carotid artery. Treatment modalities may be categorized as ablative or preservative on the basis of postoperative maintenance of carotid artery patency.

Carotid Ablative Procedures

CAROTID LIGATION (CERVICAL). Proximal vessel ligation (cervical internal or common carotid artery) is a generally unsatisfactory treatment for carotid-cavernous fistula. The development of collateral circulation usually allows the fistula to remain patent (Fig. 51–8). After cervical ligation, a "steal" syndrome may occur as blood flow from the opposite carotid is shunted into the fistula rather than supplying the brain. More blood from the ophthalmic circulation may also be diverted into the fistula. Further cerebral and ocular ischemia may result.

TRAPPING. The trapping procedure introduced by Hamby and Gardner involves ligation of the intracranial and cervical internal carotid arteries during one operation.[34] The intracranial vessel is occluded first to avoid cerebral steal. Intercavernous

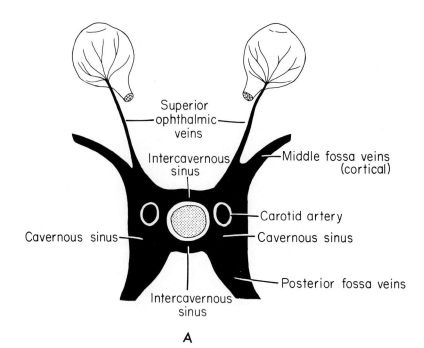

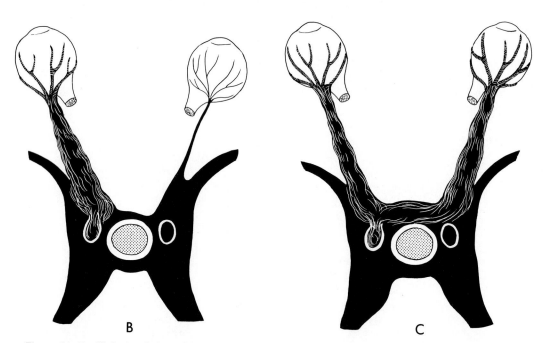

Figure 51–7   Clinical variations of cavernous sinus fistulae. *A*. Normal. *B*. The fistula drains into the ipsilateral ophthalmic veins, producing unilateral and ipsilateral ocular abnormalities. *C*. A patent anterior intercavernous sinus allows venous drainage into both ophthalmic veins. Ocular abnormalities appear bilaterally from a unilateral fistula.

Illustration continued on opposite page

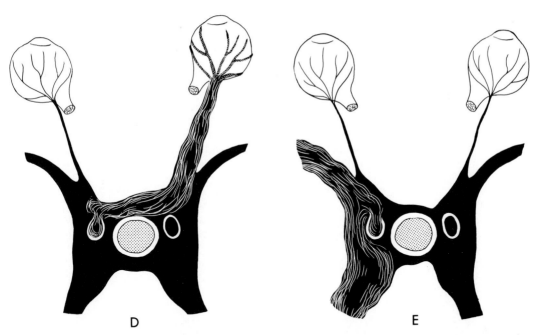

D   E

Figure 51–7 (*continued*)   *D*. Occluded (or congenitally absent) ipsilateral ophthalmic veins with patent anterior intercavernous sinus allow contralateral ophthalmic venous drainage. Ocular signs are contralateral to the fistula. *E*. Atypical fistula in which venous drainage proceeds through middle fossa or posterior fossa channels. Ocular signs may be minimal or absent, and symptoms of cerebral or posterior fossa dysfunction may be prominent.

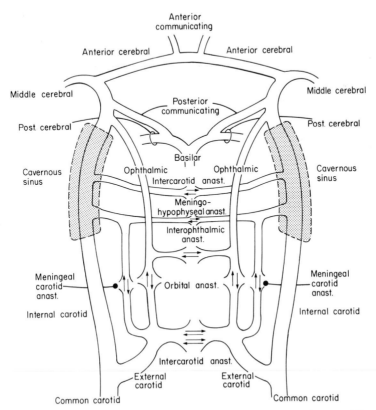

Figure 51–8   Arterial collateral circulation of the cavernous sinus region. Inadequate obliteration of a fistula may allow continued patency through extensive ipsilateral and contralateral arterial communications.

and meningeal collaterals to the isolated carotid segment, however, may allow persistence of the fistula, especially if the ophthalmic artery is not clipped. Staged ligations fail with even higher frequency because collateral circulation increases during the interim between the two procedures.

EMBOLIZATION WITH LIGATION. In 1931, Brooks successfully obliterated a carotid-cavernous fistula by introducing a muscle embolus into the cervical carotid artery and then ligating that vessel.[12,54] This procedure as originally described never gained widespread acceptance, primarily because of inability to control the ultimate location of the embolus.[69] A large muscle strip may not reach the fistula, while a small muscle strip may embolize the cerebral or systemic circulation. Arutinov and co-workers improved this control by marking the muscle embolus with a silver clip and securing it with a checkrein suture.[3] The muscle could then be followed radiographically into the cavernous region while the suture prevented distal propagation. When the fistula was occluded, the suture was firmly anchored, and the opened cervical vessel was ligated. Isamat and Black and their associates have successfully obliterated fistulae by using this technique without occluding the internal carotid artery.[10,43] Gelfoam, porcelain beads, and polyurethane foam have also been effective embolic agents.[44,51,84]

TRAPPING COMBINED WITH EMBOLIZATION. In 1942 Jaeger combined trapping with muscle embolization to obliterate a carotid-cavernous fistula.[45] Hamby subsequently popularized this method, and the technique became known as the Jaeger-Hamby procedure.[74] The recommended technique for trapping and muscle embolization is illustrated in Figure 51–9. The head is slightly elevated, and the cervical and cranial portions are draped into a common field. Intraoperative x-ray monitoring with an image intensifier or conventional films should be available. The ipsilateral orbit should be exposed for auscultation by the anesthesiologist. Because venous hypertension and secondary cerebral swelling may make intracranial conditions unfavorable, adjunctive hyperventilation, osmotic agents, preoperative steroids, and spinal drainage should be considered.

The common carotid bifurcation is exposed first, allowing room for clamping and embolization. A standard frontotemporal craniotomy follows. If the brain is tight and exposure is difficult, temporary occlusion of the cervical internal carotid artery may be advantageous. The intracranial internal carotid artery is identified by following the sphenoid ridge medially beyond the anterior clinoid process. This artery is followed proximally to the point where it first exits from the dura.

The carotid artery should be ligated prox-

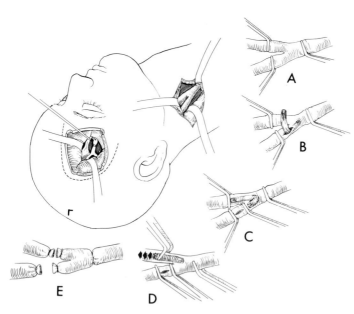

Figure 51–9 Jaeger-Hamby technique of muscle embolization combined with trapping. Intracranial carotid and ophthalmic artery ligations are performed prior to embolization. *A*. Clamping of common carotid artery and its two major branches. *B*. Arteriotomy of external carotid artery for insertion of muscle embolus. *C*. The embolus is manipulated into the internal carotid artery, and the external carotid is clamped proximal to the arteriotomy. *D*. Release of the clamps on the common and internal carotid arteries allows distal propagation of the muscle embolus. *E*. Double ligation and excision of the common carotid artery and its branches.

imal to the origin of the ophthalmic artery. This branch usually arises from the internal carotid artery just as it penetrates the dura. It generally courses inferior and medial to the optic nerve on its way to the optic foramen. Removal of the anterior clinoid and the roof of the optic canal may facilitate exposure. When vision is totally absent, the optic nerve may be sectioned. If the carotid artery cannot be ligated proximal to the ophthalmic origin, the ophthalmic artery should be ligated separately. The posterior communicating artery and its distal carotid communications must be carefully preserved.

Attention is then redirected to the cervical exposure. The common carotid and its two branches are occluded with clamps. An incision is made into the external carotid artery, leaving room between the arteriotomy and the vessel origin to place another clamp. A muscle strip prepared from the sternocleidomastoid muscle is marked with metal clips for radiographic localization. The strip should be about 3 cm long and 0.3 cm wide (the size of a paper book match). The muscle is introduced through the arteriotomy into the internal carotid artery. After a clamp has been placed across the proximal portion of the external carotid artery, the clamps on the internal and common carotid arteries are released, thus allowing the blood flow to embolize the muscle strip toward the fistula. Auscultation of the orbit verifies disappearance of the bruit. An x-ray image documents that the clips have reached the appropriate parasellar area. The common, external, and internal carotid arteries are then doubly ligated and divided to prevent recanalization.

Hamby and Dohn reported a 93 per cent cure rate among 28 patients who received a trapping procedure with or without embolization as their primary operation.[23,33] Dott and Morley introduce muscle directly into the cavernous carotid through an arteriotomy of the intracranial carotid artery.[24,74] This variation has produced excellent results in their small series.

The Jaeger-Hamby procedure is currently the most commonly employed operation for carotid-cavernous fistula. Favorable results, however, are not enjoyed by all surgeons.[74] Intracranial carotid and ophthalmic ligations may be technically very difficult, especially in long-standing fistulae

with markedly enlarged arterialized veins. The fistula may persist despite apparently successful trapping, particularly if the ophthalmic artery is not completely occluded. Some patients whose initial eye signs and visual loss are contralateral to the fistula risk total blindness with this approach. Attempts to improve the effectiveness and safety of this procedure have included intraoperative blood flow measurements and orbital Doppler ultrasonic recordings.[5,55,68,81]

Any ablative procedure of the internal carotid artery may cause significant morbidity or death. Stern and associates reported that 4 of their 15 patients developed serious postoperative ischemic complications in spite of a comprehensive analysis of the intracranial circulatory dynamics.[107] Postoperative visual failure may occur in a high percentage of patients, even if the fistula is obliterated.[100,114]

CATHETER PROCEDURES. Prolo has developed a double-lumen catheter that is especially designed for treatment of this disease (Fig. 51–10). One lumen allows angiographic visualization of the carotid circulation, while the other self-sealing lumen allows inflation of a balloon on the catheter tip. The catheter is introduced into the internal carotid artery through an open cervical exposure. As the catheter tip is advanced toward the cavernous sinus, the balloon is intermittently inflated and deflated. When intraoperative arteriography and orbital Doppler monitoring document an ideal position overlying the fistula, the balloon is fully inflated with contrast medium. The internal carotid artery is then ligated, and the free ends of the catheter are buried beneath the sternocleidomastoid muscle. This method has produced excellent results in 8 of 12 patients, with the failures occurring early in the series. Similar results have been obtained by several other authors.[4,15,65,91] Intraluminal carotid occlusion has the advantages of direct fistula occlusion and avoidance of an intracranial procedure. Preliminary extracranial-intracranial bypass procedures may further reduce the incidence of postocclusion neurological deficits.[31,104]

Carotid Preservation Techniques

DIRECT CAVERNOUS SINUS APPROACH. In 1936, Browder successfully obliterated a

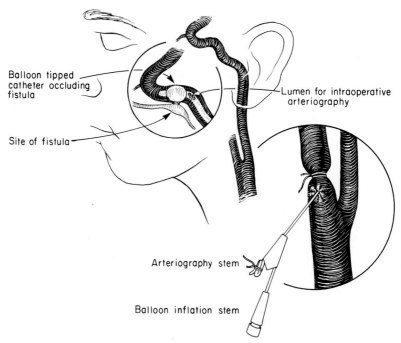

Balloon tipped catheter occluding fistula

Lumen for intraoperative arteriography

Site of fistula

Arteriography stem

Balloon inflation stem

Figure 51–10   Prolo catheter technique. The double-lumen balloon-tipped catheter is introduced into the internal carotid artery and advanced into the cavernous sinus region. The balloon is positioned at the orifice of the fistula and inflated. Complete obliteration is documented by intraoperative arteriography and Doppler monitoring. The arteriography catheter stem is then amputated and ligated to prevent retrograde flow from cavernous collateral arteries. The internal carotid artery is ligated, while patency is maintained in the external and common carotid arteries. The residual catheter body is buried beneath the sternocleidomastoid muscle.

carotid-cavernous fistula by opening the engorged cavernous sinus and stuffing muscle directly into it.[13] In 1968, Riechert induced thrombosis of a carotid-cavernous fistula by direct tamponade, using a specially fashioned tantalum plate tacked to the floor of the middle fossa.[96]

The most innovative direct approach, however, was conceived by Parkinson. On the basis of intraoperative observation and corrosion studies, Parkinson described the cavernous sinus as a plexus of various-sized veins that incompletely surround the carotid artery. He suggested that this portion of the carotid could be approached operatively without entering either the arterial or venous compartments. He also thought that a fistula in this region could be repaired with a single clip while preserving the carotid artery.[86] Parkinson and his colleagues applied these concepts to nine patients with previously untreated carotid-cavernous fistulae. Using adjunctive hypothermia and circulatory arrest, he exposed the intracavernous carotid artery through a triangular space in the lateral cavernous sinus dura (see Fig. 51–4). He was able to obliterate

the fistula and preserve the carotid artery in all nine patients. Six of these patients have since returned to work, while two are partially disabled and one is dead.[90] The carotid artery is apparently very difficult to distinguish from the surrounding arterialized veins, and identification of the exact fistula site may be extremely tedious. Because of technical difficulties of this approach, the procedure requires further investigation and refinement before it can become more useful.[88]

STEREOTAXIC AND WIRE THROMBOSIS. Three methods of stereotaxic thrombosis of a carotid-cavernous fistula have been investigated: direct current electrical thrombosis, stereotaxic copper electric needle thrombosis, and intracavernous insertion of thrombogenic wire. Focal arterial spasm has been noted when electric current was applied, and thrombogenic wire is preferred.[40,77] The wire is introduced into the cavernous sinus directly through Parkinson's triangle or by retrograde threading through a draining vein. Mullan has treated 31 fistula patients with variations of this method. There has been very little morbidity, and the carotid artery was sacrificed in only one case. Visual loss, diplopia, proptosis, and exophthalmos were reversed.[78] Success with this technique has also been reported in the treatment of a bilateral fistula.[16]

Mullan's technique of copper-wire thrombosis is a complex procedure that is continually being improved and modified. The materials, methods, and judgment required for this technique, however, are not available to most surgeons. The newer catheter techniques are probably superior to this approach in most cases of post-traumatic fistulae.

CATHETER TECHNIQUES. Serbinenko has recently developed a small, highly flexible catheter for use in selective catheterization of intracranial vessels.[103] His catheter has a small, detachable balloon tip that can be placed directly in the fistulous orifice. Once positioned, the balloon is filled with a silicone fixative and detached from the catheter. The catheter is then removed, and carotid arterial patency is maintained.

Using a similar catheter, Debrun and co-workers successfully cannulated the fistula in 14 of 17 patients with post-traumatic fistulae.[20] Postcatheterization carotid patency was maintained in 12 of these patients, while 2 patients experienced asymptomatic delayed carotid thrombosis. The three remaining fistulae were too small to allow catheter introduction, and the Prolo technique was utilized. All 17 patients were successfully treated without untoward neurological problems. As the availability of these catheters increases, this technique may become the preferred treatment for most post-traumatic fistulae.

Spontaneous Fistulae

Clinical Features

Spontaneous carotid cavernous fistulae are less common than the traumatic variety. The typical patient is a middle-aged, postmenopausal woman, although symptoms may arise throughout adulthood. Mild unilateral headache or abducens nerve paresis may antedate orbital signs by many months. Dilated conjunctival vessels and proptosis may develop later, and are generally much less striking than with post-traumatic fistulae. Bruit is absent in almost half the patients. The milder symptoms allow more frequent error or delay in diagnosis.

This disorder has a striking prevalence among women. Earlier literature reported a high degree of correlation between pregnancy and the onset of symptoms.[17,101] Walker and Allegre found that 25 to 30 per cent of women with this disease develop it during the latter half of pregnancy or during delivery.[114] These authors postulated that rupture of a pre-existing aneurysm was facilitated by increased blood pressure associated with gestation. Other reports have failed to support this association with pregnancy or to verify the pathological changes.

Most spontaneous carotid-cavernous fistulae were originally presumed to arise from ruptured intracavernous aneurysms.[83] The existence of such aneurysms, however, is seldom demonstrated by arteriography or autopsy. The unclear pathological changes in some cases may be explained by aneurysmal disintegration following rupture, or by aneurysmal obscuration by the adjacent arterialized veins. Recent refinements in arteriography, including rapid-sequence filming and magnification-subtraction techniques, have allowed better classification of these lesions. It is now apparent that many spontaneous carotid-cavernous fistulae are actually dural arteriovenous shunts.[2,26,74,80,108] Lie believed that these shunts were congenital lesions that enlarged slowly to produce symptoms in adulthood.[57] Newton and Hoyt were of the opinion that predisposing vascular disease, straining, or minor trauma might initiate fistula formation.[80] The increased vascular fragility and the high incidence of fistulae in such collagen vascular disorders as Ehlers-Danlos syndrome, fibromuscular dysplasia, and pseudoxanthoma elastica lend support to the concept of an acquired degenerative vascular origin in "normal" patients.[30,50,97,102,120]

Roentgenographic Features

Plain skull radiographs are usually normal in spontaneous carotid cavernous fistulae. A large calcified intracavernous aneurysm is not likely to rupture to produce a fistula. Computed tomography is usually normal, but may aid in the differential diagnosis. Arteriography is the diagnostic procedure of choice.

Fistulae arising from aneurysm rupture are usually high-flow, high-pressure lesions that angiographically resemble the post-traumatic variety. Many spontaneous fistulae, however, are low-flow, low-pressure dural shunts that permit excellent angiographic opacification of the intracranial arteries. Complete vertebral and selective internal and external carotid injections are essential because the fistula may receive blood from several sources. The external carotid artery frequently supplies this type of fistula and is often its exclusive source of blood. Terminal meningeal vessels of the internal maxillary artery are the most commonly observed external carotid feeding channels. Other contributing external carotid branches include the ascending pharyngeal and pterygopalatine arteries. The meningohypophyseal trunk is the usual feeding branch when the internal carotid artery supplies the fistula.[80] Contralateral arterial dural contributions are also frequent. Venous drainage is usually through the ipsilateral ophthalmic veins, although variations are not uncommon.

Prognosis and Treatment

Recent reports suggest that spontaneous resolution is much more common in this type of fistula than with the post-traumatic variety, particularly in patients with dural arteriovenous shunts.[2,59] Newton and Hoyt reported that 5 of 11 such fistulae resolved completely without operative intervention. Three of their "cures" occurred immediately after angiography.[80] Other reports also indicate that these lesions have a tendency to thrombose following contrast injection.[8,59,113] Possible explanations include reactive systemic hypotension following dye injection, direct irritating or vasoconstrictive activity of the dye, embolization during arteriography, and carotid artery compression during or following the procedure. Small changes in the hemodynamics of these low-flow lesions are apparently sufficient to initiate thrombosis.

The more benign symptoms, lesser likelihood of major visual complications, and greater tendency for spontaneous thrombosis justify conservative management of most spontaneous fistulae. When operation is indicated, less aggressive procedures may yield excellent results. External carotid embolization or ligation has resulted

in several reported cures.[36,64,94,108] More aggressive intervention is probably indicated in high-flow spontaneous fistulae.

REFERENCES

1. Ambler, M. W., Moon, A. C., and Sturner, W. Q.: Bilateral carotid-cavernous fistulae of mixed types with unusual radiological and neuropathological findings: Case report. J. Neurosurg., *48*: 117–124, 1978.
2. Aminoff, M. J.: Anomalies in the intracranial dura mater. Brain., 96:601–612, 1973.
3. Arutinov, A. I., Serbinenko, F. A., and Shlykov, A. A.: Surgical treatment of carotid-cavernous fistulae. Cere. Circ., *30*:441–444, 1968.
4. Bahuleyau, K., Nelson, L. R., and Peck, F. C.: Occlusion of carotid-cavernous fistula with a balloon catheter. Surg. Neurol., *3*:283–287, 1975.
5. Barnes, B. D., Rosenblum, M. L., Pitts, L. H., et al.: Carotid-cavernous fistula: Demonstration of asymptomatic vascular "steal." J. Neurosurg., 49:49–55, 1978.
6. Bartlow, B., and Penn, R. D.: Carotid-cavernous sinus fistula presenting as a posterior fossa mass: Case report. J. Neurosurg., *42*:585–588, 1975.
7. Bedford, M. A.: The "cavernous" sinus. Brit. J. Ophthal., *50*:41–46, 1966.
8. Bennett, D. R., Van Pyk, H. J. L., and Davis, D. O.: Carotid cavernous sinus fistula closure following angiography. J.A.M.A., *224*:1637–1638, 1973.
9. Bickerstaff, E. R.: Mechanisms of presentation of caratico-cavernous fistulae. Brit. J. Ophthal., *54*:186–190, 1970.
10. Black, P., Uematsu, S., Perovic, M., and Walker, A. E.: Carotid-cavernous fistula: A controlled embolus technique for occlusion of fistula with preservation of carotid blood flow (technical note). J. Neurosurg., *38*:113–118, 1973.
11. Bonnet, P.: Cited in Bedford, M. A.: The "cavernous" sinus. Brit. J. Ophthal., *50*:41–46, 1966.
12. Brooks, B.: Discussion: Noland, L., and Taylor, A. S.: Trans. South. Surg. Ass., *43*:176–177, 1931.
13. Browder, J.: Treatment of carotid artery-cavernous sinus fistula: Report of a case. Arch. Ophthal. (Chicago), *18*:95–102, 1937.
14. Bynke, H. G., and Efsing, H. O.: Carotid-cavernous fistula with contralateral exophthalmos. Acta Ophthal. (Kobenhavn), *48*:971–978, 1970.
15. Cares, H. L., Roberson, G. H., Grand, W., et al.: A safe technique for the precise localization of carotid-cavernous fistula during balloon obliteration (technical note). J. Neurosurg., *49*:146–149, 1978.
16. Conley, F. K., Hamilton, R. D., and Hosobuchi, Y.: Successful surgical treatment of bilateral carotid-cavernous fistulae: Case report. J. Neurosurg., *43*:357–361, 1975.
17. Dandy, W. E.: Carotid cavernous aneurysms

(pulsating exophthalmos). Z bl. Neurochir., 2:77–206, 1937.

18. Dandy, W. E.: Intracranial Arterial Aneurysms. Ithaca, N. Y., Comstock Publishing Co., 1944, p. 147.

19. Dandy, W. E.: The treatment of carotid cavernous arteriovenous aneurysms. In Troland, C. E., and Otenasek, F. J., eds.: Selected Writings of Walter E. Dandy. Springfield, Ill., Charles C Thomas, 1957.

20. Debrun, G., La Cour, P., Caron, J., et al.: Detachable balloon and calibrated balloon techniques in the treatments of cerebral vascular lesions. J. Neurosurg., 49:635–649, 1978.

21. De Schweinitz, G. E., and Holloway, T. B.: Pulsating Exophthalmos. Philadelphia, W. B. Saunders Co., 1908.

22. Djindjian, R., Picard, L., and Manelfe, C.: Fistules artério-veineuses carotide interne–sinus caverneux. Aspects radio-anatomiques actuels et perspectives thérapeutiques. Neurochirurgie, 19:75–90, 1973.

23. Dohn, D. F.: Carotid aneurysms and arteriovenous fistulae of the cavernous sinus. In Youmans, J. R., ed.: Neurological Surgery. Philadelphia, W. B. Saunders Co., 1973.

24. Dott, N. M.: Carotid-cavernous arteriovenous fistula. Clin. Neurosurg., 16:17–21, 1969.

25. Echols, D. H., and Jackson, J. D.: Carotid-cavernous fistula: A perplexing surgical problem. J. Neurosurg., 16:619–627, 1959.

26. Edwards, M. S., and Connolly, E. S.: Cavernous sinus syndrome produced by communication between the external carotid artery and cavernous sinus. J. Neurosurg., 46:92–96, 1977.

27. Enomoto, T., Sato, A., and Maki, Y.: Carotid-cavernous sinus fistula caused by rupture of a primitive trigeminal artery aneurysm: Case report. J. Neurosurg., 46:373–376, 1977.

28. Galbraith, J. G., and Clark, R. M.: Role of carotid ligation in the management of intracranial carotid aneurysms. Clin. Neurosurg., 21:171–181, 1973.

29. Gerlach, J., Jensen, H. P., Spuler, H., et al.: Case reports: Traumatic carotico-cavernous fistula combined with persisting primitive hypoglossal artery. J. Neurosurg., 20:885–887, 1963.

30. Graf, C. J.: Spontaneous carotid-cavernous fistula: Ehlers-Danlos syndrome and related conditions. Arch. Neurol. (Chicago), 13:662–672, 1965.

31. Guegan, Y., Javalet, A., Eon, J. Y., et al.: Extra-intracranial anastomosis preliminary to treatment of carotid artery-cavernous sinus fistula. Surg. Neurol., 10:85–88, 1978.

32. Hamby, W. B.: Carotid-cavernous fistula: Report of 32 surgically treated cases and suggestions for definitive operation. J. Neurosurg., 21:859–866, 1964.

33. Hamby, W. B.: Carotid Cavernous Fistulae. Springfield, Ill., Charles C Thomas, 1966.

34. Hamby, W. B., and Gardner, W. J.: Treatment of pulsating exophthalmos with report of 2 cases. Arch. Surg. (Chicago), 27:676–685, 1933.

35. Handa, J., and Handa, H.: Severe epistaxis caused by traumatic aneurysm of cavernous carotid artery. Surg. Neurol., 5:241–243, 1976.

36. Hardy, R. W., Costin, J. A., Weinstein, M., et al.: External carotid cavernous fistula treated by transfemoral embolization. Surg. Neurol., 9:255–256, 1978.

37. Harris, F. S., and Rhoton, A. L.: Anatomy of the cavernous sinus. J. Neurosurg., 45:169–180, 1976.

38. Henderson, J. W., and Schneider, R. C.: The ocular findings in carotid cavernous fistula in a series of 17 cases. Trans. Amer. Ophthal. Soc., 56:123–144, 1958.

39. Higazi, I., and El-Banhawy, A.: The value of angiography in the differential diagnosis of pulsating exophthalmos: A report of 3 cases. J. Neurosurg., 21:561–567, 1964.

40. Hosobuchi, Y.: Electrothrombosis of carotid-cavernous fistula. J. Neurosurg., 42:76–85, 1975.

41. Huber, P.: A technical contribution to the exact angiographic localization of carotid cavernous fistula. Neuroradiology, 10:239–241, 1976.

42. Hunter, W.: Further observations upon a particular species of aneurysm. Med. Observ. Inquiries, 2:390–414, 1762.

43. Isamat, F., Salleras, V., and Miranda, A. M.: Artificial embolization of carotid-cavernous fistula with postoperative patency of internal carotid artery. J. Neurol. Neurosurg. Psychiat., 33:674–678, 1970.

44. Ishimori, S., Hattori, M., Shibata, Y., et al.: Treatment of carotid-cavernous fistula by Gelfoam embolization. J. Neurosurg., 27:315–319, 1967.

45. Jaeger, R.: Intracranial aneurysms. South. Surg., 15:205–217, 1949.

46. Jefferson, G.: On the saccular aneurysms of the internal carotid artery in the cavernous sinus. Brit. J. Surg., 26:267–302, 1938.

47. Jefferson, G.: The Bowman Lecture: Concerning injuries, aneurysms, and tumours involving the cavernous sinus. Trans. Opthal. Soc. U.K., 73:117–152, 1953.

48. Kaplan, H. A., Browder, J., and Krieger, A. J.: Intercavernous connections of the cavernous sinuses: The superior and inferior circular sinuses. J. Neurosurg., 45:166–168, 1976.

49. Katsiotis, P., Kiriakopoulos, C., and Taptas, J.: Carotid-cavernous sinus fistulae and dural arteriovenous shunts. Vasc. Surg., 8:60–69, 1974.

50. Kaufman, H. H., Lind, T. A., and Mullan, S.: Spontaneous carotid-cavernous fistula with fibromuscular dysplasia. Acta Neurochir. (Wien), 40:123–129, 1978.

51. Kosary, I. Z., Lerner, M. A., Mozes, M., et al.: Artificial embolic occlusion of the terminal internal carotid artery in the treatment of carotid-cavernous fistula (technical note). J. Neurosurg., 28:605–608, 1968.

52. Krayenbühl, H.: Klassifikation und klinische Symptomatologie der zerebralen Aneurysmen. Ophthalmologica (Basel), 167:122–164, 1973.

53. Krayenbühl, H., and Yasargil, M. G.: Diagnosis and therapy of intracranial aneurysms. Surg. Annu., 2:327–343, 1970.

54. Land, E. R., and Bucy, P. C.: Treatment of carotid-cavernous fistula by muscle embolization alone: The Brooks method. J. Neurosurg., 22:387–392, 1965.

55. Larson, S. J., and Worman, L. W.: Internal ca-

rotid artery flow rate during craniotomy and muscle embolization for carotid cavernous fistula: Report of four cases. J. Neurosurg., *29*:60 –64, 1968.

56. Lee, S. H., Burton, C. V., and Chan, G. H.: Post-traumatic ophthalmic vein arterialization. Surg. Neurol., *4*:483–484, 1974.

57. Lie, T. A.: Congenital Anomalies of the Carotid Arteries Including the Carotid-Basilar and Carotid-Vertebral Anastomoses: An Angiographic Study and Review of the Literature. Amsterdam, New York, Excerpta Medica Foundation, 1968.

58. Lister, J. R., and Sypert, G. W.: Traumatic false aneurysm and carotid-cavernous fistula: A complication of sphenoidotomy. Neurosurgery, *5*:473–475, 1979.

59. Lobato, R. D., Escudero, L., and Lamas, E.: Bilateral dural arteriovenous fistula in the region of the cavernous sinus. Neuroradiology, *15*:39 –43, 1978.

60. Locke, C. E., Jr.: Internal carotid arteriovenous aneurysm, or pulsating exophthalmos. Ann. Surg., *80*:1–24, 285, 1924.

61. Locksley, H. B.: Natural history of subarachnoid hemorrhage, intracranial aneurysms, and arteriovenous malformation. J. Neurosurg., *25*:219–239, 1966.

62. Lombardi, G., Passerini, A., and Migliavacca, F.: Intracavernous aneurysms of the internal carotid artery. Amer. J. Roentgen., *89*:361– 371, 1963.

63. Love, L., and Maisan, R. E.: Carotid cavernous fistula. Angiology, *25*:231–236, 1974.

64. Mahalley, M. S., and Boone, S. C.: External carotid-cavernous fistula treated by arterial embolization: Case report. J. Neurosurg., *40*:110– 114, 1974.

65. Markham, J. W.: Carotid-cavernous sinus fistula treated by intravascular occlusion with a balloon catheter: Report of two cases. J. Neurosurg., *40*:535–538, 1974.

66. Martin, J. D., Jr., and Mabon, R. F.: Pulsating exophthalmos: Review of all reported cases. J.A.M.A., *121*:330–334, 1943.

67. Matas, R.: Testing the efficiency of the collateral circulation as a preliminary to the occlusion of the great surgical arteries. J.A.M.A., *63*:1141, 1914.

68. Matjasko, M. J., Williams, J. P., and Fontanilla, M.: Intraoperative use of Doppler to detect successful obliteration of carotid-cavernous fistulae. J. Neurosurg., *43*:634–636, 1975.

69. McCormick, W. F., Kelly, P. J., and Sarwar, M.: Fatal paradoxical muscle embolization in traumatic carotid-cavernous fistula repair: Case report. J. Neurosurg., *44*:513–516, 1976.

70. Meadows, S. P.: Aneurysms of the internal carotid artery. Trans. Ophthal. Soc. U.K., *69*:137–155, 1949.

71. Meadows, S. P.: Intracavernous aneurysms of the internal carotid artery: Their clinical features and natural history. Arch. Ophthal. (Chicago), *65*: 566–574, 1959.

72. Miller, J. D., Jawad, K., and Jennett, B.: Safety of carotid ligation and its role in the management of intracranial aneurysms. J. Neurol. Neurosurg. Psychiat., *40*:64–72, 1977.

73. Mingrino, S., and Moro, F.: Fistula between the external carotid artery and cavernous sinus: Case report. J. Neurosurg., *27*:157–160, 1967.

74. Morley, T. P.: Appraisal of various forms of management in 41 cases of carotid cavernous fistula. *In* Morley, T. P., ed.: Current Controversies in Neurosurgery. Philadelphia, W. B. Saunders Co. 1976.

75. Morley, T. P., and Barr, H. W. K.: Giant intracranial aneurysms: Diagnosis, course, and management. Clin. Neurosurg., *16*:73–94, 1968.

76. Motarjeme, A., and Keifer, J. W.: Carotid-cavernous sinus fistula as a complication of carotid endarterectomy: A case report. Radiology, *108*:83–84, 1973.

77. Mullan, S.: Experiences with surgical thrombosis of intracranial berry aneurysms and carotid cavernous fistulae. J. Neurosurg., *41*:657–670, 1974.

78. Mullan, S.: Treatment of carotid-cavernous fistulae by cavernous sinus occlusion. J. Neurosurg., *50*:131–144, 1979.

79. Nashioka, H.: Report on the Cooperative Study of Intracranial Aneurysms and Subarachnoid Hemorrhage. Results of the treatment of intracranial aneurysms by occlusion of the carotid artery in the neck. J. Neurosurg., *25*:660–682, 1966.

80. Newton, T. H., and Hoyt, W. F.: Dural arteriovenous shunts in the region of the cavernous sinus. Neuroradiology, *1*:71–81, 1970.

81. Nornes, H.: Hemodynamic aspects in the management of carotid-cavernous fistula. J. Neurosurg., *37*:687–694, 1972.

82. Nutik, S.: Carotid paraclinoid aneurysms with intradural origin and intracavernous location. J. Neurosurg., *48*:526–533, 1978.

83. Obrador, S., Gomez-Bueno, J., and Silvela, J.: Spontaneous carotid-cavernous fistula produced by ruptured aneurysm of the meningohypophyseal branch of the internal carotid artery: Case report. J. Neurosurg., *40*:539–543, 1974.

84. Ohta, T., Nishimura, S., Kikuchi, H., et al.: Closure of carotid-cavernous fistula by polyurethane foam embolus (technical note). J. Neurosurg., *38*:107–112, 1973.

85. Parkinson, D.: Cavernous circulation of cavernous carotid artery: Anatomy. Canada. J. Surg., *7*:251–268, 1964.

86. Parkinson, D.: A surgical approach to the cavernous portion of the carotid artery: Anatomical studies and case report. J. Neurosurg., *23*:474–483, 1965.

87. Parkinson, D.: Carotid-cavernous fistula: Direct repair with preservation of the carotid artery. J. Neurosurg., *38*:99–106, 1973.

88. Parkinson, D.: Carotid-cavernous fistula: Direct approach and repair of fistula and preservation of the artery. Morley, T. P., ed.: Current Controversies in Neurosurgery. Philadelphia, W. B. Saunders Co., 1976.

89. Parkinson, D., and Shields, C. B.: Persistent trigeminal artery: Its relationship to the normal branches of the cavernous carotid artery. J. Neurosurg., *40*:244–248, 1974.

90. Parkinson, D., Downs, A. R., Whytehead, L. L.,

et al.: Carotid cavernous fistula: Direct repair with preservation of carotid. Surgery, *76*:882–889, 1974.

91. Picard, L., LePoire, J., Montaut, J., et al.: Endarterial occlusion of carotid-cavernous sinus fistulae using a balloon tipped catheter. Neuroradiology, *8*:5–10, 1974.

92. Pool, J. L., and Potts, D. G.: Aneurysms and Arteriovenous Anomalies of the Brain: Diagnosis and Treatment. New York, Harper & Row, 1965.

93. Prolo, D. J., Burres, K. P., and Hanberry, J. W.: Balloon occlusion of carotid-cavernous fistula: Introduction of a new catheter. Surg. Neurol., *7*:209–214, 1977.

94. Pugatch, R. P., and Wolpert, S. M.: Transfemoral embolization of an external carotid-cavernous fistula: Case report. J. Neurosurg., *42*:94–97, 1975.

95. Renn, W. H., and Rhoton, A. L.: Microsurgical anatomy of the sellar region. J. Neurosurg., *43*:288–298, 1975.

96. Riechert, T.: A new surgical method for treatment of pulsating exophthalmus. Cereb. Circ., *30*:445–449, 1968.

97. Rios-Montenegro, E. N., Behrens, M. M., and Hoyt, W. F.: Pseudoxanthoma elasticum: Association with bilateral carotid rete mirabile and unilateral carotid-cavernous sinus fistula. Arch. Neurol. (Chicago), *26*:151–155, 1972.

98. Robbins, J. B., Fitz-Hugh, G. S., and Jane, J. A.: Intracranial carotid catastrophes encountered by the otolaryngologist. Laryngoscope, *86*:893–902, 1976.

99. Sahs, A. L., Perret, G. E., Locksley, H. B., and Nishioka, H.: Intracranial Aneurysms and Subarachnoid Hemorrhage: A Cooperative Study. Philadelphia, J. B. Lippincott Co., 1969, p. 296.

100. Sanders, M. D., and Hoyt, W. F.: Hypoxic ocular sequelae of carotid-cavernous fistulae. Study of the causes of visual failure before and after neurosurgical treatment in a series of 25 cases. Brit. J. Ophthal., *53*:82–97, 1969.

101 Sattler, C. H.: Pulsierender Exophthalmus, Handbuch der Gesamten Augenheilkunde. Berlin, Julius Springer, 1920.

102. Schoolman, A., and Kepes, J. J.: Bilateral spontaneous carotid-cavernous fistulae in Ehlers-Danlos syndrome: Case report. J. Neurosurg., *26*:82–86, 1967.

103. Serbinenko, F. A.: Balloon catheterization and occlusion of major cerebral vessels. J. Neurosurg., *41*:125–145, 1974.

104. Shen, A. L.: Superficial temporal-middle cerebral artery anastomosis in the treatment of a carotid-cavernous fistula. J. Neurosurg., *49*:760–763, 1978.

105. Shirai, S., Tomono, Y., Owada, T., et al.: Traumatic aneurysm of the internal carotid artery: Report of a case with late severe epistaxis. Europ. Neurol., *15*:212–216, 1977.

106. Smith, R. W., and Alksne, J. F.: Stereotaxic thrombosis of unaccessible intracranial aneurysms. J. Neurosurg., *47*:833–839, 1977.

107. Stern, W. E., Brown, W. D., and Alksne, J. F.: The surgical challenge of carotid-cavernous fistula: The critical role of intracranial circulatory dynamics. J. Neurosurg., *27*:298–308, 1967.

108. Taniguchi, R. M., Goree, J. A., and Odom, G. L.: Spontaneous carotid-cavernous shunts presenting diagnostic problems. J. Neurosurg., *35*:384–391, 1971.

109. Taptas, J. N.: Arteriovenous Aneurysm in Pulsating Exophthalmos: A New Conception of the Mechanism. Excerpta Medica International Congress Series 60. Amsterdam, Excerpta Medica Foundation, 1963, pp. 98–99.

110. Thomas, J. E., and Yoss, R. E.: The parasellar syndrome: Problems in determining etiology. Mayo Clin. Proc., *45*:617–623, 1970.

111. Trobe, J. D., Glaser, J. S., and Post, J. D.: Meningiomas and aneurysms of the cavernous sinus—neuro-ophthalmological features. Arch. Opthal. (Chicago), *96*:457–467, 1978.

112. Van Beusekom, G. T., Leyendijk, W., and Huizing, E. H.: Severe epistaxis caused by rupture of a non-traumatic infraclinoid aneurysm of the internal carotid artery. Acta Neurochir. (Wien), *15*:269–284, 1966.

113. Voigt, K., Saver, M., and Dichgans, J.: Spontaneous occlusion of a bilateral caroticocavernous fistula studied by serial angiography. Neuroradiology, *2*:207–211, 1971.

114. Walker, A. E., and Allegre, G. E.: Carotid-cavernous fistulae. Surgery, *39*:411–422, 1956.

115. Wallace, S., Goldberg, H. I., Leeds, N. E., et al.: The cavernous branches of the internal carotid artery. Amer. J. Roentgen., *101*:34–46, 1967.

116. Wepsic, J. G., Pruett, R. C., and Tarlov, E.: Carotid-cavernous fistula due to extradural subtemporal retrogasserian rhizotomy: Case report. J. Neurosurg., *37*:498–500, 1972.

117. White, J. C., and Adams, R. D.: Combined supra- and infraclinoid aneurysms of internal carotid artery: Report of a case of unusual congenital dilatation of intracranial portion of carotid artery and injuries to visual, oculomotor, sensory, and taste fibres. J. Neurosurg., *12*:450–459, 1955.

118. White, J. C., and Ballantine, H. T.: Intrasellar aneurysms simulating hypophyseal tumors. J. Neurosurg., *18*:34–50, 1961.

119. Winslow, J. B.: Exposition Anatomique de la Structure du Corps Humaine. Vol. 2. London, Prevost, 1732, p. 31.

120. Zimmerman, R., Leeds, N. E., and Naidich, T. P.: Carotid-cavernous fistula associated with intracranial fibromuscular dysplasia. Radiology, *122*:725–726, 1977.

52

ARTERIOVENOUS MALFORMATIONS OF THE BRAIN

Arteriovenous malformations of the brain are characterized by direct shunts from artery to vein. The arterial supply consists of the normal arteries of the area plus virtually every possible collateral artery, all enlarged to provide the required shunt flow. The venous drainage also is by way of the normal venous channels as well as all available collateral drainage, again with enlargement sufficient for the shunt flow.

HISTORICAL BACKGROUND

John Hunter first described traumatic arteriovenous fistulae of the extremities in 1757. Although Steinhill, in 1895, is generally quoted as the first to describe cerebral arteriovenous malformations, these vascular lesions had been discussed by Luschka in 1854 and by Virchow in 1867. Giordano, in 1905, and Krause, in 1908, published operative descriptions. Worster-Drought and Ballance, in 1922, added additional case material. Not until 1928, however, did definitive reviews appear with the publication of Cushing and Bailey's monograph and Dandy's report of his own 8 cases plus 22 from the literature.[9,10]

At this point, the process was considered incurable; Dandy had been able to achieve a curative excision in only one case in which an apparently simple fistula was occluded by a single ligature. He noted improvement after vertebral or carotid ligation in three cases. The first reported cases of successful removal were those of Pen-field and Erickson in 1941.[43] Pilcher, in 1946, reported three cases, in all of which the patients recovered and in two of which the patients' seizures were completely controlled postoperatively.[45]

Angiography had been invented by Moniz in the 1930's, and by 1941, after Gross's introduction of organic iodides for the contrast material, was more regularly used to study these lesions.[16] Dott, in a personal communication to Olivecrona, described seven successful cases of complete resection that were still unpublished by 1948. Olivecrona and Riives, in 1948, were able to report 43 total excisions with four deaths, and Norlén added 10 additional successful removals by 1949.[37,38]

Ley's monograph in 1957 reviewed the European and English literature and gave an excellent description of the surgical state of the art but was published only in Spanish.[28] Krayenbühl and Yaşargil's monograph in 1958 was equally divided between the subjects of intracranial aneurysms and arteriovenous malformations.[21] This remarkable review with its many illustrations in color had a bibliography of almost 900 references. Parkinson, in 1958, pointed out the still too often neglected concept of the final feeding arteries and the importance of opening the arachnoid and working in the subarachnoid space. He also regularly used induced hypotension as early as 1952, and stressed the value of stereoangiography in preoperative analysis and planning. This innovative paper reads as though it had been written 20 years later.[41]

In 1969, Yaşargil reported the first use of

L. I. MALIS

the operating microscope in the radical resection of cerebral arteriovenous malformations.[56] He reported 14 cases, 13 of which had been considered inoperable by the usual operative methods. With the use of microtechniques, all the malformations were completely resected, with excellent results in 11 cases, thereby ushering in a revolution in operative techniques and the present approach to these lesions.

The original classification of the lesions as arterial, venous, and arteriovenous was supported by Cushing and Bailey.[9] Dandy quite correctly though arbitrarily stated that they were all arteriovenous.[10] McCormick in 1966, classified them as: (1) telangiectasia, (2) varix, (3) cavernous angioma, (4) arteriovenous malformation, and (5) venous malformation.[34]

The telangiectasias, including Sturge-Weber's disease, are not further considered in this chapter. Most of the telangiectasias are incidental autopsy findings, appearing grossly as a small red spot resembling a fresh petechial area. Microscopic examination reveals an area of gliotic brain interlaced with a network of capillaries that lack elastic or muscle fibers.

Olivecrona and Riives in their 1948 review noted that arterial malformations simply do not exist.[38] They further stated that most venous malformations described in the literature were really arteriovenous and that the distinction could only be made in vivo, confirming the failure of pathological examination. Potter, in his 1955 Hunterian Lecture, noted that despite cases in which the appearance was venous—blue color and lack of pulsation—all showed arteriovenous shunts on angiography.[48]

ETIOLOGY AND PATHOPHYSIOLOGY

The arterial feeding vessels to the area of an arteriovenous shunt are found to be enlarged at the time the angiographic diagnostic study is first performed. While there are well documented cases of rapidly progressive enlargement of cerebral arteriovenous malformations, this is a rare phenomenon.[50] Unlike the traumatic arteriovenous malformations of the extremities, the cerebral malformations appear to achieve a relatively stable state, and there is little further increase in the arterial supply. While in most individually followed cases it seems that little or no progressive enlargement occurs, it is also true that the older the patient at the time of angiography, the larger the malformation is likely to be, thus indicating the probability that over the long life history, enlargement does occur.[11]

Within the short time span of a year or two of observation and evaluation, the malformations appear not to change in size. The shunt system remains constant while the arterial supply increases to fill the added demand of the shunt as well as that of the normal circulation. Blood flow is redistributed, as for example, when a lateral surface malformation is fed by the enlarged middle cerebral artery with a proportionally large carotid artery. Both anterior cerebral arteries will then generally fill from the opposite carotid. This redistribution has been described as a vascular steal. The opportunity for further increase in arterial size is not utilized, however, suggesting that sufficient flow is already available. If an arteriovenous shunt does increase in size, the feeding vessels also increase, confirming their ability to provide the necessary circulation. Conversely, when the shunt has been closed or significantly decreased, the arterial supply vessels then progressively decrease in size until they are appropriate to the new requirements, as noted by Norlén.[37]

It is therefore suggested that the concept of steal may be applicable only in the presence of a stenotic arterial lesion that cannot expand to meet the demand. Decreased tissue perfusion, elegantly documented for the adjacent cerebral substance by Feindel and co-workers, may be caused by the marked increase in venous pressure in the shared venous drain, as noted by Aminoff and associates for the spinal arteriovenous malformations.[3,12–14]

If the decreased perfusion were actually the result of "steal," carotid ligation or proximal ligation or even embolization of some of the feeding arteries would be expected to produce catastrophic results. In actual practice, however, results of proximal ligation have not been regularly bad and frequently have been temporarily beneficial, which would be expected if decreased flow through the shunt did decrease the venous pressure in the drainage system, at least until the unligated portion of the supply increased to meet the need of the shunt again and become stabilized at the original level. Paterson and McKissock had ligated only some surface feeders in 16 of their cases; none of these was made worse and some were better.[42] Dott and Maccabe had noted the long-term benefit of ligation of some close feeding arteries in unresectable malformations.[11]

Potter discussed this problem most logically more than 20 years ago when he noted that after feeder ligation the shunt remains the same size and will invite arterial blood from somewhere on the "easy terms" of low resistance. This would only be at the expense of normal brain and via the collateral supply vessels unless, of course, further compensatory changes occurred, in which case the situation would get back to much the same as it was before.[48] Potter's conception has been amply confirmed with demonstration of the compensatory enlargement of the residual supply.

Decreased capillary perfusion (whether caused by steal, thrombosis, or increased venous pressure), pulsatile compression of brain by the tense coils of the malformation, increased intracranial pressure, and hemorrhages (both clinical and subclinical) are all probable causes of progressive symptoms and deterioration. The role of small hemorrhages may well be more important than previously recognized, as suggested by Paterson and McKissock in 1956.[42] In operating on patients whose arteriovenous malformations have apparently produced only seizures, Yaşargil found that there was hemosiderin staining and reaction indicative of slight localized bleeding; and the author has confirmed this observation.[57]

PATHOLOGY

Hamby, in 1958, stated that a fresh brain specimen injected with latex would be ideal to demonstrate the pathological anatomy but was only able to get a fixed, uninjected, partly sectioned specimen for dissection.[17] Nevertheless, his reconstruction of the plexus of multiple arteriovenous connections is a classic study. He reviewed Padget's contributions to the understanding of the development of the cranial venous system in man and its relations to the arteries. Padget had demonstrated the embryologi-

cal basis for the filling and drainage patterns of arteriovenous malformation in adults.[39] Kaplan and co-workers, in 1961, reported the latex injection of a whole brain removed at autopsy after sudden hemorrhagic death.[18] Careful dissection revealed the large supplying arteries to empty directly into veins of comparable diameter. The distinct circulation of the superficial venous system and of the transcerebral venous drainage and deep system was demonstrated with its relationship to the location of the arteriovenous shunts, so providing an adequate anatomical explanation of the tendency of the malformations to have a wedged shape pointing toward the ventricular system. The presence of a multiplicity of shunts has been well documented for cerebral arteriovenous malformations, unlike the spinal lesions. Post-resection angiograms have occasionally demonstrated a tiny residual shunt of only arteriolar diameter with flow directly into a venous drain, left over when a little corner of the malformation was missed after resection of the main shunting tangle.

Burger and Vogel's description of the microscopic structure seems eminently quotable.

The microscopic characteristics of the vessels confirm the chaotic composition of this blunder of angiogenesis. Thus, some vessels have the thin collagenous walls of veins, others the muscular and elastic laminae of arteries, while many are structural hybrids.[5]

About three fourths of all arteriovenous malformations are on the lateral surface. Of the remaining fourth, half are on the medial surface, and the rest are in deep structures, in the ventricles, or in the posterior fossa. Approximately 1 in 20 has an associated aneurysm, while 1 aneurysm in 75 has an associated arteriovenous malformation. The relative frequency of arteriovenous malformations as compared with aneurysms varies in different series from less than 10 per cent to as high as 25 per cent.[4] The earlier series (Dandy, Olivecrona and Riives, Tonnis and co-workers) suggested almost a 2 to 1 predominance of arteriovenous malformations in males, but reviews of the last 20 years have indicated no significant difference in sexual incidence.[10,38,52] About two thirds produce symptoms prior to the age of 30.

DIAGNOSIS

About 50 per cent of all patients have onset with a seizure. About half of these seizures will at some time be focal, though most will be generalized during the course of the disease. Todd's paralysis is rare compared with sudden prolonged paralysis due to intracerebral bleeding, which is the mode of onset for 10 to 15 per cent of the patients. Another 10 to 15 per cent have progressive hemiparesis, while virtually all the remainder begin with an uncomplicated subarachnoid hemorrhage. Headache is frequent, and in 20 per cent it is severe and disabling. Organic mental impairment is rare as a presenting sign and is usually associated with hydrocephalus. This type of onset is most often seen with obstructive lesions of the posterior fossa or tentorial notch, while progressive organic mental syndromes late in the disease process are more likely to be associated with hydrocephalus due to obliteration of the subarachnoid spaces by repeated subarachnoid hemorrhage. Bruit was considered a common sign in the historical series; its rarity today, except in children, is evidence of the better technical methods that demonstrate the previously undiagnosed lesions that so vastly outnumber those with obvious bruit. High-output cardiac failure is very rare in adult patients but all too frequent in the newborn with the anomaly of the vein of Galen.

Olivecrona and Riives noted that the diagnosis was made eight times as frequently after the introduction of angiography.[38] The precept that every progressive neurological syndrome should now be studied by a definitive neuroradiological procedure applies well to the cerebral arteriovenous malformations. Those patients presenting with subarachnoid hemorrhage regularly come to angiography early in their course. Those presenting with seizures or progressive neurological deterioration have been less likely to be so studied. The difference in incidence of type of onset between the United States and England was striking in the cooperative study; the London center reported 1 arteriovenous malformation to 13.8 aneurysms, while in the United States the ratio was 1 to 5.3. In the London series, in 91 per cent of cases, the onset was with hemorrhage.[49] Apparently patients who present with seizures or progressive deterioration are less likely to be studied radiologically in England, and the diagnosis is not made as readily as in the United States unless subarachnoid hemorrhage occurs.

The advent of computed tomography has further improved early diagnosis of these lesions, as it has of virtually all other neurological states. Except for the very smallest arteriovenous malformations, the contrast-enhanced CT scan is ordinarily diagnostic of the site and size of the lesion and leads to performance of definitive angiography.

Four-vessel angiography is the routine roentgenological procedure, as it is for aneurysms. The circulatory alterations resulting from pressure changes and differing vessel diameters can best be evaluated if all the intracranial vessels are filled. Stereoangiography, as recommended by Penfield and Erickson and by Parkinson, is the ideal way to study the lesion.[41,43] When unilateral or simple carotid angiography alone is done, the malformation virtually always appears to be smaller than its actual size. Four-vessel study is much more accurate anatomically in delineating the operative problem and permits analysis of the differential flow to the normal tissues. Often, what appears to be a significant cerebral area of inadequate perfusion can be seen to be well supplied from a collateral source and to reflect merely the compensatory redistribution of the blood supply.

TREATMENT

Risk and Results of Therapy

The understanding of the natural course of the disease is clouded by a number of factors. First, failure to diagnose the non-bleeding case leads to the omission from the studies of patients otherwise neurologically disabled by the malformation. Second, the selection of good-risk patients for operation, rather than prospective randomization, alters the results for both operative and nonoperative care. Indeed, for randomization to be meaningful, it is obvious that only patients whose lesions are considered operable should be included in such studies. This, however, has not been done adequately.

It is possible that surgical selection

would not, in fact, make an appreciable difference in the results that a randomized study would show, since there is no good reason to presume that operability is correlated with the morbidity or mortality rates in nonoperative care. While the largest lesions deep in the dominant hemisphere may correlate with progressive neurological disability, the smallest lesions have the highest incidence of severe bleeding. After Margolis and co-workers' original study of massive hemorrhages from cryptic arteriovenous malformations in 1951, Crawford and Russell, in 1956, reviewed 20 cases in which the cause of the hemorrhage could be found only by microscopic examination of the autopsy material.[7,33] Papatheodoru, Gross, and Hollin reported similar findings in the biopsy material from the hematomas in their series of cryptic arteriovenous malformations in 1961.[40] In Potter's series, 18 of 19 small lesions bled.[48] Krayenbühl and Seibenmann, in 1965, reviewed this literature and added 24 cases of their own, in 15 of which there was angiographic or operative demonstration of the lesion, while in the other 9 the arteriovenous malformation was presumably destroyed by the hemorrhage.[20] Waltimo's study in 1973 put a statistical perspective on this incidence of bleeding. He reported that of 45 patients, 23 had had seizures and 22 had hemorrhaged. In this group, two thirds of those with lesions under 3 cm in diameter bled, and two thirds of those with lesions over 3 cm in diameter had seizures.[55]

Despite the serious questions of diagnosis and sampling, a number of authors have attempted to evaluate prognosis for the patient who is not operated on. Svien and McRae's study in 1965, most widely quoted, reviewed 68 patients who were not operated on out of an original series of 95. Of the 68, 4 died from other causes, making 64 at risk. Of the 64, 17 per cent died of their arteriovenous malformations, 5 were invalids, 12 were in fair condition, and 36, or 56 per cent, were considered in good condition.[51]

Pool's 1962 review of the literature yielded 220 patients who were not operated on in whom the results were about the same with 17 per cent dead owing to the malformation and 60 per cent living essentially normal lives with some having occasional seizures.[46] Troup, writing in support of the nonoperative viewpoint and using data from his own 1970 report of 137 nonoperative cases, listed 10 per cent of his patients dead from the malformation but only 40 per cent who could be considered well.[53] In Morello and Borghi's 1973 group of conservatively treated patients 20 per cent died of the hemorrhage.[36]

It would appear that operative treatment would be indicated if the morbidity and mortality rates were significantly improved. This was not achieved in the cooperative study, in which among 119 resections there were 13 deaths (11 per cent). Of the 85 patients who could be followed, 53 (62 per cent) were well.[44] On the other hand, Amacher, Allcock, and Drake in 1972 reported 55 resections with one death. These operations were done with magnification but without the use of the microscope.[2] Yaşargil's early results with the microscope in cases previously considered inoperable further indicated that the morbidity and mortality rates could be well below those of the natural course of the disease, even when the more difficult cases were operated on.[56] Kunc, in 1974, reported 57 resections from the dominant hemisphere and rolandic region.[23] Twelve of the patients were hemiplegic and fourteen aphasic preoperatively, while only three were hemiplegic and four aphasic postoperatively. None were made hemiplegic or aphasic by the operative procedure. Of U and Wilson's 31 cases, the malformations were excised in 25.[54] Only 1 patient was capable of working at full capacity preoperatively, while 17 were able to work at full capacity postoperatively.

Nevertheless, Leussenhopp, whose pioneering work in embolization of these lesions was first reported in 1960, after so many years of experience with operative, embolic, and conservative approaches, is less optimistic.[31] He has stated that approximately 50 per cent of all cerebral arteriovenous malformations can be excised with fewer deaths and less morbidity than is possible with nonoperative treatment. He has suggested that embolization would benefit about half the inoperable cases but has noted that embolization does not avert the likelihood of recurrent hemorrhage. Luessenhopp has also suggested a grading system based on the number of arterial feeders to predict the probable operative morbidity and mortality rates.[32]

While certain cases clearly fall into a high-risk category or indeed may be truly inoperable, this group is becoming progressively smaller. The use of the microscope permits the regular removal of lesions both large and small, virtually anywhere on the hemispheres, including their medial surfaces. Very large, deep, and extensive lesions of the midportion of the dominant hemisphere are still avoided by many surgeons with wide experience unless repeated bleeding has forced the issue, although Kunc has recommended that these be done electively and has reported excellent results.[23] While the lesions of the head of the caudate nucleus are removable, those involving the capsule, thalamus, and brain stem, a very small proportion of the total spectrum, are not yet resectable.[6,24,26]

In summary, except for the less than 10 to 15 per cent of all arteriovenous malformations that offer too high an operative risk, total resection of arteriovenous malformations can be carried out with the expectation of operative morbidity and mortality rates less than 5 per cent and with a high percentage of recovery of preoperative deficit.

General Aspects of Operative Therapy

It is obvious that the operative approach to arteriovenous malformations will be different for the various areas of involvement and vascular connections. A classification of the various lesions or at least a categorization is necessary to permit a reasonable discussion of methods. Certain concepts are fairly basic and can be discussed in general terms.

Since the arteriovenous malformations consist of an area of direct communication from arterial supply to venous drainage without an interposed capillary bed the purpose of definitive operation is the removal of the shunt. The feeding arteries and draining veins are not included in the removal. Though grossly enlarged, tortuous, and abnormal in appearance, they are merely dilated parts of the normal circulatory tree. The arteries continue past the malformation to supply more distal neural tissue, while the huge draining veins receive branches from normal areas as well. Accordingly, when excision of the malformation is to be carried out, ligation of the feeding arteries is permissible only for those short branches

entering totally into the shunt and not for the feeding artery at a distance from the arteriovenous malformation.

Many of the larger arteriovenous malformations are virtually tumor masses. They contain neural parenchyma within the interstices, but this is gliotic nonfunctional tissue; no deficit has been shown from its removal. Accordingly, the mass may be resected within its plane of cleavage without concern for interstitial material.

Unless a hematoma, intracerebral or occasionally subdural, demands early intervention, the operation on an arteriovenous malformation is elective and should await the patient's recovery from the acute phase of a subarachnoid hemorrhage. There is adequate time for careful neuroradiological evaluation. The difficulties and challenges that these lesions present leave little tolerance for surprises. Four-vessel angiography with the largest possible number of arterial phase films, preferably stereoscopic as well as with high-resolution magnification, gives the most complete information on the anatomy and circulation of the arteriovenous malformation as well as the collateralization and redistribution that has provided the brain circulation. This foreknowledge not only permits adequate planning but also provides the information needed to alter a plan that is not going according to expectations.

Operative Technique

The author's patients are operated upon with controlled ventilation and monitoring of blood gases. Intravenous urea or mannitol, given one to two hours prior to the expected time of dural opening, has produced a soft, relaxed brain, permitted easy opening of a slack dura, and regularly decreased the need for brain retraction. The head is always fixed in the Gardner or Mayfield pinned headrest. As well as providing the fixation required for microscopic visualization, the position avoids stress on neck muscles and skin and resultant jugular compression. While these adjuncts are important for any intracranial micro-operative work, they are crucial in operations for arteriovenous malformations.

The most serious problem in removal of a major arteriovenous malformation is rupture of a large vessel with severe bleeding.

Fragility of the vascular walls is the expected state wherever arterial pressure is confined only by thin vessels that often lack significant elastic or muscular layers. The use of hypotension with mean pressure between 60 and 70 mm of mercury has greatly eased the problem of this fragility, and the ability to drop the pressure suddenly to 30 or 40 mm of mercury for a few minutes has occasionally warded off a catastrophe.

Temporary clips may be useful on large proximal arteries if used for short periods in order to ascertain flow characteristics or to help in getting out of trouble. A few Mayfield clips that have been squeezed open a number of times, although thereby rendered useless as permanent clips, are gentle enough for use for temporary occlusion without likelihood of injury to the vessel wall.

The use of the bipolar coagulator is an essential part of the microtechnique. A coagulator unit with reproducible power and correct wave form that permits smooth gentle shrinkage and progressive thickening and coagulation of a vessel wall and has minimal tendency to perforate or stick is needed. This should be accompanied by a selection of forceps, from modified jewelers' shapes for surface vessels to long bayonets for work in the depths. Forceps tips 0.2 mm in diameter are excellent for sealing tiny arterioles but would regularly burn holes in a large vessel, while a 2-mm forceps would spread the current over a sufficient area to coagulate smoothly. Of course, since the power requirement for coagulation is in terms of current density per volume, the 0.2-mm forceps require less than 1 per cent of the electrical power that the 2-mm forceps should apply. Whether large or small, the forceps must be scrupulously clean and smooth to avoid sticking and should be used under saline irrigation at the lowest effective settings of the generator.

The general technique for removal of an arteriovenous malformation consists in opening the arachnoid along the margin by using the bipolar coagulator and a razor blade as well as regulated soft suction to begin a cleavage plane. The plane is continued by using the bipolar coagulation to shrink the vessels of the malformation away from the adjacent brain, continuously decreasing the size of the lesion.

It is possible with this technique to enter a false plane between vessels of the malformation and so to cut across the lesion, leaving a small portion unresected. Such areas left in place contain small remaining arteriovenous shunts and must not be simply left attached to the arterial or the venous components. The major mass of the malformation is indeed made up of multiple shunts, rather than merely a tangled network of collateral arteries and veins leading to and draining from a single shunt. Because of this characteristic, postoperative angiography is necessary to evaluate final results reasonably. Should a significant portion of the malformation be left in place by such a false plane, all major draining veins might be interrupted while a large arterial vessel was still connected. This situation would be almost certain to lead to explosive distention of the remaining malformation and to immediate postoperative hemorrhage. Yet, the absence of shunt flow in this remnant would prevent its detection by observation of venous blood, sterile stethoscope, Doppler probe, or intraoperative angiography. Prevention by exacting anatomical correlation of angiographic and operative anatomy is preferable, though the operative constraints and the abnormalities of the exposed vessels may make such anatomical accuracy impossible.

While most surgeons with wide experience in these lesions have clipped feeding arteries first, the author believes that this approach makes it more difficult to preserve the "arteries of passage."[15] These are vessels, often quite large arterial trunks, that will branch adjacent to or on the surface of the arteriovenous malformation, one branch going to the malformation and the other, often smaller, branch continuing to the more distal neural distribution. Accordingly, he usually approaches the arteriovenous malformation draining vein first. One requisite is the presence of more than one draining vein, since rarely would it be possible to close a solitary large drain first without provoking a disaster. Most arteriovenous malformations have a number of large drains, one of which may be ligated and cut and then used as a handle to mobilize the mass (Fig. 52–1). Working from the venous end, the arterial feeders that actually end in the malformation may be more readily visualized as the separation of the cleavage plane progresses. These feeders are sealed with the bipolar coagulator, with

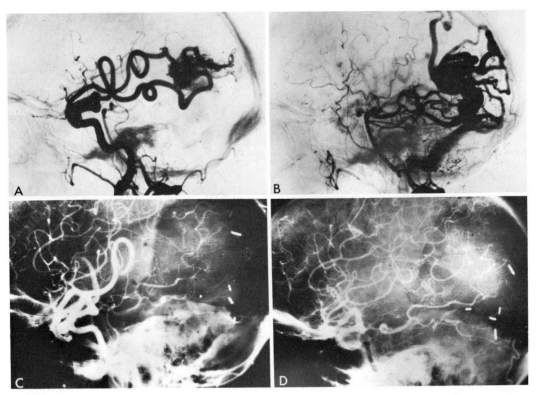

Figure 52–1 The more rapid carotid flow to the malformation through the two greatly enlarged middle cerebral branches in *A* is followed by the slower basilar circulation and venous drainage in *B*. *C*. Postoperative angiogram at one week shows slow flow with partial filling of these enlarged vessels because of their relatively constricted outflow. *D*. In angiogram one month later, the vessels have been reduced to normal size and flow rate has been restored to normal.

care to seal a fairly long segment of the vessel (three to five times the vessel diameter) before cutting it. Vessels feeding an arteriovenous malformation that are more than 1 mm in diameter should also be clipped. The reduction in the outflow channel after removal of the arteriovenous malformation will allow a serious water-hammer pulsation on the sealed ends until the supply arteries have decreased to normal size.

The progressive decline in arterial size may, indeed, take place quite slowly. Serial angiography has demonstrated the difference in flow rates in the residual large arteries in the first two weeks after operation. In postoperative angiography done in the first few days, the radiopaque material can be seen reaching the distal end of normal arteries, while the two major trunks that previously fed the malformation remain enlarged and the flow is restricted by the size of the residual normal branching, which can only accept a small proportion of the capacity of the still unchanged feeder. By the end

of several weeks, the arterial channels come down to normal size (Fig. 52–2). While the flow rate in the arterial trunks that are still enlarged early in the postoperative period may be slowed sufficiently to cause arterial occlusion, this would appear to be a rare complication.

A related problem in venous drainage after removal of the arteriovenous malformation may be illustrated by a case example. The drainage of a large malformation is by a huge vein of Labbé (Fig. 52–3). At least two normal cerebral veins of major caliber also drain to the lateral sinus by way of the vein of Labbé. When the malformation has been removed, this main trunk will have been closed at the malformation, leaving the two cortical veins still flowing through its terminal portion into the sinus. This tremendous size disparity between the venous outflow channel and the veins draining through it suggests that the flow may be insufficient to prevent spontaneous postoperative thrombosis of the major vein.

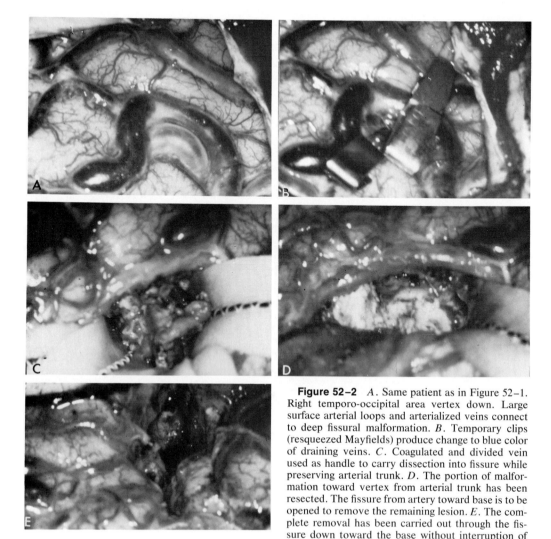

Figure 52–2 *A*. Same patient as in Figure 52–1. Right temporo-occipital area vertex down. Large surface arterial loops and arterialized veins connect to deep fissural malformation. *B*. Temporary clips (resqueezed Mayfields) produce change to blue color of draining veins. *C*. Coagulated and divided vein used as handle to carry dissection into fissure while preserving arterial trunk. *D*. The portion of malformation toward vertex from arterial trunk has been resected. The fissure from artery toward base is to be opened to remove the remaining lesion. *E*. The complete removal has been carried out through the fissure down toward the base without interruption of the artery.

Such veins do not decrease in size nearly so quickly and efficiently as the arterial feeders. In several cases, postoperative temporal lobe venous infarctions have occurred after postoperative spontaneous occlusion of such a vein of Labbé. These have been treated vigorously with removal of a bone flap and infarcted temporal lobe. So far these patients have recovered and have subsequently had cranioplastic repair, though in two cases there was a residual visual field defect. As a question of balanced risks, the number who will have such venous occlusion is small, and while the question of postoperative use of anticoagulant therapy has been discussed, the risk of immediate postoperative anticoagulation has appeared to be too great for serious consideration.

Medial Surface Malformations

The medial surface arteriovenous malformations have been approached along the falx, usually with the patient supine and the head fixed brow-up (Figs. 52–4 and 52–5). The flap is made well across the midline, and the dural flap is opened with its base at the sinus. Two self-retaining brain retractors are used, one against the falx, retracting and deviating falx and sagittal sinus, while the other supports the medial surface of the hemisphere. The use of one of the draining veins for the retrograde dissection

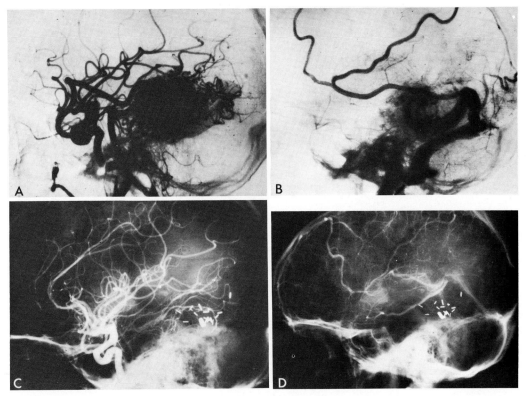

Figure 52–3 *A* and *B*. Temporo-occipital malformation with huge draining vein into lateral sinus. *C* and *D*. Postoperative angiogram shows preservation of arteries of passage but occlusion of the draining vein.

has made preservation of major anterior cerebral arterial trunks much easier. These malformations go through the corpus callosum and enter the ventricle, often with lateral vessels coming in from the middle cerebral artery, and regularly with choroidal supply. Because of the tendency for the cerebrospinal fluid to lyse small clots, more reinforcing clips are used than in malformations that do not enter the ventricles.

If recognized reasonably early, postoperative intraventricular bleeding can be evacuated, the bleeding point clipped, and the patient rescued from this otherwise most serious complication. Emergency computed tomography on any patient not awake from anesthesia by the expected time has been a lifesaving diagnostic measure.

Sylvian Fissure Lesions

Small lesions within the dominant sylvian fissure usually produce aphasic disturbances, whether they present with seizures or with bleeding (Fig. 52–6). The ability to save the "arteries of passage" that give off the feeding branches to such lesions permits recovery without language disturbance. Here the approach is made by opening the fissural arachnoid and following vessels medially within the subarachnoid space (Fig. 52–7). Frequently these lesions have both superficial and deep venous drainage, and the superficial vein, after ligation and division, becomes the dissecting handle. Some of these small lesions have true aneurysmal sacs arising at the junction point where the arterial feeding branch leaves the "artery of passage." Here permanent aneurysm clips are usually required, since just as in ordinary aneurysm procedures, they can be placed exactly or replaced until the precise occlusion is achieved without damage to the main trunk. It is in this group of malformations, in which the only preoperative indication may have been seizures, that hemosiderin staining most frequently proves that undiagnosed subarachnoid hemorrhage has indeed occurred.

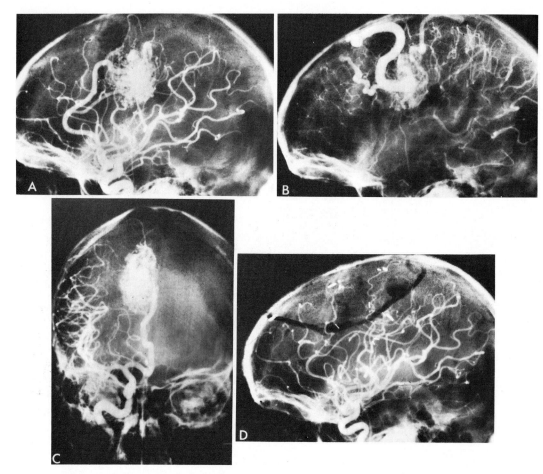

Figure 52–4   *A, B,* and *C.* Angiography of a right-sided malformation involving the corpus callosum and lateral ventricle. *D.* The postoperative film shows reduction of size of anterior cerebral artery to normal and preservation of the callosomarginal artery.

Lesions of Floor of Posterolateral Lobes

Malformations lying along the floor of the temporal and occipital lobes, particularly on the dominant hemisphere, seem best approached along the tentorial surface (Figs. 52–8 and 52–9). Here veins of the inferior temporal surface drain toward the lateral sinus, and the admixture of arterial blood permits the recognition of one of the drains of the arteriovenous malformation. This may now be ligated and cut to provide the line of dissection while sparing the portion of the vein carrying nonarterialized blood from uninvolved brain to the lateral sinus. Arteriovenous malformations of this area tend to extend into the artrium of the lateral ventricle, and complete removal generally requires that the ventricle be opened.

Galenic System Malformations

Arteriovenous malformations of the vein of Galen are often referred to as aneurysms of the galenic system, since in the classic type little else is seen. Arterial vessels from anterior cerebral branches, perforating thalamic branches from the posterior cerebral arteries, branches of superior cerebellar arteries, and choroidal arteries empty directly into the vein of Galen and drain into the straight sinus and torcular. A second type of vein of Galen malformation has the shunt vessels in the parenchyma of the quadrigeminal area, as shown in Figure 52–10, and the draining veins then enter the vein of Galen, which enlarges in quite the same manner as in the classic first type. The malformations of the quadrigeminal

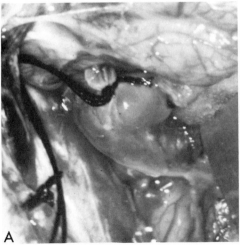
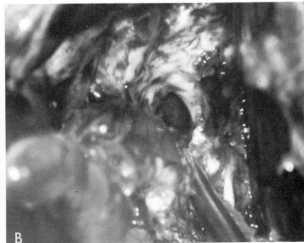

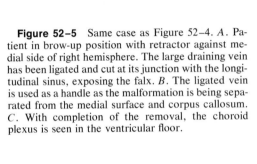

Figure 52–5 Same case as Figure 52–4. *A*. Patient in brow-up position with retractor against medial side of right hemisphere. The large draining vein has been ligated and cut at its junction with the longitudinal sinus, exposing the falx. *B*. The ligated vein is used as a handle as the malformation is being separated from the medial surface and corpus callosum. *C*. With completion of the removal, the choroid plexus is seen in the ventricular floor.

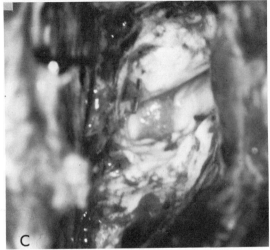

plate are apparently still inoperable; there is no evidence available to the author's knowledge that indicates better results from treatment, in terms of functional survival, than from inactivity.

When any major arteriovenous malformation appears in infancy, it presents by uncontrollable cardiac failure and, unless the cranial bruit is listened for, may not be recognized until angiocardiac study is attempted. The most frequent arteriovenous malformation of infancy is that of the vein of Galen, leading to a justifiably pessimistic outlook. Virtually all newborns presenting with the malformation and requiring immediate intervention because of the uncorrectible cardiac state are really too severely ill to permit the required operation and circulatory readjustment. As much as three or

four times the normal cardiac output may course through the malformation alone. Despite the utmost care in slow stepwise obliteration of the shunts and reduction of blood volume, cardiac decompensation cannot be managed in the largest majority. Without operation, all will die, while rarely will an operative salvage be possible.[8,27,29] Galenic malformations appearing later during the first year of life generally are accompanied by cardiac failure as part of the picture and an enlarging head as well as a cranial bruit. When the onset is still later in childhood, the enlarging head is the usual presenting problem without serious cardiac difficulty.[30]

The arterial pressure in the galenic system may prevent deep venous return from the internal cerebral veins through the

Text continued on page 1802

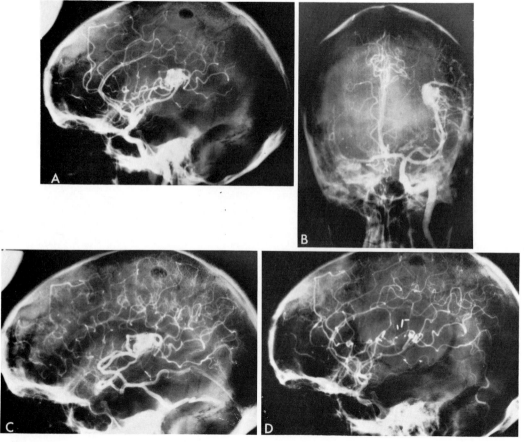

Figure 52–6   *A*, *B*, and *C*. Malformation in left sylvian fissure with superficial and deep venous drainage. *D*. After resection, all "vessels of passage" are intact. An aneurysmal sac in the malformation has been clipped with a Heifetz clip.

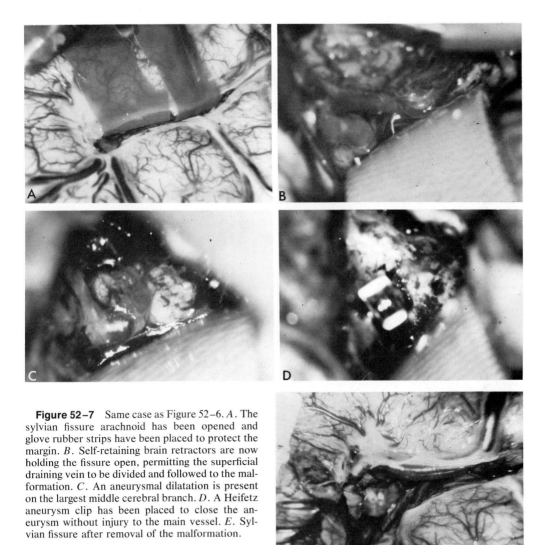

Figure 52-7 Same case as Figure 52–6. *A*. The sylvian fissure arachnoid has been opened and glove rubber strips have been placed to protect the margin. *B*. Self-retaining brain retractors are now holding the fissure open, permitting the superficial draining vein to be divided and followed to the malformation. *C*. An aneurysmal dilatation is present on the largest middle cerebral branch. *D*. A Heifetz aneurysm clip has been placed to close the aneurysm without injury to the main vessel. *E*. Sylvian fissure after removal of the malformation.

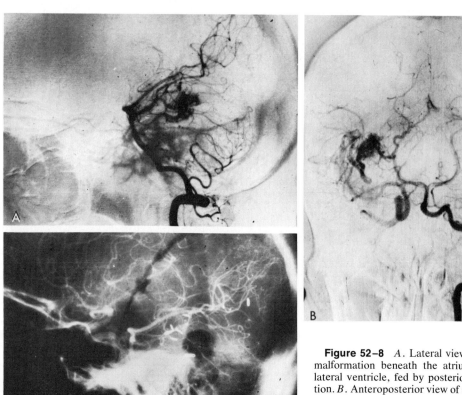

Figure 52–8 *A*. Lateral view of small malformation beneath the atrium of the lateral ventricle, fed by posterior circulation. *B*. Anteroposterior view of same malformation. *C*. Postoperative angiogram shows preservation of vessels of passage.

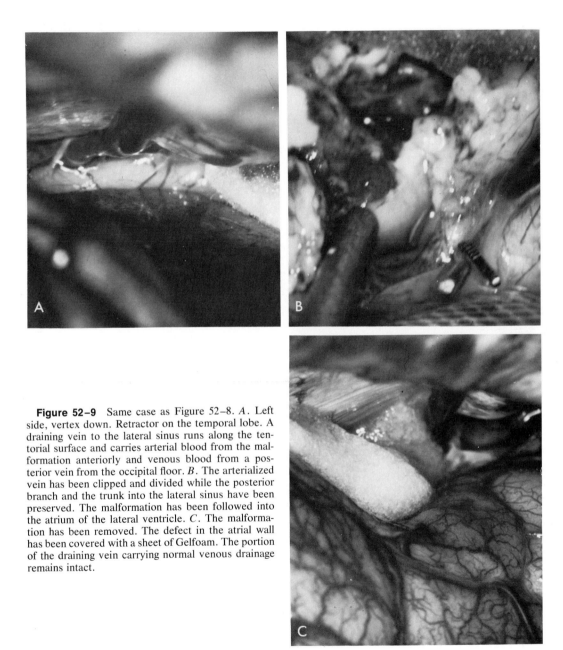

Figure 52–9 Same case as Figure 52–8. *A*. Left side, vertex down. Retractor on the temporal lobe. A draining vein to the lateral sinus runs along the tentorial surface and carries arterial blood from the malformation anteriorly and venous blood from a posterior vein from the occipital floor. *B*. The arterialized vein has been clipped and divided while the posterior branch and the trunk into the lateral sinus have been preserved. The malformation has been followed into the atrium of the lateral ventricle. *C*. The malformation has been removed. The defect in the atrial wall has been covered with a sheet of Gelfoam. The portion of the draining vein carrying normal venous drainage remains intact.

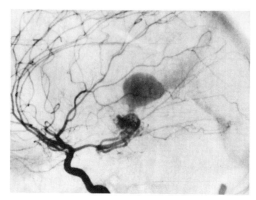

Figure 52–10 An aneurysmal dilatation of the vein of Galen, fed by an arteriovenous malformation of the quadrigeminal region. The large artery to the malformation is the posterior medial choroidal.

straight sinus and necessitate development of collateral venous drainage. This state of venous hypertension may lead to an enlarged head without enlarged ventricles. Obstruction of the subarachnoid pathways at the tentorial notch or of the aqueduct, however, will more often produce ventricular enlargement, an obstructive hydrocephalus, while posthemorrhagic arachnoid adhesions may lead to communicating hydrocephalus. Rarely, spontaneous occlusion of the anomaly has occurred, producing a calcific density that does not fill angiographically. When it is thus occluded, operative resection of the vein of Galen and its contained thrombus would appear indicated if mass effect and obstruction are not relieved by ventricular shunting.[27]

The preferred operative approach for malformations of the vein of Galen has been meticulously described by Yaşargil and associates.[58] A right posterior parasagittal craniotomy with visualization of the area between falx and medial surface exposes the straight sinus and the malformation. The arachnoid is opened, and the dissection of the feeding arteries and their closure at the vein of Galen are carried out progressively. Yaşargil has preserved the vein of Galen aneurysm intact as part of the normal venous drainage, once all feeders have been removed. Resection with ligation at the straight sinus will be tolerated, since collateral drainage of the deep veins will have developed if the arteriovenous shunt has been significant. Indeed, Poppen's case of successful resection was carried out vein first, beginning with ligation of the straight sinus.[47]

Dural Malformations

The dural malformations are a rare group that vary from the most unusual lesions in which virtually every dural artery manages to find a vein in which to empty to the better-described arteriovenous malformations draining into one lateral sinus.[19,22,25,35] They generally present with syndromes related to increased intracranial pressure as a result of the arterial pressure increasing the pressure in draining sinuses. Those of the lateral and sigmoid sinuses may produce reversal of flow in the straight sinus and internal cerebral veins, and development of collateral drainage of the deep venous system,

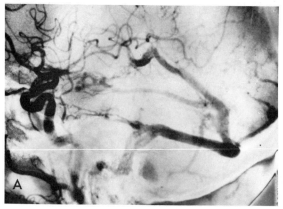
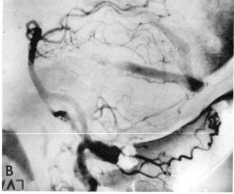

Figure 52–11 *A*. Carotid angiogram showing tentoriomeningeal artery feeding dural arteriovenous malformation of lateral sinus. The arterial pressure has reversed the flow in the deep venous system. *B*. Vertebral angiogram shows occipital and dural arteries contributing to the shunt into the lateral sinus.

a requisite for survival (Fig. 52–11). These remarkable lesions have a multiple arterial supply with external branches from occipital arteries and ascending pharyngeal branches, and internal feeders from the posterior meningeal and the tentoriomeningeal arteries. Total isolation of the sinus from attachments to bone, superficial dura, and tentorium will avail only if there are no additional arterial vessels entering along the torcular or below the jugular foramen. Sparing of the communicating veins to the occipital lobe and cerebellum would be required if this procedure were to be of value and would be particularly necessary if the sinus of the opposite side were not patent.

Ligation and resection of the entire sigmoid and lateral sinus from torcular to jugular foramen may be required and will ordinarily be tolerated in view of the collateral drainage already present. If isolation of the sinus is performed, the incision and closure of dural vessels beneath the ninth, tenth, and eleventh cranial nerves medial to the jugular foramen may be particularly awkward. Placing an aneurysm clip with one blade epidurally and one blade intradurally may secure this area (Fig. 52–12).

Ophthalmofacial-Hypothalamic Malformations

The syndrome of ophthalmofacial-hypothalamic arteriovenous malformation is another rare anomaly, sometimes referred to as the Bounet-Dechoume-Blanc syndrome. Here multiple shunts and aneurysmal dilatations occur, fortunately unilaterally in the orbit, maxilla, and nasal cavity, and intracranially in the pericarotid and hypothalamic area (Fig. 52–13). These patients may present with almost intractable epistaxis that unfortunately requires external carotid ligation for control. Such a ligation, so far proximal to the lesion, leads to development of a tremendous bilateral collateral arterial supply, involving everything from the thyrocervical and pharyngeal arteries to multiple vertebral branches as well as all of the opposite external carotid branching.

The intracranial portion of the malformation needs to be resected, though its connections at the internal carotid require precarious removal of the anterior clinoid process (Fig. 52–14). The external portion of the lesion has not been amenable to operative removal, since the shunts are so widespread through the facial soft tissues, though reasonable response and control has been achieved by operation in multiple stages in which external feeding vessels were dissected, ligated, filled with emboli, and divided. Embarking upon the definitive course of treatment of such an extensive process requires the understanding of the patient and the commitment of all involved to a long series of procedures without assurance of more than palliation.

CONCLUSIONS

While it is now reasonably established that most arteriovenous malformations are best treated by operative excision, these lesions still require great surgical circumspection, and catastrophic hemorrhage is always possible and often only a hairbreadth away. No lesion is as likely to give the surgeon sleepless nights—the anticipatory night before as well as the night after the operation, when the changed circulatory dynamics are responsible for the highest incidence of postoperative hemorrhage of any intracranial procedure. The present degree of satisfactorily low morbidity and mortality figures reflects in part a measurable number of patients rescued by prompt re-exploration, and there clearly exists a need for further improvement in method, if only to decrease the stress of the procedures.

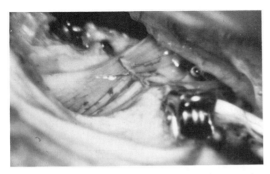

Figure 52–12 Left suboccipital craniectomy in same case as Figure 52–11. View of the ninth, tenth, and eleventh nerves at the jugular foramen. A Heifetz clip has been placed on the dura beneath the nerves to interrupt a group of dural arteries draining into the sigmoid sinus at the jugular foramen.

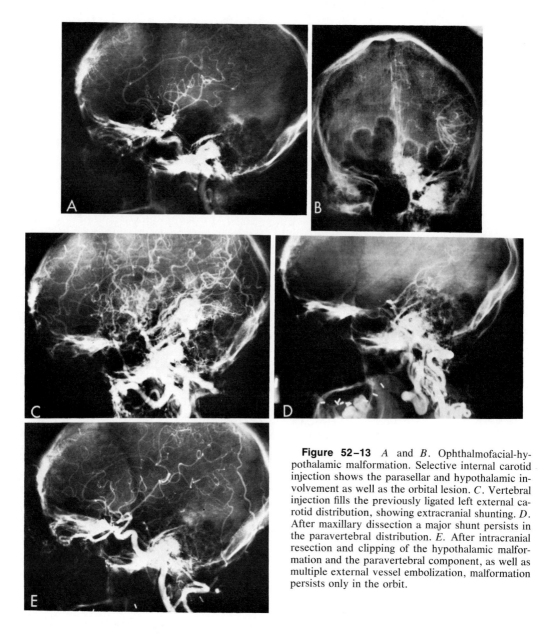

Figure 52-13 *A* and *B*. Ophthalmofacial-hypothalamic malformation. Selective internal carotid injection shows the parasellar and hypothalamic involvement as well as the orbital lesion. *C*. Vertebral injection fills the previously ligated left external carotid distribution, showing extracranial shunting. *D*. After maxillary dissection a major shunt persists in the paravertebral distribution. *E*. After intracranial resection and clipping of the hypothalamic malformation and the paravertebral component, as well as multiple external vessel embolization, malformation persists only in the orbit.

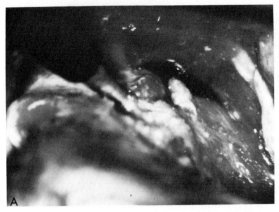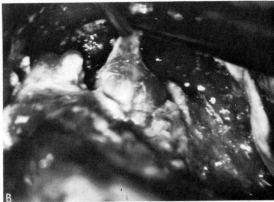

Figure 52–14. Ophthalmofacial-hypothalamic malformation. Vertex up, left side. The high-speed diamond burr is being used to remove the anterior clinoid process, unroofing an aneurysmal dilatation of the feeding artery to the hypothalamic malformation.

REFERENCES

1. Amacher, A. L., and Shillito, J., Jr.: The syndromes and surgical treatment of aneurysms of the great vein of Galen. J. Neurosurg., *39*:89–98, 1973.
2. Amacher, A. L., Allcock, J. M., and Drake, C. G.: Cerebral angiomas: The sequelae of surgical treatment. J. Neurosurg. *37*:571–575, 1972.
3. Aminoff, M. J., Barnard, R. O., and Logue, V.: The pathophysiology of spinal vascular malformations. J. Neurol. Sci., *23*:255–263, 1974.
4. Boyd-Wilson, J. S.: The association of cerebral angiomas with intracranial aneurysms. J. Neurol. Neurosurg. Psychiat., *22*:218–223, 1959.
5. Burger, P. C., and Vogel, F. S.: Surgical Pathology of the Nervous System and Its Coverings. New York, John Wiley & Sons, Inc., 1976, pp. 330–336.
6. Carton, C. A., and Hickey, W. C.: Arteriovenous malformation of the head of the caudate nucleus. J. Neurosurg., *12*:414–418, 1955.
7. Crawford, J. V., and Russell, D. S.: Cryptic arteriovenous and venous hamartomas of the brain. J. Neurol. Neurosurg. Psychiat., *19*:1–11, 1956.
8. Cronqvist, S., Granholm, L., and Lundstrom, N.: Hydrocephalus and congestive heart failure caused by intracranial arteriovenous malformations in infants. J. Neurosurg., *36*:249–254, 1972.
9. Cushing, H., and Bailey, P.: Tumors Arising From the Blood Vessels of the Brain. Springfield, Ill., C Thomas, 1928.
10. Dandy, W. E.: Arteriovenous aneurysm of the brain. Arch. Surg., *17*:190–243, 1928.
11. Dott, N. M., and Maccabe, J.: The arteriovenous malformations of the brain. Acta Chir. Acad. Sci. Hung., *7*: 111–128, 1966.
12. Feindel, W., and Perot, P.: Red cerebral veins. J. Neurosurg., *22*:315–325, 1965.
13. Feindel, W., Yamamoto, Y. L., and Hodge, C. P.: Red cerebral veins and the cerebral steal syndrome. J. Neurosurg., *35*:167–180, 1971.
14. Feindel, W., Yamamoto, Y. L., Hodge, C. P., Branan, R., and Meyer, E.: Reversal of cerebral steal during surgery of arteriovenous malformations: Evidence from fluorescein angiography and focal cortical blood flow measurement. Presented at meeting of American Association of Neurological Surgeons, Toronto, April, 1977.
15. French, L. A., and Seljeskog, E. L.: Arteriovenous malformations of the brain. In Youmans, J., ed.: Neurological Surgery. Philadelphia, W. B. Saunders Co., 1973, pp. 827–835.
16. Gross, S. W.: Cerebral arteriography. Arch. Neurol. Psychiat., *46*:704–714, 1941.
17. Hamby, W. B.: The pathology of supratentorial angiomas. J. Neurosurg., *15*:65–75, 1958.
18. Kaplan, H. A., Aronson, S. M., and Browder, E. J.: Vascular malformations of the brain. J. Neurosurg., *18*:630–635, 1961.
19. Kosnik, E. J., Hunt, W. E., and Miller, C. A.: Dural arteriovenous malformations. J. Neurosurg., *40*:322–329, 1974.
20. Krayenbühl, H., and Siebenmann, R.: Small vascular malformations as a cause of primary intracerebral hemorrhage. J. Neurosurg., *22*:7–20, 1965.
21. Krayenbühl, H., and Yasargil, M. G.: Das Hirnaneurysma. Documenta Geigy Series Chirurgica No. 4. Basel, J. R. Geigy, 1958, pp. 1–143.
22. Kuhner, A., Krastel, A., and Stoll, W.: Arteriovenous malformations of the transverse dural sinus. J. Neurosurg., *45*:12–19, 1976.
23. Kunc, Z.: Surgery of arteriovenous malformations in the speech and motor-sensory regions. J. Neurosurg., *40*:293–303, 1974.
24. Laine, E., Delandsheer, J.-M., Pruvot, P., Jomin, M., Christiaens, J.-L., Andreussi, L., Clarisse, J., and Delcoor, J.: Les anévrysmes cirsoïdes choroïdiens antérieurs et les anévrysmes cirsoïdes striés. Neurochirurgie, *16*:383–396, 1970.
25. Lamas, E., Lobato, R. D., Esparza, J., and Escudero, L.: Dural posterior fossa AVM producing

raised sagittal sinus pressure. J. Neurosurg., 46:804–810, 1977.

26. Lapras, C., Bochu, M., Russel, F., and Sindou, M.: Les angiomes de la tête du noyau caude. Neurochirurgie, 18:471–483, 1972.

27. Lazar, M. L.: Vein of Galen aneurysm: Successful excision of a completely thrombosed aneurysm in an infant. Surg. Neurol., 2:22–24, 1974.

28. Ley, A.: Aneurismas Arteriovenosos Congenitos Intracraneales. Barcelona, Tipografía la Academica de Herederos de Serra y Russell, 1957.

29. Litvak, J., Yahr, M. D., and Ransohoff, J.: Aneurysms of the great vein of Galen and midline cerebral arteriovenous anomalies. J. Neurosurg., 17:945–954, 1960.

30. Long, D. M., Seljeskog, E. L., Chou, S. N., and French, L. A.: Giant arteriovenous malformations of infancy and childhood. J. Neurosurg., 40:304–312, 1974.

31. Luessenhop, A. J.: Operative treatment of arteriovenous malformations of the brain. In Morley, T. P., ed.: Current Controversies in Neurosurgery. Philadelphia, W. B. Saunders Co., 1976, pp. 203–209.

32. Luessenhop, A. J., and Gennarelli, T. A.: Anatomical grading of supratentorial arteriovenous malformations for determining operability. Neurosurgery, 1:30–35, 1977.

33. Margolis, G., Odom, G. L., Woodhall, B., and Bloor, B. M.: The role of small angiomatous malformations in the production of intracerebral hematomas. J. Neurosurg., 8:564–575, 1951.

34. McCormick, W. F.: The pathology of vascular ("arteriovenous") malformations. J. Neurosurg., 24:807–816, 1966.

35. McCormick, W. F., and Boulter, T. R.: Vascular malformations ("angiomas") of the dura mater. J. Neurosurg., 25:309–311, 1966.

36. Morello, G., and Borghi, G. P.: Cerebral angiomas. Acta Neurochir. (Wien), 28:135–155, 1973.

37. Norlén G.: Arteriovenous aneurysms of the brain: Report of 10 cases of total removal of lesion. J. Neurosurg., 6:475–494, 1949.

38. Olivecrona, H., and Riives, J.: Arteriovenous aneurysms of the brain. Arch. Neurol. Psychiat., 59:567–602, 1948.

39. Padget, D. H.: The cranial venous system in man in reference to development, adult configuration, and relation to the arteries. Amer. J. Anat., 98:307–355, 1956.

40. Papatheodoru, C., Gross, S., and Hollin, S.: Small arteriovenous malformations of the brain. Arch. Neurol., 5:666–672, 1961.

41. Parkinson, D.: Cerebral arteriovenous aneurysms: Surgical management. Canad. J. Surg., 1:313–324, 1958.

42. Paterson, J. H., and McKissock, W.: A clinical survey of intracranial angiomas with special reference to their mode of progression and surgical treatment: A report of 110 cases. Brain, 79:223–265, 1956.

43. Penfield, W., and Erickson, T. C.: Epilepsy and cerebral localization. Springfield, Ill., Charles C Thomas, 1941, pp. 165–169, 254–255, 378–379.

44. Perret, G., and Nishioka, H.: Report on the cooperative study of intracranial aneurysms and subarachnoid hemorrhage. J. Neurosurg., 25:467–490, 1966.

45. Pilcher, C.: Vascular anomalies of brain. In Bancroft, F. W., and Pilcher, C., eds.: Surgical Treatment of the Nervous System. Philadelphia. J. B. Lippincott Co., 1946, pp. 239–246.

46. Pool, J. L.: Treatment of arteriovenous malformations of the cerebral hemisphere. J. Neurosurg., 19:136–141, 1962.

47. Poppen, J. L., and Avman, N.: Aneurysms of the great vein of Galen. J. Neurosurg., 17:238–244, 1960.

48. Potter, J. M.: Angiomatous malformations of the brain: Their nature and prognosis. Ann. Roy. Coll. Surg., 16:227–243, 1955.

49. Sahs, A. L., Perret, G. E., Locksley, H. B., et al.: Intracranial Aneurysms and Subarachnoid Hemorrhage. Philadelphia, J. B. Lippincott Co., 1969, p. 203.

50. Spetzler, R. F., and Wilson, C. B.: Enlargement of an arteriovenous malformation documented by angiography. J. Neurosurg., 43:767–769, 1975.

51. Svien, H. J., and McRae, J. A.: Arteriovenous anomalies of the brain. J. Neurosurg., 23:23–28, 1965.

52. Tonnis, W., Schiefer, W., and Walter, W.: Signs and symptoms of supratentorial arteriovenous aneurysms. J. Neurosurg., 15:471–480, 1958.

53. Troupp, H.: Arteriovenous malformations of the brain: What are the indications for operation? In Morley, T. P., ed.: Current Controversies in Neurosurgery. Philadelphia, W. B. Saunders Co., 1976, pp. 210–216.

54. U, H. S., and Wilson, C. B.: Surgical treatment of intracranial vascular malformations. West. J. Med., 123:175–183, 1975.

55. Waltimo, O.: The relationship of size, density and localization of intracranial arteriovenous malformations to the type of initial symptom. J. Neurol. Sci., 19:13–19, 1973.

56. Yasargil, G.: Operations on intracranial arteriovenous malformations. In Microsurgery Applied to Neurosurgery. Stuttgart, Georg Thieme, 1969, pp. 143–148.

57. Yasargil, G.: Personal communication, 1974.

58. Yasargil, M. G., Antic, J., Laciga, R., Jain, K. K., and Boone, S. C.: Arteriovenous malformations of vein of Galen: Microsurgical treatment. Surg. Neurol., 6:195–200, 1976.

53

SPECIAL PROBLEMS ASSOCIATED WITH SUBARACHNOID HEMORRHAGE

There are a number of special problems confronting the physician dealing with sub-arachnoid hemorrhage. Prominent among these special problems are: (1) the association of cerebral aneurysm, coarctation of the aorta, polycystic kidney, and the Ehlers-Danlos syndrome; (2) subarachnoid hemorrhage occurring in pregnancy; (3) subarachnoid hemorrhage caused by traumatic, mycotic, giant, and multiple aneurysms; (4) aneurysms associated with brain tumors; and (5) hydrocephalus following subarachnoid hemorrhage.

Since the initial descriptions by Eppinger of the association of cerebral aneurysm and coarctation of the aorta, there have appeared a number of reports proposing the association of a long list of congenital defects with cerebral aneurysm.[6,7] Stehbens, however, in a review of the literature and a careful autopsy study of 215 patients who had died of cerebral aneurysm compared to a control series of 849 noncerebral hemorrhage patients and 351 patients who had died of nonaneurysmal cerebral hemorrhage, found no significant difference in the incidence of associated congenital abnormalities.[2] Indeed, apart from polycystic kidney and coarctation of the aorta, the incidence of congenital abnormalities with cerebral aneurysm was not higher than in the general population. From analysis of the data, both Stehbens and Walton suggest that the association of aneurysm with coarctation of the aorta and polycystic kidney may be due to the hypertension and vascular changes found in the latter two conditions.[2,3] Nevertheless, the cases re-ported by Forster and Alpers and by Matson of these coincidental defects in very young children, possibly before there has been time for secondary hypertension to have had an effect, give credence to the postulate that the arterial defects may be associated.[9,16] The various lines of evidence supporting the theories of congenital medial defects, secondary changes in the internal elastic membrane, and changes secondary to hypertension and atherosclerosis in the formation of cerebral aneurysm have been recently reviewed by Sahs.[1] (See also Chapters 46 and 47.)

COARCTATION OF THE AORTA

The neurological complications of coarctation of the aorta have been most recently reviewed by LeBlanc and co-workers.[8] The literature relating to the association with cerebral aneurysm has been reviewed by Walton, by Schwartz and Baronofsky, by Matson and by Robinson.[3,9–11]

The incidence of cerebral aneurysm with coarctation is about four times as great as without. The age of cerebral aneurysmal rupture is earlier (average 25 years) than in patients without coarctation (average 50 to 54 years). The incidence of multiple aneurysms is higher (30 per cent) than in non-coarctation cases (19 per cent). Further, the mortality rate of cerebral aneurysmal rupture in patients with coarctation of the aorta is much higher than in those without (75 versus 40 per cent, approximately). Seventy-five per cent of patients with uncor-

C. E. BRACKETT AND R. A. MORANTZ

rected coarctation of the aorta will be dead before the age of 40, dying of cardiac failure, aortic rupture, endocarditis, or cerebral hemorrhage. It is therefore apparent that the combination of coarctation of the aorta and cerebral aneurysm is a highly fatal one early in life, demanding early recognition and aggressive treatment. It has been postulated that the multiplicity of aneurysms, the early age of rupture, and the high mortality rate are the results of hypertension and associated vascular changes resulting from the coarctation. It has been further suggested that the early recognition and correction of the aortic coarctation may retard the degenerative changes important in cerebral aneurysm development and prevent rupture.

The presence of hypertension in the young or evidences of severe chronic hypertension in a person with subarachnoid hemorrhage suggests the diagnosis. Confirmation is found in weakness or absence of leg pulses, discrepancy in arm and leg blood pressures, and notching of the ribs on x-ray. The diagnosis of the two lesions is established by brachial angiography. Cerebral visualization must be complete because of the high incidence of multiple aneurysms.

Treatment should begin with immediate careful reduction of the elevated blood pressure to reasonable levels by medical means. As soon as angiography and cardiac evaluation are complete, operative repair of the coarctation and the cerebral aneurysm should be undertaken. Whether these procedures should be done simultaneously or serially will depend on the severity of the hypertension, its response to drug therapy, the presence of intracranial clot or spasm, and similar considerations. If an unruptured aneurysm is encountered in a patient with coarctation, the aortic abnormality should be repaired first, and elective operative obliteration of the cerebral aneurysm should follow.[12] These considerations require careful consultation between the cardiac and neurological surgeon. The importance of this aggressive approach is supported by the experience of Matson, who reported three cases of coarctation in a series of 14 cerebral aneurysms occurring in children.[9] All three had both defects repaired; two survived. This report, along with others, underlines the importance of aggressive treatment in a combination of diseases in which the mortality rate of each is potentiated by the other and reaches high levels at an early age.

POLYCYSTIC KIDNEY

The literature regarding the association of polycystic kidney and cerebral aneurysm has been reviewed by Brown and by Walton.[3,15] On the basis of Sahs' calculated incidence for 205,000 hospital admissions and Brown's review of 11,245 autopsies (not all of which included brain examinations), it is suggested that there is a greater association of aneurysm and polycystic kidney than chance would dictate (Table 53–1).[18] Bigelow also noted a 6.4 per cent incidence of aneurysm in polycystic kidney disease.[13]

It must, however, be emphasized that at the present time no statistically reliable data are available on the incidence of cerebral aneurysm and subarachnoid hemorrhage due to cerebral aneurysm for specific ages and the like, and thus no determination of correlative significance can be made.

Thus, it may be seen that approximately 4 per cent of patients with cerebral aneurysm may be expected to have polycystic kidney disease. As in coarctation of the aorta, the incidence of multiple cerebral aneurysms is also higher than in the general population. As with coarctation, the increased incidence suggests a common developmental defect to Brown, but the importance of the associated hypertension has been stressed by Stehbens and by Walton.[2,3,15] The finding of the association at 13 weeks by Forster and Alpers, however, and the cases reported by Brown suggest the

TABLE 53–1 ASSOCIATION OF CEREBRAL ANEURYSM AND POLYCYSTIC KIDNEY

	SAHS (Per Cent)*	BROWN (Per Cent)†
Polycystic kidney	.026	.32
Aneurysms	.962	1.3
Aneurysms in polycystic kidney disease	7.3	16.6
Polycystic kidneys in aneurysm patients	3.1	4.0

* Sahs, A. L., and Myers, R.: Trans. Amer. Neurol. Ass., 76:147–150, 1951.

†Brown, R. A. P.: Glasg. Med. J., 32:33, 1951.

possibility of association of congenital defects.[16]

The diagnosis will be suggested by the presence of hypertension, renal mass, albuminuria, hematuria, casts, and azotemia. Confirmation is obtained by pyelography.

The prognosis for bilateral polycystic disease with the associated hypertension and cerebral aneurysm is poor, with early cerebral rupture and high death rate the rule. In 21 cases from the literature and 1 personal case, Walton reported that 14 died in the first attack of cerebral bleeding and 2 from bleeding recurrences, a mortality rate of 74 per cent at an early age of 25 years' average.[3] Unfortunately, the renal disease is not susceptible to definitive therapy, and the relief of hypertension with medical therapy not only is incomplete but may potentiate the renal failure. Therefore, the early diagnosis of the cerebral aneurysm by angiography, temporary reduction of hypertension by medical means, and early surgical obliteration of the cerebral aneurysm by standard methods is indicated.

EHLERS-DANLOS SYNDROME

The association of this rare syndrome with intracranial bleeding is mentioned here to warn the neurosurgeon of the extreme hazards of dealing with the condition. These are due to the excessive fragility of the arterial vasculature. Rubinstein and Cohen reported the association of multiple aneurysms, and Graf and Schoolman and Kepes the association with spontaneous arteriovenous fistula, presumably secondary to carotid aneurysmal rupture in the cavernous sinus.[19–21]

Rubinstein suggested that the defect was a lack of collagen in the adventitia, while Schoolman and Kepes stressed the fragmentation or absence of the elastic tissue in small arteries, aortic arch, veins, epiglottis, lungs, bronchi, and skin. The relation of these findings to the possible etiology of cerebral aneurysms, reviewed by Sahs and by Walton, requires further consideration.[1,3] Much evidence has been brought forth to suggest that the finding of medial defects is widespread in cases without as well as those with aneurysm and that they may not be of congenital origin. Further, the fragmentation of the internal elastic membrane seen in cerebral aneurysm is of unknown etiology, but the possible association with early changes related to arteriosclerosis secondary to hypertension has been stressed by a number of authors. This fragmentation of the elastic membrane occurring in the Ehlers-Danlos syndrome without evidence of associated hypertension or arteriosclerosis may provide an important clue to the etiology of cerebral aneurysms.

The clinical picture is characteristic: hyperelasticity of skin, increased joint mobility, subcutaneous nodules, heart defects, bowel and lung rupture, and easy bruisability due to marked vessel fragility.

Therapy is hazardous. Schoolman's patient died of aortic dissection during arteriography to search for multiple aneurysms, while Rubinstein's patient died of tearing of the intracranial carotid artery that could not be ligated because of excessive vascular fragility. It is difficult to suggest appropriate therapy other than perhaps encasement of the aneurysm with plastic. It would appear that even this mode of treatment is hazardous, and it may be that conservative therapy is best.

PREGNANCY

The incidence of subarachnoid hemorrhage in pregnancy is reported to vary between 1 in 2700 and 1 in 8700. Approximately half of these hemorrhages will be due to a ruptured aneurysm and the remainder to a ruptured arteriovenous malformation. In pregnancy, rupture obviously occurs in an earlier age group during the childbearing period than it does in the general population, in which the average age of rupture is 50 to 54 years.[1] Since age-specific data are not available as to the incidence of subarachnoid hemorrhage due to ruptured aneurysm in the general population, no conclusions can be drawn regarding the effect of pregnancy on the incidence of rupture of cerebral aneurysms.

Subarachnoid bleeding occurs more frequently in the pre-eclamptic than in the noneclamptic woman. The peak time of bleeding is during the third trimester (thirtieth week) of pregnancy. The incidence of subarachnoid hemorrhage during the stages of pregnancy is about the same for proved and unproved cases of cerebral aneurysm except that that of bleeding due to proved aneurysms appears to be lower during the period of labor than that in unproved cases. The reason for this is not clear. Summarizing the data from the literature, the percentage of subarachnoid hemorrhages due to proved and unproved cases of cerebral aneurysm during the stages of pregnancy is, approximately:

First trimester	3 per cent
Second trimester	20 per cent
Third trimester	40 per cent
Labor	13 per cent
First postpartum day	13 per cent
Later	13 per cent

Approximately 60 per cent occur in primiparous women, but it is significant that 40 per cent of pregnant patients have had one or more previous pregnancies before rupture of the intracranial aneurysm occurred.

There has been speculation as to the mechanisms that produce the peak incidence of rupture during the thirtieth week of pregnancy. Increases of blood volume, increased cardiac output, and other mechanisms have been proposed, but no convincing data are available at the present time.

The history of a pregnant woman with a subarachnoid hemorrhage due to an arteriovenous malformation often is different from that of one whose hemorrhage is due to a ruptured intracranial aneurysm. Typically, she will be a primipara between 18 and 25 years old. If, however, she has had a previous pregnancy, there is a 50-50 chance that it was complicated by either her own neurological symptoms or an obstetrical complication involving the fetus. Subarachnoid hemorrhage will usually occur between the sixteenth and twenty-fourth week of pregnancy, shortly before labor, during delivery, or in the early puerperium. In contrast, the typical patient with a subarachnoid hemorrhage due to a ruptured aneurysm will bleed between the thirtieth and fortieth week of gestation, and it is quite rare for hemorrhage to occur during labor or the puerperium.[31]

The clinical picture of subarachnoid hemorrhage during pregnancy is the same as that occurring in a nonpregnant individual. The chief differential diagnosis lies between subarachnoid hemorrhage secondary to eclampsia and that due to cerebral aneurysm. The previous prenatal history of the present and past pregnancies regarding the presence of eclamptic symptoms is

helpful. Severe hypertension, enlarged heart, generalized edema, epigastric pain, retinal exudates, and severe proteinuria will suggest a diagnosis of eclampsia, whereas the sudden onset of lesser degrees of the same symptoms, especially in the third trimester in association with severe subarachnoid hemorrhage, will suggest the presence of a ruptured cerebral aneurysm. It is in this type of case, especially, that further diagnostic procedures are indicated.

The diagnosis is confirmed by angiography, to which there is no known obstetrical contraindication. Obviously, strict precautions to protect the fetus (e.g., radiation shielding, low dye dosage) are in order, especially during the first trimester of pregnancy.

When an aneurysm is identified, it should be managed as in the nonpregnant patient.[25,28] Most authors have recommended direct operative treatment. If it can be avoided, hypotension should not be used, since it can be followed by premature labor and fetal distress. Hypothermia usually is well tolerated.[31]

Although recommendations in the literature vary, there is no evidence to suggest that delivery should not proceed as indicated obstetrically irrespective of the presence of cerebral aneurysm. Some authors have suggested that ligation of the aneurysm followed by normal vaginal delivery gives protection against the increased intracranial pressures associated with delivery. McCausland and Holmes showed that there is no increase in the cerebrospinal fluid pressure during labor pains and that it increases to a range of 300 to 700 mm of water during bearing down.[26] It must be pointed out, however, that there is no evidence to suggest that increased intracranial pressure leads to increased incidence of cerebral aneurysmal rupture. A pregnant patient with subarachnoid hemorrhage due to a ruptured aneurysm or arteriovenous malformation should be treated in the same manner as if she were not pregnant. If possible, hypotension and osmotic diuretics should be avoided.[30] With respect to obstetrical management, most authors recommend normal vaginal delivery utilizing lumbar epidural anesthesia, and forceps for the second stage of labor in those patients with aneurysms. In this case there appears to be no indication for elective cesarean section. In contrast, some authors have recommended that for patients with arteriovenous malformations, delivery by elective lower cesarean section at 38 weeks is the procedure of choice.[31]

TRAUMATIC ANEURYSMS

Cerebral aneurysms are usually classified as congenital, arteriosclerotic, mycotic, or traumatic. Of these categories, aneurysms due to trauma constitute the smallest group.

Traumatic intracerebral aneurysms may be classified in two general ways: by pathological characteristics or by location. Thus, a "true" traumatic aneurysm occurs when an arterial injury fails to penetrate the arterial wall completely. In this case, the essential damage is to the internal elastic lamina, whose destruction allows for the subsequent vascular dilatation and aneurysm formation. In a "false" traumatic aneurysm, there is a full-thickness tear through the wall of the artery, but the hemorrhage produced is adequately contained and the fibrous capsule produced by the hematoma then communicates with the arterial lumen. A "mixed" traumatic aneurysm is the rarest type of all and is caused by the rupture of a true traumatic aneurysm that then gives rise to a secondary false aneurysm.[35] With respect to location, traumatic aneurysms may be located extracranially on the scalp vessels, extradurally on the middle meningeal artery, on the internal carotid artery on either its extradural or supraclinoid portions, or on the distal intracerebral branches.

Burton and co-workers have classified trauma to the cerebral vessels as either direct or indirect.[35] The most frequently described direct cause of traumatic aneurysms is a penetrating wound, usually a gunshot wound. In several cases, however, the injury to the cerebral vessel was presumably iatrogenic secondary to intracranial operation—those developing after the placement of a temporary arterial clip or following repeated subdural taps.[32,42] Indirect arterial trauma can occur with closed head injuries.[43] In this case, the vessel may be damaged by striking the falx, tentorium, or bony prominences such as the sphenoid wing. In addition, Drake has postulated, surface arteries that are densely adherent to the dura mater may be injured during the rotary brain movements that occur with closed head injury.[36]

Two examples of the production of experimental intracranial arterial aneurysms by means of artificial vascular injury have been reported. White and associates injected hypertonic saline solution into the arterial walls of cortical vessels.[44] One third of the vessels developed the histological picture of a berry aneurysm, although a gross aneurysm was not produced. Harvey and Downer reported the inadvertent production of a grossly visible aneurysm by means of a needle puncture of the internal carotid artery of the monkey.[40]

Although more than 50 cases of traumatic intracerebral aneurysm have been reported in the literature since the turn of the century, these lesions are decidedly rare. Although 2.8 per cent of patients in the cooperative study of intracranial aneurysms in subarachnoid hemorrhage reported prior head trauma, trauma was not incriminated as a cause of aneurysm formation.[44]

Benoit and Wortzman found trauma to be the etiological agent in approximately 0.5 per cent of 850 cases of intracranial aneurysm treated at the Toronto General Hospital.[34] Ferry and Kempe, however, were able to find only two cases of false aneurysm formation among 2187 cases of penetrating wounds of the brain.[37]

Symptoms of patients with traumatic intracerebral aneurysms will vary depending upon whether the lesion is located on the internal carotid artery at the base of the skull or on a peripheral vessel. In the former case, a rather consistent clinical picture is presented. The typical history is that of a young man who has sustained major head trauma leading to an anterior basal skull fracture. Unilateral blindness is noted by the patient when he regains consciousness, and dysfunction of the third, fourth, fifth, and sixth cranial nerves is evident either immediately after injury or within a short time thereafter. Over the following weeks to months, the patient experiences multiple nosebleeds of increasing severity. Although the initial nosebleed is rarely fatal, in more than half the cases reported, death as a result of profuse hemorrhage has occurred before treatment could be accomplished.

Approximately half of those with traumatic aneurysms on peripheral vessels will present with the syndrome of delayed subarachnoid hemorrhage following head injury. Eighty-eight per cent of the hemorrhages occur less than three weeks after injury.[38] In the remaining patients, the diagnosis will be incidental to contrast procedures performed after a head injury.

The differential diagnosis is between those lesions occurring at the base and those at the periphery. Epistaxis occurs quite frequently following head injuries. In the great majority of cases, however, this hemorrhage rises from abrasion of the nasal mucosa or from trauma to branches of either the anterior ethmoidal or the sphenopalatine artery. More rarely, such hemorrhage may be due to frank rupture of the internal carotid artery itself. Patients whose epistaxis is due to traumatic extradural aneurysm will usually have monocular blindness and deficits of cranial nerves III to VI in addition to delayed epistaxis.[39] In addition, the majority will have basilar skull fractures. The definitive diagnostic procedure is cerebral angiography. In all cases this study will reveal an aneurysm that has arisen in the cavernous sinus and eroded medially and inferiorly into the sphenoid sinus.

In the differential diagnosis of traumatic cortical aneurysms, traumatic middle meningeal artery aneurysms can be excluded by the fact that they are usually adjacent to the inner table of the skull and occur along the course of the middle meningeal artery. Mycotic aneurysms frequently occur on the cortical surface. They are, however, often multiple and not associated with a history of trauma. Traumatic aneurysms of the scalp vessels occur quite frequently and can be quite misleading if only a lateral arteriogram is obtained. The anteroposterior angiogram will demonstrate the aneurysm lying outside the cranial cavity. Finally, congenital aneurysms usually occur at the base of the brain at areas of vessel bifurcation or branching. Here again a history of trauma will usually be lacking.

Although the first episode of epistaxis in patients with traumatic aneurysms of the internal carotid artery will rarely be fatal, the chances of exsanguination increase with each subsequent hemorrhage. Therefore, operative treatment must be undertaken immediately. Given the severity of the hemorrhage, local treatment such as anterior or posterior nasal packs is to no avail. The procedure of choice is ligation of the ipsilateral internal carotid artery in the neck with concomitant clipping of the internal carotid artery intracranially. Even after such a trapping procedure has been completed, the aneurysm may still fill through collateral channels between the external carotid artery and the ophthalmic artery. Consequently, if the superclinoid carotid artery cannot be clipped proximal to the origin of the ophthalmic artery, ophthalmic artery ligation is justified.

Traumatic aneurysms of the peripheral intracranial vessels have a marked tendency to rupture. Burton and associates found a mortality rate greater than 50 per cent in those cases of peripheral traumatic aneurysms that had been reported prior to 1968.[35] Asari and co-workers reported a 20 per cent mortality rate in cases treated by operation.[33] The treatment of choice is direct obliteration of the aneurysm. Since many of these lesions are likely to change in size even over a short period of time, cerebral angiography should be performed immediately prior to operation. There is a great tendency for rupture to occur during operation, especially in the case of "false" traumatic aneurysms. Consequently, one must insure that adequate exposure of both the distal and proximal parent artery is obtained prior to dissection near the aneurysm. As in the treatment of congenital aneurysms, the operating microscope offers a distinct aid in the dissection. Since in many cases a discrete neck of the aneurysm cannot be identified at the time of operation, one should be prepared to perform a coating or trapping procedure if clipping is not possible.

Although the overall mortality rate for all patients with traumatic aneurysm of peripheral intracerebral arteries is approximately 25 per cent, it would appear that the chance for survival is improved after operative therapy, since the overall mortality rate reported in the literature is approximately 18 per cent for those treated by operations, while for those treated nonoperatively it is 41 per cent.[38]

MYCOTIC ANEURYSMS

A mycotic aneurysm develops secondary to infection in the arterial wall. This infection may come either from the tissues surrounding the vessel wall (as in meningitis) or, more commonly, from an infected embolus that lodges in the vasa vasorum and results in subsequent outpouching. In 1885 Osler originated the term "mycotic" aneurysm to describe such inflammatory lesions, and although the word "mycotic" should more properly be reserved for *fungally* produced lesions, common usage through the years has applied the term "mycotic" to an aneurysm that is produced by any infectious agent. These constitute 2 to 6 per cent of all intracranial aneurysms.[47,48]

Reports indicate that 2 to 10 per cent of patients with bacterial endocarditis, acute or subacute, will develop intracranial mycotic aneurysms. There has been no significant decrease in this incidence since the beginning of the antibiotic era.[51]

Eppinger was the first to emphasize that a septic embolus lodging in the vasa vasorum is the cause of this condition.[7] Since that time, both clinical and experimental data would support the embolism being the primary mechanism.[46] The ensuing inflammatory reaction damages the elastica and media. The vessel may become occluded, or a saccular aneurysm can occur. More rarely, mycotic aneurysms may be secondary to an extravascular infectious process, such as thrombophlebitis of the cavernous sinus or purulent meningitis.[49] By far the most common underlying disease leading to septic embolism is bacterial endocarditis, although bacterial emboli from noncardiac sources such as the lungs may also occur. The organisms responsible for mycotic aneurysms usually are of low virulence. This is true because the more virulent pyogenic organisms usually tend to cause a more rapid infectious process with resultant meningoencephalitis or brain abscess.

The most common site of mycotic aneurysm formation is on the peripheral branches of the cerebral arteries, especially the middle cerebral artery. The aneurysm is usually fusiform, but saccular aneurysms do occur. They usually are small in size, which may be explained by their great tendency to rupture early. In some cases they rupture within a month from the time of the septic embolization.

The embolic episode that eventually leads to the aneurysm formation may occur without accompanying symptoms, although local spasm may lead to transient neurological deficit. If secondary thrombosis occurs during aneurysm formation, then infarction may occur. As in other aneurysms, pressure effects of the lesion may produce focal neurological deficit such as a cranial nerve palsy, but more commonly, there will be no clinical symptoms until a subarachnoid hemorrhage occurs. In most cases the diagnosis of bacterial endocarditis will have been made prior to the onset of neurological symptoms. The diagnosis of a mycotic aneurysm should be suspected in any patient with an aneurysm in an unusual site or with obvious infection, heart murmur, splenomegaly, petechiae, microscopic hematuria, fever, or elevated sedimentation rate.

Several authors have stressed the need for repeated angiography, since this can demonstrate a rapid change in aneurysm size, or even complete resolution of the lesion.[49]

The first step in the treatment of this condition is massive appropriate intravenous antibiotic therapy. Although both radiological and pathological reports indicate that not all mycotic aneurysms will rupture, it appears that in the majority of cases rupture *will* occur. Consequently, operative intervention is the procedure of choice. The question of operative timing is controversial. Prompt intervention is warranted when there is a significant intracerebral hematoma, or where the peripheral location of a lesion would allow for minimal deficit even if the parent vessel is occluded. If the aneurysm arises from a major vessel, such as the bifurcation of the middle cerebral artery, then operation should be deferred until antibiotic therapy has been accomplished. At this time (usually about one month after diagnosis) angiography should be repeated. If the aneurysm is larger in size, then operation is indicated. If, however, the lesion is smaller in size, or multiple lesions are demonstrated, then operation again should be deferred. In some instances, repeat arteriography will reveal the disappearance of a previously demonstrated aneurysm. Even if operation is required, it appears logical that during the interval of antibiotic therapy a degree of reparative fibrosis will occur, so that a clip can be more safely applied. One should be fully prepared to perform an alternative procedure such as coating or trapping if no aneurysm neck can be demonstrated. The prognosis for the patient with a mycotic aneurysm depends upon his preoperative status; however, one reviewer reported good results in 8 of 10 patients treated by operation.[50]

MULTIPLE ANEURYSMS

A significant number of patients undergoing diagnostic work-up after a subarachnoid hemorrhage will be found to harbor multiple aneurysms. The treatment of such patients offers a particular challenge for the neurosurgeon; whereas it is widely accepted that operative treatment is the choice for the lesion that has ruptured, there is no unanimity of opinion as to the proper treatment of the lesion that has not ruptured. Furthermore, even though operative obliteration of the unruptured aneurysm is to be attempted, the optimal timing for such a procedure has not been established.

The reported incidence of multiple intracranial aneurysms has varied, depending first on whether the series is based on autopsy or on angiographic demonstration of multiple lesions, and second upon whether four-vessel angiography has been performed. Thus, in *autopsy* series, Bigelow showed an incidence of 23 per cent and McKissock reported an incidence of 28 per cent, while the Cooperative Study reported an incidence of 22 per cent.[52,60,63] On the other hand, these same authors have reported incidence rates for multiple intracranial aneurysms of 10, 14, and 19 per cent respectively, *based on cerebral angiography alone.* All studies show a marked female predominance. McKissock reported 68 per cent of patients with multiple aneurysms were women, whereas Mount and Brisman reported that 83 per cent of such patients were women.[58,60] The age distribution was essentially the same as that for patients with single aneurysms, i.e., approximately 60 per cent occur between the ages of 40 and 60.

Multiple aneurysms can best be classified with respect to location as: (1) those that are bilaterally symmetrical; (2) those that are nonsymmetrically situated on more than one artery; and (3) those with more than one aneurysm on the same artery.[53] If this classification is adhered to, then approximately 40 per cent of multiple aneurysms will be in each of the first two categories, with only 20 per cent in the third category. With respect to individual vessels, most patients with multiple aneurysms will have them on the internal carotid artery; the second most common site will be the middle cerebral artery.[58] With respect to etiology, except in the case of mycotic aneurysms, for which the incidence of multiple aneurysms is approximately 20 per cent, and in patients with associated coarctation of the aorta or polycystic kidney disease, the same etiological factors that apply to the formation of a single aneurysm would appear to be operative.[52]

An important consideration in the patient with multiple aneurysms is the determination of which lesion has been responsible for the subarachnoid hemorrhage. In general, the most important angiographic factors in this regard are: (1) localized hematoma; (2) localized spasm; (3) an irregular outline to the aneurysm; and (4) size, the larger aneurysm being the one most likely to have bled in over 80 per cent of cases.[65]

Computed tomography may occasionally help in this differentiation by indicating a small hematoma, localized cerebral edema, or the like. If angiographic findings are combined with evidence of initial focal neurological deficit, then the bleeding aneurysm can be correctly identified in approximately 90 per cent of cases.[55]

Controversy has arisen in regard to the natural history of the unruptured aneurysm. If data from three studies are combined, it is seen that over a follow-up period of up to 11 years, approximately 10 per cent of patients harboring an unruptured aneurysm will experience a subarachnoid hemorrhage due to this aneurysm.[58] Four per cent of the group will eventually die from their subarachnoid hemorrhage.

The question of what treatment should be attempted on the unruptured aneurysm has been an area of controversy for many years. Bjorkesten and Troupp, McKissock and associates, and Paterson and Bond all have indicated that treatment should be limited to the aneurysm that has ruptured.[53,60,61] On the other hand, Hamby, Pool and Potts, Moyes, and Mount and Brisman have advocated the operative treatment of all intracranial aneurysms that have been demonstrated.[54,57,59,62] A middle position has been taken by Heiskanen and Marttila, who have suggested operative obliteration of an unruptured cranial aneurysm only if the asymptomatic aneurysm could be reached through the same operative field that was being used to treat the symptomatic lesion.[56] Most recently, Samson and co-workers have presented a series in which 24 patients harboring multiple aneurysms had an operation performed upon their asymptomatic aneurysms during a second elective procedure.[64] Using the operative microscope, this group has been able to report no operative mortality and only minimal morbidity. In the light of present-day data such as these, it would seem that in the absence of extenuating circumstances such as coexisting risk factors, elective prophylactic operative obliteration is the treatment of choice in the patient with multiple aneurysms.

GIANT ANEURYSMS

A giant aneurysm is usually defined as one that is larger than 2.5 cm in its greatest diameter. Such lesions are relatively rare; in an autopsy study of over 3000 brains, Stehbens discovered 128 aneurysms, of which only 8 were more than 3 cm in diameter.[76]

Giant aneurysms may arise in three distinct locations: on the supraclinoid portion of the internal carotid artery, on the peripheral intracranial arteries, especially the middle cerebral artery, and on the vessels of the posterior circulation. Since large aneurysms usually produce symptoms because of mass effect, regional anatomy dictates that the clinical presentation will be different in each of these locations.

There are two main theories about the etiology of these lesions. One holds that they form from a hematoma in communication with a smaller aneurysm, and that the hematoma then undergoes organization and is incorporated into the wall of the aneurysm, which thereby increases in size.[70,71] Others have postulated that giant aneurysms may be a separate entity from the more usual saccular or berry aneurysms, i.e., that they may be congenital in origin and quite large from the beginning.[66] This interpretation is supported by the fact that cases of giant aneurysms have been reported in infancy and childhood.[73]

Most patients with giant aneurysms are over 50 years of age, and most series show a female predominance.

The mode of clinical presentation varies widely, depending upon whether the presenting feature is subarachnoid hemorrhage or local mass effect. Most authors consider rupture of a giant aneurysm to be rare. In the series reported by Morley and Barr, subarachnoid hemorrhage occurred in 6 of 28 cases, while in Bull's series of 22 cases a probable hemorrhage had occurred in 6.[69,75] In those patients with giant aneurysms of the supraclinoid carotid artery, the presenting symptom is usually painless, gradual loss of vision in one eye. There is usually no extraocular palsy, but there is a variable visual field defect.[67,68] More rarely, a giant aneurysm may present as an intrasellar mass lesion, causing hypopituitarism.[72] If the aneurysm is on the middle cerebral artery, the patient will most likely present with seizures or evidence of increased intracranial pressure.[75] If the lesion is on a vessel of the posterior circulation, the patient most commonly presents with palsy of cranial nerves III to X, ataxia, long-tract signs, or an organic mental syndrome. The seventh and eighth cranial nerves are frequently involved, producing symptoms that may mimic those of a cerebellopontine angle tumor.[74]

Plain skull x-rays may show a calcification that is characteristically curvilinear and quite thin. In addition, bone erosion may occur at the base of the skull in proximity to the lesion. The erosion is best shown by tomography. Cerebral angiography is the neuroradiological procedure of choice. In addition to showing the mass effect, it is the best procedure for demonstrating the lesion itself. One must be aware, however, that thrombus within the lumen will many times prevent the demonstration of the full size of the aneurysm. Computed tomography frequently will show the partially thrombosed aneurysmal mass.

The treatment of this condition depends upon the location of the lesion and the severity of the clinical symptoms. Since several cases of spontaneous thrombosis have been reported, a conservative approach utilizing follow-up angiography is warranted in some cases. For supraclinoid giant aneurysms, most authors advocate common carotid occlusion.[75] The prognosis in the case of large vertebral-basilar aneurysms is poor, and therefore a direct approach should be considered whenever feasible. Sundt has reported successfully removing a large basilar aneurysm by utilizing profound hyperthermia and circulatory arrest.[77] In the case of a giant aneurysm of the middle cerebral artery, a direct approach is indicated, although total excision usually is not feasible without sacrificing the parent artery from which the aneurysm originates. Consequently, the microscopic anastomosis of an extracerebral vessel to a branch distal to the lesion may decrease the chance of postoperative neurological deficit.

BRAIN TUMORS

Although there have been over 100 reports of patients harboring both intracranial aneurysms and brain tumors, careful autopsy studies indicate that the occurrence of these two lesions in the same patient is coincidental. Taylor found only 5 saccular aneurysms in 1500 cases of verified primary intracranial neoplasms (0.3 per cent), and Handa reported 7 in 956 patients with brain tumors (0.7 per cent).[79,82]

There have been reports of aneurysms occurring in association with cardiac myxoma as well as with metastatic carcinoma of the brain.[78,81] In these cases there has been direct damage to the wall of the blood vessel by the tumor cells and the cause has been apparent. In the great majority of cases, however, the associated tumors were gliomas, meningiomas, and pituitary adenomas.[80] If the figures are corrected to reflect the greater incidence of gliomas in the general population, it is seen that there is a disproportionately frequent association between aneurysms and meningiomas and pituitary adenomas. Several factors may explain this association. Two important ones appear to be the basal location of these lesions and the increased blood flow that develops in the area of the meningioma. This interpretation is supported by the fact that these patients show a predominance of aneurysms ipsilateral to the tumor and on vessels that supply the tumor.

The most common site of aneurysmal localization in patients with a brain tumor is on the middle cerebral artery. It is of interest that there have been five cases of *giant* middle cerebral artery aneurysms associated with brain tumors. In each of them, severe atherosclerotic changes were found in the cerebral vessels. Although one author suggested a metabolic defect as the cause for both the severe atherosclerosis and aneurysm formation, this mechanism is entirely speculative.

The clinical symptoms presented by the patient usually are related to the tumor. Aneurysmal symptoms were the complaint in less than 25 per cent of the cases reported to date.[80]

Whenever possible, it is advisable to treat both lesions simultaneously, especially when a benign basal tumor such as a meningioma is associated with a basal aneurysm that can be visualized in the same operative field. In order to prevent rupture secondary to brain retraction, it is wise to expose the aneurysm before the tumor is approached. The reported operative mortality rate is almost 40 per cent, but it would appear that with modern operative techniques this rate can be substantially reduced. Of course, the prognosis is dependent upon the nature of the associated neoplasm. The combination of aneurysm and a benign tumor such as a meningioma should have a relatively good prognosis if sufficient care is taken in treating both lesions.

HYDROCEPHALUS

Since the initial work of Bagley, a number of investigators have clarified the clinical and experimental correlates of subarachnoid bleeding and hydrocephalus.[84] Hydrocephalus follows subarachnoid hemorrhage as an acute complication in approximately 15 per cent of cases, and as a late complication in at least 10 per cent of cases.[91,96] The presumed mechanisms of early and late hydrocephalus following subarachnoid hemorrhage differ.

Hydrocephalus may follow subarachnoid hemorrhage due to arteriovenous malformation or aneurysm.[83,87,90-94] Following aneurysmal rupture there is formation of clot in the various compartments of the subarachnoid space: arachnoid villi, lateral cisterns and sulci, and basal cisterns.[86,95] When the bleeding is severe and when a significant portion of the subarachnoid pathways are occluded by blood, acute hydrocephalus may result. The effect of blood in blocking the absorption of spinal fluid has been confirmed experimentally.[85]

Under usual conditions the blood is absorbed within one to two weeks. Residuals of blood breakdown, however, especially hemosiderin, may remain and, owing to mechanisms not understood, lead to scarring of arachnoid villi and adhesions and obstructions of the subarachnoid space. This adhesive process leads to blocking of the flow of cerebrospinal fluid at the basal cisterns, producing the picture of communicating hydrocephalus coming on late after subarachnoid hemorrhage.

Clinically, acute obstruction may contribute to the symptoms of headache, nausea, vomiting, decreased level of consciousness, and changes in vital signs, subsiding as blood is absorbed and cerebrospinal fluid pathways are re-established. The differentiation of hydrocephalus from cerebral edema and decreased cerebral function due to vascular spasm as the cause of these symptoms is difficult.

Late hydrocephalus becomes symptomatic six days to 12 weeks after bleeding, depending on the severity of the adhesive process. In over 50 per cent of the cases there have been multiple episodes of subarachnoid bleeding. Further, while the usual symptoms of headache, confusion, and decreased level of consciousness are commonly associated with a measurable increase in spinal fluid pressure, papilledema is usually absent, presumably because of associated fibrosis of the perioptic subarachnoid space.[87]

Theander and Granholm have emphasized a 20 per cent incidence of mental symptoms, including Korsakoff's syndrome, following subarachnoid hemorrhage.[94] Of 12 such cases, 5 proved to have hydrocephalus, of which 3 were examples of normal-pressure hydrocephalus. Four of the five cases of hydrocephalus presented with Korsakoff's syndrome, and most responded to shunting.

Foltz has estimated that 10 per cent of cases of subarachnoid hemorrhage develop late hydrocephalus and 5 per cent require shunting.[87]

In the series of Yaşargil and associates, 10 per cent of cases developed hydrocephalus, all required shunting procedures, and approximately 70 per cent improved postoperatively, in many cases within one week of operation.

The differential diagnosis of acute hydrocephalus from cerebral swelling secondary to vasospasm is difficult, but may be suggested by the appearance of the usual signs of hydrocephalus in the arteriogram taken to delineate the site of bleeding.

In the chronic phase, the onset of headache, personality change, confusion, and decreased level of consciousness in the absence of papilledema, coming on 1 to 12 weeks after one or more episodes of subarachnoid hemorrhage, will strongly suggest the diagnosis of hydrocephalus. CT scanning will indicate ventricular enlargement, and a pneumoencephalogram will indicate in addition a failure of filling of the basal and lateral cisterns. Cisternography with radioiodinated serum albumin may be used to confirm the diagnosis.

Treatment consists of cerebrospinal fluid shunting procedure.[88] Since the patient may have low-pressure hydrocephalus, it is important that appropriate shunting systems be used. The results following therapy should be good.

In summary, it appears that although many abnormalities have been associated with cerebral aneurysm, only polycystic kidney and coarctation of the aorta occur more than by chance. These produce hypertension and cerebral hemorrhage in the young, have high mortality rates, and require early diagnosis and aggressive operative management. Subarachnoid hemorrhage during pregnancy occurs at about the same incidence rate as in the general population and reaches its peak incidence early in the third trimester of gestation. The management of the cerebral hemorrhage and the delivery should both proceed as indicated individually—with due regard for the safety of the fetus. Finally, in a small percentage of cases of midline aneurysms, hydrocephalus may occur and responds well to ordinary shunting procedures.

REFERENCES

Congenital Malformations and the Etiology of Cerebral Aneurysms

1. Sahs, A. L.: Observations on the Pathology of Saccular Aneurysms in Intracranial Aneurysms and Subarachnoid Hemorrhage—A Cooperative Study. Philadelphia, J. B. Lippincott Co., 1969.
2. Stehbens, W. E.: Cerebral aneurysms and congenital abnormalities. Aust. Ann. Med., *11*:102–112, 1962.
3. Walton, J. N.: Subarachnoid Hemorrhage. Edinburgh, E. & S. Livingstone, Ltd., 1956.

Coarctation of the Aorta

4. Abbott, M. D.: Coarctation of the aorta of adult type. Amer. Heart J., *3*:392–421, 574–618, 1928.
5. Bigelow, N.: Multiple intracranial aneurysms. Arch. Neurol. Psychiat. *73*:76–99, 1955.
6. Eppinger, H.: Stenosis aortae congenita seu isthmus persistens. Vjschr. Prakt. Heilk., *112*:31–67, 1871. (Quoted by Matson, see ref. 9.)
7. Eppinger, H.: Pathogenesis (Histogenesis und Aeriologie) der Aneurysmen einschliesslich des Aneurysma equi verminosum. Pathologisch-anatomische Studien. Arch. Klin. Chir., *35*:suppl. 1, 1887. (Quoted by Matson, see ref. 9.)
8. LeBlanc, F. E., Charrette, E. P., Dobell, A. R. C., and Branch, C. L.: Neurological Complications of Coarctation of the Aorta. Canad. Med. Ass. J., *99*:299–303, 1968.
9. Matson, D.: Intracranial aneurysms in childhood. J. Neurosurg., *23*:578–583, 1965.
10. Robinson, R. G.: Coarctation of the aorta and cerebral aneurysm. J. Neurosurg., *26*:527–531, 1967.
11. Schwartz, M. J., and Baronofsky, I. D.: Ruptured intracranial aneurysm associated with coarctation of the aorta. Report of a patient treated by hypothermia and surgical repair of the coarctation. Amer. J. Cardiol., *6*:982–988, 1960.
12. Sedzimir, C. G., Jones, E. W., Hamilton, D., et al.: Management of coarctation of aorta and bleeding intracranial aneurysm in pediatric cases. Neuropaediatrie, *4*:124–133, 1973.

Polycystic Kidney

13. Bigelow, N. H.: The association of polycystic kidneys with intracranial aneurysms and other related disorders. Amer. J. Med. Sci., *255*:485–494, 1953.
14. Bigelow, N. H.: Multiple intracranial arterial aneurysms. An analysis of their significance. Arch. Neurol. Psychiat., *79*:76–99, 1955.
15. Brown, R. A. P.: Polycystic disease of the kidneys and intracranial aneurysms: Aetiology and inter-relationship of these conditions: Review of recent literature and report of severe cases in which both conditions coexisted. Glasg. Med. J., *32*:33, 1951.
16. Forster, F. M., and Alpers, B. J.: Aneurysms of the circle of Willis associated with congenital polycystic disease of the kidneys. Arch. Neurol. Psychiat., *50*:669, 1943.
17. Sahs, A. L.: Intracranial aneurysms and polycystic kidneys. Arch. Neurol. Psychiat., *63*:524, 1950.
18. Sahs, A. L., and Myers, R.: The coexistence of intracranial aneurysms and polycystic kidney disease. Trans. Amer. Neurol. Ass., *76*:147–150, 1951.

Ehlers-Danlos Syndrome

19. Graf, C. J.: Spontaneous carotid cavernous fistula. Ehlers-Danlos syndrome and related conditions. Arch. Neurol., *15*:662–672, 1965.
20. Rubinstein, M., and Cohen, N. H.: Ehlers-Danlos syndrome associated with multiple intracranial aneurysms. Neurology (Minneap.), *14*:125–132, 1964.
21. Schoolman, A., and Kepes, J.: Bilateral spontaneous carotid-cavernous fistula in Ehlers-Danlos syndrome. J. Neurosurg., *26*:82–86, 1967.

Pregnancy

22. Cannell, D. E., and Botterell, E. H.: Subarachnoid hemorrhage and pregnancy. Amer. J. Obstet. Gynec., *72*:844–855, 1956.
23. Copelan, E. L., and Mabon, R. F.: Spontaneous intracranial bleeding in pregnancy. Obstet. Gynec., *20*:373–378, 1962.
24. Daane, T. A., and Tandy, R. W.: Rupture of congenital aneurysm in pregnancy. Obstet. Gynec., *15*:305, 1960.
25. Herskanen, O., and Nikki, P.: Rupture of intracranial arterial aneurysms during pregnancy. Acta Neurol. Scand., *39*:202–208, 1963.
26. McCausland, A. M., and Holmes, F.: Spinal fluid pressure during labor. Western J. Surg., *65*:220–233, 1957.
27. Pedowitz, P., and Perell, A.: Aneurysms complicated by pregnancy. Part II. Aneurysms of the cerebral vessels. Amer. J. Obstet. Gynec., *73*:736, 1957.
28. Pool, J. L.: Treatment of intracranial aneurysms during pregnancy. J.A.M.A., *192*:209–214, 1965.
29. Pool, J. L., and Potts, D. G.: Aneurysms and Arteriovenous Malformations of the Brain. Diagnosis and Treatment. New York, Hoeber Medical Div., Harper & Row, 1965.
30. Robinson, J. L., Hall, C. S., and Sedzimir, C. B.: Subarachnoid hemorrhage in pregnancy. J.Neurosurg., *36*:27–33, 1972.
31. Robinson, J. L., Hall, C. S., and Sedzimir, C. B.: Arteriovenous malformations, aneurysms, and pregnancy. J. Neurosurg., *41*:63–70, 1974.

Traumatic Aneurysms

32. Alexander, E., Adams, J. E., and Davis, C. H.: Complications in the use of temporary intracranial arterial clip. J. Neurosurg., *20*:810–811, 1963.
33. Asari, S., Nakamura, S., Yamada, O., et al.: Traumatic aneurysm of peripheral cerebral arteries. Report of two cases. J. Neurosurg., *46*:795–803, 1977.
34. Benoit, B. G., and Wortzman, G.: Traumatic cerebral aneurysms. J. Neurol. Neurosurg. Psychiat., *36*:127–138, 1973.
35. Burton, C., Velasco, F., and Dorman, J.: Traumatic aneurysms of a peripheral cerebral artery. J. Neurosurg., *28*:468–474, 1968.
36. Drake, C. G.: Subdural hematoma from arterial rupture. J. Neurosurg., *18*:597–601, 1961.
37. Ferry, D. J., and Kempe, L. G.: False aneurysms secondary to penetration of the brain through orbitofacial wounds. J. Neurosurg., *36*:503–506, 1972.
38. Fleisher, A. S., Patton, J. M., and Tindall, G. T.: Cerebral aneurysms of traumatic origin. Surg. Neurol., *4*:233–239, 1975.
39. Handa, J., Kikuchi, H., Iwayana, K., et al.: Traumatic aneurysms of the internal carotid artery. Acta Neurochir., *17*:161–177, 1967.

40. Harvey, F. H., and Downer, J. L.: Traumatic production of an intracranial berry-like aneurysm in a monkey. Acta Neuropath., *31*:263–266, 1975.
41. Locksley, H. B.: Report on the cooperative study of intracranial aneurysms, subarachnoid hemorrhage, and arteriovenous malformations. Based on 6368 cases in the cooperative study. J. Neurosurg., 25:219–235, 1966.
42. Overton, M. C., and Calvin, T. H.: Iatrogenic cerebral cortical aneurysm. J. Neurosurg., *24*:672–675, 1966.
43. Smith, K. R., and Bardenheier, J. A.: Aneurysm of the pericallosal artery caused by closed cranial trauma. J. Neurosurg., 29:551–554, 1968.
44. White, J. C., Sayre, G. P., and Whisnant, J. P.: Experimental destruction of the media for the production of intracranial cerebral aneurysms. J. Neurosurg., *18*:741–745, 1961.

Mycotic Aneurysms

45. Cantu, R. C., LeMay, M., and Wilkerson, H. A.: The importance of repeated angiography in the treatment of mycotic-embolic intracranial aneurysms. J. Neurosurg., 25:189–193, 1966.
46. Molinari, G., Smith, L., Goldstein, M. N., et al.: Pathogenesis of cerebral mycotic aneurysms. Neurology (Minneap.), 23:325–332, 1973.
47. McDonald, C. A., and Korb, M.: Intracranial aneurysms. Arch. Neurol. (Chicago), *42*:298, 1939.
48. Roach, M. R., and Drake, C. G.: Ruptured cerebral aneurysms caused by micro-organisms. New Eng. J. Med., 273:240–244, 1965.
49. Suwanwela, C., Suwanwela, N., Charuchinda, S., et al.: Intracranial mycotic aneurysms of extravascular origin. J. Neurosurg., *36*:552–559, 1972.
50. Takahashi, M., Killeffer, F., and Wilson, G.: Cerebral mycotic aneurysms. Nippon Acta Radiol., *30*:489–499, 1970.
51. Ziment, I.: Nervous system complications in bacterial endocarditis. Amer. J. Med., *47*:593–607, 1969.

Multiple Aneurysms

52. Bigelow, N. H.: Multiple intracranial arterial aneurysms. AMA Arch. Neurol. Psychiat., *73*:76–98, 1955.
53. Bjorkesten, G., and Troupp, H.: Multiple intracranial arterial aneurysms. Acta Chir. Scand., *118*:387–391, 1959/60.
54. Hamby, W. B.: Multiple intracranial aneurysms. J. Neurosurg., *16*:558–563, 1959.
55. Heiskanen, O.: The identification of ruptured aneurysm in patients with multiple intracranial aneurysms. Neurochirurgia, 8:102–107, 1965.
56. Heiskanen, O., and Marttila, I.: Risk of rupture of a second aneurysm in patients with multiple aneurysms. J. Neurosurg., *32*:295–299, 1970.
57. Mount, L. A., and Brisman, R.: Treatment of multiple intracranial aneurysms. J. Neurosurg., *35*:728–730, 1971.
58. Mount, L. A., and Brisman, R.: Treatment of multiple aneurysms—symptomatic and asymptomatic. Clin. Neurosurg., *20*:166–170, 1973.
59. Moyes, P. D.: Surgical treatment of multiple aneurysms and of incidentally-discovered unrup-

60. McKissock, W., Richardson, A., Walsh, L., et al.: Multiple intracranial aneurysms. Lancet, *1*:623–626, 1964.
61. Paterson, A., and Bond, M. R.: Treatment of multiple intracranial arterial aneurysms. Lancet, *1*:1302–1304, 1973.
62. Pool, J. L., and Potts, D. G.: Aneurysms and Arteriovenous Anomalies of the Brain. Diagnosis and Treatment. New York, Harper & Row, 1965.
63. Sahs, A. L., Perret, G. E., Locksley, H. B., and Nishioka, H.: Intracranial Aneurysms and Subarachnoid Hemorrhage. A Cooperative Study. Philadelphia, J. B. Lippincott Co., 1969.
64. Samson, D. S., Hodosh, R. M., and Clark, W. K.: Surgical management of unruptured asymptomatic aneurysms. J. Neurosurg., *46*:731–734, 1977.
65. Wood, E. H.: Angiographic identification of the ruptured lesion in patients with multiple cerebral aneurysms. J. Neurosurg., *21*:182–198, 1964.

Giant Aneurysms

66. Adams, R. D.: Case records of the Massachusetts General Hospital. Case 22—1963. New Eng. J. Med., *268*:724–731, 1963.
67. Berson, E. L., Freeman, M. I., and Gay, A. J.: Visual field defects in giant suprasellar aneurysms of the internal carotid. Arch. Ophthal., *76*:52–58, 1966.
68. Bird, A. C., Nolan, B., Garbano, F. P., et al.: Unruptured aneurysm of the supraclinoid carotid artery. Neurology (Minneap.), *20*:445–454, 1970.
69. Bull, J.: Massive aneurysms at the base of the brain. Brain, *92*:535–570, 1969.
70. Crompton, M. R.: Mechanism of growth and rupture in cerebral artery aneurysms. Brit. Med. J., *1*:1138–1142, 1966.
71. Fried, L. C., and Ybalk, A.: Rapid formation of giant aneurysm: Case report. J. Neurol. Neurosurg. Psychiat., *35*:527–530, 1972.
72. Hoff, W. F., Hornabrook, R. W., and Marks, V.: Hypopituitarism associated with intracranial aneurysms. Brit. Med. J., *2*:1190–1193, 1961.
73. Jane, J. A.: A large aneurysm of the posterior inferior cerebellar artery in a 1-year-old child. J. Neurosurg., *18*:245–247, 1961.
74. Michael, W. F.: Posterior fossa aneurysms simulating tumors. J. Neurol. Neurosurg. Psychiat., *37*:218–223, 1974.
75. Morley, T. P., and Barr, H. W. K.: Giant intracranial aneurysms: Diagnosis, course, and management. Clin. Neurosurg., *16*:73–94, 1969.
76. Stehbens, W. E.: Intracranial arterial aneurysms. Aust. Ann. Med., *3*:214–220, 1954.
77. Sundt, T. M., Jr., Pluth, J. R., and Gronert, G. A.: Excision of giant basilar aneurysm under profound hypothermia. Report of case. Mayo Clin. Proc., *47*:631–634, 1972.

Brain Tumors

78. Damásio, H., Seabra-Gomes, R., da Silva, J. P.,

et al.: Multiple cerebral aneurysms and cardiac myxoma. Arch. Neurol., *32*:269–270, 1975.

79. Handa, J., Matsuda, I., and Handa, H.: Association of brain tumor and intracranial aneurysms. Surg. Neurol., *6*:25–29, 1976.

80. Pia, H. W., Obrador, S., and Martin, J. G.: Association of brain tumors and arterial intracranial aneurysms. Acta Neurochir., *27*:189–204, 1972.

81. Reina, A., and Seal, R. B.: False cerebral aneurysm associated with metastatic carcinoma of the brain. J. Neurosurg., *41*:380–382, 1974.

82. Taylor, P. E.: Delayed postoperative hemorrhage from intracranial aneurysm after craniotomy for tumor. Neurology (Minneap.), *11*:225–231, 1961.

Hydrocephalus

83. Askenaszy, H. M., Herzberger, E. E., and Wijsenbeck, H. S.: Hydrocephalus with vascular malformations of the brain: A preliminary report. Neurology (Minneap.), *3*:213–220, 1953.

84. Bagley, C. J.: Functional and organic alterations following the introduction of blood into the cerebrospinal fluid. Res. Publ. Ass. Nerv. Ment. Dis., *8*:217–244, 1929.

85. Bradford, F. K., and Sharkey, P. C.: Physiologic effects from introduction of blood and other substances into the subarachnoid space of dogs. J. Neurosurg., *19*:1017–1022, 1962.

86. Ellington, E., and Margolis, T.: Block of arachnoid villus by subarachnoid hemorrhage. J. Neurosurg., *30*:651–657, 1969.

87. Foltz, E. L., and Ward, A. A., Jr.: Communicating hydrocephalus from subarachnoid bleeding. J. Neurosurg., *13*:546–566, 1956.

88. Foltz, E. L.: Hydrocephalus—the value of treatment. Southern Med. J., *61*:443–454, 1968.

89. Hammes. E. M., Jr.: The reactions of the meninges to blood. Arch. Neurol. Psychiat., *52*:505–514, 1944.

90. Kibler, R. F., Couch, R. S. C., and Crompton, M. R. Hydrocephalus in the adult following spontaneous subarachnoid hemorrhage. Brain, *84*:45–61, 1961.

91. Raimondi, A. J., and Torres, H.: Acute hydrocephalus as a complication of subarachnoid hemorrhage. Surg. Neurol., *1*:23–26, 1973.

92. Shulman, K., Martin, B. F., Popoff, N., and Ransohoff, J.: Recognition and treatment of hydrocephalus following spontaneous subarachnoid hemorrhage. J. Neurosurg., *20*:1040–1049, 1963.

93. Strain, R. E.: Progressive communicating hydrocephalus following subarachnoid hemorrhage—a neurosurgical emergency. Southern Med. J., *56*:613–618, 1963.

94. Theander, S., and Granholm, L.: Sequelae after spontaneous subarachnoid hemorrhage, with special reference to hydrocephalus and Korsakoff's syndrome. Acta Neurol. Scand., *43*:479–488, 1967.

95. Tomlinson, B. E.: Brain changes in ruptured intracranial aneurysm. J. Clin. Path., *12*:391–399, 1959.

96. Yasargil, M. G., Yonekawa, Y., Zumstein, B., et al.: Hydrocephalus following spontaneous subarachnoid hemorrhage. J. Neurosurg., *39*:474–479, 1973.

54

SPONTANEOUS INTRACEREBRAL AND INTRACEREBELLAR HEMORRHAGE

Spontaneous hemorrhage into the substance of the brain is usually the result of systemic hypertension.[32,53,151] Although the pathological changes and the order of treatment of intracerebral hemorrhage may differ with the cause, the clinical pictures presented by hemorrhages into the specific areas of the brain are similar. Hypertensive hemorrhages are, therefore, the subject of primary consideration in this chapter after a review of other causes of intracerebral hemorrhage.

Local causes of intracerebral hemorrhage include saccular aneurysms and vascular anomalies, the diagnosis, treatment, and complications of which are described in Chapters 48 through 52.* Intracranial hemorrhage also results from septic emboli, the hemorrhage often originating at the site of mycotic aneurysms that are usually located distally on intracranial vessels.[87,144,185]

Hemorrhage may occur into areas of infarction. Although areas of infarction are often infiltrated with blood cells, Fisher indicates, major hemorrhage into an area of previous infarction is rare; he found only one such in 52 cases of hemorrhagic infarction.[53] Intracerebral hemorrhage is, however, frequently found adjacent to areas of infarction, a point that is expanded later in the discussion of the pathogenesis of hypertensive hemorrhages.

Hemorrhage may occur in intracranial tumors, both primary and metastatic.† Small hemorrhages occur frequently in malignant gliomas and, indeed, account for the variation in the color of glioblastomas from which the name "multiforme" is derived.[65,66,187] Occasionally hemorrhages of clinical significance are seen in glioblastomas and also with oligodendrogliomas and papillomas of the choroid plexus.[1,47,65] Hemorrhages are also seen in association with meningiomas and other primary brain tumors.[13,69,165] Of the metastatic tumors, bronchogenic carcinoma, melanoma, chorioepithelioma, and renal cell carcinoma are most commonly subject to hemorrhage.‡ Hemorrhage into the brain stem may follow transtentorial herniation.[28,84,91,122,154] Such secondary hemorrhages are found in association with supratentorial mass lesions, including tumors and previous hemorrhage. These lesions are most likely to occur in the median or paramedian planes.[124]

Intracerebral hemorrhage may result from lesions of intracranial vessels of a hyperimmune nature, from acute intracranial infectious processes, and from venous thromboses.[79,99,124,151] It may also result from rupture of dilated anastomotic vessels between the external and internal carotid systems resulting from aplasia or previous

---

* See also references 37, 50, 74, 110, 111, 138, 179 for aneurysms; 93, 105, 108 for vascular anomalies.

† See references 13, 65, 66, 69, 82, 86, 99, 156, 158, 164, 165, 169, 177, 178, 187.

‡ See references 156, 158, 169, 177, 178, 187.

M. B. ALLEN, JR., F. YAGHMAI, AND T. EL GAMMAL

occlusion of the major vessels in the neck and at the base of the brain.[51,52,98,166]

Systemic causes of intracerebral hemorrhages include hemorrhagic disorders such as leukemia, hemophilia, aplastic anemia, thrombocytopenic purpura, liver disease, complications of anticoagulation, hypofibrinogenemia, and hypertensive encephalopathy.* Intracerebral hemorrhages are also reported following the use of vasopressor drugs, after angiography, and following certain painful operative procedures.[53] Hemorrhages have been reported recently following open cardiac operations, some cases resulting from emboli or excessive use of anticoagulants.[78] Fisher and others report a few cases of intracerebral hemorrhages in which the cause is not apparent despite careful investigations.[53,99]

HYPERTENSIVE HEMORRHAGES

Pathology

Reports of anatomical localization of hypertensive hemorrhages vary primarily in that hemorrhages of the putamen and thala-

---

* See references 16, 53, 79, 89, 97, 107, 163, 168, 179.

mus are lumped together as lesions of the "basal ganglia" or "capsule" in many.[8,83] Fisher has separated hemorrhages in the region of the basal ganglia into those of the putamen and those of the thalamus, which represent 55 per cent and 10 per cent respectively of all intracerebral hemorrhages of hypertensive origin (Figs. 54–1 and 54–2).[57] Another 15 per cent occur at the junction of the cerebral cortex and white matter, and 20 per cent are divided between the pons and the cerebellum (Figs. 54–3, 54–4, and 54–5). While ratios recorded by other authors vary in minor degrees, this distribution generally prevails.† Hemorrhage may extend into the adjacent structures, i.e., the internal capsule and thalamus, from the putamen or perhaps into the temporal lobe.

A hemorrhage in the putamen may extend along the fibers of the internal capsule in an anterior-posterior direction. Hemorrhages from the putamen may extend into the midbrain. Large supratentorial hemorrhages may be complicated by secondary hemorrhages in the pons and lower midbrain, a complication rarely seen with hemorrhages in the cerebellum.[57,58] Sometimes it is difficult to differentiate hemorrhages of the midbrain that are extensions of supra-

---

† See references 61, 109, 124, 127, 129, 143, 151.

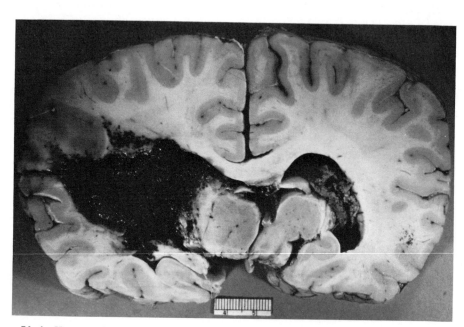

Figure 54–1 Hypertensive hemorrhage probably originating in the putamen and extensively involving the thalamus.

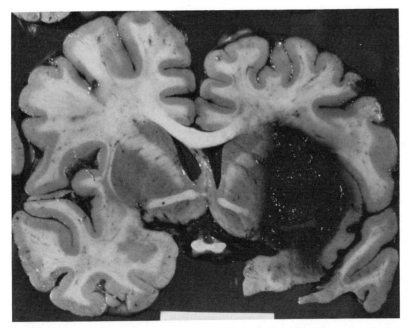

Figure 54–2   Hematoma centered in the putamen. This 57-year-old man had long-standing history of moderately severe hypertension.

tentorial lesions from hemorrhages secondary to herniation unless very discrete dissections are performed. Hemorrhages into the thalamus spread transversely, while those at the base of the cortex tend to separate the cortex from the white matter.

Intracerebral hemorrhages vary widely in size; the size that can be tolerated varies considerably according to anatomical location. Small hemorrhages in the pons may be more devastating than larger ones in the putamen, which in turn are tolerated less well

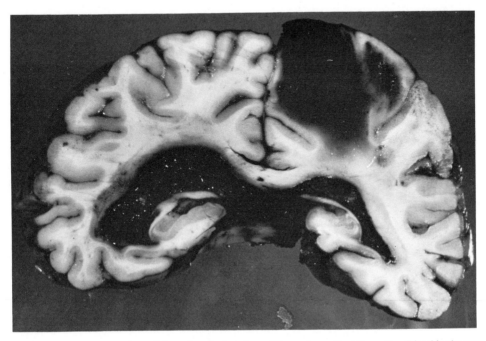

Figure 54–3   Hemorrhage that originated at the junction of the cortex and white matter. Blood in the ventricle is secondary to rupture after dissection through the entire thickness of white matter (at another site).

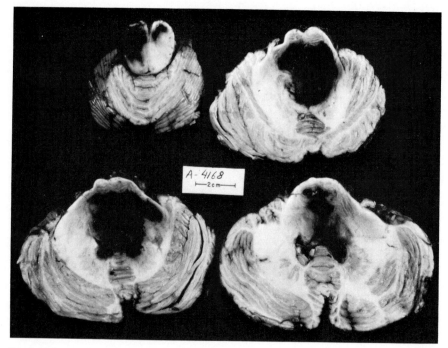

Figure 54–4 Primary pontine hemorrhage. This 37-year-old man had malignant hypertension diagnosed three months previously. The hemorrhage has destroyed the major part of the basis pontis and the tegmentum. It is extending into the midbrain and the fourth ventricle.

than subcortical hemorrhages. Large hemorrhages are often surrounded by petechiae (see Fig. 54–1). Hemorrhages in the region of the pons are likely to destroy surrounding tissue in an explosive fashion.[53]

Tolerance is also influenced by the age of the patient. Older patients tolerate hemorrhages less well than young patients. Initially, a localized blood clot may displace but usually does not destroy surrounding

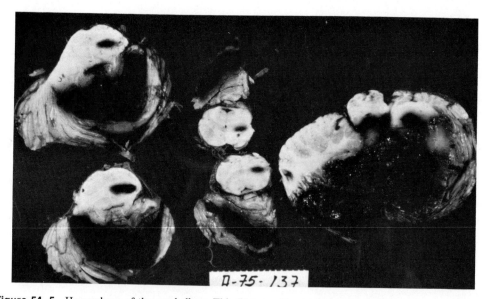

Figure 54–5 Hemorrhage of the cerebellum. This 55-year-old man had long-standing history of moderately severe untreated hypertension. The hemorrhage has destroyed major parts of both cerebellar hemispheres and the vermis. Note the small secondary hematoma in the lateral pons in association with hemorrhage of the cerebellum.

structures as does hemorrhage into areas of infarction. Hemorrhage near the ventricles may "rupture" or, at least, "leak" into the ventricular cavity (cf. Figs. 54–3, 54–10, and 54–11). It is by this route that blood most commonly enters the subarachnoid space. Hemorrhage rarely ruptures through the cortex and pia into the subarachnoid space, although it may occasionally, and cases have been reported in which penetration has extended into the subdural space.[53]

Following hemorrhage, clotting and organization occur. Clots undergo fibrinolysis and liquefaction within a few days. Some authors have postulated that hematomas enlarge in the process, the enlargement being due to influx of fluid into the cavity.[33,43,73,137] It has been supposed that fluid is drawn from a nearby ventricle.[32] The evidence that hematomas expand appears questionable and indeed, Fisher questions whether the tissue surrounding a hematoma is distended by edema as has been suggested.[53] At any rate, following liquefaction, particles of the blood clot are gradually phagocytized and removed.[53] New blood vessels form in the wall.[145] Connective tissue reaction may be followed by calcium deposition.[137] The wall of the cavity becomes lined with rust-colored macrophages.[32,53] The cavity gradually retracts, smaller cavities at the base of the cortex progressing to a characteristic slitlike space.[53]

Pathogenesis

The pathogenesis of intracerebral hemorrhage has remained a topic of controversy since Charcot and Bouchard, over 100 years ago, proposed that bleeding is the result of rupture of miliary aneurysms.[25] Their conclusions were based on examination of brains that had been immersed in running water. Blood vessels were examined under the microscope. Apparently, at least some of the lesions they identified were pseudoaneurysms produced by dissection of blood along the outer walls of blood vessels rather than luminal distentions.[30,70] Some may have been lesions of the blood vessel wall due to atheromatous plaques or degeneration, more recently called lipohyalinosis, hyaloid degeneration, or fibrinoid necrosis.[45,56,70] A number of investigators have questioned the existence

of aneurysmal dilatations on the small penetrating vessels. The presence of microaneurysms, or "miliary" aneurysms, at the bifurcation of the small perforating vessels has been confirmed, and interestingly enough, these minute aneurysms occur in roughly the same distribution as intracerebral hemorrhages.[29,152] Microaneurysms are seen occasionally in normotensive individuals, but they are much more common in hypertensive patients.[152] Hypertension seems to be their cause in a significant proportion of cases.

Other etiologies for intracerebral hemorrhage have been hypothesized.[104,147] Among the more prominent hypotheses is that hemorrhage occurs in areas of infarction due to occlusion.[49,67] Diapedesis is a common occurrence in areas of infarction. Vascular occlusion with resultant infarction is often found in areas adjacent to intracerebral hemorrhage.[55] Major hemorrhage, although rare, occurs in areas of recent cerebral infarction; however, when it does, there is significant destruction of the tissue surrounding the area of hemorrhage, a finding not seen when intracerebral hemorrhage occurs in the absence of previous infarction.[53] Careful pathological examinations have demonstrated many hemorrhages without occlusions of major vessels of the cerebrum.

Vascular spasm was advanced as an explanation for cerebral infarction leading to cerebral hemorrhage.[181] Coexistence of inflammatory or allergic lesions of the vessels of the brain has been hypothesized; and, indeed, vasculitis occasionally coexists with intracerebral hemorrhage, but inflammatory lesions do not appear to be a logical explanation for a large portion of spontaneous intracranial hemorrhages.[10,80,82,99]

It is now clear that factors that make penetrating vessels of the brain vulnerable to rupture and hemorrhage include systemic hypertension and lipohyalinosis, or degeneration, of the vessel walls (Figs. 54–6 through 54–9).[49] Microaneurysms, while often present, are not always the source of bleeding. Hyalinosis of the vessel walls often coexists with microaneurysms in the same or adjacent vessels but is not invariably present in the wall of the aneurysm.[153] Lipohyalinosis produces thickening of the walls of blood vessels. Changes may proceed to the point of vascular occlusion, or the vessel wall may be penetrated, with re-

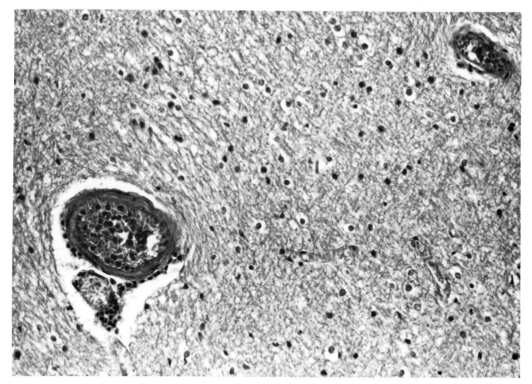

Figure 54–6 Early hypertensive changes of the cerebral vessels. Two arterioles show mild hypertrophy of the media. Hematoxylin and eosin, 125×.

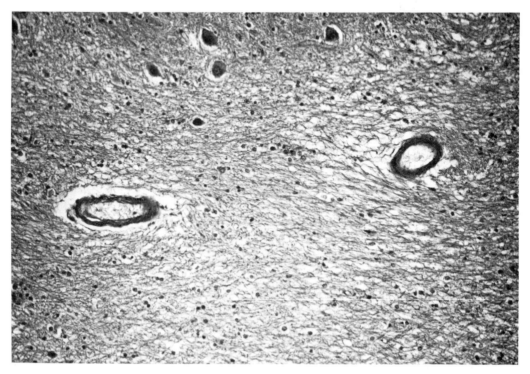

Figure 54–7 Mild hyaline sclerosis. The two arterioles show thickening attributed to hypertension. Hematoxylin and eosin, 65×.

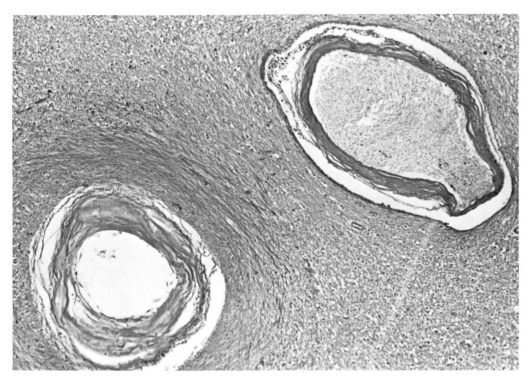

Figure 54–8   Marked hyaline sclerosis. The changes result from long-standing hypertension. The lower vessel shows marked narrowing of the lumen. Note the thinning of the wall of the upper vessel producing an aneurysmal dilatation. Hematoxylin and eosin. 25×.

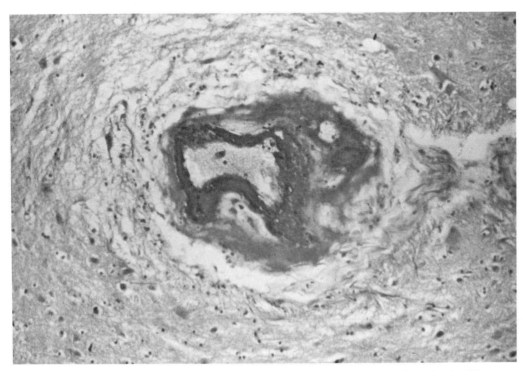

Figure 54–9   Arteriolar lipohyalinosis due to severe hypertension. Hematoxylin and eosin, 100×.

sulting major hemorrhage.[172] If the degeneration causes occlusion of the vessel, there may result an area of infarction that later converts into a lacuna.[55] Lacunae are often coexistent with hemorrhages in the same brain.[49,56] The same or adjacent vessels may be subject to hemorrhage and occlusion. Areas of infarction and hemorrhage are often adjacent, but the infarction is not routinely the cause of hemorrhage.[53]

Most hemorrhages result from rupture of a single vessel. Often, putaminal hemorrhage follows rupture of the largest and most lateral penetrating branch of the middle cerebral artery. Usually the source of intracerebral hemorrhage is a small penetrating vessel that branches directly from a major cerebral vessel. It has been proposed that the small penetrating vessels are subjected to pressures that are disproportionately high for their size because the usual "stepdown" in pressure resulting from progressive branching is missing.[53]

Clinical Presentation

Age distribution of hypertensive hemorrhages extends from the third to the ninth decade, with the great majority occurring between 40 and 70 years of age.[19,83,143] Sex distribution has varied from report to report, the Scandinavians reporting a predominance among women, while American authors have reported a fairly equal distribution.* Davidoff found a predominance in females in his own series, but stated that hemorrhages occurred predominantly in males, two to one, in the literature that he had reviewed.[38] Generally, the sex differences are insignificant.

Fisher described in detail clinical findings in a series of patients with hypertensive intracerebral hemorrhages in 1961.[54] More recently, he discretely categorized the clinical syndromes.[57] Most of this section is drawn from Fisher's reports. These clinical descriptions are, however, generalizations. Individual cases may present less typically when hemorrhages are small or in unusual locations. Fortunately, with the current availability of computed tomography, diagnosis of intracerebral hemorrhage can be readily made.

*See references 9, 27, 36, 83, 141, 186.

By definition, hypertensive hemorrhages occur in patients with hypertension, usually in the range of 200/100 mm of mercury, although intracerebral hemorrhages are seen in patients with systolic pressures as low as 160 mm of mercury. Although the syndromes described are found in patients with typical hypertensive hemorrhages, they may also be seen in patients with intracerebral hemorrhage from other causes.

Supratentorial hemorrhages may be painless unless they occur near the surface of the brain, in which case they are likely to be associated with frontal headache lateralized to the side of the hemorrhage.[57] Blood in the subarachnoid fluid usually results from penetration of the hematoma into a ventricle. Neurological deficits usually commence without warning and progress gradually. Most intracerebral hemorrhages occur during waking hours and during or following periods of strong exertion.

Putaminal Hemorrhage

Early symptoms associated with hemorrhages in the region of the putamen are due to impairment of function of the posterior limb of the internal capsule. A progressive hemiparesis or hemiplegia is usually associated with sensory loss. Visual field defects may be prominent, and dysphasia occurs if the dominant hemisphere is involved. Recognition and control of the contralateral limbs are likely to be absent if the nondominant hemisphere is affected. The eyes usually deviate toward the side of the lesion, but eye movements will be full on rotation of the neck or tilting of the head. Epileptic seizures in association with putaminal hemorrhage may involve only the paralyzed side. Deficits may progress over a few minutes or for as much as a couple of days. Signs of subarachnoid hemorrhage may develop while the patient remains alert. If the hemorrhage dissects along the internal capsule into the midbrain, a third nerve palsy may result.

If hemorrhage extends into the ventricle, the cerebrospinal fluid pressure may become quite high even when the quantity of blood in the brain tissue is small. Coma occurs early, eyes deviating toward the side of the paralysis. Brain stem compression may cause the contralateral pupil to dilate first.

According to Fisher, a paradoxical state

may develop in which the patient is in coma from a putaminal hemorrhage while retaining reflex extraocular movements. He ascribes this paradoxical state to compression and displacement of the subthalamic area or anterior midbrain that spare the third nerve complexes.

After the patient has reached the hemiplegic stage, his clinical picture may remain stable for several hours before signs of brain stem compression appear, and this may produce a false sense of security before the course progresses to its ultimate fatal outcome. Diabetes insipidus or inappropriate secretion of antidiuretic hormone may occur.

Thalamic Hemorrhage

Hemorrhage may occur into any part of the thalamus and may vary in size from less than 1 cm to 3 to 4 cm in diameter. It may originate in the thalamus primarily or extend across the internal capsule from the putamen. Blood may find its way into the third or lateral ventricles. Neurological deficits develop more slowly than those associated with putaminal hemorrhages. Thalamic hemorrhages are usually associated with progressive hemiparesis because of pressure on the internal capsule. Contralateral sensory loss results from involvement of the sensory nuclei in the thalamus. Numbness may be an early symptom. Symptoms are very similar to those produced by lesions in the putamen except for ocular signs. Patients with hemorrhage into the thalamus may demonstrate paresis of vertical gaze, upward gaze usually being impaired before downward gaze. Patients, at rest, usually have a mild downward and inward deviation of the eyes. The hemorrhage may produce a small pupil ipsilaterally. In some cases, the eyes deviate toward the side of the paresis. This is attributed to extension of blood into the third ventricle with dilatation. A "pseudoparalysis" of the sixth nerve may develop in which the eyes fail to move bilaterally unless caloric stimulation is applied. According to Fisher, homonymous hemianopia occurs only when the hemorrhages are situated far inferiorly. Drowsiness is an almost constant finding. Mutism is common with large hemorrhages. Patients with thalamic hemorrhages may linger on in stupor for prolonged periods. They may develop acute hydrocephalus due to compression or occlusion of the third ventricle, necessitating some sort of shunting procedure.

Cortical and Subcortical Hemorrhage

Fisher includes under this category all hemorrhages in the cerebral hemisphere outside the basal ganglia and thalamus. Most hemispheric hemorrhages originate beneath the cortex. Some apparently begin in the depths of the white matter. A rare one appears in the subependymal area. Many hematomas, located beneath the ependyma, originate in the deep nuclear structures. It may be difficult to determine whether some hemorrhages originate in the subcortical region or in the basal ganglia. Most subcortical hemorrhages originate in the temporal, parietal, and occipital lobes, but the frontal lobes are not excluded. As size and location vary, so do the clinical signs.

Headache may be prominent, even as the initial complaint. Headaches are usually lateralized to the side of the hemorrhage. Lesions in the posterior half of the brain lead to appropriately lateralized hemianopia and sensory deficits. Aphasia, dyslexia, and memory deficits may be prominent with a hemorrhage in the dominant hemisphere, while constructional apraxia and minor apractic agnosia may be prominent with a hemorrhage in the nondominant hemisphere.

Frontal hemorrhages may produce varying degrees of paresis. Dysphasia may be a major complaint with lateral lesions in the dominant hemisphere. Medial frontal lesions are more likely to be associated with incontinence, grasping and sucking reflexes, and abulia.

Seizures may play a prominent role in subcortical hemorrhages. They usually are focal. Large hemorrhages may extend into the ventricles, producing bloody cerebrospinal fluid, but smaller ones may remain fixed within the cerebral tissue. While the symptoms of small hemorrhages remain focalized, larger hemorrhages may produce brain stem compression with progressive drowsiness and stupor.

Pontine Hemorrhage

Hemorrhage into the pons is usually devastating, often being associated with sudden onset of headache, progressive stupor, and coma with total paralysis. Cessation of respiration may occur within a few hours of the initial symptoms. Initially, respirations may be increased, but prior to death, respiration becomes slow and gasping. In the interim, the pupils usually become small but continue to react. Spontaneous eye movement may be lost early. The eyes are usually fixed slightly upward, and "eye bobbing" is typical. With loss of sympathetic activity, sweating ceases and body temperatures may rise to above 106°F before death.

In a few cases, pontine hemorrhages remain small. The authors have observed two cases in which there was evidence of spontaneous evacuation of hematomas within the pons and have found two reports of operative evacuation of pontine hemorrhages.[11,44,92] Patients with such limited lesions typically have unilateral cranial nerve palsies with contralateral hemiparesis, nystagmus, ataxia associated with internuclear ophthalmoplegia, and dysarthria. The small lesions may have an insidious onset, leading to an erroneous diagnosis of neoplasm. Fisher reports that some pontine hemorrhages dissect through the cerebellar peduncles.[57]

Cerebellar Hemorrhage

Spontaneous hemorrhage into the parenchyma of the cerebellum usually occurs in the region of a dentate nucleus. Beginning in one cerebellar hemisphere, hemorrhage may extend across the midline. With rare exception, severe headaches accompany the ictus, the headache being located usually in the occipital region but occasionally in the frontal area.

Paresis is rarely an early sign of cerebellar hemorrhage. There is usually severe ataxia leading to inability to stand or walk, the patient falling to the side of the lesion. Owing to clumsiness of the ipsilateral extremities, patients often feel that they are paralyzed. Vomiting may be prominent. Dysarthria is often present. Lumbar puncture, if performed, will usually produce bloody cerebrospinal fluid within a few hours of the hemorrhage. Nuchal rigidity may be late in appearing but gradually progressive.

Eye signs are among the most important clinical diagnostic features. There is often paralysis of the ipsilateral sixth nerve producing paresis of lateral gaze to the side of the lesion and forced deviation of the eyes to the contralateral side. There may also be transient deviation of the eyes to the side of the lesion when they are initially opened. Internuclear ophthalmoplegia may be unilateral or bilateral, and there may be diplopia and oscillopsia. Eyes will still move in a full range on caloric stimulation, however. Horizontal nystagmus is almost constant.

Signs of cerebellar hemorrhage progress at variable rates. According to Fisher, about 75 per cent of patients with hemorrhage into the cerebellum will go on to death if not treated operatively, but at least 25 per cent will experience spontaneous recovery. Progression may be heralded by an ipsilateral facial palsy. Drowsiness may develop, although this is a fairly late sign. A Babinski sign may appear on the contralateral side, followed by a similar sign on the ipsilateral side. Fisher describes vertical deviation of the eyes in which the ipsilateral eye is lower than the contralateral one. He also has noted limitation of upward and downward gaze and involuntary closure of one eye.

As symptoms progress, the patient becomes restless and may become incontinent. Tremors and flapping movements may appear. Respiratory arrest may occur suddenly and with little warning. Respiratory arrest is ascribed to pressure at the pontomedullary junction. The cerebellar tonsils rarely show pressure cones in postmortem examinations of patients with cerebellar hemorrhage.

Fisher describes atypical cases in which there is inability to move any one or two of the four limbs. He also mentions that aphasia may occur either as an isolated deficit or in combination with paresis. In a few cases of small hemorrhages, the clots may not reach the cerebrospinal fluid. Such patients complain of dizziness, nausea, and vomiting, and they have unilateral cerebellar signs.

DIAGNOSTIC PROCEDURES

Ultrasound

Echoencephalography has proved to be helpful in diagnosing supratentorial mass lesions by demonstrating evidence of shift of midline structures and the size of the lateral ventricles.[59,171] Sophisticated techniques have been developed whereby echoencephalography may be used to demonstrate size and location of specific mass lesions and even to determine some of their characteristics, i.e., density and shape. Echoencephalography may demonstrate pulsatile masses. Such techniques require complete familiarity with the technical procedures. When personnel remain constant, over 90 per cent of intracranial masses can be accurately diagnosed. Unfortunately, ultrasonic techniques do not outline blood vessels. The recent development of computed tomography has rendered the diagnostic capabilities of ultrasound almost obsolete when applied to intracerebral hemorrhage. Ultrasound, however, remains an inexpensive and noninvasive method of following patients who have had previous intracranial operations for lesions above the tentorium when there is some concern regarding their clinical status.

Radionuclide Scanning

Early reports on radionuclide scanning suggested that techniques using isotopes were helpful in outlining vascular lesions of the brain. Deland reported that in 50 per cent of hemorrhagic lesions brain scans were positive within a week of the onset of the symptoms and that 75 per cent of such lesions could be demonstrated within four weeks of the hemorrhage.[41] Ciric, Quinn, and Bucy reported that 5 of 13 brain scans in patients with intracerebral hematomas were abnormal.[26] Overton and Glasgow and their co-workers reported that isotopic brain scans were routinely positive or, at least, questionable in their cases of intracranial hematoma.[64,131] Allen and his colleagues were able to find only one positive and two suspicious scans of four performed on patients with intracranial hematomas.[3] Most of the scans in these series were performed with isotopes of iodine or mercury, isotopes rarely used for brain scanning today.

Scans with technetium pertechnetate are not reliably positive in a high percentage of cases, but the diagnostic capabilities of radionuclide scanning may be improved by demonstrating vascular displacement when the displacement is marked.[146,159,161] At best, radionuclide scanning provides suggestive evidence of intracerebral hemorrhages.

Computed Tomography

Computed tomography (CT), where available, is now the investigation of choice in diagnosing intracerebral collections of blood. An intracerebral hemorrhage was identified in the first report on the clinical application of the technique.[133] Computed tomography has been reported to be capable of routinely identifying intracerebral blood in two large series of patients[133,151] This diagnostic capability is based upon a comparison of characteristics of different intracranial structures.[76] Not only the location of intracerebral hemorrhages but the size of such lesions and the point at which they most closely approximate the surface can be identified. Computed tomography indicates which intracranial structures are likely to be involved by the hemorrhage. Evidence of surrounding edema may also be demonstrated. It has now been shown that the capability of computed tomography far exceeds that of angiography in demonstrating the location of intracerebral hemorrhage (Fig. 54–10).[22,157]

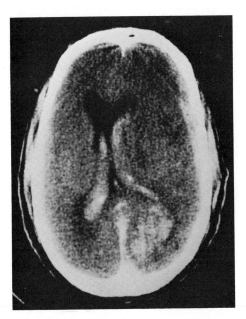

Figure 54–10 Spontaneous hemorrhage into right occipital lobe with extension into the lateral ventricles is shown in CT scan. Note the shift of the ventricles due to the mass effect of the intracerebral hematoma.

Identification of intracerebral hemorrhage is based upon high attenuation of
blood, which varies between 22 and 45 EMI
units. While the initial impression was that
the high attenuation was a characteristic of
clotted blood, it has now been determined
that the attenuation of blood in liquid form
is as high as that of clotted blood.[22,125,157] This
laboratory finding is confirmed clinically by
the demonstration of high attenuation produced by liquefied blood within ventricles
(Fig. 54–11). Also, normal carotid and basilar arteries may be demonstrated without
enhancement. Clotting is not essential to
the demonstration of intracerebral hemorrhage by computed tomography. Further
investigations have shown that it is the high
concentration of the protein segment of hemoglobin that accounts principally for the
high attenuation of blood.[125]

There is considerable variation in the rate
at which the features of intracerebral hemorrhage demonstrated on the CT scan are
dissipated. Cases have been seen in which
areas of high attenuation have persisted for
as much as three months after the ictus. In
the majority of cases, however, the high
attenuation disappears within a few
weeks. Significant change can sometimes
be detected as early as one week after hemorrhage. The decrease in attenuation does
not necessarily indicate that the blood has
been resorbed. Two cases have been reported in which the attenuation had returned to normal before postmortem examinations revealed persistent intracerebral

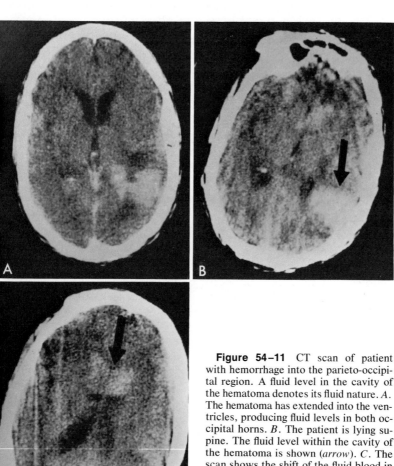

Figure 54–11 CT scan of patient
with hemorrhage into the parieto-occipital region. A fluid level in the cavity of
the hematoma denotes its fluid nature. *A*.
The hematoma has extended into the ventricles, producing fluid levels in both occipital horns. *B*. The patient is lying supine. The fluid level within the cavity of
the hematoma is shown (*arrow*). *C*. The
scan shows the shift of the fluid blood in
the frontal horns (*arrow*).

blood.[117] Other studies have demonstrated that areas of increased attenuation seen by computed tomography may disappear before the hemorrhagic mass resolves, but the limits of a residual hemorrhage may be outlined with contrast enhancement, evidenced by a ring surrounding the area of hemorrhage.[116]

Contrast Enhancement

Intravenous injection of an iodinated compound will result in increased attenuation of those structures in which the iodine remains concentrated. Blood vessels and areas of breakdown in the "blood-brain barrier" as in tumors or areas of infarction, may be identified by "enhancement." Indications for contrast-enhanced computed tomography in patients suspected of having an intracranial hemorrhage include evidence of an arteriovenous malformation and suggestion of a neoplastic lesion or cerebral infarction. Evidence of an arteriovenous malformation includes intracranial bruit, intracerebral hemorrhage in a child or young adult, an irregularly shaped or "mottled" hematoma on the CT scan, or hemorrhage near the surface of the brain. Mottling may be produced by large blood vessels of an arteriovenous malformation and constitutes a strong indication for contrast enhancement. Likewise, hemorrhages near the surface of the brain are more likely to be the result of a vascular malformation, aneurysm, or tumor than are deep lesions.

A history of, a physical examination suggestive of, or radiographic evidence of a neoplasm, and computed tomographic evidence of a large area of diminished attenuation surrounding an area of hemorrhage are other indications for contrast enhancement. Large areas of decreased attenuation surrounding hemorrhage are rare unless the hemorrhage is complicating another lesion such as a neoplasm or infarction (Fig. 54–12).

Angiography may be required to differentiate hemorrhagic lesions identified by computed tomography. Indications include (1) hemorrhages in children suggesting an arteriovenous malformation; (2) subarachnoid hemorrhage suggesting aneurysm, as shown in Figure 54–13; (3) evidence of neoplasm, especially meningioma; (4) hemorrhagic infarction; and (5) giant aneurysms. The differentiation of primary intracerebral hemorrhage from hemorrhagic infarction may be difficult. Although in initial reports differentiation was made by the finding of an irregular area of high attenuation lying within a large area of decreased attenuation, hemorrhages have been found to be so diffuse that differentiation cannot easily be made by computed tomography (Fig. 54–14). Angiographic demonstration of absence or displacement of vessels may be required to differentiate the two.

Angiography

Kristiansen described the advantages of carotid angiography in diagnosing intracranial hematomas as early as 1948.[94] Most of the hemorrhages reported in his paper resulted from trauma and produced significant displacement of surface vessels. Angiography became the accepted mode of diagnosis of intracranial hemorrhage of traumatic etiology. Its advantages in the diagnosis of saccular aneurysms and vascular anomalies led to its routine performance for diagnosing vascular lesions in most neurosurgical services. In the diagnosis of deep intracerebral hematomas, however, it has limitations because the shifts of large surface vessels are limited.

Ten years after Kristiansen's demonstration of the advantages of angiography for diagnosing surface hemorrhage, Andersen reported on the diagnostic value of examining the lenticulostriate arteries and deep veins in the search for deep cerebral hemorrhage.[6] He expanded this report in 1963, discussing the angiographic localization of small intracerebral hematomas.[7] Another report in 1966 by Westberg took issue with some of the anatomical findings of Andersen, but each of these reports demonstrated the advantages of discretely investigating the lenticulostriate vessels to localize deep intracerebral hemorrhages.[180]

The small penetrating vessels that supply the basal ganglia are branches of the anterior and middle cerebral arteries. In the angiogram made in the frontal projection, vessels take an initial medialward course, but subsequently turn lateralward to pass into the region below the lateral ventricle. Hemorrhage in the lateral putamen or temporal lobe may displace these vessels medially, while more medial hemorrhages displace

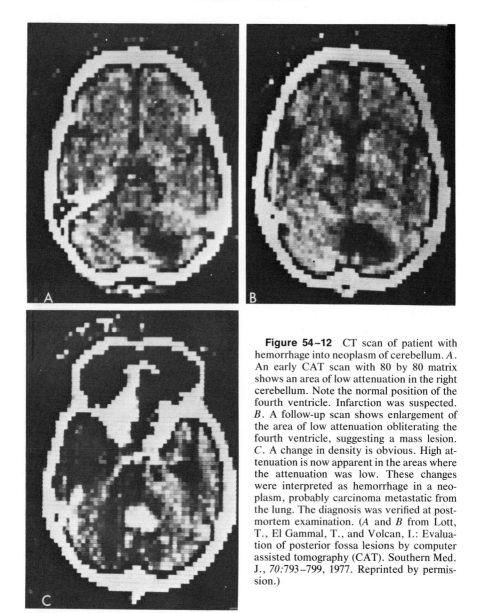

Figure 54–12 CT scan of patient with hemorrhage into neoplasm of cerebellum. *A*. An early CAT scan with 80 by 80 matrix shows an area of low attenuation in the right cerebellum. Note the normal position of the fourth ventricle. Infarction was suspected. *B*. A follow-up scan shows enlargement of the area of low attenuation obliterating the fourth ventricle, suggesting a mass lesion. *C*. A change in density is obvious. High attenuation is now apparent in the areas where the attenuation was low. These changes were interpreted as hemorrhage in a neoplasm, probably carcinoma metastatic from the lung. The diagnosis was verified at postmortem examination. (*A* and *B* from Lott, T., El Gammal, T., and Volcan, I.: Evaluation of posterior fossa lesions by computer assisted tomography (CAT). Southern Med. J., *70:*793–799, 1977. Reprinted by permission.)

them lateralward as shown in Figure 54–15 or, in some cases, separate them. Similarly, in the lateral view, the vessels may be elevated by temporal lesions. Hemorrhages at the base of the lateral ventricle may cause depression. Dilatation of the lateral ventricle resulting from rupture of hemorrhage into the ventricular system may cause lateral displacement of these deep vessels.

Subcortical hemorrhages tend to displace larger vessels over the surface of the brain, especially when these hemorrhages are located in the frontal or temporal lobes. Large hemorrhages, located more pos-

teriorly, likewise may produce shifts of the midline vessels while producing milder displacements of surface vessels. Paraventricular lesions may be difficult to demonstrate by angiography, however.[86]

Angiography of the posterior fossa permits the diagnosis of deep intracerebellar lesions if they have shifted the vermial vessels or elevated the superior cerebellar arteries.[106] Likewise, angiograms revealing pontine hemorrhage have been carefully described.[123] *In summary,* angiography is most important in demonstrating gross lesions of blood vessels that cause intracere-

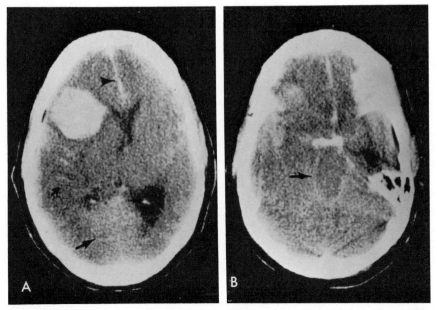

Figure 54-13   CT scan of patient with a left temporal hematoma secondary to an intracranial aneurysm. *A*. There is evidence of subarachnoid hemorrhage along the shifted anterior falx (*anterior arrow*). There is also evidence of subarachnoid bleeding around the tentorium (*posterior arrow*) and in the sylvian fissure (*middle arrow*). There is also a shift of the midline structures to the right. *B*. Subarachnoid hemorrhage around the brain stem (*arrow*), which appears flattened and elongated owing to tentorial herniation.

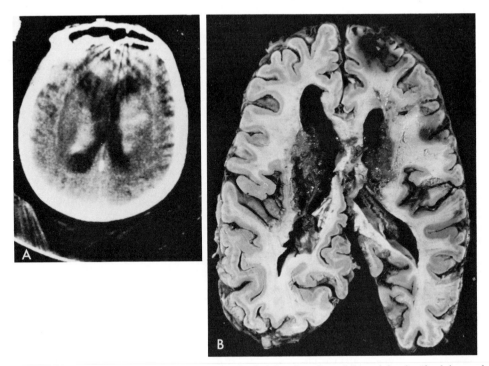

Figure 54-14   *A*. CT scan of a patient with hemorrhagic infarction shows bilateral density (fresh hemorrhage) in the basal ganglia. It was taken two months prior to the death of this 80-year-old man. *B*. A horizontal section through the basal ganglia of the same patient shows that the hemorrhage and part of the infarcted basal ganglia have been removed during the two months that the patient survived. The lesion grossly and microscopically was a "hemorrhagic infarction."

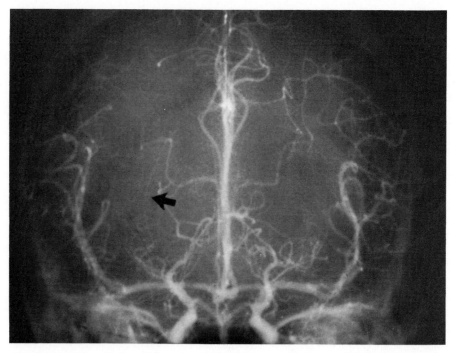

Figure 54–15   Frontal projection of bilateral carotid arteriogram (simultaneous injection) showing no displacement of the anterior cerebral arteries. The sylvian fissures appear asymmetrical, the right one being displaced laterally. Note stretching of one of the lenticulostriate arteries (*arrow*). This appearance is consistent with a deep ganglia mass such as is seen in deep cerebral hemorrhage. In this particular patient, the deep veins were shifted, as was shown on a later film.

bral hemorrhage, but in the case of hypertensive hemorrhages, the technique has limitations.[121] Angiography is helpful in differentiating primary intracerebral hemorrhage from hemorrhagic infarction and it helps to demonstrate associated lesions such as neoplasms, but computed tomography is replacing angiography as a primary diagnostic study for deep intracerebral hemorrhages.

Air Encephalography

Classically, angiography has been considered the primary contrast study for patients with intracranial vascular lesions. McKissock and co-workers, however, reported that angiograms were considered normal in 30 per cent of cases of deep-seated hematoma, and Arseni and associates, in 1967, indicated the need for additional diagnostic studies after angiography in patients with deep hematomas.[12,113]

It has been pointed out that as many as 80 per cent of deep cerebral hemorrhages rupture into the ventricles. Whereas it was formerly thought that rupture of intracerebral hemorrhages into the ventricles was usually lethal, it is now known that the extension of hemorrhage into the ventricular cavities may be associated with very little clinical change.[15,57,157] The outcome is not necessarily ominous; intraventricular extensions of hematomas are often resorbed.[24,44,100,130]

Air encephalography outlines the form of the ventricles and their contents better than other contrast examinations. Polytome pneumography outlines small defects in the walls of the ventricles. Air may be used to advantage to outline hematomas that are deforming or extruding into the ventricles. Repeat studies may be used to follow mass lesions due to hemorrhage (Figs. 54–16 and 54–17). Follow-up studies may be necessary to rule out neoplastic lesions whose radiographic pictures may mimic those of hematomas.[15] Some authors have also reported the use of air to outline deep cerebral cavities at the time hematomas were evacuated by aspiration.[12]

Pneumography is preferable to diagnostic ventriculography and it can be safely performed after an angiogram has ruled out

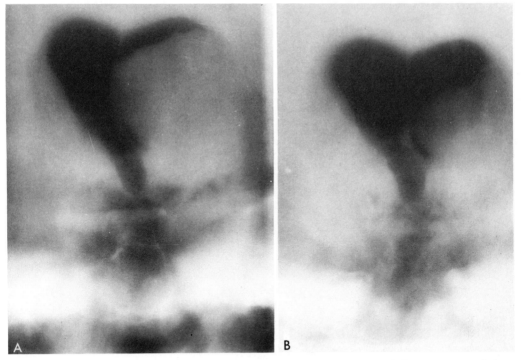

Figure 54–16 Frontal tomogram with the patient positioned with the brow up during pneumoencephalography. *A.* A large mass is protruding into the left lateral ventricle. *B.* A follow-up polytome pneumoencephalogram at the same level (at the foramen of Monro) shows marked regression of the previously diagnosed intracerebral hematoma.

a midline shift; one should, however, be prepared to perform ventricular puncture in the event of an increase in cerebrospinal fluid pressure.

Air studies have clearly offered a refinement in the diagnosis of deep-seated hemorrhage, but with the advent of computed tomography, their use has become limited to the definition of small lesions or lesions in the posterior fossa where computed tomography may be less sensitive than it is in the diagnosis of lesions located above the tentorium.

MANAGEMENT OF THE PATIENT WITH INTRACEREBRAL OR INTRACEREBELLAR HEMORRHAGE

It is customary to divide the treatment of hemorrhage into the brain into medical and surgical aspects. All patients with intracerebral hemorrhage should receive medical therapy and be evaluated for operative evacuation of the mass. The two types of treatment must be integrated and not considered to be competitive.

An excellent review on the management of stroke patients has been published recently by Toole and co-workers, representing the clinical management study committee for stroke.[174]

Emergency Evaluation

Initially, patients who have sustained intracerebral hemorrhage require assurance of adequate respiratory and circulatory functions. Once such functions have been assured, an adequate history, a physical examination, and appropriate diagnostic investigations should be accomplished.

History and Examination

The history frequently reveals an insidious onset of neurological deficits, which may be followed by headache. The neurological deficits and even the headaches are modified by the location of the hemorrhage.

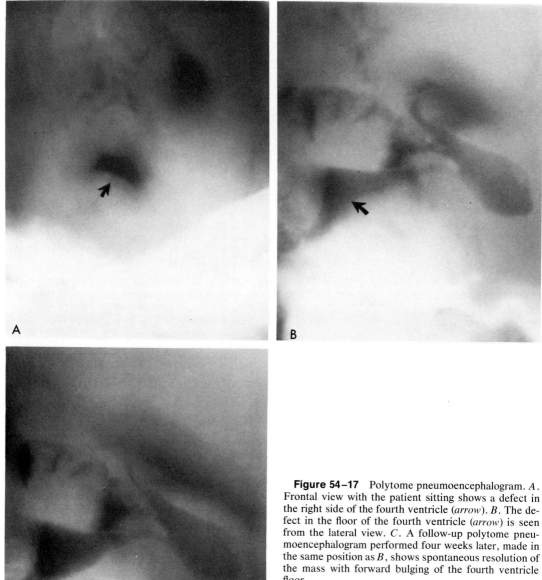

Figure 54–17 Polytome pneumoencephalogram. *A*. Frontal view with the patient sitting shows a defect in the right side of the fourth ventricle (*arrow*). *B*. The defect in the floor of the fourth ventricle (*arrow*) is seen from the lateral view. *C*. A follow-up polytome pneumoencephalogram performed four weeks later, made in the same position as *B*, shows spontaneous resolution of the mass with forward bulging of the fourth ventricle floor.

Headache is more prominent with hemorrhages near the surface of the brain.

History taking should include inquiries into previous episodes of hemorrhage, both intracranial and systemic, and indications of systemic hypertension and medications taken.

Neurological examination should determine, in addition to the state of consciousness, evidence of paresis or loss of specific sensibilities. Tests of cerebellar function are particularly important when hemorrhage in the posterior fossa is considered. Ocular findings may give evidence of long-standing hypertension, and eye signs are of great help in differentiating between lesions of the putamen, thalamus, and cerebellum.

Diagnostic Evaluation

Initial clinical diagnostic investigations should include tests of the components of blood required to control bleeding and bleeding tendencies, accomplished by obtaining the prothrombin time, the partial thromboplastin time, and a determination of the adequacy of platelets. A normal prothrombin time assures adequacy of extrinsic factors that bear on bleeding, while deficiency of any intrinsic factors will alter the partial thromboplastin time. Adequacy of platelets may be determined by smear or count and confirmed by a normal bleeding time.

Computed tomography is the initial diagnostic procedure of choice and may be the only one necessary to identify the location of intraparenchymatous hemorrhage. If available, a CT scan should be performed prior to lumbar puncture, which will reveal the presence of subarachnoid blood in about 80 per cent of cases.

The location of an intraparenchymatous hemorrhage often suggests its etiology. Subarachnoid collections of blood suggest rupture of a saccular aneurysm, but arteriovenous malformations may produce hemorrhages that can be confused with the spontaneous hemorrhage due to hypertension Differentiation may be accomplished by intravenous injection of iodinated enhancement compounds.

Angiography should be accomplished in those cases in which an arteriovenous malformation, a saccular aneurysm, or a tumor is considered a likely source of the bleeding. Brain scans and air studies are now rarely necessary but may be required to evaluate patients where computed tomography is not available.

Medical Therapy

Medical therapy includes: (1) administration of appropriate amounts of fluid, electrolytes, and nutrients; (2) maintenance of elimination; (3) adequate care of skin and lungs; (4) control of fever; (5) therapy for headache and restlessness; (6) antihypertensive medication; and (7) control of intracranial pressure.

Administration of Fluids and Nutrients

Fluid maintenance for the average adult requires 1600 to 2000 ml per day, and most adults with normal kidney function can tolerate this level of fluids without difficulty. This quantity must be adjusted in cases of inappropriate antidiuretic hormone secretion or diabetes insipidus, either of which may accompany intracranial hemorrhage.

Fluids usually should be administered intravenously in the early postictal period, especially in stuporous patients whose state of consciousness is depressed. Vomiting is often troublesome after an intracranial hemorrhage, and intravenous administration of fluids during this period is mandatory. Fluids may be administered by mouth in alert patients after vomiting has subsided or by nasogastric tube in stuporous patients. A cuffed endotracheal tube is necessary initially in the stuporous patient, however, to protect him from aspiration pneumonia.

Restriction of fluids is recommended by some authors, but this is probably not necessary if adequate quantities of electrolytes are administered and careful monitoring of electrolytes (at least twice daily) is maintained. Fluids should be restricted if the serum concentration of sodium is decreasing. Saline or lactated Ringer's solution is less likely to produce cerebral edema than are hypotonic solutions. Administration of electrolytes must be adjusted according to their concentrations in the blood.

Nutrition may not be of great concern initially, but depending upon the weight of the patient, administration of about 1000 calories per day should be begun by the fourth to fifth day after the ictus. Nourishment is usually administered by nasogastric feeding tube if it cannot be taken by mouth and, desirably, some of it is provided in the form of milk at intervals of two to three hours if steroids are being administered.

Maintenance of Elimination

Adequate means of managing elimination must be provided in order to protect the skin from decubitus ulcers. Condom catheters are usually adequate to collect urine from men, but indwelling catheters are usually necessary for women. Periodic examination of the urine and monitoring with cultures and sensitivity studies of any invading organisms are necessary to determine appropriate antibiotic therapy.

Bowel movements may be insignificant during the period when patients are not being fed. Frequent rectal examinations should be performed when oral feedings are begun and maintenance of adequate elimination assured by use of stool softeners, suppositories, or enemas.

Care of Skin and Lungs

Assuming adequate elimination of urine and feces, care of the skin is rarely a problem in the alert and mobile patient, but depression of consciousness or severe neurological deficits result in immobility that may lead to decubitus ulcers unless the dependent parts are relieved of pressure periodically. Stuporous patients should be turned no less frequently than every two hours, a schedule that should be extended, in alert patients, to paralyzed parts that might rest on a bed or chair. Paralyzed limbs must be elevated for major portions of the day to avoid development of dependent edema.

Frequent turning will reduce the chances of bronchopneumonia, which may develop in dependent parts of the lungs of a stuporous patient. Frequent massage or patting of the chest will provide similar advantages. Maintenance of an open airway and pulmonary toilet are mandatory, and respiratory assistance may be required in stuporous patients.

Control of Fever

Most victims of intracranial hemorrhage experience a mild to moderate rise in body temperature for several days. Such eleva-tions may be exaggerated when the patients are stuporous.

Depression of temperatures below the normal range by artificial means is rarely utilized over a prolonged period; however, measures that may be used to maintain temperature near normal include the use of a cooling blanket and administration of salicylates. In addition, frequent investigations should be made for sites of possible infection.

Therapy for Pain and Restlessness

Headache, a frequent complaint following intracranial hemorrhage, may require salicylates and codeine on occasion. The headaches occasionally persist and are difficult to treat. Narcotics should be avoided. Patients are often restless, and mild sedation may be required. Chlorpromazine in quantities of 200 to 300 mg per day may be used to quiet them. It often makes patients slightly drowsy, a factor that should be considered when serially evaluating the state of consciousness. Chlorpromazine may reduce the blood pressure, which could be an added advantage in hypertensive patients.

Antihypertensive Medications

Studies have shown that the survival of neurologically normal patients suffering from systemic hypertension will be prolonged by control of the systemic pressure.[20,162] Other studies have documented improved survival rates when the systemic pressure of patients who have sustained strokes associated with hypertension is adequately controlled.[18] It is mandatory, however, to maintain cerebral perfusion. A number of factors alter the cerebral blood flow in patients who have recently sustained intracerebral hemorrhage. The mass of a hematoma increases local tissue pressure and may increase the total cerebrospinal fluid pressure, which automatically lowers perfusion pressure. Frequently following intracranial hemorrhage, vasospasm becomes prominent. In addition, the walls of penetrating vessels of the brain are usually thickened and the lumina narrowed.[153] Because of these factors, greater intra-arterial blood pressure is required to maintain flow. As a consequence, great care must be taken in lowering the blood pressure of patients who have recently experienced intracerebral hemorrhage. If patients are alert, monitoring of the state of consciousness must be used as a guide to the degree to which the systolic blood pressure may be safely lowered. If consciousness is impaired, pressure should not be lowered more than 20 to 30 per cent when the systolic pressure exceeds 200 mm of mercury, or 15 to 20 per cent when the systolic pressure is recorded between 160 and 200 mm of mercury, or the diastolic pressure is above 100 mm of mercury.

A review of the medical management of systemic hypertension is beyond the scope of this chapter. A few comments and suggestions regarding basic drugs appear appropriate, however.

Medical reduction of blood pressure in patients with marked hypertension should be accomplished in two stages, immediate and long-term. In most instances, at least the initial reduction of pressure in patients who have recently sustained intracerebral hemorrhage should be accomplished at once. Several drugs are available, the most consistently effective being sodium nitroprusside, which can be administered intravenously.[75] The administration of sodium nitroprusside must be carefully controlled, since the drug is extremely potent. It is usually administered at the rate of about 0.5 μg per kilogram per minute initially, with the infusion rate being increased to as much as 3 μg per kilogram per minute if necessary to obtain an adequate response. Thiocyanate intoxication can develop if the medication is used for prolonged periods and in patients with chronic renal failure or on diets low in sodium. The medication should be discontinued if the thiocyanate concentration exceeds 12 μg per 100 ml of blood. The blood pressure returns toward its premedication level once the sodium nitroprusside infusion is discontinued.

An alternate medication that may be used is trimethaphan, which produces a similar blood pressure response but is apparently associated with a higher incidence of serious complications than sodium nitroprusside.

For long-term control of systemic blood pressure, many drugs or combinations of drugs are available from which the practitioner might choose. Three of the more commonly successful include methyldopa, hydralazine, and guanethidine. Methyldopa can be administered intramuscularly or orally in divided doses totaling 750 mg to as much as 3 gm daily. Hydralazine (Apresoline) may be given intramuscularly and orally also. It is administered in single doses of up to 200 mg per day. Guanethidine is administered orally, and doses range from 10 to 100 mg.

Control of Intracranial Pressure

Intracranial hypertension may lead to decompensation following intracerebral hemorrhage. The hypertension may be the result of the mass effect of the hematoma, of edema of the adjacent brain, or of hydrocephalus in the event of obstruction of cerebrospinal fluid flow. Treatment may be medical, surgical, or often a combination of the two. Administration of steroids, dexamethasone or methylprednisolone, significantly reduces intracranial pressure in conjunction with intracranial neoplasms and in the presence of subdural hematoma. Clinical improvement as a result of steroid administration following head injury or intracerebral hemorrhage is unproved, but steroids appear to be effective in some cases. Antacids should be administered concurrently with steroids.

Administration of hyperosmolar solutions may significantly reduce intracranial pressure. Mannitol, urea, or glycerol may be administered repeatedly as necessary to control pressure.* Ideally, for long-term administration, the intracranial pressure is monitored and the medication given when the cerebrospinal fluid pressure exceeds 300 mm of mercury. For monitoring, a catheter must be placed in a ventricle or a monitoring apparatus placed in the subarachnoid, subdural, or epidural space. In either event, penetration of the cranium is required. Optimally, intracranial pressure may be reduced by evacuation of the hematoma. This is usually accomplished by open craniotomy or craniectomy. Drainage of cerebrospinal fluid by ventriculostomy or shunt may also help.[118]

Operative Therapy

The operative management of spontaneous hematomas within the substance of the

---

* See references 23, 81, 115, 118, 160, 170.

brain has proved to be no less controversial than the pathogenesis of such lesions. Wernicke, according to Penfield, suggested trephination for "ingravescent apoplexy."[134] Macewan, in his address, Surgery of the Brain and Spinal Cord, briefly described one patient in whom he had successfully evacuated a spontaneous intracerebral hemorrhage from beneath the motor strip.[103] Cushing reported on the evacuation of spontaneous intracerebral hematomas in two patients, both of whom died of complications of the craniotomies.[35] Another successful evacuation of an intracerebral hematoma was described by Russell and Sargent in 1909, but the patient remained dysphasic and severely hemiparetic.[150] Subsequently, numerous reports appeared describing the evacuation of hematomas from the parenchyma of the brain. Bagley made it clear in 1932 that such evacuations met with varying degrees of success according to the location of the hematoma within the brain.[14] In brief, he achieved an acceptance rate of success when evacuating hematomas from the periphery of the cerebrum, but his results when dealing with hematomas deep within the nuclear substances of the brain were unacceptable.

Others have noted poor results when evacuating hematomas from the nuclear structures of the brain. Luessenhop and co-workers, who were generally optimistic regarding the results of evacuation of intracerebral hematomas, recorded a mortality rate of 89 per cent when "capsular" lesions were encountered.[102] Richardson stated that obviously many deep-seated hematomas were unsuitable for operation, and Scott said that "hemorrhages into the capsule were more serious than hemorrhages into . . . the temporal lobe."[142,155] To the contrary, Paillas and Alliez noted an insignificant difference between the mortality rates of patients with deep and those with superficial hematomas, and Tedeschi and associates state that the site of a hematoma made no difference in the outcome.[132,173]

Generally, in the past, it was widely thought that few patients with intracerebral hemorrhage survived. A number of authors saw little to lose by evacuation of intracerebral hemorrhages.[48,72,88] It has now become apparent, however, that many patients with intraparenchymal hemorrhages experience spontaneous recovery. McKissock and his colleagues began to question the advantages of evacuation and in a controlled study found that 49 per cent of their patients with proved deep-seated lesions survived the acute ictus.[112,113] According to Ojemann, these figures are similar to those obtained at the Massachusetts General Hospital when lesions of the brain stem producing early coma and severe neurological deficits are excluded.[128] McKissock and co-workers found no group of operatively treated patients for whom the outcome was better than that of patients treated more conservatively.[112] Indeed, there were groups in which the operative results appeared disastrous. Their statistical study placed the advantages of any operative therapy for intracerebral hemorrhage in question.

Many surgeons, both before and since the time of McKissock's statistical study, have tried to identify specific factors that might indicate areas in which an operation would improve the results. Most reports indicate that the occurrence of coma soon after the onset of the ictus is often associated with an extremely poor prognosis, although there are reports of satisfactory outcome of a few cases following evacuation of hematomas in deeply stuporous patients.[19,34,68,167] It is generally stated that age has little influence on the outcome, although Lazorthes was insistent that operative procedures were particularly indicated in young and middle-aged patients.[34,96,173]

Hypertension is present in most cases, and some authors have indicated that the prognosis is particularly grave when hypertension is coexistent, but others feel that the presence of hypertension should not influence the decision to evacuate hematomas.[34,77,96,102]

Timing for the evacuation has been the subject of a number of reports. Cook and co-workers, in 1965, reported that evacuation of hematomas immediately after hemorrhage was particularly unrewarding, while several authors have indicated a preference for delay in the evacuation for two to five or more days after the onset of symptoms.[31,90,132,142,173] Snodgrass, in his report in 1961, stated that there was no general agreement on the timing of the operation.[167]

There seems to be general agreement that patients who have a rather insidious onset of symptoms and progressively increasing neurological deficits have a better prognosis following evacuation of the hematoma than patients whose initial ictus is accompanied by stupor or coma.[173] Curatico and co-workers stated that the volume of the hematoma had no effect on the outcome, provided the hematoma had not caused damage by pressure on contiguous structures, but Beneš and associates report that operative treatment of a hematoma that "crushes the surrounding tissue, tamponades the ventricles, and produces fatal increase in intracranial pressure" does not improve the results.[19,34]

Detailed clinical descriptions of the syndromes related to hemorrhages in specific areas and the development of computed tomography have provided more discrete diagnosis than has been possible with intracerebral hemorrhages in the past. It may be that results of patients treated operatively, in comparison with results of those receiving only medical care, in the future will be more favorable. There can be little doubt of the advantages of relieving acute hydrocephalus associated with deep-seated intracerebral hematomas. There can also be very little doubt about the advantages of evacuating a hematoma when the patient has had an initial apoplectic episode followed by improvement and subsequent neurological deterioration that has been associated with evidence of increasing intracranial pressure such as papilledema, increasing stupor, paresis, and the like. Such patients often show dramatic improvement after evacuation of their mass lesions.

The outcome for patients with intracerebellar hematomas is clearly improved by evacuation of their lesions.[58,114,128,129,142] Patients with hemorrhage into the cerebellum often experience acute hydrocephalus due to occlusion of the fourth ventricle and compression of the medulla, probably in the region of the pontomedullary junction. A high percentage of such patients will survive with minimal deficits if they undergo early evacuation of their hematomas. Contrarily, delay in evacuaton results in death in a high percentage of cases. Hemorrhage into the cerebellum constitutes an indication for early intervention. Subcortical hemorrhage in an anterior temporal lobe leaves minimal deficits when evacuated early but may be devastating when left alone. There can be little question of the advantages of evacuation of lesions in this area.

Technique

Early reports suggested that simple aspiration by a cannula inserted into the parenchyma of the brain through burr holes was adequate for evacuation of hematomas, but there is now almost universal agreement that craniectomy or craniotomy and evacuation of hematomas under direct observation offers optimal benefit.[21,77,96,120] This method permits complete removal of the blood clot and provides the best opportunity for control of sites of hemorrhage.

Operative evacuation of an intracerebral hematoma is accomplished through a cortical incision at a point where the lesion most closely approximates the surface. Aspiration through an exploratory needle will confirm the diagnosis, reduce intracerebral tension, blood clots are evacuated by aspiration tion or manually. Care must be taken not to ting its removal with minimal destruction of the brain tissue. Following the cortical incision, blood clots are evacuated by aspiration or manually. Care must be taken not to traumatize the surfaces of the brain. Small fragments of clot may be left attached to the walls in order to avoid disturbing potential bleeding points.

Hemostasis must be meticulous. Magnification and bipolar electrocautery are utilized to occlude all bleeding points. If hypotensive medications are used during the operation, blood pressure should be allowed to rise to near normal levels before the wound is closed, and during the postoperative period, care must be taken to avoid return of blood pressure to elevated levels that could result in recurrent hemorrhage. Intra-arterial monitoring of blood pressure may be helpful in controlling the systemic pressure.

As computed tomography has added a new dimension to the initial diagnosis of intraparenchymatous hemorrhage of the brain, so it has also found a place in the postoperative care of patients. Performed early after an operative evacuation, it will demonstrate the amount and location of any residual hematoma. Serial CT scans may show evidence of recurrent hemorrhage before such is clinically apparent. They may likewise demonstrate decreasing size of hematomas before clinical improvement is apparent.

Reaccumulation of a hematoma is a frequent postoperative problem and a major cause of morbidity and death.[102] Since it is now well known that intracerebral hematomas are often resorbed, it follows that small residual hematomas do not require re-exploration of the wound provided the patient is clinically improving. An aggressive attack should be considered for a large residual hematoma, however, in the event that a patient is slow to recover. Re-exploration should be accomplished quickly whenever there is significant recurrent hemorrhage.

CONCLUSION

Much progress has been made in understanding the etiology of intraparenchymatous hemorrhages of the brain within the last 20 years. Most cases result from rupture of a penetrating vessel that has been subjected to systemic hypertension and has undergone consequent degenerative changes. The most common sites for spontaneous intracerebral hemorrhages are the putamen, the junction between the cortex and the white matter, the thalamus, the pons, and the cerebellum.

Most lesions above the tentorium produce hemiparesis with unilateral sensory changes. Visual field deficits are not produced by hemorrhages involving the frontal cortex, the upper parts of the thalamus, or structures in the posterior fossa, but are common with the lesions of the putamen or lower thalamus. Eye signs are helpful in localizing the lesions. Clinical onset of symptoms with lesions of the cerebellum usually include nausea, vomiting, and ataxia, more prominent on the side of the lesion. Operative treatment of lesions of the cerebellum is often urgent, and evacuation may be of benefit to many patients with supratentorial hemorrhage, especially hemorrhage beneath the cortex.

Computed tomography has proved to be an excellent diagnostic tool because of the rapidity with which it localizes intraparenchymatous lesions of the brain and the advantages it provides by demonstrating the point at which a hematoma most closely approximates the surface of the brain.

Medical therapy is required for each patient who has had an intraparenchymatous hemorrhage. Patients must be evaluated for defects in coagulation, and appropriate therapy must be administered. Antihypertensive drugs may be helpful at the time of the acute ictus as well as subsequently in patients with hemorrhages of hypertensive origin. Drugs to reduce parenchymatous fluid content are often of great aid. All patients with devastating neurological deficits require supportive care in the form of control of fluid and electrolytes. Appropriate methods of caring for elimination of body wastes and appropriate care of the skin and pulmonary toilet are important aspects of the medical therapy. Physical therapy is also important in the rehabilitation of patients whether treated by operation or solely by medications.

REFERENCES

1. Abbott, K. H., Rollas, Z. H., and Meagher, J. N.: Choroid plexus papilloma causing spontaneous subarachnoid hemorrhage. Report of case and review of literature. J. Neurosurg., 14:566–570, 1957.
2. Adams, R. D., and Vander Eecken, H. M.: Vascular diseases of the brain. Ann. Rev. Med., 4:213–252, 1953.
3. Allen, M. B., Jr., Dick, D. A. L., Hightower, S. J., and Brown, M.: The value and limitations of brain scanning: A review of 401 consecutive cases. Clin. Radiol., 18:19–27, 1967.
4. Ambrose, J.: Computerized transverse axial scanning (tomography): Part 2. Clinical application. Brit. J. Radiol., 46:1023–1047, 1973.
5. Anders, H. E., and Eicke, W. J.: Über Veranderungen an Gehirngefassen bei Hypertonie. Z. Ges. Neurol. Psychiat., 167:562–575, 1939.
6. Andersen, P. E.: The lenticulo-striate arteries and their diagnostic value; a preliminary report. Acta Radiol., 50:84–91, 1958.
7. Andersen, P. E.: Angiographic localization of small intracerebral hematomas. Acta Radiol. (Diagn.), 1:173–181, 1963.
8. Aring, C. D.: Intracerebral hemorrhage (primary). Int. J. Neurol., 1:129–135, 1960.
9. Aring, C. D., and Merritt, H. H.: Differential diagnosis between cerebral hemorrhage and cerebral thrombosis. A clinical and pathologic study of 245 cases. Arch. Intern. Med., 56:435–456, 1935.
10. Arkin, A.: A clinical and pathological study of periarteritis nodosa. A report of five cases, one histologically healed. Amer. J. Path., 6:401–426, 1930.
11. Arseni, C., and Stanciu, M.: Primary hematomas of the brain stem. Acta Neurochir., 28:323–330, 1973.
12. Arseni, C., Ionescu, S., Maretsis, M., and Ghitescu, M.: Primary intraparenchymatous hematomas. J. Neurosurg., 27:207–215, 1967.

13. Askenasy, H. M., and Behmoaram, A. D.: Subarachnoid hemorrhage in meningiomas of the lateral ventricle. Neurology (Minneap.), *10*: 484–489, 1960.

14. Bagley, C., Jr.: Spontaneous cerebral hemorrhage. Discussion of four types, with surgical considerations. Arch. Neurol. Psychiat., *27*:1133–1174, 1932.

15. Banna, M., Gryspeerdt, G. L., and Lavelle, M. I.: Some specific features of primary cerebral haematomas which may be seen on air-ventriculography. Clin. Radiol., *23*:417–421, 1972.

16. Barron, K. D., and Fergusson, G.: Intracranial hemorrhage as a complication of anticoagulant therapy. Neurology (Minneap.), *9*:447–455, 1959.

17. Beck, D. J. K.: Operable intracranial haemorrhage. Proc. Roy. Soc. Med., *47*:700–701, 1954.

18. Beevers, D. G., Fairman, M. J., Hamilton, M., and Harpur, J. E.: Antihypertensive treatment and the course of established cerebral vascular disease. Lancet, *1*:1407–1409, 1973.

19. Beneš, V., Koukolík, F., and Obrovská, D.: Two types of spontaneous intracerebral hemorrhage due to hypertension. J. Neurosurg., *37*:509–513, 1972.

20. Breckenridge, A., Dollery, C. T., and Parry, E. H. O.: Prognosis of treated hypertension. Changes in life expectancy and causes of death between 1952 and 1967. Quart. J. Med., *39*: 411–429, 1970.

21. Browder, E. J., and Corradini, E. W.: Surgical treatment of intracerebral hematomas. Arch. Neurol. Psychiat., *65*:112–113, 1951.

22. Butzer, J. F., Cancilla, P. A., and Cornell, S. H.: Computerized axial tomography of intracerebral hematoma. A clinical and neuropathological study. Arch. Neurol., *33*:206–214, 1976.

23. Cantore, G., Guidetti, B., and Virno, M.: Oral glycerol for the reduction of intracranial pressure. J. Neurosurg., *21*:278–283, 1964.

24. Carton, C. A., and Alvord, E. C., Jr.: Localized intra-ventricular hematoma. J. Neuropath. Exp. Neurol., *16*:113–114, 1957.

25. Charcot, J. M., and Bouchard, C.: Nouvelles recherches sur la pathogénie de l'hémorrhagie cérébrale. Arch. Physiol. Norm. Path. Paris, *1*:110–127, 643–665, 1868.

26. Ciric, I. S., Quinn, J. L., III, and Bucy, P. C.: Mercury 197 and technetium 99m brain scans in the diagnosis of non-neoplastic intracranial lesions. J. Neurosurg., *27*:119–125, 1967.

27. Cohen, M. M.: Cerebrovascular accidents. A study of 200 cases. Arch. Path. (Chicago), *60*:296–307, 1955.

28. Cohen, S. I., and Aronson, S. M.: Secondary brain stem hemorrhages. Predisposing and modifying factors. Arch. Neurol. (Chicago), *19*:257–263, 1968.

29. Cole, F. M., and Yates, P. O.: The occurrence and significance of intracerebral micro-aneurysms. J. Path. Bact., *93*:393–411, 1967.

30. Cole, F. M., and Yates, P. O.: Pseudo-aneurysms in relationship to massive cerebral haemorrhage. J. Neurol. Neurosurg. Psychiat., *30*:61–66, 1967.

31. Cook, A. W., Plaut, M., and Browder, J.: Spontaneous intracerebral hemorrhage. Factors related to surgical results. Arch. Neurol. (Chicago), *13*:25–29, 1965.

32. Courville, C. B.: Intracerebral hematoma, its pathology and pathogenesis. Arch. Neurol. Psychiat., *77*:464–472, 1957.

33. Craig, W. M., and Adson, A. W.: Spontaneous intracerebral hemorrhage: Etiology and surgical treatment, with a report of nine cases. Arch. Neurol. Psychiat., *35*:701–715, 1936.

34. Cuatico, W., Adib, S., and Gaston, P.: Spontaneous intracerebral hematomas, a surgical appraisal. J. Neurosurg., *22*:569–575, 1965.

35. Cushing, H.: The blood-pressure reaction of acute cerebral compression, illustrated by cases of intracranial hemorrhage. Amer. J. Med. Sci., *125*:1017–1044, 1903.

36. Dalsgaard-Nielson, T.: Survey of 1000 cases of apoplexi cerebri. Acta Psychiat. Neurol. Scand., *30*:169–185, 1955.

37. Dandy, W. E.: Intracranial Arterial Aneurysms. Ithaca, N.Y., Comstock Publishing Co., Inc., 1944, pp. 1–147.

38. Davidoff, L. M.: Intracerebral hemorrhage associated with hypertension and arteriosclerosis. J. Neurosurg., *15*:322–328, 1958.

39. Davis, D. O., and Pressman, B. D.: Computerized tomography of the brain. Radiol. Clin. N. Amer., *12*:297–313, 1974.

40. Davis, K. R., Taveras, J. M., New, P. F. J., Schnur, J. A., and Roberson, G. H.: Cerebral infarction diagnosis by computerized tomography: Analysis and evaluation of findings. Amer. J. Roentgen., *124*:643–660, 1975.

41. Deland, F. H.: Nuclear medicine in diseases of the central nervous system. Hospital Practice, *6*:57–66, 1971.

42. Dhar, S. K., and Freedman, P.: Clinical management of hypertensive emergencies. Heart Lung, *5*:571–575, 1976.

43. Douglas, R. G.: Case of recent and old haemorrhages of the brain. Canad. Med. Ass. J., *15*:638–639, 1925.

44. El Gammal, T., and Allen, M. B.: Hypocycloid tomography in encephalography to demonstrate deep hemorrhage of the brain. Acta Radiol. [Diagn.], suppl. 347:301–312, 1975.

45. Ellis, A. G.: The pathogenesis of spontaneous cerebral hemorrhage. Proc. Path. Soc. Phil., *12*:197–235, 1909.

46. Eppinger: Pathogenesis, Histogenesis und Actiologie der Aneurysmen. Arch. Klin. Chir., *35*:suppl. 1, 1887.

47. Ernsting, J.: Choroid plexus papilloma causing spontaneous subarachnoid haemorrhage. J. Neurol. Neurosurg. Psychiat., *18*:134–136. 1955.

48. Fazio, C.: A neurologist's study of the problem concerning surgical treatment of spontaneous cerebral hemorrhage. Sci. Med. Ital., *1*:101–110, 1950.

49. Feigin, I., and Prose, P.: Hypertensive fibrinoid arteritis of the brain and gross cerebral hemorrhage. A form of "hyalinosis." Arch. Neurol., *1*:98–110, 1959.

50. Fields, W. S., and Sahs, A. L.: Intracranial Aneurysms and Subarachnoid Hemorrhage. Springfield, Ill., Charles C Thomas, 1965.

51. Fisher, A. G. T.: A case of complete absence of

both internal carotid arteries, with a preliminary note on the developmental history of the stapedial artery. J. Anat. Physiol., *48*:37–46, 1913.

52. Fisher, C. M.: Early-life carotid-artery occlusion associated with late intracranial hemorrhage. Observations on the ischemic pathogenesis of mantle sclerosis. Lab. Invest., *8*:680–700, 1959.

53. Fisher, C. M.: The pathology and pathogenesis of intracerebral hemorrhage. *In* Fields, W. S., ed.: Pathogenesis and Treatment of Cerebrovascular Disease. Springfield, Ill., Charles C Thomas, 1961, pp. 295–342.

54. Fisher, C. M.: Clinical syndromes in cerebral hemorrhage. *In* Fields, W. S., ed.: Pathogenesis and Treatment of Cerebrovascular Disease. Springfield, Ill., Charles C Thomas, 1961, pp. 318–342.

55. Fisher, C. M.: Lacunes: Small, deep cerebral infarcts. Neurology (Minneap.), *15*:774–789, 1965.

56. Fisher, C. M.: The arterial lesions underlying lacunes. Acta Neuropath. (Berlin), *12*:1–15, 1969.

57. Fisher, C. M.: Clinical syndromes in cerebral thrombosis, hypertensive hemorrhage, and ruptured saccular aneurysm. Clin. Neurosurg., *22*:117–147, 1975.

58. Fisher, C. M., Picard, E. H., Polak, A., Dalal, P., Ojemann, R. G.: Acute hypertensive cerebellar hemorrhage: Diagnosis and surgical treatment. J. Nerv. Ment. Dis., *140*:38–57, 1965.

59. Ford, R., and Ambrose, J.: Echoencephalography. The measurement of the position of midline structures in the skull with high frequency pulsed ultrasound. Brain, *86*:189–196, 1963.

60. French, L. A., and Galicich, J. H.: The use of steroids for control of cerebral edema. Clin. Neurosurg., *10*:212–223, 1964.

61. Freytag, E.: Fatal hypertensive intracerebral haematomas: A survey of the pathological anatomy of 393 cases. J. Neurol. Neurosurg. Psychiat., *31*:616–620, 1968.

62. Furlow, L. T., Carr, A. D., and Wattenberg, C.: Spontaneous cerebral hemorrhage, the surgical treatment of selected cases. Surgery, *9*:758–770, 1941.

63. Gildersleeve, N., Koo, A. H., and McDonald, C. J.: Metastatic tumor presenting as intracerebral hemorrhage, report of 6 cases examined by computed tomography. Radiology, *124*:109–112, 1977.

64. Glasgow, J. L., Currier, R. D., Goodrich, J. K., and Tutor, F. T.: Brain scans of cerebral infarcts with radioactive mercury. Radiology, *88*:1086–1091, 1967.

65. Glass, B., and Abbott, K. H.: Subarachnoid hemorrhage consequent to intracranial tumors, review of literature and report of seven cases. Arch. Neurol. Psychiat., *73*:369–379, 1955.

66. Globus, J. H., and Sapirstein, M.: Massive hemorrhage into brain tumor, its significance and probable relationship to rapidly fatal termination and antecedent trauma. J.A.M.A., *120*:348–352, 1942.

67. Globus, J. H., and Strauss, I.: Massive cerebral hemorrhage, its relation to pre-existing cerebral softening. Arch. Neurol. Psychiat., *18*:215–239, 1927.

68. Gol, A., Ehni, G., and Leavens, M. E.: The surgery of intracerebral hemorrhage. Texas State J. Med., *56*:783–785, 1960.

69. Goran, A., Ciminello, V. J., and Fisher, R. G.: Hemorrhage into meningiomas. Arch. Neurol., *13*:65–69, 1965.

70. Green, F. H. K.: Miliary aneurysms in the brain. J. Path. Bact., *33*:71–77, 1930.

71. Grinker, R. R., Bucy, P., and Sahs, A. L.: Neurology. 5th Ed. Springfield, Ill., Charles C Thomas, 1960.

72. Guillaume, J., Ribadeau-Dumas, C. H., and Mazars, G.: Hémorrhagie cérébrale aiguë guérie chirurgicalement. Rev. Neurol. (Paris), *78*:30–32, 1946.

73. Hamby, W. B.: Gross intracerebral hematomas, report of 16 surgically treated cases. New York J. Med., *45*:866–876, 1945.

74. Hamby, W. B.: Intracranial Aneurysms. Springfield, Ill., Charles C Thomas, 1952.

75. Harker, L. A.: Hemostasis Manual. 2d Ed. Philadelphia, F. A. Davis Co., 1974.

76. Hounsfield, G. N.: Computerized transverse axial scanning (tomography): Part 1. Description of system. Brit. J. Radiol., *46*:1016–1022, 1973.

77. Howell, D. A.: The surgical treatment of massive cerebral haemorrhage, a report of 33 cases. Canad. Med. Ass. J., *77*:542–555, 1957.

78. Humphreys, R. P., Hoffman, H. J., Mustard, W. T., and Trusler, G. A.: Cerebral hemorrhage following heart surgery. J. Neurosurg., *43*:671–675, 1975.

79. Hyland, H. H.: Nonaneurysmal intracranial hemorrhage. Neurology (Minneap.), *11*:Pt. 2:165–168, 1961.

80. Ingvar, S.: Sur les hémorragies méningées. Nouv. Iconogr. Salpêt. (Paris), *28*:313–342, 1916–18.

81. Javid, M., and Sattlage, P.: Effect of urea on cerebrospinal fluid pressure in human subjects. Preliminary report. J.A.M.A., *160*:943–949, 1956.

82. Jewesbury, E. C. O.: Atypical intracerebral haemorrhage, with special reference to cerebral haematoma. Brain, *70*:274–303, 1947.

83. Johansson, S. H., and Melin, H. S.: Spontaneous cerebral haemorrhage and encephalomalacia, a clinico-pathological study of 263 cases with special reference to cardiovascular diseases and cerebral atherosclerosis. Acta Psychiat. Neurol. Scand., *35*:457–479, 1960.

84. Johnson, R. T., and Yates, P. O.: Brain stem haemorrhages in expanding supratentorial conditions. Acta Radiol., *46*:250–256, 1956.

85. Johnston, I. H., and Jennett, B.: The place of continuous intracranial pressure monitoring in neurosurgical practice. Acta Neurochir., *29*:53–63, 1973.

86. Kalbag, R. M.: Recurrent subarachnoid haemorrhage from paraventricular lesions with normal angiography. J. Neurol. Neurosurg. Psychiat., *27*:435–439, 1964.

87. Katz, R. I., Goldberg, H. I., and Selzer, M. E.: Mycotic aneurysm, case report with novel sequential angiographic findings. Arch. Intern. Med., *134*:939–942, 1974.

88. Kelly, R.: Discussion: Intracerebral hemorrhage—diagnosis and treatment. Proc. Roy. Soc. Med., *51*:213–217, 1957.

89. Kerr, C. B.: Intracranial haemorrhage in haemophilia. J. Neurol. Neurosurg. Psychiat., *27*: 166–173, 1964.

90. King, R. B.: Neurosurgery in management of patients with cerebral vascular disease. New York J. Med., *62*:3908–3912, 1962.

91. Klintworth, G. K.: Evaluation of the role of neurosurgical procedures in the pathogenesis of secondary brain-stem haemorrhages. J. Neurol. Neurosurg. Psychiat., *29*:423–425, 1966.

92. Koos, W. T., Sunder-Plassmann, M., and Salah, S.: Successful removal of a large intrapontine hematoma. Case report. J. Neurosurg., *31*: 690–694, 1969.

93. Krayenbühl, H., and Siebenmann, R.: Small vascular malformations as a cause of primary intracerebral hemorrhage. J. Neurosurg., *22*:7–20, 1965.

94. Kristiansen, K.: Cerebral angiography in the diagnosis of intracranial hematomas. Surgery, *24*:755–768, 1948.

95. Kullberg, G., and West, K. A.: Influence of corticosteroids on the ventricular fluid pressure. Acta Neurol. Scand., suppl. 13, 445–452, 1965.

96. Lazorthes, G.: Surgery of cerebral hemorrhage, report on the results of 52 surgically treated cases. J. Neurosurg., *16*:355–364, 1959.

97. Lévy, A., and Stula, D.: Neurochirurgische Aspekte bei Antikoagulantienblutungen im Zentralnervensystem. Deutsch. Med. Wschr., *96*:1043–1048, 1971.

98. Lhermitte, F., Gautier, J.-C., Poirier, J., and Tyrer, J. H.: Hypoplasia of the internal carotid artery. Neurology (Minneap.), *18*:439–446, 1968.

99. Locksley, H. B., Sahs, A. L., and Sandler, R.: Subarachnoid hemorrhage unrelated to intracranial aneurysm and A-V malformation, a study of associated diseases and prognosis. J. Neurosurg., *24*:1034–1056, 1966.

100. Loeser, J. D., Stuntz, J. T., and Kelly, W. A.: Spontaneous remission of an intraventricular hemorrhage. Case report. J. Neurosurg., *28*:277–279, 1968.

101. Lott, T., El Gammal, T., and Volcan, I.: Evaluation of posterior fossa lesions by computer assisted tomography (CAT). Southern Med. J., *70*:793–799, 1977.

102. Luessenhop, A. J., Shevlin, W. A., Ferrero, A. A., McCullough, D. C., and Barone, B.M.: Surgical management of primary intracerebral hemorrhage. J. Neurosurg., *27*:419–427, 1967.

103. Macewen, W.: The surgery of the brain and spinal cord. Brit. Med. J., *2*:302–309, 1888.

104. Marburg, O.: Zur Frage der hemorrhagia cerebri bei jungeren Menschen und deren differentieller Diagnose. Deutsch. Z. Nervenheilk., *105*:22–34, 1928.

105. Margolis, G., Odom, G. L., Woodhall, B., and Bloor, B. M.: The role of small angiomatous malformations in the production of intracerebral hematomas. J. Neurosurg., *8*:564–575, 1951.

106. Massie, J. D., Haussen, S., and Gerald, B.: Angiography of cerebellar hemorrhage secondary to hypertension. Amer. J. Roentgen., *123*:22–26, 1975.

107. Mazars, G., Ribadeau-Dumas, C., and Roge, R.: Accidents hémorrhagiques cérébraux au cours des traitements anticoagulants. Indications opératoires et résultats à propos de 38 cas opérés. Marseille Méd., *104*:27–30, 1967.

108. McCormick, W. F., and Nofzinger, J. D.: "Cryptic" vascular malformations of the central nervous system. J. Neurosurg., *24*:865–875, 1966.

109. McCormick, W. F., and Rosenfield, D. B.: Massive brain hemorrhage: A review of 144 cases and an examination of their causes. Stroke, *4*:946–954, 1973.

110. McKissock, W., and Paine, K. W. E.: Subarachnoid haemorrhage. Brain, *82*:356–366, 1959.

111. McKissock, W., Paine, K., and Walsh, L.: Further observations on subarachnoid haemorrhage. J. Neurol. Neurosurg. Psychiat., *21*: 239–248, 1958.

112. McKissock, W., Richardson, A., and Taylor, J.: Primary intracerebral haemorrhage, a controlled trial of surgical and conservative treatment in 180 unselected cases. Lancet, *2*: 221–226, 1961.

113. McKissock, W., Richardson, A., and Walsh, L.: Primary intracerebral haemorrhage, results of surgical treatment in 244 consecutive cases. Lancet, *2*:683–686, 1959.

114. McKissock, W., Richardson, A., and Walsh, L.: Spontaneous cerebellar haemorrhage, a study of 34 consecutive cases treated surgically. Brain, *83*:1–9, 1960.

115. McQueen, J. D., and Jeanes, L. D.: Dehydration and rehydration of the brain with hypertonic urea and mannitol. J. Neurosurg., *21*:118–128, 1964.

116. Messina, A. V.: Computed tomography: Contrast enhancement in resolving intracerebral hemorrhage. Amer. J. Roentgen., *127*:1050–1052, 1976.

117. Messina, A. V., and Chernik, N. L.: Computed tomography: The "resolving" intracerebral hemorrhage. Radiology, *118*:609–613, 1975.

118. Miller, J. D., and Leech, P.: Effects of mannitol and steroid therapy on intracranial volume-pressure relationships in patients. J. Neurosurg., *42*:274–281, 1975.

119. Miller, R. H., Clark, E. C., and Dodge, H. W., Jr.: Treatment of intracerebral hematomas in young and middle-aged patients. Neurology (Minneap.), *5*:567–572, 1955.

120. Mitsuno, T., Kanaya, H., Shirakata, S., Ohsawa, K., and Ishikawa, Y.: Surgical treatment of hypertensive intracerebral hemorrhage. J. Neurosurg., *24*:70–76, 1966.

121. Mizukami, M., Araki, G., Mihara, H., Tomita, T., and Fujinaga, R.: Arteriographically visualized extravasation in hypertensive intracerebral hemorrhage, report of seven cases. Stroke, *3*:527–537, 1972.

122. Moore, M. T., and Stern, K.: Vascular lesions in the brain-stem and occipital lobe occurring in association with brain tumours. Brain, *61*:70–98, 1938.

123. Moscow, N. P., and Margolis, M. T.: Angiography of pontine hemorrhage. Neuroradiology, *7*:125–127, 1974.

124. Mutlu, N., Berry, R. G., and Alpers, B. J.: Mas-

sive cerebral hemorrhage. Clinical and patho-logical correlations. Arch. Neurol. (Chicago), 8:644–661, 1963.

125. New, P. F. J., and Aronow, S.: Attenuation mea-surements of whole blood and blood fractions in computed tomography. Radiology, 121:635–640, 1976.

126. New, P. F. J., Scott, W. R., Schnur, J. A., Davis, K. R., and Taveras, J. M.: Compu-terized axial tomography with the EMI scan-ner. Radiology, 110:109–123, 1974.

127. Odom, G. L., Bloor, B. M., and Woodhall, B.: Intracerebral hematomas, a survey of 106 veri-fied cases. Southern Med. J., 45:936–942, 1952.

128. Ojemann, R. G.: The surgical treatment of cere-brovascular disease. New Eng. J. Med., 274:440–448, 1966.

129. Ojemann, R. G., and Mohr, J. P.: Hypertensive brain hemorrhage. Clin. Neurosurg., 23:220–244, 1976.

130. Ojemann, R. G., and New, P. F. J.: Spontaneous resolution of an intraventricular hematoma, re-port of a case with recovery. J. Neurosurg., 20:899–902, 1963.

131. Overton, M. C., III, Haynie, T. P., and Snod-grass, S. R.: Brain scans in nonneoplastic in-tracranial lesions, scanning with chlormerodrin Hg 203 and chlormerodrin Hg 197. J.A.M.A., 191:431–436, 1965.

132. Paillas, J. E., and Alliez, B.: Surgical treatment of spontaneous intracerebral hemorrhage, im-mediate and long-term results in 250 cases. J. Neurosurg., 39:145–151, 1973.

133. Paxton, R., and Ambrose, J.: The EMI scanner. A brief review of the first 650 patients. Brit. J. Radiol., 47:530–565, 1974.

134. Penfield, W.: The operative treatment of spon-taneous intracerebral haemorrhage. Canad. Med. Ass. J., 28:369–372, 1933.

135. Pia, H. W.: Diagnose und Behandlung der spon-tanen intracerebralen Massenblutungen. Acta Neurochir., 7:425–439, 1959.

136. Pick, L.: Ueber die sogenannten miliaren An-eurysmen Hirngefässe. Berlin. Klin. Wschr., 47:325–329, 382–386, 1910.

137. Pilcher, C.: Subcortical hematoma, surgical treatment, with report of eight cases. Arch. Neurol. Psychiat., 46:416–430, 1941.

138. Pool, J. L., and Potts, D. G.: Aneurysms and Ar-teriovenous Anomalies of the Brain. New York, Hoeber Medical Division of Harper & Row, 1965.

139. Pressman, B. D., Kirkwood, J. R., and Davis, D. O.: Posterior fossa hemorrhage, localiza-tion by computerized tomography. J.A.M.A., 232:932–933, 1975.

140. Ransohoff, J.:The effects of steroids on brain edema in man. In Schuermann, K., and Reu-len, H. J., eds.: Steroids and Brain Edema. New York, Springer-Verlag, 1972, pp. 211–217.

141. Ransohoff, J., Derby, B., and Kricheff, I.: Spon-taneous intracerebral hemorrhage. Clin. Neurosurg., 18:247–266, 1971.

142. Richardson, A.: The management of primary in-tracranial hemorrhage. Mod. Trends Neurol., 3:89–107, 1962.

143. Richardson, J. C., and Einhorn, R. W.: Primary intracerebral hemorrhage. Clin. Neurosurg., 9:114–130, 1963.

144. Roach, M. R., and Drake, C. G.: Ruptured cere-bral aneurysms caused by micro-organisms. New Eng. J. Med., 273:240–244, 1965.

145. Robinson, G. W., Jr.: Encapsulated brain hemor-rhages. A study of their frequency and pathol-ogy. Arch. Neurol. Psychiat., 27:1441–1444, 1932.

146. Rockett, J. F., Kaplan, E. S., Hudson, J. S., and Moinuddin, M.: Intracerebral hemorrhage demonstrated by nuclear cerebral angiogram: Case report. J. Nucl. Med., 16:459–461, 1975.

147. Rosenblath: Uber die Entstehung der Hirnblu-tung bei dem Schlaganfall. Deutsch. Z. Nerven-heilk., 61:10–143, 1918.

148. Rosenblath: Einige Bemerkungen zür Frage der Entstehung des Schlaganfalls. Virchow Arch. Path. Anat., 259:261–268, 1926.

149. Rowbotham, G. F., and Ogilvie, A. G.: Chronic intracerebral haematomata, their pathology, diagnosis and treatment. Brit. Med. J., 1:146–149, 1945.

150. Russell, A. E., and Sargent, P.: Apoplectiform cerebral haemorrhage. Operation. Evacuation of blood. Slow improvement. Proc. Roy. Soc. Med., 2:44–51, 1909.

151. Russell, D. S.: Discussion: The pathology of spontaneous intracranial haemorrhage. Proc. Roy. Soc. Med., 47:689–693, 1954.

152. Russell, R. W. R.: Observations on intracerebral aneurysms. Brain, 86:425–442, 1963.

153. Russell, R. W. R.: How does blood-pressure cause stroke? Lancet, 2:1283–1285, 1975.

154. Scheinker, I. M.: Transtentorial herniation of the brain stem. A characteristic clinicopathologic syndrome; pathogenesis of hemorrhages in the brain stem. Arch. Neurol. Psychiat., 53:289–293, 1945.

155. Scott, M.: Neurosurgical treatment of spontane-ous intracranial hemorrhage. Importance of differential diagnosis in "cerebral apoplexy" and evaluation of long-term postoperative re-sults. J.A.M.A., 172:889–895, 1960.

156. Scott, M.: Spontaneous intracerebral hematoma caused by cerebral neoplasms, report of eight verified cases. J. Neurosurg., 42:338–342, 1975.

157. Scott, W. R., New, P. F. J., Davis, K. R., and Schnur, J. A.: Computerized axial tomography of intracerebral and intraventricular hemor-rhage. Radiology, 112:73–80, 1974.

158. Seal, R. M. E., and Millard, A. H.: A case of chorionepithelioma presenting with subarach-noid haemorrhage. J. Obstet. Gynaec. Brit. Emp., 62:932–934, 1955.

159. Sharma, S. M., and Quinn, J. L.: Brain scans in autopsy proved cases of intracerebral hemor-rhage. Arch. Neurol. (Chicago), 28:270–271, 1973.

160. Shenkin, H. A., Goluboff, B., and Haft, H.: The use of mannitol for the reduction of intracranial pressure in intracranial surgery. J. Neurosurg., 19:897–901, 1962.

161. Shivers, J. A., Adcock, D. F., Guinto, F. C., and Radcliffe, W. B.: Radionuclide imaging in pri-mary intracerebral hemorrhage. Radiology, 111:211–212, 1974.

162. Shurtleff, D.: The Framingham Study, 16 Year Follow-up. Washington, D.C., U.S. Govern-ment Printing Office, 1970.

163. Silverstein, A.: Intracranial bleeding in hemo-

philia. Arch. Neurol. (Chicago), *3*:141–156, 1960.

164. Simonsen, J.: Fatal subarachnoid haemorrhage originating in an intracranial chordoma. Acta Path. Microbiol. Scand., *59*:13–20, 1963.

165. Skultety, F. M.: Meningioma simulating ruptured aneurysm, case report. J. Neurosurg., *28*:380–382, 1968.

166. Smith, K. R., Jr., Nelson, J. S., and Dooley, J. M., Jr.: Bilateral "hypoplasia" of the internal carotid arteries. Neurology (Minneap.), *18*:1149–1156, 1968.

167. Snodgrass, S. R.: The surgical treatment of spontaneous intracerebral hemorrhage. *In* Fields, W. S., ed.: Pathogenesis and Treatment of Cerebrovascular Disease. Springfield, Ill., Charles C Thomas, 1961, pp. 343–364.

168. Sreerama, V., Ivan, L. P., Dennery, J. M., and Richard, M. T.: Neurosurgical complications of anticoagulant therapy. Canad. Med. Ass. J., *108*:305–307, 1973.

169. Strang, R. R., and Ljungdahl, T. I.: Carcinoma of the lung with a cerebral metastasis presenting as subarachnoid haemorrhage. Med. J. Aust., *49*:90–91, 1962.

170. Suzuki, J., and Takaku, A.: Nonsurgical treatment of chronic subdural hematoma. J. Neurosurg., *33*:548–553, 1970.

171. Taylor, J. C., Newell, J. A., and Karvounis, P.: Ultrasonics in the diagnosis of intracranial space-occupying lesions. Lancet, *1*:1197–1199, 1961.

172. Tavcar, D.: Hyalinosis as the cause of massive cerebral hemorrhage. Acta Med. Iugosl., *28*:403–420, 1974.

173. Tedeschi, G. Bernini, F. P., and Cerillo, A.: Indications for surgical treatment of intracerebral hemorrhage. J. Neurosurg., *43*:590–595, 1975.

174. Toole, J. F., Truscott, B. L., Anderson, W. W., Aronson, P. R., Blaisdell, W., Dustan, H. P., Dyken, M. L., Foley, A. R., Halsey, J. H. Jr., Langfitt, T. W., Lawrence, M. S., and Mullan, J. F.: Medical and surgical management of stroke. Stroke, *4*:273–320, 1973.

175. Turnbull, H. M.: Alterations in arterial structure and their relation to syphilis. Quart. J. Med., *8*:201–254, 1915.

176. VanderArk, G. D., and Kahn, E. A.: Spontaneous intracerebral hematoma. J. Neurosurg., *28*:252–256, 1968.

177. Vaughan, H. G., Jr., and Howard, R. G.: Intracranial hemorrhage due to metastatic chorionepithelioma. Neurology (Minneap.), *12*:771–777, 1962.

178. Walton, J. N.: Subarachnoid haemorrhage of unusual aetiology. Neurology (Minneap.), *3*:517–543, 1953.

179. Walton, J. N.: Subarachnoid Hemorrhage. London, E. N. S. Livingstone, Ltd., 1956.

180. Westberg, G.: Arteries of the basal ganglia. Acta Radiol. [Diagn.] (Stockholm), *5*:581–596, 1966.

181. Westphal, K., and Bar, R.: Uber die Entstehung des Schlaganfalles. I. Pathologisch-anatomische Untersuchungen zür Frage der Entstehung des Schlaganfalles. Deutsch. Arch. Klin. Med., *151*:1–30, 1926.

182. Wing, S. D., Norman, D., Pollock, J. A., and Newton, T. H.: Contrast enhancement of cerebral infarcts in computed tomography. Radiology, *121*:89–92, 1976,

183. Wise, B. L., and Chater, N.: The value of hypertonic mannitol solution in decreasing brain mass and lowering cerebrospinal-fluid pressure. J. Neurosurg., *19*:1038–1043, 1962.

184. Wright, R. L., Ojemann, R. G., and Drew, J. H.: Hemorrhage into pituitary adenomata. Arch. Neurol. (Chicago), *12*:326–331, 1965.

185. Ziment, I., and Johnson, B. L., Jr.: Angiography in the management of intracranial mycotic aneurysms. Arch. Intern. Med., *122*:349–352, 1968.

186. Zimmerman, H. M.: Cerebral apoplexy: Mechanism and differential diagnosis. New York J. Med., *49*:2153–2157, 1949.

187. Zülch, K. J.: Neuropathology of intracranial haemorrhage. Progr. Brain Res., *30*:151–165, 1968.

55

ARTERIOVENOUS MALFORMATIONS OF THE SPINAL CORD

Arteriovenous malformations of the spinal cord are relatively rare lesions. They occur with a frequency about equal to 4 per cent of that of primary intraspinal tumors. Men have them four times as frequently as women. While they may occur at any age, 80 per cent are seen between the ages of 20 and 60. They have excited interest out of proportion to their numbers. Debates about their anatomy, natural course, pathophysiology, diagnosis, and treatment have led to almost as many papers as cases. Only in the past 10 years has some of the controversy been settled. Many questions still remain to be answered, and there is sharp disagreement among various writers on the subject.

Little is known about the etiology of arteriovenous malformations. It is speculated that they are congenital in origin. There also is little information about the rate of vascular change. While usually considered to be of slow development, in some cases they show great enlargement within a single year (Fig. 55–1).

In 1925 Sargent reviewed all the literature from the time of Gaupp's first case report in 1888 and added four cases of his own for a total of 21 cases.[22,45] In all but two the lesion was considered to be a venous angioma. Only the case of Raymond and Cestan in 1904 and one of Sargent's cases were considered to have arterial components.[43] He miscited one of Elsberg's cases, however, in which the lesion was clearly described, was called by Elsberg "an arteriovenous aneurysm," and was illustrated by a classic picture.[19] Sargent stressed the fluctuating course of the symptoms with intermittent remissions and exacerbations in the progression of neurological difficulty.

In his famous monograph, Wyburn-Mason noted that the literature indicated that angioma racemosum venosum, a purely venous anomaly, was the common type.[55] He said, however, that in his experience arteriovenous anomalies were at least as common as venous. He was able to collect 80 cases from the literature, of which 61 were considered venous and 19 arteriovenous. He added 14 venous cases and 16 arteriovenous cases from his own materials. Wyburn-Mason recognized that purely arterial malformations did not exist and also believed that many of the cases that had been considered as venous in character were actually arteriovenous, a conclusion that was fully confirmed years later.

ANATOMICAL AND PHYSIOLOGICAL CONSIDERATIONS

Vascular Anatomy of the Spinal Cord

All arteries entering the spinal canal enter with a nerve root and follow the root to the cord. Accordingly, arteries to the lowest part of the cord must have a long ascending path, while midthoracic arteries have a correspondingly shorter path. Cervical cord arteries have a virtually horizontal entrance.

L. I. MALIS

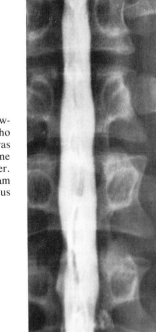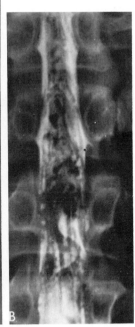

Figure 55-1 *A*. Prone lumbar myelogram showing the area from T11 through L2 in a patient who complained of sciatica. One curvilinear shadow was interpreted as a probable swollen root. *B*. Prone myelogram covering the same area one year later. The patient now is paraparetic, and the myelogram shows the canal to be filled with an arteriovenous malformation later confirmed at operation.

The ventral root arteries are few in number, usually from three to seven. They join the anterior spinal artery, which has a predominantly downward flow and a lumen that tapers to a quite narrow diameter until the next inferior ventral root artery enters. The anterior spinal artery then widens abruptly and again tapers downward. Angiographically, this produces a hairpin or hooklike appearance in each ventral entering artery. The downward limb of the hook is the anterior spinal artery.

In contrast, the dorsolateral arteries have a rather constant diameter, with dorsal entering arteries at almost every level and a very complete collateral network. The dorsal entering arteries are much smaller than the ventral arteries and normally are demonstrated angiographically only with difficulty if at all. As would be expected, when the dorsal entering artery is visualized, it takes the same ascending course as a ventral entering artery. The hook or hairpin appearance of the ventral entering artery is replaced by a simple end-to-side junction when the dorsolateral spinal artery is also visualized.

When an arteriovenous malformation is fed by either a dorsal or a ventral entering artery, the upward course of the entering artery is determined only by the spinal level.[3] Just as in intracranial arteriovenous malformations, the artery will enlarge because of the increased flow through the arteriovenous shunt.

Normally, the largest ventral entering artery, the great radicular artery, also called the artery of Adamkiewicz, supplies the lumbar cord and conus. It enters more often from the left side, usually between T6 and T12.[1] Its relative importance is in part determined by the size and contribution of the ascending artery originating from an iliac artery branch, which accompanies the filum terminale up to the conus. It must be noted that the definition of the artery of Adamkiewicz depends upon size, its position being quite variable. If an arteriovenous malformation is present, the major arterial feeder will have become the largest artery, but this may not warrant being called the artery of Adamkiewicz. A few segments away, the artery of Adamkiewicz may be present, providing adequate circulation to the cord. In this situation the huge hooked vessel supplying the malformation could be sacrificed without damage.

Bergstrand and co-workers described the

pathological findings.[5] The larger pial arteries are markedly abnormal. The veins usually are as wide as the arteries. The vessels have thickened walls, mainly of collagenous connective tissue. The intima is thickened, owing to endothelial proliferation, and often there are organized thrombi. Small penetrating vessels to the cord also are greatly thickened, their walls made up predominantly of hyalinized connective tissue. Elastic substance is completely lacking. A distinction between arteries and veins usually is not possible.

Pathophysiological Mechanisms

Steal Phenomena

The concept of stealing of blood has been promulgated to explain the neural dysfunction accompanying both cerebral and spinal arteriovenous malformations. Probably this is the most widely accepted explanation. Several logical problems raise questions about it. Most obvious is the improvement, at least temporarily, when the proximal feeder vessel or vessels are ligated. This ligation leaves the shunt and venous drain intact and should greatly increase the steal phenomenon, which in turn should lead to a marked increase in symptoms. Since an increase in symptoms does not occur, another explanation is required. The same is true for embolization. Doppman, DiChiro, and Ommaya emphasize that emboli lodge at the arterial narrowing that apparently is at the site of arterial penetration of the dura.[17] Again, this is a proximal occlusion that leaves the drain and the shunt intact and should increase the steal from any other zones of arterial supply.

Indeed, if steal were a factor, obliteration of the shunt, presumably by thrombosis, would have to follow proximal vessel ligation in order to provide benefit and avoid catastrophe. It is well known that occlusion of the shunt does not occur with proximal occlusion unless all the arteries are ligated or embolized. Yet, the patients may show considerable improvement until the remaining arteries again enlarge. The use of the term "siphoning" as a synonymn for "steal" appears to be particularly suspect, since pressure in the arteriovenous malformation venous drain is increased rather than decreased as compared with normal

veins. Perhaps the decreased flow in the adjacent normal areas is the result of the increased venous pressure in the draining system. The only gradient to move blood from the normal arterial supply network into the arteriovenous malformation is the pressure difference between the arterial feeder and the venous drain. Rate of shunt flow will be determined by a complex of pressure differences and vessel diameters and lengths, with the supplying arteries dilating rapidly (within weeks) to make up the shunt requirement if some arteries are closed. In like manner, if the shunt can be occluded, the size of the enlarged arteries decreases proximally to reach normal within a few weeks. Again, the compensatory change in arterial size militates against acceptance of the concept of a steal phenomenon.

The concept of stealing of blood arose from the study of occlusive disease in which inability to enlarge or maintain the size of a diseased vascular lumen led to flow reversal in remaining arteries and indeed produced a vascular steal. In an open system with a shunt, the hydrodynamic basis for a steal is not present. Further, empirical observations with proximal ligation tend to negate this explanation of the problem.

Thrombosis

Another mechanism to account for the progressive symptoms is thrombosis. Perhaps it is more difficult to understand why thrombosis should occur than to recognize that it does occur. Why thrombosis should produce catastrophic symptoms is also difficult to understand, but again it undeniably may do so. Possibly spontaneous thrombosis occurs more often without symptoms and produces damage only if it involves vascular channels to the spinal cord rather than (or in addition to) the malformation.

Compression

In the older literature, compression was the mechanism most often considered responsible for symptoms. Yet, the number of arteriovenous malformations with block is exceedingly small. Also, the result of simple decompressive procedures has been significantly worse than the natural course of the disease. These results are hardly to be expected if compression from the mass of the lesion is a major cause of the symptoms. There are cases, however, in which a huge vascular glomus does produce block and true cord compression. This concept will not, however, explain the deterioration in the great majority of clinical cases.

Two additional possible mechanisms come to mind. Pulsatile compression is a particular sort of neural trauma. The coils of the arteriovenous malformation are bound to the cord by multiple pial-arachnoid bands, and their undersurfaces are deeply grooved into a thickened, shiny pial layer. With each cardiac pulsation, these loops expand. Each heartbeat brings another water hammer striking against the cord. The impressive vigor and firmness of the pulsatile movement is seen when a looping vessel of this type is dissected from the cord while it is still in continuity with its arterial supply. The movement is particularly marked in the more proximal parts of the lesion. The thinning of the cord in the grooves made by the malformation testifies to the underlying damage. This explanation will fit a great deal of the data that have been observed. Simple posterior decompression will not release the pulsatile coils, which are bound to the cord by multiple bands. Perhaps the improvement following dentate ligament section noted in Teng and Papatheodoru's unconfirmed report could have resulted from the freer movement of the cord with the vessel pulsation that decreased the force of each pulsatile impact.[50] Also, proximal ligation or embolization in the absence of or prior to collateral revascularization would decrease the pulsatile movement and its pressure on the cord and would be expected to improve the neurological status. Obviously, removal of the arteriovenous malformation or closure of the shunt would totally protect the cord from further pulsatile trauma.

Venous Pressure Increase

Finally, chronic increase of venous pressure will be present in the small venules draining the local capillary bed if they have collaterals to the arteriovenous malformation drain.[2] This increased venous pressure may prevent normal capillary membrane transfer. Since it is a quite local phenomenon rather than a generalized pressure increase, as evidenced by normal cerebrospinal fluid pressure, arterial pressure compensation will not occur, and the normal capillary gradient will be decreased or obliterated. This hypothesis could explain the progressive myelomalacia. The improvement produced by proximal ligation would follow, since any decrease of arterial flow in the malformation would cause a marked drop in venous pressure and so permit a capillary gradient to be re-established.

SYNDROMES AND NATURAL HISTORY

While most patients do not present with any specific picture that will differentiate their disease from other intraspinal lesions, some will be found with characteristic syndromes. About 15 per cent present with subarachnoid hemorrhage.[4,25,51,55] The diagnosis is obvious when the hemorrhage is accompanied by paraplegia or quadriplegia. Frequently, however, there will not be any associated clear cord manifestations, and diagnosis of the spinal origin may be difficult. Onset of subarachnoid hemorrhage with sudden excruciating back pain (coup de poignard of Michon) is strongly indicative of an arteriovenous malformation of the spinal cord.[35]

Very rarely, auscultation of a bruit over the spine is diagnostic of an arteriovenous shunt or other high-velocity flow that suddenly meets a point of altered resistance.[26] Most often heard over huge juvenile arteriovenous malformations, such a bruit has also occurred in extraspinal lesions.

Occasionally, the presence of an associated cutaneous vascular angioma will lead to the diagnosis of a spinal arteriovenous malformation. The two lesions will be fed by the same arterial metamere, although their circulation is independent. The cutaneous lesion will expand and darken during a Valsalva maneuver.[18]

A small percentage of patients present with catastrophic onset of paraplegia or quadriplegia without subarachnoid hemorrhage. This acute necrotizing myelitis, the syndrome of Foix-Alajouanine, is the result of spontaneous occlusion in an arteriovenous malformation and infarction of the spinal cord.[21] While some improvement has occurred in some patients, this complication is essentially untreatable and often is fatal.

About 85 per cent of patients present with progressive neurological loss, and in 50 per cent of these it is intermittent and recurrent. Pain is frequent, often dysesthetic, usually radicular, and relatively severe. It tends to be worse with exertion or application of heat, and may be worse on recumbency; however, the pattern is not consistent from patient to patient.[36,55] Rarely, the pain is altered by cough or strain. Pregnancy nearly always makes the pain and the neurological defect worse.

Gait disturbance tends to be the most common early neurological complaint. It often resembles claudication and can be increased by walking. After the patient rests briefly, the gait may improve markedly, only to become again impaired as walking is resumed. At this stage, bladder dysfunction with occasional incontinence or retention begins.

Following the early period of pain, gait disturbance, and bladder dysfunction, the onset of weakness in one or more limbs presages rapid deterioration. During the next phase, averaging about two years from the onset of significant weakness, the patient develops progressive spastic paraparesis and sensory loss. Impairment of bladder and bowel control becomes severe, and finally there is a syndrome of total transection of the cord. The paraplegia usually is flaccid, probably because there is destruction of a large area of the cord rather than transection at a single level. In the past, the mortality rate has been high, with an average survival time of only seven years.[36]

RADIOLOGICAL INVESTIGATION

In this era of neuroradiology, every patient with progressive neurological disease should have an appropriate definitive study at least once. A surprising number of patients with tumors and arteriovenous malformations will be separated from those whose disorders have been diagnosed clinically as multiple sclerosis and other diseases.

Most of the patients should be studied first by myelography. In 1924 Guillain and Alajouanine clearly described the myelographic picture of the tortuous channels as shown by the drops of Lipiodol enmeshed in the vascular network.[23] They did not recognize the lesion, but found the explanation by operative exploration. In 1927 Perthes made the diagnosis by myelography preoperatively and successfully performed a resection.[40] Since most of the malformations are on the dorsal surface of the cord, it is more usual now to do supine Pantopaque myelography for these lesions. The author prefers prone myelography with enough oil to fill the canal in the entire area of interest. With the patient prone and with the sac full of oil, the cord floats up against the dorsal surface and outlines the vessels. Metrizamide myelography has the advantage of not obscuring subsequent spinal angiography. Because of normal dorsal kyphosis, there may be difficulty in filling the thoracic canal with the contrast material in the prone position, but the problem is readily overcome by using larger quantities of the medium. As much as 30 or 40 ml or more is frequently used. The normal midline irregular defect seen in most supine thoracic myelograms is thought to represent the arachnoid bands associated with the dorsal midline raphe, the so-called septum posticum. This filling defect may make recognition of the malformation difficult when the study is performed in the supine position, but it does not appear in prone myelography (Fig. 55–2).

In either the prone or supine position, cross-table x-ray projections give the best information below the full-column fluid level.[33] Complete compression block is unusual. Repeated hemorrhage, however, with arachnoid sealing and scarring, may produce an apparent block. A vascular mass sufficient to cause block is unusual. Expansion of the cord with or without block is more likely due to intramedullary tumor with accompanying dilation of vessels, though it occurs in some malformations with intramedullary extensions.

In 1958 Hook and Lidvall reported two cervical lesions demonstrated by vertebral angiography.[26] They noted that angiography should settle the question of arterial, arteriovenous, or venous origin. Djindjian and co-workers introduced the use of aortography for spinal angiography in 1962 with the first of a series of papers delineating this subject.[12] In 1967 DiChiro, Doppman, and Ommaya stressed the importance of selective spinal angiography, the tech-

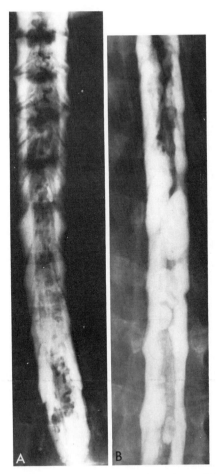

Figure 55–2 *A*. Prone upper thoracic myelogram performed with 42 ml of Pantopaque clearly shows the arteriovenous malformation. Lateral myelography and later operation demonstrated this lesion to be on the dorsal surface. *B*. In the myelogram in the supine position and covering the same area, the characteristic midline defect of the "septum posticum" is seen and the appearance of the malformation is obscured.

nique of which they had pioneered since 1964. This method requires experience and skill on the part of the angiographer. Part of the skill consists in making certain that the correct branch of the spinal artery is injected and in filling the spinal circulation around the rib cage. If the little blush of vessels in the paravertebral muscle is not seen, the catheter must be repositioned.

The process of catheterizing each individual aortic or iliac branch that might contribute to the circulation of the lesion as well as the carotid and vertebral systems demands a long detailed study. In addition, the patient suffers discomfort over many hours and receives a large amount of radia-

tion and radiopaque material. While the risk has been decreased with more modern equipment and techniques, there is still morbidity that increases with multiple injections of dye and the taking of lateral, stereoscopic, and magnified views. Small-vessel identification as well as magnification may require general anesthesia to permit control of all movement, particularly respiratory excursions.

Even with a skilled and experienced angiographic team, it is unusual for the study to demonstrate the arteriovenous malformation as well as it is seen at operation. Occasionally, it will be impossible to demonstrate angiographically a malformation that has been demonstrated by myelography. For instance, a feeding vessel may be seen on the myelogram, yet repeated repositioning and reinjection at this intercostal space may never fill the cord circulation (Fig. 55–3). DiChiro and co-workers reported failure to demonstrate 3 out of 23 lesions of this type.[10] It must be assumed that there may have been an anomalous take-off of the spinal vessel through a separate aortic branch; even intra-aortic injection directed at the intercostal ostium in an effort to prevent spinal branch occlusion by the catheter had failed to solve the problem.

Luessenhop and Cruz had reported inability to demonstrate angiographically the three myelographically diagnosed lesions they successfully excised.[32] Pool noted the malformations to be more extensive at operation than they appeared on the angiograms.[42]

While angiography has demonstrated much about the dynamic flow patterns and flow rates and has given clear delineation of the extent of the lesion in the cervical area, its preoperative value remains in question in thoracic lesions. In the majority of cases there will be findings at operation that are unpredicted by the angiograms. In the most common lesions, the long racemose arteriovenous malformation, operation could be performed as well without the angiogram as with it. In the thoracic glomus lesion, angiography should be most valuable. Here, however, the usually incomplete information provided by most studies can be quite misleading. With the best available myelographic and angiographic guidance, the surgeon still may have no certainty that a particular feeding vessel may be safely closed. As the complexity of the lesion increases,

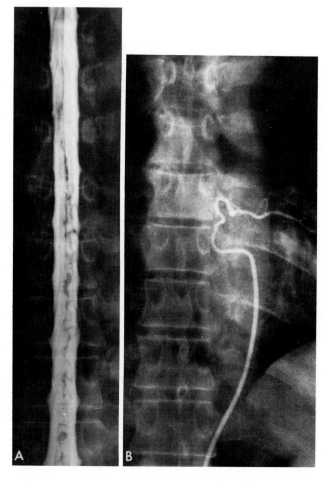

Figure 55-3 *A*. Myelographic demonstration of a thoracic arteriovenous malformation shows outlining of the feeding vessel on the right at T8. *B*. Selective angiography repeatedly failed to demonstrate circulation to the malformation. Aortic flush injection also failed to demonstrate this lesion. Operative exploration confirmed that this vessel was indeed the largest arterial pedicle.

so does its operative difficulty. Unfortunately, in this situation, angiography gives progressively less help.

A major criticism of spinal angiography as compared with cerebral angiography is the inability to demonstrate the normal vasculature of the cord except in the most rudimentary way. The circulation in intramedullary glial tumors, even with concomitant markedly dilated vessels, is not visualized angiographically.[8] It appears that there would be little value in performing a postoperative angiogram in an attempt to confirm the complete resection of a lesion whose arterial feeders were so poorly demonstrated preoperatively.

CLASSIFICATION OF MALFORMATIONS

These lesions tend, fairly consistently, to take certain patterns. All appear to be arteriovenous shunts. It would seem that Wyburn-Mason's "angioma racemosum venosum" does not exist. None has ever been demonstrated angiographically, nor has any lesion found in the modern era failed to have an arteriovenous shunt.

The concept of a purely arterial malformation also has been rejected for the same reasons. There is one type of completely arterial lesion with hugely enlarged anterior spinal and segmental arteries in the lower cervical and upper dorsal regions that may be accompanied by severe neurological damage. This arterial dilatation is produced by the huge collateral enlargement in an uncorrected coarctation of the aorta. In this situation, diagnosis of the coarctation and its correction will avoid potentially embarrassing neurosurgical involvement.[52-54]

Long Dorsal Lesion

The most common spinal cord arteriovenous malformation is the posteriorly placed long lesion. Also it is the easiest to resect. Since Wyburn-Mason's material was mostly derived from autopsy study, the inability to demonstrate the arterial shunt is readily understood. His angioma racemosum venosum probably corresponds to this long dorsal lesion and could be called simply angioma racemosum, as suggested by H. Bergstrand and by Krayenbühl, Yaşargil, and McClintock, or the single coiled-vessel malformation, as suggested by Doppman, DiChiro, and Ommaya.[6,16,29] The author prefers the name "long dorsal arteriovenous malformation" (Fig. 55-4).

The lesions receive at least two or three major feeders coming in along with corresponding dorsal roots. At each dorsal root, there is normally a small arteriole, entering to feed into the pair of dorsolateral spinal arteries. Where a large dorsal artery feeds into the malformation, it is nearly always a separate vessel, implying a separate circulation, with a normal smaller vessel on the same dorsal root going to the dorsolateral chain.[30,37,47] There are multiple anastomoses between the two normal dorsolateral arteries, forming a fine dorsal arterial plexus, with penetrating branches along the midline raphe. Multiple communications

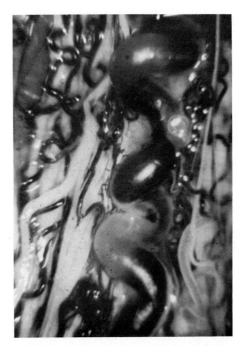

Figure 55-5 Sedimentation of red cells and separation of serum appears as typical dark sediment beneath a golden layer of fluid, indicating cessation of flow within the malformation. This strongly suggests that the shunt has been occluded.

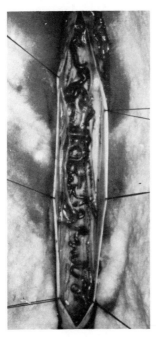

Figure 55-4 Typical operative appearance of a long dorsal arteriovenous malformation. The vessels were bright red and were pulsatile, though the pressure within them was only about 30 mm of mercury.

pass between the dorsolateral arterial plexus and the malformation. These communications have been described as providing the opportunity for the steal phenomenon, which has been thought to produce the progressive neurological deficit. Eventually, these communications become less frequent, and finally an area is reached where the drain is purely venous with no further new arterial input. While sometimes some drainage exits laterally to join the epidural venous plexus, most of the drainage tends to travel cephalad. There are less frequent long caudal drains as well. When ligated at this point, the entire long drain above will cease to flow, and sedimentation of the red cells from the serum will occur within its lumen (Fig. 55-5).

The long dorsal lesions are the only ones with little or no ventral arterial communication. Even when a loop penetrates into the cord, if the loop is isolated and cut, no blood will drain from the intramedullary segment. Finally, this type of malformation is the only one in which the intravascular pressure is relatively low, averaging 20 to 30 mm of mercury, despite the clearly arterial blood they contain.

"Glomus" Malformation

Another type of lesion is the so-called glomus malformation.[39] Unlike the long dorsal racemose malformations, these tend to have only one or two major feeders and a high pressure. They will have numerous small collaterals. Although often located posteriorly, the glomus malformation regularly is fed by a major arterial trunk that is more likely to be a ventral rather than a dorsal entering artery. Either artery may loop around the lateral surface of the cord. If the entering artery is truly a ventral artery, it may supply a main branch to the malformation before continuing on to supply the anterior spinal artery, but it is more likely to give off the branch to the anterior spinal artery and then continue on to be the major feeder of the malformation. While these lesions may have a long drain ascending or descending the cord, they are marked by the presence of the "glomus," a relatively small mass of strongly pulsating tangled vessels, usually becoming intramedullary at least in part. When intramedullary, they regularly have feeder vessels from the anterior spinal artery.

These glomus lesions are not usually ventral lesions. Most of their substance is posterior to the dentate ligament, as is the major loop of arterial supply. They frequently have aneurysmal dilatations, usually incorporating the point from which bleeding occurs and usually at the arterial junction of feeding vessels.

Cervical Intramedullary Lesions

There are two special types of cervical intramedullary lesions. The entirely intramedullary lesion is more common. It resembles the glomus lesion of the lower cord, except that it is almost completely within the cord. While there are one or more feeders entering with ventral or dorsal roots (perhaps from the costocervical trunk or a thyroid or pharyngeal artery), there is virtually always a line of fine arteries extending directly posteriorly through the cord from the enlarged anterior spinal artery to enter the ventral surface of the intramedullary malformation. Intravascular pressure is close to systemic arterial pressure in these lesions.

Another group of cervical lesions occur at the cervicomedullary junction. These lesions are dorsally placed. Usually they have some intramedullary extension and are directly fed by vertebral artery branches, which divide into an enlarged posterior division that goes to the malformation and a smaller normal ventral division that continues on to form the anterior spinal artery. Also regularly associated with thin-walled aneurysmal sacs, these formidable lesions may continue cephalad onto the brain stem. Frequently they can be operated on easily, owing to the fortunate circumstance that most, if not all, of the shunting vessels are dorsal or dorsolateral.

While these two types of cervical lesions might be classified as subgroups of glomus lesions, it is important to recognize the difference between both forms of cervical lesions and the thoracic glomus lesions, because that difference greatly alters the operative procedures.

Juvenile Malformations

Fortunately, the malformations classified as juvenile by DiChiro, Doppman, and Ommaya are the rarest.[10] Their large feeding arteries may be more than 1 cm in diameter. They surround the cord for many segments. Other anomalies such as a tethered cord reaching the sacrum or a duplicated anomalous cord with huge vascular channels between the two halves may accompany them (Fig. 55–6). Frequently, there are associated collateral vessels in huge tangles in the mediastinum, the pelvis, or the retroperitoneal space. Anomalous vessels may perforate the bone to enter the lesion instead of just enlarging the normal trunks. These patients have a significantly increased cardiac output requirement, usually secondary to the extraspinal component. Scoliosis, maldevelopment of extremities, paralysis, and recurrent bleeding regularly coexist in these unfortunate patients. Bruit, often audible at a modest distance, is common.

Also there is a group of extradural malformations without intradural arterial connections. Sometimes they have the widespread massive involvement of the juvenile lesion. Pia reported a high incidence of the latter type.[41]

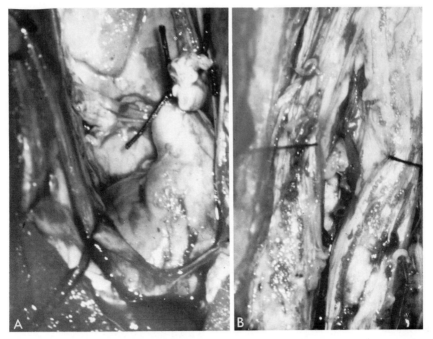

Figure 55–6 *A*. Lower end of laminectomy at L5, showing a huge aneurysmal sac fed by a perforating transsacral branch of the iliac artery. The connection from the aneurysmal sac to the ascending malformation in the cauda equina has been ligated with braided silk. The cauda equina has been parted by the vascular mass. *B*. The photograph taken at the L3 level shows that the spinal cord is duplicated and reaches past the L3 level, in fact ending at L4. The two halves of the cord are held apart by pial traction sutures. The extensive arteriovenous malformation between the two halves of the cord has been shrunk by bipolar coagulation preparatory to resection.

TREATMENT

As has been demonstrated for many years in cerebral arteriovenous malformations, the only proved successful treatment is obliteration of the lesion. Decompression serves no purpose except perhaps in the rare case in which a juvenile lesion may actually cause cord compression. Indeed, decompression has produced poorer results than a nonoperative approach.

Proximal Ligation

Houdart and co-workers stated that much of the complexity and size of some of the arteriovenous malformations was due to the presence of a long venous pedicle that is not really part of the malformation.[27] They advocated ligation of the arterial pedicles. Although they recognized the inability to demonstrate all of them, or to expose all of them operatively, they thought that their ligation would decrease the flow and benefit the patient. DiChiro, Doppman, and Ommaya stressed feeder ligation and reported good results.[9,39] Bailey and Sperl reported two cases of cervical intramedullary arteriovenous malformations proved by angiography and treated by feeder ligation.[3] Postoperative angiography was done in one of the cases, however, and demonstrated that early collateral enlargement had already occurred.

In summary, proximal ligation may give initial improvement in some cases, particularly those in which repeated bleeding has been the major problem, but often it will lead to an increase in other collateral pathways and to revascularization. Recently Ommaya withdrew his advocacy of the technique.[38]

Embolization

Newton and Adams reported the first case of embolization of an arteriovenous malformation with recovery from paraplegia.[37] Their case is of particular interest, since the major supply appeared to come from the artery of Adamkiewicz. This vessel was completely occluded by the procedure. Houdart and co-workers stated that occlusion of even a few of the afferent arteries may diminish the pressure and thus reduce the risk of subsequent subarachnoid hemorrhage.[27]

Doppman, DiChiro, and Ommaya reported on their technique of percutaneous embolization of arteriovenous cord malformations.[15,17] They emphasized that there is a focal area of narrowing of the arterial feeders just inside the spinal canal. They believed that this narrowing is the point where the artery penetrates the dura and is the ideal site for embolic impaction. Their report concerned five patients, of whom three had progressive improvement and two were unchanged.

Embolization remains as a developing technique. Obliteration of the arteriovenous shunt is required if the method is to be completely effective. Embolization of feeder vessels is likely to be permanently effective only if sufficient slowing of total flow occurs to allow thrombotic occlusion of the shunting lesion. It will be safe only if sufficient spinal vascular supply is preserved to prevent cord ischemia. Further discussion of embolization techniques is given in Chapter 33. With the glomus lesions at least, this technique would appear to hold considerable promise. It may constitute either complete therapy or preparation for an operative approach.

Operative Excision

The first operative exposure of a spinal cord arteriovenous malformation was reported by Krause in 1911.[28] The patient was paraplegic and did not improve after partial ligation of the vessels of the lesion. The first successful removal of what may have been arteriovenous malformation was performed by Elsberg in 1914.[19] His patient had severe spastic paresis of the left leg and marked sensory loss up to T9 on the right. A left posterior spinal vein as large as the nerve root accompanied the eighth dorsal root and ran up the cord. Unfortunately, the artist's drawing of the operative appearance is not very convincing. A 2-cm segment of the vein was excised, and complete neurological recovery occurred. Elsberg stated that the recovery might have been due simply to the laminectomy or to "the

free entrance of air into the subdural space."

In 1927, Perthes used Lipiodol to make the diagnosis of a spinal cord arteriovenous malformation by myelography.[40] He radically removed the lesion, and the patient recovered. Since this well-illustrated malformation would now be considered a typical lesion, Perthes's case probably is the first clear operative success as well. Scoville performed the first successful removal of an intramedullary arteriovenous malformation in 1941.[46] The procedure included clipping of the anterior spinal artery. The patient was paraplegic immediately after the operation but recovered excellent function.

Newman reported operation on 11 cases with no successes.[36] Svien and Baker reviewed 23 cases operated upon at the Mayo Clinic, in none of which was there improvement.[49] Bergstrand and co-workers reported 11 cases treated by operation, all with poor results.[5] On the other hand, in 1965 Shepard reported 11 cases that he had operated on, and 7 had improved after the resection.[48]

Krayenbühl and associates reported on 17 cases, of which 11 had total removal and 6 had subtotal removal.[29] Results were excellent in 5, good or fair in 8, and poor in 3. Later, Yaşargil reported 24 cases with 13 radical removals, 7 subtotal removals with coagulation and obliteration of the remaining vessels, and 4 subtotal removals of the lesion.[56,57] All 13 total resections produced excellent results. Yaşargil noted that in these 24 cases, two malformations were intramedullary, one in the lateral aspect of the cervical cord and one in the ventrolateral aspect of the thoracic cord. None lay ventral to the cord; the other 22 were located posteriorly. He emphasized the operability of the malformations when micro-operative technique was used and the importance of bipolar coagulation. He demonstrated the multiple connections of the pial anastomosis and the dorsolateral arterial chain. These multiple connections need to be sealed if the shunt and steal are to be cured.

Guidetti reported on 26 cases of spinal arteriovenous malformation, 15 of which were operated upon. Six patients had decompression, only two of whom had slight reduction of their spastic paraparesis, and two had ligation of feeders with no improvement; but seven had total removal, and four of these had marked benefit. He drew the straightforward conclusion that the best results are obtained if the motor defect is mild, the lesion is extramedullary and posterior, and total removal is accomplished.[23]

Yaşargil, DeLong, and Guarnaschelli reported on their unique series of 11 cervical arteriovenous malformations, representing 16 per cent of the 76 cases of arteriovenous malformations Yaşargil had then operated on under the microscope.[59] All 11 lesions were totally excised, and nine patients had good results.

Unfortunately, the relatively ineffectual nature of operative treatment in the premicroscope era has not been countered by reeducation. Too many patients are still referred after they develop severe paresis and bladder dysfunction. Their lesions are already of large size, making the operation more difficult, the hazard greater, and the result less likely to be satisfactory. Even then, operation is still the only chance the patient has for any long-term preservation of function.

Contraindications to operative intervention are relative. The most difficult patient to assess is the one who has had a laminectomy and may have scarring that will make it impossible to remove the malformation completely. If a wide laminectomy to decompress the entire lesion was performed and the dura was left open, re-exploration is more likely to be ineffectual. If artificial or natural dural substitutes were used, the scarring and adhesive process may be even worse. Sometimes the cord and malformation will look as if they had been coated with opaque glue. In this situation, the dissection is impossible (Fig. 55–7). Closure of the dura, or the use of fat or a Gelfoam layer when complete closure was not possible, has more frequently permitted reoperation with reasonable success.

If not too severe, repeated bleeding episodes will be lysed by the spinal fluid without a marked arachnoidal reaction. If massive bleeding occurs, as it does in some of the high-pressure lesions, particularly of the juvenile group, the entire spinal subarachnoid space may fill with a clot that prevents lysis of the blood by the cerebrospinal fluid, leading to the formation of an impenetrable scar. Usually subarachnoid

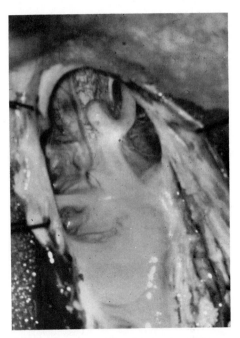

Figure 55–7 Re-exploration one year after a previous exploration at which the dura had been left open for decompression. The exposure that has been achieved has already taken several hours of microdissection. It is clearly impossible to visualize the malformation in a manner permitting micro-operative excision, and only fragmentary pedicle ligation is feasible.

hemorrhage from a spinal arteriovenous malformation indicates the need for an early operation. Preferably, the operation should be done as soon as the patient's post-hemorrhage state permits and before organization of scar is likely to have occurred (Fig. 55–8).

A special problem and possibly a contraindication to operation has developed that is unique to the United States. The patient who enters the operating room still able to walk and who leaves it as a paraplegic is extremely likely to enter a malpractice claim. This is true regardless of the degree of hazard to the patient if the operation is not performed, the nature of the informed consent, or the skill and experience of the surgeon. For lesions with ventral connections, and others with greater than average risk, particularly in patients who appear to have questionable personality traits or to be hostile, the risk to the surgeon rather than that to the patient may have to be the determining factor. It may be necessary to inform the patient that the surgeon cannot carry out the procedure because of this

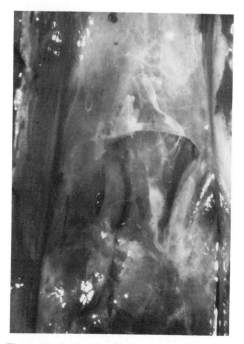

Figure 55-8 Exploration two weeks after massive subarachnoid hemorrhage filled the spinal canal. The subarachnoid space is filled with golden-brown, partially organized blood clot, its consistency resembling that of an intracranial subdural hematoma. It was still possible to remove the clot in order to proceed with resection of the malformation. The later stages of this patient's operation appeared in Figure 55-6.

risk, though he believes that the patient requires the operation. Such patients should be given an explanation of the problem and the names of neurosurgeons (almost certainly from outside the United States) who might be willing to make the attempt.

Operative Technique

While there may well be surgeons of sufficient skill and technical proficiency to achieve excellent results without magnification, the author has performed all removals under the Zeiss OPMI operating microscope. Usually the 16 × magnification changer setting is used with occasional shifts up to 25 × or down to 10 ×. With the 300-mm objective, the 125-mm binocular, and the 20 × oculars, the actual magnification is half of that on the magnification changer.

Adequate positioning for removal of a spinal arteriovenous malformation requires that the spine be fixed so that respiratory movement does not alter the position of the cord and move it out of the focus of the mi-

croscope. Also, there must be access to the field for the surgeon's arms, which should be supported in a comfortable manner.

For the operative exposure from the suboccipital region down through T3, the semi-sitting position can be used. It must be appropriately modified to permit an easy approach for the microscope and the surgeon, who is seated. The head should be fixed in the Gardner or Mayfield pinned headrest, and the patient should be wrapped in an inner thermal circulating blanket and an outer Gardner pressure suit. Because of the progressive fall in body temperature during the long operation, supportive heating should be used to keep the temperature above 35°C. Doppler monitoring of the right side of the heart and a transvenous endocardiac catheter should be used routinely. Controlled respiration should be used for all patients, and usually hypotension of 70 mm of mercury mean is maintained.

The oblique position is used for the thoracic and lumbar arteriovenous malformations. The patient is placed in flexion with his back close to the edge of the table. The table should be flexed to straighten the slight scoliotic curve that is induced by the lateral position. Next the patient is tilted forward to about 45 degrees. The underneath arm should be brought forward, and care must be taken to prevent obstruction of brachial venous return. When the lesion extends above T2, the head may be raised and fixed in a proper position with the pinned headrest. This technique allows access all the way up the cervical spine. With the patient in the oblique position, the surgeon is physically comfortable, and the use of a padded armrest adds to his dexterity. Because of the 45-degree angle, some anatomical reorientation is required. The ease with which the reorientation is achieved differs greatly, even among experienced surgeons.

There is no perfect position, particularly when operative procedures last more than 10 to 14 hours. Decubiti can form despite padding, and the opportunity to turn the patient periodically is not available. The use of alternating-pressure pneumatic pads prevents maintenance of fixation of the field and focus, both of which are essential to micro-operative procedures. Thick soft foam padding also causes loss of fixation. The use of silicone gel pads will protect the patient from skin pressure but leave him so mobile that operation under the microscope cannot be done.

Staging the longest operation into two or more procedures obviously is easier on the surgeon. It appears, however to carry additional risk because of reaction, edema, and alteration in the lesion at the junction between the first and second procedures. More rapid operative technique could be even more of a hazard, particularly in some of the complex lesions, which require meticulous dissection with precise hemostasis.

When the wide laminectomy has been completed (usually starting at the lowest level at which the malformation is present), the dura is opened and sewn back over the laminar cut edges with traction sutures. This controls hemorrhage from epidural veins and provides the maximum exposure. Preserving the arachnoid will prevent epidural bleeding while the dural sutures are being placed. Also, the intact arachnoid will protect the malformation from damage while it is still inadequately exposed. At this point, it may be obvious that the malformation continues cephalad or caudad past the level of the laminectomy. If six or eight segments have already been exposed, it is best not to extend the laminectomy, since the apparent continuation may be only a draining vein without further arteriovenous communication.

Long Dorsal Lesions

The long dorsal lesion is common, and it will have feeding vessels coming in with the dorsal roots. If the feeding vessels have been visualized myelographically or angiographically, the surgeon may proceed directly to them. If a total excision is to be done and dissection of the arachnoid will be required over the entire lesion, however, the arachnoid dissection may be done without first ligating the feeding vessels. Sharp dissection with fine pointed microscissors, pointed freshly cut razor blade bits, or the diamond knife is required. Blunt dissection must be avoided; it will tear the malformation away from the small communicating vessels of the cord circulation and lead to hemorrhage and cord trauma. The malformation may loop upon itself or have T connections, some to feeding arteries and some to draining veins. These connections are difficult or impossible to tell apart.

Occasionally an unusual looking structure, the so-called "white vessel," is encountered. It is a thick-walled artery with an extremely fine threadlike lumen and virtually no flow. How these vessels develop or function is not known. The author has seen them most often in cases with rapid loss of function. Their presence usually is followed by a poor postoperative result. Perhaps they represent a stage in vascular occlusion leading to myelomalacia (Fig. 55–9).

Except in the cauda equina, the drainage usually is upward. As a result, it usually is easier to begin at the most caudal feeding vessel. If a large feeding vessel comes in more cephalad, however, there is no hesitation in closing it first. The arachnoid dissection should be precise and should free the feeding artery from the attached root fibers. Since these are not part of the malformation, any arteries going to the tortuous and enlarged but nevertheless normal dorsal lateral arteries should be freed by dissection. The feeding vessel should then be slowly coagulated with the lowest power of the bipolar coagulator that will produce a slow shrinkage. This coagulation is done under

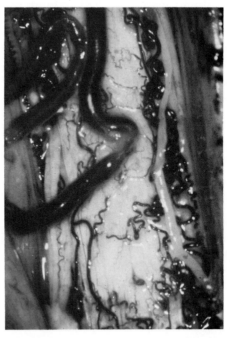

Figure 55–9 The loops of a partly resected arteriovenous malformation are seen on the left side of the picture. Running along the right side of the cord is a so-called "white vessel." A very tiny threadlike lumen appears to be present in at least some areas within this smooth, shiny, thick-walled vascular structure.

sufficient saline irrigation to prevent heating of the adjacent neural fibers. When the feeding vessel is rather well occluded, it is doubly clipped and cut between clips. At this point there may be a change in the malformation, with arterialized blood turning dark, at least for a short while. Since these malformations are low-pressure lesions, closing a major venous drain instead of a feeding artery will only lead to enlargement of some of the vessels and increased pulsation, and while it may increase the difficulty of dissection, it will not be serious. When in doubt, it is easy to put a temporary clip on the apparent feeding vessel and observe the result before permanently closing it. If a draining vessel is clipped and there is no other drain for a significant distance, flow may cease in that segment, and the blood may lose its bright color, even though pulsation increases with higher pressure, and this can be misleading.

After a feeding vessel has been clipped, removal of the malformation consists of cutting all the little trabeculae of arachnoid that bind the vessels to the pia. Each of the fine communicating branches from the cord circulation to the malformation must be isolated and closed with a very fine, sharp bipolar forceps. The forceps should be at the very lowest possible setting and under continuous saline irrigation. With these precautions, the tiny communicating vessels may be cut while the essential dorsolateral arteries are preserved (Fig. 55–10).

Even very complex coiled malformations may be removed in one very long piece. It is usually easier, however, to close off segments 3 to 6 cm in length with the bipolar coagulator and to remove them one segment after another. A tear into the thinwalled channel will bleed profusely, but since the intraluminal pressure is relatively low, the vessel may easily be closed above and below the tear with the bipolar coagulator used under saline irrigation. As long as there are connections to the dorsolateral arterial chain, the flow to the malformation can be re-established (Fig. 55–11).

Finally, the area will be reached where no further small communication vessels enter the malformation, and it becomes only a draining vein. This situation can be confirmed by closing the malformation with the bipolar coagulator or a clip. In the entire area distal to the clip, flow should cease and sedimentation should begin. This re-

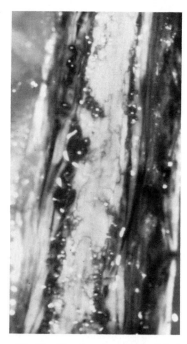

Figure 55–10 The dorsolateral arterial chain with its intercommunications is preserved after the removal of a typical long dorsal arteriovenous malformation. The dorsolateral arteries are dilated and tortuous, since they participated in the collateral supply to the main arteriovenous malformation.

maining draining vessel need not be removed; it will collapse and become occluded spontaneously (Fig. 55–12).

Continuation of the long dorsal arteriovenous malformations into the cauda equina is relatively common. If, after removal of the most caudal portion of the malformation on the cord, there is cessation of flow and sedimentation of the blood in the vessels of the malformation in the cauda, they may be accepted as venous drains and left in situ. If, however, these vessels remain tense and pulsatile, there is still arterial connection and they may require resection. The characteristic corkscrew appearance of these vessels in the caudal roots is shown in Figure 55–13. By gently spreading the finest microforceps, the surgeon can separate the individual roots into fascicles, and then the anomalous vessels can be freed segment by segment until the cauda equina has been cleared. When the operative procedure is the primary one, the separation of these elements is readily accomplished, as shown in Figure 55–13*B*. Adhesions and organized scar from prior operations will make it difficult

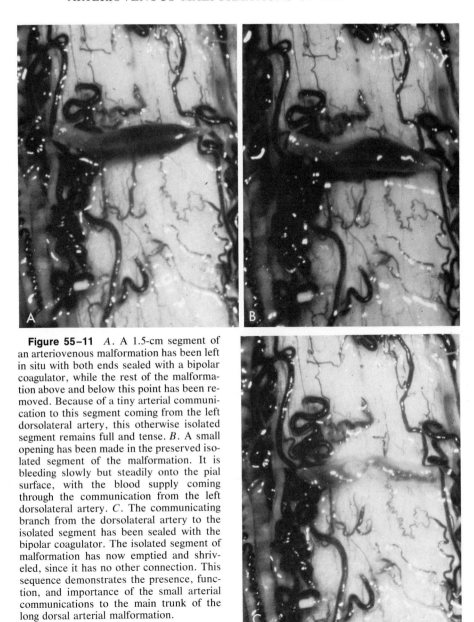

Figure 55-11 *A.* A 1.5-cm segment of an arteriovenous malformation has been left in situ with both ends sealed with a bipolar coagulator, while the rest of the malformation above and below this point has been removed. Because of a tiny arterial communication to this segment coming from the left dorsolateral artery, this otherwise isolated segment remains full and tense. *B.* A small opening has been made in the preserved isolated segment of the malformation. It is bleeding slowly but steadily onto the pial surface, with the blood supply coming through the communication from the left dorsolateral artery. *C.* The communicating branch from the dorsolateral artery to the isolated segment has been sealed with the bipolar coagulator. The isolated segment of malformation has now emptied and shriveled, since it has no other connection. This sequence demonstrates the presence, function, and importance of the small arterial communications to the main trunk of the long dorsal arterial malformation.

or impossible. Again, earlier recognition and earlier operation make the procedure much easier and safer to perform. Delay of definitive resection has permitted lesions to develop many additional segments of collateral flow as well as increased complexity. These longer lesions may require laminectomy of most of the spinal canal for alleviation of the problem. Yet, the lesion may still remain a simple long dorsal malformation, relatively easily removed in any area, and difficult only because of its extent.

In contrast to the foregoing approach, Doppman suggested that angiograms usually show a vascular nidus that is the site of shunting.[14] He considered it the point toward which multiple feeding arteries converge and from which enlarged veins drain. Since he considered that most of the apparent malformation was simply enlarged venous drainage, he suggested removal of the nidus rather than "stripping" as an adequate operative treatment. He also suggested that the nidus could be recognized angiographically. Salient features

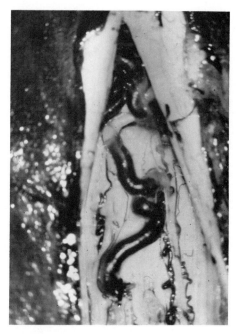

Figure 55–12 Closure of the main trunk above the highest level at which arterial communications enter it will lead to cessation of flow in the ascending venous drain and progressive sedimentation and separation of the red cells from the serum. This malformation had extended six segments above the highest level of the laminectomy and was easily demonstrable on preoperative myelograms or angiograms. Postoperative myelography two weeks later demonstrated a completely open system and total obliteration of the residual malformation, indicating that it was indeed merely an ascending venous drain with no further shunt.

of the nidus point are the converging of multiple arterial feeding vessels, the divergence of multiple venous draining vessels, the abrupt increase in the vessel diameter (venous transition), and the vessels of the tightly coiled nidus itself.

Doppman's important contribution was essentially rejected on the basis of microscopic visualization of the multiple arterial communications between the dorsolateral arterial chain and the long malformation and the recognition that if these arterial communications were not resected, revascularizaton would occur.

The author believes that in the long dorsal racemose arteriovenous malformations there is a single point of shunting from arterial to venous vessels. The shunt is along the course of the long vessel at the area where the communicating arterioles between the dorsolateral arterial chain and the malformation end. The so-called "nidus" is not necessarily the point of shunt but only the junction of enlarged collateral arterial circulation. If the idea of a single shunt point is correct, the malformation must indeed be arterial as long as it receives communications from the dorsolateral chain and venous beyond that level. Other than absence of further small arterial communications, there may be no change in diameter or appearance of the lesion at this level.

If the lesion were to be clipped only at the point of the presumed shunt, there would be sedimentation in the venous drain above, yet the multiple coiled segments below would probably change little in appearance. It would have been converted to a large artery with much of its drainage cut off and only the tiny vessels to the dorsolateral arterial chain to carry away its flow. Probably it would pulsate more strongly and seem more tense. Perhaps, in the next few weeks, the entire lesion would decrease to the size of a normal posterior artery with no further shunt. Unfortunately, without more definitive data such as is available for intracranial lesions, it still appears too dangerous to leave the tense, pulsating, enlarged coiled artery in place.

"Glomus" Malformations

Removal of a glomus lesion may be a difficult problem. It is unlikely that its relationship to the anterior spinal artery circulation can be determined preoperatively. While one major feeding vessel is the rule, others may be present. A high arterial pressure is invariable, and if the vessel is opened, hemorrhage from these thin-walled high-pressure channels is difficult to control. A venous drain of variable length, usually but not always shorter than in the long dorsal malformations, will often extend upward and have small communications to the pial arteries. These communications will finally have to be dissected as well but should generally be allowed to remain until the nidus has been removed.

Meticulous arachnoidal dissection permits an attempt to demonstrate the route of flow into the nidus. Some nidi are fed entirely by looped vessels that conform to the description of an Adamkiewicz loop, but yet are purely dorsal. Others do not appear particularly different, but will have a dorsal loop and then turn ventrally to reach the anterior spinal artery. In a few cases, the an-

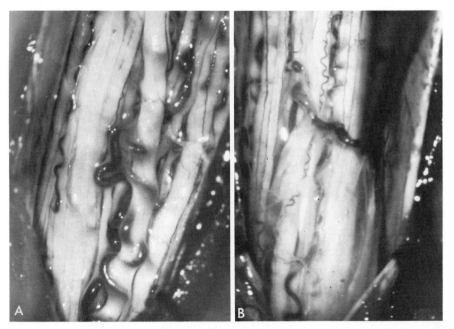

Figure 55–13 *A*. Typical corkscrew appearance of arteriovenous malformation within the nerve roots of the cauda equina. *B*. The removal of the intraradicular malformation by intrafascicular separation is demonstrated.

terior spinal artery has enlarged, and flow is outward from it to feed the malformation.

Some glomus malformations may require clipping of what appears to be a major radicular tributary to the anterior spinal artery. This maneuver could produce cord devascularization if the flow were in the other direction. As yet, no magnetic flowmeter or Doppler unit has proved delicate enough to use in determining flow direction in a single vessel in among the complex group of vessels that usually are present. Temporary clips may be applied briefly in an attempt to make the determination. The closer the vessel to be occluded is to the malformation glomus, the safer the maneuver is likely to be. In resecting a glomus lesion, no vessel should be clipped just as it enters the spinal canal. This situation is in sharp contrast to the clipping of entering vessels at the dorsal root when a long dorsal arteriovenous malformation is resected or to proximal ligation when that is recommended.

In a normal individual, closure of the artery of Adamkiewicz is said to entail a significant probability of paraplegia. The number of times this artery must have been sacrificed in the removal of extramedullary tumors without producing significant damage, however, suggests that the collateral circulation is usually adequate, either through the ascending sacral artery or the narrow descending watershed zone of the anterior spinal artery.

Larson and co-workers, in discussing operative treatment of spinal cord trauma, stated that spinal cord angiography prior to anterior vertebral resection has been advocated to identify the artery of Adamkiewicz so that it could be protected.[31] They also stated, however, that their observations and those of Martin indicated that the hazards of interrupting the artery of Adamkiewicz may be more apparent than real.[34] They believed that they must have divided the artery in at least some instances in their cases because of the levels at which they worked and the fact that they worked on the left side. Yet none of these probable cases were made worse.

The level of risk in closure of the large ventral entering artery in the treatment of glomus lesions is most difficult to assess. What has been designated as the artery of Adamkiewicz has been completely embolized without producing deficit by Decker and ligated in the approach to an arteriovenous malformation with an excellent result in Fischer's two cases.[7,20]

The resection of the glomus is accomplished by the same technique as the removal of the previously discussed long dorsal malformations. The low power of the bipolar coagulator under saline irrigation may be used to slowly shrink large dilated thin-walled vessels into smaller tougher ones, permitting easier manipulation (Fig. 55–14).

The intramedullary portion of such a malformation, if present, may be aneurysmal and may require longitudinal splitting of the cord for visualization. Using the bipolar current to shrink the aneurysm dome car-ries a significant risk of perforation, but blunt forceps, low current, and large amounts of saline give increased safety. Shrinkage of the aneurysm gives room for dissection without cord trauma. Small per-forating vessels from the anterior spinal ar-tery may enter the aneurysm from the ante-rior raphe. Sectioning these branches requires room that would not be readily

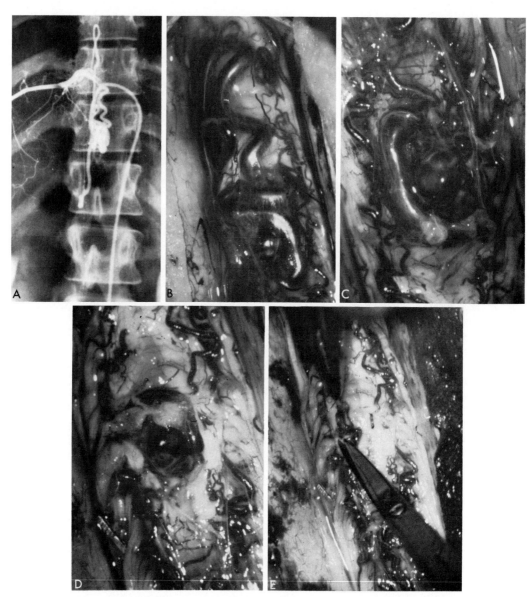

Figure 55–14 *A.* A large hooked vessel above and to the left feeds a glomus malformation of the lower tho-racic cord. Just below the catheter, a recurrent loop of malformation extends from the lower portion of the body of T10 down to the midportion of T11, where it joins an aneurysmal dilatation. *B.* The T11 area, at the micro-opera-tive procedure. The hooked feeding artery above the field was left undisturbed, and the resection began with the looped vessel at T11. *C.* The aneurysmal sac is still tense and pulsating despite the removal of the upper loop. *D.* The aneurysmal loop being followed into the cord by myelotomy. *E.* Final completion of the resection with the coagulation and cutting of the sulcal branches coming up to the aneurysmal dilatation from the anterior spinal artery.

achieved if the aneurysms were not reduced in size.

Intramedullary Cervical Lesions

With intramedullary cervical lesions, the perforating vessels from the anterior spinal artery present the major operative problem. These lesions usually come to the surface somewhere, thus providing a zone in which to start the separation from the surrounding cord. When a large arterial feeding vessel has been identified, its occlusion may make the procedure easier but may also deprive the anterior spinal artery of needed supply. The venous drain in such lesions may afford the only solution to resection of the malformation without damage to cord supply.

With a mean systemic hypotension of 50 to 60 mm of mercury, the draining vein may be the first vessel to be ligated and cut and then used as a handle for retrograde dissection. In these high-pressure malformations, temporary occlusion would be required first, since it must be demonstrated that engorgement of the lesion will be sufficiently controlled by hypotension to allow its dissection, manipulation, and coagulation shrinkage. With this technique, only those arterial vessels entering the shunt are sealed and cut, and vessels of passage are more readily isolated and preserved. Usually this method has been reserved for lesions in which more than one draining vein was present. In a high cervical lesion to which all of the arterial supply appeared to be from anterior spinal circulation, the technique was used successfully even though only one venous drain was present (Fig. 55–15).

Fortunately, the lesions of the cervicomedullary junction tend to be posterior in location, often including large thin-walled aneurysmal sacs. These high-pressure lesions usually present with severe subarachnoid hemorrhages. Major feeding vessels usually enter from the vertebral arteries and turn posteriorly around the dentate attachment to reach the lesion. This posterior feeding trunk is often a much enlarged branch of the vessel, the smaller primary segment of which will join with that of the other side to form the anterior spinal artery. As long as the clip is applied distal to this anterior branch, clipping of the large feeding trunks can facilitate the rest of the procedure. Again, sedimentation in the remaining vessels will indicate the completion of the resection that is required.

Juvenile Malformations

The juvenile malformations are the most formidable of all. Complete operative resection will rarely be possible, and the multiplicity of very large-caliber feeding arteries can produce massive bleeding, even under hypotension. The large transosseous channels, the epidural communications, and the association with extension into mediastinal, retroperitoneal, and abdominal areas may be beyond any reasonable operative approach. In the author's experience, the attempts to resect these lesions have been unsatisfactory, with only two cases in which the malformation appeared to be completely removed (Fig. 55–16). One of these two unfortunate patients, long bedridden preoperatively, died of a pulmonary embolus on the third postoperative day. The other came through the spinal resection well, only to become paraplegic after a separate operation for resection of the retroperitoneal and pelvic components of the malformation (Fig. 55–17). Obviously, aortic or iliac branches necessary for spinal cord circulation were resected in the abdominal procedure. Their rarity is perhaps the only favorable aspect of these lesions.

Epidural Malformations

The final group of lesions comprises the epidural malformations. These relatively unusual lesions may be quite large, with vessels over a centimeter in diameter. Most often they are fed by large branches of the spinomedullary arteries proximal to the radicular arteries. Also they have feeding vessels from the arterial supply of the vertebral bodies. There is also a large collateral circulation through the paravertebral muscles and, on occasion, from the occipital branch of the external carotid or from branches of the vertebral artery at the arch of the atlas. Removal of these lesions is less difficult than might be expected. The external vessels are thick-walled and easier to handle and identify, permitting ligation of major supply with sparing of the radicular branches. Resection of the shunting area leads to collapse of the remaining venous channels and return of the arterial trunks to normal size (Fig. 55–18).

The absolute requirement for safe dissec-

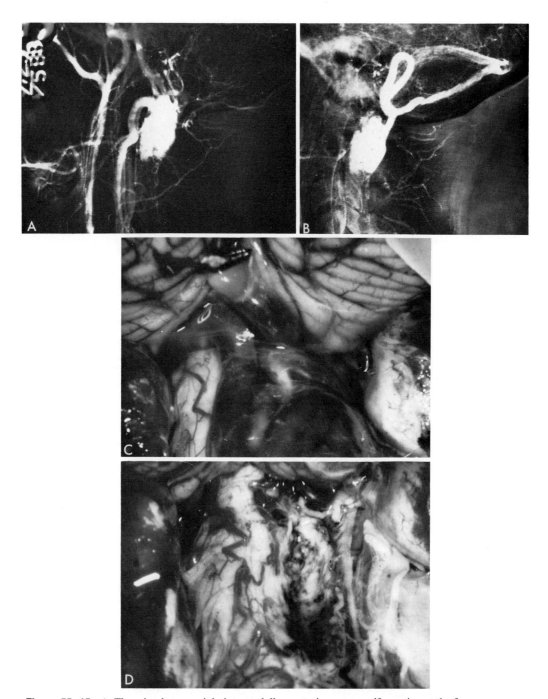

Figure 55–15 *A*. There is a large, mainly intramedullary arteriovenous malformation at the foramen magnum down through C2. Its major blood supply is from branches of the two vertebral arteries, which join to form the anterior spinal artery, as well as from transsulcal branches from the anterior spinal artery. *B*. The presence of only one large venous drain is shown. *C*. The large venous drain has been clipped and is being used as a handle for the backward resection of the malformation in order to spare any arterial vessels that may be continuing to the spinal cord after giving off branches to the malformation. *D*. The intramedullary cavity after resection of the malformation.

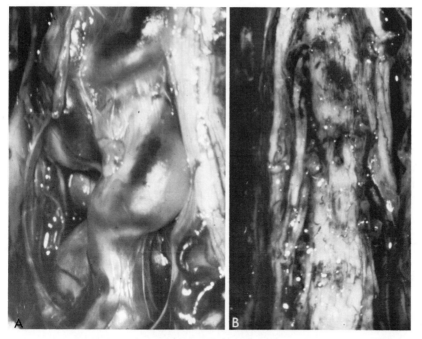

Figure 55–16 *A*. In this juvenile malformation, the spinal cord is completely covered by a tangle of high-pressure, relatively thin-walled arterial trunks, each more than 1 cm in diameter. These trunks seem to engulf the entire spinal cord. *B*. Appearance of the cord after removal of the malformation. The cord itself is small and atrophic compared with the nerve roots, which occupy more of the canal than the remaining cord.

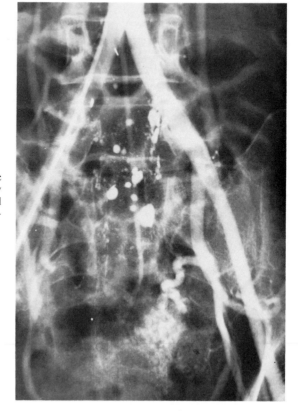

Figure 55–17 The presence of an intrapelvic arteriovenous malformation is angiographically demonstrated after the removal of the intraspinal malformation, indicating the presence of an additional shunt.

tion is systemic hypotension that permits control of osseous perforators and, by decreasing vascular tension and rigidity, prevents the unexpected tear and massive hemorrhage. Even though evidence of intradural extension has been present on preoperative myelography or angiography, it is preferable not to open the dura, on the assumption that the intradural component will be purely venous drainage. Postoperative study has confirmed the disappearance of the abnormality in all six of the author's cases of this type.

CONCLUSIONS

Spinal arteriovenous malformations are relatively rare lesions. Nevertheless, the

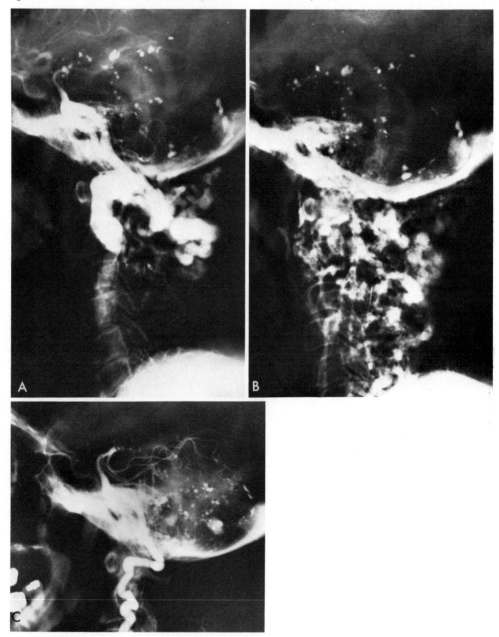

Figure 55–18 *A*. An extradural cervical arteriovenous malformation is fed by tremendously dilated vertebral arteries that become normal in size intracranially and go on to a normal basilar arterial circulation. *B*. The extensive extraspinal venous drainage of the malformation. *C*. After resection of the shunt, the vertebral arteries have returned to virtually normal size, though they remain extremely tortuous. The basilar circulation remains unchanged.

prognosis is so serious when they are left untreated that definitive attempts to make the diagnosis by myelography or angiography are indicated. The long dorsal malformations, the cervical intramedullary lesions, the foramen magnum lesions, and the epidural malformations can be resected by micro-operative technique. Usually the results are good and are much better than those of nonoperative treatment. The ventrally placed glomus lesions and the juvenile malformations carry a greater operative risk. The risk is still significantly less, however, than that of the natural course of the disease. Embolization does not produce as high a percentage of satisfactory results as resection in primary cases. It should be reserved for those patients in whom an operation is contraindicated.

REFERENCES

1. Adamkiewicz, A.: Die Blutgefasse des menschlichen Rückenmarkes. S. Ber. Akad. Wiss., Wien, III:*85*:101–130, 1882.
2. Aminoff, M. J., Barnard, R. O., and Logue, V.: The pathophysiology of spinal vascular malformations. J. Neurol. Sci., *23*:255–263, 1974.
3. Bailey, W. L., and Sperl, M. P.: Angiomas of the cervical spinal cord. J. Neurosurg., *30*:560–568, 1969.
4. Balck, C. A., and Harman, W. M.: A case of angioma of the spinal cord with recurrent hemorrhages. Brit. Med. J., *2*:1707–1708, 1900.
5. Bergstrand, A., Hook, O., and Lidvall, H.: Vascular malformations of the spinal cord. Acta Neurol. Scand., *40*:169–183, 1964.
6. Bergstrand, H.: On the classification of the haemangiomatous tumours and malformations of the central nervous system. Acta Path. Microbiol. Scand., Suppl. *26*:89–95, 1936.
7. Decker, R.: Complete embolization of artery of Adamkiewicz to obliterate an intramedullary arteriovenous aneurysm. J. Neurosurg., *43*:486–489, 1975.
8. DiChiro, G., and Wener, L.: Angiography of the spinal cord—a review of contemporary techniques and applications. J. Neurosurg., *39*:1–29, 1973.
9. DiChiro, G., Doppman, J., and Ommaya, A. K.: Selective arteriography of arteriovenous aneurysms of the spinal cord. Radiology, *88*:1065–1077, 1967.
10. DiChiro, G., Doppman, J. L., and Ommaya, A. K.: Radiology of spinal cord arteriovenous malformations. Progr. Neurol. Surg., *4*:329–354, 1971.
11. Djindjian, R., Cophignon, J., Theron, J., Merland, J., and Houdart, R.: Embolization by superselective arteriography from the femoral route in neuroradiology. Neuroradiology, *6*:20–26, 1973.
12. Djindjian, R., Dumesnil, M., Faure, C., LeFebvre, J., and Leveque, B.: Etude angiographique d'un angiome intra-rachidien. Rev. Neurol., *106*:278–285, 1962.
13. Djindjian, R., Cophignon, J., Rey, A., Theron, J., Merland, J., and Houdart, R.: Superselective arteriographic embolization by the femoral route in neuroradiology. Neuroradiology, *6*:132–42, 1973.
14. Doppman, J. L.: The nidus concept of spinal cord arteriovenous malformations. Brit. J. Radiol., *44*:758–763, 1971.
15. Doppman, J. L., DiChiro, G., and Ommaya, A. K.: Obliteration of spinal cord arteriovenous malformation by percutaneous embolization. Lancet, *1*:477–478, 1968.
16. Doppman, J. L., DiChiro, G., and Ommaya, A. K.: Selective Arteriography of the Spinal Cord. St. Louis, Warren H. Green, Inc., 1969.
17. Doppman, J. L., DiChiro, G., and Ommaya, A. K.: Percutaneous embolization of spinal cord arteriovenous malformations. J. Neurosurg., *34*:48–55, 1971.
18. Doppman, J. L., Wirth, F. P., DiChiro, G., and Ommaya, A. K.: Value of cutaneous angiomas in the arteriographic localization of spinal-cord arteriovenous malformations. New Eng. J. Med., *281*:1440–1444, 1969.
19. Elsberg, C. A.: Diagnosis and Treatment of Surgical Diseases of the Spinal Cord and Its Membranes. (Chapter XV—Abnormalities and diseases of the spinal vessels.) Philadelphia and London, W. B. Saunders Co., 1916.
20. Fischer, G.: Personal communication, 1974.
21. Foix, C., and Alajouanine, T.: La myélite nécrotique subaiguë. Rev. Neurol., *2*:1–42, 1926.
22. Gaupp, J.: Hamorrhoiden der Pia mater spinalis im Gebiete des Lendenmarkes. Bietr. Path. Anat., *2*:516–518, 1888.
23. Guidetti, B.: Surgical treatment of vascular tumors and vascular malformations of the spinal cord. Vasc. Surg., *4*:179–185, 1970.
24. Guillain, G., and Alajouanine, T.: Travaux originaux. J. Neurol. Psychiat. (Brux.) *11*:689–697, 1925.
25. Henson, R. A., and Croft, P. B.: Spontaneous spinal subarachnoid hemorrhage. Quart. J. Med., *25*:53–66, 1956.
26. Hook, O., and Lidvall, H.: Arteriovenous aneurysms of the spinal cord. J. Neurosurg., *15*:84–91, 1958.
27. Houdart, R., Djindjian, R., and Hurth, M.: Vascular malformations of the spinal cord. J. Neurosurg., *24*:583–594, 1966.
28. Krause, F.: Surgery of the Brain and Spinal Cord. Vol. III. New York, Rebman Company, 1912, pp. 1129–1130.
29. Krayenbühl, H., Yasargil, M. G., and McClintock, H. G.: Treatment of spinal cord vascular malformations by surgical excision. J. Neurosurg., *30*:427–435, 1969.
30. Kunc, A., and Bret, J.: Diagnosis and treatment of vascular malformations of the spinal cord. J. Neurosurg., *30*:436–445, 1969.
31. Larson, S. J., Holst, R. A., Hemmy, D. C., and Sances, A.: Lateral extracavitary approach to traumatic lesions of the thoracic and lumbar spine. J. Neurosurg., *45*:628–637, 1976.
32. Luessenhop, A. J., and Cruz, T. D.: The surgical excision of spinal intradural vascular malformations. J. Neurosurg., *30*:552–559, 1969.

33. Malis, L. I.: The myelographic examination of the foramen magnum. Radiology, 70:196–221, 1958.

34. Martin, N. S.: Pott's paraplegia. A report on 120 cases. J. Bone Joint Surg., 53B:596–608, 1971.

35. Michon, R.: Le coup de poignard rachidien. Presse Méd., 36:964–967, 1928.

36. Newman, M. J. D.: Racemose angioma of the spinal cord. Quart. J. Med., 28:97–109, 1959.

37. Newton, T. H., and Adams, J. E.: Angiographic demonstration and nonsurgical embolization of spinal cord angioma. Radiology, 91:873–876, 1968.

38. Ommaya, A. K.: Personal communication, 1976.

39. Ommaya, A. K., DiChiro, G., and Doppman, J.: Ligation of arterial supply in the treatment of spinal cord arteriovenous malformations. J. Neurosurg., 30:679–692, 1969.

40. Perthes, G.: Über das Rankenangiom der weichen Häute des Gehirns und Rückenmarks. Dtsch. Z. Chir., 203/204:93–103, 1927.

41. Pia, H. W.: Diagnosis and treatment of spinal angiomas. Acta Neurochir. (Wien), 28:1–12, 1973.

42. Pool, J. L.: Discussion (on p. 265) in Yasargil, M. G.: Surgery of vascular lesions of the spinal cord with the microsurgical technique. Clin. Neurosurg., 17:257–265, 1969.

43. Raymond, E., and Cestan, R.: Un cas d'anevrisme cirsoïde probable de la moëlle cervicale. Rev. Neurol., 12:457–463, 1904.

44. Sano, K., Jimbo, M., and Saito, I.: Artificial embolization with liquid plastic. Neurol. Medicochir. (Tokyo), 8:198–201, 1966.

45. Sargent, P.: Hemangioma of the pia mater causing compression paraplegia. Brain, 48:259–267, 1925.

46. Scoville, W. B.: Intramedullary arteriovenous aneurysms of the spinal cord. J. Neurosurg., 5:307–312, 1948.

47. Shephard, R. H.: Observations on intradural spinal angioma: Treatment by excision. Neurochirurgia (Stuttgart), 6:58–74, 1963.

48. Shephard, R. H.: Some new concepts in intradural spinal angioma. Riv. Pat. Nerv. Ment., 86:276–283, 1965.

49. Svien, H. J., and Baker, H. L., Jr.: Roentgenographic and surgical aspects of vascular anomalies of the spinal cord. Surg. Gynec. Obstet. 112:729–735, 1961.

50. Teng, P., and Papatheodoru, C.: Myelographic appearance of vascular anomalies of the spinal cord. Brit. J. Radiol., 37:358–366, 1964.

51. Trupp, M., and Sachs, E.: Vascular tumors of the brain and spinal cord and their treatment. J. Neurosurg., 5:354–571, 1948.

52. Tyler, H. R., and Clark, D. B.: Neurological complications in patients with coarctation of aorta. Neurology (Minneap.), 8:712–718, 1958.

53. Weenink, H. R., and Smilde, J.: Spinal cord lesions due to coarctatio aortae. Psychiat. Neurol. Neurochir., 67:259–269, 1964.

54. Woltman, H. W., and Shelden, W. D.: Neurological complications associated with congenital stenosis of the isthmus of the aorta. Arch. Neurol. Psychiat., 17:303–316, 1927.

55. Wyburn-Mason, R.: The Vascular Abnormalities and Tumors of the Spinal Cord and Its Membranes. London, Henry Kimpton, 1943.

56. Yasargil, M. G.: Surgery of vascular lesions of the spinal cord with the microsurgical technique. Clin. Neurosurg., 17:257–265, 1969.

57. Yasargil, M. G.: Vertebral column and spinal cord lesions. In Microsurgery Applied to Neurosurgery. New York, Academic Press, 1969, pp. 167–177.

58. Yasargil, M. G.: Diagnosis and treatment of spinal cord arteriovenous malformations. Progr. Neurol. Surg., 4:355–428, 1971.

59. Yasargil, M. G., DeLong, W. B., and Guarnaschelli, J. J.: Complete microsurgical excision of cervical extramedullary and intramedullary vascular malformations. Surg. Neurol., 4:211–224, 1975.

Index

In this index page numbers set in *italics* indicate illustrations. Page numbers followed by (t) refer to tabular material. Drugs are indexed under their generic names when dosage or action or special use is given. The abbreviation vs. is used to indicate differential diagnosis.

Abdomen, distention of, postoperative, 1106
  ganglioneuroma of, 3310
  in head injury in children, 2093
  in multiple trauma, 2520–2521
  in thoracic spinal injury, 2346
  pain in, in cancer, 3630, 3630(t)
    of unknown origin, 3631
Abdominal cutaneous nerve syndrome, 2463
Abducens nerve, anatomy of, orbital, 3027
  clinical examination of, 20
    in infants and children, 46, 56
    in percutaneous trigeminal rhizotomy, 3569, *3571*
  palsy of, 657, *657*
    in pseudotumor cerebri, 896
    increased intracranial pressure and, 878
Ablative procedures, 3769–3786
  in refractory pain, 3763–3765
ABLB test, 697, 2974
Abnormal movement disorders, 3821–3857. See also *Dyskinesias.*
Abscess. See also names of specific abscesses.
  actinomycotic, 3399
  brain, 3343–3355
    brain scanning in, 155(t), 159
    computed tomography in, 116, *118,* 3346, *3348,* 3355
    ultrasound in, 190
  epidural, 3333
    in head injury, 1915
  spinal, epidural, vs. viral encephalitis, 3360
    extradural, 3449–3451, *3450, 3451*
    subdural, 3451–3452, *3451*
  spinal cord, *3451,* 3452–3453, *3452*
  stitch, 1088
  subgaleal, 3328
Absence status, treatment of, 3878
Abulic trait, in normal-pressure hydrocephalus, 1424
Acceleration-deceleration injury, cervical, 2320, 2330–2332, 2338–2343, *2339*
Accident(s), care of spine in, cervical,
  thoracic, 2345
  cerebrovascular. See *Cerebrovascular accident* and *Stroke.*
Acetazolamide, cerebral blood flow and, 810(t)
  in pseudotumor cerebri, 3192
Acetylcholine, cerebral blood flow and, 808(t)
  metabolism of, 770
Achondroplasia, genetic aspects of, 1229, *1230, 1231*
  narrow spinal canal in, 2554
Acid-base balance, in multiple trauma, 2497–2500, *2498,* 2499(t)
Acid cholesteryl ester hydrolase deficiency, diagnosis of, 385(t)
Acidosis, metabolic, in multiple trauma, 2499
  respiratory, in head injury, in children, 2121
    in multiple trauma, 2500

Acoustic neuromas, 2967–3003
  angiography in, *317,* 2979–2985, *2982–2984*
  brain scanning in, 146, 150(t), 152, *153*
  computed tomography in, 122, *122,* 2976, *2977*
  diagnosis of, 2971–2992, *2974*
  operation(s) for, development of, 2968
    posterior fossa transmeatal, 2992–2997, *2992–2997*
    results of, *2998, 2999,* 2999–3000
  postoperative care in, 2997–2999
Acoustic reflex test, 700
Acrocephalopolysyndactyly, 1212–1213
Acrocephalosyndactyly, 1212–1213
Acrodysostosis, 1214
Acromegaloid appearance, vs. early acromegaly, 956
Acromegaly, 952–958
  diagnosis of, differential, 956
    potential pitfalls in, 955
  galactorrhea with, hormone secretion and, 964
  headache in, 3129
  histological study in, *3118*
  laboratory examination in, 953
  microadenoma in, 3124, *3125*
  pituitary tumor and, 952
  radiation therapy for, 3165, *3166*
  skull in, 3251
  study schedule for, 957
  treatment of, 956, 957(t)
    results of, 3146
  tumor herniation in, *3132*
Acrylic resin, cranioplasty with, 2236–2239, *2238–2240*
  advantages and complications of, 2241, *2241*
ACTH. See *Adrenocorticotropic hormone.*
Actinomycosis, 3398–3401
  meningitic, cerebrospinal fluid in, 462
Activities of daily living, in rehabilitation, 3996
Adamkiewicz, artery of, 553, *554, 556, 557, 561, 565*
Addison's disease, pseudotumor cerebri and, 3181(t)
Adenocarcinoma, ethmoid sinus, *3278,* 3279
  metastatic, tumor complexes of, *189*
  paranasal sinus, 3277
  scalp, 3319
Adenohypophysis, 935–970. See also *Anterior pituitary.*
  anatomy of, 3108
Adenoid cystic carcinoma, of paranasal sinuses, 3277
Adenoma, chromophobe, brain scanning in, *154*
  facial sebaceous, *1228*
  nonfunctioning chromophobe, radiation therapy of, 3164
  pituitary. See *Pituitary adenoma.*
Adenosine, cerebral blood flow and, 812(t)
Adenosine arabinoside, in herpes simplex encephalitis, 3363
Adenosine triphosphate, cerebral blood flow and, 812(t)

INDEX

Intracranial pressure (*Continued*)
  increased, clinical diagnosis of, 17, 876–880
    definition of, 900
    disturbed brain function and, 860, *860*
    hyperbaric oxygen in, 903
    hypertonic solutions in, 905
    hyperventilation in, 901
    hypothermia in, 912
    incidence and significance of, 880–897
    in brain ischemia and anoxia, 894
    in brain tumors, 889
      of posterior fossa, in children, 2734–2735
      supratentorial, in children, 2704
    in comatose patient, 898
    in head injury, 880, 881(t), 882(t), 885(t), *886–888,*
      1922–1927, 1922–1924, 2045–2048
      in children, 2119, *2120*
    in normal-pressure hydrocephalus, 895, 1426
    in pseudotumor cerebri, 896
    in Reye's syndrome, 895
    in subarachnoid hemorrhage, 891, *892*
    lumbar puncture in, 850
    nitrous oxide and, 1121
    operative decompression in, 916
    pathology of, 860–876
    pressure waves of, 875
    prognosis after head injury and, 2150–2152, *2151, 2152*
    pulmonary edema with, 864
    respiratory failure and, 1016
    signs and symptoms of, 876
    sinus occlusion and, in cerebral infarction, 1539, 1540
    steroids in, 910
    tentorial pressure cone in, 878
    treatment of, 897–916
    vital signs and, 861
  intracranial volume and, 853, *854–856*
  measurement of, in head injury, 1989–1992
    methods of, 850
  monitoring of, postoperative, in closed head injury,
    2037–2042, *2038–2042*
  neuroleptanalgesia and, 1121
  normal, 847, *848–850*
    pressure/volume index of, 855
  tests for, in cerebral death, 755(t)
  transmission of, 857
Intracranial space, pain-sensitive structures in, 877
  volume/pressure response for elastance of, 854
Intracranial tap, percutaneous, in pediatric hydrocephalus, 1400,
  1400
Intracranial tumors, enlarged ventricles and, 1429
  increased intracranial pressure in, 889
  vs. trigeminal neuralgia, 3557
Intracranial vascular disease, postoperative vasospasm and, 1092
Intracranial vessels, manipulation of, in operative procedures,
  1080
Intracranial volume, reduction of, for operation, 1667
Intradiploic cyst, 3245
Intravenous pyelogram, in urinary bladder malfunction, 1038
Intravenous thiopental test, 3492
Intraventricular foramen, *353*
Intraventricular space, measurement of intracranial pressure from,
  852
Intubation, in multiple trauma, endotracheal, 2476–2477
  nasogastric, 2526–2528
Iophendylate, in ventriculography, 3788
IQ. See *Intelligence quotient.*
Iron, in cerebrospinal fluid, 450
Iron deficiency anemia, and pseudotumor cerebri, 3181(t), 3187
  skull involvement in, 3261
Irradiation necrosis, delayed, ultrasound in, 190
Irrigation, in cerebral resections, 1146
Ischemia. See also *Ischemic vascular disease.*
  brain damage in, in head injury, 1927–1928
  cerebral, definition of, 774

Ischemia (*Continued*)
  cerebral, diffuse, 1540–1549, *1541,* 1543–1545(t)
    increased intracranial pressure and, 876, 894–895
    metabolism in, 774–781
    pathophysiology of, 1513–1516, 1515(t)
    transient, carotid, 1520–1530
      cerebral blood flow in, 828, *829*
      vertebrobasilar, 1530–1531
  complete, 777, *778, 779*
  coronary, pain in, dorsal rhizotomy in, 3668
  in peripheral nerve entrapment, 2433–2435, *2433–2437*
  in peripheral nerve injury, 2367, *2367, 2368*
  incomplete, 775, *776*
  postoperative, in carotid ligation, 1708
  recovery following, factors affecting, 780
Ischemic stroke, acute, operative management of, 1619–1626
Ischemic vascular disease, cerebral, 1511–1553
  clinical evaluation of, 1516–1520, *1517,* 1519(t)
  definitions and classification of, 1511–1513
  epidemiology of, 1513
  focal, 1514, 1520–1534
  kinking of carotid artery and, 816
  management of, 1534–1538
  mechanisms of, 1512, 1512(t), 1513(t), 1515–1516
  pain management in, 3632
  pathophysiology of, 1513, 1515(t)
  time course of, 1512
  unusual arterial disorders in, 1549–1553
  venous infarction in, 1538–1540
Isoproterenol, cerebral blood flow and, 808(t)
Isotope scan. See *Brain scan* and *Radionuclide imaging.*
Isoxsuprine hydrochloride, cerebral blood flow and, 808(t)

Jakob-Creutzfeldt disease, brain biopsy in, 386(t)
  cerebrospinal fluid in, 465
  electroencephalography in, 207, *213,* 222
Jaundice, neonatal, 40
  postoperative, 1107
Jefferson's fracture, 500, 2324
Joints, range of motion of, in rehabilitation, 4000
Juvenile malformations, of spinal cord, 1858, *1859,* 1869

Kanamycin, in bacterial infections, 3327
  in cerebral vasospasm, 821
  inner ear damage and, 691, 691(t)
Katzman cerebrospinal fluid absorption test, 455
Keratinitis, in lower facial weakness, 47
Keratitis, exposure, tarsorrhaphy in, 643, *643*
  post-craniotomy for trigeminal neuralgia, 3583
Kernig test, 2542
Kernohan notch, supratentorial mass lesion and, 879
Ketamine, as general anesthetic, 1122
  cerebral blood flow and, 805
  in increased intracranial pressure, 901
Ketoacidosis, diabetic, intracranial hypertension in, 3180(t)
Ketone bodies, in cerebral metabolism, 767
Kidney(s), hypothermia and, 1129
  pain in, 3632
  polycystic, cerebral aneurysm and, 1808–1809, 1808(t)
  spinal metastasis from, 512
Kiloh-Nevin syndrome, 659, *660*
Kindling, 3862
Kinetron machine, 3995
Kinking, vascular, angiography in, *288,* 289, *289*
  cerebral blood flow and, 815–816
Klippel-Feil syndrome, 491, *494,* 1215
Klippel-Trenaunay syndrome, 565, *568, 569*
Klumpke's palsy, in neonate, 49
Klüver-Bucy syndrome, clinical examination in, 15
Knee, peroneal nerve injury at, 2402–2404